AIDS and the Nervous System

Second Edition

AIDS and the Nervous System

Second Edition

Editors

Joseph R. Berger, M.D.
Professor and Chairman, Department of Neurology
Professor, Department of Internal Medicine
University of Kentucky Medical Center
Lexington, Kentucky

Robert M. Levy, M.D., Ph.D.
Associate Professor of Neurological Surgery and Physiology
Department of Surgery
Northwestern University Medical School
Chicago, Illinois

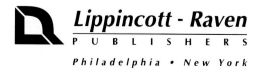

Lippincott - Raven
PUBLISHERS
Philadelphia • New York

Lippincott-Raven Publishers, 227 East Washington Square, Philadelphia, Pennsylvania 19106

Printed in the United States of America

9 8 7 6 5 4 3 2 1

Library of Congress Cataloging-in-Publication Data

AIDS and the nervous system / editors, Joseph R. Berger, Robert M. Levy.
  —2nd ed.
      p.   cm.
    Includes bibliographical references and index.
    ISBN 0-7817-0309-3
    1. Nervous system—Infections.   2. AIDS (Disease)—Complications.
  I. Berger, Joseph R. 1951–   . II. Levy, Robert M.
    [DNLM: 1. Acquired Immunodeficiency Syndrome—complications.
  2. Nervous System Diseases—complications.   WC 503.5 A288   1996]
  RC359.5.A33   1996
  616.8—dc20
  DNLM/DLC
  for Library of Congress   96-2020

To my parents, Motzi and Marty Berger,
My wife, Sandy,
And my children, Aaron, Michael, and Rachel

J. R. B.

To my sons, Benjamin and Samuel

R. M. L.

Contents

Section I. Introduction

Section II. HIV Neuropathogenesis

Section III. Clinical Neurological Syndromes and Diagnosis

Section VI. Patient Care Issues

Contributing Authors

J. Hampton Atkinson, M.D.
Adjunct Professor
Department of Psychiatry
University of California, San Diego
9500 Gilman Drive
La Jolla, California 92093

Anita L. Belman, M.D.
Associate Professor of Neurology and
    Pediatrics
Department of Neurology
State University of New York at Stony Brook
Stony Brook, New York 11794

Bernard Bendok, M.D.
Division of Neurological Surgery
Northwestern University Medical School
233 East Erie Street
Chicago, Illinois 60611

Joseph R. Berger, M.D.
Professor and Chairman
Department of Neurology
Professor, Department of Internal Medicine
University of Kentucky Medical Center
Room 228E
820 South Limestone, Annex 4 (Chambers
    Building)
Lexington, Kentucky 40536-2226

Benjamin M. Blumberg, Ph.D.
Associate Professor of Neurology,
    Microbiology, and Immunology
Department of Neurology
University of Rochester School of Medicine
601 Elmwood Avenue
Rochester, New York 14642

Elizabeth Bosler, M.P.H.
Infectious Disease Epidemiologist (Research
    Associate)
Department of Medicine
State University of New York at Stony Brook
T-16, Room 020
Stony Brook, New York 11794

**Bruce J. Brew, M.B.B.S., M.B.,
    F.R.A.C.P.**
Associate Professor
Department of HIV Medicine and Neurology
University of New South Wales
St. Vincent's Hospital
376 Victoria Street
Darlinghurst
Sydney 2010
Australia

Herbert Budka, M.D.
Professor of Clinical Neuropathology
Department of Neuropathology
Clinical Institute of Neurology
University of Vienna
Währinger Gürtel 18-20, Neues AKH 04J
POB 48
A-1097 Wien
Austria

**Andrew D. Carr, M.B.B.S., F.R.A.C.P.,
    F.R.C.P.A.**
Department of HIV Medicine
St. Vincent's Hospital
University of New South Wales
376 Victoria Street
Darlinghurst
Sydney 2010
Australia

Yahia Chebloune, Ph.D.
Visiting Scientist
University of Kansas Medical Center
3901 Rainbow Boulevard
Kansas City, Kansas 66160; and
Department of Microbiology
Institute National de la Recherche
    Agronomigue
Ecole Vétèrincure de Lyon
1 Rue Bourgelat
Marcy L'Etoile 69630
France

Bruce A. Cohen, M.D.
Associate Professor
Department of Neurology
Northwestern University Medical School
645 North Michigan Avenue
Chicago, Illinois 60611

Katherine E. Conant, M.D.
Senior Staff Fellow
Laboratory of Molecular Medicine and
Neuroscience
National Institutes of Health
Building 36, Room 5C13
9000 Rockville Pike
Bethesda, Maryland 20892

Mauricio Concha, M.D.
Department of Neurology
University of Miami School of Medicine
Miami, Florida, 33136

David A. Cooper, M.D., F.R.A.C.P.,
F.R.C.P.A., D.Sc.
Professor of Medicine
National Centre in HIV Epidemiology and
Clinical Research
University of New South Wales
Victoria Street
Sydney 2010
Australia

Gerald J. Dal Pan, M.D., M.H.S.
Instructor
Department of Neurology
The Johns Hopkins University School of
Medicine
Meyer 6-109
600 North Wolfe Street
Baltimore, Maryland 21287-7609

Janet L. Davis, M.D.
Associate Professor
Department of Ophthalmology
University of Miami School of Medicine
Bascom Eye Institute
Ann Bates Leach Hospital
900 Northwest 17th Street
Miami, Florida 33136

Gordon Dickinson, M.D.
Professor of Medicine
Division of Infectious Diseases and
Immunology
Department of Internal Medicine
University of Miami Medical School
Veterans Administration Medical Center
1201 Northwest 16th Street
Miami, Florida 33125

Richard D. Dix, Ph.D.
Associate Professor
Departments of Ophthalmology, Microbiology
and Immunology, and Neurology
University of Miami School of Medicine
Bascom Palmer Eye Institute
1638 Northwest 10th Avenue
Miami, Florida 33136

Leon G. Epstein, M.D.
Professor of Neurology, Pediatrics,
Microbiology, and Immunology
Department of Neurology
University of Rochester School of Medicine
601 Elmwood Avenue, Box 631
Rochester, New York 14642

Bruno V. Gallo, M.D.
Chief Resident
Department of Neurology
Jackson Memorial Hospital
1611 Northwest 12th Avenue
Miami, Florida 33136

Howard E. Gendelman, M.D.
Professor
Departments of Medicine, Surgery, Pathology,
and Microbiology
University of Nebraska Medical Center
600 South 42nd Street
Omaha, Nebraska 68198-5215

Igor Grant, M.D., F.R.C.P.
Professor
Department of Psychiatry
University of California, San Diego
Veterans Affairs Medical Center
9500 Gilman Drive
La Jolla, California 92093-0680

Johann A. Hainfellner, M.D.
Clinical Institute of Neurology
University of Vienna
Währinger Gürtel 18-20, Neues AKH 04J
POB 48
A-1097 Wien
Austria

Colin D. Hall, M.B., Ch.B.
Professor and Interim Chair of Neurology
Professor of Medicine
Department of Neurology
University of North Carolina School of
Medicine
CB # 7025
Manning Drive
Chapel Hill, North Carolina 27599

Michael J. G. Harrison, D.M., F.R.C.P.
Professor of Clinical Neurology
University College London Medical School
Martimer Street
London WIN 8AA
United Kingdom

Harry Hollander, M.D.
Professor of Clinical Medicine
University of California, San Francisco
Box 0378
San Francisco, California 94143

Sidney A. Houff, M.D., Ph.D.
Chief
Department of Neurology Service
Washington Veterans Administration Medical
*   Center*
50 Irving Street Northwest
Washington, D.C. 20422

Robert S. Janssen, M.D.
Acting Chief
HIV Seroepidemiology Branch
Division of HIV/AIDS Prevention
National Center for HIV, STD, and TB
*   Prevention*
1600 Clifton Road
Atlanta, Georgia 30333

Sanjay V. Joag, M.D., Ph.D., M.B.B.S.
Research Assistant Professor
Departments of Microbiology, Molecular
*   Genetics, and Immunology*
University of Kansas Medical Center
3901 Rainbow Boulevard
Kansas City, Kansas 66160

Robert M. Levy, M.D., Ph.D.
Associate Professor of Neurological Surgery
*   and Physiology*
Department of Surgery
Northwestern University Medical School
250 East Superior Street, Suite 928
Chicago, Illinois 60611

Stuart A. Lipton, M.D., Ph.D.
Associate Professor
Department of Neurology
Program in Neuroscience
Harvard Medical School
300 Longwood Avenue
Enders Building, Suite 361
Boston, Massachusetts 02115

Benjamin J. Luft, M.D.
Professor
Department of Medicine
State University of New York at Stony Brook
T-16, Room 020
Stony Brook, New York 11794

Peter Mariuz, M.D.
Assistant Professor
Department of Medicine
State University of New York at Stony Brook
T-15, Room 080
Stony Brook, New York 11794

Christina M. Marra, M.D.
Assistant Professor of Medicine, Neurology,
*   and Infectious Diseases*
Departments of Neurology and Medicine
University of Washington School of Medicine
Harborview Medical Center
325 9th Avenue
Seattle, Washington 98104-2499

Eugene O. Major, Ph.D.
Chief
Laboratory of Molecular Medicine and
*   Neuroscience*
National Institute of Neurological Disorders
*   and Stroke*
Building 36, Room 5W21
Bethesda, Maryland 20892

Justin C. McArthur, M.B., B.S., M.P.H.
Associate Professor of Neurology and
*   Epidemiology*
Department of Neurology
The Johns Hopkins University School of
*   Medicine*
600 North Wolfe Street
Baltimore, Maryland 21287-7609

John A. Messenheimer, M.D.
Professor
Department of Neurology
University of North Carolina School of
*   Medicine*
CB #7025
Manning Drive
Chapel Hill, North Carolina 27599

Mariachiara G. Monaco, Ph.D.
Visiting Fellow
Laboratory of Molecular Medicine and
*   Neuroscience*
National Institutes of Health
36 Convent Drive
Bethesda, Maryland 20892

Victor E. Mulanovich, M.D.
1749 Northeast 26th Street
Suite F
Fort Lauderdale, Florida 33305

Opendra Narayan, D.U.M., Ph.D.
Professor
Department of Microbiology and Molecular
Genetics
University of Kansas Medical Center
3901 Rainbow Boulevard
Kansas City, Kansas 66160

Carol K. Petito, M.D.
Professor
Department of Pathology
University of Miami School of Medicine
Papanicolaou Research Building
Room 417
1550 Northwest 10th Avenue
Miami, Florida 33136

M. Judith Donovan Post, M.D.,
F.A.C.R.
Professor of Radiology, Neurological Surgery,
and Ophthalmology
Department of Radiology
University of Miami School of Medicine
Jackson Memorial Medical Center
1115 Northwest 14th Street
Miami, Florida 33136

Michael S. Saag, M.D.
Associate Professor
Department of Medicine
The University of Alabama at Birmingham
908 20th Street South
Birmingham, Alabama 35294

Yoshihiro Saito, M.D.
Research Scientist
PAF Scholar
Department of Neurology
University of Rochester School of Medicine
601 Elmwood Avenue
Rochester, New York 14642

Frederick A. Schmitt, Ph.D.
Associate Professor
Departments of Neurology, Psychiatry, and
Psychology
Sanders-Brown Center of Aging
University of Kentucky Medical Center
800 Rose Street
Lexington, Kentucky 40536

Ola A. Selnes, Ph.D.
Associate Professor
Department of Neurology
The Johns Hopkins University School of
Medicine
600 North Wolfe Street
Baltimore, Maryland 21287-7609

Leroy R. Sharer, M.D.
Professor
Department of Pathology and Laboratory
Medicine
New Jersey Medical School
185 South Orange Avenue
Newark, New Jersey 07103

David M. Simpson, M.D.
Associate Professor and Director
Department of Neurology
Clinical Neurophysiology Laboratories
The Mount Sinai Medical Center
Box 1052
One Gustave L. Levy Place
New York, New York 10029

Elyse J. Singer, M.D.
Associate Professor
Department of Neurology
University of California Los Angeles Medical
Center
Veterans Administration Medical Center, West
Los Angeles
11301 Wilshire Boulevard
Los Angeles, California 90073

Evelyn M. L. Sklar, M.D.
Associate Professor of Clinical Radiology and
Neurological Surgery
Department of Radiology
University of Miami School of Medicine
Jackson Memorial Hospital
1115 Northwest 14th Street
Miami, Florida 33136

Edward B. Stephens, Ph.D.
Associate Professor
Departments of Microbiology, Molecular
Genetics, and Immunology
University of Kansas Medical Center
3901 Rainbow Boulevard
Kansas City, Kansas 66160

Yaakov Stern, Ph.D.
Associate Professor of Clinical
Neuropsychology
Department of Neurology and Psychiatry
Columbia University College of Physicians
and Surgeons
The Presbyterian Hospital in the City of New
York
Sergievsky Center
630 West 168th Street
New York, New York 10032

Karl Syndulko, Ph.D.
Research Neurologist
Department of Neurology
University of California at Los Angeles
Los Angeles, California 90024

Michele Tagliati, M.D.
Research Fellow in Neurology and Clinical
*   Neurophysiology*
The Mount Sinai Medical Center
One Gustave L. Levy Place
New York, New York 10029

Michael L. Tapper, M.D.
Clinical Professor of Medicine
New York University School of Medicine
Chief, Section of Infectious Diseases
Medical Director, AIDS Program
Lennox Hill Hospital
100 East 77th Street
New York, New York 10021-1883

Claudia Tellez, M.D.
Fellow in Training
Department of Hematology/Oncology
Northwestern University Medical School
233 East Erie, Suite 700
Chicago, Illinois 60611

Bret Tindall, Bapp.Sc., Ph.D.
Senior Project Scientist
National Centre in HIV Epidemiology and
*   Clinical Research*
University of New South Wales, and
Research Fellow
Centre for Immunology
St. Vincent's Hospital
Sydney 2020
Australia

Wallace W. Tourtellotte, M.D., Ph.D.
Department of Neurology
University of California Los Angeles School of
*   Medicine*
Veterans Administration Medical Center West
*   Los Angeles*
11301 Wilshire Boulevard
Los Angeles, California 90073

Bradley V. Vaughn, M.D.
Assistant Professor
Department of Neurology
University of North Carolina School of
*   Medicine*
University of North Carolina Hospitals
738 Burnett Womack Building, CB #7025
Chapel Hill, North Carolina 27599

Jamie VonRoenn, M.D.
Associate Professor
Department of Medicine
Division of Hematology/Oncology
Northwestern University Medical School
Chicago, Illinois 60611

Mary M. Wetherby, Ph.D.
Department of Neurology
Sanders-Brown Center on Aging
University of Kentucky Medical Center
800 Rose Street
Lexington, Kentucky 40536

Michelle L. Hansman Whiteman, M.D.
Assistant Professor of Clinical Radiology,
*   Otolaryngology, and Neurological Surgery*
Department of Radiology
Neuroradiology Section
University of Miami School of Medicine
Jackson Memorial Center
MRI Center
1115 Northwest 14th Street
Miami, Florida 33136

Foreword

The First Edition of *AIDS and the Nervous System* published in 1988 was one of the first compilations of the diseases of the brain, spinal cord, and peripheral nerve associated with human immunodeficiency virus (HIV) infections. Since that publication, the virus has continued to spread worldwide, making it the most prevalent viral infection of the nervous system in history. Furthermore, numerous clinical neurological syndromes have been associated with HIV infection making it unique among neurotropic viruses in its diversity of clinical presentations.

In 1983, the isolation of HIV in activated lymphocyte cultures led to a simple scenario: HIV infected cells of the immune system that expressed CD4 markers. This infection led to CD4 cell destruction and resultant immunodeficiency, and this immunodeficiency resulted in fatal opportunistic infections. Early neurological interest focused on the unusual opportunistic infections and lymphomas that affected the nervous system. In 1985, the isolation of HIV from brain, spinal cord, cerebrospinal fluid, and peripheral nerves of patients dying with neurological complications of AIDS, the demonstration of HIV RNA and DNA in the brains of patients, and the demonstration of intrathecal synthesis of antibody against HIV in patients with AIDS focused instead on primary infection of the nervous system. Initially, some postulated that this infection might occur as a terminal event with the infiltration of inflammatory cells in response to opportunistic infections, but it was subsequently shown in a number of studies that infection occurred early during the long asymptomatic phase of HIV infection and that this infection occurred in the majority of healthy seropositive people. As the epidemic continues to evolve with rising numbers in Africa, with greater involvement of the intravenous drug-using populations of Europe and the United States, their sexual partners and progeny, and the new explosive epidemic spread in south and southeast Asia, it is probable that over 15 million people now are infected with the virus. It is estimated that over 30 million people will be infected by the year 2000. The majority of infected patients already have nervous system infections making this the most prevalent viral infection of the nervous system in history. Furthermore, the majority of those infected will develop dementia, myelopathy and/ or neuropathies in the later phases of the infection, and these serious neurological complications will pose an enormous public health burden over the next two decades.

The second unique aspect of HIV infections of the nervous system is the diversity of clinical syndromes. These complications occur at different times during infection and show varied neuropathological findings. For example, in the peripheral nerve alone, acute inflammatory, demyelinating neuropathy (which is presumably an autoimmune disease) is seen early during the infectious process; mononeuritis multiplex, which probably represents a vasculitis, occurs later in infection; and predominantly sensory painful neuropathy with axonal degeneration is common among patients with severe immunodeficiency. Most viral syndromes depend on the selective vulnerability of specific cell populations to specific viral infections. Thus, paralytic poliomyelitis results from selected infection of motor neurons by polioviruses, and their destruction leads to flaccid paralysis; progressive multifocal leukoencephalopathy results from selective infection of oligodendrocytes by JC virus leading to multifocal demyelination. Although HIV is clearly highly neuroinvasive, its neurotropism seems to be limited largely to macrophages and microglia, and infection of these cells has been demonstrated in healthy seropositive persons, as well as in fatal cases of AIDS without neurological complications. The diverse neurological complications of HIV infection suggested varied mechanism of pathogenesis, and the failure to correlate virulence with neuronal infection suggests indirect effects of viral proteins, cytokines, or toxins.

The pace of knowledge about AIDS has been unprecedented. In 1983 the virus was recovered within two years of the clinical description, the total sequence was available in 1985, and in 1987 the first effective antiviral drug was developed, tested, and licensed. There is over 100,000 literature citations about AIDS and HIV. Despite this extraordinary collection of data, many questions remain unanswered regarding HIV-associated neurological diseases. This volume provides an update on the opportunistic infections of the nervous system and the diseases thought to be related to primary HIV infections. This book covers the diagnosis, treatment, and prevention of these diseases, and it defines the areas where important questions still await solutions.

> *Richard T. Johnson, M.D.*
> *Professor and Director, Department of Neurology*
> *The Johns Hopkins University School of Medicine*
> *Baltimore, Maryland*

Preface

Since the publication of the first edition of *AIDS and the Nervous System* in 1988, the human immunodeficiency virus-type 1 (HIV-1) has continued its relentless progression. Although rates of infection have plateaued in some populations, such as homosexual men in the United States, in others it has continued to demonstrate frightening increases. As of October 1995, more than 500,000 persons with acquired immunodeficiency syndrome (AIDS) have been reported to the Centers for Disease Control. Ten percent of these cases had been reported from 1981–1987, 41% from 1988–1992, and 49% from 1993 to October 31, 1995. The illness in the United States is no longer confined to large metropolitan areas, but may be found in even the most remote rural regions of the country. In other parts of the world, particularly in some Third World countries of Africa and Southeast Asia, the disease has taken a staggering toll, affecting a significant percentage of the population. On an encouraging note, the increase in the number of persons with AIDS has been coupled with an unparalleled increase in our understanding of the virus and its manifold presentations.

Not unexpectedly, an increase in the numbers of persons with HIV-associated neurological complications has occurred in tandem with the increase in the number of persons with AIDS in the general population. Careful examination at autopsy reveals neuropathological abnormalities in virtually all HIV-infected persons. At least 50% to 60% of all HIV-infected persons develop clinically significant neurological disease, and these disorders are frequently the heralding manifestations of AIDS. Another potential contributing factor to the incresed frequency with which these disorders are observed is the greatest length of survival of HIV-infected persons as a consequence of the development and application of improved antiretroviral regimens and standards of care. Previously, rare neurological disorders, such as progressive multifocal leukoencephalopathy and primary central nervous system lymphoma, are now increasingly commonplace. There is a strong possibility that the increase in the frequency of these and possibly other HIV-associated neurological complications are the consequences of longer survivals of patients with advanced cellular immunosuppression.

Although mirroring the First Edition, the Second Edition of *AIDS and the Nervous System* has been greatly expanded. This book is intended for all healthcare workers who deal with HIV-infected patients and others interested in understanding these disorders. It is meant to have a broad scope. Although emphasis is on the diagnosis and management of these disorders, thorough discussions of HIV neuropathogenesis, pathology, and related patient care issues are meant to reinforce its value as a comprehensive reference. We hope that this effort helps improve the quality of life of those infected with HIV.

Joseph R. Berger, M.D.
Robert M. Levy, M.D., Ph.D.

Acknowledgments

Dr. Berger thanks his parents for imbuing all their children with a ''can do'' spirit, and his wife and children for their support and indulgence during this project.

Dr. Levy thanks his colleagues Drs. Bruce Cohen, Jamie VonRoenn, Robert Murphy, and John Phair for their support and collaboration; Mary Martin Rogers and Elizabeth Greenspan at Lippincott-Raven Publishers for their persistence and energy during this project; and his patients whose spirit and courage are an inspiration.

AIDS and the Nervous System

Second Edition

AIDS and the Nervous System, Second Edition,
edited by J. R. Berger and R. M. Levy.
Lippincott-Raven Publishers, Philadelphia © 1997.

1

Acquired Immunodeficiency Syndrome and the Nervous System: Fifteen Years of Progress

An Overview to the Second Edition of *AIDS and the Nervous System*

[†]Bernard Bendok, [°]Joseph R. Berger, and [†]Robert M. Levy

*[°]Department of Neurology, University of Kentucky Medical Center,
Lexington, Kentucky 40536, and [†]Department of Surgery,
Northwestern University Medical School, Chicago, Illinois 60611*

No longer a rare disease afflicting only a small segment of the population, the acquired immunodeficiency syndrome (AIDS) has been observed throughout the United States and in 194 other countries in the world (13). At the time of our writing of the first edition of this book in 1986, 13,189 new cases of AIDS were reported to the U.S. Centers for Disease Control and prevention (CDC); 7,787 patients diagnosed as having AIDS in 1985 and earlier years were still alive for at least part of 1986. Therefore, 20,976 patients were treated for AIDS during 1986, and there were 8,320 deaths (9). By the beginning of 1987, a total of 29,137 cases and 16,481 deaths had been reported.

Through October, 1995, only 8 years later, 501,310 cases of AIDS and 311,381 (63%) deaths due to AIDS in the United States had been reported to the CDC (1). In the single year from July 1993 to June 1994, >85,000 cases of AIDS were reported (1). The World Health Organization (WHO) estimates there have been 4.5 million AIDS cases worldwide and that 18 million adults and 1.5 million children are infected with the human immunodeficiency virus (HIV) (3). In its cost of human lives and financial productivity, the AIDS epidemic has confirmed many of the worst fears that were projected at the time that the first edition of this book was published.

Since the first publication of this book, the CDC (2) has revised its classification of HIV infection several times. In 1987, the CDC redefined AIDS as a disabling or life-threatening illness caused by HIV and included HIV encephalopathy, among other illnesses, as an AIDS-defining condition. In 1993, the CDC further included CD4+ T-lymphocyte counts (CD4+ counts) as a measure of immunodeficiency; people with HIV infection and CD4+ counts of $<200/mm^3$ were defined as having AIDS.

The risk groups defined by the CDC are presented in Chapter 2. As was the case at the time of the first edition of this volume, the largest risk group in the United States is that of homosexual or bisexual men; this group now represents only 53% of the cumulative total of patients with AIDS as opposed to 72% in 1986. Intravenous (IV) drug abusers now make up 24% of AIDS cases; this has increased from 17% in the past 8 years. In 6% of AIDS cases, both homosexual/bisexual activity and IV drug use are risk factors. Heterosexual transmission of HIV has increased from 1–2% to 7% of cases. The remaining cases have been patients in whom blood transfusions were the only possible risk factor (2%), hemophiliacs who regularly received infusions of concentrated blood products (1%), and children of mothers infected with HIV (1%); these figures have remained stable over the past decade. Approximately 6% of patients have no known risk factors (1). The CDC has said that AIDS ''continues to affect blacks and Hispanics disproportionately.'' The rate of AIDS is 17 per 100,000 whites, whereas it is 51 per 100,000 Hispanics and 101 per 100,000 blacks.

The neurological manifestations of AIDS and HIV infection are being observed with an increasing frequency that parallels the increasing number of AIDS cases. Neurological syndromes occur in patients across the spectrum of HIV disease. At least 10% of all patients with AIDS first present with a neurologic complaint, 40–60% develop significant neurological signs or symptoms during their lifetime, and 80% have significant neuropathological abnormalities on autopsy. Thus, nervous system disease is both common and often clinically unrecognized. As patients survive longer, this subclinical disease may become evident and the frequency of neurologic complaints may increase.

The symptoms and signs of many AIDS-associated neurological syndromes overlap extensively, making bedside diagnosis nearly impossible. Computerized tomographic (CT) scanning demonstrates abnormalities in 60% of patients, but the findings are usually nonspecific, even with double-dose contrast enhancement (7). Magnetic resonance imaging (MRI) is more sensitive than CT and is the radiographic study of choice for identifying and following intracranial lesions in patients with AIDS (5); however, even with gadolinium enhancement, MRI findings are not specific for particular diseases. Because serological and cerebrospinal fluid (CSF) studies are usually not helpful in establishing the etiology of intracranial masses, histological verification of the type of intracranial lesions may be necessary. This is usually best accomplished by image-guided stereotactic brain biopsy, which has a diagnostic efficacy of 95% in patients with HIV infection (6). The observation that seropositive patients in high-risk groups may have neurological diseases that are not causally associated with AIDS, such as malignant gliomas, benign tumors, and herniated lumbar disks, further supports the need for operative confirmation of neurological processes in certain circumstances.

CHAPTER HIGHLIGHTS

The epidemiology and neuroepidemiology of HIV infection are detailed in Chapter 2. As noted above, by June 1994 >400,000 cases of AIDS and 243,000 deaths due to AIDS in the United States were reported to the CDC, and in the single year from July 1993 to June 1994 >85,000 cases of AIDS were reported. Worldwide, over 1 million cases of AIDS have been reported to the WHO; due to underreporting, the true number of AIDS cases is thought to be ~4 million and over 16 million people are thought to be HIV infected. By the end of the century, there will have been roughly 10 million AIDS cases and as many as 40 million HIV infected people. As many as one in every 160 people in the world between the ages of 15 and 49 may be HIV infected.

The biology and neurotropism of HIV is discussed in Chapter 3. Since the publication of the first edition of *AIDS and the Nervous System*, research in this area has been the most active and productive. Although the pathological effects of HIV on the brain can be diffuse, the virus has thus far been found in limited cell numbers and types, although newer techniques are allowing for identification of HIV in greater cell numbers and types than once thought. Our knowledge of HIV biology has grown to include the isolation and characterization of neurotropic strains of the virus and has led to greater understanding of the possible mechanisms of HIV-induced neuropathogenicity.

It is this issue of HIV-1 neuropathogenicity that is the focus of Chapter 4. Three of the leading researchers in this field have combined the efforts of their laboratories with those of other investigators to provide a rigorous review of the proposed mechanisms whereby HIV-1 infection of the brain results in neurologic damage and dysfunction. The authors critically review the theories and supporting data for both direct and indirect mechanisms for neural damage (neurovirulence). These theories include the direct viral infection of neural cells, indirect toxicity of HIV-1 proteins on neural cells, HIV-infected macrophage-glial cell interactions producing neural damage, proinflammatory cytokines, platelet activating factor and arachidonic acid metabolites contributing to HIV-related neural damage and the possibility that the NMDA receptor serves as a final common pathway for HIV-related neural damage.

As several critical issues of HIV-1 neurotropism and neuropathogenicity involve the interactions between HIV-1 and the brain's immune system, the discussion in Chapter 5 of the neuroimmunology of HIV-1 infection is particularly relevant. This state of the art review of neuroimmunology as it applies to HIV-1 infection covers the broad spectrum of systemic and CNS immunologic responses to HIV-1 infection and the pathologic implications of these responses. Of particular interest is the discussion of the blood brain barrier in HIV-1 infection.

Almost unknown at the time of the first edition of the book, animal models used to study HIV infection are presented in Chapter 6. Infection with the simian immunodeficiency virus in macaques (SIVmac) appears to be the best current animal model for AIDS. Of great interest are those animal studies that indicate that the development and clinical expression of HIV encephalitis requires a two-step process. Typically, only after immunosuppression occurs does replication of a macrophage tropic virus in the brain take place. Although HIV-related cognitive motor dysfunction rarely occurs in the setting of immune competence, these animal findings are of great import to the usual human case of immunosuppression predating the clinical onset of HIV encephalopathy.

The great number and breadth of neurologic symptoms associated with HIV infection are discussed in Chapter 7. As experience increases over time, the list of possible HIV-associated neurologic disease grows and becomes better defined. The relative importance of various adjunctive diagnostic measures has been much better characterized in the past decade. Thus, the degree of immunosuppression as shown by CD4+ count can be of significant diagnostic utility; cytomegalovirus (CMV) encephalitis, for example, rarely develops unless the CD4+ count falls below 50 cells/ mm^3.

The spinal cord diseases associated with HIV infection are presented in Chapter 8. Our increased knowledge of myelopathy in the setting of HIV infection has warranted the inclusion of a separate chapter in the current volume. Although the most common spinal cord disease seen in HIV-infected individuals remains vacuolar myelopathy, myelopathies due to infectious, metabolic, vascular, and neoplastic causes need to be excluded before this diagnosis can be established.

The neuromuscular syndromes in HIV disease are presented in Chapter 9. Considered a curiosity at the time of the first edition of this volume, myopathy is now a well-characterized entity that has profound implications to patients' quality of life. Myopathy may be related to HIV infection or due to antiretroviral therapy; there may well be effective treatment for this disorder. Although myopathy can occur equally at all stages of HIV infection, different peripheral neuropathies tend to present preferentially during certain stages of infection and immunosuppression. Inflammatory polyneuropathies tend to occur during periods of immune competence, whereas CMV nerve infections typically present in patients with CD4+ counts of <50 cells/mm^3. The diagnosis and treatment for these peripheral neuropathies have been well investigated over the past several years.

HIV infection in infants, children, and adolescents is discussed in Chapter 10. As the number of women infected with HIV has risen, so has the number of infected children. Twenty percent of all HIV-infected people are 13–29 years of age; >6,000 cases of pediatric AIDS have been reported in the United States. The most frequent signs of HIV-1–associated central nervous system (CNS) disease in the pediatric population are cognitive impairment, poor brain growth, and abnormalities of tone and motor function.

The prognostic and diagnostic utility of CSF analysis in the setting of HIV infection is presented in Chapter 11. Because a variety of diagnostic tests have been developed and validated since the publication of the first edition, their relative value must be discussed and put into perspective. The role of assaying p24 antigen, cytokines, intrathecal antibody synthesis, beta-2 microglobulin, neopterin, excitotoxic metabolites, and tryptophan in assessing disease progression and response to therapy is discussed.

The value of neurophysiological testing is discussed in Chapter 12. Over the past decade, a number of such noninvasive neurophysiological tests have been applied to HIV-infected subjects. Quantitative electroencephalography can be used as a research tool to monitor AIDS-associated neurologic disease progression and possibly predict neurologic dysfunction. Somatosensory evoked potentials show the greatest abnormalities of all evoked potentials in HIV infection but are not specific. Study of autonomic function shows abnormalities early in the course of AIDS. Sleep studies on both symptomatic and asymptomatic HIV-infected individuals show abnormalities of various sleep parameters. Because these tests are both highly sensitive and noninvasive, they may well play an important role in the neurodiagnostics of HIV-related nervous system illnesses.

Diagnostic neuroimaging of HIV-related neurological illnesses is presented in Chapter 13. CT and MRI are the most commonly used imaging modalities for HIV-infected individuals. Delayed double-dose contrast enhancement increases the sensitivity of CT scanning, whereas gadolinium enhancement improves the sensitivity and specificity of MRI. MRI is the diagnostic imaging modality of choice for patients with HIV infection. Angiography may rarely be useful in the setting of vasculitis; MR angiography may well be an alternative to conventional angiography in this setting. Of great promise is thallium-201 brain SPECT imaging, which may help to differentiate inflammatory processes such as toxoplasmosis from neoplastic lesions such as lymphoma; further developments in this area may limit the need for brain biopsy in the future.

The neuroophthalmology of AIDS is presented in Chapter 14. Most of the visual morbidity in HIV-infected individuals is due to infections; most of these infections are related to CMV. CMV has a greater predilection for the eye over the brain, whereas other infecting organisms tend to infect the brain preferentially. Ocular neoplasms are rare and may be difficult to distinguish from infection. There has been considerable progress over the past several years in the treatment of ocular CMV in the setting of AIDS.

The neuropsychological assessment of patients with HIV infection is discussed in Chapter 15. Although the neuropsychological impact of early HIV infection was a great source of dissention, a general consensus has been reached in this area since the publication of the first edition of *AIDS and the Nervous System*. Although cognitive impairment in seropositive, otherwise asymptomatic individuals does occur, it is a rare event and may be a marker for CNS involvement with HIV. In general, the severity of cognitive dysfunction correlates with disease progression. Most significantly, this cognitive impairment may respond to pharmacological therapy.

The neuropsychiatry of HIV infection is discussed in Chapter 16. As the number of HIV infected individuals continues to grow, and as the impact of HIV infection on the practice of psychiatry becomes significant, awareness of the unique psychiatric aspects of this disease becomes critical. Three models for interpreting psychiatric problems during HIV infection are presented: the biologic model, the transition model, and the background model. Well-considered psychiatric interventions may be of considerable impact on the quality of life of patients with HIV infection and AIDS.

A single chapter in the first edition of the book, the neuropathology of AIDS has grown to cover three chapters in this second edition. Chapter 17 reviews the HIV-related pathology of the spinal cord. Postmortem studies show a high incidence of spinal cord abnormalities in HIV-infected individuals, including vacuolar myelopathy, opportunistic infections, primary HIV infection, and neoplasms. The neuropathology of primary HIV-1 infection of the brain is presented in Chapter 18. Atrophy and white matter changes may characterize the gross neuropathologic examination of the HIV-1–infected brain. The interaction of HIV-1 with other viruses in the CNS may facilitate neurotropism and disease progression. The chapter highlights studies on neuronal loss in HIV infection and the effect of antiretroviral therapy on brain pathology. The neuropathological changes associated with HIV-related opportunistic infections and neoplasms are discussed in Chapter 19. Neuropathological changes are seen in the brains of up to 95% of HIV-1–infected patients; opportunistic infections may account for up to two thirds of these findings. These findings, and their relative infrequency in the pediatric HIV population, are carefully documented and reviewed. The neurologic manifestations of primary HIV-1 infection are discussed in Chapter 20. Seventy percent of individuals infected with HIV-1 will develop an acute illness characterized by nonspecific systemic symptoms such as fever and adenopathy. Occasionally, primary HIV-1 infection manifests neurologically with headaches, meningo-encephalitis, seizures, or myelopathy. Primary HIV-1 infection should therefore be considered in the differential diagnosis of a wide range of acute neurologic syndromes.

Of the neurologic manifestations of primary HIV-1 infection, HIV-associated dementia is, of course, the most common and well studied. As such, the entirety of Chapter 21 is devoted to this subject. The chapter begins by addressing the problems of terminology and taxonomy which have profoundly complicated the field. This is followed by a discussion of HIV-1 associated minor cognitive-motor disorder and neuropsychological studies in asymptomatic and symptomatic HIV infection; the controversies which surround the neurocognitive deficits possibly associated with asymptomatic HIV infection are carefully presented and discussed. Then presented are the clinical features, epidemiology, neuropsychological assessment, natural history, diagnosis, neuropathology and treatment of HIV-associated dementia.

Progressive multifocal leukencephalopathy (PML) is discussed in Chapter 22. Before the AIDS epidemic, PML was a rare entity, mostly seen in patients with lymphoproliferative disorders. Now, up to 5% of patients with AIDS develop PML; this represents a significant increase over the past 8 years. PML results from infection with the papovavirus JC. However, HIV-induced immunosuppression alone is not sufficient for the development of PML in JC-infected patients. There appear to be multiple factors that increase the likelihood for the development of PML in AIDS including the molecular interaction between virus and HIV-1 JC. Despite over a decade of experience, PML remains a largely untreatable illness with a median life expectancy of only a few months. Clinical trials are underway and in development; by the next edition of this book, there is hope that some therapeutic impact will become possible.

The impact of herpesviruses in AIDS is outlined in Chapter 23. CMV is a major cause of morbidity and mortality in AIDS. Largely unrecognized as an important nervous system pathogen at the time of the first edition of this volume, CMV has become the focus of considerable clinical and basic science investigation. CMV appears to be a significant nervous system pathogen in AIDS. The use of CMV polymerase chain reaction diagnostic testing on the serum and cerebrospinal fluid has allowed for the definitive diagnosis of nervous system CMV infection; the availability of effective antiviral agents against CMV has made therapy possible. Recent research has implicated Epstein-Barr virus (EBV) as a cause of primary central nervous system lymphoma, the most common brain tumor in AIDS. Furthermore, herpesviruses may act as cofactors that facilitate the progression of HIV infection.

Toxoplasmosis is discussed in Chapter 24. In the United States, 40% of adults with AIDS are latently infected with toxoplasmosis, and 30% will develop toxoplasmosis encephalitis (TE). Infection with toxoplasmosis can range from a well-localized indolent granulomatous process to a widely diffuse necrotizing encephalitis. Immunoglobulin G antibodies are present in 100% of patients with AIDS who have TE. Absence of the antibody makes the diagnosis unlikely but not impossible. Therapy is empirically started based on clinical presentation and typical radiological findings, and the response to therapy is monitored. In selected cases, with equivocal antibody test results, solitary lesions on MRI, or inadequate responses to empiric therapy, biopsy may be required to definitively establish the diagnosis of toxoplasmosis. Although first-line drug treatment remains pyrimethamine and sulfadiazine, several alternative agents have been tested and appear to be effective in this patient population.

Cryptococcal meningitis is discussed in Chapter 25. *Cryptococcus neoformans* is the most common cause of meningitis in AIDS. Clinical presentation is often nonspecific, with most patients presenting only with lethargy and headache. The majority of patients with AIDS-related cryptococcal meningitis have normal CSF parameters. India ink preparations and cryptococcal antigen assays allow for accurate diagnosis. Therapy includes amphotericin B with or without flucytosine, and fluconazole. The use of fluconazole for both primary and maintenance therapy for cryptococcal meningitis has been a significant advance since the first edition of the book. Initial response rates have been high (>70%), with initial morbidity and mortality reserved largely for those patients first presenting with alterations in mental status. Recurrence remains a significant problem, although it has lessened with oral fluconazole maintenance therapy.

The manifestations of syphilis in HIV-infected patients is discussed in Chapter 26. In the past decade, HIV infection has been found to alter the course of syphilis. Neurosyphilis and ocular syphilis are more likely to develop in the presence of HIV infection after standard therapy for early syphilis. The cutaneous manifestations of primary syphilis are also more severe with HIV infection. The chapter outlines recommendations for diagnosis and therapy of this newly epidemic disease.

A discussion of less common opportunistic infections is presented in Chapter 27. Aside from the more common HIV-related infections, various bacteria, viruses, parasites, and fungi can cause illness in patients with AIDS. A careful travel history may help with the differential diagnosis. Because most of these unusual pathogens are treatable, early diagnosis and therapy can be lifesaving. CNS neoplasms in patients with AIDS are discussed in Chapter 28. CNS involvement with Kaposi's sarcoma is rare, whereas primary CNS lymphoma occurs in up to 5% of all HIV-infected patients. This represents a significant increase over the past decade. Lymphoma is the most common CNS mass lesion in HIV-infected children and only second to toxoplasmosis in adults. Brain biopsy is usually needed to establish the diagnosis of primary CNS lymphoma. Although these tumors do respond to radiotherapy, the response is often incomplete and increases survival only from about 1 to 4 months. There may thus be a role for chemotherapy either alone or in conjunction with radiotherapy.

The hospital epidemiology and infection control strategies are presented in Chapter 29. Although the likelihood of physician-to-patient and patient-to-physician transmission of HIV was largely unknown a decade ago, exhaustive epidemiologic studies have defined the risks of HIV transmission in the health-care setting. Universal precautions, based on the principle of presuming all patients to be potentially infected with HIV-1 and guarding against contact with bodily fluids, is recommended. Needles are never to be recapped, and mouth pieces should be used during cardiopulmonary resuscitation. Health-care workers with exudative lesions should refrain from direct patient contact. The seroconversion of health-care workers exposed to HIV through needle sticks is rare. With the full knowledge available through epidemiologic studies, both patients and health-care workers can function in an informed and responsible manner.

Future directions for research and therapy of AIDS-associated neurological disease are discussed in Chapter 30. There remains a need for better diagnostic modalities and more effective and safer drugs in addition to better diagnostic modalities. A better way to assay for JC virus, for example, would simplify the diagnosis and therapy of PML. Because of the association between EBV and primary cerebral lymphoma, prophylaxis against EBV may reduce the incidence of cerebral lymphoma.

Chapter 31 outlines algorithms for the diagnosis and treatment of HIV-infected individuals with signs and symptoms of peripheral nerve, cranial nerve, or CNS dysfunction. Although the algorithms presented in the first edition of the book have proven to be vigorous, several advances have led to refinements in our recommendations. The adjunctive value of toxoplasma titers is now better understood, and thallium SPECT scanning, for example, may well limit the need for brain biopsy in the future.

IMPACT OF AIDS ON THE PRACTICE OF NEUROLOGY AND NEUROSURGERY

In the first edition of this volume, we made predictions concerning the impact of HIV-related neurologic disease on the practice of the clinical neurosciences. Unfortunately, the reality of the AIDS epidemic has served to confirm these predictions. Over the past 8 years, HIV-related neurologic disease has proven to have an important impact on the practice of neurology, neurosurgery, and psychiatry. To again predict the scope of AIDS-related neurological problems and their impact on medicine, we took the recent neuroepidemiologic data from the CDC (Chapter 2) and compared it with our 1986 estimates. Unfortunately, estimating the number of cases of AIDS with neurologic conditions has become extremely more complicated due largely to the 1993 change in the AIDS surveillance case definition. This new case definition added persons with CD4+ counts of less than 200; thus the number of AIDS cases in 1993 and 1994 was much higher than before the change in the definition, because there were a large number of HIV infected people with CD4+ counts below 200 who hadn't yet had an opportunistic infection. With those people identified as having AIDS in 1993 and 1994, the number of AIDS cases has been flattening. The issue is further complicated by the fact that opportunistic infection or neoplasm, as an AIDS defining condition, was reported at the time of AIDS diagnosis until the new definition in 1993. Since that time, as CD4+ counts below 200 are sufficient for the surveillance case definition of AIDS and longitudinal reporting is not requried, opportunistic infections and neoplasms are less frequently reported to the CDC.

In light of these reporting problems, we present here a range of numbers for each HIV-related neurologic disease. On the low end of the range, as suggested by the CDC, we report the number of cases as determined by the proportion of AIDS cases with that disease reported to the CDC times the total number of AIDS cases times that percentage of AIDS cases with opportunistic infections. For 1991, for example, there were 50,400 cases of AIDS diagnosed with an opportunistic infection in the United States; in 1994, there were 62,300. At the high end of the range, we report the number of cases as determined by the proportion of AIDS cases with that disease reported in the most recent clinical series times the total number of AIDS cases. The number of new cases, the number of yearly deaths, and the cumulative number of cases and deaths are presented in Table 1.

TABLE 1. *AIDS cases and AIDS deaths in the United States*

	1986	1994
New cases	13,189	80,691
Deaths	8,320	32,330
Cumulative		
Cases	29,137	501,310[a]
Deaths	16,481	311,381[a]

[a] Reported as of October 1995.

TABLE 2. *Predicted number of HIV-related neurologic disorders*

	1986	1991	1994
Primary CNS lymphoma	266	1000–1848	1200–3400
Progressive multifocal leukoencephalopathy (PML)	141	978–1100	1400–3400
AIDS dementia	1,817	5200–7500	6450–9300

The large number of HIV-infected individuals has significantly affected the prevalence of several specific diseases. Primary CNS lymphoma, for example, accounted for 1–1.5% of all brain tumors in the pre-AIDS era. Because reporting of AIDS-related diseases to the CDC is required only at the time of the initial diagnosis of AIDS and follow-up reports are infrequent, the yearly incidence of specific diseases can be estimated only from epidemiological studies. From the relative frequency of lymphomas in our study of 1,286 patients with AIDS (0.6% at presentation and 1.3% after AIDS diagnosis) and from CDC statistics (9), we estimated that 266 cases of primary AIDS-associated CNS lymphomas occurred in 1986, compared with ~225 cases not related to AIDS that were reported yearly before 1979 (8) (Table 2). By 1991, we predicted 1,848 cases of primary CNS lymphoma would be observed annually in patients with AIDS; this incidence exceeded that of low-grade astrocytomas and approached that of meningiomas (10) (Table 3). Using the newer case definitions and numbers supplied by the CDC, we now estimate that roughly 1000 and 1200 cases of primary brain lymphoma occurred in AIDS patients in 1991 and 1994, respectively. Using the more recent clinical series which report that about 4% of all AIDS patients develop PCNSL, we estimate that as many as 3400 cases occurred in 1994.

Similarly, we estimated that there were 141 cases of AIDS-associated PML in 1986; by 1991, the annual number of cases of PML was estimated to be 978 (Table 2), which is equivalent to the yearly number of cases of Huntington's disease and myasthenia gravis (Table 4). Using the CDC model described above, we now estimate that roughly 1100 cases of PML occurred in the United States in 1991 and 1400 cases occurred in 1994. Using the more recent clinical series which report that about 4% of all AIDS patients develop PML, we estimate that as many as 3400 cases of PML occurred in 1994.

Finally, in 1986 we estimated that there were 1,817 such cases of HIV-related encephalopathy as determined by clinical criteria; our predictions suggested that

TABLE 3. *The possible number of HIV-related primary CNS lymphomas in comparison with the yearly incidence of primary brain tumors in the United States*

Tumor	Yearly incidence[a]	HIV-related CNS lymphomas
Malignant astrocytoma	6,000	1994
Meningioma	2,250	1991
Astrocytoma	1,500	
Pituitary tumor	1,500	
Neurinoma/fibroma	750	
Medulloblastoma	600	
Congenital	600	
Ependymoma	300	1986
Lymphoma	225	

Data from Schoenberg BS. The epidemiology of CNS tumors. In: Walker MD, ed. *Oncology of the Nervous System*. Boston: Martinus-Nijhoff, 1983:1–29.

TABLE 4. *The possible number of HIV-related PML and HIV-related encephalopathy cases in comparison with the yearly incidence of selected neurological diseases*

Neurological disease	Yearly incidence[a]	PML	HIV-related encephalopathy
			1994
Multiple sclerosis	7,200		1991
Guillain-Barré syndrome	4,800		
Motor neuron disease	4,800		
Polymyositis	1,920	1994	
Muscular dystrophies	1,680		1986
Myasthenia gravis	960	1991	
Huntington's disease	960	1986	

Data from Kurtzke JF, Kurland LT. The epidemiology of neurologic disease. In: Baker AB, Baker LH, eds. *Clinical Neurology.* Philadelphia: Harper & Row, 1983:1–14.

there were 13,144 such cases in 1991 (Table 2). This number is significantly larger than the yearly incidence of multiple sclerosis and approaches the total yearly incidence of all primary brain tumors (Table 4). In the interval since the publication of the first edition of this volume, the definitions of HIV-related cognitive dysfunction and dementia have been changed considerably. Using current diagnostic criteria, we predict in 1995 that there will be 22,248 cases of HIV-1–associated minor cognitive/motor disorder and 6,459 cases of AIDS dementia. The CDC does not provide for estimation of the number of cases of minor cognitive/motor disorder. Using the data from the Multicenter AIDS Cohort Study (MACS) and from the CDC sponsored study at San Francisco General Hospital (11), the CDC suggests that 15% of AIDS patients will develop AIDS dementia. Thus, it would be predicted that there were 7500 demented AIDS patients in 1991 and 9300 in 1994 (11).

In 1988 we illustrated the impact of AIDS on the practice of neurosurgery by estimating the possible number of brain biopsies that would be performed in patients without a prior diagnosis of AIDS who present with CNS mass lesions and in those in whom empirical treatment for CNS masses fails (9). These two groups of patients could have accounted for 920 biopsies in 1986 and for 5,978 biopsies in 1991; the latter figure equalled the yearly incidence of malignant astrocytoma in the United States (10).

At present, we use the following criteria to direct image-guided stereotactic brain biopsy: the presence of a solitary CNS lesion on MRI, the failure of multiple CNS lesions to respond to antitoxoplasmosis therapy, the presence of CNS lesions in a patient allergic to agents used to treat toxoplasmosis, or the presence of CNS lesions in a patient whose illness is felt to be so severe that he or she is unable to tolerate a 2- to 3-week course of empiric therapy for toxoplasmosis. Using these criteria, we predict that in 1995 a maximum of 13,290 biopsy cases will be indicated.

The number of operations performed will probably be much lower because physicians may be reluctant to suggest an operation for patients who are faced with a debilitating, invariably fatal disease. Furthermore, some investigators do not favor the biopsy of low-intensity white matter lesions without mass effect. Increased awareness of the low mortality and morbidity rates associated with stereotactic biopsy procedures should minimize that reluctance.

It is our fervent hope that current efforts will prove effective and decrease both the number of patients with AIDS and the frequency of their neurological complications. Unfortunately, the CDC predictions, which were based on the lack of an effective intervention for HIV infection, have proven to be vigorous. Furthermore, although research on the development of new antiretroviral agents and on a vaccine that will protect against infection with HIV is active, recent failures have suggested that there will be no major epidemiologic impact in the near future. Even if effective treatment for AIDS is developed in the next several years, it is clear that the neurological manifestations of HIV infection will have a significant impact on neurology, neurosurgery, psychiatry, infectious disease, and ultimately all medical specialties for a long time to come.

REFERENCES

1. Centers for Disease Control and Prevention. First 500,000 AIDS cases—United States, 1995. *MMWR* 1995;44:849–853.
2. Centers for Disease Control and Prevention. 1993 revised classification system for HIV infection and expanded surveillance case definition for AIDS among adolescents and adults. *MMWR* 1992; 41(RR-18):1–29.
3. *Chicago Tribune.* 1995 Dec.
4. Kurtzke JF, Kurland LT. The epidemiology of neurologic disease. In: Baker AB, Baker LH, eds. *Clinical Neurology.* Philadelphia: Harper & Row, 1983:1–143.
5. Levy R, Mills C, Posin J, et al. The efficacy and clinical impact of brain imaging in neurologically symptomatic AIDS patients: a prospective CT/MRI study. *J AIDS* 1990;3:461–471.
6. Levy RM, Russell E, Yungbluth M, et al. The efficacy of image-guided stereotactic brain biopsy in neurologically symptomatic acquired immunodeficiency syndrome patients. *Neurosurgery* 1992;30: 186–190.
7. Post MJD, Kursunoglu SJ, Hensley GT, et al. Cranial CT in acquired immunodeficiency syndrome: spectrum of diseases and optimal contrast enhancement technique. *AJNR* 1985;6:743–754.
8. Rosenblum ML, Levy RM, Bredesen DE. Neurosurgical implications of the acquired immunodeficiency syndrome (AIDS). *Clin Neurosurg* 1988;34:419–445.
9. Rosenblum ML, Levy RM, Bredesen DE. *Overview of AIDS and the nervous system.* In: Rosenblum ML, Levy RM, Bredesen DE, eds. *AIDS and the Nervous System.* New York: Raven, 1988:1–12.
10. Schoenberg BS. The epidemiology of CNS tumors. In: Walker MD, ed. *Oncology of the Nervous System.* Boston: Martinus-Nijhoff, 1983:1–29.
11. Wong, JAIDS, 1994
12. World Health Organization. *The Current Global Situation of the HIV/AIDS Pandemic.* Geneva: World Health Organization Gobal Programme on AIDS, July 1994:1–11.
13. World Health Organization. *The HIV/AIDS Pandemic: 1993 Overview.* Geneva: World Health Organization Global Programme on AIDS, July 1993:1–17.

AIDS and the Nervous System, Second Edition,
edited by J. R. Berger and R. M. Levy.
Lippincott-Raven Publishers, Philadelphia © 1997.

2

Epidemiology and Neuroepidemiology of Human Immunodeficiency Virus Infection

Robert S. Janssen

*Division of HIV/AIDS Prevention, National Center for Infectious Diseases,
Centers for Disease Control and Prevention, Public Health Service, U.S.
Department of Health and Human Services, Atlanta, Georgia 30333*

Since June 1981, when five gay men in Los Angeles were reported to have developed *Pneumocystis carinii* pneumonia (38), acquired immunodeficiency syndrome (AIDS) has rapidly become one of the most important health problems in the United States and in the world. Although human immunodeficiency virus (HIV), the cause of AIDS (12,95), has been detected in banked sera from central Africa from 1959 (169), where HIV may have been present in rural areas at stable low rates (176) and in sera from the United States from 1968 (96), HIV did not cause large-scale health problems until the early 1980s. In the past 13 years, an estimated 4.0 million persons have developed AIDS worldwide (240), and an estimated one of every 250 persons 15–49 years of age is now infected with HIV (239). Although 194 countries have reported at least one case of AIDS, HIV has not affected the world's population uniformly (240). The pandemic consists of several separate epidemics, separate even within certain countries (239).

Nervous system disease was not widely noted in the early years of the epidemic; however, it is now recognized that almost every part of the nervous system can be affected not only by opportunistic infections but directly or indirectly by HIV itself (93,122,146). Neurologic complications have been described in patients with AIDS from every group at risk for HIV infection and in every part of the world.

EPIDEMIOLOGY OF HIV INFECTION

Classification of HIV Infection and Case Definition of AIDS

In 1993, the U.S. Centers for Disease Control and Prevention (CDC) revised its classification for HIV infection to include CD4+ T-lymphocyte counts (CD4+ counts) as a measure of immunodeficiency (Table 1) (44). This revision replaced the 1986 classification system, which included only clinical disease criteria (43). The new classification system divides asymptomatic infection into three categories based on CD4+ counts and more clearly distinguishes asymptomatic infection from symptomatic infection (categories B and C, Table 1).

TABLE 1. *1993 Revised classification system for HIV infection and expanded AIDS surveillance case definition for adolescents and adults*

	Clinical categories		
CD4$^+$ T-cell categories	A. Asymptomatic, acute (primary) HIV, or PGL	B. Symptomatic, not (A) or (C) conditions	C. AIDS-indicator conditions
(1) ≥500/μL	A1	B1	**C1**
(2) 200–499/μL	A2	B2	**C2**
(3) <200/μL AIDS-indicator T-cell count	**A3**	**B3**	**C3**

The boldfaced values illustrate the expanded AIDS surveillance case definition. Persons with AIDS-indicator conditions (category C) as well as those with CD4$^+$ T-lymphocyte counts <200/μL (categories A3 or B3) will be reportable as AIDS cases in the United States and Territories, effective January 1, 1993.

Data From the CDC. Projections of the number of persons diagnosed with AIDS and the number of immunosuppressed, HIV-infected persons—United States, 1992–1994. *MMWR* 1992; 41 (RR-17):1–4.

PGL, persistent generalized lymphadenopathy.

For national surveillance purposes, in 1987 the CDC revised its 1985 AIDS case definition to define AIDS as a disabling or life-threatening illness caused by HIV and included HIV encephalopathy, HIV wasting syndrome, and certain diseases associated with immunodeficiency in the list of AIDS-defining conditions (39). Studies have suggested that reporting of AIDS according to the 1987 case definition includes >80% of all AIDS cases in the United States (198). In 1993, the CDC also expanded the case definition for AIDS to include pulmonary tuberculosis, invasive cervical carcinoma, recurrent bacterial pneumonia, and CD4+ counts of <200/mm^3. To ascertain AIDS cases worldwide, the World Health Organization (WHO) uses a clinical case definition because facilities and personnel for establishing laboratory diagnoses are limited in developing countries (231).

Modes of Transmission of HIV

HIV is transmitted by sexual contact, by parenteral inoculation of blood or body fluids, and from mother to infant. There remains no epidemiologic evidence for transmission of HIV by insect bite, saliva, tears, urine, or casual contact (148).

Sexual Transmission: Homosexual Contact

In the United States, the majority of AIDS cases have occurred among men infected with HIV through sex with other men (Table 2) (49), particularly through receptive anal intercourse. Transmission of HIV by men having sex with men is also the predominant mode of infection in countries in western Europe, in Australia, and in some countries in Latin America, where the population seroprevalence is low and the ratio of infected men to women is high. These countries account for an estimated 2.5 million infected persons (51).

Sexual Transmission: Heterosexual Contact

In the United States, persons infected through heterosexual contact with someone known to be HIV positive have accounted for a small but growing proportion of

TABLE 2. *AIDS cases by sex, race/ethnicity, and HIV exposure group reported to the CDC between July 1993 and June 1994, and cumulative totals from 1981 through June 1994*

	July 1993–June 1994		Cumulative totals	
	n	%	n	%
Sex				
Males	70,442	83	347,767	87
Females	14,814	17	53,978	13
Race/ethnicity				
White	36,134	42	198,130	49
Black	32,108	38	130,184	33
Hispanic	15,996	19	68,903	17
Other	888	1	3,650	1
HIV exposure group[a]				
Homosexual/bisexual males	37,991	45	211,779	53
Injecting drug users	23,581	28	98,367	24
Homosexual/bisexual males who inject drugs	4,165	5	25,447	6
Hemophilia	603	1	3,404	1
Heterosexual contact	8,296	10	27,281	7
Recipient of blood transfusion of organ transplant	873	1	6,548	2
Adult/adolescent undetermined risk	8,759	10	23,189	6
Pediatric hemophilia	15	0	214	0
Mother HIV+ or at risk for HIV	908	1	5,095	1
Pediatric recipient of blood transfusion	29	0	348	0
Pediatric undetermined risk	40	0	77	0

Data from the CDC. *HIV/AIDS surveillance report.* Mid-year edition 1994;6:1–27.
[a] Categories are hierarchical and mutually exclusive.

AIDS cases (49). However, as of 1992, WHO estimated that 75% of the cumulative HIV infections worldwide were a result of heterosexual contact (238). Heterosexual transmission predominates primarily in sub-Saharan Africa and the Caribbean, where population seroprevalence rates are >1% and the male-to-female ratio of infection is approximately 1:1. In Africa, seroprevalence studies in some areas have shown that 5–29% of blood donors and pregnant women are already infected with HIV (3,27). African countries account for >10 million infected persons (240).

In Thailand, where HIV infection began independently among injecting drug users (IDUs) and prostitutes (178), heterosexual transmission has played an important role in the rapid increase in the number of persons infected, from a few thousand in 1987 to an estimated 50,000 in 1990 and to 450,000 by the end of 1992 (239). Heterosexual contact is also an important factor in spreading HIV in India, where the epidemic is also growing rapidly (237).

Parenteral Exposure to Blood or Blood Products

Sharing of contaminated needles or injecting equipment is the major mode of spread of HIV by IDUs. In the United States, western Europe, and Latin America, injecting drug use is a major mode of transmission of HIV (49,238). HIV seroprevalence among IDUs varies markedly across the United States; rates are as high as 49% in metropolitan areas in the Northeast, particularly in New York and New Jersey (48).

Reuse of contaminated needles can also be a mode of iatrogenic spread of HIV. In Romania, for example, in the late 1980s, several hundred children were likely to have been iatrogenically infected with HIV through injections from reused, contaminated needles (111).

Transmission of HIV by transfusion of blood or blood products in developed countries is now rare (68,229). However, in developing countries where not all blood is screened, blood transfusion is thought to account for as much as 10% of all HIV transmission (238).

Occupational exposure to HIV has concerned health-care workers since the beginning of the epidemic. Numerous studies have evaluated the risk of transmission of HIV from HIV-positive patients to health-care workers through parenteral exposure (e.g., needle stick injuries). Although the risk is low, transmission has occurred (153,223); through the end of June 1994, 42 health-care workers had documented HIV infection acquired through occupational exposure (49). The American Academy of Neurology has published guidelines to reduce the risk of transmission of HIV in neurological practice (123).

Although the transmission of HIV from an infected dentist to six of his patients during dental procedures has been documented (40,46), the risk of health-care worker–to–patient transmission is estimated to be extremely low. In the United States, no other transmissions from HIV-positive health-care workers to their patients have been documented, even though >19,000 patients of 57 HIV-positive health-care workers have been investigated (46).

Perinatal Transmission

Perinatal transmission from mother to infant is responsible for most pediatric HIV infection and is thought to occur intrautero or intrapartum. Current data suggest that 13–35% of children born to infected women are infected (25,86,118,179), but zidovudine has been shown to decrease the risk of transmission (61). Transmission by breast-feeding also has been documented, and the estimated risk of transmission is 29% (79). In the United States, an estimated 1,500–2,000 children are born each year with perinatally acquired HIV infection (106). WHO estimates that a million infants worldwide had been infected through perinatal transmission by mid-1994. About 80–90% of perinatal infections occur in sub-Saharan Africa (238).

Cofactors for HIV Transmission

Multiple sexual partners, the presence of ulcerative genital lesions or exudative genital infection, and injecting drug use have all been associated with increased transmission of HIV (27). In addition, there is evidence that HIV-infected persons with very recent HIV infection or severe immune deficiency (AIDS) have high titers of HIV in their blood and body fluids and may be more likely to transmit HIV than other HIV-infected persons (98,112). Such high viral load in recently infected persons might account for some of the explosive growth of the HIV epidemic in Thailand (158).

Natural History of HIV Infection

Within 4–6 weeks after infection with HIV, the virus can be detected in blood, and antibody to HIV is detectable shortly thereafter (2). Most HIV-infected persons develop persisting antibody to HIV within 6 months of exposure (116). A few weeks after primary HIV infection, up to 70% of persons develop an acute viral syndrome that can include fever, myalgia, arthralgia, maculopapular rash, lymphadenopathy, and aseptic meningitis (63,89). From ~6 months to several years, conditions associated with progressive immune deficiency (94) or HIV itself may develop in HIV-infected persons; these include herpes zoster, generalized lymphadenopathy, chronic diarrhea, fever, night sweats, weight loss, fatigue, oral thrush, and oral hairy leukoplakia. These conditions are manifestations of mild to moderate HIV infection and precede the development of AIDS in most patients. In some HIV-infected persons, however, AIDS may be the initial manifestation of HIV infection.

The period between HIV infection and the development of AIDS is usually long and variable, with AIDS developing in 50% of perinatally infected children within 3 years of birth (CDC, unpublished observation) and developing in 50% of adults within ~10 years after infection (1,23,150). Zidovudine therapy and prophylaxis for opportunistic infections prolong the period between infection and development of AIDS (90,204,228). Age seems to be an important factor in determining the time from HIV infection to AIDS; in young children and older adults, AIDS develops faster than in adolescents and young adults (87,183). Viral factors also may influence the time from infection to AIDS (62,137).

What proportion of infected persons will eventually develop AIDS is not known, but the risk of developing AIDS increases as the duration of HIV infection increases. In one study of adults with known date of HIV infection, HIV-related disease (not all of it AIDS) had developed in 80% after 7.3 years of follow-up (69). One statistical model suggested that up to 99% of HIV-infected persons eventually develop AIDS, although the effect of treatment was not considered (150).

Incidence of AIDS

Of the 189 cases of AIDS reported to the CDC in 1981, 97% were in men and none were in children (41). Between July 1993 and June 1994, >85,000 cases of AIDS were reported to the CDC; >83% were in men and >1% were in children (49). Between June 1981 and June 1994, more than 400,000 cases of AIDS and 243,000 (60%) deaths due to AIDS were reported to CDC (49). Recent AIDS cases comprise progressively larger proportions of women, African-Americans, Hispanics, IDUs, and persons infected by heterosexual contact (Table 2). Because AIDS incidence is indicative of HIV incidence ~10 years earlier, these data are consistent with a statistical model of HIV transmission in the United States that suggests that transmission peaked among gay men in 1984 and among IDUs between 1984 and 1986. Transmission by heterosexual contact is stable or increasing (31).

The incidence of AIDS varies greatly across the United States. By 1990, cases were reported from every state, the District of Columbia, and the U.S. territories (41). Within states, rates are highest in metropolitan areas. The highest incidences have been in San Francisco (213/100,000 population/year) and New York (160/100,000 population/year) and the lowest incidence in nonmetropolitan areas of the

United States (8.9/100,000 population/year) (49). In contrast, the annual incidence of multiple sclerosis in the United States is 0.1 to 3/100,000 population (141).

Worldwide, by mid-1994, >985,000 AIDS cases had been reported to WHO (240). Because of reporting difficulties in many countries, the true number of AIDS cases is not known but is thought to be ~4.0 million. Although >50% of reported cases are from developed countries, more than two thirds of estimated cases are from developing countries, mostly in sub-Saharan Africa (240).

Prevalence of HIV Infection

Soon after HIV was discovered in 1983, antibody assays were developed to identify infected persons. Serologic studies showed that most infected persons were asymptomatic. Usually, AIDS-defining conditions occur in patients with <200 CD4+ cells/mm^3 (235), and in the United States <20% of HIV-seropositive persons are estimated to have CD4+ counts that low (42). Therefore, the AIDS case count represents a fraction of the entire spectrum of HIV infection. For example, in 1992 in the United States, an estimated 150,000 persons had AIDS, but an estimated 1 million persons were HIV positive (42). Worldwide, by mid-1994 an estimated 16 million persons worldwide had been infected with HIV (240), but only an estimated one quarter of the cumulative total of HIV-infected adults had developed symptomatic HIV infection or AIDS (51).

Mortality

Before zidovudine was widely available, >55% of persons reported with AIDS died within a year of diagnosis (199); however, with zidovudine therapy, 55% die within 2 years of diagnosis (225). In 1993, ~39,000 deaths in the United States were due to AIDS (49), compared with >140,000 deaths due to stroke (170). However, 1992 data indicate that AIDS has become the leading cause of death among men 25–44 years of age in the United States, accounting for 19.9% of all deaths in this age group (47), whereas stroke was eighth, accounting for 1.9% of deaths in this age group (170). In 1992, among women 25–44 years of age, AIDS was the fourth leading cause of death, accounting for 7.3% of deaths (47).

The Future

By the year 2000, an estimated 10 million AIDS cases will have occurred worldwide, and 30–40 million persons, including 10 million children, will be infected with HIV (239). As many as one in every 160 persons 15–49 years of age in the world may be infected. Moreover, in the 1990s, an additional 10 million children will be orphaned as their mothers or both parents die of AIDS (239).

EPIDEMIOLOGY OF NEUROLOGIC COMPLICATIONS OF HIV INFECTION

Results of numerous studies on the neurologic complications of HIV infection have varied widely. In epidemiologic studies, there are four important considerations in determining the validity of research results. The first is representativeness, or the extent to which the study participants are representative of the population to which investigators want to generalize their results. For example, patients with AIDS included in studies of consecutive autopsies are representative of all patients with AIDS who had autopsies but not necessarily of all patients with AIDS because all or even a random sample of patients with AIDS are unlikely to have autopsies. The second important consideration is the accuracy of diagnosis, which includes how well the conditions of interest are defined; what symptoms, signs, and laboratory results are needed to establish the diagnosis; and how they are evaluated. In an effort to standardize results from research studies, the American Academy of Neurology has proposed nomenclature and research case definitions for the neurologic complications of HIV infection (4). In addition, criteria also have been proposed for neuropathology-based terminology (35). The third consideration is the completeness of information ascertained about the condition of interest. For example, review of medical records is limited in its ability to determine the proportion of patients with a particular physical sign because not all patients have the same physical examination. A neurologic examination by a neurologist is likely to be more thorough than that by a non-neurologist. The fourth consideration is the evaluation of confounding factors. For example, to determine the etiology of cognitive impairment in HIV-infected persons, investigators must be certain that other causes of cognitive impairment, such as head injury or drug use, have been considered. Even the results of the most sophisticated data analysis are no better than the quality of the original data (203).

General Neurologic Complications

Although the true frequency of the various neurologic diseases over the course of HIV infection is currently unknown, the natural history of such conditions is becoming better understood. During acute HIV infection, a self-limited aseptic meningitis (113), acute encephalopathy (36), myelopathy (74), or neuropathy (187) may occur. In persons with mild immunodeficiency or immune dysfunction, asymptomatic aseptic meningitis or symptomatic inflammatory demyelinating polyradiculoneuropathy, myopathy, or herpes zoster radiculitis may occur. In persons with moderate to severe immunodeficiency, cognitive dysfunction, dementia, myelopathy, sensory neuropathy, myopathy, and neurologic opportunistic infections and cancers are most likely to occur (123,160,186).

Neurologic diseases have been reported as the initial manifestation of AIDS in 7–20% of patients (21,37,105,146,147). In cross-sectional studies of patients with AIDS or symptomatic HIV infection, the range of prevalence of neurologic complications increases to 39–70% (21,105,146,160,212). Of the approximately 154,000 persons with AIDS alive in 1992 in the United States (42), 55,000–118,000 had a neurologic complication.

Prevalence of HIV Among Neurologic Patients

To determine the frequency of HIV infection among hospital patients with various medical conditions, the CDC conducted an unlinked seroprevalence survey of 195,000 patients in 20 acute-care U.S. hospitals (127). Among patients with neurologic conditions, hospital-specific seroprevalence ranged from 0% to 13% and was highly correlated with the seroprevalence among all patients in the hospital. Most importantly, an estimated two thirds of HIV-positive patients in these hospitals had undiagnosed HIV infection, suggesting that neurologists in hospitals where HIV prevalence is high should routinely offer HIV counseling and testing to their 15- to 54-year-old patients (45).

HIV-1–Associated Meningitis

An acute self-limited aseptic meningitis sometimes associated with cranial nerve abnormalities has been described at the time of seroconversion to HIV (113). In addition to this acute, symptomatic meningitis, a chronic asymptomatic meningitis has been described. Pleocytosis or elevated protein in the cerebrospinal fluid (CSF) has been noted in as many as 59% of asymptomatic HIV-seropositive persons (156), whereas as many as 45% of asymptomatic persons may have antibodies to HIV in the CNS (218,224). Intrathecal synthesis of antibodies to HIV increases as duration of infection and immunosuppression increase (82,155,218,224). HIV has been identified in the CSF by polymerase chain reaction or virus culture techniques in all stages of HIV infection, but particularly late in infection (29,53,195,208,216,217,219).

Neuropsychologic and Electrophysiologic Dysfunction in HIV Infection

Cognitive impairment in late HIV infection has been well documented (172), but results of neuropsychologic and electrophysiologic studies defining the natural history of cognitive impairment remain controversial. Because HIV can reach the brain quickly after intravenous injection (70) and because a high proportion of asymptomatic HIV-infected persons have intrathecal synthesis of antibodies to HIV, cognitive impairment early in HIV infection might be expected. However, many cross-sectional and longitudinal studies have found few or no neurologic, neuropsychologic, or neuroimaging abnormalities in persons with asymptomatic HIV infection compared with controls (55,58,60,76,80,91,99,125,128,138,159,160,162,164,166,175,180,200, 206,207,215). Others have suggested that such persons might have subclinical CNS disease, with abnormal results on some neuropsychologic tests (102,131,136,151, 154,182,192,211,220,226,233), electrophysiologic tests (100,138,165,196), or neuroimaging studies (102,108,177). The differences in these studies are probably due to differences in sample size, sample selection, exclusion criteria (particularly regarding non-HIV risk factors such as drug and alcohol use), assessment methodology, and definitions of impairment (119,175). Nonetheless, the neuropsychologic and electrophysiologic abnormalities described in otherwise asymptomatic HIV-infected persons are usually not clinically manifest (236). Most studies suggest that cognitive impairment and electrophysiologic abnormalities are more likely to occur in HIV-infected persons with symptomatic HIV infection or moderate to severe immunodeficiency (28,80,99,100,102,125,131,136,154,166,172,180,196,209,215).

Risk Factors for Neuropsychologic or Electrophysiologic Abnormalities

Few studies have identified risk factors for impaired performance on neuropsychologic tests or abnormalities on electrophysiologic tests. Lower cognitive reserve capacity has been reported as a possible risk factor for impaired performance on neuropsychologic tests (201), and in one study, HIV-positive persons with a history of head injury with loss of consciousness were more likely to have abnormalities on neuropsychologic tests than were HIV-negative persons with a history of head injury with loss of consciousness (154). Although vitamin B12 deficiency (15) has been reported to be associated with diminished performance on neuropsychologic tests in one study, no association with vitamin B12 deficiency was found in another (197).

HIV-1–Associated Minor Cognitive/Motor Disorder

The American Academy of Neurology has developed criteria for diagnosis of cognitive impairment that is not severe enough to warrant a diagnosis of dementia (4). The criteria for HIV-1–associated minor cognitive/motor disorder are similar to those for stage 1 AIDS dementia complex (193).

Few studies have reported on these mild, symptomatic cognitive problems. Among patients with AIDS-related complex or AIDS with only Kaposi's sarcoma, an estimated one third have mild AIDS dementia complex (Price stage 1), and one quarter have very mild, nonspecific cognitive symptoms (Price stage 0.5) (193). In the only other study to focus on symptomatic minor cognitive impairment, an estimated 3% of 74 participants with CDC group II or III infection and 31% of 26 patients with CDC group IVA or IVC2 infection (43) had mild, symptomatic cognitive dysfunction (125). Although some patients with minor cognitive disorder become demented, others have stable or slowly progressive dysfunction (202).

Dementia Associated with HIV Infection in Adults

Prevalence of Dementia

The epidemiology of dementia associated with HIV infection is becoming better defined. HIV dementia has been estimated to be the initial manifestation of AIDS in 0.8–5.5% of patients (21,124,146,204,225). The lower estimates are from studies conducted before dementia was widely recognized as a manifestation of AIDS. The prevalence of dementia in patients with AIDS in western Europe and North America has been reported to be 7–11% (Table 3) (105,146,212) and is similar in other parts of the world. In a multicenter study of outpatients conducted by WHO, using ICD-10 criteria, the point prevalence of dementia among patients with symptomatic HIV infection was 0% in Bangkok, Thailand, and ranged from 4.4% to 6.5% in centers in Zaire, Kenya, and Brazil (152). Dementia was absent in Thailand because the onset of the epidemic in Thailand is more recent than that in sub-Saharan Africa and Brazil, and dementia is a late complication of HIV infection. In a study of hospitalized patients with AIDS in Zaire, the prevalence of probable HIV dementia was 9% (181), but a study of hospitalized patients in Tanzania using less specific diagnostic criteria found dementia in 19% of patients with AIDS (117).

The higher estimates of the prevalence of dementia in autopsy studies than in clinical studies suggest that cognitive impairment may frequently be subclinical. In most autopsy series, the incidence of HIV encephalitis, the neuropathologic correlate of dementia, ranged from 11% to 30% (34,85,104,134,140,142,143,157,184,232). However, in the original autopsy description of AIDS dementia complex, which used

TABLE 3. *Prevalence of the major neurologic complications of HIV infection among persons with AIDS*

Disease	Prevalence in clinical studies (%)	References	Prevalence in autopsy studies (%)	References
HIV dementia	7–11	105,146,152, 212	11–66	34,85,104,134,140, 142,157, 172,185,232
Progressive encephalopathy of childhood	23	205		
Myelopathy			22–55	7,172,184
Sensory neuropathy	10–35	65,92,212,214		
Inflammatory demyelinating neuropathy	Rare	11,92		
Myopathy	<1–26	72,103,146,212	26–73	59,241
Cryptococcal meningitis	1–9	20,37,72,75,83, 105,146,243	3–13	5,34,140,142,185
Toxoplasma encephalitis	3–25	20,37,72,191, 212,234	5–26	5,34,140,142,185
Cytomegalovirus encephalitis	2	72,105	10–33	5,34,140,142,185,232
Progressive multifocal leukoencephalopathy	0.4–5	19,20,72,105, 139,146,212	2–7	5,34,140,142,185
Primary lymphoma of the brain	1.5–2.5	20,37,105,146, 212	3–8	5,34,140,142,185
Tuberculous meningitis	0.8–2.4	20,24,105,140		

broader diagnostic criteria than the American Academy of Neurology criteria (4), the prevalence was 66% (171). The range in prevalence in these autopsy studies is much broader than that in clinical studies, probably because of the wide spectrum of neuropathologic abnormalities in AIDS (157), the proportion of cases at different stages of HIV infection, different criteria for abnormalities, and different selection criteria for cases.

Incidence of Dementia

The incidence rate is the number of new cases of a disease occurring in a population during a specified period of time divided by the number of persons in the population at risk of developing the disease during that time. Thus, it is an estimate of the risk or probability of developing the disease during a specified period of time (135). Prevalence rates do not estimate such risk or probability.

In the United States, HIV-associated dementia is one of the most common causes of dementia in young persons. In 1990, among persons 20–59 years of age, the incidence rate of HIV encephalopathy (1.9 per 100,000 population) was nearly one third the hospital discharge rate of patients with non–HIV-associated dementia in 1988 (6.3 per 100,000 population). The hospital discharge data probably overestimated the incidence of non–HIV-associated dementia because it included patients admitted more than once in 1988 and some patients with dementia diagnosed before 1988 (124). Among HIV-positive men in the Multicenter AIDS Cohort Study (MACS), the incidence of HIV dementia was 1.5 per 100 person-years (9).

Although several studies have estimated the frequency or point prevalence of HIV-associated dementia, few studies have estimated the cumulative incidence of dementia. In a small prospective study of 32 patients with AIDS-related complex or

AIDS, 28% developed dementia during a 2-year follow-up period (71). However, among 492 gay men with AIDS in the MACS, the cumulative incidence of HIV-associated dementia was estimated to be 3.3% at the time of diagnosis of AIDS, 10.4% at 1 year after diagnosis, and 15% at 2 years (163). In a retrospective longitudinal cohort study at San Francisco General Hospital, medical records for 487 patients with AIDS hospitalized in 1988 were reviewed. In this study, like in the MACS, the probability of HIV-associated dementia was estimated to be 3% at the time of diagnosis of AIDS, 10% at 1 year after diagnosis, and 18% at 2 years (Wang F, personal communication). These data demonstrate that dementia is a late complication of HIV infection. Survival after diagnosis of dementia has been estimated to be as short as 3–7 months in patients with AIDS (163,173) but may be longer in those treated with zidovudine (190).

Risk Factors for Dementia

Older HIV-infected persons are more likely to develop dementia than are younger HIV-infected persons (124,163; Wang F, personal communication). In addition, analysis of cases reported to the CDC indicates that very young HIV-infected children are more likely to develop progressive encephalopathy than are adolescents and young adults (Fig. 1). Among persons in the MACS, having anemia, lower body mass index, and more constitutional symptoms before AIDS were all predictive of more rapid development of HIV-associated dementia after AIDS. Two studies have suggested that dementia may occur more frequently in IDUs than in gay men (204; Wang F, personal communication); however, among AIDS cases reported to the CDC, dementia has been reported with similar frequency among all risk groups,

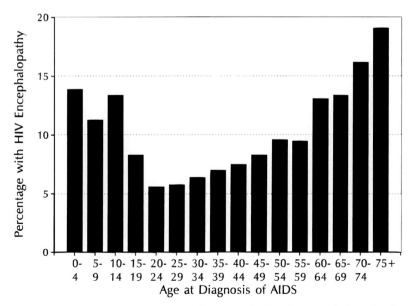

FIG. 1. The percentage of persons with AIDS reported with HIV encephalopathy, September 1, 1987, through August 31, 1991, by age at diagnosis of AIDS. (From Janssen RS, Nwanyanwu OC, Selik RK, et al. Epidemiology of human immunodeficiency virus encephalopathy in the United States. *Neurology* 1992;42:1472–1476.)

among men and women, among all racial and ethnic groups, and in all regions of the country (124).

Whether zidovudine affects the incidence of dementia remains unclear. In The Netherlands, zidovudine has been reported to have a prophylactic effect; as zidovudine use has increased, the frequency of diagnosis of dementia among patients with AIDS has decreased (189,190). In addition, high doses of zidovudine may be more effective for dementia than low doses of zidovudine (174). However, among persons in the MACS, zidovudine did not protect against development of dementia (9,163).

Progressive Encephalopathy of Childhood

Progressive encephalopathy due to HIV is a common and severe manifestation of AIDS in children. HIV encephalopathy is the initial manifestation of AIDS in 12–18% of perinatally infected children with AIDS (26,205; Lobato M, personal communication). Early studies of children with symptomatic HIV infection or AIDS estimated that 33–76% (16,17,84) developed progressive encephalopathy. However, two recent longitudinal studies of 172 and 766 children both estimated that 23% of perinatally infected children with AIDS developed progressive encephalopathy (Table 3) (205; Lobato M, personal communication).

Among perinatally infected children, the incidence of progressive encephalopathy in the first year of life is 4.5% (Lobato M, personal communication), with a median age of 9–18 months at diagnosis (84,205; Lobato M, personal communication). Estimated median survival after diagnosis, 11–22 months (205; Lobato M, personal communication), is similar to that of children with *P. carinii* pneumonia and is much shorter than survival after lymphoid interstitial pneumonitis (Lobato M, personal communication). Median survival from birth for children with progressive encephalopathy has been estimated to be ~53 months (Lobato M, personal communication). No risk factors for developing progressive encephalopathy of childhood have been identified.

Myelopathy

The epidemiology of HIV-1–associated myelopathy has not been well described. The pathologic entity of vacuolar myelopathy (35) probably accounts for the majority of conditions that meet the definition of HIV-1–associated myelopathy (4). Electrophysiologic studies suggest that structural spinal cord dysfunction may occur in otherwise neurologically asymptomatic and HIV-asymptomatic persons (110,121), but most studies have been of autopsy cases. From 22% to 55% of patients with AIDS at autopsy have vacuolar myelopathy (7,171,185). In one study, 90% of those with vacuolar myelopathy had AIDS dementia complex (171).

Peripheral Nervous System Conditions

Several distinct diseases affect the peripheral nerves and muscles of persons infected with HIV. Inflammatory demyelinating neuropathies, mononeuritis multiplex, distal symmetric polyneuropathy, polyradiculoneuropathy, mononeuropathy, toxic neuropathies, and inflammatory myopathies have been reported in HIV-infected persons. Electrophysiologic abnormalities may occur in persons with early HIV infection (121), but symptomatic disease and electrophysiologic abnormalities become more frequent with advanced HIV disease (107). In a retrospective review of medical records of 7,636 HIV-infected patients, peripheral neuropathy was noted in 2% of those with CD4+ counts >500/mm^3, in 4% of those with counts of 200–499/mm^3, and in 10% of those with counts <200/mm^3 (88). In a study of 798 HIV-positive men, peripheral neuropathy was rare in early infection but occurred in 17% of those with AIDS (11). In one pathologic study, 19 (95%) of 20 peripheral nerves examined in a group of patients with symptomatic HIV infection or AIDS had histopathologic changes (73).

Distal Symmetric Polyneuropathy

Sensory neuropathy (10,64) or HIV-1–associated predominantly sensory polyneuropathy (4) is a distal symmetric polyneuropathy. It is the most common peripheral nervous system manifestation of HIV infection, and the incidence of sensory neuropathy increased 50% per year between 1988 and 1992 among men in the MACS (9). Sensory neuropathy usually occurs in patients with severe immune deficiency (11,64,92,145,161). In small clinical series, sensory neuropathy has been reported in up to 35% of patients with AIDS (212,214), but larger series suggest the frequency is closer to 10% (64,92). Sensory neuropathies with and without painful dysesthesias have been described (10,64,92,214) and perhaps represent different entities (92). Cytomegalovirus infection has been associated with the painful neuropathy, suggesting that it perhaps should not be a subdivision of HIV-1–associated predominantly sensory neuropathy (92).

Inflammatory Demyelinating Neuropathies

Acute (Guillain-Barré syndrome [GBS]) and chronic inflammatory demyelinating polyneuropathy (IDP) (8,65) are associated with HIV infection (92,222). Unlike other HIV-associated neuropathies, the inflammatory neuropathies occur primarily in patients who do not have AIDS (64,66,67,145,161). The frequency of IDP is unknown but thought to be rare (11,92). Because GBS in persons infected with HIV is similar to GBS in persons not infected with HIV, patients with GBS who have risk factors for HIV exposure should be screened for HIV (66).

Myopathy

Although myopathy can be related to HIV infection or to treatment with zidovudine (109), the epidemiology of myopathy in HIV infection has not been clearly defined. The frequent clinical findings of fatigue and generalized weakness in persons with severe HIV infection make it difficult to delineate the myopathic component (210).

Myopathy, which may occur in any stage of HIV infection (210), has rarely been found (<1%) in cross-sectional studies (72,146,212). However, in a study of 50 unselected HIV-infected persons at all stages of HIV infection, 26% had myopathies related to HIV infection. None of the patients taking zidovudine had a symptomatic myopathy thought to be related to zidovudine therapy, but two thirds had morphologic changes attributed to zidovudine (103).

Subclinical pathologic changes in muscles of HIV-infected persons seem to be common; in a study of 15 unselected patients with AIDS, 11 had electrophysiologic abnormalities, and four of seven had myopathy on biopsy (59). However, in an autopsy study of 92 persons with AIDS, 24 had skeletal muscle pathology ascribed to the direct or indirect action of HIV (241).

Opportunistic Infections and Cancers

Cryptococcal Meningitis

Cryptococcal meningitis, one of the most frequent opportunistic infections of the CNS in patients with AIDS in the United States, has been reported in ~5% of patients at the time of diagnosis of AIDS (21,147; Wong F, personal communication), and prevalence estimates from cross-sectional studies in the United States, Europe, and Africa range from 1% to 9% (21,37,72,75,83,105,146,243). In autopsy studies of patients dying with AIDS, the estimates range from 3% to 13% (5,34,140,142,184).

Among men in the MACS with CD4 counts $\leq$200/mm^3, the incidence of cryptococcal meningitis was 2.4 per 100 person-years (9). In a retrospective chart review of patients with AIDS at San Francisco General Hospital, 5% of patients had cryptococcal meningitis as their first AIDS illness; the cumulative incidence was 10% at 1 year and 14% at 2 years after AIDS diagnosis (Wong F, personal communication). The median survival from first symptoms of cryptococcal meningitis is 6–9 months (54,230).

In the United States, cryptococcal meningitis has been reported most frequently among African Americans and among IDUs (147).

Toxoplasma Encephalitis

Among patients with AIDS, 95% of toxoplasma encephalitis is due to recrudescence of latent infection in an immunosuppressed host (149), and its incidence is proportional to the prevalence of antibodies to *Toxoplasma gondii* in the population. Like the prevalence of toxoplasma antibodies in the general population, toxoplasma encephalitis is more common in Africa, Europe, the Caribbean, and Latin America than in the United States (149). In the United States, it is more common in Florida (147) than in other parts of the country.

Toxoplasma encephalitis is the most common CNS mass lesion in patients with AIDS. In the United States, in cases of AIDS diagnosed between September 1987 and January 1993 and reported to the CDC by July 1993, it was reported in 10,837 (4.7%) of 231,332 cases (CDC, unpublished data). Toxoplasma encephalitis was reported in 3% of cases of AIDS through 1986 (147), but presumptive diagnoses added to the 1987 CDC case definition for AIDS probably account for the increased frequency of reported cases. In New York and San Francisco, toxoplasma encephalitis has been reported in 3–7% of patients with AIDS (191,212,234), whereas in Florida, toxoplasmosis was the initial diagnosis in 13% of patients with AIDS and occurred in up to 25% of patients with AIDS (21). In Europe, toxoplasma encephalitis has been reported as the initial AIDS condition in 13% of cases in Spain (37) and, in a cross-sectional study, in 21% of patients in The Netherlands (72). However, only 4% of patients with AIDS had toxoplasmosis in a study in the United Kingdom (105). Autopsy studies have found toxoplasma encephalitis in 5–26% of patients with AIDS, with the highest rates in Europe (5,34,140,142,184).

Among men in the MACS with CD4+ counts ≤200/mm^3, the incidence of toxoplasma encephalitis was 2.5 per 100 person-years (9). In a study in San Francisco, the incidence of toxoplasma encephalitis was 3% at the time of diagnosis of AIDS, 10% at 1 year after AIDS diagnosis, and 19% after 2 years (Wang F, personal communication). These data suggest that toxoplasma encephalitis is a very late complication of HIV infection.

Less than half of all HIV-infected persons with antibodies to toxoplasmosis will develop encephalitis (149). In a study in the United States, an estimated 6–12% of those with antibody to *T. gondii* developed toxoplasma encephalitis (234), but in a study in Austria, 47% of patients with AIDS with antibodies to *T. gondii* developed toxoplasma encephalitis (242).

The median survival after onset of symptoms of toxoplasma encephalitis is 4–10 months (105,191,194) and does not differ from survival after *P. carinii* pneumonia (Wang F, personal communication).

Cytomegalovirus

Although approximately 50% of the general population has antibodies to cytomegalovirus (CMV) by 50 years of age (77), up to 100% of HIV-infected gay men have antibodies (144) acquired before they were infected with HIV (77). Thus, CMV-induced disease is a result of reactivation of latent CMV. Clinical manifestations of CMV infection occur in the late stages of AIDS (56,167) and include encephalitis (129,227,232), myelopathy (101), polyradiculomyelopathy (81,133), and peripheral neuropathy (101). CNS disease due to CMV is frequently associated with disseminated CMV disease including retinitis and pneumonia (129,133,227).

Both CMV encephalitis and polyradiculomyelopathy have been reported in up to 2% of patients with AIDS (72,105) but do not necessarily occur in the same patients (133). They are much less common than CMV retinitis, which occurs in 15–28% of patients with AIDS (50,120). No estimates for CMV peripheral neuropathy are available. At autopsy, 10–33% of patients with AIDS have evidence of CMV infection (5,34,140,142,184,232).

Progressive Multifocal Leukoencephalopathy

Progressive multifocal leukoencephalopathy (PML) is a rare CNS condition in immunocompromised patients caused by infection with a JC papovavirus. Although PML has been reported in <1% of AIDS cases reported to the CDC through mid-1993 (CDC, unpublished observation), it occurs more frequently in patients with AIDS than in patients with any other disease (221).

The frequency of PML as the first indicator disease of AIDS varies from 0.8% to 1.6% (21,37,97). Of those patients with AIDS with PML, 25–77% have PML as their first AIDS indicator disease (20,97,130). In cross-sectional studies, the prevalence of PML has ranged from 0.5% to 4% (20,21,72,105,139,146,212). PML at autopsy has been reported in 2–7% of AIDS cases (5,34,140,142,184). PML is a rapidly progressive disease: median survival after onset of symptoms is ~4 months (20,97,130), compared with median survival after *P. carinii* pneumonia of 10 months (97). However, prolonged survival with PML has been reported (22).

Examination of death certificates between 1979 and 1987 in the United States (114) demonstrated a fourfold increase in PML-related deaths, most of which were attributed to AIDS. PML mortality in 1987 (5.7 per 10,000,000 persons) was similar to that for Creutzfeldt-Jakob disease (4.3–10.0 per 10,000,000 persons per year [32]).

Primary Lymphoma of the Brain

Primary lymphoma of the brain is a rare disease and an uncommon complication of AIDS. It is the initial AIDS-defining condition in up to 0.6% of patients with AIDS (37,146). In cross-sectional studies, primary lymphoma of the brain has been reported in 1.5–2.5% of patients with AIDS (21,105,146,212), and in autopsy series of patients with AIDS, primary lymphoma of the brain has been found in 3–8% of cases (5,34,140,142,184). In the only longitudinal study reported, 9% of patients with AIDS receiving zidovudine therapy for 3 years developed primary lymphoma of the brain (188). In the general population, the incidence of primary lymphoma of the brain in HIV-infected persons now exceeds that of low-grade astrocytomas (14).

Primary lymphoma of the brain is a late complication of AIDS. In a study in San Francisco, 13 of 20 cases occurred after other AIDS diseases, and an additional three were incidental findings at autopsy (213). Median survival is 2–3 months after onset of symptoms (213). No risk factors have been identified for primary brain lymphoma, but the finding that Epstein-Barr virus proteins are expressed in tumor cells in the CNS suggests that Epstein-Barr virus–infected B cells may give rise to primary brain lymphoma (13).

Tuberculous Meningitis

A higher proportion of HIV-positive patients with tuberculosis have meningitis (10%) than do HIV-negative patients with tuberculosis (2%) (18). Tuberculous meningitis has been reported in 0.8–2.4% of patients with symptomatic HIV infection or AIDS (21,24,105,140). Although tuberculous meningitis in HIV-infected patients is remarkably similar to tuberculous meningitis in HIV-negative patients (18,78), a higher proportion of HIV-positive patients with meningitis have tuberculous brain masses than do HIV-negative patients with meningitis (18,78).

Neurosyphilis

Syphilis infection has been reported in 23–31% of HIV-infected persons (30,115). Several studies have estimated that asymptomatic neurosyphilis, defined by a positive CSF Venereal Disease Research Laboratory test, occurs in 1–2% of HIV-positive patients (6,19,30,115,132). Among those with a history of syphilis, 4.2% have asymptomatic neurosyphilis (19). Neurosyphilis can be diagnosed in any stage of HIV infection; a review of 38 patients reported in the medical literature found that 47%

had AIDS, 18% had symptomatic HIV infection, and 34% had asymptomatic HIV infection (168).

Other Neurologic Conditions

Several other neurologic conditions have been reported among HIV-infected persons. Herpes zoster radiculopathy has been reported in 11–23% of HIV-infected persons (57,105,125,126). A cohort study of 287 HIV-positive and 499 HIV-negative homosexual men found that the incidence of herpes zoster was significantly higher among the HIV-infected men (29.4 per 1,000 person-years) than among the uninfected men (2.0 per 1,000 person-years) (33). Herpes zoster radiculopathy was not associated with duration of HIV infection and did not predict faster progression to AIDS (33).

Neurologic conditions occurring in <1% of patients with AIDS include herpes simplex virus encephalitis, CNS candidiasis, aspergillosis, histoplasmosis, and herpes zoster virus encephalitis (21,105,140,146).

CONCLUSION

In just over a decade, the HIV pandemic has mushroomed from a cluster of an unusual type of pneumonia among five gay men in Los Angeles to 2.5 million cases of AIDS in 173 countries with a case fatality rate of >65%. In the United States, transmission of HIV through homosexual contact and injecting drug use may have peaked in the mid-1980s, but HIV transmission through heterosexual contact is continuing to increase. Worldwide, heterosexual transmission is responsible for most infections. Although incidence rates may now be stable in some areas of sub-Saharan Africa, where prevalence is high, the rapid increases in transmission seen in Thailand are thought to be occurring now in India. WHO estimates that transmission of HIV will continue unabated, with an estimated threefold increase in the number of infected persons between 1993 and the year 2000.

Both the central and peripheral nervous systems can be affected directly by HIV or indirectly as a result of immunosuppression caused by HIV. Nervous system involvement becomes increasingly more frequent as immunodeficiency worsens and occurs most frequently in patients with AIDS. As the number of patients with AIDS increases, physicians can expect to see more HIV-infected patients with neurologic complications.

REFERENCES

1. Alcabes P, Munoz A, Vlahov D, Friendland GH. The incubation period of human immunodeficiency virus. *Epidemiol Rev* 1993;15:305–318.
2. Allain JP, Paul DA, Laurian Y, Senn D. Serologic markers in early stages of human immunodeficiency virus infection in haemophiliacs. *Lancet* 1986;2:1233–1236.
3. Allen S, Van de Perre P, Serufilira A, et al. Human immunodeficiency virus and malaria in a representative sample of childbearing women in Kigali, Rwanda. *J Infect Dis* 1991;164:67–71.
4. American Academy of Neurology. Nomenclature and research case definitions for neurologic manifestations of human immunodeficiency virus-type 1 (HIV-1) infection: report of a working group of the American Academy of Neurology AIDS Task Force. *Neurology* 1991;41:778–785.
5. Anders KH, Guerra WF, Tomiyasu U, et al. The neuropathology of AIDS. UCLA experience and review. *Am J Pathol* 1986;124:537–538.

6. Appelman ME, Marshall DW, Brey RL, et al. Cerebrospinal fluid abnormalities in patients without AIDS who are seropositive for the human immunodeficiency virus. *J Infect Dis* 1988;158:193–199.
7. Artigas J, Grosse G, Niedobitek F. Vacuolar myelopathy in AIDS. A morphological analysis. *Pathol Res Pract* 1990;186:228–237.
8. Asbury AK, Cornblath DR. Assessment of current diagnostic criteria for Guillain-Barré Syndrome. *Ann Neurol* 1990;27(suppl):21–24.
9. Bacellar H, Munoz A, Miller EN, et al. Temporal trends in the incidence of HIV-1-related neurologic diseases: Multicenter AIDS Cohort Study, 1985–1992. *Neurology* 1994;44:1892–1900.
10. Bailey R, Baltch A, Venkatesh R, Singh J, Bishop M. Sensory motor neuropathy associated with AIDS. *Neurology* 1988;38:886–891.
11. Barohn RJ, Gronseth GS, LeForce BR, et al. Peripheral nervous system involvement in a large cohort of human immunodeficiency virus-infected individuals. *Arch Neurol* 1993;50:167–171.
12. Barre-Sinoussi F, Chermann JC, Rey F, et al. Isolation of a T-lymphotropic retrovirus from a patient at risk for AIDS. *Science* 1983;220:868–870.
13. Bashir R, Luka J, Cheloha K, Chamberlain M, Hochberg F. Expression of Epstein-Barr virus proteins in primary CNS lymphoma in AIDS patients. *Neurology* 1993;43:2358–2362.
14. Baumgartner JE, Rachlin JR, Beckstead JH, et al. Primarycentral nervous system lymphomas: natural history and response to radiation therapy in 55 patients with acquired immunodeficiency syndrome. *J Neurosurg* 1990;73:206–211.
15. Beach RS, Morgan R, Wilkie F, et al. Plasma vitamin B12 level as a potential cofactor in studies of human immunodeficiency virus type 1-related cognitive changes. *Arch Neurol* 1992;49:501–506.
16. Belman AL, Ultmann MH, Horoupian D, et al. Neurological complications in infants and children with acquired immune deficiency syndrome. *Ann Neurol* 1985;18:560–566.
17. Belman AL, Diamond G, Dickson D, et al. Pediatric acquired immunodeficiency syndrome: neurologic syndromes. *Am J Dis Child* 1988;142:29–35.
18. Berenguer J, Moreno S, Laguna F, et al. Tuberculous meningitis in patients infected with the human immunodeficiency virus. *N Engl J Med* 1992;326:668–672.
19. Berger JR. Neurosyphilis in human immunodeficiency virus type 1-seropositive individuals. A prospective study. *Arch Neurol* 1991;48:700–702.
20. Berger JR, Kaszovitz B, Post MJD, Dickinson G. Progressive multifocal leukoencephalopathy associated with human immunodeficiency virus infection. *Ann Intern Med* 1987;107:78–87.
21. Berger JR, Moskowitz L, Fischl M, et al. Neurologic disease as the presenting manifestation of acquired immunodeficiency syndrome. *South Med J* 1987;80:683–686.
22. Berger JR, Mucke L. Prolonged survival and partial recovery in AIDS-associated progressive multifocal leukoencephalopathy. *Neurology* 1988;38:1060–1065.
23. Biggar RJ, International Registry of Seroconverters. AIDS incubation in 1891 HIV-seroconverters from different exposure groups. *AIDS* 1990;4:1059–1066.
24. Bishburg E, Sunderam G, Reichman LB, Kapila R. Central nervous system tuberculosis with the acquired immunodeficiency syndrome and its related complex. *Ann Intern Med* 1986;105:210–213.
25. Blanche S, Rouzioux C, Moscato M-L, et al. A prospective study of infants born to women seropositive for human immunodeficiency virus type 1. *N Engl J Med* 1989;320:1643–1648.
26. Blanche S, Tardieu M, Duliege A, et al. Longitudinal study of 94 symptomatic infants with perinatally acquired human immunodeficiency virus infection. Evidence for a bimodal expression of clinical and biological symptoms. *Am J Dis Child* 1990;144:1210–1215.
27. Blattner WA. HIV epidemiology: past, present, and future. *FASEB J* 1991;5:2340–2348.
28. Boccellari AA, Dilley JW, Yingling CD, et al. Relationship of CD4 counts to neurophysiological function in HIV-1-infected homosexual men. *Arch Neurol* 1993;50:517–521.
29. Böni J, Emmerich BS, Leib SL, Wiestler OD, Schüpbach J, Kleihues P. PCR identification of HIV-1 DNA sequences in brain tissue of patients with AIDS encephalopathy. *Neurology* 1993;43:1813–1817.
30. Brandon WR, Boulos LM, Morse A. Determining the prevalence of neurosyphilis in a cohort co-infected with HIV. *Int J STD AIDS* 1993;4:99–101.
31. Brookmeyer R. Reconstruction and future trends of the AIDS epidemic in the United States. *Science* 1991;253:37–42.
32. Brown P. An epidemiologic critique of Creutzfeldt-Jakob disease. *Epidemiol Rev* 1980;2:113–135.
33. Buchbinder SP, Katz MH, Hessol NA, et al. Herpes zoster and human immunodeficiency virus infection. *J Infect Dis* 1992;166:1153–1156.
34. Budka H, Costanzi G, Cristina S, et al. Brain pathology induced by infection with the human immunodeficiency virus (HIV). A histological, immunocytochemical, and electron microscopical study of 100 autopsy cases. *Acta Neuropathol (Berl)* 1987;75:185–198.
35. Budka H, Wiley CA, Kleihues, et al. HIV-associated disease of the nervous system: review of nomenclature and proposal for neuropathology-based terminology. *Brain Pathol* 1991;1:143–152.
36. Carne CA, Tedder RS, Smith A, et al. Acute encephalopathy coincident with seroconversion for anti-HTLV-III. *Lancet* 1985;2:1206–1208.

37. Casabona J, Sanchez E, Graus F, et al. Trends and survival for AIDS patients presenting with indicative neurologic diseases. *Acta Neurol Scand* 1991;84:51–55.
38. Centers for Disease Control. Pneumocystis pneumonia—Los Angeles. *MMWR* 1981;30:250–252.
39. Centers for Disease Control. Revision of the CDC surveillance case definition for acquired immunodeficiency syndrome. *MMWR* 1987;36(suppl 1S):1–15.
40. Centers for Disease Control. Possible transmission of human immunodeficiency virus to a patient during an invasive dental procedure. *MMWR* 1990;39:489–493.
41. Centers for Disease Control. Update: acquired immunodeficiency syndrome—United States, 1981–1990. *MMWR* 1991;40:358–363,369.
42. Centers for Disease Control. Projections of the number of persons diagnosed with AIDS and the number of immunosuppressed HIV-infected persons—United States, 1992–1994. *MMWR* 1992; 41(RR-18):1–29.
43. Centers for Disease Control and Prevention. Classification system for human T-lymphotropic virus type III/lymphadenopathy-associated virus infections. *MMWR* 1986;35:334–339.
44. Centers for Disease Control and Prevention. 1993 revised classification system for HIV infection and expanded surveillance case definition for AIDS among adolescents and adults. *MMWR* 1992; 41(RR-17):1–4.
45. Centers for Disease Control and Prevention. Recommendations for HIV testing services for inpatients and outpatients in acute-care hospital settings. *MMWR* 1993;42(RR-2):1–6.
46. Centers for Disease Control and Prevention. Update: investigations of persons treated by HIV-infected health-care workers—United States. *MMWR* 1993;42:329–331,337.
47. Centers for Disease Control and Prevention. Update: mortality attributable to HIV infection among persons aged 25–44 years—United States, 1991 and 1992. *MMWR* 1993;42:869–872.
48. Centers for Disease Control and Prevention. *National HIV serosurveillance summary. Results through 1992.* Washington, DC: U.S. Department of Health and Human Services, 1993;3:1–51.
49. Centers for Disease Control and Prevention. *HIV/AIDS Surveillance Report.* Mid-year edition 1994; 6:1–27.
50. Cheong I, Flegg PJ, Brettle RP, et al. Cytomegalovirus disease in AIDS: the Edinburgh experience. *Int J STD AIDS* 1992;3:324–328.
51. Chin J, Remenyi MA, Morrison F, Bulatao R. The global epidemiology of the HIV/AIDS pandemic and its projected demographic impact in Africa. *World Health Stat Q* 1992;45:220–227.
52. Chin J, Sato PA, Mann JM. Projections of HIV infections and AIDS cases to the year 2000. *Bull WHO* 1990;68:1–11.
53. Chiodi F, Keys B, Albert J, et al. Human immunodeficiency virus type 1 is present in the cerebrospinal fluid of a majority of infected individuals. *J Clin Microbiol* 1992;30:1768–1771.
54. Chuck SL, Sande MA. Infections with *Cryptococcus neoformans* in the acquired immunodeficiency syndrome. *N Engl J Med* 1989;321:794–799.
55. Clifford DB, Jacoby RG, Miller JP, Seyfried WR, Glicksman M. Neuropsychometric performance of asymptomatic HIV-infected subjects. *AIDS* 1990;4:767–774.
56. Cohen BA, McArthur JC, Grohman S, et al. Neurologic prognosis of cytomegalovirus polyradiculomyelopathy in AIDS. *Neurology* 1993;43:493–499.
57. Colebunders R, Mann JM, Francis H, et al. Herpes zoster in African patients: a clinical predictor of human immunodeficiency virus infection. *J Infect Dis* 1988;157:314–318.
58. Collier AC, Marra C, Coombs RW, et al. Central nervous system manifestations in human immunodeficiency virus infection without AIDS. *J AIDS* 1992;5:229–241.
59. Comi F, Madaglin S, Galardi J, et al. Subclinical neuromuscular involvement in AIDS. *Muscle Nerve* 1985;9:665.
60. Connolly S, Manji H, McAllister RH, et al. Long-latency event-related potentials in asymptomatic human immunodeficiency virus type 1 infection. *Ann Neurol* 1994;35:189–196.
61. Connor EM, Sperling RS, Gelber R, et al. Reduction of maternal-infant transmission of human immunodeficiency virus type 1 with zidovudine treatment. *N Engl J Med* 1994;331:1173–1180.
62. Connor RI, Mohri H, Cao Y, Ho DD. Increased viral burden and cytopathicity correlate temporally with CD4 + T-lymphocyte decline and clinical progression in human immunodeficiency virus type-1 infected individuals. *J Virol* 1993;67:1772–1777.
63. Cooper DA, Gold J, Maclean P, et al. Acute AIDS retrovirus infection: definition of clinical illness associated with seroconversion. *Lancet* 1985;1:537–540.
64. Cornblath D, McArthur J. Predominantly sensory neuropathy in patients with AIDS and AIDS-related complex. *Neurology* 1988;38:794–796.
65. Cornblath D, Asbury A, Albers JW, et al. Research criteria for diagnosis of chronic inflammatory demyelinating polyneuropathy (CIDP). *Neurology* 1991;41:617–618.
66. Cornblath D, McArthur J, Kennedy P, et al. Inflammatory demyelinating peripheral neuropathies associated with human T cell lymphotropic virus type III infection. *Ann Neurol* 1987;21:32–40.
67. Cruz Martinez A, Villoslada C. Electrophysiologic study in peripheral neuropathy associated with HIV infection. *J Electromyogr Clin Neurophysiol* 1991;31:407–414.
68. Cumming PD, Wallace EL, Schorr JB, Dodd RY. Exposure of patients to human immunodeficiency

virus through the transfusion of blood components that test antibody-negative. *N Engl J Med* 1990; 321:941–946.

69. Curran JW, Jaffe HW, Hardy AM, Morgan WM, Selik RM, Dondero TJ. Epidemiology of HIV infection and AIDS in the United States. *Science* 1988;239:610–616.

70. Davis LE, Hjelle BL, Miller VE, et al. Early viral brain invasion in iatrogenic human immunodeficiency virus infection. *Neurology* 1992;42:1736–1739.

71. Day JJ, Grant I, Atkinson JH, et al. Incidence of AIDS dementia in a two-year follow-up of AIDS and ARC patients on an initial phase II AZT placebo-controlled study: San Diego cohort. *J Neuropsychiatry Clin Neurosci* 1992;4:15–20.

72. De Gans J, Portegies P. Neurological complications of infection with human immunodeficiency virus type 1. A review of literature and 241 cases. *Clin Neurol Neurosurg* 1989;91:199–219.

73. De la Monte S, Gabuzda D, Ho D, et al. Peripheral neuropathy in the acquired immunodeficiency syndrome. *Ann Neurol* 1988;23:485–492.

74. Denning DW, Anderson J, Rudge P, et al. Acute myelopathy associated with primary infection with human immunodeficiency virus. *Br Med J* 1987;294:143–144.

75. Desmet P, Kayembe KD, De Vroey C. The value of cryptococcal serum antigen screening among HIV-positive/AIDS patients in Kinshasa, Zaire. *J AIDS* 1989;3:77–78.

76. Dooneief G, Bello J, Todak G, et al. A prospective controlled study of magnetic resonance imaging of the brain in gay men and parenteral drug users with human immunodeficiency virus infection. *Arch Neurol* 1992;49:38–43.

77. Drew WL. Cytomegalovirus infection in patients with AIDS. *J Infect Dis* 1988;158:449–456.

78. Dube MP, Holtom PD, Larsen RA. Tuberculous meningitis in patients with and without human immunodeficiency virus infection. *Am J Med* 1992;93:520–524.

79. Dunn DT, Newell ML, Ades AE, Peckham CS. Risk of human immunodeficiency virus type 1 transmission through breastfeeding. *Lancet* 340;1992:585–588.

80. Egan V, Brettle RP, Goodwin GM. The Edinburgh cohort of HIV-positive drug users: pattern of cognitive impairment in relation to progression of disease. *Br J Psychiatry* 1992;161:522–531.

81. Eidelberg D, Sotrel A, Vogel H, Walker P, Kleefield J, Crumpacker CS III. Progressive polyradiculopathy in acquired immune deficiency syndrome. *Neurology* 1986;36:912–916.

82. Elovaara I, Nykyri E, Poutiainen E, Hokkanen L, Raininko R, Suni J. CSF follow-up in HIV-1 infection: intrathecal production of HIV-specific and unspecific IGG, and beta-2-microglobulin increase with duration of HIV-1 infection. *Acta Neurol Scand* 1993;87:388–396.

83. Eng RHK, Bishburg E, Smith SM, Kapila R. Cryptococcal infections in patients with acquired immunodeficiency syndrome. *Am J Med* 1986;81:19–23.

84. Epstein LG, Sharer LR, Oleske JM, et al. Neurologic manifestations of HIV infection in children. *Pediatrics* 1986;78:678–687.

85. Esiri MM, Scaravilli F, Millard PR, et al. Neuropathology of HIV infection in haemophiliacs: comparative necropsy study. *Br Med J* 1989;299:1312–1315.

86. European Collaborative Study. Children born to women with HIV-1 infection: natural history and risk of transmission. *Lancet* 1991;337:243–260.

87. Eyster ME, Gail MH, Ballard JO, et al. Natural history of human immunodeficiency virus infections in hemophilics: effects of T cell subsets, platelet counts, and age. *Ann Intern Med* 1987;107:1–6.

88. Farizo KM, Buehler JW, Chamberland ME, et al. Spectrum of disease in persons with human immunodeficiency virus infection in the United States. *JAMA* 1992;267:1798–1805.

89. Fauci AS. Multifactorial nature of human immunodeficiency virus disease: implications for therapy. *Science* 1993;262:1011–1018.

90. Fischl MA, Richman DD, Grieco MH, et al. The efficacy of azidothymidine (AZT) in the treatment of patients with AIDS and AIDS-related complex. *N Engl J Med* 1987;317:185–191.

91. Franzblau A, Letz R, Hershman D, Mason P, Wallace JI, Bekesi G. Quantitative neurologic and neurobehavioral testing of persons infected with human immunodeficiency virus type 1. *Arch Neurol* 1991;48:263–268.

92. Fuller GN, Jacobs JM, Guiloff RJ. Nature and incidence of peripheral nerve syndromes in HIV infection. *J Neurol Neurosurg Psychiatry* 1993;56:372–381.

93. Gabuzda DH, Hirsch MS. Neurologic manifestations of infection with human immunodeficiency virus: clinical features and pathogenesis. *Ann Intern Med* 1987;107:383–391.

94. Gallo RC. Mechanism of disease induction of HIV. *J AIDS* 1990;3:380–389.

95. Gallo RC, Salahuddin SZ, Popovic M, et al. Frequent detection and isolation of cytopathic retrovirus (HTLV-III) from patients with AIDS and at risk for AIDS. *Science* 1984;224:500–504.

96. Garry RF, Witte MH, Gottlieb AA, et al. Documentation of an AIDS virus infection in the United States in 1968. *JAMA* 1988;260:2085–2087.

97. Gillespie S, Chang Y, Lemp G, et al. Progressive multifocal leukoencephalopathy in persons infected with human immunodeficiency virus, San Francisco, 1981–1989. *Ann Neurol* 1991;30:597–604.

98. Goedert JJ, Eyster ME, Biggar RJ, Blattner WA. Heterosexual transmission of human immunodeficiency virus: association with severe depletion of T-helper lymphocytes in men with hemophilia. *AIDS Res Hum Retrovir* 1987;3:355–361.

99. Goethe KE, Mitchell JE, Marshall DW, et al. Neuropsychological and neurological function of human immunodeficiency virus seropositive asymptomatic individuals. *Arch Neurol* 1989;46: 129–133.
100. Goodin DS, Aminoff MJ, Chernoff DN, Hollander H. Long latency event-related potentials in patients infected with human immunodeficiency virus. *Ann Neurol* 1990;27:414–419.
101. Grafe MR, Wiley CA. Spinal cord and peripheral nerve pathology in AIDS: the roles of cytomegalovirus and human immunodeficiency virus. *Ann Neurol* 1989;5:561–566.
102. Grant I, Atkinson J, Hesselink J, et al. Evidence for early central nervous system involvement in the acquired immunodeficiency syndrome (AIDS) and other human immunodeficiency virus (HIV) infections. *Ann Intern Med* 1987;107:828–836.
103. Grau JM, Masanes F, Pedrol E. Human immunodeficiency virus type 1 infection and myopathy: clinical relevance of zidovudine therapy. *Ann Neurol* 1993;34:206–211.
104. Gray F, Gherardi R, Keohane C, Favolini M, Sobel A, Poirier J. Pathology of the central nervous system in 40 cases of acquired immune deficiency syndrome (AIDS). *Neuropathol Appl Neurobiol* 1988;14:365–380.
105. Guiloff RJ, Fuller GN, Roberts A, et al. Nature, incidence and prognosis of neurological involvement in the acquired immunodeficiency syndrome in central London. *Postgrad Med J* 1988;64:919–925.
106. Gwinn M, Pappaioanou M, George JR, et al. Prevalence of HIV infection in childbearing women in the United States. *JAMA* 1991;265:1704–1708.
107. Hall CD, Snyder CR, Messenheimer JA, et al. Peripheral neuropathy in a cohort of human immunodeficiency virus-infected patients. Incidence and relationship to other nervous system dysfunction. *Arch Neurol* 1991;48:1273–1274.
108. Handelsman L, Song IS, Losonczy M, et al. Magnetic resonance abnormalities in HIV infection: a study in the drug-user risk group. *Psychiatry Res* 1993;47:175–186.
109. Helbert M, Fletcher T, Peddle B, Harris JRW, Pinching AJ. Zidovudine-associated myopathy. *Lancet* 1988;2:689–690.
110. Helweg-Larsen S, Jakobsen J, Boesen F, et al. Myelopathy in AIDS. A clinical and electrophysiological study of 23 Danish patients. *Acta Neurol Scand* 1988;77:64–73.
111. Hersh BS, Popovici F, Apetrei RC, et al. Acquired immunodeficiency syndrome in Romania. *Lancet* 1991;338:645–649.
112. Ho DD, Moudgil T, Alam M. Quantitation of human immunodeficiency virus type 1 in the blood of infected persons. *N Engl J Med* 1989;321:1621–1625.
113. Ho DD, Sarngadharan MG, Resnick L, diMarzo-Veronese F, Rota TR, Hirsch MS. Primary human T-lymphotropic virus type III infection. *Ann Intern Med* 1985;103:880–883.
114. Holman RC, Janssen RS, Buehler JW, Zelasky MT, Hooper WC. Epidemiology of progressive multifocal leukoencephalopathy in the United States: analysis of national mortality and AIDS surveillance data. *Neurology* 1991;41:1733–1736.
115. Holtom PD, Larsen RA, Leal ME, Leedom JM. Prevalence of neurosyphilis in human immunodeficiency virus-infected patients with latent syphilis. *Am J Med* 1992;93:9–12.
116. Horsburgh CR, Ou CY, Jason J, et al. Duration of human immunodeficiency virus infection before detection of antibody. *Lancet* 1989;2:637–640.
117. Howlett WP, Nkya WM, Mmuni KA, Missalek WR. Neurological disorders in AIDS and HIV disease in the northern zone of Tanzania. *AIDS* 1989;3:289–296.
118. Hutto C, Parks WP, Lai SH, et al. A hospital-based prospective study of perinatal infection with human immunodeficiency virus type 1. *J Pediatr* 1991;118:347–353.
119. Ingraham LJ, Bridge TP, Janssen RS, Stover E, Mirsky AF. Neuropsychological effects of early HIV-1 infection: assessment and methodology. *J Neuropsychiatry Clin Neurosci* 1990;2:174–182.
120. Jabs DA, Green WR, Fox R, Polk BF, Bartlett JG. Ocular manifestations of acquired immune deficiency syndrome. *Ophthalmology* 1989;96:1092–1099.
121. Jakobsen J, Smith T, Gaub J, Helweg-Larsen S, Trojaborg. Progressive neurological dysfunction during latent HIV infection. *Br Med J* 1989;299:225–228.
122. Janssen RS. Epidemiology of human immunodeficiency virus infection and the neurologic complications of the infection. *Semin Neurol* 1992;12:10–17.
123. Janssen RS, Cornblath DR, Epstein LG, McArthur JC, Price RW. Human immunodeficiency virus (HIV) infection and the nervous system: report from the American Academy of Neurology AIDS Task Force. *Neurology* 1989;39:119–122.
124. Janssen RS, Nwanyanwu OC, Selik RK, et al. Epidemiology of human immunodeficiency virus encephalopathy in the United States. *Neurology* 1992;42:1472–1476.
125. Janssen RS, Saykin AJ, Cannon L, et al. Neurological and neuropsychological manifestations of HIV-1 infection: association with AIDS-related complex but not asymptomatic HIV-1 infection. *Ann Neurol* 1989;26:592–600.
126. Janssen R, Saykin A, Kaplan J, et al. Neurologic complications of human immunodeficiency virus infection in patients with lymphadenopathy syndrome. *Ann Neurol* 1988;23:49–55.
127. Janssen RS, St. Louis ME, Satten G, et al. HIV infection among patients in U.S. acute-care hospitals: strategies for the counseling and testing of hospital patients. *N Engl J Med* 1992;327:445–452.

128. Jernigan TL, Archibald S, Hesselink JR, et al. Magnetic resonance imaging morphometric analysis of cerebral volume loss in human immunodeficiency virus infection. *Arch Neurol* 1993;50:250–255.

129. Kalayjian RC, Cohen ML, Bonomo RA, Flanigan TP. Cytomegalovirus ventriculoencephalitis in AIDS. A syndrome with distinct clinical and pathologic features. *Medicine* 1993;72:67–77.

130. Karahalios D, Breit R, Dal Canto M, Levy RM. Progressive multifocal leukoencephalopathy in patients with HIV infection: lack of impact of early diagnosis by stereotactic brain biopsy. *J AIDS* 1992;5:1030–1038.

131. Karlsen NR, Reinvang I, Froland SS. Slowed reaction time in asymptomatic HIV-positive patients. *Acta Neurol Scand* 1992;86:242–246.

132. Katz DA, Berger JR. Neurosyphilis in acquired immunodeficiency syndrome. *Arch Neurol* 1989; 46:895–898.

133. Kim YS, Hollander H. Polyradiculopathy due to cytomegalovirus: report of two cases in which improvement occurred after prolonged therapy and review of the literature. *Clin Infect Dis* 1993; 17:32–37.

134. Kleihues P, Leib SL, Strittmatter C, Wiestler OD, Lang W. HIV encephalopathy: incidence, definition and pathogenesis. Results of a Swiss collaborative study. *Acta Pathol Jpn* 1991;41:197–205.

135. Kleinbaum DG, Kupper LL, Morgenstern H. *Epidemiologic Research*. New York: Van Nostrand Reinhold, 1982.

136. Kokkevi A, Hatzakis A, Maillis A, et al. Neuropsychological assessment of HIV-seropositive haemophiliacs. *AIDS* 1991;5:1223–1229.

137. Koot M, Keet IP, Vos AH, et al. Prognostic value of HIV-1 syncytium-inducing phenotype for rate of CD4- cell depletion and progression to AIDS. *Ann Intern Med* 1993;118:681–688.

138. Koralnik IJ, Beaumanoir A, Häusler R, et al. A controlled study of early neurologic abnormalities in men with asymptomatic human immunodeficiency virus infection. *N Engl J Med* 1990;323: 864–870.

139. Krupp LB, Lipton RB, Swerdlow ML, Leeds NE, Llena J. Progressive multifocal leukoencephalopathy: clinical and radiographic features. *Ann Neurol* 1985;17:344–349.

140. Kure K, Llena JF, Lyman WD, et al. Human immunodeficiency virus-1 infection of the nervous system: an autopsy study of 268 adult, pediatric, and fetal brains. *Hum Pathol* 1991;22:700–710.

141. Kurtzke JF. Epidemiology of multiple sclerosis. In: Hallpike JF, Adams CMW, Tourtellotte WW, eds. *Multiple Sclerosis—Pathology, Diagnosis, and Management*. London: Chapman & Hall, 1983: 47–95.

142. Lang W, Miklossy J, Deruaz JP, et al. Neuropathology of the acquired immunodeficiency syndrome (AIDS): a report of 135 consecutive autopsy cases from Switzerland. *Acta Neuropathol* 1989;77: 379–390.

143. Lantos PL, McLaughlin JE, Scholtz CL, Berry CL, Tighe JR. Neuropathology of the brain in HIV infection. *Lancet* 1989;1:309–311.

144. Leach CT, Cherry JD, English PA, et al. The relationship between T cell levels and CMV infection in asymptomatic HIV-1 antibody-positive homosexual men. *J AIDS* 1993;6:407–413.

145. Leger JM, Bouche P, Bolgert F, et al. The spectrum of polyneuropathies in patients infected with HIV. *J Neurol Neurosurg Psychiatry* 1989;52:1369–1374.

146. Levy RM, Bredesen DE, Rosenblum ML. Neurological manifestations of the acquired immunodeficiency syndrome (AIDS): experience at UCSF and review of the literature. *J Neurosurg* 1985;62: 475–495.

147. Levy RM, Janssen RS, Bush TJ, Rosenblum ML. Neuroepidemiology of acquired immunodeficiency syndrome. *J AIDS* 1988;1:31–40.

148. Lifson AR. Do alternate modes for transmission of human immunodeficiency virus exist? A review. *JAMA* 1988;259:1353–1356.

149. Luft BJ, Remington JS. Toxoplasmic encephalitis in AIDS. *Clin Infect Dis* 1992;15:211–222.

150. Lui K-J, Darrow WW, Rutherford GW. A model-based estimate of the mean incubation period for AIDS in homosexual men. *Science* 1988;240:1333–1335.

151. Lunn S, Skydsbjerg M, Schulsinger H, Parnas J, Pedersen C, Mathiesen L. A preliminary report on the neuropsychologic sequelae of human immunodeficiency virus. *Arch Gen Psychiatry* 1991; 48:139–142.

152. Maj M, Satz P, Janssen R, et al. WHO neuropsychiatric AIDS Study, cross-sectional phase. II. Neuropsychological and neurological findings. *Arch Gen Psychiatry* 1994;51:51–61.

153. Marcus R, CDC Cooperative Needlestick Surveillance Group. Surveillance of health-care workers exposed to blood from patients infected with the human immunodeficiency virus. *N Engl J Med* 1988;319:1118–1123.

154. Marder K, Stern Y, Malouf R, et al. Neurologic and neuropsychological manifestations of human immunodeficiency virus infection in intravenous drug users without acquired immunodeficiency syndrome: relationship to head injury. *Arch Neurol* 1992;49:1169–1175.

155. Marshall DW, Brey RL, Butzin CA, Lucey DR, Abbadessa SM, Boswell RN. CSF changes in a longitudinal study of 124 neurologically normal HIV-1-infected U.S. Air Force personnel. *J AIDS* 1991;4:777–781.

156. Marshall DW, Brey RL, Cahill WT, Houk RW, Zajac RA, Boswell RN. Spectrum of cerebrospinal fluid findings in various stages of human immunodeficiency virus infection. *Arch Neurol* 1988;45: 954–958.
157. Masliah E, Achim CL, Ge N, DeTeresa R, Terry RD, Wiley CA. Spectrum of human immunodeficiency virus-associated neocortical damage. *Ann Neurol* 1992;32:321–329.
158. Mastro TD, Satten GA, Nopkesorn T, Sangkharomya S, Longini IM. High probability of female-to-male transmission of HIV-1 in Thailand. *Lancet* 1994;343:204–207.
159. Mauri M, Sinforiani E, Muratori S, Zerboni R, Bono G. Three-year neuropsychological follow-up in a selected group of HIV-infected homosexual men. *AIDS* 1993;7:241–245.
160. McAllister RH, Herns MV, Harrison MJG, et al. Neurological and neuropsychological performance in HIV seropositive men without symptoms. *J Neurol Neurosurg Psychiatry* 1992;55:143–148.
161. McArthur JC. Neurologic manifestations of AIDS. *Medicine* 1987;66:407–437.
162. McArthur JC, Cohen BA, Selnes OA, et al. Low prevalence of neurological and neuropsychological abnormalities in otherwise healthy HIV-1-infected individuals: results from the multicenter AIDS cohort study. *Ann Neurol* 1989;26:601–611.
163. McArthur JC, Hoover DR, Bacellar H, et al. Dementia in AIDS patients: incidence and risk factors. *Neurology* 1993;43:2245–2252.
164. McArthur JC, Kumar AJ, Johnson DW, et al. Incidental white matter hyperintensities on magnetic resonance imaging in HIV-1 infection. Multicenter AIDS Cohort Study. *J AIDS* 1990;3:252–259.
165. Messenheimer JA, Robertson KR, Wilkins JW, Kalkowski JC, Hall CD. Event-related potentials in human immunodeficiency virus infection: a prospective study. *Arch Neurol* 1992;49:396–400.
166. Miller EN, Selnes OA, McArthur JC, et al. Neuropsychological performance in HIV-1-infected homosexual men: the Multicenter AIDS Cohort Study (MACS). *Neurology* 1990;40:197–203.
167. Miller RG, Storey JR, Greco CM. Ganciclovir in the treatment of progressive AIDS-related polyradiculopathy. *Neurology* 1990;40:569–574.
168. Musher DM, Hamill RJ, Baughn RE. Effect of human immunodeficiency virus (HIV) infection on the course of syphilis and on the response to treatment. *Ann Intern Med* 1990;113:872–881.
169. Nahmias AJ, Weiss J, Yao X, et al. Evidence for human infection with HTLV-III/LAV-like virus in central Africa, 1959. *Lancet* 1986;1:1279–1280.
170. National Center for Health Statistics. Annual summary of births, marriages, divorces, and deaths: United States, 1992. *Monthly Vital Stat Rep* 1993;41:17.
171. Navia BA, Cho ES, Petito CK, Price RW. The AIDS dementia complex: II. Neuropathology. *Ann Neurol* 1986;19:525–535.
172. Navia BA, Jordan BD, Price RW. The AIDS dementia complex: I. Clinical features. *Ann Neurol* 1986;19:517–524.
173. Navia B, Price RW. The acquired immunodeficiency syndrome dementia complex as the presenting or sole manifestation of human immunodeficiency virus infection. *Arch Neurol* 1987;44:65–69.
174. Nordic Medical Research Councils HIV Therapy Group. Double blind, dose-response study of zidovudine in AIDS and advanced HIV infection. *Br Med J* 1992;304:13–17.
175. Nuwer MR, Miller EN, Visscher BR, et al. EEG findings in asymptomatic HIV (reply from authors). *Neurology* 1993;43:635–636.
176. Nzilambi N, De Cock KM, Forthal DN, et al. The prevalence of infection with human immunodeficiency virus over a 10-year period in rural Zaire. *N Engl J Med* 1988;318:276–279.
177. Ollo C, Johnson R, Grafman J. Signs of cognitive change in HIV disease: an event-related brain potential study. *Neurology* 1991;41:209–215.
178. Ou C-Y, Takebe Y, Weniger BG, et al. Independent introduction of two major HIV-1 genotypes into distinct high-risk populations in Thailand. *Lancet* 1993;341:1171–1174.
179. Oxtoby MJ. Perinatally acquired human immunodeficiency virus infection. In: Pizzo P, Wilfert C, eds. *Pediatric AIDS: The Challenge of HIV Infection in Infants, Children, and Adolescents.* Baltimore, MD: Williams & Wilkins, 1991:3–21.
180. Perdices M, Cooper DA. Simple and choice reaction time in patients with human immunodeficiency virus infection. *Ann Neurol* 1989;24:460–467.
181. Perriëns J, Mussa M, Luabeya M, et al. Neurological complications of HIV-1 seropositive internal medicine inpatients in Kinshasa, Zaire. *J AIDS* 1992;5:333–340.
182. Perry S, Belsky-Barr D, Barr WB, Jacobsberg L. Neuropsychological function in physically asymptomatic, HIV-seropositive men. *J Neuropsychiatry* 1989;1:296–302.
183. Peterman TA, Jaffe HW, Feorino PM, et al. Transfusion-associated acquired immunodeficiency syndrome in the United States. *JAMA* 1985;254:2913–2917.
184. Petito CK, Cho ES, Lemann W, Navia BA, Price RW. Neuropathology of acquired immunodeficiency syndrome (AIDS): an autopsy review. *J Neuropathol Exp Neurol* 1986;45:635–646.
185. Petito CK, Navia BA, Cho ES, Jordan BD, George DC, Price RW. Vacuolar myelopathy pathologically resembling subacute combined degeneration in patients with the acquired immunodeficiency syndrome. *N Engl J Med* 1985;312:874–879.
186. Petty RK, Kennedy PG. The neurological features of HIV-positive patients in Glasgow—a retrospective study of 90 cases. *Q J Med* 1992;82:223–234.

187. Piette AM, Tusseau F, Vignon D, et al. Acute neuropathy coincident with seroconversion for anti-LAV/HTLV-III [Letter]. *Lancet* 1986;1:852.
188. Pluda JM, Yarchoan R, Jaffe ES, et al. Development of non-Hodgkin lymphoma in a cohort of patients with severe human immunodeficiency virus (HIV) infection on long-term antiretroviral therapy. *Ann Intern Med* 1990;113:276–282.
189. Portegies P, de Gans J, Lange JMA, et al. Declining incidence of AIDS dementia complex after introduction of zidovudine treatment. *Br Med J* 1989;299:819–821.
190. Portegies P, Enting RH, de Gans J, et al. Presentation and course of AIDS dementia complex: 10 years of follow-up in Amsterdam, The Netherlands. *AIDS* 1993;7:669–675.
191. Porter SF, Sande MA. Toxoplasmosis of the central nervous system in the acquired immunodeficiency syndrome. *N Engl J Med* 1992;327:1643–1648.
192. Poutiainen E, Elovaara I, Raininko R, et al. Cognitive performance in HIV-1 infection: relationship to severity of disease and brain atrophy. *Acta Neurol Scand* 1993;87:88–94.
193. Price R, Brew BJ. The AIDS dementia complex. *J Infect Dis* 1988;158:1079–1083.
194. Renold C, Sugar A, Chave JP, et al. Toxoplasma encephalitis in patients with the acquired immunodeficiency syndrome. *Medicine* 1992;71:224–239.
195. Resnick L, Berger J, Shapshack P, Tourtellotte W. Early penetration of the blood-brain-barrier by HIV. *Neurology* 1988;38:9–14.
196. Riedel RR, Helmstaedter C, Bülau P, et al. Early signs of cognitive deficits among human immunodeficiency virus-positive hemophiliacs. *Acta Psychiatr Scand* 1992;85:321–326.
197. Robertson KR, Stern RA, Hall CD, et al. Vitamin B12 deficiency and nervous system disease in HIV infection. *Arch Neurol* 1993;50:807–811.
198. Rosenblum L, Buehler JW, Morgan MW, et al. The completeness of AIDS case reporting, 1988: a multisite collaborative surveillance project. *Am J Public Health* 1992;82:1495–1499.
199. Rothenberg R, Woelfel M, Stoneburner R, Milberg J, Parker R, Truman B. Survival with the acquired immunodeficiency syndrome: experience with 5833 cases in New York City. *N Engl J Med* 1987;317:1297–1302.
200. Royal W, Updike M, Selnes OA, et al. HIV-1 infection and nervous system abnormalities among a cohort of intravenous drug users. *Neurology* 1991;41:1905–1910.
201. Satz P, Morgenstern H, Miller EN, et al. Low education as a possible risk factor for cognitive abnormalities in HIV-1: findings from the multicenter AIDS Cohort Study (MACS). *J AIDS* 1993;6:503–511.
202. Saykin AJ, Janssen RS, Sprehn GC, Kaplan JE, Spira TJ, O'Connor B. Longitudinal evaluation of neuropsychological function in homosexual men with HIV infection:18-month follow-up. *J Neuropsychiatry Clin Neurosci* 1991;3:286–298.
203. Schoenberg BS. General considerations. In: Schoenberg BS, ed. *Advances in Neurology.* Vol. 19. New York: Raven, 1978:13.
204. Schwartländer B, Horsburgh CR Jr, Hamouda O, et al. Changes in the spectrum of AIDS-defining conditions and decrease in CD4- lymphocyte counts at AIDS manifestation in Germany from 1986 to 1991. *AIDS* 1992;6:413–420.
205. Scott GB, Hutto C, Makuch RW, et al. Survival in children with perinatally acquired human immunodeficiency virus type 1 infection. *N Engl J Med* 1989;321:1791–1796.
206. Selnes OA, McArthur JC, Royal W III, et al. HIV-1 infection and intravenous drug use: longitudinal neuropsychological evaluation of asymptomatic subjects. *Neurology* 1992;42:1924–1930.
207. Selnes OA, Miller E, McArthur J, et al. HIV-1 infection: no evidence of cognitive decline during the asymptomatic stages. *Neurology* 1990;40:204–208.
208. Shaunak S, Albright RE, Klotman ME, Henry SC, Bartlett JA, Hamilton JD. Amplification of HIV-1 provirus from cerebrospinal fluid and its correlation with neurologic disease. *J Infect Dis* 1990;161:1068–1072.
209. Silberstein CH, O'Dowd MA, Chartock P, et al. A prospective four-year follow-up of neuropsychological function in HIV seropositive and seronegative methadone-maintained patients. *Gen Hosp Psychiatry* 1993;15:351–359.
210. Simpson DM, Citak KA, Godfrey E, Godbold J, Wolfe DE. Myopathies associated with human immunodeficiency virus and zidovudine: can their effects be distinguished? *Neurology* 1993;43:971–976.
211. Sinforiani E, Mauri M, Bono G, Muratori S, Alessi E, Minoli L. Cognitive abnormalities and disease progression in a selected population of asymptomatic HIV-positive subjects. *AIDS* 1991;5:1117–1120.
212. Snider WD, Simpson DM, Nielsen S, Gold JWM, Metroka CE, Posner JB. Neurological complications of acquired immunodeficiency syndrome: analysis of 50 patients. *Ann Neurol* 1983;14:403–418.
213. So YT, Beckstead JH, Davis RL. Primary central nervous system lymphoma in acquired immunodeficiency syndrome: a clinical and pathological study. *Ann Neurol* 1986;20:566–572.
214. So YT, Holtzman DM, Abrams DI, Olney RK. Peripheral neuropathy associated with acquired

immunodeficiency syndrome. Prevalence and clinical features from a population-based survey. *Arch Neurol* 1988;45:945–948.

215. Sönnerborg A, Saaf J, Alexius B, Strannegard Ö, Wahlund LO, Wetterberg L. Quantitative detection of brain aberrations in human immunodeficiency virus type 1-infected individuals by magnetic resonance imaging. *J Infect Dis* 1990;162:1245–1251.

216. Sönnerborg A, Johansson B, Strannegard Ö. Detection of HIV-1 DNA and infectious virus in cerebrospinal fluid. *AIDS Res Hum Retrovir* 1991;7:369–373.

217. Sönnerborg AB, Ehrnst AC, Bergdahl SKM, Pehrson P-O, Sköldenberg BR, Strannegård Ö. HIV isolation from cerebrospinal fluid in relation to immunological deficiency and neurological symptoms. *AIDS* 1988;2:89–93.

218. Sönnerborg AB, von Sydow MA, Forsgren M, Strannegard Ö. Association between intrathecal anti-HIV-1 immunoglobulin G synthesis and occurrence of HIV-1 in cerebrospinal fluid. *AIDS* 1989;3: 701–705.

219. Spector SA, Hsia K, Pratt D, et al. Virologic markers of human immunodeficiency virus type 1 in cerebrospinal fluid. *J Infect Dis* 1993;168:68–74.

220. Stern Y, Marder K, Bell K, et al. Multidisciplinary baseline assessment of homosexual men with and without human immunodeficiency virus infection. *Arch Gen Psychiatry* 1991;48:131–138.

221. Stoner GL, Ryschkewitsch CF, Walker DL, Webster HdeF. JC papovavirus large tumor (T)-antigen expression in brain tissue of acquired immunodeficiency syndrome (AIDS) and non-AIDS patients with progressive multifocal leukoencephalopathy. *Proc Natl Acad Sci USA* 1986;83:2271–2275.

222. Thornton CA, Latif AS, Emmanuel JC. Guillain-Barre syndrome associated with human immunodeficiency virus infection in Zimbabwe. *Neurology* 1991;41:812–815.

223. Tokars JI, Marcus R, Culver DH, et al. Surveillance of HIV infection and zidovudine use among health care workers after occupational exposure to HIV-infected blood. *Ann Intern Med* 1993;118: 913–919.

224. Van Wielink G, McArthur JC, Moench T, et al. Intrathecal synthesis of anti-HIVIgG: correlation with increasing duration of HIV-1 infection. *Neurology* 1990;40:816–819.

225. Vella S, Giuliano M, Pezzotti P, et al. Survival of zidovudine-treated patients with AIDS compared with that of contemporary untreated patients. *JAMA* 1992;267:1232–1236.

226. Villa G, Monteleone D, Marra C, et al. Neuropsychological abnormalities in AIDS and asymptomatic HIV seropositive patients. *J Neurol Neurosurg Psychiatry* 1993;56:878–884.

227. Vinters HV, Kwok MK, Ho HW, et al. Cytomegalovirus in the nervous system of patients with the acquired immunodeficiency syndrome. *Brain* 1989;112:245–268.

228. Volberding PA, Lagakos SW, Kock MA, et al. Zidovudine in asymptomatic human immunodeficiency virus infection: a controlled trial in persons with fewer than 500 CD4-positive cells per cubic millimeter. *N Engl J Med* 1990;322:941–949.

229. Ward JW, Holmberg SD, Allen JR, et al. Transmission of human immunodeficiency virus (HIV) by blood transfusions screened as negative for HIV antibody. *N Engl J Med* 1988;318:473–478.

230. White M, Cirrincione C, Blevins A, Armstrong D. Cryptococcal meningitis: outcome in patients with AIDS and patients with neoplastic disease. *J Infect Dis* 1992;165:960–963.

231. Widy-Wirski R, Berkley S, Downing R, et al. Evaluation of WHO clinical case definition for AIDS in Uganda. *JAMA* 1988;260:3286–3289.

232. Wiley CA, Nelson JA. Role of human immunodeficiency virus and cytomegalovirus in AIDS encephalitis. *Am J Pathol* 1988;133:73–81.

233. Wilkie FL, Eisdorfer C, Morgan R, Loewenstein DA, Szapocznik J. Cognition in early human immunodeficiency virus infection. *Arch Neurol* 1990;47:433–440.

234. Wong B, Gold JWM, Brown AE, et al. Central nervous system toxoplasmosis in homosexual men and parenteral drug abusers. *Ann Intern Med* 1984;100:36–42.

235. World Health Organization. Acquired immunodeficiency syndrome (AIDS): interim proposal for a WHO staging system for HIV infection and disease. *Wkly Epidemiol Rec* 1990;65:221–224.

236. World Health Organization. *Report on the Consultation on the Neuropsychiatric Aspects of HIV-1 Infection: An Update.* Geneva: World Health Organization, January 1990.

237. World Health Organization. *In Point of Fact.* Geneva: World Health Organization, May 1991 (no. 74).

238. World Health Organization. *Current and Future Dimensions of the HIV/AIDS Pandemic: A Capsule Summary.* Geneva: World Health Organization, January 1992:1–15.

239. World Health Organization. *The HIV/AIDS Pandemic: 1993 Overview.* Geneva: World Health Organization, 1993:1–17.

240. World Health Organization. *The Current Global Situation of the HIV/AIDS Pandemic.* Geneva: World Health Organization Global Programme on AIDS, July 1994:1–11.

241. Wrzolek MA, Sher JH, Kozlowski PB, Rao C. Skeletal muscle pathology in AIDS: an autopsy study. *Muscle Nerve* 1990;13:508–515.

242. Zangerle R, Allenberger F, Pohl P, Fritsch P, Dierich MP. High risk of developing toxoplasmic encephalitis in AIDS patients seropositive for *Toxoplasma gondii*. *Med Microbiol Immunol* 1991; 180:59–66.

243. Zuger A, Louie E, Holzman RS, Simberkoff MS, Rahal JJ. Cryptococcal disease in patients with the acquired immunodeficiency syndrome. *Ann Intern Med* 1986;104:234–240.

AIDS and the Nervous System, Second Edition,
edited by J. R. Berger and R. M. Levy.
Lippincott-Raven Publishers, Philadelphia © 1997.

3

The Biology and Tropism of Human Immunodeficiency Virus-1 in the Nervous System

Katherine E. Conant, Mariachiara G. Monaco,
and Eugene O. Major

*Laboratory of Molecular Medicine and Neuroscience, National Institutes of
Health, Bethesda, Maryland 20892*

Human immunodeficiency virus-1 (HIV-1)–associated neuropathology is notable for a discrepancy between the small number of demonstrably infected brain cells and the widespread pathological changes. Because of this discrepancy, indirect mechanisms of neuronal damage, such as those related to cytokines and HIV-1 gene products, have been invoked to account for the major part of the associated neurological disease. As more sensitive and specific viral detection techniques emerge, however, an increase in both the absolute number of infected cells and the number of infected cell types is becoming evident. Consequently, direct infection of cells of the central nervous system (CNS) may contribute more to the neurological manifestations of acquired immunodeficiency syndrome (AIDS) than is presently considered.

THE LENTIVIRINAE

HIV-1 belongs to the lentivirus genus of the retroviridae family. In addition to both HIV-1 and HIV-2, viruses belonging to this subgroup include equine infectious anemia virus, Maedi-visna virus, caprine arthritis-encephalitis virus, bovine immunodeficiency virus, feline immunodeficiency virus, and simian immunodeficiency virus (SIV). Characteristics common to this genus include a long incubation period, infection of cells of the immune system, and viral invasion of the central nervous system. Disease results both from direct viral multiplication in cells and tissues as well as from opportunistic infections resulting from immune suppression in the host. Clinical manifestations include glomerulonephritis, hemolytic anemia, cachexia, and encephalitis.

Certain infected cells may demonstrate a latent or persistent type of infection, whereas others demonstrate cytopathic effect. Additionally, there may be an accumulation of unintegrated viral DNA in certain cells. A schematic representation of an HIV-1 virion is depicted in Fig. 1. The viral genome is depicted in Fig. 2.

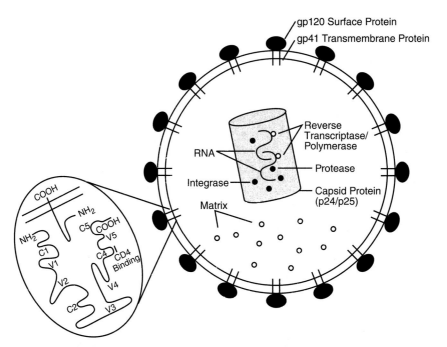

FIG. 1. Schematic representation of an HIV-1 Virion.

IN VIVO INFECTION OF THE CNS BY HIV-1

Early in the AIDS epidemic, there was uncertainty as to whether any cells of the central nervous system were infected with HIV-1. Neurological symptoms often were attributed either to depression, to the effects of opportunistic CNS infections, or to the debilitating effects of severe systemic disease. In 1985, however, HIV-1 nucleic acids were detected by Southern blot and *in situ* hybridization in the brains of five patients with AIDS (143). In this same year, Epstein et al. demonstrated retroviruslike particles in the brains of three patients with AIDS by electron microscopy. These particles were localized to multinucleated giant cells and occasionally to astrocytes (41). In 1986, Koenig et al. demonstrated that mononucleated and multinucleated giant cells were the major cell types synthesizing HIV-1 in the brains of the two patients examined in their study (84). Another study in 1986 examined the brains

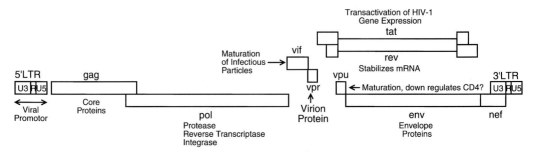

FIG. 2. Genomic organization of HIV-1.

of 12 patients with AIDS by *in situ* hybridization and immunocytochemistry using an antibody to HIV-1 *gag*–encoded proteins. In this study HIV-1 was detected not only in mononuclear and giant cells but in capillary endothelial cells as well. Additionally, in one of the 12 cases, HIV-1 was demonstrated in astrocytes and neurons. This was a case that had demonstrated severe encephalopathy (169). Other early studies also detected HIV-1 in cells that were not of macrophage/monocyte lineage, such as capillary endothelial cells (50,135,160,169), astrocytes (59,149,160), and neurons (149). Nonetheless, controversy remained as to whether infection of such cell types was significant. For example, in a large study by Kure et al., brain tissue from 102 patients was examined with a probe to the HIV-1 structural protein gp41. In this study, HIV-1 was again detected in cells of the macrophage/microglial lineage but not in neurons, astrocytes or endothelial cells (87).

These early studies suggested what has become apparent from *in vitro* work as well: that cells of the macrophage/microglial lineage are the predominant productively infected cell types in the CNS. However, many of the early studies relied on structural protein probes. Such probes were not ideal for the detection of a possible latent or restricted viral infection in other cell types. Recently two groups published results from studies that had been designed to specifically improve conditions that would allow detection of a restricted infection (136,153). In a restricted infection, viral regulatory proteins are often expressed at a time when structural proteins are not (136,154). Tornatore et al. identified HIV-1–infected astrocytes in the brains of pediatric patients with AIDS by immunocytochemistry with an antibody to the Nef regulatory protein. Additionally, four of 12 pediatric AIDS cases demonstrated HIV-1 nucleic acid by *in situ* hybridization in cells that had stained positive for glial fibrillary acidic protein, an astrocyte marker (153). In a simultaneously reported study, Saito et al. noted that most prior *in situ* studies had used a proviral DNA (pGemmBenn), which contains the entire Gag, Pol, and Env encoding sequences but lacks the entire Nef encoding sequence. Because Nef may be overexpressed in a restricted infection, this group designed *nef*-specific probes for *in situ* hybridization and found that up to 20% of astrocytes were positive (136).

Although infection of the astrocyte may generally be nonproductive, it may have serious consequences not only because such cells may serve as a viral reservoir but because these cells are support cells for the neuron.

The astrocyte is not the only cell type in which HIV-1 infection may have been underestimated. As *in situ* polymerase chain reaction (PCR) techniques improve, infection in other cell types such as the neuron is being reported. Nuovo et al. used *in situ* gene amplification techniques (PCR) to examine brain tissue from 7 HIV-1–positive and seven HIV-1–negative cases (115). PCR was used because standard *in situ* hybridization often fails to detect infected cells having less than 10–20 copies/cell threshold (114,116,117). In fact, in this study HIV-1 was rarely detected by the standard technique. In contrast, with *in situ* PCR, seven of seven HIV-1–positive cases demonstrated HIV-1–infected brain cells, whereas none of the controls did so. Furthermore, in those cases with severe dementia, many astrocytes and neurons demonstrated HIV-1 infection (115). This observation is consistent with the works of Tornatore (153) and Wiley (169) in that in each of these studies, infection of astrocytes is correlated with severe neuropathology (153,169). These studies suggest that direct infection of such cell types could contribute to the clinical manifestations of AIDS.

IN VITRO INFECTION OF CNS-DERIVED CELLS BY HIV-1

In vitro, HIV-1 has been shown to infect a variety of primary brain-derived cells as well as a large number of CNS-derived cell lines. For example, that microglial cells are infectable *in vitro* has been demonstrated by Watkins et al. (161). Macrophage-tropic strains were shown to be capable of infecting these cells, whereas two T-cell–tropic strains were not. Infection of microglial cells was subsequently demonstrated to be CD4 + -T lymphocyte dependent (75). However, contrasting data were reported in another study that separated microglial cells from monocytes/macrophages based on the expression of F_c, CD68/KiM7, and CD11b/CR3 receptors and a lack of expression of CD4, CD14, and CD68/KiM6. This study failed to detect HIV-1 infection of microglia (124).

Several laboratories have reported infection of human glial cells. Primary human fetal dorsal root ganglia–derived cells have been infected (86,168), as have several glial cell lines (7,11,21,26,37,157). Additionally, primary human astrocytes can be infected (11,155). Infection in glial cells is typically much less productive than is infection in T cells or microglia. However, in the presence of various cytokines or uninfected T cells, latently infected astrocytes have been demonstrated to release infectious virions (155). This suggests that such cells could serve as a viral reservoir, contributing to viral spread in the presence of infiltrating lymphocytes or macrophages.

Neural derived cells also have been demonstrated to be infectable by HIV-1 (93), and neural cells have been shown to contain the transcription factors necessary for activation of a CNS-derived HIV-1 LTR (31).

Finally, endothelial cells also have been infected *in vitro*. Moses et al. demonstrated that primary brain endothelial cells can be infected by HIV-1 (108). This study suggested that brain endothelial cells could be productively infected in a galactosyl-ceramide, CD4 + -T lymphocyte-independent manner. Infection of such cells could potentially affect blood–brain barrier function and thus contribute to the neurological manifestations of AIDS.

SPECIFIC DETERMINANTS OF TROPISM

Given that cells of the CNS are directly infected by HIV-1, it is necessary to explore the specific determinants of this tropism. The literature indicates that several factors are involved. These include the viral sequence itself, the specific cell type infected (including receptor[s] expressed), as well as the presence of intracellular cofactors, the particular host immune response, and environmental factors such as opportunistic viral infections and other antigenic stimuli.

ENTRY: CELLULAR DETERMINANTS

The demonstration in 1986 that the CD4 + -T lymphocyte molecule can bind the AIDS virus provided an explanation for the T cell tropism of this virus (34,83,99). It was subsequently determined that other cell types that undergo *in vivo* infection also display this receptor. For example, macrophages and monocytes express a CD4 molecule that has the same mobility by sodium dodecyl sulfate–polyacrylamide gel electrophoresis as does the lymphocyte CD4 + -T lymphocyte molecule (30).

Furthermore, both anti–Leu 3a, which binds CD4, as well as recombinant soluble CD4 (RSCD4) can block infection of macrophages by several macrophage-tropic strains of HIV-1 (30).

Additionally, the level of CD4 expression may influence the level of viral expression in certain situations. Volsky et al. demonstrated that transfection of neuroglioma cells with a CD4 expression vector produced a cell line that had viral expression, at 3 days postinfection, which was comparable with that measured under the same conditions for HIV-1–infected T cells (157). Others have demonstrated that in four T cell lines the rate and efficiency of viral uptake is correlated with the degree of permissiveness (147).

Although CD4 can indeed influence permissiveness, there are other factors that can affect replication in an equally significant manner. For example, viral replication in activated versus nonactivated T cells was found to be independent of HIV-1 binding to CD4 (102). Furthermore, despite the importance of the CD4 molecule in efficient viral entry, the presence of this receptor is not necessarily associated with efficient HIV-1 expression. There are cells that express high levels of CD4 and yet are resistant to infection with certain HIV-1 strains (42,80). Additionally, it is now well established that the CD4 receptor is not essential for viral entry. Many cells and cell lines that do not express CD4 can be infected with HIV-1 (18,21,26,28,37, 65,93,151). CD4-independent entry is further supported by evidence from several investigators that antibodies to CD4 as well as RS CD4 can block HIV-1 infection of lymphoid cells but cannot block HIV-1 infection of neural cells (28,86,163,168). In fact, clinically, RS CD4 has failed (76,139). *In vitro* results may not have predicted *in vivo* results because of viral strain differences (118). Primary HIV-1 isolates are more resistant to neutralization by RS CD4 than are cell line–adapted isolates (33). Another of the many possible reasons for the clinical failure of RS CD4 is that this compound may strip glycoprotein (gp)120 from HIV-1, thereby triggering or enhancing a fusion epitope of gp41 (35,105). This fusion epitope may be important in the second of a probable two-step entry of HIV-1 into the host cell (92). The first step of this process, viral/cell surface juxtaposition, may be made more efficient by the presence of CD4 or an alternate receptor but also could occur independent of such receptors. The second step, viral fusion with the cell membrane, possibly mediated by gp41, may require a fusion receptor (92). Results of one study do suggest that HIV-1 enters the cell by direct fusion rather than by endocytosis of CD4 (100). Work by Haggerty et al. supports a two-step process in that certain mutations in the HIV-1 *env* sequence were shown to affect the ability of the virus to enter CD4+ cells but not to enter CD4− cells (60).

Alternative molecules that bind HIV-1 and may thus be involved in entry have been identified (64). Gonzales-Scarano et al. demonstrated that antibodies to galactosylceramide (GalC) inhibited viral internalization and infection in two cell lines from the nervous system (64).

In primary astrocytes, HIV-1 entry is independent of CD4 as well as GalC (unpublished observations). However, Ma et al. have identified an astrocyte-associated 260-kDa protein that binds HIV-1 gp120 and could act as a receptor on these cells (98).

Additional factors that may enhance entry and thus affect tropism include the CD26 molecule. This is a serine protease that cleaves at specific motifs that happen to be highly conserved in the V3 loop of HIV-1 (16). In one study, entry of HIV-1 into certain T-lymphoblastoid and monocytoid cell lines could be inhibited by a monoclonal antibody to CD26 as well as by inhibition of its protease activity (16).

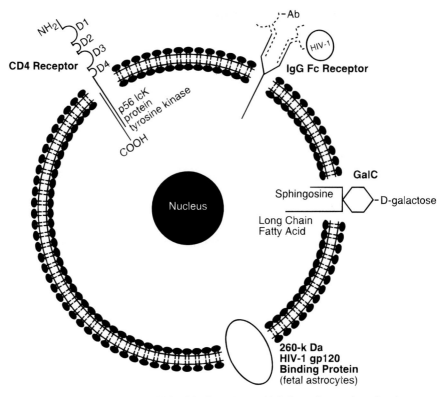

FIG. 3. Cell surface HIV-1 binding sites which have been described.

However, there is controversy as to the role of CD26 in HIV-1 fusion (3,12,15,17,122).

Finally, cofactors may affect tropism in that they can sometimes enhance viral entry. The ubiquitous human herpesvirus 6, which is a common infectious agent of childhood, has been shown to induce expression of CD4 molecules in cells that do not normally express this molecule (96,97). Furthermore, other members of the herpesvirus family, herpes simplex virus 1 (HSV-1) and cytomegalovirus (CMV), have been implicated in one of the two described *in vitro* mechanisms for antibody-dependent enhancement of HIV-1 infection. Both HSV-1 and CMV can induce expression of immunoglobulin G F_c receptors (47,49,77,162,166,167). F_c receptors have been shown to bind HIV-1–antibody complexes (68,69,150). CMV-induced F_c receptors were associated with HIV-1 infection of otherwise nonpermissive fibroblasts (103). The second described form of antibody-dependent enhancement is complement dependent. This form requires both CD4 and complement receptor type 2 (132,133). It has been demonstrated that antibodies to an immunodominant peptide in gp41 can be associated with this complement-dependent form of antibody-mediated enhancement (131). Figure 3 is a pictorial representation of some of the HIV-1 binding proteins and receptors that have been described.

ENTRY: VIRAL DETERMINANTS

Because different viral strains have differing abilities to infect a given cell type, it is apparent that factors specific to the virus affect tropism. These differences may result as a consequence of chance mutations that lead to strains that are then selected for, or infected cells may influence viral phenotype in a more direct manner.

In vitro, one study demonstrated that passage of viral isolates through different cell types was associated with changes in the level of viral expression as well as host cell tropism (22). This study demonstrated an associated change in the size of an envelope glycoprotein, a posttranslational effect that others have also implicated as possibly influencing tropism (60). Because the virus had been passaged short term, it was unlikely that there had been selection of a genetic variant (22).

In vivo, as disease progresses there is a general emergence of viral strains that are more cytopathic and have an increased ability to replicate in a wide variety of cell types (23). This may be related to selection of various mutants. Selection pressure is also evident at the level of specific isolates. Specific isolates recovered from different sites *in vivo* do indeed display marked differences. These differences are evident in their ability to infect certain cell types, to replicate efficiently, to undergo serum neutralization, to modify CD4 expression, and to cause cytopathic effect (24). In one study, a frontal lobe isolate was determined to replicate well in both macrophages and peripheral blood lymphocytes, whereas an isolate from the cerebrospinal fluid (CSF) of the same patient was determined to replicate well in lymphocytes but not in macrophages (85). Additionally, only the CSF isolate was able to infect a brain glioma explant culture (85). In another study, blood-derived isolates replicated more efficiently in T cell and glioma cell lines, whereas CNS isolates replicated more efficiently in primary macrophages (24). In general, microglia are infected by macrophage-tropic strains of HIV-1 (161), whereas astrocytes also may be infected with both macrophage-tropic (79) and lymphotropic strains (155). In fact, the tropism of HIV-1 for microglia has been shown to be controlled by regions of the HIV-1 envelope that also determine macrophage tropism (142,161).

As to which viral elements are primarily involved in the entry determinants of tropism, much attention has focused on the viral envelope because this region not only displays considerable heterogeneity but also is responsible for CD4 binding. Studies using recombinant viruses have indeed demonstrated that the envelope region contains many of the determinants of T cell versus macrophage tropism. Additionally, the specific regions of envelope (gp120) that are necessary for CD4 binding have been defined (32,89). However, sites that are actually outside of the CD4 binding domain have been shown to be important determinants of tropism (70,71,94,119). The V3 loop is one such region. This region may be the major determinant of macrophage tropism (94,144,165). In fact, the V3 loops of macrophage-tropic strains have been found to be quite homogenous as compared with T cell–specific V3 sequences (25). Although T cell tropism may depend on several regions such as V1, V2, V4, and the CD4 binding domain, V3 is important as well (144). One study, using reciprocal DNA fragment exchange between a monocyte-tropic and two non-monocyte-tropic HIV-1 clones, identified a 283–base pair (bp) sequence that conferred monocyte tropism (165). Examination of this region in a number of published HIV-1 sequences suggested that six amino acids in particular may be important in this tropism (165). The 94 amino acids that this 283-bp sequence encoded were noted to include the entire third variable domain but only two of the 11 amino acids that have been implicated in CD4 binding. Because these two amino acids were identical among the three strains examined, it was unlikely that they were responsible for the tropic differences. As to the quality of V3 that may determine monocyte versus lymphocyte tropism, several features have been noted (121,165). In general, strains having more positively charged amino acids in V3 are less efficient at replicating in monocytes (121).

Although certain regions of V3 vary among diverse HIV-1 isolates and generally this region displays considerable variability, it should be noted that the tip of the V3 loop, Gly-Pro-Gly-Arg (G-P-G-R) or the principal neutralizing determinant, tends to be highly conserved (88).

Because small amino acid changes in the V3 loop can affect T cell versus macrophage tropism, the actual conformation of the V3 loop may be important (145). The V3 loop may serve as a substrate for a cell surface protease that acts to assist the viral fusion process. It could be that a change in V3 affects tropism by changing the recognition site for this protease (29,54).

Another viral region that may be important in tropism resides in the 41-kDa transmembrane protein that is associated with gp120. This protein probably functions in fusion. Changes in this region have been associated with a change in the host range of HIV-1 (48).

NEUROINVASIVENESS, NEUROTROPISM, AND NEUROVIRULENCE

In addition to its importance in tropism, the V3 loop may play a critical role in neurovirulence. One study examined 22 HIV-infected patients premortem and classified them as demented (n = 14) or nondemented (n = 8) (128). At autopsy, virus was isolated from the brains of these patients, and it was noted that two amino acid

TABLE 1. *HIV-1 strains isolated from neural tissues or blood*

Isolate	Neuroinvasive[a]	Neurovirulent[b]	Neurotropic[c]	Reference
CSF				
JR-CSF	+	+	+ −	85
SF 185A	+	+	+ −	24
L23	+	+	−	79
2815 CSF	+	+ −	+ −	51
2844 CSF	+	+ −	+ −	79
SF 161B	+	+	−	21
Brain Tissue				
JR-FL	+	+	−	85
CNS-1	+	+	+ −	79
BR	+	+	−	4
SF 301A	+	+	+	21
Spinal cord				
SF 128A	+	+	−	21
Blood				
SF 2	−	−	+	21,138
SF 117	−	−	+	21
NL4-3	−	−	+	1,153
Ba-L	−	−	+ −	53,79,161
IIIB	−	−	+ −	11,64,65,86,125,126,129,161,168
RF	−	−	+ −	11,93
N1T	−	−	+ −	37,157
LAV	−	−	−	108,129

[a] Invasive, isolated from neural tissue.
[b] Virulent, associated with histopathology.
[c] Tropic, able to infect neural derived cells, e.g., glial, neuron.

positions within the V3 region showed significant divergence between the two groups. Additionally, the demented group was noted to have 21 amino acid residues at specific positions that were unique relative to the nondemented group. Although the strains isolated in this study may have differed in their ability to cause neuropathology, they were similar in that they demonstrated homology to the macrophage-tropic consensus sequence within the V3 loop (128). This information taken together with that of other studies emphasizes the idea that a distinction must be made between neuroinvasive, neurotropic, and neurovirulent. Although a particular strain of HIV-1 may be isolated from brain tissue or CSF and thus considered neuroinvasive, it is not necessarily neurotropic in that it may enter and/or replicate as well or better in non–CNS-derived cells. Similarly, a strain that is neurotropic in that it can enter and possibly replicate well in neurally derived cells is not necessarily more virulent than a less neurotropic strain; neurovirulence does not necessarily imply neurotropism. Table 1 summarizes this point.

LEVEL OF HIV-1 EXPRESSION: VIRAL DETERMINANTS

Although it has been demonstrated that the rate and efficiency of entry can significantly impact on permissiveness (147,157), entry should not be considered the sole factor influencing replication efficiency. The ability to replicate efficiently is also controlled by viral sequences outside of *env* as well as by both intracellular and extracellular factors.

The viral promotor for HIV-1, or long terminal repeat (LTR), pictured in Fig. 4 contains binding sites for several transcription factors. Important among these sites are the TATAA motif, which binds TFIID, as well as binding sites for NF-kB, SP-1, and the viral transactivator Tat. Mutation of the TATAA motif is associated with a loss of both basal and induced HIV-1 LTR activity (109). Mutations of the binding sites for the cellular protein Sp1, especially sites 2 and 3, lead to a significant diminution of LTR activity (66,74,91,109,134). Mutations of the binding sites for the inducible transcription factor NF-kB also decrease LTR activity. However, the effect of LTR mutations at this motif can be overcome, and in certain cells LTR NF-kB

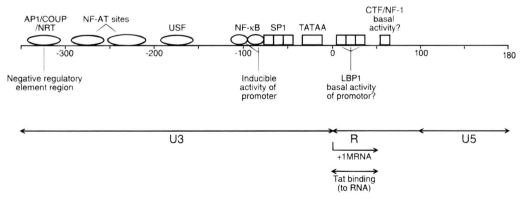

FIG. 4. Schematic organization of the HIV-1 LTR. Approximate binding sites for some of proteins which may interact with the LTR are indicated. See text for further information on selected binding proteins.

mutants replicate as efficiently as do wild-type viral strains (91). *In vivo*, binding sites for SP1 and NF-kB tend to be highly conserved (110). Work by Perkins et al. has demonstrated that a cooperation between SP1 binding to the SP1 III site and NF-kB binding to the adjacent kB site may be necessary for efficient transactivation (123). Other LTR sites that bind transcription factors have been described and include those for NFAT-1, AP-1, UBP-1, EBP-1, NF-1, LBP, and Myb (130).

Studies that have examined the effect of various substitutions in the viral promotor include one that replaced the NF-kB, SP-1, and TATAA motifs with the CMV immediate early enhancer (19). The resulting virus exhibited infectious kinetics similar to wild-type HIV-1 in peripheral blood lymphocytes and AA2 cells but replicated less efficiently in H9 and CEM cells. It has been noted that various HIV-1 isolates have considerable variation not only in the *env* sequence but in the LTR (146,159,170). Given the effect of the LTR on viral expression, it would be expected that *in vivo* strains differing in this region may display varied replication kinetics. Interestingly, an SIV strain that is associated with assymptomatic infection in African Sykes' monkeys has been isolated and found to lack NF-kB binding sites in the LTR (67).

Other elements that influence the level of viral expression include the viral regulatory protein products of the genes for *tat*, *rev*, and *nef*. The *tat* gene product, in cooperation with cellular factors, is a viral transactivator (5). Initial production of Tat is dependent on the activity of the viral promotor. Once induced, Tat may then serve to amplify HIV-1 expression. In certain cases the amount of Tat protein expressed may limit viral expression. For example, in the latently infected U1 cell line, Tat was associated with a release from latency characterized by an increase in promotor distal transcripts (2). Furthermore, the addition of a Tat expression vector can lead to an increase in HIV-1 expression from cells that had been relatively resistant to replication with certain HIV-1 strains (141). Several studies suggest that Tat may function to increase the efficiency of transcriptional elongation (43,95,101). Additionally, Tat may in certain circumstances function in the initiation complex because it may interact with elements 5′ to its TAR binding region (10).

The *rev* gene product is essential for the production of HIV-1 structural proteins. Thus, a viral strain that had a significant defect in the *rev* gene or the binding site for its protein, the RRE, may not have the ability to produce infectious virions and would thus be at a selection disadvantage. Indeed, both the sequence of the Rev protein and that of the RRE are highly conserved among HIV isolates (90). The function of the *nef* gene product is poorly understood. In some *in vitro* studies the *nef* gene product can inhibit replication of certain HIV-1 strains (20,92,111–113), an effect that may be mediated by downregulation of the CD4 receptor (58,127). However, whereas in some *in vitro* experimental situations the *nef* gene product has been associated with an inhibition of HIV-1 replication, in others *nef* not only failed to inhibit HIV-1 replication (27,62,81), but it was associated with enhanced infectivity (27). Furthermore, in SIV studies *nef* has been associated with increased pathogenicity (36,78). *In vivo* the gene tends to be highly conserved, whereas *in vitro* the sequence may be dispensable (45,152). It is likely that because different selection pressures exist *in vivo* and *in vitro*, *nef* may offer an *in vivo* selection advantage that does not always apply *in vitro*.

Like *nef*, the accessory genes *vpr*, *vpu*, and *vif* were initially believed to be nonessential because in certain *in vitro* systems elimination of such genes was not fatal to viral replication. However, their conservation suggests that they may have a necessary role in HIV-1 pathogenesis.

The requirement for *vif*, an effector of viral infectivity (44), varies depending on the system and cell type studied. It may be indispensable for HIV-1 replication in certain cells such as the primary T-lymphocyte (51). The method by which this gene product may increase progeny virion infectivity is not yet clear. Vif may affect the gp120 content of newly synthesized virions (137). In another study, *vif*-defective viruses were impaired in their ability to complete proviral DNA synthesis once in an infected cell (158).

Like *vif*, the necessity of *vpr* and *vpu* also may be dependent on cell type. These gene products may impact on viral replication. In one study, mutations in *vpr* or *vpu* reduced viral antigen production in the macrophage to a much greater extent than in the lymphocyte (8). Among other studies, one that used antisense oligodeoxynucleotides to *vpr* messenger RNA (mRNA) also suggested that this gene might be important in the modulation of HIV-1 expression in macrophages (9).

LEVEL OF EXPRESSION: CELLULAR DETERMINANTS

Similar viral strains, when expressed in different cell types, can have different replication rates. This suggests that cells vary in whether they have the necessary quality or quantity of cofactors for viral replication. It is now well established that viral regulatory proteins such as Tat and Rev depend on cellular cofactors if they are to function efficiently. In addition, the process of viral integration uses cellular cofactors (57). Certain cell types may fail to display a high level of viral replication because they are either lacking in or possess insufficient quantities of necessary cofactors. For example, the primary astrocyte can be infected with HIV-1, but after several days the level of viral production is very low, and although mRNA transcripts for regulatory proteins can be detected, those for structural proteins cannot (154). This could be due to several mechanisms, including insufficient Tat or Rev expression as well as an inhibition of Tat or Rev function. If such an inhibition exists, it could be because the astrocyte contains a factor that interferes with the function of such regulatory gene products or it could be that the astrocyte lacks a sufficient quantity of a necessary cofactor. Once structural proteins are no longer detectable, cocultivation of the astrocyte with uninfected lymphocytes or stimulation with certain cytokines will lead to the release of fully infectious virions (155).

Several stimuli that increase HIV-1 expression also increase the activity of protein kinase C. In one study, depletion of PKC may have been responsible for a decrease in Tat transactivation that was not associated with a decrease in the amount of Tat protein (72). In another study, the binding of a cellular factor to TAR suggested phosphorylation dependence (63).

In association with the activation of certain protein kinases, stimuli such as tumor necrosis factor-alpha (TNF-α) also have been demonstrated to increase the nuclear translocation of the transcriptional activator NF-kB (39). This transcription factor can increase HIV-1 expression by binding to its consensus sequence on the viral promotor (39). However, this transcription factor may have other effects as well. It was recently demonstrated that an excess of the inhibitor IkB-α, which sequesters the transactivating p50/p65 form of NF-kB in the cytoplasm, is associated with the expression of regulatory protein-encoding mRNAs and a lack of expression of structural protein mRNAs (171). One suggestion was that NF-kB may be necessary for the expression of a cellular cofactor for Rev. Thus, although efficient HIV-1 expression may in certain situations occur despite a lack of NF-kB binding to its sites on the LTR (91), the possibility remains that this transcription factor is required for efficient virion production.

The expression of NF-kB is variable. Although SP-1 may be constitutively expressed and is typically noninducible, in many cell types NF-kB can be induced and its binding independently increased by a wide variety of stimuli that are associated with an increase in HIV-1 expression. For example, it is known from previous work that the astrocyte typically has little nuclear NF-kB. It is also known that TNF-α, which increases HIV-1 expression in the astrocyte is associated with an increase in NF-kB binding in this cell type (6). Additionally it is known that cell types that demonstrate relatively high levels of nuclear NF-kB, such as macrophages and activated T-lymphocytes, display productive infection with HIV-1. Thus, although there are several prerequisites for efficient viral production, in certain cell types it may be that an insufficient quantity of transcription factors, because they are required for the expression of necessary cellular cofactors, precludes productive infection.

In certain studies, productive infection has been shown to depend on additional factors. One of these is viral integration. Although both activated and unactivated T cells can be infected with HIV-1, integration occurs only in the activated T cell and may be essential for productive HIV-1 expression in this cell type (148). Integration depends on several factors, including efficient reverse transcription. In certain situations an insufficiency of nucleotide precursors may limit reverse transcription and thus integration (52,120). Integration also may depend on host cell active transport processes in order to bring the viral preintegration complex to the nucleus in nondividing cells such as the macrophage (13). It has been demonstrated that the simian virus 40 T protein nuclear localization signal (NLS) could reduce nuclear import of HIV-1 preintegration complexes (57). Because nuclear localization signals from proteins of different viruses may be similar (38), the T protein NLS was presumably competing with the HIV-1 preintegration complex NLS for the cellular receptor for this signal.

THE EFFECT OF HOST AND ENVIRONMENTAL FACTORS

It is clear from this discussion that replication is dependent on events external to the infected cell. For example, Stevenson has suggested that HIV-1 spread is influenced by events leading to T cell activation such as antigenic stimulation (14). Other investigators have suggested that viral cofactors may be involved in AIDS progression. For example, much attention has focused on coinfection with HIV-1 and herpesviruses. There is evidence that herpesviruses may activate the HIV-1 LTR (55,106,107). Such activation may, in certain cases, be related to a herpesvirus-associated increase in kB binding proteins (40,61,156). In at least one study, however, dual infection of certain cell lines with HIV-1 and CMV was actually associated with an inhibition of HIV-1 gene expression (73). Although the effect of cofactors may be situation dependent, it is clear nonetheless that they can influence HIV-1 gene expression.

Additionally, work has focused on the role of cytokines in HIV-1 infection. Not only is HIV-1 infection associated with changes in the level of expression of various cytokines (56,104,164), but certain cytokines are associated with an increase in HIV-1 expression (39,46,82,121,155).

Even the genetics of the particular host may influence AIDS progression. Individuals demonstrate diverse immunological responses to infection. These differences may affect not only the rate of progression but the propensity to develop neurologic sequelae. For example, certain human leukocyte antigen (HLA) types may be associated with a lower immune response to CMV and an associated higher probability of developing CMV encephalitis (140). Potentially, HLA type could also influence the probability of developing HIV encephalitis.

CONCLUSIONS

The CNS can be directly infected by HIV-1. Cells of macrophage/microglial lineage are the predominant productively infected cell types. However, because the CD4 molecule is not essential for viral entry and because HIV-1 has been shown to infect many cell types *in vitro*, it is not surprising that with improved detection techniques an increase in the number of infected cells and cell types is becoming apparent. Infected cells include astrocytes, endothelial cells, and possibly neurons. HIV-1 expression in such cells may be limited for several reasons, including inefficient viral entry as well as insufficient cellular cofactors. However, as disease progresses, the number of infected cells and the level of HIV-1 expression in such cells may increase. This may be due to many factors, including those that serve to increase cellular cofactors such as opportunistic infections and cytokines as well as to the emergence of more virulent HIV-1 strains. The exact mechanisms responsible not only for a possible increase in HIV-1 expression as disease progresses but for the typically restricted nature of HIV-1 expression in certain cell types remains under investigation. Understanding such mechanisms is important in that it may provide insight for novel anti-HIV-1 therapies.

Although HIV-1 expression may be limited in many of the cell types of the CNS, even a nonproductive infection could perturb cell function in a manner sufficient to contribute to the neurological manifestations of AIDS. Thus, although it is likely that indirect mechanisms contribute significantly to the neuropathology of AIDS, it remains premature to attribute most of the neurologic manifestations of HIV-1 disease to such indirect mechanisms.

REFERENCES

1. Adachi A, Gendelman HE, Koenig S, Folks T, Willey R, Rabson A, Martin MA. Production of acquired immunodeficiency syndrome-associated retrovirus in human and nonhuman cells transfected with an infectious molecular clone. *J Virol* 1986;59:284–291.
2. Adams M, Sharmeen L, Kimpton J, et al. Cellular latency in human immunodeficiency virus-infected individuals with high CD4 levels can be detected by the presence of promotor-proximal transcripts. *Proc Natl Acad Sci U S A* 1994;91:3862–3866.
3. Alizon M, Dragic T. CD26 antigen and HIV fusion? *Science* 1994;264:1161–1162.
4. Anand R, Thayer R, Srinivasan A, et al. Biological and molecular characterization of human immunodeficiency virus (HIV-1Br) from the brain of a patient with progressive dementia. *Virology* 1989; 168:79–89.
5. Arya SK, Guo C, Josephs SF, Wong-Staal F. Trans-activator gene of human T-lymphotropic virus type III (HTLV-III). *Science* 1985;229: 69–73.
6. Atwood W, Tornatore C, Traub R, Conant K, Major EO. Stimulation of HIV-1 gene expression

and induction of NF-kB (p50/p65) binding activity in TNF-alpha treated human fetal glial cells. *AIDS Res Hum Retrovir* 1994 (in press).

7. Atwood WJ, Norkin LC. Class I major histocompatability proteins as cell surface receptors for simian virus 40. *J Virol* 1989;63:4474–4477.
8. Balliet JW, Kolson DL, Eiger G, et al. Distinct effects in primary macrophages and lymphocytes of the human immunodeficiency virus type 1 accessory genes *vpr, vpu,* and *nef:* mutational analysis of a primary HIV-1 isolate. *Virology* 1994;200:623–631.
9. Balotta C, Lusso P, Crowley R, Gallo RC, Franchini G. Antisense phosphorothioate oligodeoxynucle-otides targeted to the vpr gene inhibit human immunodeficiency virus type 1 replication in primary human macrophages. *J Virol* 1993;67:4409–4414.
10. Berkhout B, Gatignol A, Rabson AB, Jeang KT. TAR independent activation of the HIV-1 LTR: evidence that Tat requires specific regions of the promotor. *Cell* 1990;62:757–767.
11. Brack-Werner R, Kleinschmidt A, Ludvigsen A, et al. Infection of human brain cells by HIV-1: restricted virus production in chronically infected human glial cell lines. *AIDS* 1991;6:273–285.
12. Broder CC, Nussbaum O, Gutheil WG, Bachovchin WW, Berger EA. CD26 antigen and HIV fusion? *Science* 1994;264:1156–1159.
13. Bukrinsky MI, Sharova N, Dempsey MP, et al. Active nuclear import of human immunodeficiency virus type 1 preintegration complexes. *Proc Natl Acad Sci USA* 1992;89:6580–6584.
14. Bukrinsky MI, Stanwick TL, Dempsey MP, Stevenson M. Quiescent T lymphocytes as an inducible virus resevoir in HIV-1 infection. *Science* 1991;254:423–427.
15. Callebaut C, Jacotot E, Krust B, Hovanessian AG. CD26 antigen and HIV fusion? *Science* 1994; 264:1162–1165.
16. Callebaut C, Krust B, Jacotot E, Hovanessian AG. T cell activation antigen, CD26, as a cofactor for entry of HIV in CD4- cells. *Science* 1993;262:2045–2050.
17. Camerini D, Planelles V, Chen ISY. CD26 antigen and HIV fusion? *Science* 1994;264:1160–1161.
18. Cao Y, Friedman-Kien AE, Huang Y, et al. CD4-independent, productive human immunodeficiency virus type 1 infection of hepatoma cell lines *in vitro. J Virol* 1990;64:2553–2559.
19. Chang L, McNulty E, Martin M. Human immunodeficiency viruses containing heterologous enhan-cer/promoters are replication competent and exhibit different l lymphocyte tropisms. *J Virol* 1993; 67:743–752.
20. Cheng-Mayer C, Ianello P, Shaw K, Luciw P, Levy JA. Differential effects of *nef* on HIV replication: implications for viral pathogenesis in the host. *Science* 1989;246:1629.
21. Cheng-Mayer C, Rutka JT, Rosenblum ML, McHugh T, Stites DP, Levy JA. Human immunodefi-ciency virus can productively infect cultured human glial cells. *Proc Natl Acad Sci USA* 1987;84: 3526–3530.
22. Cheng-Mayer C, Seto D, Levy JA. Altered host range of HIV-1 after passage through various human cell types. *Virology* 1991;181:288–294.
23. Cheng-Mayer C, Seto D, Tateno M, Levy JA. Biological features of HIV-1 that correlate with virulence in the host. *Science* 1988;240:80–82.
24. Cheng-Mayer C, Weiss C, Seto D, Levy JA. Isolates of human immunodeficiency virus type 1 from the brain may constitute a special group of the AIDS virus. *Proc Natl Acad Sci USA* 1989;86: 8575–8579.
25. Chesebro B, Wehrly K, Nishio J, Perryman S. Macrophage-tropic human immunodeficiency virus isolates from different patients exhibit unusual V3 envelope sequence homogeneity in comparison with T cell-tropic isolates: definition of critical amino acids involved in cell tropism. *J Virol* 1992; 66:6547–6554.
26. Chiodi F, Fuerstenberg S, Gidlund M, Asjo B, Fenyo EM. Infection of brain-derived cells with the human immunodeficiency virus. *J Virol* 1987;61:1244–1247.
27. Chowers MY, Spina CA, Kwoh TJ, Finch NJS, Richman DD, Guatelli JC. Optimal infectivity *in vitro* of human immunodeficiency virus type 1 requires an intact *nef* gene. *J Virol* 1994;68: 2906–2914.
28. Clapham PR, Weber JN, Whitby D, et al. Soluble CD4 block the infectivity of diverse strains of HIV and SIV for T cells and monocytes but not for brain and muscle cells. *Nature* 1989;337: 368–370.
29. Clements GJ, Price-Jones MJ, Stephens PE, et al. The V3 loops of the HIV-1 and HIV-2 surface glycoproteins contain proteolytic cleavage sites: a possible function in viral fusion. *AIDS Res Hum Retrovir* 1991;7:3–10.
30. Collman R. Human immunodeficiency type 1 tropism for human macrophages. *Pathobiology* 1992; 60:213–218.
31. Corboy JR, Buzy JM, Zink MC, Clements JE. Expression directed from HIV long terminal repeats in the central nervous system of transgenic mice. *Science* 1992;258:1804–1808.
32. Cordonnier A, Montagnier L, Emerman M. Single amino acid changes in HIV envelope affect viral tropism and receptor binding. *Nature* 1989;340:571–574.
33. Daar ES, Li XL, Moudgil T, Ho D. High concentrations of recombinant soluble CD4 are required

to neutralize primary human immunodeficiency virus type 1 isolates. *Proc Natl Acad Sci U S A* 1990;87:6574–6578.

34. Dalgliesh A, Beverly P, Clapham P, et al. The CD4 antigen is an essential component of the receptor for the AIDS retrovirus. *Nature* 1984;312:763–767.
35. Dalgleish AG, Habeshaw J, Manca F. HIV and tropism: implications for pathogenesis. *Mol Aspects Med* 1991;12:267–292.
36. Daniel MD, Kirchhoff F, Czajak SC, Seghal PK, Desrosiers RC. Protective effects of a live attenuated SIV vaccine with a deletion of the *nef* gene. *Science* 1992;258:1938–1941.
37. Dewhurst S, Sakai K, Bresser J, Stevenson M, Evinger-Hodges MJ, Volsky DJ. Persistent productive infection of human glial cells by human immunodeficiency virus (HIV) and by infectious molecular clones of HIV. *J Virol* 1987;61:3774–3782.
38. Dingwall C, Laskey RA. Nuclear targeting sequences—a consensus? *Trends Biochem Sci* 1991;16: 478–481.
39. Duh EJ, Maury WJ, Folks TM, Fauci AS, Rabson AB. Tumor necrosis factor-alpha activates human immunodeficiency virus type 1 through induction of nuclear factor binding to the NF-kB sites in the long terminal repeat. *Proc Natl Acad Sci U S A* 1989;86:5974–5978.
40. Ensoli B, Lusso P, Schachter F, et al. Human herpes virus-6 increases HIV-1 expression in co-infected T cells via nuclear factors binding to the HIV-1 enhancer. *EMBO J* 1986;8:3019–3027.
41. Epstein LG, Sharer LR, Cho ES, Meyenhofer M, Navia BA, Price RW. HTLVIII/LAV-like retrovirus particles in the brains of patients with AIDS encephalopathy. *AIDS Res* 1985;1:447–454.
42. Evans LA, McHugh TM, Stites DP, Levy JA. Differential ability of human immunodeficiency virus isolates to productively infect human cells. *J Immunol* 1987;138:3415–3418.
43. Feinberg MB, Baltimore D, Frankel AD. The role of Tat in the human immunodeficiency virus life cycle indicates a primary effect on transcriptional elongation. *Proc Natl Acad Sci U S A* 1991;88: 4045–4049.
44. Fisher AG, Ensoli B, Ivanoff L, et al. The sor gene of HIV-1 is required for efficient virus transmission *in vitro*. *Science* 1987;237:888–892.
45. Fisher AG, Ratner L, Mitsuya H, et al. Infectious mutants of HTLV-III with changes in the 3′ region and markedly reduced cytopathic effects. *Science* 1986;233:655–659.
46. Folks TM, Justement J, Kinter A, Dinarello CA, Fauci AS. Cytokine-induced expression of HIV-1 in a chronically infected promonocyte cell line. *Science* 1987;238:800–802.
47. Frey J, Einsfelder B. Induction of surface IgG receptors in cytomegalovirus-infected human fibroblasts. *Eur J Biochem* 1984;138:213–216.
48. Fujita K, Silver J, Peden K. Changes in both gp120 and gp41 can account for increased growth potential and expanded host range of human immunodeficiency virus type 1. *J Virol* 1992;66: 4445–4451.
49. Furukawa T, Hornberger E, Sakuma S, Plotkin SA. Demonstration of immunoglobulin G receptors induced by human cytomegalovirus. *J Clin Microbiol* 1975;2:332–336.
50. Gabuzda DH, Ho DD, De La Monte SM, Hirsch MS, Rota TR, RA Sobel. Immunohistochemical identification of HTLV-III antigen in grains of patients with AIDS. *Ann Neurol* 1986;20:289–295.
51. Gabuzda DH, Lawrence K, Langhoff E, et al. Role of vif in replication of human immunodeficiency virus type 1 in CD4 + T lymphocytes. *J Virol* 1992;66:6489–6495.
52. Gao W, Cara A, Gallo RC, Lori F. Low levels of deoxynucleotides in peripheral blood lymphocytes: a strategy to inhibit human immunodeficiency virus type 1 replication. *Proc Natl Acad Sci U S A* 1993;90:8925–8928.
53. Gartner S, Markovits P, Markovitz DM, Betts RF, Popovic M. Virus isolation from and identification of HTLV-III/LAV-producing cells in brain tissue from a patient with AIDS. *JAMA* 1986;256: 2365–2371.
54. Gartner S, Ohashi K, Popovic M. Virus-host cell interactions in human immunodeficiency virus infections. *Adv Exp Med Biol* 1991;300:45–55.
55. Gendelman HE, Phelps W, Feigenbaum L, et al. Trans-activation of the human immunodeficiency virus long terminal repeat sequence by DNA viruses. *Proc Natl Acad Sci U S A* 1986;83:9759–9763.
56. Genis P, Jett M, Bernton EW, et al. Cytokines and arachidonic metabolites produced during human immunodeficiency virus (HIV)-infected macrophage-astroglia interactions: implications for the neuropathogenesis of HIV disease. *J Exp Med* 1992;176:1703–1718.
57. Gulizia J, Dempsey MP, Sharova N, et al. Reduced nuclear import of human immunodeficiency virus type-1 preintegration complexes in the presence of a prototypic nuclear targeting signal. *J Virol* 1994;68:2021–2025.
58. Guy B, Kieny MP, Riviere Y, et al. HIV F/3′ orf encodes a phosphorylated GTP-binding protein resembling an oncogene product. *Nature* 1987;330:266.
59. Gyorkey F, Melnick JL, Gyorkey P. Human immunodeficiency virus in brain biopsies of patients with AIDS and progressive encephalopathy. *J Infect Dis* 1987;155:870–876.
60. Haggerty S, Dempsey MP, Bukrinsky MI, Guo L, Stevenson M. Posttranslational modifications within the HIV-1 envelope glycoprotein which restrict virus assembly and CD-4 dependent infection. *AIDS Res Hum Retrovir* 1991;7:501–510.

61. Hammarskjold M, Simurda MC. Epstein-Barr virus latent membrane protein transactivates the human immunodeficiency virus type-1 long terminal repeat through induction of NF-kB activity. *J Virol* 1992;66:6496–6501.
62. Hammes SR, Dixon EP, Malim MH, Cullen BR, Greene WC. Nef protein of human immunodeficiency virus type 1: evidence against its role as a transcriptional inhibitor. *Proc Natl Acad Sci U S A* 1989;86:9549–9553.
63. Han X, Laras A, Rounseville MP, Kumar A, Shank PR. Human immunodeficiency type-1 Tat-mediated transactivation correlates with the phosphorylation state of a cellular Tar RNA stem-binding factor. *J Virol* 1992;66:4065–4072.
64. Harouse JM, Bhat S, Spitalnik SL, et al. Inhibition of entry of HIV-1 in neural cell lines by antibodies against galactosyl ceramide. *Science* 1991;253:320–323.
65. Harouse JM, Kunsch C, Hartle HT, et al. CD4-independent infection of human neural cells by human immunodeficiency virus type 1. *J Virol* 1989;63:2527–2533.
66. Harrich D, Garcia J, Wu F, Mitsuyasu R, Gonazalez J, Gaynor R. Role of SP1-binding domains in *in vivo* transcriptional regulation of the human immunodeficiency virus type 1 long terminal repeat. *J Virol* 1989;63:2585–2591.
67. Hirsch VM, Dapolito GA, Goldstein S, et al. A distinct African lentivirus from Sykes' monkeys. *J Virol* 1993;67:1517–1528.
68. Homsy J, Meyer M, Tateno M, Clarkson S, Levy JA. The FC and not CD4 receptor mediates antibody enhancement of HIV infection in human cells. *Science* 1989;244:1357–1360.
69. Homsy J, Meyer M, Levy JA. Serum enhancement of human immunodeficiency virus (HIV) infection correlates with disease in HIV-infected individuals. *J Virol* 1990;64:1437–1440.
70. Hwang SS, Boyle TJ, Lyerly HK, Cullen BR. Identification of the envelope V3 loop as the primary determinant of cell tropism in HIV-1. *Science* 1991;253:71–74.
71. Ivanoff LA, Dubay JW, Morris JF, et al. V3 loop region of the HIV-1 gp120 envelope protein is essential for virus infectivity. *Virology* 1992;187:423–432.
72. Jacobovits A, Rosenthal A, Capon DJ. Trans-activation of HIV-1 LTR-directed gene expression by tat requires protein kinase C. *EMBO J* 1990;9:1165–1170.
73. Jault FM, Spector SA, Spector DH. The effects of cytomegalovirus on human immunodeficiency virus replication in brain-derived cells correlate with permissiveness of the cells for each virus. *J Virol* 1994;68:959–973.
74. Jones KA, Kadonaga JT, Luciw PJ, Tijian R. Activation of the AIDS retrovirus promoter by the cellular transcription factor Sp1. *Science* 1986;232:755–759.
75. Jordan CA, Watkins BA, Kufta C, Dubois-Dalcq M. Infection of brain microglial cells by human immunodeficiency virus type 1 is CD4 dependent. *J Virol* 1991;65:736–742.
76. Kahn JO. The safety and pharmacokinetics of recombinant soluble CD4 in subjects with the acquired immunodeficiency syndrome and AIDS-related complex: a phase 1 study. *Ann Intern Med* 1990; 112:254–261.
77. Keller R, Peitchel R, Goldman JN, Goldman M. An IgG-FC receptor induced in cytomegalovirus-infected human fibroblasts. *J Immunol* 1976;116:772–777.
78. Kestler HW III, Ringler DJ, Mori K, et al. Importance of the *nef* gene for maintenance of high virus loads and for development of AIDS. *Cell* 1991;65:651–662.
79. Keys B, Albert J, Kovamees J, Chiodi F. Brain-derived cells can be infected with HIV isolates derived from both blood and brain. *Virology* 1991;183:834–839.
80. Kikukawa R, Yoyanagi Y, Harada S, Kobayashi N, Hatanaka M, Yamamoto N. Differential susceptibility to the acquired immunodeficiency syndrome retrovirus in cloned cells of human leukemic T cell lines Molt-4. *J Virol* 1986;57:1159–1162.
81. Kim S, Ikeuchi K, Byrn R, Groopman J, Baltimore D. Lack of a negative influence on viral growth by the *nef* gene of human immunodeficiency virus type 1. *Proc Natl Acad Sci U S A* 1989;86: 9544–9548.
82. Kinter AL, Poli G, Maury W, Folks TM, Fauci AS. Direct and cytokine-mediated activation of protein kinase C induces human immunodeficiency virus expression in chronically infected promonocytic cells. *J Virol* 1990;64:4306–4312.
83. Klatzman D, Champagne E, Camaret S, et al. T-lymphocyte T4 molecule behaves as the receptor for human retrovirus LAV. *Nature* 1984;312:767–769.
84. Koenig S, Gendelman HE, Orenstein JM, et al. Detection of AIDS virus in macrophages in brain tissue from AIDS patients with encephalopathy. *Science* 1986;233:1089–1093.
85. Koyanagi Y, Miles S, Mitsuyasu RT, Merrill JE, Vinters HV, Chen ISY. Dual infection of the central nervous system by AIDS viruses with distinct cellular tropisms. *Science* 1987;236:819–822.
86. Kunsch C, Hartle HT, Wigdahl B. Infection of human fetal dorsal root ganglion cells with human Immunodeficiency virus type I involves an entry mechanism independent of the CD4 T4A epitope. *J Virol* 1989;63:5054–5061.
87. Kure K, Lyman WD, Weidenheim KM, Dickson DW. Cellular localization of an HIV-1 antigen in subacute AIDS encephalitis using an improved double-labeling immunohistochemical method. *Am J Pathol* 1990;136:1085–1092.

88. LaRosa GJ, Davide JP, Weinhold K, et al. Conserved sequence and structural elements in the HIV-1 principal neutralizing determinant. *Science* 1990;249:932–935.

89. Lasky LA, Nakamura G, Smith DH, et al. Delineation of a region of the human immunodeficiency virus type I gp120 glycoprotein critical for interaction with the CD4 receptor. *Cell* 1987;50:975–985.

90. Le S-Y, Malim MH, Cullen BR, Maizel JV. A highly conserved RNA folding region coincident with the Rev response element of primate immunodeficiency viruses. *Nucleic Acids Res* 1990;18: 1613–1623.

91. Leonard J, Parrott C, Buckler-White AJ, et al. The NF-kappa B binding sites in the human immunodeficiency virus type 1 long terminal repeat are not required for virus infectivity. *J Virol* 1989;63: 4919–4924.

92. Levy JA. Viral and cellular factors influencing HIV tropism. In: Duzgunes N, ed. *Mechanisms and Specificity of HIV Entry into Host Cells.* New York: Plenum, 1991:1–15.

93. Li XL, Moudgil T, Vinters HV, Ho DD. CD4-independent, productive infection of a neuronal cell line by human immunodeficiency virus type 1. *J Virol* 1990;64(3):1383–1387.

94. Liu ZQ, Wood C, Levy JA, Cheng-Mayer C. The viral envelope gene is involved in macrophage tropism of a human immunodeficiency virus type 1 strain isolated from brain tissue. *J Virol* 1990; 64:6148–6153.

95. Lu X, Welsh TM, Peterlin BM. The human immunodeficiency type-1 long terminal repeat specifies two different transcriptional complexes, only one of which is regulated by Tat. *J Virol* 1993;67: 1752–1760.

96. Lusso P, De Maria A, Malnati M, et al. Induction of CD4 and susceptibility to HIV-1 infection in human CD8 + T lymphocytes by human herpesvirus 6. *Nature* 1991;349:533–535.

97. Lusso P, Malnati MS, Garzino-Demo A, Crowley RW, Long EO, Gallo RC. Infection of natural killer cells by human herpesvirus 6. *Nature* 1993;362:458–462.

98. Ma M, Geiger JD, Nath A. Characterization of a novel binding site for the human immunodeficiency virus type-1 envelope protein gp120 on human fetal astrocytes. *J Virol* 1994;68:6824–6828.

99. Maddon PJ, Dalgleish AG, McDougal JS, Clapham PR, Weiss RA, Axel R. The T4 gene encodes the AIDS virus receptor and is expressed in the immune system and the brain. *Cell* 1986;47:333–348.

100. Maddon PJ, McDougal JS, Clapham PR, et al. HIV infection does not require endocytosis of its receptor, CD4. *Cell* 1988;54:865–874.

101. Marciniak RA, Calnan BJ, Frankel AD, Sharp PA. HIV-1 Tat protein transactivates transcription *in vitro. Cell* 1990;63:791–802.

102. McDougal JS, Mawle A, Cort SP, et al. Cellular tropism of the human retrovirus HTLV-III/LAV. *J Immunol* 1985;135:3151–3162.

103. McKeating JA, Griffiths PD, Weiss RA. HIV susceptibility conferred to human fibroblasts by cytomegalovirus-induced Fc receptor. *Nature* 1990;343:659–661.

104. Merrill JE, Koyanagi Y, Zack J, Thomas L, Martin F, Chen ISY. Induction of interleukin-1 and tumor necrosis factor alpha in brain cultures by human immunodeficiency virus type 1. *J Virol* 1992;66:2217.

105. Moore J, McKeating JA, Weiss RA, Sattentau QJ. Disassociation of gp120 from HIV-1 virions. *Science* 1990;250:1139–1142.

106. Mosca JD, Bednarik DP, Raj NBK, et al. Activation of human immunodeficiency virus by herpesvirus infection: identification of a region within the long terminal repeat that responds to a trans-acting factor encoded by herpes simplex virus 1. *Proc Natl Acad Sci U S A* 1987;84:7408–7412.

107. Mosca JD, Bednarik DP, Raj NBK, et al. Herpes simple virus type-1 can reactivate transcription of latent human immunodeficiency virus. *Nature* 1987;325:67–70.

108. Moses AV, Bloom FE, Pauza CD, Nelson JA. Human immunodeficiency virus infection of human brain capillary endothelial cells occurs via a CD4/galactosylceramide-independent mechanism. *Proc Natl Acad Sci U S A* 1993;90:10474–10478.

109. Nabel GJ, Rice SA, Knipe DM, Baltimore D. Alternative mechanisms for activation of human immunodeficiency virus enhancer in T cells. *Science* 1988;239:1299–1302.

110. Nagashunmugan T, Velpandi A, Otsuka T, Cartas M, Srinivasan A. Analysis of the viral determinants underlying replication kinetics and cellular tropism of human immunodeficiency virus. *Pathobiology* 1992;60:234–245.

111. Niederman TMJ, Garcia JV, Hastings WR, Luria S, Ratner L. Human immunodeficiency virus type 1 Nef protein inhibits NF-kB induction in human T cells. *J Virol* 1992;66:3243–3249.

112. Niederman TMJ, Hastings WR, Luria S, Bandres JC, Ratner L. HIV-1 Nef protein inhibits the recruitment of AP-1 DNA binding activity in human T cells. *Virology* 1993;194:338–344.

113. Niederman TMJ, Thielan BJ, Ratner L. Human immunodeficiency virus type 1 negative factor is a transcriptional silencer. *Proc Natl Acad Sci U S A* 1989;86:1128–1132.

114. Nuovo GJ. *PCR In Situ Hybridization: Protocols and Applications.* New York: Raven, 1992.

115. Nuovo GJ, Gallery F, MacConnell P, Braun A. *In situ* detection of polymerase chain reaction-amplified HIV-1 nucleic acids and tumor necrosis factor-alpha RNA in the central nervous system. *Am J Pathol* 1994;144:659–666.

116. Nuovo GJ, Lidonocci K, MacConnell P, Lane B. Intracellular localization of PCR-amplified hepatitis C cDNA. *Am J Surg Pathol* 1993;17:683–690.
117. Nuovo GJ, Margiotta M, McConnell P, Becker J. Rapid *in situ* detection of PCR-amplified HIV-1 DNA. *Diagn Mol Pathol* 1992;1:98–102.
118. O'Brien WA. Genetic and biological basis of HIV-1 neurotropism. In: Price RW, Perry SW III, eds. *HIV, AIDS, and the Brain.* New York: Raven, 1994:47–70.
119. O'Brien WA, Koyanagi Y, Namazie A, et al. HIV-1 tropism for mononuclear phagocytes can be determined by regions of gp120 outside the CD4-binding domain. *Nature* 1990;348:69–73.
120. O'Brien WA, Namazi A, Kalhor H, Mao S, Zack JA, Chen ISY. Kinetics of human immunodeficiency virus type 1 reverse transcription in blood mononuclear phagocytes are slowed by limitations of nucleotide precursors. *J Virol* 1994;68:1258–1263.
121. Osborne L, Kunkel S, Nabel GJ. Tumor necrosis factor alpha and interleukin 1 stimulate the human immunodeficiency virus enhancer by activation of the nuclear factor kB. *Proc Natl Acad Sci USA* 1989;86:2336–2340.
122. Patience C, McKnight A, Clapham PR, Boyd MT, Weiss RA, Schulz TF. CD26 antigen and HIV fusion? *Science* 1994;264:1159–1160.
123. Perkins ND, Edwards NL, Duckett CS, Agranoff AB, Schmid RM, Nabel GJ. A cooperative interaction between NF-kB and Sp1 is required for HIV-1 enhancer activation. *EMBO J* 1993;12:3551–3558.
124. Peudenier S, Hery C, Montagnier L, Tardieu M. Human microglial cells: characterization in cerebral tissue and in primary culture, and study of their susceptibility to HIV-1 infection. *Ann Neurol* 1991;29:152–161.
125. Popovic M, Sarngadharan MG, Read E, Vollo RC. Detection, isolation, and continuous production of cytopathic retroviruses (HTLV-III) from patients with AIDS and pre-AIDS. *Science* 1984;224:497.
126. Popovic M, Read-Connole E, Gallo R. T4 positive human neoplastic cell lines susceptible to and permissive for HTLV-III. *Lancet* 1984;2:1472.
127. Poulin L, Levy JA. *In vitro* expression of a functional HIV-*nef* gene product. *V International Congress on AIDS,* Montreal. 1989:58.
128. Power C, McArthur JC, Johnson RT, et al. Demented and nondemented patients with AIDS differ in brain-derived human immunodeficiency virus type 1 envelope sequences. *J Virol* 1994;68:4643–4649.
129. Ratner L, Haseltine W, Patarca R, et al. Complete nucleotide sequence of the AIDS virus, HTLV-III. *Nature* 1985;313:277.
130. Reddy EP, Dasgupta P. Regulation of HIV-1 gene expression by cellular transcription factors. *Pathobiology* 1992;60:219–224.
131. Robinson WE Jr, Kawamura T, Lake D, Masuho Y, Mitchell WM, Hersh EM. Antibodies to the primary immunodominant domain of human immunodeficiency virus type 1 (HIV-1) glycoprotein gp41 enhance HIV-1 infection *in vitro. J Virol* 1990;64:5301–5305.
132. Robinson WE Jr, Montefiori DC, Gillespie DH, Mitchell WM. Complement-mediated antibody-dependent enhancement of HIV-1 infection *in vitro* is characterized by increased protein and RNA synthesis and infectious virus release. *J AIDS* 1989;2:33–42.
133. Robinson WE Jr, Montefiori DC, Mitchell WM. Complement-mediated antibody-dependent enhancement of HIV-1 infection requires CD4 and complement receptors. *Virology* 1990;175:600–604.
134. Ross EK, Buckler-White AJ, Rabson AB, Englund G, Martin MA. Contribution of NF-kB and Sp1 binding motifs to the replicative capacity of human immunodeficiency virus type 1: distinct patterns of viral growth are determined by T cell types. *J Virol* 1991;65:4350–4358.
135. Rostad SW, Sumi SM, Shaw CM, Olson K, McDougall JK. Human immunodeficiency virus (HIV) infection in brains with AIDS-related leukoencephalopathy. *AIDS Res Hum Retrovir* 1987;3:4–10.
136. Saito Y, Sharer LR, Epstein LG, et al. Overexpression of *nef* as a marker for restricted HIV-1 infection of astrocytes in postmortem pediatric central nervous system tissues. *Neurology* 1993;4:474–481.
137. Sakai H, Shibata R, Sakuragi J, Sakuragi S, Kawamura M, Adachi A. Cell-dependent requirement of human immunodeficiency virus type-1 vif protein for maturation of virus particles. *J Virol* 1993;67:1663–1666.
138. Sanchez-Pescador R, Power MD, Barr PJ, et al. *Science* 1985;227:484–492.
139. Schooley RT. Recombinant soluble CD4 therapy in patients with the acquired immunodeficiency syndrome and AIDS-related complex: a phase I-II escalating dosage trial. *Ann Intern Med* 1990;112:247–253.
140. Schrier RD, Freeman WR, Wiley CA, McCutchan JA, HNRC group. CMV-specific immune responses and HLA phenotypes of AIDS patients who develop CMV retinitis. *Adv Neuroimmunol* 1994;4:327–336.
141. Schwartz S, Felber BK, Fenyo EM, Pavlakis GN. Rapidly and slowly replicating human immunodeficiency virus type 1 isolates can be distinguished according to target-cell tropism in T cell and monocyte cell lines. *Proc Natl Acad Sci U S A* 1989;86:7200.
142. Sharpless NE, O'Brien WA, Verdin E, Kufta CV, Chen ISY, Dubois-Dalcq M. Human immunodefi-

ciency virus type 1 tropism for brain microglial cells is determined by a region of the env glycoprotein that also controls macrophage tropism. *J Virol* 1992;66:2588–2593.

143. Shaw GM, Harper ME, Hahn BH, et al. HTLV-III infection in brains of children and adults with AIDS encephalopathy. *Science* 1985;227:177–182.

144. Shioda T, Levy JA, Cheng-Mayer C. Macrophage and T cell-line tropisms of HIV-1 are determined by specific regions of the envelope gp120 gene. *Nature* 1991;349:167–169.

145. Shioda T, Levy JA, Cheng-Mayer C. Small amino acid changes in the V3 hypervariable region of gp120 can affect the T cell-line and macrophage tropism of human immunodeficiency virus type 1. *Proc Natl Acad Sci U S A* 1992;89:9434–9438.

146. Srinivasan A, York D, Ranganathan P, et al. Transfusion associated AIDS: donor-recipient human immunodeficiency virus exhibits genetic heterogeneity. *Blood* 1987;69:1766–1770.

147. Srivastava KK, Fernandez-Larsson R, Zinkus DM, Robinson HL. Human immunodeficiency type 1 NL4-3 replication in four T cell lines: rate and efficiency of entry, a major determinant of permissiveness. *J Virol* 1991;65:3900–3902.

148. Stevenson M, Stanwick TL, Dempsey MP, Lamonica CA. HIV-1 replication is controlled at the level of T cell activation and proviral integration. *EMBO J* 1990;9:1551–1560.

149. Stoler MH, Eskin TA, Benn S, Angerer RC, Angerer LM. Human T cell lymphotropic virus type III infection of the central nervous system. *JAMA* 1986;256:2360–2364.

150. Takeda A, Tuazon CU, Ennis FA. Antibody-enhanced infection by HIV-1 via fc receptor-mediated entry. *Science* 1988;242:580–583.

151. Tateno M, Gonzalez-Scarano F, Levy JA. The human immunodeficiency virus can infect CD4-negative human fibroblastoid cells. *Proc Natl Acad Sci U S A* 1989;86:4287.

152. Terwilliger EF, Langhoff E, Gabuzda D, Zazopoulos E, Hazeltine WA. Allelic variation in the effects of the *nef* gene on replication of human immunodeficiency virus type 1. *Proc Natl Acad Sci U S A* 1991;88:10971–10975.

153. Tornatore C, Chandra R, Berger JR, Major EO. HIV-1 infection of subcortical astrocytes in the pediatric central nervous system. *Neurology* 1994;44:481–487.

154. Tornatore C, Meyers K, Atwood W, Conant K, Major E. Temporal characteristics of human immunodeficiency virus-1 transcripts in human fetal astrocytes. *J Virol* 1994;68:93–102.

155. Tornatore C, Nath A, Amemiya K, Major EO. Persistent human immunodeficiency virus type 1 infection in human fetal glial cells reactivated by T cell factors or by the cytokines tumor necrosis factor alpha and interleukin-1 beta. *J Virol* 1991;65:6094–6100.

156. Vlach J, Pitha PM. Herpes simplex virus type 1-mediated induction of human immunodeficiency virus type 1 provirus correlates with binding of nuclear proteins to the NF-kB enhancer and leader sequence. *J Virol* 1992;66:3616–3623.

157. Volsky B, Sakai K, Reddy MM, Volsky DJ. A system for high efficiency relication of HIV-1 in neural cells and its application to anti-viral evaluation. *Virology* 1992;186:303–308.

158. Von Schwedler U, Song J, Aiken C, Trono D. vif is critical for human immunodeficiency virus type 1 proviral DNA synthesis in infected cells. *J Virol* 1993;67:4945–4955.

159. Wain-Hobson S. HIV genome variability *in vivo*. *AIDS* 1989;3(suppl 1):13–18.

160. Ward JM, O'Leary TJ, Baskin GB, et al. Immunohistochemical localization of human and simian immunodeficiency viral antigens in fixed tissue sections. *Am J Pathol* 1987;127:199–205.

161. Watkins BA, Dorn HH, Kelly WB, et al. Specific tropism of HIV-1 for microglial cells in primary human brain cultures. *Science* 1990;249:549–552.

162. Watkins JF. Nature 1964;202:1364–1365.

163. Weber J, Clapham P, McKeating J, Stratton M, Robey E, Weiss R. Infection of brain cells by diverse human immunodeficiency virus isolates: role of CD4 as receptor. *J Gen Virol* 1989;70(Pt10):2653–2660.

164. Wesselingh SL, Power C, Glass JD, et al. Intracerebral cytokine messenger RNA expression in acquired immunodeficiency syndrome dementia. *Ann Neurol* 1993;33:576–582.

165. Westervelt P, Gendelman HE, Ratner L. Identification of a determinant within the human immunodeficiency virus 1 surface envelope glycoprotein critical for productive infection of primary monocytes. *Proc Natl Acad Sci U S A* 1991;88:3097–3101.

166. Westmoreland D, St. Jeor S, Rapp F. *J Immunol* 1976;116:1566–1570.

167. Westmoreland D, Watkins JF. *J Gen Virol* 1974;24:167–178.

168. Wigdahl B, Guyton RA, Sarin PS. Human immunodeficiency virus infection of the developing human nervous system. *Virology* 1987;159:440–445.

169. Wiley CA, Schrier RD, Nelson JA, Lampert PW, Oldstone MBA. Cellular localization of human immunodeficiency virus infection within the brains of acquired immune deficiency syndrome patients. *Proc Natl Acad Sci U S A* 1986;83:7089–7093.

170. Wong-Staal F, Shaw GM, Hahn BH, et al. Genomic diversity of human T-lymphotropic virus type III (HTLV-III). *Science* 1985;229:759–762

171. Wu B-Y, Woffendin C, Duckett CS, Ohno T, Nabel GJ. Regulation of human retroviral latency by the NF-kB/IkB family: inhibition of HIV replication by IkB through a Rev-dependent mechanism. *Proc Natl Acad Sci U S A* 1995;92:1480–1484.

AIDS and the Nervous System, Second Edition,
edited by J. R. Berger and R. M. Levy.
Lippincott-Raven Publishers, Philadelphia © 1997.

4

Human Immunodeficiency Virus-1 Neuropathogenesis

*Leon G. Epstein, †Howard E. Gendelman, and ‡Stuart A. Lipton

*Department of Neurology, University of Rochester School of Medicine,
Rochester, New York 14642; †Departments of Medicine, Surgery, Pathology, and
Microbiology, University of Nebraska Medical Center, Omaha, Nebraska,
68198–5215; and ‡Department of Neurology, Program in Neuroscience,
Harvard Medical School, Boston, Massachusetts 02115

Human immunodeficiency virus-1 (HIV-1) infection of the central nervous system (CNS) results in neural tissue damage (76,81,101,104,132). Although this process occurs in both adults and children, pathologic findings due to HIV-1 are particularly apparent in children, in whom secondary or reactivated opportunistic infections are rare (4,14,31,32,76,101,104). The preeminent neuropathological finding in HIV-1 encephalitis is productive infection of blood-derived macrophages, resident microglia, and multinucleated giant cells (14,30,57,101,102,104,132). Signs of neural tissue damage associated with HIV-1 infection include widespread myelin pallor, reactive astrogliosis, neuronal loss, and subtle alterations of neocortical dendritic processes (34,35,56,125,131). The deep gray matter structures have the most severe neuronal damage, which correlates to some degree with the localization of greatest HIV-1 burden in postmortem brain (131). Progressive clinical sequelae including a subcortical dementia or less severe cognitive and motor abnormalities often parallel this neuropathologic process (55,82) (see Chapters 18 and 19). These clinical features suggest cell death, or damage, to selected neuronal populations. Neurons do not appear to be targets of HIV-1 infection, although one recent report, discussed in detail below, challenges this statement (84). Furthermore, the predominant localization of productive HIV-1 infection to a relatively small number of macrophage/microglia cannot completely explain the marked neurocognitive dysfunction and brain pathology (28,89,118). These observations support an evolving and popularly held theory that diffusible viral and/or cellular gene products mediate neurotoxicity (28,43, 73,89).

An emerging body of evidence indicates that virus-infected macrophages secrete neurotoxins, which may be amplified or attenuated through a complex web of intracellular interactions between macrophages (or microglia), astrocytes, and neurons (25,28,43,60). HIV-1 infection primes macrophages (or microglia) to produce high levels of cytokines, including tumor necrosis factor-alpha (TNF-α) and interleukin-1-beta (IL-1β) after cell activation (43,83). The activation of HIV-1–infected macrophages results in the overproduction of eicosanoids, i.e., arachidonic acid and its metabolites, including platelet-activating factor (PAF) (28,43) (Fig. 1). Recent studies

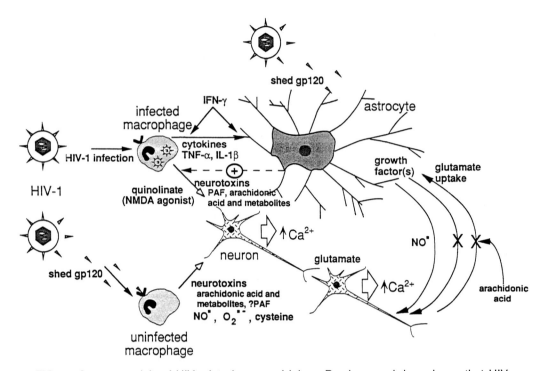

FIG. 1. Current models of HIV-related neuronal injury. Previous work has shown that HIV-infected macrophages/microglia, especially when previously activated or in conjunction with astrocytes, release factors that lead to neurotoxicity. These factors include PAF, arachidonic acid and its metabolites, as well as cytokines and other as yet unidentified substances. Macrophages and astrocytes have mutual feedback loops (signified by the reciprocal *arrows*). The excitatory action of the macrophage factors may lead to an increase in neuronal Ca^{2+} and the consequent release of glutamate. In turn, glutamate overexcites neighboring neurons, leading to an increase in intracellular Ca^{2+}, neuronal injury, and subsequent further release of glutamate. This final common pathway of neurotoxic action can be blocked by NMDA antagonists. For certain neurons, depending on their exact repertoire of ionic channels, this form of damage also can be ameliorated to some degree by calcium channel antagonists or non-NMDA receptor antagonists. A major pathway of entry of HIV-1 into monocytoid cells is via gp120 binding; therefore, it is not surprising that gp120 (or a fragment thereof) can activate uninfected macrophages to release similar factors to those secreted in response to frank HIV infection. Cytokines participate in this cellular network in several ways. For example, HIV infection or gp120 stimulation of macrophages enhances their production of TNF-α and IL-1β *(solid arrow)*. The TNF-α and IL-1β produced by macrophages stimulate astrocytosis. Astrocytes appear to feed back *(dashed arrow)* onto monocytic cells by an as yet unknown mechanism to increase the macrophage production of these cytokines. TNF-α also may increase voltage-dependent calcium currents in neurons. IFN-τ, known to be elevated in the CNS of patients with AIDS, can induce macrophage/microgliosis and macrophage production of quinolinate (an NMDA-like agonist) and PAF; in conjunction with IL-1β, IFN-τ can induce nitric oxide synthase (NOS) expression with consequent NO· production in cultured astrocytes, and in this manner may potentiate NMDA receptor-mediated neurotoxicity in mixed neuronal–glial cultures. NO· has recently been shown to react with O_2·⁻ to yield a neurotoxic substance, probably in the form of ONOO⁻ (peroxynitrite). It is possible that such cytokine stimulation of the inducible form of NOS in macrophages or astrocytes may thereby contribute to HIV-related neurotoxicity. In addition, the constitutive form of NOS (cNOS) has been implicated in gp120 neurotoxicity; the neuronal form of the enzyme (cNOS) is activated by a rise in intracellular CA^{2+} after stimulation of the NMDA receptor, and inhibitors of this enzyme have been reported to prevent gp120 neurotoxicity. the coat protein gp120 may have additional direct or indirect effects on astrocysts, e.g., to decrease growth factor production or to inhibit glutamate reuptake, for example, via arachidonic

demonstrate that the secretion of one or more of these factors from HIV-infected macrophages results in neuronal death (43,45,90). Some monocyte-produced neurotoxin(s) are heat stable and protease-resistant and act by way of N-methyl-D-aspartate (NMDA) receptors (40,45).

Excitotoxicity may be a final common pathway for neuronal damage or death. This mechanism involves the activation of voltage-dependent calcium channels and NMDA receptor–operated channels (25,60,62) and has been implicated as a cause of neuronal death in a wide range of neurologic disorders, including stroke, trauma, epilepsy, Huntington's disease, Parkinson's disease, and amyotrophic lateral sclerosis (1,66). This chapter discusses our current understanding of the mechanisms underlying HIV-1 damage to the CNS and how this knowledge may suggest therapeutic strategies to block proinflammatory cell factors or excitatory amino acid–mediated neurotoxicity.

NEUROINVASION

There is substantial evidence for invasion of the nervous system by HIV-1 during the primary viremia that accompanies seroconversion (47,76). During this time period HIV-1 and its gene products are present in the cerebrospinal fluid (CSF) (47,54). In addition, an acute encephalopathy or meningoencephalitis can occur (76). Similarly, after experimental inoculation of simian immunodeficiency virus (SIV) into rhesus macaques, infected cells invaded brain tissue within 2 weeks of systemic virus challenge (105). These findings, taken together, indicate that virus invasion into the CNS occurs early after infection.

However, questions remain about the degree of virus persistence in the nervous system. Two recent studies, using polymerase chain reaction (PCR) to examine postmortem brain tissue from adult intravenous drug users who died from causes not due to HIV-1 or immunodeficiency, found that HIV-1 was not detected in the brain in most cases or was present at low levels in only a few cases at this asymptomatic stage (3,110). Similarly, Gray et al. were unable to detect HIV-1 antigens in the CNS postmortem in asymptomatic cases (48). Using more powerful PCR *in situ* hybridization, Nuovo et al. were able to detect HIV-1 proviral DNA, suggesting latent infection in a small number of perivascular microglial cells in the absence of brain pathology (84). CSF from asymptomatic patients contains elevated protein or intra–blood-brain barrier HIV-1–specific immunoglobulin G, indicating that small amounts of virus persist in the absence of neurologic disease (29,71,92). However, an alternative explanation for these CSF findings may be immune complex deposition in the choroid plexus (36). Most postmortem studies of patients with acquired immunodeficiency syndrome (AIDS) who are found to have substantial pathologic evidence of disease demonstrated that brain tissue is a reservoir for large amounts of HIV-1 by Southern blot analysis or PCR (85,108), although other investigators have

---

acid. Arachidonate has also been recently reported to enhance NMDA-evoked currents and therefore could contribute to neurotoxicity not only by enhancing net glutamate efflux but also by increasing its effectiveness at the NMDA receptor. Also, it has recently been shown that gp120 enhances cysteine secretion from human macrophages. Cysteine is a known NMDA agonist and could therefore represent at least one of the neurotoxic substances released from stimulated macrophages.

found only low levels of HIV-1 in pediatric postmortem brain using similar methodology (118).

The fact that HIV-1 is frequently found postmortem in brains of individuals with end-stage disease does not resolve whether virus persists in the CNS, or alternatively, whether additional HIV-1 neuroinvasion is a late event. It is likely that substantial recruitment of HIV-1–infected macrophages into the brain occurs during the late stages of disease, as has been described in other lentiviral infections (80,86). Studies in SIV-infected rhesus macaques have demonstrated upregulation of adhesion molecules, including intracellular adhesion molecules or VCAMs in blood vessel walls (96). These observations are consistent with the generalized chronic inflammation and activation of cytokines present in the late stages of disease, as described below.

How HIV-1 preferentially infects macrophages and enters the brain is beginning to be understood. Virus-infected brain macrophages likely originate from expansion of peripherally infected monocytes that carry HIV-1 into the brain (the "Trojan horse" hypothesis) (86). HIV-1 and SIV, like other lentiviruses, require macrophage tropism for tissue invasion (23,80,107,128,129). This HIV-1 tropism for macrophages is determined in large part by the V3 domain of the viral envelope glycoprotein (107,128,129). However, macrophage tropism is necessary but not sufficient for invasions of brain tissue by HIV-1 or SIV (23,107). These reports indicate that only a subset of macrophage-tropic virus can invade the CNS and produce disease (23,107).

Alternatively, virus also may penetrate the brain through a disrupted blood–brain barrier as free viral particles or via normal trafficking by infected T-lymphocytes (76). This may be particularly relevant to infection of brain astrocytes, which may be more susceptible to lymphocyte-tropic strains of HIV-1 (Nath A, personal communication). Astrocyte foot processes are in extensive contact with endothelial cells in the walls of cerebral blood vessels. HIV-1 infection of endothelial cells in postmortem brain has been observed (132) and Moses et al. recently found convincing HIV-1 infection of primary human brain capillary endothelial cells that is productive but noncytopathic (77). Choroid plexus cells (50) may be susceptible to HIV-1 infection *in vitro*. Flangola et al. reported finding HIV-immunoreactive T-lymphocytes and monocytes in the stroma of the choroid plexus in 11 of 25 patients with AIDS (37). These data suggest that hematogenous dissemination of HIV-1–infected cells may occur through the choroid plexus to the CSF and periventricular regions of the brain (37). A ventriculo-fugal spread of HIV infection has previously been hypothesized as an explanation for the distribution of HIV-1–associated pathology with a predominance of lesions in deep gray matter, cerebral white matter, and brain stem (27).

MECHANISMS FOR CNS TISSUE DAMAGE (NEUROVIRULENCE)

Direct Mechanisms for Neural Damage: Evidence for Virus Infection of Neurons, Oligodendrocytes, and Astrocytes

Previous postmortem studies of brain tissues did not convincingly identify HIV-1 in cells of neuroectoderm origin (neurons, astrocytes, and/or oligodendrocytes), which constitute the major cell populations (14,31,101,132). Immunohistochemical and *in situ* hybridization assays consistently found selective, productive HIV-1 infection in mesoderm-derived brain macrophages, microglia, and multinucleated giant cells (75,76,102,103,111,132). However, the numbers and distribution of these productively infected cells often do not correlate with the degree of tissue pathology and fail to explain the observed neuronal damage, the probable substrate for the clinical neurological impairments. These data suggested that either available techniques were unable to detect low levels of neuronal/glial infection or that the major, if not exclusive, mechanism for neuropathology in HIV disease was indirect.

In support of the former explanation are several reports of *in vitro* nonproductive infection of neuronal or glial cell lines (9,24,76). Using *in situ* PCR to probe postmortem tissue, one investigator identified HIV-1 proviral DNA in a small number astrocytes and neurons, as well as in macrophages and microglia, in brains from demented patients (84). In the same study, reverse transcriptase (RT) PCR co-localized HIV-1 messenger RNA (mRNA) to neurons and astrocytes in the few cases with severe pathology (84). Other investigators using similar methods have not found HIV-1–infected neurons (106). Still other recent reports showed that nonproductive HIV-1 infection restricted to early regulatory gene products, such as *nef*, occurs in astrocytes in pediatric postmortem brain tissue (7,8,95,115) Immunocytochemical studies of brain tissue surprisingly identified reactive astrocytes as the predominant cell type harboring the *nef* gene product, and *in situ* hybridization studies using HIV-1 *nef*-specific RNA probes demonstrated overexpression of *nef* in these cells (95,115). Hence, *nef* may serve as a marker for restricted HIV-1 infection due to overexpression from early multiply spliced mRNAs (8,98). These observations complement *in vitro* studies suggesting that cellular factors in glial cells may interfere with the action of the HIV-1 regulatory protein *rev* and thus block the later steps in HIV-1 transcription (9,33). These data, although provocative, may help explain the large amounts of HIV-1 DNA present in brain tissue (108,85) and suggest a direct role for HIV-1–infected astrocytes or, conceivably, neurons in neuropathogenesis (8,28,84).

Indirect Mechanisms for Neural Damage: HIV-1 Proteins Can Damage Neural Cells

HIV-1 may produce cellular pathology through interaction with neuronal and/or glial cell membranes with or without subsequent viral entry. Indeed, HIV-1 may interact with primary neural cells via galactosylceramide (gal-C) (49). Other investigators have found that HIV-1 binds to astrocytes by a novel 240-kDa receptor distinct from gal-C or CD4 + -T lymphocyte (Nath A, personal communication).

Several HIV-1 gene products have been implicated as neurotoxins. HIV-1 *nef* has sequence homology with the scorpion peptide neurotoxins (126) and with a T cell surface protein (97). Similarly, HIV-1 *tat* specifically binds rat brain synaptosomal membranes, as well as glioma and neuroblastoma cell lines (94). The neurotoxicity of *tat* may be due to its well-defined basic region (amino acids [aa] 49–57) (94). Similar neurotoxic basic domains have been identified on the HIV and SIV *rev* proteins (69). Although at least one form of *nef* is likely to remain membrane bound, *tat* has been shown to be secreted and taken up by neighboring cells (38). Synthetic *tat* is neurotoxic in mice (94). In isolated axons, *tat* induces large depolarizations and decreased cell membrane permeability (94).

The HIV-1 envelope glycoprotein (gp)120 or a smaller peptide fragment of this protein is toxic to primary rodent neurons (10,25,61). Neuronal death occurs subsequent to excessive calcium influx (25). This gp120 neurotoxicity is mediated through factors released by activated macrophages/microglia and astrocytes (Fig. 1) (46,61). Recently, Toggas et al. reported that expression of HIV-1 gp120 in the CNS of transgenic mice results in pathology similar to that seen in HIV-1 infection (114). In these studies the HIV-1 *env* sequence coding for a truncated gp120 was placed under the control of a murine glial fibrillary acidic protein promoter. Although intact gp120 protein was not detected, the localization of gp120 mRNA correlated with regional pathology (114). In these regions, vacuolization of dendrites, decrease in synaptodendritic complexity, and loss of neuronal subpopulations (large pyramidal neurons) were observed (114). The brains of these transgenic mice expressing gp120 also showed widespread reactive astrocytosis and microglial activation. These studies provide *in vivo* evidence that gp120, even at low levels, can cause CNS damage in the absence of viral infection (or other HIV-1 proteins), but leaves unresolved which cellular factors released by astrocytes or activated microglia may contribute to the pathologic process (63,114).

Secretory Products from HIV-1–Infected Cells Can Damage Neurons

Additionally, several reports suggest that brain dysfunction is related to cell-encoded toxins generated from virus-infected macrophages (45,74,90). Cellular factors released from HIV-1–infected monocytes were toxic in human brain aggregates (90) and to chick (45) and rodent (74) neurons in culture. The monocyte-produced neurotoxin(s) were heat stable and protease resistant and acted by way of NMDA receptors (45). One report failed to confirm these observations (6), and another study demonstrated neurotoxicity only after cell-to-cell contact between HIV-infected monocytic and human neural cells (113). This could reflect differences between the individual experimental systems, the viral isolates, and/or neuronal receptors. Cumulatively, these studies suggest that if the macrophage plays a role in virus-induced neuropathology, it most likely acts in conjunction with other neural cells to produce CNS tissue damage.

HIV-Infected Macrophage–Glial Cell Interactions Are Required for Neural Damage

Early observations by Gendelman et al. demonstrated that HIV-1 infection of monocytes does not alter constitutive phagocytic or monocyte effector cell function (6). Indeed, after HIV-1 infection of monocytes, phagocytosis, antigen presentation, and cytokine production are similar, if not identical, to those of uninfected cells (6). The absence of neurotoxic activity in supernatant from steady-state HIV-1–infected macrophages suggests that the production of neurotoxins likely requires cooperation of other cells in brain or perhaps coincident or previous macrophage activators (opportunistic infection and/or immune stimuli). Previous observations that interactions between HIV-1–infected monocytes and PBMCs result in interferon alpha (IFNα) production in PBMCs appeared to support such a notion (41). Could similar mechanisms occur in the CNS and be responsible for the observed cytokine response? Because both microglia (brain macrophages) and macroglia (astrocytes/oligodendrocytes) produce IL-1β and TNFα after stimulation, astrocytes could amplify the monokine response-associated HIV-1 infection. Previous work seemed to support such a theory, but the mechanism(s) involved in neural cytokine regulation is distinct from those observed with IFNα (42).

Proinflammatory Cytokines TNF-α and IL-1β, PAF, and Arachidonic Acid Metabolites Contribute to Neural Damage

Two cytokines, IL-1β and TNF-α, are associated with glial proliferation, neurotoxicity, and myelin damage (18,39,93,99,100). Interestingly, these pathologic changes associated with cytokines are all prominent features of HIV-related encephalopathy (28,101). TNF-α is found in postmortem brains of patients with HIV encephalitis (117,127). Moreover, TNF-α is toxic to neurons in a dose-dependent manner (39). In contrast, however, other investigators report that TNF-α at even higher concentrations is neuroprotective from glutamate toxicity, suggesting that changes in local concentrations may be critical (16). TNF-α may act on neurons indirectly by affecting intracellular signalling or transcription activation (58,68,91). Human astrocytes proliferate in response to TNF-α and IL-1β, and conditioned medium from LPS-treated astrocytes stimulates HIV-1 gene expression in monocytic cells (18,99,119). Conversely, monokines can activate HIV-1 expression in astrocytes (116).

An important lead into understanding the mechanisms of HIV encephalitis came through studies of cell-to-cell interactions associated with macrophage activation. HIV-1–infected monocytes cocultured with human astrocytoma (U251 MG) cells synthesized TNF-α and IL-1β, PAF, free arachidonic acid, and its metabolites, including the leukotrienes LTB$_4$, LTD$_4$, and lipoxin A4 (43). All are candidate neurotoxins. Synthesis of the same or similar factors occurred during coculture of HIV-1–infected monocytes with human fetal astrocytes, but here macrophage priming/activation was required in primary cell systems. Importantly, in this system the HIV-1–infected monocytes produce increased levels of TNF-α after activation (43).

Astrocytes May Attenuate CNS Inflammation but Increase Virus Burden

HIV-induced damage to the brain and its coincident cognitive/motor changes appear to be chronic manifestations of persistent brain infection and inflammation that could result from competing pro- and antiinflammatory cytokine productions. If the HIV-1–infected macrophage produces neurotoxins in response to activation, then what factors control their production and explain the subacute nature of HIV-1–associated encephalopathy? Various immunoregulatory cytokines are produced in the CNS during HIV-1 infection, and all potentially serve as autocrine or paracrine mediators of viral replication and tissue injury. Two such candidates that may control chronic CNS inflammation include IL-10 and transforming growth factor-beta (TGF-β). IL-10 is produced from activated macrophages at high levels and is a potent deactivator in an autocrine manner for proinflammatory cytokine production. Moreover, human fetal astrocytes constitutively produce TGF-β2, which has been shown to markedly downregulate cytokine production by macrophages in murine systems.

Therefore, studies were performed to determined whether IL-10 and /or TGF-β might be responsible for the astrocyte-induced downregulation of proinflammatory cytokines in the brain (83). IL-10 produced by activated macrophages in an autocrine and very potent manner markedly downregulates TNF production in macrophages. Although high levels of TGF-β are produced by astrocytes, the addition of recombinant TGF-β to activated HIV-infected monocytes did not affect the levels of TNF secretion (83). Moreover, all TGF-β detected from astrocytes was found in an inactive form. Nevertheless, TGF-β likely plays an important role in other regulatory responses in the brain. Indeed, TGF-β suppresses interferon-gamma (IFN-τ)–induced suppression of class II major histocompatibility complex (MHC) and macrophages (112). Moreover, TGF-β in the brain is an important chemotactic factor for recruitment of additional macrophages into the brain, providing mechanisms for more efficient viral spread and an expanding cellular reservoir in the brain. Indeed, TGF-β gene expression is localized to monocytes and astrocytes in areas of HIV-1 brain pathology (121). However, taken together these observations provide evidence that astrocytes can control the level of proinflammatory cytokines by mechanisms that are likely independent from TGF-β. Macrophages, on the other hand, supply their own autocrine factors, including IL-10, which may serve to deactivate prolonged neurotoxin production in the brain. These data provide evidence to support the hypothesis that complex interactions between HIV-1–infected monocytes and astrocytes are responsible for components of the neural damage associated with HIV-1 infection.

The NMDA Receptor as a Final Common Pathway

Lipton et al. have proposed that HIV-1–associated neuronal damage is mediated via activation of the NMDA subtype of glutamate receptor (25,61,67), a mechanism previously implicated in neuronal loss in a number of diverse neuropathologic processes. The details of excitotoxicity via glutamate receptors have been extensively reviewed (2,66). Support for this theory, that HIV-1 neurotoxicity ultimately occurs via an excitotoxic mechanism, comes from the observation that neuronal death induced by soluble HIV-1 gp120 can be blocked pharmacologically by antagonists of the L-type, voltage-dependent Ca^{2+} channel, such as nimodipine and nifedipine (25), and by antagonists of the NMDA receptor channel complex such as D-2-amino-5-phosphonovalerate and dizocilpine (MK-801) (67). Moreover, the effects of the neurotoxic substances released from HIV-1–infected monocytoid cells are also inhibited by NMDA antagonists *in vitro* (45). In patch-clamp experiments, soluble HIV-1 gp120 itself does not appear to be a glutamate-like agonist of the NMDA receptor (60,61). However, depletion of endogenous glutamate from the cultures protects neurons from gp120-induced toxicity (67). Nitric oxide (NO·) contributes to NMDA receptor–mediated neurotoxicity (21). NO· has been implicated in HIV-1–associated neuronal death based on the finding that L-nitroarginine, an inhibitor of nitric oxide synthase, prevents gp120-induced toxicity in primary cortical neurons (22). Such excitatory amino acid–mediated neurotoxicity may be further enhanced as injured neurons release glutamate, thus damaging neighboring neurons (17,62), or by the failure of astrocytes to adequately take up excessive glutamate (Fig. 1) (66,120). Of particular interest is that arachidonic acid specifically inhibits the high-affinity glutamate uptake system in neurons (synaptosomes) and astrocytes (120). HIV-1 coat protein gp120 can also inhibit glutamate uptake by astrocytes (5), and preliminary data suggest that this effect is mediated, at least in part, by gp120-induced release of arachionic acid from macrophages (122) (Dreyer and Lipton, manuscript in preparation). In addition, IFN-τ–induced stimulation of macrophages induces release of the glutamate-like agonist quinolinate (53). Heyes et al. reported that the concentration of quinolinate, a weak NMDA agonist, is markedly elevated in the CSF of adults (51) and children (12) with HIV-1–associated dementia complex, as well as in SIV-infected macaques (52), suggesting that excitotoxicity may be biologically relevant to HIV-1–induced neurotoxicity *in vivo*. The quinolinate concentration correlates with the severity of the dementia and diminishes coincident with antiviral therapy and clinical improvement in neurological signs (12,51).

It is important to recognize that excitotoxicity can be implicated in chronic as well as acute neuronal death. Albin and Greeenamyre (1) hypothesized that alterations in cellular energy metabolism, membrane potential, or receptor sensitivity can result in weak excitotoxic damage. This could explain intra- and inter-regional variations in neuronal loss in neurodegenerative disorders such as Huntington's disease (1,2) and may be relevant to neuronal injury and death due to HIV-1.

Arachidonic Acid, PAF, and TNF Amplify Excitotoxicity

It is possible that interactions between HIV-1–infected monocytes and astrocytes represent an amplification of paracrine cytokine production. Autocrine loops between arachidonic acid metabolites and cytokines (and *vice versa*) could amplify macrophage–glial cell interactions. HIV-1 gp120 induces arachidonic acid metabolites, IL-1β, and TNF-α in monocytes (74,122), and TNF causes amplification of arachidonic acid metabolites in response to IL-1 (20), whereas PAF enhances TNF production (26,87). TNF-α upregulates class I and II MHC antigens and likely facilitates the production of inflammatory cell infiltrates in brain parenchyma and the penetration of virus-infected monocytes through the blood–brain barrier (70). The ultimate result is the overproduction of cytokines and other products of inflammation that act directly as neurotoxins or synergistically with glutamate and other excitotoxic molecules.

Both TNF-α and PAF are reported to be toxic to primary human fetal neurons in a dose-dependent manner (40,39). The neurotoxicity of TNF-α is reduced by 6-cyano-7-hydroxy-5-methyl-2,3-dione, which blocks the α-amino-3-hydroxy-5-methyl-isoxazole-4-proprionic acid glutamate receptor (39). PAF neurotoxicity is blocked by MK-801 or memantine, uncompetitive NMDA receptor antagonists (40). In addition, PAF acts directly on neurons as a potent modulator of excitatory synaptic transmission (19), apparently by increasing Ca^{2+} and consequently glutamate release. Arachidonic acid inhibits high-affinity glutamate reuptake by astrocytes at synaptic clefts (120). All these mechanisms favor excitotoxic neuronal damage.

Cytokines May Lead to Myelin Damage

Most recent investigations have attempted to better understand the mechanisms underlying neuronal damage or death; however, excessive cytokine production also could be responsible for damage to myelin by causing oligodendrocyte dysfunction or death (93,100). Alternatively, chronic inflammation and cytokine activation may result in disruption of the blood–brain barrier. The latter explanation is favored by a recent report that found no ultrastuctural evidence of primary or secondary immune-mediated destruction of myelin in the brain of HIV-1–infected individuals (88).

Therapeutic Strategies

Because HIV-1–infected macrophages/microglia probably initiate the inflammatory cascade leading to neuronal damage, any therapeutic strategy must include the use of antiretroviral agents to decrease CNS virus load. To date, zidovudine has been the most effective antiviral medication used to treat HIV-1 infection in the CNS. Zidovudine in sufficient doses produces clinical improvement in neurocognitive function in both children (13) and adults (109). Coincident with this improved neurological status is a decline in CSF quinolinate (12,51) and β2-microglobulin (11). Quinolinate is a potential excitotoxin, and β2-microglobulin is a reliable marker of immune activation/inflammation in the CNS.

Additionally, compounds that block the actions of proinflammatory cytokines or PAF may prove beneficial. A clinical trial of pentoxyfilline, a potent inhibitor of TNF-α, is currently in progress (McArthur J, personal communication). The corticosteroids such as dexamethasone and prednisone are known to inhibit the arachidonic acid cascade, but their use could be problematic in patients with severe immunodeficiency. Other more specific compounds that block PAF are in development or being used in clinical trials for other conditions such as asthma.

To be useful in the treatment of HIV-1–associated neurocognitive deficits, a candidate compound must have a favorable safety profile to allow long-term administration and should not worsen other AIDS-associated conditions. We have already described how cytokines including TGF-β may cause additional recruitment of HIV-1–infected macrophages into the CNS in the later stages of disease. Although the initial neuroinvasion that occurs during primary infection may be not be easily blocked, it is possible that a better understanding of cytokine regulation and endothelial cell adhesion molecules might provide opportunities to impede this later neuroinvasion.

Last are strategies to protect neurons from a final common pathway of excitotoxic injury. The potential sites for pharmacologic intervention targeting excitotoxicity are reviewed in detail by Lipton and Rosenberg (66). Antagonists of voltage-dependent Ca^{2+} channels, such as nimodipine, can in some circumstances ameliorate NMDA receptor–mediated neurotoxicity by decreasing the calcium burden of neurons (59). In fact, gp120-induced neurotoxicity has been shown to be decreased *in vitro* and *in vivo* by nimodipine (25,65). For these reasons, the AIDS Clinical Trials Group (ACTG) has completed a phase I/II trial of nimodipine for AIDS dementia, and the results are currently being analyzed.

A number of glutamate receptor antagonists are also available that competitively block the glutamate binding site. However, competitive antagonists also impair the normal physiologic activity of the glutamate receptor and are therefore probably not useful. There are, however, a number of modulatory sites that are accessible and may be inhibited without totally blocking physiologic activity. Certain compounds block NMDA receptor activity by entering the channel when it is open. These open channel blockers have the advantage of being most likely to enter the channel and block it in the presence of excessive glutamate but are less likely to do so in the presence of physiologic levels of glutamate. The reason for this is simple: the ion channels are on average open for a greater fraction of time when activated by greater concentrations of glutamate or other agonist such as quinolinate. Still, many of these drugs, (phencyclidine and dizocilpine [MK-801]) have adverse neuropsychiatric side effects because they remain in the NMDA-associated channels for too long. The most promising compound in the category of NMDA open-channel blockers is memantine, which appears to be neuroprotective at concentrations known to be clinically tolerated in humans (15,66). Unlike MK-801, memantine exits NMDA-associated channels quickly, thus permitting nearly physiological (but not excessive) Ca^{2+} entry. The ACTG is currently considering a clinical study for AIDS dementia using memantine.

An additional strategy to block excitotoxicity is based on the novel redox modulatory site(s) of the NMDA receptor (64). Nitroglycerin, a well-established medication, may be capable of blocking NMDA receptor–mediated neurotoxicity by reacting with sulfhydryl groups at this site(s) (64). Felbamate is an anticonvulsant medication reported to be a competitive antagonist at the glycine-binding site of NMDA receptors (72,123,130). Felbamate has been shown to be neuroprotective in animal models of hypoxia-ischemia (123), in which neuronal damage is thought to be due to excitoxicity. Alternatively, it may be possible to protect neurons from "weak" excitotoxicity by blocking oxidative stress using compounds such as alpha-lipoic acid (1).

CONCLUSIONS

HIV-1–associated neural damage is most likely initiated by HIV-1–infected and primed macrophages/microglia. The HIV-1–infected macrophage appears to be hyper-responsive to activation stimuli. Both viral proteins and cellular products of HIV-1–infected cells may act as neurotoxins. A complex interaction occurs between HIV-1–infected macrophages/microglia and astrocytes that results in the release of proinflammatory cytokines TNF-α and IL-1β, as well as PAF and arachidonic acid metabolites. Furthermore, opportunistic infection might trigger abnormalities in cytokine production within infected macrophages. Ultimately, the cytokines upregulate HIV-1 infection in the brain. Although these products amplify neurotoxic and glial proliferatory effects of a small number of productively HIV-1–infected cells, astrocytes produce TGF-β and macrophages release IL-10, which independently downregulate proinflammatory cytokines. This may lead to chronic low-level inflammation, viral replication, and tissue pathology

There is an emerging and increased understanding of the role of the astrocyte in HIV-1 neuropathogenesis (8,28). The demonstration of restricted HIV-1 infection of astrocytes *in vivo* (95,115) adds biologic significance to prior *in vitro* studies. Astrocyte expression of HIV-1 gp120 in transgenic mice results in neuronal damage and astroglial and microglial activation. Interestingly, functional deficits (in trained cognitive motor behaviors) in SIV-infected monkeys were not accompanied by dramatic neuropathological findings (79) but did correlate with cortical astrogliosis (124). Astrocytes have classically been viewed as protecting against neuronal injury, whereas the microglia have been proposed as the major source of neuron-killing molecules (44,178). It is likely, however, that the role of the astrocyte in pathologic processes is more complex. In particular, the failure of astrocytes to perform their "normal" functions, such as releasing TGF-β or sequestering glutamate at synaptic junctions (120), could lead to further neuronal damage.

Complex interactions also occur between cytokines and HIV-1. HIV-1–infected and primed macrophages and microglia secrete excessive TNFα and IL-1β, which in turn upregulates HIV-1 replication in monocytes and astroglia *in vitro*, and possibly *in vivo*.

Lastly, it appears that an excitotoxic mechanism may underlie neuronal injury and death in HIV-1 encephalitis. This final common pathway could be the result of production or release of excessive amounts of glutamate, PAF, or NMDA agonists such as quinolinate. Alternatively, weak excitotoxic neuronal damage (1) may occur over a longer duration due to indirect "insults" to neurons from cytokines or other inflammatory factors (arachidonic acid, leukotrienes) that could potentially impair cell energy metabolism or membrane intregrity, resulting in increased sensitivity to physiological concentrations of glutamate (1).

Above all, recent insights and understanding of the persistent nature of HIV-1 infection and resulting inflammation of cell–cell interactions in the CNS, as well as of excitotoxic neuronal injury, may allow significant pharmacologic interventions to treat the neurocognitive deficits in this condition or to provide prophylactic neuro-protection.

ACKNOWLEDGMENT

These studies were supported under Public Health Service Grants R01 NS 28754 (L.G.E.), R01 AI32305 (L.G.E.) P01 NS 31492 (L.G.E., H.E.G.), R01 EY09024 (S.A.L.), P01 HD29587 (S.A.L.), and the American Foundation for AIDS Research (S.A.L.). Dr. Gendelman is a Carter-Wallace fellow of the Department of Pathology and Microbiology, University of Nebraska Medical Center. We thank Ben Blumberg, Ph.D., for help in editing, Corrine Gartland for assistance in preparing the manuscript, and Harris Gelbard, M.D., Ph.D., for thoughtful discussions and his willingness to share unpublished data.

REFERENCES

1. Albin RL, Greenamyre JT. Alternative excitotoxic hypotheses. *Neurology* 1992;42:733–738.
2. Beal MF. Role of excitotoxicity in human neurological disease. *Curr Opin Neurobiol* 1992;2: 657–662.
3. Bell JE, Busuttil A, Ironside JW, Rebus S, Donaldson YK, Simmonds P. Human immunodeficiency virus and the brain: investigation of virus load and neuropathologic changes in pre-AIDS subjects. *J Infect Dis* 1993;168:818–824.
4. Belman AL, Lantos G, Horoupian D, et al. AIDS: calcification of the basal ganglia in infants and children. *Neurology* 1986;36:1192–1199.
5. Benos DJ, Hahn BH, Bubien JK, et al. Envelope glycoprotein gp120 of human immunodeficiency virus type 1 alters ion transport in astrocytes: implications for AIDS dementia complex. *Proc Natl Acad Sci U S A* 1994;91:494–498.
6. Bernton EW, Bryant HU, Decoster MA, et al. No direct neuronotoxicity by HIV-1 virions or culture fluids from HIV-1–infected T cells or monocytes. *AIDS Res Hum Retrovir* 1992;8:495–503.
7. Blumberg BM, Epstein LG, Saito Y, Chen D, Sharer LR, Anand R. Human immunodeficiency virus type 1 nef quasispecies in pathological tissue. *J Virol* 1992;66:5256–5264.
8. Blumberg BM, Gelbard HA, Epstein LG. HIV-1 infection of the developing nervous system: central role of astrocytes in pathogenesis. *Virus Res* 1994;32(2):253–267.
9. Brack-Werner R, Kleinschmidt A, Ludvigsen A, et al. Infection of human brain cells by HIV-1: restricted virus production in chronically infected human glial cell lines. *AIDS* 1992;6:273–285.
10. Brenneman DE, Westbrook GL, Fitzgerald SP, et al. Neuronal cell killing by the envelope protein of HIV and its prevention by vasoactive intestinal peptide. *Nature* 1988;335:639–642.
11. Brew BJ, Bhalla RB, Paul M, et al. Cerebrospinal fluid beta 2-microglobulin in patients with AIDS dementia complex: an expanded series including response to zidovudine treatment. *AIDS* 1992;6: 461–465.
12. Brouwers P, Heyes MP, Moss HA, Wolters PL, Poplack DG, Markey SP. Quinolinic acid in the cerebrospinal fluid of children with symptomatic human immunodeficiency virus type 1 disease: relationships to clinical status and therapeutic response. *J Infect Dis* 1993;168:1380–1386.
13. Brouwers P, Moss H, Wolters P, et al. Effect of continuous-infusion zidovudine therapy on neuropsychologic functioning in children with symptomatic human immunodeficiency virus infection. *J Pediatr* 1990;117:980–985.
14. Budka H, Wiley CA, Kleihues P, et al. HIV-associated disease of the nervous system: review of nomenclature and proposal for neuropathology based terminology. *Brain Pathol* 1991;1:143–152.
15. Chen HS, Pellegrini JW, Aggarwal SK, et al. Open-channel block of N-methyl-D-aspartate (NMDA)

responses by memantine: therapeutic advantage against NMDA receptor-mediated neurotoxicity. *J Neurosci* 1992;12:4427–4436.

16. Cheng B, Christakos S, Mattson MP: Tumor necrosis factors protect neurons against metabolic excitotoxic insults and promote maintenance of calcium homeostasis. *Neuron* 1994;12:139–153.
17. Choi DW, Rothman SM. The role of glutamate neurotoxicity in hypoxic-ischemic neuronal death. *Ann Rev Neurosci* 1990;13:171–182.
18. Chung IY, Benveniste EN. Tumor necrosis factor-alpha production by astrocytes. Induction by lipopolysaccharide, IFN-gamma, and IL-1 beta. *J Immunol* 1990;144:2999–3007.
19. Clark GD, Happel LT, Zorumski CF, Bazan NG. Enhancement of hippocampal excitatory synaptic transmission by platelet-activating factor. *Neuron* 1992;9:1211–1216.
20. Conti P, Reale M, Barbacane RC, Bongrazio M, Panara MR, Fiore S. The combination of interleukin 1 plus tumor necrosis factor causes greater generation of LTB4, thromboxanes and aggregation of human macrophages than these compounds alone. *Prog Clin Biol Res* 1989;301:541–545.
21. Dawson VL, Dawson TM, London ED, Bredt DS, Snyder SH. Nitric oxide mediates glutamate neurotoxicity in primary cortical cultures. *Proc Natl Acad Sci U S A* 1991;88:6368–6371.
22. Dawson VL, Dawson TM, Uhl GR, Snyder SH. Human immunodeficiency virus type 1 coat protein neurotoxicity mediated by nitric oxide in primary cortical cultures. *Proc Natl Acad Sci U S A* 1993;90:3256–3259.
23. Desrosiers RC, Hansen-Moosa A, Mori K, et al. Macrophage-tropic variants of SIV are associated with specific AIDS-related lesions but are not essential for the development of AIDS. *Am J Pathol* 1991;139:29–35.
24. Dewhurst S, Sakai K, Bresser J, Stevenson M, Evinger-Hodges MJ, Volsky DJ. Persistent productive infection of human glial cells by human immunodeficiency virus (HIV) and by infectious molecular clones of HIV. *J Virol* 1987;61:3774–3782.
25. Dreyer EB, Kaiser PK, Offermann JT, Lipton SA. HIV-1 coat protein neurotoxicity prevented by calcium channel antagonists. *Science* 1990;248:364–367.
26. Dubois C, Bissonnette E, Rola-Pleszczynski M. Platelet-activating factor (PAF) enhances tumor necrosis factor production by alveolar macrophages. Prevention by PAF receptor antagonists and lipoxygenase inhibitors. *J Immunol* 1989;143:964–970.
27. Epstein LG. Human immunodeficiency virus (HIV) brain infection in infants and children. In: Johnson RT, Lyon G, eds. *Virus Infections and the Developing Nervous System*. Dordrecht, The Netherlands: Kluwer Academic, 1988:57–67.
28. Epstein LG, Gendelman HE. Human immunodeficiency virus type 1 infection of the nervous system: pathogenetic mechanisms [Review]. *Ann Neurol* 1993;33:429–436.
29. Epstein LG, Goudsmit J, Paul DA, et al. Expression of human immunodeficiency virus in cerebrospinal fluid of children with progressive encephalopathy. *Ann Neurol* 1987;21:397–401.
30. Epstein LG, Sharer LR, Cho ES, Myenhofer M, Navia B, Price RW. HTLV-III/LAV-like retrovirus particles in the brains of patients with AIDS encephalopathy. *AIDS Res* 1984;1:447–454.
31. Epstein LG, Sharer LR, Joshi VV, Fojas M, Koenigsberger MR, Oleske JM. Progressive encephalopathy in children with acquired immune deficiency syndrome. *Ann Neurol* 1985;17:488–496.
32. Epstein LG, Sharer LR, Oleske JM, et al. Neurologic manifestations of human immunodeficiency virus infection in children. *Pediatrics* 1986;78:678–687.
33. Erfle V, Stoeckbauer P, Kleinschmidt A, et al. Target cells for HIV in the central nervous system: macrophages or glial cells? *Res Virol* 1991;142:139–144.
34. Everall I, Luthert P, Lantos P. A review of neuronal damage in human immunodeficiency virus infection: its assessment, possible mechanism and relationship to dementia. *J Neuropathol Exp Neurol* 1993;52:561–566.
35. Everall IP, Luthert PJ, Lantos PL. Neuronal loss in the frontal cortex in HIV infection. *Lancet* 1991;337:1119–1121.
36. Falangola MF, Castro-Filho BG, Petito CK. Immune complex deposition in the choroid plexus of AIDS patients. *Ann Neurol* 1994;36(3):437–440.
37. Falangola MF, Hanly A, Galvao-Castro B, Petito CK. HIV infection of human choroid plexus: a possible mechanism of viral entry into the CNS. *J Neuropathol Exp Neurol* 1995;54(4):497–503.
38. Frankel AD, Pabo CO. Cellular uptake of the Tat protein from human immunodeficiency virus. *Cell* 1988;55:1189–1193.
39. Gelbard HA, Dzenko K, Diloreto D, Delcerro C, Delcerro M, Epstein LG. Neurotoxic effects of tumor necrosis factor in primary human neuronal cultures are mediated by activation of the glutamate AMPA receptor subtype: implications for AIDS neuropathogenesis. *Dev Neurosci* 1994;15:418–422.
40. Gelbard HA, Nottet HSLM, Swindells S, et al. Platelet activating factor: a candidate HIV-1-induced neurotoxin. *J Virol* 1994;68(7):4628–4635.
41. Gendelman HE, Baca LM, Kubrak CA, et al. Induction of IFN-alpha in peripheral blood mononuclear cells by HIV-infected monocytes. Restricted antiviral activity of the HIV-induced IFN. *J Immunol* 1992;148:422–429.
42. Gendelman HE, Friedman RM, Joe S, et al. A selective defect of interferon alpha production in

human immunodeficiency virus-infected monocytes [erratum in *J Exp Med* 1991;173:277]. *J Exp Med* 1990;172:1433–1442.

43. Genis P, Jett M, Bernton EW, et al. Cytokines and arachidonic metabolites produced during human immunodeficiency virus (HIV)-infected macrophage-astroglia interactions: implications for the neuropathogenesis of HIV disease. *J Exp Med* 1992;176:1703–1718.
44. Giulian D, Vaca K, Corpuz M. Brain glia release factors with opposing actions upon neuronal survival. *J Neurosci* 1993;13:29–37.
45. Giulian D, Vaca K, Noonan CA. Secretion of neurotoxins by mononuclear phagocytes infected with HIV-1. *Science* 1990;250:1593–1596.
46. Giulian D, Wendt E, Vaca K, Noonan CA. The envelope glycoprotein of human immunodeficiency virus type 1 stimulates release of neurotoxins from monocytes. *Proc Natl Acad Sci U S A* 1993; 90:2769–2773.
47. Goudsmit J, de Wolf F, Paul DA, et al. Expression of human immunodeficiency virus antigen (HIV-Ag) in serum and cerebrospinal fluid during acute and chronic infection. *Lancet* 1986;2:177–180.
48. Gray F, Lescs MC, Keohane C, et al. Early brain changes in HIV infection: neuropathological study of 11 HIV seropositive, non-AIDS cases. *J Neuropathol Exp Neurol* 1992;51:177–185.
49. Harouse JM, Bhat S, Spitalnik SL, et al. Inhibition of entry of HIV-1 in neural cell lines by antibodies against galactosyl ceramide. *Science* 1991;253:320–323.
50. Harouse JM, Wroblewska Z, Laughlin MA, Hickey WF, Schonwetter BS, Gonzalez-Scarano F. Human chorioid plexus cells can be latently infected with human immunodeficiency virus. *Ann Neurol* 1989;25:406–411.
51. Heyes MP, Brew BJ, Martin A, et al. Quinolinic acid in cerebrospinal fluid and serum in HIV-1 infection: relationship to clinical and neurological status. *Ann Neurol* 1991;29:202–209.
52. Heyes MP, Jordan EK, Lee K, et al. Relationship of neurologic status in macaques infected with the simian immunodeficiency virus to cerebrospinal fluid quinolinic acid and kynurenic acid. *Brain Res* 1992;570:237–250.
53. Heyes MP, Saito K, Markey SP. Human macrohages convert L-tryptophan into the neurotoxin quinolinic acid. *Biochem J* 1992;283:633–635.
54. Ho DD, Rota TR, Schooley RT, et al. Isolation of HTLV-III from cerebrospinal fluid and neural tissues of patients with neurologic syndromes related to the acquired immunodeficiency syndrome. *N Engl J Med* 1985;313:1493–1497.
55. Janssen RS, Cornblath DR, Epstein LG, McArthur J, Price RW. Human immunodeficiency virus (HIV) infection and the nervous system: report from the American Academy of Neurology AIDS Task Force. *Neurology* 1989;39:119–122.
56. Ketzler S, Weis S, Haug H, Budka H. Loss of neurons in the frontal cortex in AIDS brains. *Acta Neuropathol* 1990;80:92–94.
57. Koenig S, Gendelman HE, Orenstein JM, et al. Detection of AIDS virus in macrophages in brain tissue from AIDS patients with encephalopathy. *Science* 1986;233:1089–1093.
58. Kolesnick R, Golde DW. The sphingomyelin pathway in tumor necrosis factor and interleukin-1 signaling. *Cell* 1994;77:325–328.
59. Lei SZ, Zhang D, Abele AE, Lipton SA. Blockade of NMDA receptor-mediated mobilization of intracellular Ca^{2+} prevents neurotoxicity. *Brain Res* 1992;598:196–202.
60. Lipton SA. Models of neuronal injury in AIDS: another role for the NMDA receptor? *Trends Neurosci* 1992;15:75–79.
61. Lipton SA. Requirement for macrophages in neuronal injury induced by HIV envelope protein gp120. *Neuroreport* 1992;3:913–915.
62. Lipton SA. Human immunodeficiency virus-infected macrophages, gp120, and N-methyl-D-aspartate receptor-mediated neurotoxicity. *Ann Neurol* 1993;33:227–228.
63. Lipton SA. HIV displays its coat of arms. *Nature* 1994;367:113–114.
64. Lipton SA, Choi YB, Pan ZH, et al. A redox-based mechanism for the neuroprotective and neurodestructive effects of nitric oxide and related nitroso-compounds. *Nature* 1993;364:626–632.
65. Lipton SA, Jensen FE. Memantine, a clinically tolerated NMDA open-channel blocker, prevents HIV coat protein-induced neuronal injury *in vitro* and *in vivo*. *Soc Neurosci Abstr* 1992;18:757.
66. Lipton SA, Rosenberg PA. Excitatory amino acids as a final common pathway for neurologic disorders. *N Engl J Med* 1994;330:613–622.
67. Lipton SA, Sucher NJ, Kaiser PK, Dreyer EB. Synergistic effects of HIV coat protein and NMDA receptor-mediated neurotoxicity. *Neuron* 1991;7:111–118.
68. Liscovitch M, Cantley LC. Lipid second messengers. *Cell* 1994;77:329–334.
69. Mabrouk K, Van Rietschoten J, Vives E, Darbon H, Rochat H, Sabatier JM. Lethal neurotoxicity in mice of the basic domains of HIV and SIV Rev proteins. Study of these regions by circular dichroism. *FEBS Lett* 1991;289:13–17.
70. Mauerhoff T, Pujol-Borrell R, Mirakian R, Bottazzo GF. Differential expression and regulation of major histocompatibility complex (MHC) products in neural and glial cells of the human fetal brain. *J Neuroimmunol* 1988;18:271–289.

71. McArthur JC, Cohen BA, Farzedegan H, et al. Cerebrospinal fluid abnormalities in homosexual men with and without neuropsychiatric findings. *Ann Neurol* 1988;23(suppl):34–37.
72. McCabe RT, Wasterlain CG, Kucharczyk N, Sofia RD, Vogel JR. Evidence for anticonvulsant and neuroprotectant action of felbamate mediated by strychnine-insensitive glycine receptors. *J Pharmacol Exp Ther* 1993;264:1248–1252.
73. Merrill JE, Chen IS. HIV-1, macrophages, glial cells, and cytokines in AIDS nervous system disease [Review]. *FASEB J* 1991;5:2391–2397.
74. Merrill JE, Koyanagi Y, Zack J, Thomas L, Martin F, Chen IS. Induction of interleukin-1 and tumor necrosis factor alpha in brain cultures by human immunodeficiency virus type 1. *J Virol* 1992;66:2217–2225.
75. Michaels J, Price RW, Rosenblum MK. Microglia in the giant cell encephalitis of acquired immune deficiency syndrome: proliferation, infection and fusion. *Acta Neuropathologica* 1988;76:373–379.
76. Michaels J, Sharer LR, Epstein LG. Human immunodeficiency virus type 1 (HIV-1) infection of the nervous system: a review. *Immunodefic Rev* 1988;1:71–104.
77. Moses AV, Bloom FE, Pauza CD, Nelson JA. Human immunodeficiency virus infection of human brain capillary endothelial cells occurs via a CD4/galactosylceramide-independent mechanism. *Proc Natl Acad Sci U S A* 1993;90:10474–10478.
78. Mucke L, Eddleston M. Astrocytes in infectious and immune-mediated diseases of the central nervous system [Review]. *FASEB J* 1993;7:1226–1232.
79. Murray EA, Rausch DM, Lendvay J, Sharer LR, Eiden LE. Cognitive and motor impairments associated with SIV infection in rhesus monkeys. *Science* 1992;255:1246–1249.
80. Narayan O, Clements JE. Biology and pathogenesis of lentiviruses. *J Gen Virol* 1989;70:1617–1639.
81. Navia BA, Cho ES, Petito CK, Price RW. The AIDS dementia complex: II. Neuropathology. *Ann Neurol* 1986;19:525–535.
82. Navia BA, Jordan BD, Price RW. The AIDS dementia complex: I. Clinical features. *Ann Neurol* 1986;19:517–524.
83. Nottet HSLM, Jett M, Flanagan CR, et al. A regulatory role for astrocytes in HIV-1 encephalitis. An overexpression of eicosanoids, platelet-activating factor, and tumor necrosis factor alpha by activated HIV-1–infected monocytes is attenuated by primary human astrocytes. *J Immunol* 1995;154(7):3567–3581.
84. Nuovo G. *In situ* detection of polymerase chain reaction-amplified HIV-1 nucleic acids and tumor necrosis factor-alpha RNA in the central nervous system. *Am J Pathol* 1994;144:659–666.
85. Pang S, Koyanagi Y, Miles S, Wiley C, Vinters HV, Chen I. High levels of unintegrated HIV-1 DNA in brain tissue of AIDS dementia patients. *Nature* 1990;343:85–89.
86. Peluso R, Haase A, Stowring L, Edwards M, Ventura P. A Trojan horse mechanism for the spread of visna virus in monocytes. *Virology* 1985;147:231–236.
87. Poubelle PE, Gingras D, Demers C, Dubois C, Harbour D, Grassi J. Platelet-activating factor (PAF-acether) enhances the concomitant production of tumour necrosis factor-alpha and interleukin-1 by subsets of human monocytes. *Immunology* 1991;72:181–187.
88. Power C, Kong PA, Crawford TO, et al. Cerebral white matter changes in acquired immunodeficiency syndrome dementia: alterations of the blood-brain barrier. *Ann Neurol* 1993;34:339–350.
89. Price RW, Brew B, Sidtis J, Rosenblum M, Scheck AC, Cleary P. The brain in AIDS: central nervous system HIV-1 infection and AIDS dementia complex. *Science* 1988;239:586–592.
90. Pulliam L, Herndier BG, Tang NM, McGrath MS. HIV-infected macrophages produce soluble factors that cause histological and neurochemical alterations in cultured human brains. *J Clin Invest* 1991;87:503
91. Rattner A, Korner M, Walker MD, Citri Y. NF-kB activates the HIV promoter in neurons. *EMBO J* 1993;12:4261–4267.
92. Resnick L, diMarzo-Veronese F, Schupbach J, et al. Intra-blood-brain-barrier synthesis of HTLV-III–specific IgG in patients with neurologic symptoms associated with AIDS or AIDS-related complex. *N Engl J Med* 1985;313:1498–1504.
93. Robbins DS, Shirazi Y, Drysdale BE, Lieberman A, Shin HS, Shin ML. Production of cytotoxic factor for oligodendrocytes by stimulated astrocytes. *J Immunol* 1987;139:2593–2597.
94. Sabatier JM, Vives E, Mabrouk K, et al. Evidence for neurotoxic activity of tat from human immunodeficiency virus type 1. *J Virol* 1991;65:961–967.
95. Saito Y, Sharer LR, Epstein LG, et al. Overexpression of Nef as a marker for restricted HIV-1 infection of astrocytes in post-mortem pediatric central nervous tissue. *Neurology* 1994;44:474–481.
96. Sasseville VG, Newman WA, Lackner AA, et al. Elevated vascular cell adhesion molecule-1 in AIDS encephalitis induced by simian immunodeficiency virus. *Am J Pathol* 1992;141:1021–1030.
97. Scheider T, Beck A, Ropke C, et al. The HIV-1 Nef protein shares an antigenic determinant with a T cell surface protein. *AIDS* 1993;7:647–654.
98. Schwartz S, Felber BK, Benko DM, Fenyo E-M, Pavlakis GN. Cloning and functional analysis of multiply spiced mRNA species of human immunodeficiency virus type 1. *J Virol* 1990;64:2519–2529.

99. Selmaj KW, Farooq M, Norton WT, Raine CS, Brosnan CF. Proliferation of astrocytes *in vitro* in response to cytokines. A primary role for tumor necrosis factor. *J Immunol* 1990;144:129–135.

100. Selmaj KW, Raine CS. Tumor necrosis factor mediates myelin and oligodendrocyte damage *in vitro*. *Ann Neurol* 1988;23:339–346.

101. Sharer LR. Pathology of HIV-1 infection of the central nervous system. A review [Review]. *J Neuropathol Exp Neurol* 1992;51:3–11.

102. Sharer LR, Cho ES, Epstein LG. Multinucleated giant cells and HTLV-III in AIDS encephalopathy. *Hum Pathol* 1985;16:760.

103. Sharer LR, Dowling PC, Michaels J, et al. Spinal cord disease in children with HIV-1 infection: a combined molecular biological and neuropathological study. *Neuropathol Appl Neurobiol* 1990;16: 317–331.

104. Sharer LR, Epstein LG, Cho ES, et al. Pathologic features of AIDS encephalopathy in children: evidence for LAV/HTLV-III infection of brain. *Hum Pathol* 1986;17:271–284.

105. Sharer LR, Michaels J, Murphey-Corb M, Hu FS, Kuebler DJ, Martin LN. Serial pathogenesis study of SIV brain infection. *J Med Primatol* 1991;20:211–217.

106. Sharer LR, Saito Y, Epstein LG, Blumberg BM. Dectection of HIV-1 DNA in pediatric AIDS brain tissue by two-step ISPCR. *Adv Neuroimmunol* 1994;4(3):283–285.

107. Sharma DP, Zink MC, Anderson M, et al. Derivation of neurotropic simian immunodeficiency virus from exclusively lymphocytotropic parental virus: pathogenesis of infection in macaques. *J Virol* 1992;66:3550–3556.

108. Shaw GM, Harper ME, Hahn BH, et al. HTLV-III infection in brains of children and adults with AIDS encephalopathy. *Science* 1985;227:177–182.

109. Sidtis JJ, Gatsonis C, Price RW, et al. Zidovudine treatment of the AIDS dementia complex: results of a placebo-controlled trial. AIDS Clinical Trials Group. *Ann Neurol* 1993;33:343–349.

110. Sinclair E, Gray F, Ciardi A, Scaravilli F. Immunohistochemical changes and PCR detection of HIV provirus DNA in brains of asymptomatic HIV-positive patients. *J Neuropathol Exp Neurol* 1994;53:43–50.

111. Stoler MH, Eskin TA, Benn S, Angerer RC, Angerer LM. Human T cell lymphotropic virus type III infection of the central nervous system. A preliminary in situ analysis. *JAMA* 1986;256:2360–2364.

112. Suzumura A, Sawada M, Yamamoto H, Marunouchi T. Transforming growth factor-beta suppresses activation and proliferation of microglia *in vitro*. *J Immunol* 1993;151:2150–2158.

113. Tardieu M, Hery C, Peudenier S, Boespflug O, Montagnier L. Human immunodeficiency virus type 1-infected monocytic cells can destroy human neural cells after cell-to-cell adhesion. *Ann Neurol* 1992;32:11–17.

114. Toggas SM, Masliah E, Rockenstein EM, Rall GF, Abraham CR, Mucke L. Central nervous system damage produced by expression of the HIV-1 coat protein gp120 in transgenic mice. *Nature* 1994; 367:188–193.

115. Tornatore C, Chandra R, Berger J, Major E. HIV-1 infection of subcortical astrocytes in pediatric central nervous system. *Neurology* 1994;44:481–487.

116. Tornatore C, Nath A, Amemiya K, Major EO. Persistent human immunodeficiency virus type 1 infection in human fetal glial cells reactivated by T cell factor(s) or by the cytokines tumor necrosis factor alpha and interleukin-1 beta. *J Virol* 1991;65:6094–6100.

117. Tyor WR, Glass JD, Griffin JW, et al. Cytokine expression in the brain during the acquired immuno-deficiency syndrome. *Ann Neurol* 1992;31:349–360.

118. Vazeux R, Lacroix-Ciaudo C, Blanche S, et al. Low levels of human immunodeficiency virus replication in the brain tissue of children with severe acquired immunodeficiency syndrome encephalopathy. *Am J Pathol* 1992;140:137–144.

119. Vitkovic L, Kalebic T, de Cunha A, Fauci AS. Astrocyte-conditioned medium stimulates HIV-1 expression in a chronically infected promonocyte clone. *J Neuroimmunol* 1990;30:153–160.

120. Volterra A, Trotti D, Cassutti P, Tromba C, Salvaggio A, Melcangi RC. High sensitivity of glutamate uptake to extracellular free arachidonic acid levels in rat cortical synaptosomes and astrocytes. *J Neurochem* 1992;59:600–606.

121. Wahl SM, Allen JB, McCartney-Francis N, et al. Macrophage- and astrocyte-derived transforming growth factor beta as a mediator of central nervous system dysfunction in acquired immune deficiency syndrome. *J Exp Med* 1991;173:981–991.

122. Wahl LM, Corcoran ML, Pyle SW, Arthur LO, Harel-Bellan A, Farrar WL. Human immunodeficiency virus glycoprotein (gp120) induction of monocyte arachidonic acid metabolites and interleukin 1. *Proc Natl Acad Sci U S A* 1989;86:621–625.

123. Wasterlain CG, Adams LM, Hattori H, Schwartz PH. Felbamate reduces hypoxic-ischemic brain damage *in vivo*. *Eur J Pharmacol* 1992;212:275–278.

124. Weihe E, Nohr D, Sharer L, Murray E, Rausch D, Eiden L. Cortical astrocytosis in juvenile rhesus monkeys infected with simian immunodeficiency virus. *Neuroreport* 1993;4:263–266.

125. Weis S, Haug H, Budka H. Neuronal damage in the cerebral cortex of AIDS brains: a morphometric study. *Acta Neuropathol* 1993;85:185–189.

126. Werner T, Ferroni S, Saermark T, et al. HIV-1 Nef protein exhibits structural and functional similarity to scorpion peptides interacting with K+ channels. *AIDS* 1991;5:1301–1308.
127. Wesselingh SL, Power C, Glass JD, et al. Intracerebral cytokine messenger RNA expression in acquired immunodeficiency syndrome dementia. *Ann Neurol* 1993;33:576–582.
128. Westervelt P, Gendelman HE, Ratner L. Identification of a determinant within the human immunodeficiency virus 1 surface envelope glycoprotein critical for productive infection of primary monocytes. *Proc Natl Acad Sci U S A* 1991;88:3097–3101.
129. Westervelt P, Trowbridge DB, Epstein LG, et al. Macrophage tropism determinants of human immunodeficiency virus type 1 *in vivo*. *J Virol* 1992;66:2577–2582.
130. White HS, Wolf HH, Swinyard EA, Skeen GA, Sofia RD. A neuropharmacological evaluation of felbamate as a novel anticonvulsant. *Epilepsia* 1992;33:564–572.
131. Wiley CA, Masliah E, Morey M, et al. Neocortical damage during HIV infection. *Ann Neurol* 1991; 29:651–657.
132. Wiley CA, Schrier RD, Nelson JA, Lampert PW, Oldstone MB. Cellular localization of human immunodeficiency virus infection within the brains of acquired immune deficiency syndrome patients. *Proc Natl Acad Sci U S A* 1986;83:7089–7093.

AIDS and the Nervous System, Second Edition,
edited by J. R. Berger and R. M. Levy.
Lippincott-Raven Publishers, Philadelphia © 1997.

5

Neuroimmunology of Human Immunodeficiency Virus Infection

Sidney A. Houff

Neurology Service, Washington Veterans Administration Medical Center, Washington, DC 20422

Diseases of the nervous system occur throughout the course of human immunodeficiency virus (HIV) infection (108). Neuroimmune responses are implicated in the pathogenesis of HIV-related neurological diseases in two different settings. Infiltration of the brain by HIV-infected mononuclear cells, release of cytokines, and other neurotoxic metabolites of these cells have been proposed as features of the pathogenesis of HIV-induced neurologic disease, especially HIV-1–associated dementia complex and vacuolar myelopathy. Abnormalities in immune responses to opportunistic infections and cancers and autoimmune phenomena secondary to loss of immunoregulation also have figured in the understanding of neurological complications that occur throughout the course of HIV infection. This chapter examines known features of immune reactions in the central nervous system (CNS) and how alterations in these reactions may lead to opportunistic infections and cancers of the CNS. The role of the immune system in neurologic diseases resulting from HIV infection itself is considered elsewhere in this volume.

The nervous system was long considered an immune privileged site, primarily as a result of Medawar's description of diminished immune rejection of transplanted skin grafts in the brain (43,171). More recently, the immunologic privilege of the CNS has been called into question as a result of the many descriptions of immunologic reactions in the brain after CNS infections and the hypotheses of immune-related neurologic disease. At present, the CNS is at best considered a relatively immune privileged site (79). The unusual nature of the blood–brain barrier (BBB), the lack of major histocompatibility complex (MHC) antigen expression in normal brain, and the absence of professional antigen-presenting cells (APCs) lead to differences in immune reactions in the CNS compared with those that occur in systemic organs. These differences undoubtedly have effects on the immune responses to infections and cancers of the nervous system. When the immune system itself is altered, as in the case of HIV infection, the effects on neuroimmune responses to diseases of the nervous system are likely to also be altered. However, the effects on the neuroimmune system may be different than those encountered in systemic organs.

IMMUNOLOGIC RECOGNITION OF ANTIGENS PRESENT IN THE CNS

It is unclear whether initial recognition of foreign antigens by the immune system occurs within the CNS, at the level of systemic lymphoid organs, or both. One of the reasons for considering the CNS an immunologically privileged site was, in part, the lack of recognizable secondary immune organs and lymphatic system in the CNS (43). The absence of these features of the immune system suggests that activation of cognitive or memory lymphocytes is unlikely within the CNS (274). The tight endothelial cell junctions, pericytes, and astrocytic foot processes of the BBB impede entry of inflammatory cells, cytokines, and immunoregulatory molecules into the brain. Antigens of the MHC, required for presentation of foreign antigens to antigen-specific lymphocytes, are not constitutively expressed in brain as they are at systemic sites (129,140). Lastly, professional APCs, i.e., macrophages, dendritic cells, etc., are absent in the brain (109). These findings suggest that immune reactions in the CNS must differ significantly from those in systemic organs.

Neuroimmune System: Afferent Limb

The afferent limb of the immune response defines those aspects of immune recognition that result in activation of cognitive or memory lymphocytes leading to the development of antigen-specific effect lymphocytes and recruitment of inflammatory cells and molecules of the natural, antigen-nonspecific immune system. The initial recognition of foreign antigens present in the brain by cognitive or memory lymphocytes may occur by two pathways. Antigen recognition may occur in systemic lymphoid organs or at the BBB or related structures. These two pathways may not be mutually exclusive.

Experimental evidence suggests that antigens present in the brain or cerebrospinal fluid (CSF) reach systemic, secondary immune organs, where they can initiate an immune response (29,43,280). Foreign antigens introduced into the brain are transported by interstitial fluid flow to the cribiform plate, where they exit to reach deep cervical lymphatics, lymph nodes, and spleen. Antigens that reach systemic lymphoid organs elicit humoral and cellular immune responses (107). Antibody responses elicited by foreign antigens transplanted into the CNS are consistently higher than the same antigens inoculated at systemic sites (91). Transplanted antigens in the CSF may lead to immunosuppression of cellular immunity while supporting antibody synthesis (107).

Lymphocyte trafficking through the CNS may offer a second mechanism by which initial immune recognition of foreign antigens may occur. Lymphocyte trafficking into the CNS may result from lymphocyte activation in systemic lymphoid organs or activation at the level of the BBB. Lymphocytes activated in systemic sites cross the BBB regardless of their antigen specificity (184,272). Resting lymphocytes are incapable of crossing the BBB. Only activated lymphocytes that recognize foreign antigens within the CNS can elicit a second wave of immune cell infiltration, including antigen-specific and nonspecific immune cells.

Immune Recognition of Reactivated Latent Infections of the CNS in HIV-Infected Patients

Reactivation of organisms that are latent in the CNS requires that immune recognition by antigen-specific lymphocytes take place without the benefit of a systemic infection, as occurs with primary infections. In HIV-infected patients, *Toxoplasma gondii*, herpes simplex, and herpes zoster are common latent infections of the CNS whose reactivation results in CNS disease in patients with acquired immunodeficiency syndrome (AIDS). Alterations in systemic lymph nodes during HIV infection may explain, in part, the inability of patients with AIDS to respond to these infections if immune recognition of reactivated latent CNS infections occurs in systemic lymphoid organs. Alterations in systemic lymph nodes are present early and progress throughout the course of HIV infection (209). Replication of HIV in lymph nodes is followed by depletion of CD4+ T cells, involution of B cell germinal centers, and disintegration of the follicular dendritic cell network responsible for trapping and presenting antigen to lymphocytes (190). These changes result in an impaired ability to mount either cellular or humoral immune responses to foreign antigens. The "burnt out" stage found in lymph nodes at latter stages of AIDS suggests that immune recognition of reactivated latent infections in the brain would be severely impaired if systemic recognition of foreign antigens were required for immune responses to CNS infections. The destruction of peripheral lymph nodes during the later stages of HIV infection likely account, at least in part, for the development of opportunistic infections due to reactivation of latent CNS infections.

Foreign Antigen Recognition at the Level of the BBB

The type of APC encountered at the BBB may define, at least in part, the lymphocyte subset that undergoes recruitment and activation. Experimental studies suggest that cerebrovascular endothelial cells and B cells preferentially stimulate T_H2 CD4+ T-helper/inducer lymphocytes (64). Smooth muscle/pericytes (SM/Ps) and macrophages are involved in the activation of T_H1 CD4+ T-helper/inducer cells (64). Cerebrovascular endothelial cells and SM/Ps also differ in their ability to process and present antigens to T cells (65). SM/Ps process foreign antigens and undergo upregulation of class 2 antigen expression after interferon-gamma (IFN-γ) treatment. Cerebrovascular endothelial cells, on the other hand, appear incapable of processing the same antigens but can present trypsin-treated antigen to antigen-specific T cells. Both SM/Ps and endothelial cells provide the required second, costimulatory signal necessary for complete activation of CD4+ T-helper/inducer cells. The differential stimulation of CD4+ helper/inducer T cell subsets offers a molecular pathway for regulating the type of inflammatory response recruited into the CNS.

Subsets of CD4+ T-helper/inducer cells participate in different arms of the immune response and are usually defined by the cytokine profile secreted after antigen stimulation. Virgin T-lymphocytes exposed to antigen synthesize interleukin (IL)-2. Antigenic stimulation of naive T cells leads to differentiation of some lymphocytes into memory, T_H0, cells that produce a wide range of lymphokines, including IL-2, IL-3, IL-4, IL-5, IL-6, IL-10, granulocyte-macrophage colony-stimulating factor (GM-CSF), and lymphotoxin (LT) (214). T_H0 cells can be further stimulated to differentiate into T_H1 or T_H2 CD4+ subsets (207). T_H1 CD4+ helper/inducer T cells are the principal lymphocyte subset involved in immune responses to viral and other intercellular parasites. T_H1 cells trigger phagocyte-mediated natural immunity. T_H1 CD4+ helper/inducer T cells are also involved in the development of delayed hypersensitivity reactions. The cytokine profile of T_H1 T cells is made up of macrophage activators, including IFN-γ, IL-2, and LT. T_H1 T-helper cell–stimulated B cells produce antibodies capable of acting as opsonizing agents for phagocytosis and activating complement. T_H2 T cells are involved in phagocyte-independent host defenses, especially those directed against helminthic parasites. T_H2 helper/inducer T cells also are involved in mediating allergic reactions. After antigen stimulation, T_H2 T cells synthesize IL-4, IL-5, IL-6, IL-10, and IL-13. T_H2 T-helper/inducer cells preferentially stimulate B cell growth and differentiation.

The differentiation of T_H0 cells into T_H1 or T_H2 cells is a function of the types of cytokines produced early after antigen exposure, the identity of the APC stimulating T_H0 cells, and the nature and amount of antigen present. IL-12, IFN-γ, and IFN-1α promote the development of T_H1 helper/inducer T cells from T_H0 memory T cells (39,207,252). Microbes stimulate macrophages to produce IL-12 and natural killer (NK) cells to synthesize IFN-γ. Activated macrophages are especially potent stimulators of T_H1 helper/inducer T cells through the synthesis of IL-12. This pathway may be bidirectional because activated T_H1 cells produce IFN-γ, which in turn activates macrophages to upregulate IL-12 synthesis. Some T_H1 clones also synthesize IL-12, stimulating their differentiation through autocrine and paracrine mechanisms. In the absence of IFN-γ, IL-4 directs T_H0 cell differentiation into T_H2 helper/inducer T cells. T_H2 T cells secrete IL-4, IL-5, IL-6, and IL-10. T_H2 helper/inducer T cells augment humoral immune responses by their effects on B cell differentiation.

The ability of cell types at the BBB to preferentially stimulate CD4+ T cell subsets involved in response to different foreign antigens suggests they may control the types of immune responses elicited by infections of the CNS. Selective recruitment of T_H1 CD4+ T cells has been described in experimental allergic encephalomyelitis (EAE) (175). In EAE, MHC class 2 antigen expression is present on perivascular macrophages before induction of MHC antigens on cerebrovascular endothelial cells. Thus, the majority of T cells in EAE lesions express IFN-γ and IL-12, the cytokine profile of T_H1 T cell subsets (176). The absence of endothelial cell class 2 antigen expression early in EAE results in the failure to recruit significant numbers of T_H2 T cells.

Perivascular cells at the BBB share cell surface antigens with macrophages. These perivascular cells constitute another possible facultative APC (62,71,92,93). The anatomic location and immunophenotype of perivascular cells clearly differentiate these cells from SM/P cells (92,93). Perivascular cells also appear to be a distinct cell lineage from microglia. Expression of class 2 antigen by perivascular cells does not correlate with class 2 antigen expression by microglia. Furthermore, cell kinetic studies suggest that perivascular cells undergo frequent turnover, unlike microglia. Perivascular mononuclear cells are probably derived from blood monocytes. These perivascular cells have been shown to be efficient APCs for immunocompetent T cells (115). It is not known whether perivascular mononuclear cells differentiate between T-lymphocyte subsets.

The APCs that activate T cells at the BBB may determine, at least in part, the type of T cell effectors and natural immune responses recruited into the CNS during infections of the brain (41). The recruitment of a secondary wave of inflammatory cells results from the secretion of cytokines and chemotactic molecules after activation of T cells encountering foreign antigens presented by endothelial cells, SM/P cells, or perivascular macrophages.

MHC Antigen Expression at the BBB in HIV Infection

MHC antigen expression occurs at the level of the BBB in patients with HIV infection. Cerebrovascular endothelial cells in patients with AIDS express high levels of beta$_2$-microglobulin (β_2-M), the invariant chain of class 1 MHC antigens (2). Significant β_2-M staining is also present on perivascular mononuclear cells. Patients with HIV, herpes simplex, and cytomegalovirus (CMV) encephalitis have high levels of endothelial cell class 1 expression. Expression of β_2-M is highest in patients with HIV encephalitis. However, other investigators have reported only scant class 1 antigen expression by brain endothelial cells (133). The reasons for the discrepancies in these results is unclear.

Class 2 antigen expression is present on macrophages within perivascular cuffs and in perivascular regions of the BBB (2,133). Class 2 antigen is also detected on microglia. Class 2 antigen expression by endothelial cells is rare. Rhesus monkeys with simian immunodeficiency virus (SIV) encephalitis have endothelial cell class 2 antigen expression associated with areas of SIV encephalitis (15). The level of endothelial cell expression of class 2 antigen correlated with the presence of encephalitis. SIV infection of endothelial cells could not be detected.

The cell types expressing MHC antigens at the BBB may affect the type and extent of inflammatory responses to CNS infections. Class 1 antigen expression by endothelial cells could explain, in part, the preponderance of CD8+ T cells in perivascular infiltrates in the brains of patients with AIDS. CD4+ T cells are the most frequently encountered T cell subset in viral infections of the CNS and appear earlier than other T cell subsets and B cells (98). The reduction in CD4+ T cells in the perivascular infiltrates of patients with AIDS may have several explanations. Depletion of CD4+ T cells, occurring throughout the course of HIV infection, reduces the number of CD4+ T-helper/inducer cells in the peripheral circulation available for recruitment by APCs. A reduction in the percentage of CD45+ RO memory cells begins early in the course of HIV infection and continues throughout the course of infection (104,113,262). The loss of T memory cells also may alter inflammatory cell recruitment into the CNS. The results of the experiments described above suggest that the type of APC at the level of the BBB may determine which CD4+ helper/inducer subset is recruited during CNS infections. The class 2 positive APCs present in the brains of patients with AIDS may be restricted to recruitment of the CD4+ T$_H$1 helper/inducer subset. However, the switch of T$_H$1 to T$_H$2 CD4+ T cell subsets that occurs during HIV infection may reduce the number of T$_H$1 CD4+ T cells available for recruitment (39). This reduction in T$_H$1 CD4+ T cells may render antigen presentation at the level of the BBB ineffective. This is of special importance in CNS infections because T$_H$1 T-helper/inducer cells are involved as the primary T cells responding to viruses and intercellular parasites such as *Toxoplasma gondii*. Absence of class 2 antigen expression by cerebrovascular endothelial cells in the brains of patients with AIDS, along with decline in the T$_H$2 T-helper/inducer cell subset as HIV disease progresses, suggest that recruitment of this helper/inducer subset also may be impaired. Reduction in T$_H$2 T-helper/inducer cell recruitment could alter the ability to recruit and promote B cell differentiation in the second wave of immune response to CNS infections.

Regardless of whether the immune response to CNS antigens is initiated in systemic lymphoid organs or by activated lymphocytes at the level of the BBB, several unique features of the immune system specific for the CNS must be considered in assessing immune responses to infections of the brain in HIV-infected patients (98). Lymphocytes, inflammatory cells, cytokines, and immunoregulatory cells must cross specialized capillaries of the BBB. Foreign antigens in the CNS must be presented to lymphocytes in the context of the appropriate MHC antigen. APCs must be capable of providing a second signal to CD4 + T-helper/inducer subsets for T cell activation to occur (271). The phagocytic properties and synthesis of immunoregulatory cytokines by resident cells of the nervous system also must be considered in the immune responses to CNS infections.

MONONUCLEAR CELL TRAFFICKING IN THE CENTRAL NERVOUS SYSTEM

Immune surveillance of the CNS depends on mononuclear cell trafficking through the nervous system. Our current understanding of cell trafficking in the CNS has been gained primarily from animal models of autoimmune diseases and viral infections of the brain. Results of these studies provide a useful model for examining changes in cell trafficking in the CNS in patients with HIV infection.

Leukocyte trafficking through systemic organs, especially immune organs, is controlled by unique homing receptors on endothelial cells. To date, homing receptors specific for the CNS have not been described. The absence of unique homing receptors for the brain suggest that inflammatory cell trafficking in the CNS is likely the result of a combinatorial process involving several factors, including (a) the state of activation of inflammatory cells, (b) the hemodynamic properties at the site of cell adhesion to the endothelium, (c) the regional diversity of the cell adhesion molecule expression by cerebrovascular endothelial cells and their corresponding ligands on mononuclear cells, and (d) the type of APCs present at the BBB (272,273).

As yet, there are no general rules suggesting the type of inflammatory responses associated with specific cell adhesion molecules on endothelial cells and their respective ligands on inflammatory cells. Activated, but not resting, T cells cross the BBB without requiring antigen recognition at the endothelial cell surface (273). Antigen recognition by T cells is followed by a second wave of mononuclear cell infiltration occurring within 96 hours. This second wave of cellular infiltration involves both antigen-specific and antigen-nonspecific leukocytes, including lymphocytes, monocytes, and macrophages. Alterations in the BBB after antigen recognition facilitates entry of inflammatory cells through upregulation of the synthesis of inflammatory cytokines by endothelial cells and, possibly, pericytes and perivascular macrophages (272). At sites of inflammation, cerebrovascular endothelial cells express cell adhesion molecules but do not appear to develop morphologic changes consistent with high endothelial venules found at other sites of inflammation in systemic organs (203,237). These experiments suggest that activated lymphocytes likely participate in immune surveillance of the CNS. Activation of cognitive memory lymphocytes would facilitate the entry of effector lymphocytes into the CNS. Activated T and B cells have both been shown to be important in clearance of virus in viral encephalitis and preventing replication of virus in persistent viral infections in the CNS (98,151,188).

Trafficking of leukocytes out of the CNS is less well understood. Evidence suggests that lymphocytes may exit the CNS by various pathways or undergo programmed cell death. There is some morphologic evidence for lymphatic-like pathways in the brain, which may provide a route for the exit of lymphocytes from the CNS. Lymphocytes also may leave the brain by crossing the brain–CSF barrier. The phenotypic profile of CSF lymphocytes is consistent with either an activated or postactivated state, suggesting that they may have crossed the BBB before entering the CSF

(35,106,112,186). The appearance of B-lymphocytes in the CSF after their appearance in the brain during Sindbis virus encephalitis supports the parenchymal origin of CSF B-lymphocytes (99,100). Lymphocytes that enter the CNS may also undergo programmed cell death. After entering the brain, activated T cells do not persist in an activated state for long periods of time (187). DNA extracted from T cells in the brains of animals with EAE have ladderlike DNA sequences consistent with cells undergoing apoptosis (145).

CEREBROVASCULAR ENDOTHELIAL CELLS IN NEUROIMMUNE RESPONSES

Endothelial cells play an active role in modulating inflammatory responses. The immune functions of cerebrovascular endothelial cells are likely important in recruiting inflammatory cells and determining the phenotype of cellular infiltrates present in areas of inflammation. Endothelial cells in the CNS also likely contribute to neuroimmune responses through synthesis of cytokines and other immunoregulatory molecules and act as APCs.

Endothelial Cell Recruitment of Immune Cells

Recruitment of inflammatory cells is an active process that can be divided into four phases (163). Although many specific features of cerebrovascular endothelial cell/leukocyte interactions are unknown, the general features of leukocyte binding and egress from the circulation are likely to follow the same general principles found at systemic sites. However, the unique properties of cerebrovascular endothelial cells and the BBB may result in differences in expression of cell adhesion molecules, MHC antigens, synthesis of cytokines, and chemoattractants that could have effects on the type and timing of cells recruited as inflammatory infiltrates into the CNS.

Primary adhesion of leukocytes to endothelial surfaces comprises the initial event of leukocyte recruitment. Primary adhesion, or leukocyte rolling, results in transient, unstable attachment of leukocytes to endothelial cell surfaces. For firmer attachment and egress to occur, leukocytes must undergo activation, which results in firmer attachment to the endothelial surface. During the activation phase, changes in the molecular configuration of leukocyte cell adhesion molecules increase their affinity for receptors on endothelial cells. Activation of leukocytes resulting in changes in the molecular configuration of cell adhesion molecules may occur by at least three mechanisms, including (a) activation via receptors such as the TCR receptor on T cells, (b) cytokine stimulation, and (c) binding of the CD31 molecule to endothelial cell surfaces (163). CD3/TCR activation preferentially induces changes in the molecular configuration of the lymphocyte function-associated antigen 1 (LFA-1) integrin. Cytokines activate changes in the molecular structure of a variety of integrins. CD31 binding to endothelial cells preferentially changes the molecular configuration of the very late antigen-4 (VLA-4).

After activation of leukocytes, their affinity to bind to cell adhesion molecules of the immunoglobulin (Ig) superfamily expressed on endothelial cells (intracellular adhesion molecule [ICAM]-1, ICAM-2, and VCAM-1) is significantly increased. The increased affinity of binding of leukocytes to endothelial cell adhesion molecules stabilizes leukocyte adherence, allowing transendothelial migration of leukocytes across the BBB. Several molecular events have been associated with transmigration of leukocytes across the BBB. ICAM-1 binding by LFA-1 signals changes in endothelial cell cytoskeletal structures such as the actin-binding protein cortactin (60). The entry of leukocytes into the brain also has been shown to depend on release of vasoactive molecules from mast cells present at the BBB (98,101). Vasoactive molecules are released from mast cells after stimulation by cytokines from T cells, endothelial cells, perivascular macrophages, and possibly astrocytes (6). The vasoactive molecules released by mast cells open tight junctions in the BBB, facilitating entry of inflammatory cells and immunologically active circulating molecules.

The multistep process of leukocyte adhesion and migration at the endothelial cell surface provides a number of sites for the molecular regulation of recruitment of inflammatory cells. Specificity of leukocyte/endothelial cell binding is likely a result of sequential and combinatorial expression of selectins, integrins, and cell adhesion molecules of the Ig superfamily (163). The regulation of leukocyte adhesion to endothelial cells results from rapid transient upregulation of leukocyte adhesion molecules and/or endothelial adhesion molecules after receptor binding and a more persistent expression of endothelial adhesion molecules after cytokine stimulation (160). At least five receptor types with their ligands have been identified as possible participants in leukocyte interactions with vascular endothelium and extracellular matrix (98). Adhesion of leukocytes to endothelial cells involves three superfamilies of adhesion molecules: (a) the selectins or lectin-epidermal growth factor complement–related cell adhesion molecules, (b) the heterodimeric integrins, and (c) members of the Ig superfamily.

The initial step of leukocyte adhesion (leukocyte rolling) is mediated by leukocyte selectins and their ligands, the terminal structures on carbohydrate groups of glycoproteins or glycolipids on endothelial cells. Post-translational modifications of glycoproteins or glycolipids provide multiple potential binding sites for selectins. L-selectin (LAM-1, MEL-14) is constitutively expressed on neutrophils, monocytes, some myeloid cells, and a subset of T-lymphocytes (CD4 + memory T cells). L-selectins are involved in lymphocyte homing to lymph nodes and recruitment of leukocytes to sites of inflammation. Like integrins, L-selectin undergoes conformational changes after activation of neutrophils and lymphocytes, increasing the avidity of L-selectin for its glycoprotein/glycolipid receptors (239). Constitutive expression of ELAM-1 does not occur. However, endothelial cell expression of ELAM-1 is upregulated by IL-1β, tumor necrosis factor-alpha (TNF-δ), LT, IFN-γ, and substance P (26,191). P-selectin, which is also not constitutively expressed, is upregulated on endothelial cells and platelets by thrombin, histamine (a product of mast cells), and hydrogen peroxide (26). ELAM-1 binds neutrophils, monocytes, eosinophils, NK cells, and a subset of CD4 + memory T cells. P-selectin binds neutrophils and monocytes.

Stabilization of the initial adhesion of leukocytes is mediated by leukocyte integrins and endothelial cell adhesion molecules of the Ig superfamily. The integrin family of adhesion molecules consists of at least 13 alpha-beta heterodimers. Ligand specificity is determined by both the α and β chains. Three integrin subfamilies sharing a common β chain are involved in leukocyte binding. β_2 integrins are primarily involved in cell–cell adhesion by binding to members of the Ig superfamily adhesion molecules expressed on endothelial cells (36,189,240). The β_2 integrin, LFA-1, binds ICAM-1 and ICAM-2. ICAM-2 appears not to be involved in recruitment of inflammatory responses. The constitutive expression of ICAM-1 by endothelial cells is either extremely low or not expressed at all under normal circumstances.

ICAM-1 expression by endothelial cells is upregulated by cytokines, including IL-1β, TNF-α, LT, and by lipopolysaccharide (LPS). Expression of ICAM-1 is downregulated by transforming growth factor-beta (TGF-β) as part of its' role as a negative modulator of inflammatory responses (173).

The $\alpha 4 \beta 1$ integrin (VLA-4) is found on the cell surface of T- and B-lymphocytes, monocytes, NK cells, eosinophils, and a subset of CD8 + T memory cells. VLA-4 binds VCAM-1 on endothelial cells. VCAM-1 is not constitutively expressed by endothelial cells but can be upregulated by IL-1β, TNF-α, LT, and IL-4. IL-4 is unique among cytokines in selectively upregulating VCAM-1 expression by endothelial cells (219). Two forms of VCAM-1, resulting from alternate splicing of VCAM messenger RNA (mRNA), are expressed by endothelial cells. Alternate forms of VCAM-1 may play a role in defining the types of inflammatory cells recruited into inflammatory infiltrates (45). For instance, VCAM-1/VLA-4 binding results in a switch from a predominantly neutrophil to mononuclear cell infiltrate or an initial recruitment of mononuclear cell infiltrates at sites of inflammation (248).

Endothelial cell adhesion molecule expression has been examined in a limited number of diseases of the nervous system. Endothelial cells from mice with EAE express VCAM-1 and ICAM-1 adjacent to sites of inflammation (242,282). Treatment with antibodies to VCAM-1 and ICAM-1 suggests that they are involved in recruitment of autoimmune inflammatory responses. Endothelial ICAM-1 expression has been described in patients with multiple sclerosis, herpes simplex encephalitis, and progressive multifocal leukoencephalopathy (PML) (237). Numerous endothelial cells in areas of demyelination in the brains of patients with multiple sclerosis (MS) express ICAM-1. Lymphocytes from patients with acute exacerbation of MS and chronic progressive MS upregulate ICAM-1 expression by cultured brain endothelial cells, suggesting that cytokines released by lymphocytes at sites of demyelination may be responsible for ICAM-1 expression (255). Endothelial cells in patients with herpes simplex encephalitis and PML after renal transplantation express ICAM-1. The brief duration of herpes simplex encephalitis suggests that ICAM-1 expression is upregulated early in the course of CNS infections. In both herpes simplex encephalitis and PML, endothelial cell ICAM-1 expression was limited to areas of inflammatory cell infiltration, suggesting that ICAM-1/LFA-1 binding was important in recruitment of leukocytes to areas of tissue damage and foreign antigen expression.

Endothelial Cell Expression of Cell Adhesion Molecules in HIV Infection

Limited information is available concerning expression of cell adhesion molecules in HIV infection. HIV infection of T-lymphocyte and monocyte cell lines upregulates LFA-1 protein and mRNA expression (210). ICAM-1 is unaffected by HIV-1 infection of T- and monocyte cell lines. HIV-1–infected T- and monocyte cell lines have increased adherence to human umbilical vein endothelial cells compared with uninfected control cells. Cell adhesion is blocked by antibodies to both LFA-1 and ICAM-1, suggesting that LFA-1 expressed by HIV-infected mononuclear cells is functional.

Rhesus monkeys inoculated with the simian immunodeficiency virus in macaques (SIVmac) strain express VCAM-1 on endothelial cells adjacent to areas of SIV encephalitis (217). In regions of SIV encephalitis, VCAM-1 is present on arteriolar, capillary, and venular endothelial cells. VCAM-1 is not expressed by endothelial cells from uninvolved areas of the brain. ELAM-1, P-selectin, and ICAM-1 expression are associated with SIV encephalitis. Human monocytic and B cell lines show increased binding to cerebrovascular endothelial cells from the brains of monkeys with SIV encephalitis but not to endothelial cells from monkeys without encephalitis (216). Only 70% of cell binding to endothelial cells is blocked by antibodies to VCAM-1 or VLA-4. LFA-1 and selectin-mediated binding of leukocytes to cerebrovascular endothelial cells is insignificant. These findings suggest that other as yet unidentified adhesion molecules are involved in mononuclear cell adhesion in SIV infection.

Expression of VCAM-1 by cerebrovascular endothelial cells only in monkeys with SIV encephalitis suggests that VLA-4/VCAM-1 adhesion may be involved in the pathogenesis of retroviral encephalitis. VLA-4 is expressed by human monocyte/ macrophage cells, the mononuclear cell most often implicated in the pathogenesis of HIV-1–associated dementia (160). VCAM-1 also binds monocytes expressing the Mac-1 antigen, which is essential for the entry of macrophages into inflammatory lesions (208).

Cytokines likely have a role in upregulating expression of cell adhesion molecules during HIV infection. IL-1β, TNF-α, LT, and IFN-γ upregulate expression of ICAM-1, ELAM-1, and VCAM-1. TGF-β downregulates these three cell adhesion molecules but is also strongly chemotactic for monocytes and macrophages. IL-1β, TNF-α, IFN-γ, and TGF-β have been identified on cerebrovascular endothelial cells in the brains of HIV-infected patients (261,265). IL-1 and TNF-α are also present on endothelial cell surfaces of spinal cord vessels in patients with vacuolar myelopathy (260). IL-1 may play a pivotal role in the expression of cell adhesion molecules in HIV-infected patients. IL-1β stimulates IL-1β synthesis by endothelial cells via an autocrine mechanism while also upregulating synthesis of other cytokines by endothelial cells (265). The importance of IL-1β in cell adhesion is further supported by the ability of monocytes and T cells to bind to endothelial cells treated with IL-1β.

Infection of endothelial cells in the brains of HIV-infected patients may alter endothelial cell adhesion molecule expression or open the BBB by destruction of endothelial cells. Virus infection of endothelial cells may initiate an inflammatory response by increasing adherence of leukocytes to infected endothelial cells through upregulation of cell adhesion molecules, induction of C3 and Fc receptors, increased synthesis of cytokines, and/or upregulation of MHC class 1 or 2 antigen expression (14). HIV infection of endothelial cells has been reported (105,153,281). It remains unclear whether endothelial cells can support HIV replication. HIV can be rescued from brain endothelial cells infected *in vitro* by coculture with susceptible T cells. Expression of HIV regulatory proteins, i.e., Tat, Rev, and Nef, may alter expression of the cell adhesion molecules and/or cytokine synthesis by endothelial cells without requiring virus replication. Coinfection of cerebrovascular endothelial cells by HIV and CMV also has been reported (153). CMV infection of umbilical endothelial cells upregulates ICAM-1 expression within 24 hours of infection (223). VCAM-1 and ELAM-1 expression is unaffected by CMV-infected endothelial cells. These studies suggest that ICAM-1 could be expressed by cerebrovascular endothelial cells infected with CMV with or without HIV infection. Further studies of endothelial cell adhesion molecule expression in the brains of patients with HIV infection should provide a better understanding of the role of cell adhesion at the level of the cerebrovascular endothelium in the pathogenesis of AIDS-related neurological diseases.

LEUKOCYTE TRAFFICKING IN THE NERVOUS SYSTEM DURING INFECTIONS

Mononuclear cell trafficking in the CNS has been examined in both human and experimental viral infections of the CNS (98). Viral infections of the nervous system may result in inflammatory responses in the CSF, meninges, and/or brain parenchyma (98). Inflammatory responses to viral infections are usually mononuclear in character, including NK cells, lymphocytes, and macrophages. Perivascular cuffs in viral infections of the CNS vary in composition but usually include significant numbers of T- and B-lymphocytes, monocytes, and NK cells (73,128,178). T-lymphocytes are the predominant cell type during the early stages of infection (178). CD4+ T-helper/inducer cells are the earliest cells to appear in the perivascular space (157,244). CD8+ cytotoxic T cells, macrophages, and B-lymphocytes are found in perivascular cuffs later during the course of infection. The secondary infiltration by the cells is likely the result of activation of CD4+ T-helper/inducer cells either at the level of the BBB or in brain parenchyma. After activation of CD4+ T-helper/inducer cells, cytokines and chemotactic factors released by activated lymphocytes recruit other antigen-specific and -nonspecific cells of the immune system.

CSF inflammatory responses in viral infections are predominantly made up of T-lymphocytes and NK cells (99–101). The type of cells present in the CSF depends in part on the type of viral infection studied. Acute meningoencephalitis due to Sindbis virus is associated with an inflammatory response, with NK cells appearing first in the CSF before inflammation is found later in the meninges and brain. In both acute Sindbis and Japanese encephalitis, CD4+ T-helper/inducer cells are the predominant T cell subset present in CSF (127,128,178). Most T cells present in the CSF compartment express antigens consistent with an activated T cell population, including MHC class 2 antigens (98,100,112,169). During chronic viral infections of the CNS, an increased proportion of CD8+ T-lymphocytes is present in the CSF (37,46,59,172,178).

CD4+ T-helper/inducer cells in CSF appear unable to recruit B cells or macrophages (99,100). Because CD4+ T cells are unable to recognize soluble antigen, the inability to recruit B cells and macrophages may be the result of failure to produce chemotactic cytokines, which are released after successful recognition of foreign antigens. B cells are more likely to be preferentially recruited into the brain parenchyma, where viral antigens are presented to CD4+ T-helper/inducer cells by APCs either at the level of the BBB or in the brain parenchyma. The preferential recruitment of B cells into the brain would explain the correlation of antiviral antibody in the CSF with the appearance of B-lymphocytes in brain parenchyma rather than CSF as well as the lack of increased numbers of B cells in CSF during viral infections (98,99).

Leukocyte Trafficking in the Nervous System in HIV Infection

Alterations in leukocyte trafficking through the nervous system occur throughout the course of HIV infection. CSF pleocytosis has been described during primary HIV infection that was complicated by meningoencephalitis (102). Increased CSF cell counts are also present in patients who recently seroconverted to HIV (172). The CSF profile is consistent with that seen in chronic meningitis, i.e., increased percentage of CD8 + compared with CD4 + T-lymphocytes. There is also evidence for altered leukocyte trafficking in the brain early in HIV infection. Varying degrees of vasculitis and perivascular cuffing were found in brains of HIV-seropositive patients dying from unrelated causes early in the course of HIV infection (96). In a significant number, true vasculitis was present with transmural vascular inflammation and leptomeningitis. Mild perivascular cuffing and lymphocytic meningitis was found at autopsy 15 days after a patient received an intravenous injection of white cells from a patient with AIDS (53). The findings of signs of increased lymphocyte trafficking in the CNS early after HIV infection likely reflect activation of T cells, expansion of CD8 + T cell population, and retrafficking of lymphocytes between the intravascular and extravascular compartments, which occurs at the beginning of the course of HIV infection (40,249). The increased percentage of CD8 + compared with CD4 + T cells in the CSF early in HIV infection likely reflects the transient decrease in CD4 + T cells that occurs after primary infection but also may be a reflection of the antigenic stimulation associated with retrovirus infections of the CNS.

Intrathecal synthesis of antibodies to HIV consistently occurs early in HIV infection (205). The first antibody response to HIV occurs as the initial viremia decreases and B cell activation is detected (52). However, *in situ* synthesis of HIV antibody occurs without an increase in the percentage of B cells in the CSF. The presence of activated B cells in the circulation that can cross the BBB suggests that HIV antibody found in CSF may arise from HIV-specific B cells that have crossed the BBB. These findings are consistent with those from experimental Sindbis virus encephalitis, in which CSF antibody correlates with entry of B cells in the brain and not the presence of B cells in CSF (98–100).

Leukocyte trafficking in the CNS in Rhesus monkeys with simian acquired immunodeficiency syndrome (SAIDS) follows that seen in humans. Meningeal inflammation and perivascular cuffing are present early after infection with SIV (47,138,229). In monkeys with SAIDS, the early leptomeningitis, perivascular cuffing, and parenchymal inflammation overlaps the appearance of multinucleated giant cells in brain parenchyma. The appearance of multinucleated giant cells along with other signs of CNS inflammation differs from that seen in patients with HIV infection in whom multinucleated giant cells are a late finding rarely associated with significant parenchymal inflammation or leptomeningitis (230). The differences in the neuropathologic findings in SIV and HIV infection are probably related to the rapid clinical course of SIV infection in monkeys compared with the prolonged asymptomatic period in humans infected with HIV.

Lymphocyte trafficking through the CNS declines with progression of HIV infection. CSF pleocytosis is rare in late stages of HIV infection unless opportunistic infections are present (119). HIV-1–specific CD8 + cytotoxic T cells are found in the CSF of patients with HIV-1–associated dementia complex despite the reduced cellular response in the spinal fluid (124). Cytotoxic T cell clones isolated from CSF are directed against epitopes of the Gag, reverse transcriptase, envelope, and Nef proteins. If inflammatory responses are found in patients with AIDS, they consist of scant mononuclear cell infiltrates (261). Macrophages are the predominant cell type in inflammatory infiltrates and perivascular cuffs. T cells are present, located mainly in perivascular cuffs. CD8 + T cells are slightly more numerous than CD4 + T cells. B-lymphocytes are only rarely encountered. The decreased leukocyte trafficking through the CNS late in the course of HIV infection likely reflects the declining numbers of circulating T- and B-lymphocytes in the late stages of HIV infection. The preponderance of macrophages in the brains of patients with AIDS may result from several factors, including VCAM-1 expression by cerebrovascular endothelial cells and synthesis of cytokines, especially TGF-β, which are strongly chemotactic for macrophages.

NEUROGLIAL CELLS IN IMMUNE REACTIONS IN THE CNS

Neuroglial cells have a number of properties that suggest they are capable of participating in immune reactions in the CNS. Microglia synthesize cytokines, present antigen to antigen-specific T cells, can act as phagocytes, and release toxic molecules capable of killing microorganisms. Astrocytes also can present antigen to T cells, produce cytokines, form glial scars at sites of tissue injury, and probably have limited phagocytic properties. Both astrocytes and oligodendrocytes can express class 1 MHC antigens and serve as targets for CD8+ cytotoxic T-lymphocytes. However, oligodendrocytes do appear to have facultative antigen-presenting properties as found in astrocytes.

Immunologic Properties of Microglia

Microglia comprise ~10% of the total glial cell population of the CNS (194). Reactive microglial cells are associated with various types of CNS tissue injury. Microglial nodules are present in the brains of many infections of the CNS, especially viral and spirochete diseases (57,86). Microglia are believed to play a prominent role in the pathogenesis of HIV-related neurologic disease. An understanding of the immunologic properties of microglia is therefore important in examining CNS immune reactions in HIV-infected patients (Table 1).

Although the origin of microglia remains controversial, most studies suggest microglia are derived from blood monocytes that enter the CNS during embryonic development. After a period of limited proliferation, they remain quiescent until reactivated (85–87,194). Microglia are classified by morphologic appearance. Ramified microglia are highly branched cells most frequently found surrounding neurons. Ameboid microglia have either a unipolar or bipolar morphology and are the principal microglial cell type responding to tissue injury. Microglia share some, but not all, cell surface antigens expressed by monocyte/macrophage cells. CD45 and CD11b

TABLE 1. *Immunological features of microglia*

Ameboid and ramified microglia principal responding cells in immunologic reactions
Immune response of microglia is graded with predominant microglial cell reaction with intact blood-brain barrier and mixed microglial cell/macrophage reactions with disruption of the blood-brain barrier
Microglia present foreign antigen to immunocompetent T cells
Microglia express B7/BB-1 co-stimulatory signal necessary for activating T cells
Activated microglia synthesize immunoregulatory molecules including Interleukin 1, Interleukin 6, Interleukin 10, Tumor Necrosis Factor-α and Transforming Growth Factor-β
Phagocytic Properties of Microglia

CD11B (Mac1, CR3)	Adhesion, Phagocytosis of iC3b coated particles
Fc Receptors	Phagocytosis of coated particles
Proteolytic enzymes, free oxygen, arachidonic acid metabolites, lysosomal proteinases	Destruction of phagocytized microorganisms

antigens are present on resting microglia. Activated microglia express class 1 and 2 MHC antigens and Fc receptors (283). Human microglia do not have nonspecific esterase activity or synthesize nitrous oxide (148,283).

Microglia are distinct from the perivascular mononuclear cell population present at the BBB. Microglia undergo limited turnover in the normal adult nervous system, whereas perivascular monocytes at the BBB and in the meninges are slowly replaced on a continuous basis by blood-borne monocytes/macrophages (115,140,141). The turnover rate of perivascular cells is rapid during CNS infections, whereas resident microglia are replaced by blood monocytes only during illnesses with severe inflammatory responses.

The microglial cell reaction to injury, including infections, varies between a pure reaction of microglia to mixed reactions made up of activated microglia and macrophages recruited from the systemic circulation. These findings have been conceptualized as a graded response by microglia to tissue injury (243). In the graded response theory, tissue injury leaving the BBB intact results in a predominantly microglial cell response. More extensive tissue damage that disrupts the BBB results in recruitment of macrophages from the systemic circulation, leading to a mixed microglia and macrophage reaction.

Microglia can act as APCs to lymphocytes. In normal brains, class 2 MHC antigens are expressed by a small number of microglia in the white matter with increasing expression by microglia in the gray matter with advancing age (93,141,215). Class 2 antigen microglia expression is upregulated by the cytokines, IFN-γ and TNF-α, and by herpes simplex infection (86,276,284,286). Microglia have the capability of providing costimulatory, or second, signals to T cells through the expression of B7/BB-1 antigen, resulting in complete activation. Antibody to B7 inhibits microglial antigen presentation in both antigen-specific T cells and in mixed lymphocyte reactions (285). Microglia from normal human brain present *Candida albicans* antigen to antigen-specific T cells, resulting in proliferation and activation of T-lymphocytes (286). Both untreated and IFN-γ–treated microglia present antigen to T-lymphocytes, with the greatest T cell activation after exposure to IFN-γ–treated microglia. The increased T cell response using IFN-γ–treated microglia correlates with increased levels of microglial class 2 antigen expression.

Microglia constitutively express cytokine mRNAs. IL-1, IL-6, and TNF-α mRNA are present in normal microglia (284). IFN-γ treatment upregulates the expression of interleukins, resulting in synthesis and release of cytokines, including IL-1, IL-6, and TNF-α (85,86,224,284). Microglia also synthesize IL-10 after treatment with LPS (284). The synthesis of cytokines by microglia may have multiple effects on immune responses. Microglial cell cytokines promote astrocyte proliferation, formation of glial scars, and neovascularization (86,88,90). IL-1 is the principal cytokine involved in gliosis and neovascularization. TNF-α has been shown to be cytotoxic to oligodendrocytes (33,227). Activated microglia express Fc and complement receptors on the cell surface, rendering them capable of phagocytizing MBP and other antigens (295). Microglial cell infection with lymphocytic choriomeningitis virus and vesicular stomatitis virus results in upregulation of the synthesis of IL-6, a potent regulator of macrophage and B cell functions. TGF-β synthesis by microglia is upregulated by infection with HIV and CMV.

The ability of human microglia to proliferate after activation has been difficult to demonstrate (89,284). Treatment with a variety of cytokines and growth factors (IFN-γ, GM-CSF, LPS, IL-1, TNF-α, fibroblast growth factor, epidermal growth factor, insulin-like growth factor, platelet-derived growth factor, and nerve growth factor) does not result in proliferation of adult microglia (284). These studies suggest that human microglia are fully differentiated, end-stage cells without the ability to divide. Recently, human fetal microglia have been shown to divide or undergo apoptosis when stimulated via the CR3 (Mac1) receptor. The CR3 receptor binds the C3b component of the alternate complement pathway and denatured proteins that are present in significant amounts in damaged tissue, including inflammatory tissue.

Several cytotoxic pathways are known to be present in activated microglia (9). The phagocytic properties of activated microglia require direct cell-to-cell contact with damaged cells. Neuronophagia is a well-known feature of reactive microglial cell reactions. Microglia expressing Fc and complement receptors can function as nonspecific accessory cells in immune responses in the presence of antibody and complement. Microglial cell cytotoxicity also involves release of active molecules that damage tissue. Free oxygen radicals, proteolytic enzymes, arachidonic acid metabolites, and inflammatory cytokines (TNF-α) capable of damaging tissue have all been found to be released by activated microglia (176,295). Lysosomal proteinases, present in activated microglia, degrade extracellular matrix proteins which may facilitate movement of inflammatory cells in the extracellular space (292).

Microglia Cells in Immune Reactions in HIV Infection

The role of microglial cells in the pathogenesis of HIV-associated neurologic disease is considered elsewhere in this volume. Here the discussion focuses on the role of microglial cells during immune reactions to CNS infections in HIV-infected patients. Neuropathologic studies support the ability of microglial cells from HIV-infected patients to respond to tissue damage caused by CNS infections with viruses and parasites. Microglial nodules are commonly present in the brains of patients with AIDS who also have CMV encephalitis and toxoplasmosis, especially diffuse toxoplasmosis without abscess formation (34,96,131,142,195,289). Microglial nodules are also encountered in myelitis due to herpes simplex and CMV and in patients with herpes zoster encephalitis (195). Although microglial nodules are frequently found in the brains of patients with AIDS, the microglial nodules associated with CMV, *T. gondii*, herpes simplex, and herpes zoster often contain phagocytized organisms, supporting their role in the response to opportunistic infections.

Little is known about the immune functions of human microglia infected with HIV or other opportunistic infections. TGF-β synthesis is upregulated in microglia infected *in vitro* with either HIV or CMV. HIV infection of microglia could either impair or augment their immunologic functions, especially cytotoxic functions. The results of studies of HIV infection of macrophages may be suggestive of the changes expected in microglia. Although many of the functions of monocytes and macrophages are preserved in HIV infection, deficiencies in chemotaxis, monocyte-dependent T cell proliferation, Fc receptor function, C3 receptor–mediated clearance of antigens, and impaired oxidative burst in response to intracellular infections have been reported (209). Because monocytes and microglia appear to be derived from the same cell lineage and have many of the same functions, it is likely that these functions are impaired in HIV-infected microglia. HIV infection of microglia also may reduce the number of microglial cells capable of responding to tissue damage. HIV infection of microglia results in cell death (270). Because microglia are replaced by blood monocytes at a negligible rate unless there is severe inflammation, reduction in the numbers of microglia capable of responding to opportunistic infections also may impair the ability to locally control infections by phagocytosis, release of cytotoxic molecules, and induction of gliosis by IL-1.

Immunological Properties of Macroglia

Immunological properties of macroglia include MHC-restricted antigen presentation to lymphocytes and synthesis of immunoregulatory cytokines (Table 2). Macroglia also can serve as targets for cytotoxic T-lymphocytes through presenting foreign antigen in the context of class 1 MHC antigens. The cytokines synthesized by astrocytes are discussed in the next section. Here the ability of macroglia to present antigen to immunocompetent lymphocytes is reviewed as background for discussing changes in macroglial cell MHC antigen expression in HIV-infected patients.

MHC antigen expression by macroglia is under negative regulatory control at the gene transcriptional level (79). In the normal brain, constitutive MHC antigen expression is limited to cerebrovascular endothelial cells and occasional microglial cells. Endothelial cells express MHC class 1 antigen and occasionally class 2 antigens (141,234). MHC antigen expression is rarely present in normal brains except for the occasional microglial cell expressing class 2 antigens. Ultrastructural studies have shown that cerebrovascular endothelial cells have a continous staining pattern using monoclonal antibodies recognizing class 1 MHC antigens (92,93). Class 1 antigens also have been detected on scattered cells in the perivascular space in normal brains.

TABLE 2. *Immunologic properties of macroglia*

Antigen presentation of macroglia		
MHC antigen type	Cell type	Function
Class 1	Astrocyte and oligodendrocyte	Present foreign antigen to CD8 + T cytotoxic cells
Class 2	Astrocyte	Present foreign antigen to CD4 + T helper/inducer and cytotoxic

Cytokines synthesized by astrocytes		
Cytokine	Effect on macroglia	Effect on microglia
IL-1	Astrocyte proliferation ↑ synthesis of cell adhesion molecules ↑ astrocyte synthesis of C3 ↑ astrocyte synthesis of cytokines (IL-6, TNF-α, GM-CSF, G-CSF)	Unknown
TNF-α	↑ expression of MHC antigens ↑ synthesis of cell adhesion molecules ↑ astrocyte synthesis of C3 ↑ astrocyte synthesis of cytokines (IL-6, TNF-α, GM-CSF, G-CSF) ↑ expression of TNF-α receptors Oligodendroctye cytotoxicity	↑ synthesis of TNF-α
IL-6	Astrocyte proliferation ↑ Expression of NGF	Unknown

IL, interleukin; C3, complement C3; TNF, tumor necrosis factor; GM-CSF, granulocyte/macrophage colony stimulating factor; G-CSF, granulocyte colony stimulating factor; MHC, major histocompatibility complex; NGF, nerve growth factor.

Microglial cells and a distinct class of perivascular cells that share cell surface antigens with macrophages occasionally express class 2 MHC antigen (93,215). The MHC class 2–positive perivascular cells likely represent the resident macrophages derived from circulating monocytes previously described in the human CNS (62,72,93,125). MHC antigens are rarely found on the surface of astrocytes or oligodendrocytes in normal brains using ultrastructural studies (93,167). The lack of MHC antigen expression in normal brains suggests that antigen presentation in the brain requires upregulation of MHC antigen expression.

Astrocytes have been proposed as facultative APCs for CD4+ helper/inducer T cells. Class 2 antigens are spontaneously expressed by astrocytes in tissue culture, but *in vivo* expression is limited to only a minority of astrocytes that stain primarily for HLA-DR and -DQ alleles (97,117,135,159). Oligodendrocytes do not appear able to express class 2 MHC antigens. To fully activate CD4+ helper/inducer T cells, facultative APCs must be capable of processing antigen, presenting processed peptides in the context of class 2 MHC antigens, and providing a costimulatory signal, which may be either the B7/BB1 antigen or IL-1. Activated T cells upregulate astrocyte expression of class 2 antigen through stimulation by T cell–derived IFN-γ. The α and β variant chains and γ invariant chain of astrocyte class 2 molecules are identical to those present on syngeneic spleen cells (68). Human astrocytes do not express the costimulatory B7/BB-1 molecule, even after IFN-γ treatment that upregulates class 2 antigen expression (284,285). Astrocytes synthesize and release IL-1, which can also serve as a second signal for lymphocyte activation.

Astrocyte populations vary in their potential to fully activate CD4+ T cells. Astrocyte populations cloned from the same brain may act as facultative APCs, resulting in complete activation of lymphocytes, may fail to provide the required second signal resulting in incomplete T cell activation, or may induce tolerance to antigens by a yet to be defined pathway (83,274).

Macroglia expressing class 1 and 2 MHC antigens are recognized by CD8+ and CD4+ cytotoxic T cells, respectively (233). Antigen-specific CD8+ cytotoxic T cells lyse astrocytes expressing class 1 antigens in the presence of the appropriate antigen (69). Class 1–restricted allogeneic-specific T cytotoxic cells can kill MHC-matched class 1–expressing astrocytes (233). Human influenza–specific cytotoxic T cells lyse class 1–positive human adult astrocytes infected with the A/JAP influenza strain (55). Astrocyte killing is not observed with either unstimulated lymphocytes or uninfected astrocytes. Class 2 HLA-DR2–restricted CD4+ T cytotoxic cells are also capable of killing human astrocytes expressing class 2 antigens.

MHC antigen gene expression by macroglia is regulated, in part, by immunoregulatory cytokines (79,245). IFN-γ upregulates both class 1 and 2 MHC antigen expression by astrocytes and class 1 antigen expression by oligodendrocytes (10,97,111,117,170,202,257,287). TNF-α also upregulates class 1 antigen expression by both human astrocytes and oligodendrocytes (146,170). TNF-α has no direct effect on class 2 antigen expression but acts synergistically with IFN-γ in upregulating class 2 antigen expression by human astrocytes (146,170). TNF-α also acts synergistically with measles infection in upregulating class 2 antigen expression by astrocytes (166). IFN-α/β upregulates class 1 antigen expression by astrocytes (130,170,204,287). The entire repertoire of class 1 genes is not expressed by neuroglia after treatment with IFN-γ and possibly other cytokines, a feature unique to neuroglial cells. The inability to express the entire repertoire of class 1 antigens may restrict the ability of neuroglia to present some microbial antigens to antigen-specific T cells.

TGF-β_{1-3} are potent immunoregulatory molecules that terminate many immune responses by downregulating many immune functions (268). TGF-β has no effect on astrocyte expression of MHC class 1 antigens (126,220). TGF-β inhibits IFN-γ and IFN-γ/TNF-α upregulation of class 2 antigen expression by astrocytes. Astrocyte populations from various regions of the brain differ in their response to TGF-β (126). TGF-β inhibits IFN-γ–induced expression of class 2 antigens by brain stem but not forebrain astrocytes. These findings are the first to suggest that astrocytes from different regions of the brain may vary in their ability to respond to the immunoregulatory effects of cytokines. TGF-β downregulation of astrocyte class 2 antigen expression prevents antigen presentation to T-lymphocytes (220).

Macroglial Cell MHC Antigen Expression in Patients with HIV Infection

MHC antigen expression has been examined in the brains of a limited number of patients with HIV infection (2,196). Class 1 (β_2-M) was increased in all brains examined from HIV-infected patients (2). High levels of β_2-M expression were present on both endothelial cells and some unidentified parenchymal cells. Patients with HIV encephalitis tended to have higher levels of β_2-M expression compared with those without encephalitis. Class 1 antigen expression was found predominantly in the deep gray and white matter, areas where HIV antigens are most frequently detected. Oligodendrocytes frequently stained for class 1 antigens, especially in areas where myelin loss had occurred. β_2-M was rarely present on cells with astrocyte or neuronal morphology. Class 2 HLA-DR antigen was not detected on astrocytes. Macrophages, multinucleated giant cells and occasional endothelial cells were found to express class 2 HLA-DR antigens. The level of HLA-DR expression in HIV-infected patients was highest in those with HIV encephalitis.

MHC antigen expression has been reported in an even more limited number of patients with opportunistic infections. MHC antigen expression has been reported in the brains of patients with PML, with and without HIV infection (3). Oligodendrocytes infected with JC virus, the etiologic agent of PML, stained for invariant β_2-M class 1 antigen. Class 1 antigens were also present on cerebrovascular endothelial cells in demyelinating lesions and astrocytes with bizarre morphology, a frequent neuropathologic finding in PML. HLA-DR class 2 antigen expression was restricted to macrophages, microglia and endothelial cells within demyelinating lesions.

Experimental evidence also suggests that retrovirus infections can upregulate MHC antigen expression. Intraperitoneal inoculation of mice with the murine leukemia virus is followed by MHC class 1 expression localized to the meninges and choroid plexus endothelial cells early after inoculation (183). Parenchymal cells express class 1 antigen within 4 weeks of infection. The class 1 antigen–expressing cells appeared to be oligodendrocytes and astrocytes using morphological criteria. Macroglia only rarely express class 2 MHC antigens. Microglia, endothelial cells, and macrophages were the predominant cells expressing class 2 antigens. Infection of human fetal glial cells by human T-lymphotropic virus-1 (HTLV-I) is followed by upregulation of class 2 antigen expression (116,162). HTLV-I trans activator (TAX) protein upregulates MHC class 1 gene expression in rat glial cell lines (218). Whether HIV TAT protein can upregulate class 1 antigen expression is unknown.

Class 1 expression by oligodendrocytes in brains from HIV-infected patients may have several explanations. IFN-γ, TNF-α, or both are present in the brains of patients with AIDS may upregulate class 1 antigen expression by oligodendrocytes. The absence of MHC antigen expression by astrocytes may have several explanations. TNF-α would not be expected to upregulate class 2 antigen expression by astrocytes but would be expected to upregulate class 1 MHC antigen expression. IFN-γ would be expected to upregulate both class 1 and 2 MHC antigen expression by astrocytes. It is possible that MHC antigen expression by astrocytes is downregulated by neurotransmitters, especially glutamate, which blocks the ability of IFN-γ and TNF-α to upregulate MHC gene expression (80,81,134,147). Soluble TAT protein released from HIV-infected mononuclear cells may act like HTLV-I TAX protein in upregulating class 1 antigen expression by neuroglia. Whatever the mechanism, upregulation of class 1 antigen expression by oligodendrocytes would render them susceptible to CD8+ cytotoxic T cells in the presence of the appropriate antigen.

Although *in vitro* studies suggest that astrocytes are facultative APCs, available evidence suggests that astrocytes do not act as APCs in either HIV infection of the CNS or in the opportunistic infections examined to date. These findings are consistent with other studies that have failed to detect class 2 antigen expression by astrocytes in other CNS infections (235).

Cytokines and the Regulation of Immune Responses in the CNS

Cytokines are a diverse set of molecules that are involved in regulation of immune responses (1,120,211). Cytokines participate in both antigen-nonspecific natural immunity and antigen-specific, acquired immunity. Cytokine actions are normally brief in duration. The limited time during which cytokines act are a result of the short half-life of cytokine mRNAs, the lack of stored cytokines, and the burst release of cytokines from cells. TGF-β requires posttranscriptional activation by extracellular proteolytic enzymes for release of active molecules.

Cytokines initiate their action by binding to specific receptors on the cell surface. Expression of many cytokine receptors is regulated by specific signals, many of which are either another or the same cytokine. Cytokines have extremely high affinities for their respective receptors, allowing very low concentrations of cytokines to elicit responses from target cells. The regulation of cytokine receptor expression by cytokines themselves provides for a regulatory network of positive or negative amplification of cytokine actions. The target cells for cytokines may be the same cell producing the cytokine (autocrine action), an adjacent cell (paracrine action), or cells distant from the cell of origin (endocrine action).

Cytokines demonstrate considerable redundancy and pleiotropism. Individual cytokines can act on many different cell types, including nonimmune cells. Cytokines also have multiple effects on the same target cells. In addition, different cytokines may have identical effects on the same target cells. The redundancy, pleiotropism, and regulation of cytokine synthesis by cytokine networks provides the molecular basis for cytokine cascades, resulting in both positive and negative regulatory circuits in the control of immune and inflammatory responses.

Cytokine Expression in the CNS

Cytokines are expressed by intrinsic cells of the CNS. Four cell types within the brain are possible sources of cytokine synthesis: microglia, macrophages, astrocytes,

TABLE 3. *Cytokine regulation of immune responses*

| | **Source of Cytokines** | | | |
Cytokine	Principal	CNS	Effects	CNS/HIV INF
Natural Immunity				
IFN1-α/β	Monocyte Macrophage	Astrocyte Endothelial cells	Inhibition of viral replication, ↑ NK cell lytic activity ↑ MHC class 1 expression	Absent
TNF-α	Monocyte Macrophage NK cells Mast Cells	Astrocyte Microglia	↑ Permeability of BBB ↑ ICAM-1 expression ↑ MHC expression ↑ cytokine synthesis	Macrophage Microglia Astrocyte
IL-1	Monocyte Macrophage		Macrophage activation ↑ ICAM expression ↑ IL-6 synthesis	Endotheital cells Microglia
Regulation of Acquired Immunity				
IL-6	Monocyte Macrophage T cells	Astrocyte Microglia Endothelial cells	Synthesis of acute phase reactants Glia cell proliferation ↑ Astrocyte synthesis of NGF	Endothelial cells Microglia
IL-8	Macrophages T cells	Endothelial cells Platelets	Leukocyte chemotaxis Leukocyte activation	Unknown
TGF-β	T cells Macrophage	Macroglia Microglia	Macrophage chemotaxis Macrophage activation; early Macrophage inhibition; late ↓ MHC antigen expression ↓ Inflammatory response ↓ Lymphocyte & NK cell activation Astrocyte & microglia proliferation	Diffuse and focal expression
IL-2	T cells	None	Growth and differentiation of lymphocytes and NK cells	Not detected
IL-4	CD4$^+$ T cells Mast cells	Mast cells	Generation of T_H2 T cells ↑ endothelial cell VCAM-1 expression ↑ inflammatory cell entry into CNS Macrophage chemotaxis	IL-4 mRNA present, ↓ in ADC
IL-8	Monocyte Macrophage T cells	Astrocytes Microglia Endothelial cells	B cell growth & differentiation ? Co-stimulator T cells	Endothelial and microglial cells
Regulation of Immune Mediated Inflammation				
IFN-γ	T cells	NK cells	Antiviral state Macrophage activation Lymphocyte differentiation Activates neutrophils ↑ NK cell cytotoxicity ↑ Endothelial cell CAMs Promotes T_H1 T cell and macrophage Inflammatory infiltrates	Endothelial cells Microglia
CSFs	T cells Macrophage, Fibroblasts	Astrocytes Endothelial cells	Growth and differentiation of stem cells	Unknown
LT	T cells	Astrocyte Microglia	Same as TNF-α	Similar distribution to IL-6
IL-10	T cells B cells Macrophages	Mast cells	Inhibits macrophage functions by ↓ regulation of cytokine synthesis by macrophages and ↓ class 2 and B7 antigen expression B cell activation	Unknown

TABLE 3. *(Continued)*

| | Source of Cytokines | | | |
Cytokine	Principal	CNS	Effects	CNS/HIV INF
IL-12	T cells B cells Monocytes	NK cells	↑ NK cell activity Differentiation of $T_H0 \rightarrow T_H1$ $\quad$ CF4$^+$ T cell subset Stimulates CD8 differention $\quad$ into functional cytotoxic T cells	Unknown
IL-5	T_H2 CD4$^+$ T $\quad$ cells Mast cells	?	Growth and differentiation of $\quad$ eosinophils Co-stimulator of B cells	Unknown

BBB, blood brain barrier; IFN,interferon; CSFs,colony stimulating factors; LT,lymphotoxin; ICAM, intracellular cell adhesion molecule; IL, interleukin; MHC, major histocompatibility complex; NGF, nerve growth factor; NK-natural killer; CAMs-cell adhesion molecules; TGF, transforming growth factor; TNF-tumor necrosis factor; VCAM, vascular cell adhesion molecule.

and endothelial cells. The synthesis of cytokines by intrinsic cells of the CNS will be discussed in relation to their immunoregulatory properties in natural and acquired immunity. In this regard, cytokines may be classified into (a) those mediating natural immunity elicited by infectious agents, (b) those regulating lymphocyte activation and differentiation after recognition of antigen, and (c) those regulating immune-mediated inflammation (1). Several cytokines participate in more than one aspect of the immune response (Table 3).

Cytokine-Mediated Regulation of Natural Immunity

Type 1 IFN (IFN1-α/β), TNF-α, IL-1, IL-6, and IL-8 participate in natural immune responses to infections. IFN1-α/β is produced during both natural and acquired immunity (1). The monocyte/macrophage is the principal cell type that synthesizes IFN-1α/β. In the CNS, IFN-1α/β has been reported to be synthesized by astrocytes infected with Newcastle disease virus and by cerebrovascular endothelial cells. IFN-α and -β bind the same receptor on target cells. IFN-1α/β inhibits virus replication through induction of a series of enzymes interfering with viral RNA and DNA replication. The antiviral action of IFN-1α is primarily paracrine on adjacent cells. IFN-1α/β also inhibits cell proliferation, increases the lytic potential of NK cells, and upregulates class 1 MHC antigen expression while downregulating class 2 antigen expression.

TNF-α participates in both the natural and acquired immune responses. TNF-α is released from activated mononuclear cells, NK cells, and mast cells after microbial infections. IFN-γ augments the synthesis of TNF-α from macrophages. In the CNS, astrocytes synthesize TNF-α in response to multiple stimuli, including IFN-γ, IL-1β, LPS, phorbol ester, and calcium ionophore (23,24,38). Astrocyte infection by Newcastle disease virus is also associated with synthesis of TNF-α (154,155). Microglia are also capable of synthesizing TNF-α. Mouse microglia produce TNF-α after treatment with LPS and IFN-γ (78). TNF-α mRNA is present in normal human microglia, and secretion of TNF-α by human microglia follows treatment with IFN-γ (284).

TNF-α has multiple effects on target cells, which can alter immune responses in the CNS. TNF-α enhances permeability of the BBB, induces ICAM-1 expression by endothelial cells, and increases lymphocyte and monocyte adhesion to endothelial cells (31,199,201). The close proximity of astrocyte foot processes to cerebrovascular endothelial cells suggests that TNF-α released by activated astrocytes may alter mononuclear cell adhesion and permeability at the cerebrovascular endothelial cell surface, thus increasing the inflammatory response. TNF-α upregulation of astroctye ICAM-1 expression also may contribute to the ability of astrocytes to act as APCs (79). Upregulation of class 1 antigen by TNF-α would render virus-infected astrocytes and endothelial cells recognizable by CD8 + cytotoxic T cells during acquired immune responses. TNF-α has mitogenic effects on astrocytes, which may contribute to the formation of astrocytosis and glial scars, which would provide a barrier to the spread of CNS infections (23,24,139,226). TNF-α also has antiviral effects similar to interferons.

TNF-α upregulates astrocyte synthesis of cytokines, which participate in natural and acquired immunity. Astrocytes treated with TNF-α upregulate expression of IL-6 (17,18,76). IL-6 has pleiotropic effects on the immune system, including stimulation of B cell growth and differentiation during the late stages of B cell maturation (263). TNF-α also upregulates astrocyte synthesis of the colony-stimulating factors granulocyte colony-stimulating factor (G-CSF) and GM-CSF (165). G-CSF and GM-CSF participate in regulation of immune-mediated inflammation by providing chemotactic stimuli for granulocytes and macrophages, promoting their survival at sites of inflammation, and upregulating their effector functions. GM-CSF may induce proliferation of activation of microglial cells (77). Astrocytes that synthesize TNF-α express high levels of TNF-α receptors. TNF-α also upregulates astrocyte TNF-α mRNA levels. These findings suggest that the regulation of TNF-α synthesis is regulated, in part, by a positive autocrine feedback loop (17).

IL-1 is a third cytokine participating in natural immune responses to infections. Mononuclear cells stimulated by microbial antigens or macrophage-derived cytokines, including IL-1 and TNF-α, are the principal source of IL-1. IL-1, like TNF-α, augments host inflammatory responses during natural immune responses. Inflammatory properties of IL-1 that contribute to natural immune responses include macrophage activation, increased endothelial cell adhesion molecule expression, and upregulation of IL-6 synthesis. IL-1 indirectly activates other inflammatory cells through upregulation of synthesis of other cytokines by mononuclear phagocytes and endothelial cells.

Low levels of IL-1 mRNA are constitutively expressed in normal brains (265). The highest levels of IL-1 mRNA are found in the hypothalamus, whereas low levels are present in the frontal cortex. IL-1 receptors are found extensively throughout the brain, especially in areas where neurons are densely packed, such as in granule cells of the dentate gyrus, pyramidal cells of the hippocampus, neurons of the oculomotor nucleus, and granule cells in the cerebellum (67). The widespread distribution of IL-1 receptors suggests that IL-1 could play a major role in neuroimmune responses.

Astrocytes, microglia, and endothelial cells have been shown to synthesize IL-1. Astrocytes synthesize IL-1 after LPS stimulation (165). Microglia express low levels of IL-1 mRNA that can be upregulated by IFN-γ treatment (284). The constitutive expression of IL-1 mRNA suggests that microglia are the likely source of IL-1 produced during the early phases of CNS infections. IL-1 synthesis by activated astrocytes appears to occur later. IL-1 upregulates its own synthesis by microglia and astrocytes. Thus, a positive paracrine regulatory loop is present between microglia and astrocytes.

IL-1 has pleiotropic effects on a wide range of target cells. IL-1, along with TNF-α, stimulates astrocyte proliferation and glial scars, which can limit the spread of CNS infections (86,88,90). IL-1 stimulates ICAM-1 expression by astrocytes and endothelial cells (79). IL-1 is also a strong inducer of synthesis of TNF-α, IL-6, and colony-stimulating factors by astrocytes (18,24,38,76,258,259). IL-1α treatment of glial cell cultures results in upregulation of TGF-β expression. Oligodendrocytes express higher levels of TGF-β than do astrocytes after treatment with IL-1α. The upregulation of TGF-β may provide a negative feedback loop for control of immune responses elicited by the synthesis and release of inflammatory cytokines (48,49).

IL-6, like TNF-α, is involved in both natural and antigen-specific immunity. IL-6 participates in natural immunity by stimulating synthesis of acute-phase reactants. IL-6 mRNA and protein expression is upregulated by cytokines (284,286). IL-6 synthesis is upregulated in macrophages, endothelial cells, and fibroblasts after treatment by IL-1 and, to a lesser extent, TNF-α. Both human astrocytes and microglia constitutively express IL-6 (266,284). Astrocytes, microglia, and endothelial cells can upregulate the synthesis of IL-6. IL-1, TNF-α, and IFN-γ upregulate astrocyte IL-6 synthesis (18,76,154,263). Upregulation of IL-6 synthesis also has been found to occur during infections of the CNS. Patients with meningococcal meningitis have increased CSF levels of IL-6 (58). Vesicular stomatitis virus infection of astrocytes results in upregulation of IL-6 synthesis, which can be detected in CSF (76).

Astrocyte proliferation follows treatment with IL-6. Thus, IL-6 may participate along with IL-1 and TNF-α in the development of astrocyte gliosis (226). Astrocytes also produce nerve growth factor when treated with IL-6. These findings suggest that IL-6 may have a protective effect on neurons during CNS inflammation. IL-6 may also be protective by downregulating TNF-α synthesis by microglia and astrocytes (17). The downregulation of astrocyte synthesis of TNF-α by IL-6 provides a negative regulatory circuit by which IL-6 released by astrocytes downregulates an important cytokine stimulus for its own synthesis.

Cytokines Regulating Lymphocyte Activation, Growth, and Differentiation

Of the four cytokines involved in regulation of the acquired immune response, IL-6, IL-4 and TGF-β are synthesized by cells in the CNS. IL-2 is involved in the activation and proliferation of T cells. IL-2 also supports growth and differentiation of B-lymphocytes. CD4+ T cells and, to a lesser extent, CD8+ T cells are major sources of IL-2 in immune reactions. There is no evidence that intrinsic cells of the CNS synthesize IL-2. The first appearance of IL-2 in the brains of Sindbis-infected mice occurs 3 days after infection, a time when significant T cell infiltration is occurring in the CNS (278). These findings support the lack of in situ synthesis of IL-2 by intrinsic cells of the CNS.

The primary sources of IL-4 are CD4+ T-lymphocytes and mast cells. During CNS infections with Sindbis virus, *in situ* synthesis of IL-4 appears before development of CD4+ T cell infiltration. These findings suggest that mast cells are the likely source for IL-4 mRNA present in Sindbis virus encephalitis early in the course of infection (278). IL-4 is a pivotal cytokine in inflammatory reactions. IL-4 participates in the generation of T_H2 T-helper/inducer cells and upregulation of VCAM-1 expression by endothelial cells and serves as a chemotactic signal for macrophages. The requirement of mast cells for optimal entry of mononuclear cells into the brain during inflammatory responses may be related to the ability to synthesize IL-4 (101,179,198,278).

T cells and macrophages are the primary cells synthesizing TGF-β. The effects of TGF-β on immune responses depends on the target cell type and its state of activation. Expression of TGF-β early in the immune responses initiates a cascade of events pivotal to immune-mediated inflammation and repair (267,268). The early effects of TGF-β occur mainly through indirect activation of immune effector cells. TGF-β provides an extremely potent chemotactic signal for recruitment of peripheral blood monocytes during the early stages of the immune response. TGF-β activates monocytes to synthesize inflammatory mediators, including IL-1, TNF-α, platelet-derived growth factor, and fibroblast growth factor. The negative regulatory properties of TGF-β occur mainly through downregulation of T- and B-cell proliferation and IFN-γ–induced class 2 MHC antigen expression. A negative autocrine and paracrine network exists where TGF-β downregulates its own synthesis by activated lymphocytes.

TGF-β_1 mRNA, but not protein, is constitutively expressed in normal brains (49,265,279). Astrocytes, oligodendrocytes, and microglia have been identified as intrinsic sources of TGF-β in the brain. IL-1α, but not IL-1β, upregulates TGF-β_1 protein expression by macroglia and microglia (48,49,279). Similar effects are seen in macrophages where only IL-1α upregulates TGF-β expression (275). Macroglial and microglial cell TGF-β_1 mRNA levels are unchanged by treatment with cytokines. These findings are consistent with posttranscriptional modification of TGF-β as a result of cytokine stimulation. Oligodendrocytes express higher levels of TGF-β_1 protein than do astrocytes. Unlike the negative feedback loop for TGF-β synthesis in lymphocytes, TGF-β stimulates its own synthesis by astrocytes using autocrine and paracrine networks in the brain (267).

TGF-β has multiple roles in inflammatory responses to infections of the CNS. TGF-β recruits macrophages and monocytes into areas of inflammation, downregulates other portions of the natural immune response including NK cell proliferation, and promotes wound healing. TGF-β_1 and -β_2 downregulate astrocyte class 2 MHC antigen expression after stimulation with IFN-γ (220,296). TGF-β stimulates astrocyte and microglia proliferation and microglial cell recruitment into areas of tissue injury (156,180,251). TGF-β, along with IL-1 and IL-6, promote healing by facilitating development of glial scars through inducing astrocyte proliferation. TGF-β has been shown to inhibit cerebral edema in experimental meningitis through an unknown mechanism (197).

Cytokines Regulating Immune-Mediated Inflammation

IFN-γ, colony-stimulating factors, LT, IL-10, IL-12, and migration inhibitory factor (MIF) regulate immune-mediated inflammation (1). IFN-γ is synthesized by naive T cells (T$_H$0), T$_H$1 CD4+ T-helper/inducer cells, nearly all CD8+ T cells, and NK cells. IFN-γ is not synthesized by intrinsic cells of the CNS. IFN-γ has pleiotropic effects on immune reactions. IFN-γ is the principal activator of macrophages. The cytokines GM-CSF, IL-1, and TNF-α, which can be produced by intrinsic cells of the CNS, act synergestically with IFN-γ in activating macrophages. IFN-γ upregulates expression of class 1 and 2 MHC antigens, promotes differentiation of T and B cells, activates neutrophils, increases NK cell cytolytic activity, activates vascular endothelial cell synthesis of cell adhesion molecules promoting leukocyte adhesion, and induces morphologic changes in endothelial cells that facilitate lymphocyte extravasation. The presence of IFN-γ in the brain during CNS infections is evidence that activated T cells, NK cells, or both have reached the CNS.

Colony-stimulating factors are synthesized by cerebrovascular endothelial cells and astrocytes. At least two colony-stimulating factors are produced by astrocytes. Resting astrocytes express mRNA for GM-CSF and G-CSF mRNA but do not synthesize the respective proteins (165). IL-1 and TNF-α treatment of human astrocytes results in expression of GM-CSF and G-CSF protein synthesis (4,77,258,259). Colony-stimulating factors can be proliferative factors for microglia and upregulate their phagocytic activity (78,86). GM-CSF also activates macrophages that have entered the CNS.

LT and TNF-α share many functions in immune responses. LT has a 30% homology with TNF-α, and both the LT and TNF-α genes are located within the MHC complex on chromosome 6. LT is produced by activated lymphocytes, often along with IFN-γ. Microglia and astrocytes appear to synthesize LT *in vivo* (224). LT and TNF-α have essentially the same effects on target cells. LT acts in a paracrine fashion to activate neutrophils. LT also upregulates cytokine synthesis and leukocyte adhesion by endothelial cells while promoting leukocyte extravasation across endothelial cell barriers.

IL-10 is produced by a T_H2 subset of CD4+ T-helper/inducer cells, some T_H1 T cells, and activated B cell macrophages. IL-10 may be produced by cells present in the CNS. IL-10 mRNA is present in the brains of mice with Sindbis encephalitis before the occurrence of lymphocyte infiltration (278). Human astrocytes and microglia are known not to produce IL-10 (284). Perivascular mast cells appear to be the most likely source of IL-10 synthesis within the CNS during viral infections. IL-10 inhibits the synthesis of cytokines by macrophages, including TNF-α and IL-12. IL-10 also downregulates macrophage ability to present antigen to immunocompetent lymphocytes. IL-10 is involved in activation of resting B-lymphocytes.

Synthesis of IL-5 and IL-12 by macroglia or microglia has not been described. IL-5 is produced by T_H2 T-helper/inducer lymphocytes and activated mast cells. IL-5 regulates growth and differentiation of eosinophils and acts as a costimulator of B cells along with IL-2, IL-4, and IL-10. IL-12 is synthesized by T- and B-lymphocytes, NK cells, and monocytes. IL-12 is a potent inducer of IFN-γ synthesis by NK cells, participates in the differentation of T_H0 to T_H1 CD4+ helper/inducer T cell subsets, and stimulates differentiation of CD8+ T cells into functionally active cytotoxic T-lymphocytes. Only IL-5 may possibly be produced within the CNS by release from activated perivascular mast cells.

Cytokine Expression in the CNS During HIV Infection

Most studies examining the role of cytokines in HIV infection have concentrated on their possible role in the pathogenesis of HIV-1–associated dementia complex. Here we discuss the possible role of cytokines in modifying neuroimmune responses to opportunistic infections (Table 3).

An ideal immune response to CNS infections results in clearing of the infectious agent while protecting neuronal function and viability (279). The cytokine profile present in the brains of patients with HIV infection suggests a state of chronic immune activation that is present regardless of whether the patient has any neurologic disease (260,261). IL-1 is found on virtually all endothelial cells. IL-1 staining is also found on cells in the perivascular region. Stellate cells with the appearance of ameboid microglia occasionally stain for IL-1. Rarely, non–process-bearing cells stained for IL-1. TNF-α is primarily found on stellate parenchymal cells with the morphology of microglia or macrophages. Rarely, TNF-α is found on endothelial cells and astrocytes. The distribution of IFN-γ is similar to that of IL-1. Endothelial cells and stellate parenchymal cells resembling microglia most frequently stain for IFN-γ. IL-6 is found on cerebrovascular endothelial cells and occasional stellate parenchymal cells. LT is found in a similar distribution to IL-6. Fewer cells stain for LT compared with the number staining for IL-6. TGF-β_1 is detected throughout the brain of individuals with AIDS who are dying with or without neurologic diseases (47,48). TGF-β_1 expression correlates with the presence of IL-1. Astrocytes, oligodendrocytes, microglia, and multinucleated giant cells stain for TGF-β_1. In areas of multinucleated giant cells and microglia, the release of soluble TAT protein may upregulate TGF-β expression by glial cells (44).

Cytokine mRNA expression also has been examined in the brains of patients with AIDS with and without dementia (279). TGF-β mRNA is present in the subcortical white matter of most brains. The levels of mRNA for TNF-α, LIF, IL-1β, and IL-6 are more variable. TNF-α mRNA levels are significantly higher in the brains from demented patients compared with those without dementia. IL-1 mRNA levels are consistently lower in patients with dementia. Differences in the levels of mRNA levels for LIF, IL-6, TGF-β_1, or TGF-β_2 do not differ in the brains from patients with and without AIDS-related dementia. IL-2 and IL-10 mRNA are undetectable in the brains of patients with AIDS. IL-4 mRNA expression occurs in nondemented patients but is absent in those with HIV-1–associated dementia. IFN-γ mRNA is variably detected in the brains of patients with AIDS and correlates with the presence of the macrophage cytokine MIG-2.

The presence of increased TNF-α and decreased levels of expression for both IL-4 and IL-1 in patients with AIDS with dementia suggest that the normal coexpression of TNF-α mRNA and IL-1 mRNA and the respective monocyte cytokines are dissociated in the brains of patients with AIDS dementia (279). The absence of IL-4 mRNA, produced by T_H2 CD4 + helper/inducer T cells, CD8 + T cells, and possibly mast cells, in the brains of patients with AIDS with dementia may contribute to the pathogenesis of HIV-related neurologic disease because IL-4 suppresses macrophage activation and downregulates activated macrophage TNF-α expression (63,110,118,149,288).

The cytokine profile present in the brains of patients with AIDS suggests that a number of important cytokines involved in immune responses are either present in low concentrations or not expressed at all. Cytokine profiles found in the brains of HIV-infected patients may be ineffective in protecting against infections of the CNS. In experimental viral encephalitis, IL-1β, IL-4, IL-6, IL-10, LT, and TGF-β mRNAs are synthesized before the onset of the inflammatory response in the CNS (278). In patients with AIDS, TNF-α and IL-6, involved in natural immune responses, are present in the brain. The level of IL-1 mRNA is reduced, and IFN-1α/β appears not to be present. Thus, of the cytokines studied, two of the four involved in natural immune responses are absent or in low concentrations. IL-2, IL-4, IL-6, and TGF-β are involved in the regulation of lymphocyte activation and differentiation during immune responses to foreign antigens. IL-4 mRNA is markedly reduced in the brains of patients with AIDS who also have dementia, and IL-2 mRNA is not present at all. IL-6 and TGF-β are present. These findings suggest that the widespread distribution of TGF-β may downregulate immune responses to opportunistic infections, including antigen-specific and natural immunity. IL-6 may contribute to B cell responses to opportunistic infections by promoting B cell growth and differentiation. However, IL-6 also may contribute to the development of PML by activating JC virus replication in activated B cells that enter the CNS (121). Immune-mediated inflammation is dependent on the presence of IFN-γ, colony-stimulating factor, LT, IL-10, IL-12, and MIF. IFN-γ and LT are found in the brains of patients with AIDS. IL-10 mRNA is undetectable. The remaining cytokines have not been studied. The partial expression of some, but not all, cytokines involved in immune-mediated inflammatory responses may impair host responses to opportunistic infections. Studies of the expression of cytokines in the brains of patients with AIDS with opportunistic infections and lymphoma may help clarify the role of intrinsic cytokine expression in neuroimmune responses in AIDS.

The cytokine profiles present in the brains of HIV-infected patients may have other effects on the pathogenesis of neurologic disease. Cytokines are usually expressed in bursts of short periods. Chronic upregulation of cytokine expression for long periods and at high levels may result in pathologic changes in target cells, i.e., the cytotoxic effects of TNF-α on oligodendrocytes. If IL-4 and IL-10 levels are decreased in patients with opportunistic viral infections, the immune response to these infections may be altered. Of the five cytokines involved in natural immune responses to infections, TNF-α, IL-1, and IL-6 are present in the brains of HIV-infected patients. These findings suggest that antigen-nonspecific natural immune responses may play a role in controlling some opportunistic infections. However, the high level of TGF-β expression in the brains of patients with AIDS may impair NK cell and macrophage activity, thus impairing natural immune responses. IL-6, which is involved in both natural immunity and lymphocyte activation and differentiation, is present in the brains of patients with AIDS. However, IL-4 levels appear to be variable, and their is no information on the levels of IL-2, IL-4, and TGF-β during opportunistic infections. Both LT and IFN-γ, which are involved in immune-mediated inflammatory responses, are present in the brains of HIV-infected patients. The failure to mount a significant immune-mediated inflammatory response in these patients may be the result of declining levels of immunocompetent lymphocytes and changes in antigen presentation at the level of the BBB. Expression of IL-10 mRNA has been shown to be associated with recovery from experimental viral encephalitis (132,228). The absence of IL-10 expression, which is involved in immune-mediated inflammatory responses, may further impair host resistance in opportunistic infections.

AUTOIMMUNE DISEASES OF THE NERVOUS SYSTEM

A number of illnesses encountered during the course of HIV infection result from autoimmune disorders (Table 4). Autoimmune diseases have been associated with a variety of viral infections, including the retroviruses equine infectious anemia, faprine arthritis encephalitis virus, visna, and HTLV-I (50). The most common autoantibodies associated with virally induced autoimmune diseases react with nervous system antigens (247). Autoimmune diseases occurring during HIV infection may be related to (a) polyclonal B cell activation leading to the synthesis of autoantibodies,

TABLE 4. *HIV related autoimmune diseases of the nervous system*

Disease	Proposed immunopathogenesis
Neuromuscular disease	
Inflammatory demyelinating neuropathies	Declining $CD4^+$ and $CD8^+$ T immunoregulatory cells
Mononeuritis multiplex	$T_H1 \rightarrow T_H2$ $CD4^+$ helper/inducer T cells
Myasthenia gravis	Loss of T_H0 naive T cells
	$DR5^+$, $DR3^+$ MHC phenotype
Inflammatory myopathies	$CD8^+ > CD4^+$ cell infiltrates
	↑ myocyte class 1 MHC expression
Cerebrovascular diseases	
Intracranial hemorrhage	Autoimmune thrombocytopenia
CNS vasculitis	↑ T_H2 $CD4^+$ helper/inducer T cells
	Eosinophilic vasculitis
TIA/stroke	? anticardiolipin/antiphospholipid antibody
Multiple sclerosis	Oligodendrocyte expression of HSP 70
	↑ γ/δ cytotoxic T cells
	HHV-6 infection
Dementia	Anti-brain antigen antibodies

MHC, major histocompatibility complex; TIA, transient ischemic attack; HSP, 70-heat shock protein 70; HHV, human herpesvirus.

(b) upregulation of class 2 MHC antigen expression on professional and facultative APCs, (c) coating of uninfected cells with viral proteins such as glycoprotein (gp)120 and gp41, and (d) shared epitopes between HIV and host cell antigens (molecular mimicry) (50).

Autoantibodies are commonly found in HIV-infected patients (168,181,182). IgG antibodies reacting with double-stranded DNA, synthetic peptides of ubiquitinated histone H2A, SM-D antigen, U1-A RNP antigen, and 60-kDa SSA/Ro antigen are found in high titers in 44–85% of sera tested from HIV-infected patients (182). The presence or level of autoantibodies do not correlate with the stage of HIV infection or presence of disease. Autoantibodies directed against ubiquitinated histones are associated with apoptosis of regulatory T-lymphocytes which may, at least in part, contribute to the development of autoimmunity in HIV infection.

The initiating event leading to autoimmune disorders is likely HIV infection of monocytes/macrophages (181). HIV infection of monocytes is followed by upregulation of cytokine production, i.e., IL-1 and IL-6, which leads to activation of CD4 + T-helper/inducer cells and B-lymphocytes. TNF-α and LT are also secreted by HIV-infected macrophages and can activate CD8 + T-cytotoxic cells directed against self antigens. Increased synthesis of IFN-γ by lymphocytes, activated NK cells, or macrophages also can contribute to autoimmune diseases by upregulating class 2 antigen expression on T cells and APCs. Autoantibodies directed against CD8 + T-cytotoxic/suppresser cells are present and may lead to death of CD8 + regulatory T cells. CD8 + regulatory T cells are also killed by antilymphocyte antibodies that result from molecular mimicry between the shared domains of gp120 and CD8 lymphocyte antigens. Immune complexes of autoantibodies and self antigens may modulate CD8 + and B-lymphocyte functions through binding to cell surface Fc receptors.

Most autoimmune disorders of the nervous system in HIV-infected patients involve the peripheral nervous system, neuromuscular junction, or muscle. In addition, cerebrovascular diseases, myasthenia gravis, an MS-like syndrome, and HIV-1–associated dementia have been proposed as diseases associated with autoimmune reactions.

Neuromuscular Diseases

Acute, subacute, and chronic inflammatory demyelinating polyneuropathies have been encountered in patients with HIV infection (143). The onset of an inflammatory demyelinating neuropathy may be the initial illness leading to the diagnosis of HIV infection. The demyelinating polyneuropathies associated with HIV infection are associated with abnormalities of leukocyte trafficking in the CSF as evidenced by the presence of a CSF pleocytosis, which is not present in demyelinating polyneuropathies from other causes. The pathological changes are typical of those found in other inflammatory neuropathies. Peripheral nerves are infiltrated with CD8 + suppressor T cells and macrophages (54). HIV has not been found in pathologic specimens. The response of HIV patients to plasmapharesis, steroids, and intravenous Ig lends further support to the autoimmune nature of the demyelinating polyneuropathies (30,143).

Mononeuritis multiplex involving cranial, peripheral, or spinal nerves has been attributed to either immune complex deposition or vasculitis (84,232). Eosinophil infiltration has been reported in cases of mononeuritis multiplex associated with vasculitis. The switch of CD4 + T-helper/inducer cells from the T_H1 to T_H2 subsets may play a role in the development of eosinophilic vasculitis of peripheral nerves because T_H2 CD4-helper/inducer T cells are associated with recruitment of eosinophils into areas of inflammation (39).

Myasthenia gravis has been reported in HIV-infected patients (185,206,277). The disease is no different than that found in HIV-seronegative patients. In one patient, symptoms of myasthenia improved as the CD4 + T cell counts decreased and antibody titers to the acetylcholine receptor decreased (185). The investigators suggested that preferential loss of CD4 + /CD45R + naive (T_H0) T cells may have been responsible for unmasking antigen-specific autoreactive memory cells specific to epitopes on the acetylcholine receptor. Loss of naive T-lymphocytes has been reported in other autoimmune diseases. However, in HIV infection CD4 + /CD45RO + memory T-lymphocytes appear to be the first T cell subsets lost (104,262). If loss of CD45R + naive T cells is associated with autoimmunity in HIV infection, these findings may explain the relative rarity of myasthenia-like syndromes and other autoimmune diseases during the course of HIV infection. The patient's MHC phenotype may be an additional factor contributing to the development of myasthenia in this patient. The patient reported by Nath et al. had both DR3 + and DR5 + class 2 MHC alleles. DR5 positivity is more frequently encountered in HIV-infected patients than in normal seronegative control patients, and the DR3 + class 2 antigen is associated with myasthenia gravis in HIV-seronegative patients (212,238). The unique MHC phenotype of this patient also may have contributed to the development of a myasthenia gravis–like syndrome. A pseudo-myasthenic syndrome restricted to the ocular muscles has been associated with IFN-α treatment of Kaposi's sarcoma (206).

The similarities between HIV-1–related polymyositis and idiopathic polymyositis suggest that autoimmunity is involved in the pathogenesis of inflammatory myopathies in HIV-infected patients (122,232). CD8 + T cells and macrophages are the predominant cell types found in endomysial inflammatory infiltrates in both HIV-seropositive and -seronegative patients with polymyositis (61,221). The percentage of CD4 + T cells in inflammatory infiltrates is reduced in HIV-related inflammatory myositis. The reduced percentage of CD4 + T cells in HIV-related inflammatory myopathies is likely the result of changes in T-lymphocyte subsets in HIV infection

(61,209). The reduced number of CD4 + T cells in HIV-related inflammatory myopathies also may reflect decreasing numbers of T_H1 helper/inducer T cells that are responsible for delayed hypersensitivity reactions (39). Recruitment of activated CD8 + T cells in inflammatory myopathies likely follows upregulation of MHC class 1 antigen expression found on muscle cells undergoing T cell invasion. Upregulation of MHC class 1 antigen expression in polymyositis does not appear to be related to interferons that have not been detected in areas of MHC antigen expression in either HIV-related on -unrelated inflammatory myopathies (61,122). In patients with HIV-related inflammatory myopathies, increased class 1 antigen expression may be secondary to circulating TNF-α, IL-1, or both.

Cerebrovascular Diseases

Cerebrovascular diseases have multiple causes in HIV-infected patients (19). Intracranial hemorrhage has been associated with thrombocytopenia that results from antiplatelet antibodies (269). CNS vasculitis also has been described in HIV-infected patients. In several of these, an eosinophilic vasculitis is present on biopsy (222,264). The occurrence of an eosinophilic vasculitis may be related to the switch from T_H1 to T_H2 CD4 + T-helper/inducer cells known to occur during the course of HIV infection (39).

The CNS is rich in phospholipids and antiphospholipid antibodies have been implicated in the pathogenesis of a wide range of neurologic diseases, including stroke, chorea, dementia, seizures, headache, and acute demyelinating polyneuropathy (152). These findings suggest that the occurrence of these antibodies may play a role in neurologic diseases in HIV-infected patients. Antiphospholipid antibody/anticardiolipin antibodies have been proposed as a possible mechanism for stroke and TIA occurring in HIV-infected patients. However, studies of the antiphospholipid antibody/anticardiolipin antibodies in HIV-infected patients have shown that these antibodies are frequently present and have not been associated with a particular neurologic syndrome. Serum anticardiolipin antibody (ACA) is present in up to 50% of all HIV-infected patients (22,246). In one study, IgG ACA was the most common autoantibody found. The prevalence of ACA did not differ either in relation to HIV risk factors or U.S. Centers for Disease Control and Prevention (CDC) stage of disease (22). Patients with ACA do have higher titers of other autoantibodies, including anti-i and anti-single and –double-stranded DNA antibodies, as well as increases in circulating immune complexes. There are no significant differences in ACA IgM antibody titers between HIV-1–infected patients and seronegative matched controls. *In situ* synthesis of ACA occurs in the CSF of many HIV-infected patients (32). However, only one of the HIV-infected patients had symptoms of the antiphospholipid syndrome, i.e., thrombocytopenia. The incidence of stroke and TIA is not increased in patients with ACA antibodies. An association of ACA and opportunistic infections also has been proposed. However, the prevalence of ACA in asymptomatic HIV-1–infected patients and the lack of correlation with CDC stages of HIV infection suggest that ACA is not a predictor of opportunistic infections or progression to AIDS. As yet, there is no firm evidence that autoantibodies to cardiolipin/phospholipid are involved in neurologic diseases occurring in HIV-infected patients.

MS-like Syndrome

Reports of MS in HIV-infected patients have been one of the more interesting associations of an autoimmunity and HIV infection. Berger initially reported an MS-like syndrome in seven patients with HIV infection (20). All patients fulfilled the criteria of definite MS. Four patients developed MS before their HIV infection, whereas in the other three the diagnosis of HIV infection was made either concurrently or within 3 months of onset of MS. Pathologic findings in three of these patients confirmed the diagnosis of MS. Multinucleated giant cells, microglial nodules, and astrocytosis found in HIV-1–associated encephalopathy were not present. In all seven patients, the MS-like syndrome followed a florid course. Two other HIV-infected patients with fulminating MS-like leukoencephalopathy died within 2 months of the onset of their neurologic disease (95). In a subsequent report, Berger reported a 33-year-old man with a steroid-responsive, relapsing, and remitting leukoencephalopathy pathologically consistent with MS (21). We have encountered a patient with AIDS who developed a subacute progressive cerebellar syndrome with pathologic features of MS (Houff, submitted for publication). Heat shock protein (HSP)70 was present in oligodendrocytes and astrocytes at the edges of the lesions. τ/δ T-lymphocytes were scattered throughout the lesion and in perivascular cuffs.

The pathogenesis of an MS-like illness in HIV-infected patients is unknown. A direct relationship between the MS-like illness and HIV infection has been postulated because no other infections agent was detected after extensive study at autopsy. The association of MS with HIV infection may be serendipitous in some patients. However, the temporal association of MS-like illness with seroconversion for HIV-1 infection in a significant number of the reported patients suggests an association between the two illnesses. The possibility that τ/δ T cells are involved in the pathogenesis of MS in HIV-infected patients is supported by previous findings of τ/δ T cells in demyelinating lesions and CSF of patients with MS (177,225,290). Peripheral blood τ/δ T cells lyse human oligodendrocytes in the context of expression of HSPs (74,75).

Changes in τ/δ T-lymphocytes have been described in HIV infection. Early in the course of HIV infection, significant increases are found in the number of τ/δ T cells (28). The increase in τ/δ T cells is associated with an increase in the percentage of τ/δ T cells mediating T-lymphocyte cytotoxicity (16). The presence of τ/δ T cells in the CSF of patients with HIV-1 infection support the ability of τ/δ T cells to enter the CNS either across the BBB or CSF–blood barrier (193). HIV-1–infected mononuclear cells undergo upregulation of the expression of HSPs, a putative target for τ/δ T cells (200). τ/δ cytotoxic T cells lyse HIV-infected mononuclear cells expressing HSPs. HHV-6–infected target cells, including lymphocytes, are also lysed by τ/δ cytotoxic T-lymphocytes (161). This finding is of interest in view of the recent report of HHV-6 infection of oligodendrocytes, astrocytes, microglia, and neurons in children with AIDS encephalopathy (213). The decline in τ/δ T cells during the progression of HIV infection may explain the rarity of MS-like illness late in the course of HIV infection (114).

Antibrain Antibodies

Several investigators have reported autoantibodies to brain proteins in HIV-infected patients. Kumar et al. reported serum antibodies reactive to brain proteins in

14 of 18 patients with AIDS dementia and in four of 12 without neuropsychological abnormalities (137). Serum antibrain antibodies reacted to an unidentified brain protein with a molecular weight of 45,000–50,000 kDa. Trujillo reported finding antibrain antibodies in one third of all HIV-infected patients with and without dementia (254). Antibrain autoantibodies were also found in seronegative controls and in a patient with juvenile rheumatoid arthritis. However, in one patient with HIV encephalopathy, autoantibodies recognized a 50-kDa brain protein similar to that reported by Kumar. Monoclonal antibodies to the HIV-1 gp120 V3 loop, which cross-react with human brain antigens, did not block the reaction to the 50-kDa brain protein (253). Autoantibodies to a 125-kDa antigen from human fetal brain have been found in four of 49 HIV-infected patients with neurologic complications, MS patients, and normal controls. Antibodies recognizing an astrocyte-specific antigen are found in patients with dementia and vacuolar myelopathy but not in HIV-infected patients without neurologic disease or in seronegative controls (291). The astrocyte antigen shares a common determinant with the gp41 antigen of HIV-1, suggesting that molecular mimicry may explain, in part, the presence of these autoantibodies. Antibodies to myelin basic protein also have been reported in the CSF of patients with AIDS dementia (168). The importance of antibrain antibodies in the pathogenesis of neurologic diseases in patients with HIV infection is not clear. Further studies are needed to determine whether they participate in the pathogenesis of neurologic disease or are a secondary result of tissue destruction and release of self antigens from other causes.

IMMUNOLOGY OF OPPORTUNISTIC INFECTIONS OF THE CNS IN AIDS

In this section, we consider the immunologic features of opportunistic infections occurring in patients with HIV infection. The discussion is limited to immunologic responses to these diseases and how HIV infection alters patients immune response within the CNS to these diseases (Table 5).

Opportunistic infections of the CNS, with the exception of cryptococcal meningitis,

TABLE 5. *HIV-related neurologic infections*

Disease	Proposed immunopathogenesis
Toxoplasma encephalitis	↓ T_H1 CD4$^+$ helper/inducer T cells ↓ NK cell cytotoxicity IL-6 down-regulation of IFN-γ macrophage activation
Cytomegalovirus encephalitis	↓ Antiviral antibody Activation CD8$^+$ T suppressor cells ↓ T_H1 CD4$^+$ helper/inducer T cells ↓ T cell proliferation A2D44, B51 or DR7 MHC phenotype
Progressive multifocal leukoencephalopathy	? Polyclonal B cell activation ? ↓ T_H1 CD4$^+$ helper/inducer T cells ? Altered macrophage functions ? Loss of T memory cells
Cryptococcal meningitis	↓ CD4$^+$ helper/inducer T cells ↑ CD8$^+$ T suppressor cells ↓ NK cell activity ↓ Macrophage fungistatic activity

NK, natural killer; IL, 6-interleukin 6; MHC, major histocompatibility complex.

usually follow reactivation of latent infections. Reactivation of latent infections suggests that defects in immunoregulation and immune surveillance are the principal immunologic deficits leading to the development of opportunistic infections.

Toxoplasma Encephalitis

Toxoplasma encephalitis in patients with AIDS results mainly, if not exclusively, from reactivation of latent brain infection with *T. gondii* (289). T-lymphocytes are important in host resistance to primary *T. gondii* infection and control of latent infections (5). CD4+ and CD8+ T cells protect against toxoplasmosis (82). Natural immunity is also involved. Macrophages, NK cells, and lymphokine-activated killer (LAK) cells all have been shown to be involved in resistance to experimental infection with *T. gondii* (13,51,231). Depletion of CD4+ T cells during acute experimental infection results in deficient cell-mediated and humoral immunity to toxoplasma infection and disseminated disease (51,289). CD8+ T cells are directly cytotoxic to *T. gondii*–infected cells. CD8+ T cells also release cytokines, especially IFN-γ, which are protective against *T. gondii* infection (7,82). NK and LAK cells lyse *T. gondii*–infected cells. NK cells are also capable of killing extracellular *T. gondii* (51). Humoral immunity to *T. gondii* oocysts and sporozoites alone does not provide significant protection against virulent toxoplasma infections. Humoral immunity does provide limited protection against less virulent strains of *T. gondii* (192). Cytokines provide significant protection against *T. gondii* infection. IFN-γ is the major cytokine involved in protection against toxoplasmosis (13,51,82,231). TNF-α is important for IFN-γ activation of macrophage inhibition of *T. gondii* replication and paracidal activity (144). The presence of IL-6 is detrimental in experimental *T. gondii* infections. *T. gondii* replication in macrophages is increased treated with IL-6 (12). IL-6 appears to inhibit the ability of IFN-γ–treated macrophages to kill intracellular tachizoites.

Reactivation of *T. gondii* during the course of HIV infection probably results from several alterations in systemic and CNS immune functions. The experimental evidence that depletion of CD4+ T cells leads to an inability to control *T. gondii* infection during the course of HIV infection is illustrated by the experimental findings that depletion of CD4+ T cells results in loss of protection against *Toxoplasma* infection. The loss of T-lymphocyte memory cells and, especially, CD4+ T_H1 helper/inducer cells during the progression of HIV infection eliminates the CD4+ subset responsible for resistance to intracellular parasites and which secrete IFN-*ars (39,209). The need for other effector cells for resistance to toxoplasmosis is affected by immunologic abnormalities occurring in HIV infection. T_H1 helper/inducer cells trigger phagocyte-mediated host defenses important in the resistance to intracellular parasites. HIV infection of macrophages results in impaired intracellular antimicrobial activity that further impairs the ability of macrophages to kill tachyoites of *T. gondii* (8,39). NK cell cytotoxicity is also reduced in HIV-infected patients (209). Finally, the increase in IL-6 expression in the brains of HIV-infected patients may reduce the ability of IFN-*ars to effectively activate macrophage antiparasitic activity (261,279).

CMV

CMV infection in HIV-infected patients is almost invariably the result of reactivation of latent infection or reinfection. Immunity to CMV involves both humoral and cell-mediated aspects of the immune system (293). Antibody to CMV antibody can directly neutralize the virus or participate in antibody-dependent cell cytotoxicity and complement-mediated cytolysis of infected cells. During primary infection, cell-mediated immunity is depressed, as evidenced by the poor response to stimulation, and other herpesvirus antigens. CMV strongly stimulates CD8 + totoxic/ suppressor cells. The majority of cytotoxic T-lymphocytes recognize immediate early regulatory proteins involved in CMV replication. NK cells can lyse CMV-infected cells undergoing virus replication. CMV infection results in upregulation of the expression of ICAM-1 and LFA-3 *in vitro* and VCAM-1 and VLA-4 by endothelial cells and leukocytes *in vivo* (103,136). CMV antigens stimulate high FA-1 and ICAM-1 by CD4 + CD45RO + and CD8 + CD45RO + mory cells (123). CMV downregulates MHC class 1 antigen expression (103).

Impairment of several immune functions may result in reactivation or reinfection with CMV in HIV-infected patients (293). Declining levels of CMV antibodies impair antibody-mediated effector cell functions in controlling CMV infection. Impairment of the cytolytic activity of NK cells further impair the ability to kill cells undergoing CMV replication. Reactivation of CMV during the course of AIDS likely further impairs host cell immunity through its immunosuppression of cell-mediated immunity by activating CD8 + suppressor cells. Downregulation of class 1 MHC antigen expression by CMV would render cells unrecognizable by remaining T-cytotoxic cells (103). The loss of memory T cells and the T_H1 CD4 + helper/inducer lymphocytes also likely explain the occurrence of CMV retinitis and encephalitis late in the course of HIV infection (123). Patients who develop CMV retinitis and encephalitis have decreased T cell proliferation to CMV antigens before developing significant immunosuppression (221). Patients who failed to develop a proliferative response to CMV antigens had at least one of three MHC alleles, A2B44, B51, or DR7. These results suggest that the HLA phenotype of HIV-infected patients may predispose them to the development of reactivation of CMV and may provide a means of determining which patients are at risk.

PML

PML follows JC virus infection of neuroglial cells. The site of JC virus latency remains uncertain, with the brain, B-lymphocytes, and kidney proposed as possible sites of virus reactivation. Serum antibody to JC virus is present in the majority of the population (164). Antigen-specific cell-mediated immunity has not been studied. Patients with PML have been shown to have reduced T cell proliferation to mitogens, suggesting cellular immune deficiencies that lead to reactivation of JC virus replication. The immune response to PML consist primarily of macrophage infiltration of demyelinating lesions, regardless of the underlying disease. Perivascular infiltration with T cells, B cells, and macrophages is seen in patients with less severe immunodeficiencies.

The site of JC virus latency is likely to determine, at least in part, which aspects of the immune system are important in preventing PML (164). If JC virus latency occurs in the brain or kidney, reduction in T-lymphocyte surveillance through the loss of T memory cells and T_H1 CD4 + helper/inducer T cells are likely to contribute to reactivation of latent infection (39,123). Because macrophages are the primary immune effector cell response in PML, the impairment of antibody-dependent cell cytotoxicity, intracellular antimicrobicidal activity, reduced respiratory burst, and reduction in the synthesis of antiviral type 1 IFN synthesis may contribute to the extensive demyelinating lesions often found in patients with AIDS (8). The presence of IL-6 in the brains of HIV-infected patients also may effect the immune functions of macrophages in PML lesions.

Several reports suggest that JC virus may be latent in B cells (121). If this proves to be the case, several changes in immune functions in HIV-infected patients may be responsible for reactivation and promote entry of infected B cells into the brain. Polyclonal B cell activation that occurs in HIV-infected patients may secondarily reactivate JC virus as a result of loss of regulation of B-lymphocyte growth and differentiation. The switch to T_H2 CD4+ helper/inducer T cells, which promote B cell differentiation, also may play a role (39). The presence of IL-6 in the brains of HIV-infected patients provides cytokine support for B cell growth and differentiation (261,279).

Cryptococcal Meningitis

Cell-mediated immunity is the primary arm of the immune system protecting against infection with *Cryptococcus neoformans*. Cryptococcal meningitis rarely develops until there is significant depletion of CD4+ T cells, usually with counts of <100 cells/mm^3 (42). Activated macrophages in the CSF are fungostatic and correlate with recovery in experimental infections (94). The polysaccharide capsule of *C. neoformans* induces proliferation of CD8+ T-suppressor cells. NK cells also have been shown to participate in elimination of the initial infection (56). Humoral immunity plays a secondary role in resistance to cryptococcal meningitis. IgG antibody to cryptococcal capsule is opsonizing for heavily encapsulated organisms via the classical complement pathway (174). In the nonimmune host, infection with poorly encapsulated organisms activates the alternate complement pathway. Antibody-mediated killing of *C. neoformans* by monocytes/macrophages has been described, and *C. neoformans* antibody titers, especially in the CSF, correlate with outcome.

Cryptococcal meningitis in patients with AIDS follows dissemination of primary infection of the lung. Host cell immunity contributes to the formation of *C. neoformans* capsules. Patients with severe cell-mediated immune deficiencies experience disease from poorly encapsulated organisms. Poorly encapsulated cryptococci are commonly isolated from the CSF of patients with AIDS (27). This most likely impairs phagocytosis and leads to early dissemination and inability to clear infection from the CSF. Decreasing antibody titers during the stages of HIV infection may decrease levels of opsonizing antibodies. The impaired fungostatic functions of HIV-infected macrophages are also likely to lead to inability to clear cryptococci from the CSF (209). Finally, the decreased cytolytic activity of NK cells as HIV infection progresses is also likely to impair patients with AIDS immune responses during cryptococcal meningitis.

CONCLUSIONS

In this review, we have used the current understanding of neuroimmunology to examine alterations in immune reactions to neurologic diseases in patients with HIV infection. HIV infection renders the patient susceptible to CNS disease through a variety of mechanisms. In patients with HIV infection, both the systemic immune system and the immunologic functions of intrinsic cells of the nervous system are impaired, leading to failure to mount the appropriate immune response to infections of the nervous system. The autoimmune changes occurring during the course of HIV infection also lead to diseases of the neurovascular and neuromuscular systems. Future studies examining the role of the cells of the BBB, microglia, and macroglia in response to infections of the nervous system should lead to a better understanding of how HIV infection can alter the immune functions in the nervous system.

REFERENCES

1. Abbas AK, Lichtman AH, Pober JS. *Cellular and Molecular Immunology*. Philadelphia: Saunders, 1994:240–260.
2. Achim CL, Morey MK, Wiley CA. Expression of major histocompatibility complex and HIV antigens within the brains of AIDS patients. *AIDS* 1991;5:535–541.
3. Achim CL, Wiley CA. Expression of major histocompatibility complex antigens in the brains of patients with progressive multifocal leukoencephalopathy. *J Neuropathol Exp Neurol* 1992;51: 257–263.
4. Alosisi F, Borsellino G, Samoggia P, et al. Astrocytic cultures from human embryonic brain: characterization and modulation of surface molecules by inflammatory cytokines. *J Neurosci Res* 1992; 32:494–506.
5. Araujo FG. Depletion of CD4+ T cells but not inhibition of the protective activity of IFN-γ prevents cure of toxoplasmosis mediated by drug therapy in mice. *J Immunol* 1992;149:3003–3007.
6. Askenase PW, Van Loveren H. Delayed-type hypersensitivity: activation of mast cells by antigen-specific T cell factors initiates the cascade of cellular interactions. *Immunol Today* 1983;4:259–264.
7. Auzuki Y, Orellana MA, Schreiber RD, Remington JS. Interferon-γ: the major mediator or resistance against *Toxoplasma gondii*. *Science* 1988;240:516–518.
8. Baldwin GC, Fleischmann J, Chung Y, et al. Human immunodeficiency virus causes mononuclear phagocyte dysfunction. *Proc Natl Acad Sci U S A* 1990;87:3933–3937.
9. Banti RB, Gehrmann J, Schubert P, Kreutzberg GW. Cytotoxicity of Microglia. *Glia* 1993;7: 111–118.
10. Barna BP, Chou SM, Jacobs B, Ranssohoff RM. Induction of HLA-DR antigen expression in cultured human adult nonneoplastic glial cells. *Ann Neurol* 1987;22:152–158.
11. Baskin GB, Murphy-Corb M, Roberts ED, Dudier PJ, Martin LN. Correlates of SIV encephalitis in rhesus monkeys. *J Med Primatol* 1992;21:59–63.
12. Beaman MH, Remington JS. IL-6 impairs macrophage killing of *Toxoplasma gondii* and IFN-γ function [Abstract]. *Clin Res* 1991;39:176.
13. Beaman MH, Wong SY, Remington JS. Cytokines, toxoplasma, and intracellular parasitism. *Immunol Rev* 1992;127:97–117.
14. Beilke MA. Vascular endothelium in immunology and infectious disease. *Rev Infect Dis* 1989;11: 273–283.
15. Beilke MA, In DR, Hamilton R, et al. HLA-DR expression in macaque neuroendothelial cells *in vitro* and during SIV encephalitis. *J Neuroimmunol* 1991;33:129–143.
16. Bensussan A, Rabian C, Schiavon V, et al. Significant enlargement of a specific subset of CD3+ CD8+ peripheral blood leukocytes mediating cytotoxic T-lymphocyte activity during human immunodeficiency virus infection. *Proc Natl Acad Sci U S A* 1993;90:9427–9430.
17. Benveniste EN. Astrocyte-microglia Interactions. In: Murphy S, ed. *Astrocytes: Pharmacology and Function*. San Diego: Academic, 1993:355–382.
18. Benveniste EN, Sparacio SM, Norris G, Grenett HE, Fuller GM. Induction and regulation of interleukin-6 gene expression in rat astrocytes. *J Neuroimmunol* 1990;30:201–212.
19. Berger JR, Harris JO, Gregorius J, Norenberg M. Cerebrovascular disease in AIDS: a case-control study. *AIDS* 1990;4:239–244.
20. Berger JR, Shermata WA, Resnick L, Atherton S, Fletcher MA, Norenberg M. Multiple sclerosis-like illness occurring with human immunodeficiency virus infection. *Neurology* 1989;39:324–329.
21. Berger JR, Tornatore C, Major EO, et al. Relapsing and Remitting human immunodeficiency virus-associated leukoencephalomyelopathy. *Ann Neurol* 1992;31:34–38.
22. Bernard C, Exquis B, Reber G, de Moerloose P. Determination of anti-cardiolipin and other antibodies in HIV-1-infected patients. *J AIDS* 1990;3:536–539.
23. Bethea JR, Chung IY, Sparacio SM, Gillespie GY, Benveniste EN. Interleukin-1β induction of

tumor necrosis factor-alpha gene expression in human astroglioma cells. *J Neuroimmunol* 1992;36: 179–191.

24. Bethea JR, Gillespie GY, Chung IY, Benveniste EC. Tumor necrosis factor production and receptor expression by a human astroglioma cell line. *J Biol Chem* 1990;30:1–13.
25. Bevilacqua MP. Endothelial-leukocyte adhesion molecules. *Ann Rev Immunol* 1993;11:767–804.
26. Bevilacqua MP, Pober JS, Wheeler ME, Cotran RS, Gimbrone MA. Interleukin 1 acts on cultured human vascular endothelium to increase the adhesion of polymorphonuclear leukocytes, monocytes and related leukocyte lines. *J Clin Invest* 1985;76:2003–2011.
27. Bottone EJ, Toma M, Johansson BE, Wormser GP. Poorly encapsulated *Cryptococcus neoformans* from patients with AIDS. I. Preliminary observations. *AIDS Res* 1986;7:249–254.
28. Boullier S, Cochet M, Poccia F, Gougeon ML. CDR3-independent gamma delta V delta 1 + T cell expansion in the peripheral blood of HIV-infected persons. *J Immunol* 1995;154:1418–1431.
29. Bradbury MWB, Cole DF. The role of lymphatic system in drainage of cerebrospinal fluid and aqueous humor. *J Physiol* 1980;299:353–365.
30. Bredesen DE. Sticker RB, Neyman P, Wesley AM, Mahawar SK. Autoimmunity in the pathogenesis of HIV-related peripheral neuropathy. *Neurology* 1989;39(suppl 1):329.
31. Brett J, Gerlach H, Nawroth P, Steinberg S, Godman G, Stern D. Tumor necrosis factor/cachectin increases permeability of endothelial cell monolayers by a mechanism involving regulatory G proteins. *J Exp Med* 1989;169:1977–1991.
32. Brey RL, Arroyo R, Boswell RN. Cerebrospinal fluid anti-cardiolipin antibodies in patients with HIV-1 Infection. *J AIDS* 1991;4:435–441.
33. Brosnan CF, Seimaj K, Raine CS. Hypothesis: a role for tumor necrosis factor in immune-mediated demyelination and its relevance to multiple sclerosis. *J Neuroimmunol* 1988;18:87–94.
34. Budka H, Costanzi G, Cristina S, et al. Brain pathology induced by infection with the human immunodeficiency virus (HIV). A histological, immunocytochemical and electron microscopical study of 100 autopsy cases. *Acta Neuropathol* 1987;75:185–198.
35. Burns J, Zweiman B, Lisak R. Tetanus toxoid reactive T lymphocytes in the cerebrospinal fluid of multiple sclerosis patients. *Immunol Commun* 1984;13:361–369.
36. Carlos TM, Harlan JM. Membrane proteins involved in phagocyte adherence to endothelium. *Immuno Rev* 1990;114:5–28.
37. Ceredig R, Allan JE, Tabi Z, Lynch F, Doherty PC. Phenotypic analysis of the inflammatory exudate in murine lymphocytic choriomeningitis. *J Exp Med* 1987;165:1539–1551.
38. Chung IY, Benveniste EN. Tumor necrosis factor-alpha production by astrocytes: induction by lipopolysaccharide, interferon-gamma and interleukin-1. *J Immunol* 1990;144:2999–3007.
39. Clerici M, Shearer GM. A T_H1/T_H2 switch is a critical step in the etiology of HIV infection. *Immunol Today* 1993;14:107–111.
40. Cooper DA, Tindall EJ, Wilson EJ, Imrie AA, Penny R. Characterization of T lymphocyte responses during primary infection with human immunodeficiency virus. *J Infect Dis* 1988;157:889–896.
41. Cross AH, Cannella B, Crosman CF, Raine CS. Homing to central nervous system vasculature by antigen-specific lymphocytes. 1. Location of ^{14}C-labeled cells during acute chronic and relapsing experimental allergic encephalomyelitis. *Lab Invest* 1990;63:162–170.
42. Crowe SM, Carlin JB, Stewart KI, Lucas CR, Hoy JF. Predictive value of CD4 lymphocyte numbers for the development of opportunistic infections and malignancies in HIV-infected persons. *J AIDS* 1991;4:70–76.
43. Cserr HF, Knopf PM. Cervical lymphatics, the blood-brain barrier and the immunoreactivity of the brain. *Immunol Today* 1992;13:507–512.
44. Cupp C, Taylor JP, Khalili K, Amini S. Evidence for stimulation of the transforming growth factor $\beta1$ promoter by HIV-1 Tat in cells derived from the CNS. *Oncogene* 1993;8:2231–2236.
45. Cybulsky MI, Fries JWU, Williams AJ. Alternative splicing of human VCAM-1 in activated vascular endothelium. *Am J Pathol* 1991;138:815–820.
46. Czlonkowska A, Korlak JM, Iwingska B. Subacute sclerosing panencephalitis and progressive multiple sclerosis: T cell subset in blood and CSF. *Neurology* 1986;36:992–993.
47. da Cunha A, Elden LE. Neuro-AIDS: primate lentivirus infection and the brain. *Adv Neuroimmunol* 1993;3:97–127.
48. da Cunha A, Jefferson JA, Jackson RW, Vitkovic. Glial cell-specific mechanisms of TGF-$\beta1$ induction by IL-1 in cerebral cortex. *J Neuroimmunol* 1993;42:71–86.
49. da Cunha A, Vitkovic L. Transforming growth factor-beta (TGF-$\beta1$) expression and regulation in rat cortical astrocytes. *J Neuroimmunol* 1992;36:157–169.
50. Dalglesih AG. For debate: what is the role of autoimmunity in AIDS? *Autoimmunity* 1993;15: 237–244.
51. Dannemann BR, Morris VA, Araujo FG, Remington JS. Assessment of human natural killer and lymphokine-activated killer cell cytotoxicity against *Toxoplasma gondii* trophozoites and brain cysts. *J Immunol* 1989;143:2684–2691.
52. Darr ES, Moudgil T, Myer RD, Ho DD. Transient high levels of viremia in patients with primary human immunodeficiency virus type I infection. *N Engl J Med* 1991;324:961–964.

53. Davis LE, Hjelle BL, Miller VE, et al. Early viral brain invasion in iatrogenic immunodeficiency virus infection. *Neurology* 1992;42:1736–1739.

54. De la Monte SM, Gabuzda DH, Ho DD, et al. Peripheral neuropathy in the acquired immunodeficiency syndrome. *Ann Neurol* 1988;23:485–492.

55. Dhib-Jalbut S, Kufta CV, Flerlage M, Shimojo N, McFarland HF. Adult human glial cells can present target antigens to HLA-restricted cytotoxic T cells. *J. Neuroimmunol* 1990;29:203–211.

56. Diamond R, Root RK, Bennett JE. Factors influencing killing of *Cryptococcus neoformans* by human leukocytes *in vitro. J Infect Dis* 1972;125:367–376.

57. Dickson DW, Mattiace LA, Kure K, Hutchins K, Lyman WD, Brosman CF. Biology of disease. Microglia in human disease, with and emphasis on acquired immune deficiency syndrome. *Lab Invest* 1991;64:135–156.

58. Dinarello CA. Role of interleukin-1 in infectious diseases. *Immunol Rev* 1992;127:119–146.

59. Doherty PC, Allan JE, Dixon JE, Tabi Z, Ceredig R. Characteristics of the CSF inflammatory exudate in murine lymphocytic choriomeningitis. In: Lowenthal A, Raus J, eds. *Cellular and Humoral Components of Cerebrospinal Fluid in Multiple Sclerosis.* London: Plenum, 1987:351–360.

60. Durieu-Trautmann O, Chaverot N, Cazaubon S, Strosberg AD, Couraud PO. Intercellular adhesion molecule 1 activation induces tyrosine phosphorylation of the cytoskeleton-associated protein cortactin in brain microvessel endothelial cells. *J Biol Chem* 1994;269:12536–12540.

61. Engel AG, Arahata K, Emslie-Smith A. Immune effector mechanisms in inflammatory myopathies. In: Waksman BH, ed. *Immunologic Mechanisms in Neurologic and Psychiatric Disease.* New York: Raven, 1990:141–157.

62. Esiri MM, McGee JOD. Monoclonal antibody to macrophages (EBM/11) labels macrophages and microglial cells in human brain. *J Clin Pathol* 1986;39:615–621.

63. Essner R, Rhoades K, McBride WH, et al. IL-4 down-regulates IL-1 and TNF gene expression in human monocytes. *J Immunol* 1989;142:3857–3861.

64. Fabry Z, Hart MN. Antigen presentation at the cerebral microvasculature. In: Pardridge WM, ed. *The Blood-Brain Barrier: Cellular and Molecular Biology.* New York: Raven, 1993:47–66.

65. Fabry Z, Waldschmidt MM, VanDyk L, Moore SA, Hart MN. Activation of CD4 + lymphocytes by syngeneic brain microvascular smooth muscle cells. *J Immunol* 1990;145:1099–1104.

66. Fahey JL, Giorgi J, Martinez-Maza O, Detels R, Mitsuyasu T, Taylor J. Immune pathogenesis of AIDS and related syndromes. *Ann Inst Pasteur Immunol* 1987;138:245–252.

67. Farrar WL, Kilian PL, Ruff MR, Hill JM, Pert CB. Visualization and characterization of interleukin 1 receptors in brain. *J Immunol* 1987;139:459–463.

68. Fierz W, Endeler B, Reske K, Werkerle H, Fontana A. Astrocytes as antigen-presenting cells: I. Induction of Ia antigen expression on astrocytes by T cells via immune interferon and its effect on antigen presentation. *J Immunol* 1985;134:3785–3793.

69. Fontana A, Erb P, Percher H, et al. Astrocytes as antigen-presenting cells. Part II: Unlike H-2K-dependent cytotoxic T cells, H-2Ia-restricted T cells are only stimulated in the presence of interferon-γ. *J Neuroimmunol* 1986;12:15–28.

70. Fontana A, Kristensen F, Dubs R, Gemsa D, Weber E. Production of prostaglandin E and an interleukin-1 like factor by cultured astrocytes and C_6 glioma cells. *J Immunol* 1982;129:2413–2419.

71. Franklin WA, Mason DY, Pulford K, et al. Immunohistological analysis of human mononuclear phagocytes and dendritic cells by using monoclonal antibodies. *Lab Invest* 1986;54:322–335.

72. Franson P, Ronnevi LO. Myelin breakdown and elimination in the posterior funiculus of the adult cat after dorsal rhizotomy: a light and electron microscopic qualitative and quantitative study. *J Comp Neurol* 1984;223:138–151.

73. Fredrikson S, Karsson-Parra A, Olson T, Lin H. HLA-DR antigen expression of T cells from cerebrospinal fluid in multiple sclerosis and aseptic meningo-encephalitis. *Clin Exp Immunol* 1989; 9:1–9.

74. Freedman MS, Buu NN, Ruijs TCJ, Williams K, Antel JP. Differential expression of heat shock proteins by human glial cells. *J Neuroimmunol* 1992;41:231–238.

75. Freedman MS, Ruijs TCG, Selin LK, Antel JP. Peripheral blood γ/δ T cells lyse fresh human brain-derived oligodendrocytes. *Ann Neurol* 1991;30:784–800.

76. Frei K, Malipiero UV, Leist TP, Zinkernagel RM, Schwab ME, Fontana A. On the cellular source and function of interleukin 6 produced in the central nervous system in viral diseases. *Eur J Immunol* 1989;19:689–694.

77. Frei K, Piani D, Malipiero UV, Van Meir E, de Tribolet N, Fontana A. Granulocyte-macrophage colony-stimulating factor (GM-CSF) production by glioblastoma cells. *J Immunol* 1992;148:3140–3146.

78. Frei K, Siepl C, Groscurth P, Bodmer S, Schwerdel C, Fontana A. Antigen presentation and tumor cytotoxicity by interferon-γ–treated microglial cells. *Eur J Immunol* 1987;17:1271–1278.

79. Frohman EM, van den Noort S, Gupta S. Astrocytes and intracerebral immune responses. *J Clin Immunol* 1989;9:1–9.

80. Frohman EM, Vayuvegula B, Gupta S, van den Noort S. Norepinephrine inhibits γ-interferon–

induced major histocompatibility class II (Ia) antigen expression on cultured astrocytes via β_2-adrenergic signal transduction mechanisms. *Proc Natl Acad Sci U S A* 1988;85:1292–1296.

81. Frohman EM, Vayuvegula B, van den Noort S, Gupta S. Norepinephrine inhibits gamma-interferon–induced MHC class II (Ia) antigen expression on cultured brain astrocytes. *J Neuroimmunol* 1988;17:89–101.

82. Gazzinelli RT, Hakim FT, Henry S, Shearer GM, Sher A. Synergistic role of CD4 + and CD8 + T lymphocytes in IFN-γ production and protective immunity induced by an attenuated *Toxoplasma gondii* vaccine. *J Immunol* 1991;146:286–292.

83. Geppert TD, Lipsky PE. Antigen presentation by interferon-γ–treated endothelial cells and fibroblasts: differential ability to function as antigen-presenting cells despite comparable Ia expression. *J Immunol* 1985;135:3750–3762.

84. Gherardi R, Lebargy F, Galardi J, et al. Necrotizing vasculitis and HIV replication in peripheral nerves. *N Engl J Med* 1989;321:685–686.

85. Giulian D. Ameboid microglia as effectors of inflammation in the central nervous system. *J Neurosci Res* 1987;18:278–303.

86. Giulian D. Microglia and diseases of the nervous system. In: Appel SH, ed. *Current Neurology*. St Louis: Mosby Year Book, 1992;12:23–54.

87. Giulian D, Baker TJ. Characterization of ameboid microglia isolated from developing mammalian brain. *J Neurosci* 1986;6:2163–2178.

88. Giulian D, Baker TJ, Shih LN, Lachmann LB. Interleukin 1 of the central nervous system is produced by ameboid microglia. *J Exp Med* 1986;164:594–604.

89. Giulian D, Johnson B, Krebs JF, et al. Microglial mitogens are produced in the developing and injured mammalian brain. *J Cell Biol* 1991;112:323–333.

90. Giulian D, Lachman LB. Interleukin-1 stimulation of astroglial proliferation after brain injury. *Science* 1985;228:497–499.

91. Gordon LB, Knopf PM, Cserr HF. Ovalbumin is more immunogenic when introduced into brain or cerebrospinal fluid than into extracerebral sites. *J Neuroimmunol* 1992;40:81–88.

92. Graeber MB, Streit WJ, Kreutzberg GW. Toward an immunological definition of the blood-brain barrier: significance of MHC class II positive perivascular cells. In: Yonezawa T, ed. Satellite symposium on demyelination, mechanisms and background. *Proceedings of the XI International Congress of Neuropathology*. Kyoto, Japan: Japanese Society of Neuropathology, 1991:74–79.

93. Graeber MB, Streit WJ, Buringer D, Sparks L, Kreutzberg GW. Ultrastructural location of major histocompatibility complex (MHC) class II positive perivascular cells in histologically normal human brain. *J Neuropathol Exp Neurol* 1992;51:303–311.

94. Granger DL, Perfect JR, Durack DT. Macrophage-mediated fungistasis *in vitro:* requirements for intracellular and extracellular cytotoxicity. *J Immunol* 1985;131:672–680.

95. Gray F, Chimelli L, Mohr M, Clavelou P, Scaravilli F, Poirier J. Fulminating multiple sclerosis-like leukoencephalopathy revealing human immunodeficiency virus infection. *Neurology* 1991;41:105–109.

96. Gray F, Lescs M-C, Keohane C, Paraire F, Marc B, Durigon M, Gherardi R. Early brain changes in HIV infection: neuropathological study of 11 HIV seropositive, non-AIDS cases. *J Neuropathol Exp Neurol* 1992;51:177–185.

97. Grenier Y, Ruijs CG, Robitaille Y, Olivier A, Antel JP. Immunohistochemical studies of adult human glial cells. *J Neuroimmunol* 1989;21:103–115.

98. Griffin DE. The immunology of CNS viral infections. In: Tyler KL, Martin JB, eds. *Infectious Diseases of the Central Nervous System*. Philadelphia: FA Davis, 1993:23–46.

99. Griffin DE, Hess JL, Moench TR. Immune responses in the central nervous system. *Toxicol Pathol* 1987;15:294–302.

100. Griffin DE, Levine B, Tyor WR, Irani DN. The immune response in viral encephalitis. *Semin Immunol* 1992;4:111–119.

101. Griffin DE, Mendoza Q. Identification of the mononuclear cells in the brains of mast-cell deficient (W/Wv) and normal mice during Sindbis virus induced encephalitis. *Cell Immunol* 1986;97:454–458.

102. Griffin De, McArthur JC, Cornblath DR. Soluble interleukin-2 receptor and soluble CD8 in serum and cerebrospinal fluid during human immunodeficiency virus-associated neurologic disease. *J Neuroimmunol* 1990;28:97–109.

103. Grundy JE, Downes KL. Up-regulation of LFA-3 and ICAM-1 on the surface of fibroblasts infected with cytomegalovirus. *Immunology* 1993;78:405–412.

104. Gruters RA, Terpstra RG, De Jong R, et al. Selective loss of T cell functions in different stages of HIV infection: early loss of anti–CD3-induced T cell proliferation followed by decreased anti–CD3-induced cytotoxic T lymphocyte generation in AIDS-related complex and AIDS. *Eur J Immunol* 1990;20:1039–1044.

105. Gyorkey F, Melnick JL, Gyorkey P. Human immunodeficiency virus in brain biopsies of patients with AIDS and progressive encephalopathy. *J Infect Dis* 1987;155:87–876.

106. Hafler DA, Fox DA, Manning ME, Schlossman AD, Reinherz EL, Weiner HL. *In vivo* activated

T lymphocytes in the peripheral blood and cerebrospinal fluid of patients with multiple sclerosis. *N Engl J Med* 1985;312:1405–1411.

107. Harling-Berg C, Knopf PM, Merriam J, Cserr HF. Role of cervical lymph nodes in the systemic humoral immune response to human serum albumin microinfused into rat cerebrospinal fluid. *J Neuroimmunol* 1989;25:185–193.

108. Harrison MJG, McArthur JC. *AIDS and Neurology.* Edinburgh, Scotland: Churchill Livingstone, 1995.

109. Hart DN, Fabre JW. Demonstration and characterization of Ia-positive dendritic cells in the interstitial connective tissues of rat heart and other tissues, but not brain. *J Exp Med* 1981;153:347–361.

110. Hart PH, Vitti GF, Burgess DER, et al. Potential antiinflammatory effects of interleukin 4: suppression of human monocyte tumor necrosis factor alpha, interleukin-1 and prostaglandin E_2. *Proc Natl Acad Sci U S A* 1989;86:3803–3807.

111. Hartung HP, Heininger K, Toyka RV. Primary rat astroglial cultures can generate leukotriene B_4. *J Neuroimmunol* 1988;19:237–243.

112. Hedlund G, Sandberg-Wollheim M, Sjogren HO. Increased proportion of CD4+ CDw29+CD45R−UCHL-1+ lymphocytes in the cerebrospinal fluid of both multiple sclerosis patients and healthy individuals. *Cell Immunol* 1989;118:406–412.

113. Helbert MR, L'age-Stehr J, Mitchison NA. Antigen presentation, loss of immunological memory and AIDS. *Immunol Today* 1993;14:340–343.

114. Hermier F, Comby E, Delaunay A, et al. Decreased blood TCR gamma delta + lymphocytes in AIDS and p24-antigenemic HIV-1–infected patients. *Clin Immunol Immunopathol* 1993;69: 248–250.

115. Hickey WF, Kimura H. Perivascular microglial cells of the CNS are bone marrow-derived and present antigen *in vivo. Science* 1988;239:290–292.

116. Hirayama M, Miyadai T, Yokochi T, Sato K, et al. Infection of human T-lymphotrophic virus type 1 to astrocytes *in vitro* with induction of the class II MHC. *Neurosci Lett* 1988;92:34–39.

117. Hirayama M, Yokochi T, Shimokata K, Lida M, Fujika N. Induction of human leukocyte antigen A,B,C, and -DR on cultured human oligodendrocytes and astrocytes by human gamma interferon. *Neurosci Lett* 1986;72:369–374.

118. Ho JL, He SH, Rios MJC, et al. Interleukin-4 inhibits human macrophage activation by tumor necrosis factor, granulocyte-monocyte colony-stimulating factor and interleukin-3 for anti-leishmanial activity and oxidative burst capacity. *J Infect Dis* 1992;165:344–351.

119. Hollander H. Cerebrospinal fluid normalities and abnormalities in individuals infected with human immunodeficiency virus. *J Infect Dis* 1988;158:855–858.

120. Hopkins SJ, Rothwell NJ. Cytokines and the nervous system I: expression and recognition. *Trends Neurosci* 1995;18:83–88.

121. Houff SA, Major EO, Katz DA, et al. Involvement of JC virus-infected mononuclear cells from the bone marrow and spleen in the pathogenesis of progressive multifocal leukoencephalopathy. *N Engl J Med* 318:301–305.

122. Illa I, Nath A, Dalakas M. Immunocytochemical and virological characteristics of HIV-associated inflammatory myopathies: similarities with seronegative polymyositis. *Ann Neurol* 1991;29: 474–481.

123. Ito M, Watanabe M, Kamiya H, Sakuari M. Changes of adhesion molecule (LFA-1, ICAM-1) expression by memory T cells activated with cytomegalovirus antigen. *Cell Immunol* 1995;160: 8–13.

124. Jassoy C, Johnson RP, Navia BA, Worth JM, Walker BD. Detection of a vigorous HIV-1–specific cytotoxic T lymphocyte response in cerebrospinal fluid from infected persons with AIDS dementia complex. *J Immunol* 1992;149:3113–3119.

125. Jellinger K, Seitelberger F, Kozik M. Perivascular accumulation of lipids in the infant human brain. *Acta Neuropathol* 1971;19:331–342.

126. Johns LD, Babcock G, Green D, Freedman M, Sriram S, Ransohoff RM. Transforming growth factor-β_1 differentially regulates proliferation and MHC class-II antigen expression in forebrain and brainstem astrocyte primary cultures. *Brain Res* 1992;585:229–236.

127. Johnson RT, Burke DS, Elwell M, et al. Japanese encephalitis: immunocytochemical studies of viral antigen and inflammatory cells in fatal cases. *Ann Neurol* 1985;18:567–573.

128. Johnson RT, Intralawan P, Puapanwatton S. Japanese encephalitis: identification of inflammatory cells in the cerebrospinal fluid. *Ann Neurol* 1986;20:691–695.

129. Joly E, Mucke L, Oldstone MBA. Viral persistence in neurons explained by lack of major histocompatibility class I expression. *Science* 1991;253:1283–1285.

130. Joseph J, D'Imperio C, Knobler RL, Lublin FD. Down-regulation of gamma-interferon-induced class II expression of human glioma cells by recombinant beta-interferon. *Ann N Y Acad Sci* 1988; 540:475–476.

131. Kato T, Hirano A, Llena JF, Dembitzer HM. Neuropathology of acquired immune deficiency syndrome (AIDS) in 53 autopsy cases with particular emphasis on microglial modules and multinucleated giant cells. *Acta Neuropathol* 1987;73:287–294.

132. Kennedy MK, Torrance DS, Picha KS, Mohler KM. Analysis of cytokine mRNA expression in the central nervous system of mice with experimental autoimmune encephalomyelitis reveals that IL-10 mRNA expression correlates with recovery. *J Immunol* 1992;149:2496–2498.

133. Kennedy PGE, Gairns J. Major histocompatibilty complex (MHC) expression in HIV encephalitis. *Neuropathol Appl Neurobiol* 1992;18:515–523.

134. Kettenmann H, Schachner M. Pharmacological properties of γ-aminobutyric acid–, glutamate-, and aspartate-induced depolarizations in cultured astrocytes. *J Neurosci* 1985;5:3295–3301.

135. Kim SU, Moretto G, Shin DH. Expression of Ia antigens on the surface of human oligodendrocytes and astrocytes in culture. *J Neuroimmunol* 1985;10:141–149.

136. Koskinen PK. The association of the induction of vascular cell adhesion molecule-1 with cytomegalovirus antigenemia in human heart allografts. *Transplantation* 1993;56:1103–1108.

137. Kumar M, Resnick L, Lowenstein DA, Berger J, Eisdorfer G. Brain-reactive antibodies and the AIDS dementia complex. *J AIDS* 1989;2:469–471.

138. Lachner AA, Smith MO, Munn RJ, et al. Localization of simian immunodeficiency virus in the central nervous system of rhesus monkeys. *Am J Pathol* 1991;139:609–621.

139. Lachman LB, Brown DC, Finstrello VS. Growth promoting effect of recombinant human Interleukin-1 and tumor necrosis factor for a human astrocytoma cell line. *J Immunol* 1987;138:2913–2916

140. Lampson LA. Molecular bases of the immune response to neural antigens. *Trends Neurosci* 1987; 10:211–216.

141. Lampson LA, Hickey WF. Monoclonal antibody analysis of MHC expression in human brain biopsies: tissue ranging from histologically normal to that showing different levels of glial tumor involvement. *J Immunol* 1986;136:4054–4062.

142. Lang W, Miklossy J, Deruaz PJ, et al. Neuropathology of the acquired immune deficiency syndrome (AIDS): a report of 135 consecutive autopsy cases from Switzerland. *Acta Neuropathol* 1989;77:379–390.

143. Lange DJ. AAEM minimonograph 41: Neuromuscular diseases associated with HIV-1 infection. *Muscle Nerve* 1994;17:16–30.

144. Langermans JAM, Van Der Hulst MEB, Nibbering PH, et al. IFN-α induced L-arginine–dependent toxoplasmastatic activity in murine peritoneal macrophages is mediated by endogenous tumor necrosis factor-α. *J Immunol* 1992;148:568–574.

145. Lassman H, Schmied M, Vass K, Hickey WF. Bone marrow derived elements and resident microglia in brain inflammation. *Glia* 1993;7:19–24.

146. Lavi E, Suzumura A, Murasko DM, Murray EM, Silberberg DH, Weiss SR. Tumor necrosis factor induces expression of MHC class I antigens on mouse astrocytes. *J Neuroimmunol* 1988;18:245–253.

147. Lee SC, Collins M, Vanguri P, Shin ML. Glutamate differentially inhibits the expression of class II MHC antigens on astrocytes and microglia. *J Immunol* 1992;148:3391–3397.

148. Lee SC, Dickson DW, Liu W, Brosman CF. Activation of nitric oxide synthetase in human astrocytes by IL-β and IFN-γ. *J Neuroimmunol* 1993;46:19–24.

149. Lehn M, Weiser WY, Engelhorn S, et al. IL-4 inhibits H_2O_2 production and antileishmanial capacity of human mononuclear phagocytes. *J Immunol* 1989;143:3020–3024.

150. Levine B, Griffin DE. Persistence of viral RNA in mouse brains after recovery from acute alphavirus encephalitis. *J Virol* 1992;66:6429–6435

151. Levine B, Griffin DE. Molecular analysis of neurovirulent strains of Sindbis virus that evolve during persistent infection of scid mice. *J Virol* 1993;67:6872–6875.

152. Levine SR, Welch KM. The spectrum of neurologic disease associated with antiphospholipid antibodies. *Arch Neurol* 1987;44:876–883.

153. Levy JA. Pathogenesis of human immunodeficiency virus infection. *Microbiol Rev* 1993;57:183–289.

154. Lieberman AP, Pitha PM, Shin ML. 1990. Protein kinase regulates tumor necrosis factor mRNA stability in virus-stimulated astrocytes. *J Exp Med* 1990;172:989–992.

155. Lieberman AP, Pitha PM, Shin HS, Shin ML. Production of tumor necrosis factor and other cytokines by astrocytes stimulated with lipopolysaccharide or a neurotropic virus. *Proc Natl Acad Sci U S A* 1989;86:6348–6352.

156. Lindholm D, Castren E, Kiefer R, Zafra F, Thoenen H. Transforming growth factor-β1 in the rat brain: increase after injury and inhibition of astrocyte proliferation. *J Cell Biol* 1992;117:395–400.

157. Lindsley MD, Rodriguez M. Characterization of the inflammatory response in the central nervous system of mice susceptible or resistant to demyelination by Theiler's virus. *J Immunol* 1989;142:2677–2682.

158. Linsley PS, Brady W, Grosmaire L, Arufoo A, Damle NK, Ledbetter JA. Binding of the B cell activation antigen B7 to CD28 costimulates T cell proliferation and IL-2 mRNA accumulation. *J Exp Med* 1991;173:721–730.

159. Lisak R, Hirayama M, Kuchmy D, et al. Cultured human and rat oligodendrocytes and rat Schwann cells do not have immune response gene associated antigen (Ia) on their surface. *Brain Res* 1983; 289:285–292.

160. Lobb RR. Integrin-immunoglobulin superfamily interactions in endothelial-leukocyte adhesion. In:

Harlan JM, Liu DY, eds. *Adhesion: Its Role in Inflammatory Disease*. New York: SH Freeman, 1992:1–18.

161. Lusso P, Garzino-Demo A, Crowley RW, Malnati MS. Infection of gamma/delta T lymphocytes by herpesvirus 6: transcriptional induction of CD4 and susceptibility to HIV infection. *J Exp Med* 1995;181:1303–1310.

162. Macchi B, Caronti B, Cocchia D, et al. Correlation between P19 presence and MHC class II expression in human fetal astroglial cells cocultured with HTLV-1 donor cells. *Int J Dev Neurosci* 1992; 10:231–241.

163. Mackay CR, Imhof BA. Cell adhesion in the immune system. *Immunol Today* 1993;14:99–102.

164. Major EO, Amemiya K, Tornatore CS, Houff SA, Berger JR. Pathogenesis and molecular biology of progressive multifocal leukoencephalopathy, the JC virus-induced demyelinating disease of the human brain. *Clin Microbiol Rev* 1992;5:49–73.

165. Malipiero UV, Frei K, Fontana A. Production of hemopoeitic colony-stimulating factors by astrocytes. *J Immunol* 1990;144:3816–3821.

166. Massa PT, Schimph A, Wecker E, ter Meulen V. Tumor necrosis factor amplifies measles virus-mediated Ia induction on astrocytes. *Proc Natl Acad Sci U S A* 1987;84:7242–7245.

167. Mato M, Ookawara S, Mato TK, Namiki T. An attempt to differentiate further between microglial and fluorescent granular perithelial (FGP) cells by their capacity to incorporate exogenous protein. *Am J Anat* 1985;172:125–140.

168. Matsiota P, Chamaret S, Montagnier L, Avrameas S. Detection of natural autoantibodies in the serum of anti-HIV-positive individuals. *Ann Inst Pasteur Immunol* 1987;138:223–233.

169. Matusi M, Mori KJ, Salda T. Cellular immunoregulatory mechanisms in the central nervous system: characterization of non-inflammatory and inflammatory cerebrospinal fluid lymphocytes. *Ann Neurol* 1990;27:647–651.

170. Mauerhoff T, Pujol-Borrell R, Mirakian R, Botazzo GF. Differential expression and regulation of major histocompatibility complex (MHC) products in neural and glial cells of the human fetal brain. *J Neuroimmunol* 1988;18:271–289.

171. Medawar PB. Immunity to homologous grated skin. III. The fate of skin homografts transplanted in the brain, to subcutaneous tissue, and to the anterior chamber of the eye. *Br J Exp Pathol* 1948; 29:58–69.

172. McArthur JC, Sipos E, Cornblath DR, et al. Identification of mononuclear cells in CSF of patients with HIV infection. *Neurology* 1989;39:66–70.

173. McCarron RM, Wang L, Racke MK, McFarlin DE, Spatz M. Effect of cytokines on ICAM expression and T cell adhesion to cerebrovascular endothelial cells. *Adv Exp Med Biol* 1993;331:237–242.

174. McGraw TG, Kozel TR. Opsonization of *Cryptococcus neoformans* by human immunoglobulin G: masking of immunoglobulin G by cryptococcal polysaccharide. *Infect Immun* 1979;25:262–267.

175. Merrill JE, Kono DH, Clayton J, Ando DG, Hinton DR, Hofman FM. Inflammatory leukocytes and cytokines in the peptide-induced disease of experimental allergic encephalomyelitis in SJL and B10. PL mice. *Proc Natl Acad Sci U S A* 1992;89:574–578.

176. Merrill JE, Zimmermann RP. Natural and induced cytotoxicity of oligodendrocytes by microglia is inhibitable by TGF-β. *Glia* 1991;4:327–331.

177. Mix E, Olsson T, Correlae J, et al. CD4+ , CD8$^+$, and CD4 + − CD8$^-$ T cells in CSF and blood of patients with multiple sclerosis and tension headache. *Scand J Immunol* 1990;31:493–501.

178. Moench TR, Griffin DE. Immunocytochemcial identification and quantitation of mononuclear cells in cerebrospinal fluid, meninges, and brain during acute viral encephalitis. *J Exp Med* 1984;159: 77–88.

179. Mokhtarian F, Griffin DE. Role of mast cells in virus-induced CNS inflammation in the mouse. *Cell Immunol* 1984;86:941.

180. Morganti-Kossmann MC, Kossmann T, Brandes ME, Mergenhagen SE, Wald SM. Autocrine and paracrine regulation of astrocyte function by transforming growth factor-β. *J Neuroimmunol* 1992; 39:163–174.

181. Morrow WJ, Isenberg DA, Sobol RE, Stricker RB, Kieber-Emmons T. AIDS virus infection and autoimmunity: a perspective of the clinical, immunological and molecular origins of the autoallergic pathologies associated with HIV disease. *Clin Immunol Immunopathol* 1991;58:163–180.

182. Muller S, Richalet P, Laurent-Crawford A, et al. Autoantibodies typical of non-organ-specific autoimmune diseases in HIV-seropositive patients. *AIDS* 1992;6:933–942.

183. Nagra RM, Wong PKY, Wiley CA. Expression of major histocompatibility complex antigens and serum neutralizing antibody in murine retroviral encephalitis. *J Neuropathol Exp Neurol* 1993;52: 163–170.

184. Naparstek T, Ben-Nun A, Holoshitz J, et al. T lymphocyte lines producing or vaccinating against autoimmune encephalomyelitis (EAE). Functional activation induces peanut agglutinin receptors and accumulation in the brain and thymus of line cells. *Eur J Immunol* 1983;13:418–423.

185. Nath A, Kerman RHM, Novak IS, Wolinsky JS. Immune studies in human immunodeficiency virus infection with myasthenia gravis: a case report. *Neurology* 1990;40:581–583.

186. Nathason JA, Chun LLY. Immunologic function of the blood-cerebrospinal fluid barrier. *Proc Natl Acad Sci U S A* 1989;86:1648–1648.
187. Ohmori K, Hong Y, Fujiwarra M, Matsumoto Y. *In situ* demonstration of proliferating cells in the rat central nervous system during experimental autoimmune encephalomyelitis. Evidence suggesting that most infiltrating T cells do not proliferate in the target organ. *Lab Invest* 1992;66:54–62.
188. Oldstone MBA. Viral persistence. *Cell* 1989;56:517–520.
189. Osborn, L. Leukocyte adhesion to endothelium in inflammation, *Cell* 1990;62:3–6.
190. Pantaleo G, Graziosi C, Demarest JF, et al. HIV infection in active and progressive lymphoid tissue during the clinically latent stage of disease. *Nature* 1993;362:355–358.
191. Paulson JC. Selectin/carbohydrate-mediated adhesion of leukocytes. In: Harlan JM, Liu DY, eds. *Adhesion: Its Role in Inflammatory Disease*. New York: WH Freeman, 1992:19–42.
192. Pavia CS. Protection against experimental toxoplasmosis by adoptive immunotherapy. *J Immunol* 1986;137:2985–2990.
193. Peerrella O, Soscia M, Iaccarino C, Carrieri PB. Cerebrospinal fluid T cell receptor gamma/delta + lymphocyte subsets in patient with AIDS-dementia complex. *J Biol Regul Homeost Agents* 1992; 6:53–56.
194. Perry VH, Hume D, Gordon S. Immunohistochemical localization of macrophages and microglia in the adult and developing mouse brain. *Neurosciences* 1985;15:313–326.
195. Pettio CK, Cho E-S, Lemann W, Navia BA, Price RW. Neuropathology of acquired immunodeficiency syndrome (AIDS): an autopsy review. *J Neuropathol Exp Neurol* 1986;45:635–646.
196. Peudenier S, Henry C, Ng C, Tardieu M. HIV receptors within the brain: a study of CD4 and MHC-II on human neurons, astrocytes and microglial cells. *Rev Virol* 1991;142:145–149.
197. Pfister H-W, Frie K, Ottnad B, Koedel U, Tomasz A, Fontana A. Transforming growth factor beta-2 inhibits cerebrovascular changes and brain edema formation in the tumor necrosis factor alpha–independent early phase of experimental pneumococcal meningitis. *J Exp Med* 1992;176: 265–271.
198. Plaut M, Pierce JH, Watson CJ, Hanley-Hydes J, Nordan RP, Paul WE. Mast cell lines produce lymphokines in response to cross-linkage of Fc-e R1 or to calcium ionophores. *Nature* 1989;339: 64–67.
199. Pober JS, Gimbrose M, Lapierre LA, et al. Overlapping patterns of activation of human endothelial cells by interleukin 1, tumor necrosis factor and immune interferon. *J Immunol* 1986;137:1893–1896.
200. Poccia F, Placido R, Mancino G, Colizzi V. Surface heat shock proteins and V gamma 9/V delta 2 T cells are induced by HIV-1 infection [Abstract WS-A13-5]. *International Conference on AIDS.* 1993.
201. Pohlman TH, Stanness KA, Beatty PG, Ochs HD, Harlan JM. An endothelial cell surface factor(s) induced *in vitro* by lipopolysaccharide, interleukin-1, and tumor necrosis factor-Qa increases neutrophil adherence by a cd 18-dependent mechanism. *J Immunol* 1986;136:4548–4553.
202. Pulver M, Carrell S, Mach JP, de Tribolet N. Cultured human fetal astrocytes can be induced by interferon-γ to express HLA-DR. *J Neuroimmunol* 1987;14:123–133.
203. Raine CS, Cannell B, Dujvesitju AM, Cross AH. Homing to central nervous system vasculature by antigen-specific lymphocytes. II. Lymphocyte/endothelium cell adhesion during the initial stages of autoimmune demyelination. *Lab Invest* 1990;63:476–489.
204. Ransohoff RM, Devajyothi C, Estes L, et al. Interferon-β specifically inhibits interferon-α induced class II major histocompatibility complex gene transcription in a human astrocytoma cell line. *J Neuroimmunol* 1991;33:103–112.
205. Resnick L, diMarzo-Veronese F, Schupbach J, et al. Intra-blood-brain barrier synthesis of HTLV-III-specific IgG in patients with neurologic symptoms associated with AIDS or AIDS-related complex. *N Engl J Med* 1985;313:1498–1504.
206. Riedel RR, Schmitt A, Hartman A. Ocular pseudo-myasthenic reaction by interferon in an AIDS patient. *Klin Wochenschr* 1991;69:930–931.
207. Romagnani S. Induction of T_H1 and T_H2 responses: a key role for the natural immune response? *Immunol Today* 1992;13:1379–1381.
208. Rosen H, Milon G, Gordon S. Antibody to the murine type 3 complement receptor inhibits T lymphocyte-dependent recruitment of myelomonocytic cells *in vivo*. *J Exp Med* 1987;169:535–548.
209. Rosenberg ZF, Fauci AS. The immunopathogenesis of HIV infection. *Adv Immunol* 1989;47: 377–431.
210. Rossen RD, Smith CW, Laughter AH, et al. HIV-1–stimulated expression of CD11/CD18 integrins and ICAM-1: a possible mechanism for extravascular dissemination of HIV-1–infected cells. *Trans Assoc Am Physicians* 1989;102:117–130.
211. Rothwell NJ, Hopkins SJ. Cytokines and the nervous system II: actions and mechanisms of action. *Trends Neurosci* 1995;18:130–136.
212. Sachs JA. The relevance of HLA-antigens in some neurological diseases. In: Rose FC, ed. *Clinical Neuroimmunology*. Oxford: Blackwell Scientific, 1979:42–52.
213. Saito Y, Sharer LR, Dewhurst S, et al. Cellular localization of human herpesvirus-6 in the brains of children with AIDS encpehalopathy. *J Neurovirol* 1995;1:30–39.

214. Sanders ME, Makgoba MW, Shaw S. Human naive and memory T cells: reinterpretation of helper-inducer and suppressor-inducer subsets. *Immunol Today* 1988;9:195–199.

217. Sasserville VG, Newman WA, Lackner AA, et al. Elevated vascular cell adhesion molecule-1 in AIDS encephalitis induced by simian immunodeficiency virus. *Am J Pathol* 1992;141:1021–1030.

216. Sasserville VG, Newman W, Brodie SJ, Hesterberg P, Pauley D, Ringler DJ. Monocyte adhesion to endothelium in simian immunodeficiency virus-induced AIDS encephalitis is mediated by vascular cell adhesion molecule-1/alpha 4 beta1 integrin interactions. *Am J Pathol* 1994;144:27–40.

215. Saski A, Nakazato Y. The identity of cells expressing MHC class II antigens in normal and pathological human brain. *Neuropathol Appl Neurobiol* 1992;18:13–26.

218. Sawada M, Suzumura A, Yoshida M, Marunouchi T. Human T cell leukemia virus type 1 trans activator induces class I major histocompatibility complex antigen expression in glial cells. *J Virol* 1990;64:4002–4006.

219. Schleimer R, Sterbinsky P, Kaiser SA, et al. IL-4 induces adherence of human eosinophils and basophils but not neutrophils to endothelium. *J Immunol* 1992;148:1086–1092.

220. Schluesener HJ. Transforming growth factors type $_1$ and $_2$ suppress rat astrocyte autoantigen presentation and antagonize hyperinduction of class II major histocompatibility complex antigen expression by interferon-γ and tumor necrosis factor-α. *J Neuroimmunol* 1990;27:41–47.

221. Schrier RD, Freeman WR, Wiley CA, McCuthcan JA. CMV-specific CMV retinits, HNRC Group. HIV Neurobehavioral Research Center. *Adv Neuroimmunol* 1994;4:327–336.

222. Schwartz ND, So YT, Hollander H, Allen S, Frye KH. Eosinophilic vasculitis leading to amaurosis fugax in a patient with acquired immunodeficiency syndrome. *Arch Intern Med* 1986;146: 2059–2060. .

223. Sedmak DD, Knight DA, Vook NC, Waldman JW. Divergent patterns of ELAM-1, ICAM-1 and VCAM-1 expression on cytomegalovirus-infected endothelial cells. *Transplantation* 1994;58: 1379–1385.

224. Selmaj K, Raine CS, Cannellla B, Brosnana CF. Identification of lymphotoxin and tumor necrosis factor in multiple sclerosis lesions. *J Clin Invest* 1991;87:949–954.

225. Selmaj KW, Brosnan CF, Raine CS. Colocalization of lymphocytes bearing gamma-delta TCR and hsp 65$^+$ oligodendrocytes in multiple sclerosis. *Proc Natl Acad Sci U S A* 1991;88:6452–6456.

226. Selmaj KW, Farooq M, Norton WT, Raine CS, Brosnan CF. Proliferation of astrocytes *in vitro* in response to cytokines: a primary role for tumor necrosis factor. *J Immunol* 1990;144:129–135.

227. Selmaj KW, Raine CS. Tumor necrosis factor mediates myelin and oligodendrocyte damage *in vitro*. *Ann Neurol* 1988;23:339–346.

228. Shanker V, Kao M, Hamir AN, Sheng H, Koprowski H, Dietzschold B. Kinetics of virus spread and changes in levels of several cytokine mRNAs in the brain after intranasal infection of rats with Borna disease virus. *J Virol* 1992;66:992–997.

229. Sharer LR, Baskin GB, Cho E, Murphey-Corb M, Blumberg BM, Epstein LG. Comparison of simian immunodeficiency virus and human immunodeficiency virus encephalitis in the immature host. *Ann Neurol* 1988;23(suppl):108–112.

230. Sharer LR, Michaels J, Murphey-Corb M, et al. Serial pathogenesis study of SIV brain infection. *J Med Primatol* 1991;20:211–217.

231. Sibley LD, Adams LB, Fukutomi Y, Krahenbuhl JL. Tumor necrosis factor-α triggers anittoxoplasmal activity of IFN-γ primed macrophages. *J Immunol* 1991;147:2340–2345.

232. Simpson DM. Neuromuscular complications of human immunodeficiency virus infection. *Semin Neurol* 1992;12:34–42.

233. Skias DD, Kim D-K, Reder AT, Antel JP, Lancki DW, Fitch FW. Susceptibility of astrocytes to class 1 MHC antigen-specific cytotoxicity. *J Immunol* 1987;138:3254–3258.

234. Sobel RA, Ames MB. Major histocompatibility complex molecule expression in the human central nervous system: immunohistochemical analysis of 40 patients. *J Neuropathol Exp Neurol* 1988;47: 19–28.

235. Sobel RA, Collins AB, Colvin RB, Bhan AK. The *in situ* cellular immune response in acute herpes simplex encephalitis. *Am J Pathol* 1986;125:332–338.

236. Sobel RA, Mitchell ME, Fondren G. Intercellular adhesion molecule-1 (ICAM-1) in cellular immune reactions in the human central nervous system. *Am J Pathol* 1990;136:1309–1316.

237. Sobel RA, Natale JM, Schneeberger EE. The immunopathology of acute experimental allergic encephalomyelitis IV. An ultrastructural immunocytochemical study of class II major histocompatibility complex (Ia) expression. *J Neuropathol Exp Neurol* 1987;46:239–249.

238. Solinger AM, Adams LE, Friedman-Kein AE, Hess EV. Acquired immune deficiency syndrome (AIDS) and autoimmunity—mutually exclusive entities? *J Clin Immunol* 1988;8:32–42.

239. Spertini O, Kansas GS, Munro JM, Griffin JD, Tedder TF. Regulation of leukocyte migration by activation of the leukocyte migration by activation of the leukocyte adhesion molecule-1 (LAM-1) selectin. *Nature* 1991;349:691–694.

240. Springer TA. Adhesion receptors of the immune system. *Nature* 1990;346:425–434.

241. Stanley ER, Bartoccii A, Patinkin D, Rosendaal M, Bradley TR. Regulation of very primitive, multipotent hemopoietic cells by hemopoietin-1. *Cell* 1986;45:667–674.

242. Steffen BJ, Butcher EC, Engelhardt B. Evidence for involvement of ICAM-1 and VCAM-1 in lymphocyte interactions with endothelium in experimental autoimmune encephalomyelitis in the central nervous system in the SHL/J mouse. *Am J Pathol* 1994;145:189–201.

243. Streat WJ, Graeber MB, Kreutzberg GW. Functional plasticity of microglia: a review. *Glia* 1988; 1:301–307.

244. Stohlman SA, Sussman MA, Matsushima GK, Shubin RA, Erlich SS. Delayed-type hypersensitivity response in the central nervous system during JHM virus infection requires viral specificity for protection. *J Neuroimmunol* 1988;19:255–268.

245. Strelein JW, Wildbanks GA, Cousins SW. Immunoregulatory mechanisms of the eye. *J Neuroimmunol* 1992;39:185–200.

246. Taillan B, Roul C, Fuzibet J-G, et al. Circulating anticoagulant in patients seropositive for human immunodeficiency virus. *Am J Med* 1989;87:238.

247. Tardieu M, Powers ML, Hafler DA, Hauser SL, Weiner HL. Autoimmunity following viral infection: demonstration of monoclonal antibodies against normal tissue following infection of mice with reovirus and demonstration of shared antigenicity between virus and lymphocytes. *Eur J Immunol* 1984;14:561–565.

248. Thornbill MH, Wellicome SM, Mahiouz, DL, Lancbury JSS, Kyan-Aung U, Haskard DO. Tumor necrosis factor combines with IL-4 or IFN-γ to selectively enhance endothelial cell adhesiveness for T cells: the contribution of vascular cell adhesion molecule-1-dependent and -independent binding mechanisms. *J Immunol* 1991;146:592–598.

249. Tindall B, Cooper DA. Primary HIV infection: host responses and intervention strategies. *AIDS* 1991;5:1–14.

250. Tornatore C, Berger JR, Houff SA, et al. Detection of JC virus DNA in peripheral lymphocytes from patients with and without progressive multifocal leukoencephalopathy. *Ann Neurol* 1992;31: 454–462.

251. Toru-Delbauffe D, Baghdassarian-Chalaye D, Gavaret JM, Courtin F, Pomerance M, Pierce M. Effects of transforming growth factor β_1 on astroglial cells in culture. *J Neurochem* 1990;54: 1056–1061.

252. Trinchieri G. Interleukin-12 and its role in the generation of T_H1 cells. *Immunol Today* 1993;14: 335–338.

253. Trujillo JR, McLane MF, Lee T-H, Essex M. Molecular mimicry between the human immunodeficiency virus type 1 gp120 V3 loop and human brain proteins. *J Virol* 1993;67:7711–7715.

254. Trujillo JR, Navia B, McLane MF, Worth JL, Lee T-H, Essex M. Evaluation of autoantibodies to brain proteins in patients with AIDS dementia complex. *J AIDS* 1994;7:103–108

255. Tsukada N, Matsuda M, Miyagi K, Yanagisawa N. *In vitro* intercellular adhesion molecule-1 expression on brain endothelial cells in multiple sclerosis. *J Neuroimmunol* 1994;49:181–187.

256. Tunkel AR, Wispelwey B, Scheld WM. Pathogenesis and pathophysiology of meningitis. *Infect Dis Clin North Am* 1990;4:555–581.

257. Turley AM, Miller JFAP, Bartlett PF. Regulation of MHC molecules on MBP positive oligodendrocytes in mice by IFN-γ and TNF-α. *Neurosci Lett* 1991;123:45–48.

258. Tweardy DJ, Glazier EW, Mon PL, Anderson K. Modulation by tumor necrosis factor-α of human astroglial cell production of granulocyte-macrophage colony-stimulating factor (GM-CSR) and granulocyte colony-stimulating factor (G-CSR). *J Neuroimmunol* 1991;32:269–278.

259. Tweardy D, Mott P, Glazer E. Monokine modulation of human astroglial cell production of granulocyte colony-stimulating factor and granulocyte-macrophage colony stimulating factor. I. Effects of IL-1α and IL-1β. *J Immunol* 1990;144:2233–2241.

260. Tyor WR, Glass MD, Baumrind N, et al. Cytokine expression of macrophages in HIV-1–associated vacuolar myelopathy. *Neurology* 1993;43:1002–1009.

261. Tyor WR, Glass JD, Griffin JW, et al. Cytokine expression in the brain during the acquired immunodeficiency syndrome. *Ann Neurol* 1992;31:349–360.

262. van Noesel CJM, Gruters RA, Terpstra FG, Schellekens TA, van Lier RAW, Miedema F. Functional and phenotypic evidence for a selective loss of memory T cells in asymptomatic human immunodeficiency virus–infected men. *J Clin Invest* 1990;86:293–299.

263. van Snick JV. Interleukin-6: an overview. *Ann Rev Immunol* 1990;8:253–278.

264. Vinters HV, Guerra WF, Eppolito L, Keith PE. Necrotizing vasculitis of the nervous system in a patient with AIDS-related complex. *Neuropathol Appl Neurobiol* 1988;20:362–364.

265. Vitkovic L, da Cunha A, Tyor WR. Cytokine expression and pathogenesis in AIDS brain. In: Price RW, Perry SW, eds. *HIV, AIDS and the Brain*. New York: Raven, 1994:203–222.

266. Vitkovic L, Wood G, Major EO, Fauci AS. Human astrocytes stimulate HIV-1 expression in a chronically infected promonocyte clone via interleukin-6. *AIDS Res Hum Retrovir* 1991;7:723–727.

267. Wahl SM, Allen JB, McCartney-Francis N, et al. Macrophage- and astrocyte-derived transforming growth factor as a mediator of central nervous system dysfunction in acquired immune deficiency syndrome. *J Exp Med* 1991;173:981–991.

268. Wahl SM, McCartney-Francis N, Mergenhagen SE. Inflammatory and immunomodulatory roles of TGF-β. *Immunol Today* 1989;10:258–261.

269. Walsh C, Krigel R, Lennette E, Karpatkin S. Thrombocytopenia in homosexual patients: prognosis, response to therapy and prevalence of antibody to the retrovirus associated with acquired immunodeficiency syndrome. *Ann Intern Med* 1985;103:542–545.
270. Watkins BA, Dorn HH, Kelley WB, et al. Specific tropism of HIV-1 for microglial cells in primary human brain cultures. *Science* 1990;249:549–553.
271. Weaver CT, Unanue ER. The costimulatory function of antigen-presenting cells. *Immunol Today* 1990;11:49–55.
272. Wekerle H, Engelhardt B, Rissau W, Meyermann R. Interaction of T lymphocytes with cerebral endothelial cells *in vitro. Brain Pathol* 1991;1:107–114.
273. Wekerle H. Lymphocyte traffic to the brain. In: Pardridge WM, ed. *The Blood-Brain Barrier*. New York: Raven, 1993:67–85.
274. Wekerle H, Sun D, Oropeza-Wekerle RL, Meyermann R. Immune reactivity in the nervous system: modulation of T-lymphocyte activation by glial cells. *J Exp Med* 1987;132:43–57.
275. Weller M, Stevens A, Sommer N, et al. Comparative analysis of cytokines patterns in immunological, infections and other neurological disorders. *J Neurol Sci* 1991;104:215–221.
276. Wenstein DL, Walker DG. Akiyama H, McGeer PL. Herpes simplex virus type I infection of the CNS induces major histocompatibility complex antigen expression on rat microglia. *J Neurosci Res* 1990;26:55–65.
277. Wessel HB, Zitrelli BJ. Myasthenia gravis associated with human T cell lymphotrophic virus type III infection. *Pediatr Neurol* 1987;3:238–239.
278. Wesselingh SL, Levine B, Fox RJ, Choi S, Griffin DE. Intracerebral cytokine mRNA expression during fatal and nonfatal alphavirus encephalitis suggests a predominant type 2 T cell response. *J Immunol* 1994;152:1289–1297.
279. Wesselingh SL, Power C, Glass JD, et al. Intracerebral cytokine messenger RNA expression in acquired immunodeficiency syndrome dementia. *Ann Neurol* 1993;33:576–582.
280. Widner H, Moller G, Johansson BB. Immune response in deep cervical lymph nodes and spleen in the mouse after intracerebral antigen deposition. *Scand J Immunol* 1988;28:563–572.
281. Wiley CA, Schrier RD, Nelson JA, Lampert PW, Oldstone MBA. Cellular localization of human immunodeficiency virus infection within the brains of acquired immune deficiency syndrome patients. *Proc Natl Acad Sci U S A* 1986;83:7089–7093.
282. Willenborg DO, Simmons RD, Tamatani T, Miyasaka M. ICAM-1–dependent pathway is not critically involved in the inflammatory process of autoimmune encephalomyelitis or in cytokine-induced inflammation of the central nervous system. *J Neuroimmunol* 1993;45:147–154.
283. Williams K, Bar-Or A, Ulvestad E. Oliver A, Antel JP, Yong VW. Biology of adult human microglia in culture: comparisons with peripheral blood monocytes and astrocytes. *J Neuropathol Exp Neurol* 1992;51:538–549.
284. Williams K, Ulvestad E, Antel J. Immune regulatory and effector properties of human adult microglia studied *in vitro* and *in situ. Adv Neuroimmunol* 1994;4:273–281.
285. Williams K, Ulvestad E, Antel JP. B7/BB-1 antigen expression on adult human microglia *in vitro* and *in situ. Eur J Immunol* 1994;24:3031–3037.
286. Williams K, Ulvestad E, Cragg L, Blain M, Antel JP. Induction of primary T cell responses by human glial cells. *J Neurosci Res* 1993;36:382–390.
287. Wong GHW, Bartlett PF, Clark-Lewis I, McKimm-Breschkin JL, Scharder JW. Interferon-γ induces the expression of H-2 and Ia antigens on brain cells. *J Neuroimmunol* 1985;7:255–278.
288. Wong HL, Welch GR, Brandes ME, et al. IL-4 antagonizes induction of Tc-gamma-RIII (CD16) expression of transforming growth factor beta on human monocytes. *J Immunol* 1991;147:1843–1848.
289. Wong S-Y, Remington JS. Toxoplasmosis in the setting of AIDS. In: Broder S, Merigan TC, Bolognesi D, eds. *Textbook of AIDS Medicine*. Baltimore: Williams & Wilkins, 1994:223–257.
290. Wucherpfenning KW, Newcombe J, Cuzner L, et al. Analysis of α and δ T cell receptor in MS plaques. *Neurology* 1991;41(suppl 1):380.
291. Yamada M, Zurbiggen A, Oldstone MBA, Fujinami RS. Common immunologic determinant between human immunodeficiency virus type 1 gp41 and astrocytes. *J Virol* 1991;65:1370–1376.
292. Yanagishawa K, Sato S, Miyatake T, Kominami E, Katsunuma N. Degradation of myelin protein by cathepsin B and inhibition by E-64 analogue. *Neurochem Res* 1984;9:691–694.
293. Yarrish RL. Cytomegalovirus Infection in AIDS. In: Wormser GP, ed. *AIDS and Other Manifestations of HIV Infection*. New York: Raven, 1992:249–268.
294. Yasukawa K, Hirano T, Watanabe Y, et al. Structure and expression of human B cell stimulatory factor-2 (BSF-2/IL-6). *EMBO J* 1987;6:2939–2945.
295. Zajicek JP, Wing M, Scolding NJ, Compston DAS. Interactions between oligodendrocytes and microglia. *Brain* 1992;115:1611–1631.
296. Zuber P, Kupper MC, de Tribolet N. Transforming growth factor-β_2 down-regulates HLA-DR antigen expression on human malignant glioma cells. *Eur J Immunol* 1988;18:1623–1626.

AIDS and the Nervous System, Second Edition,
edited by J. R. Berger and R. M. Levy.
Lippincott-Raven Publishers, Philadelphia © 1997.

6

Animal Models of Human Immunodeficiency Virus Neurological Disease

°Opendra Narayan, °†Edward B. Stephens, °†Sanjay V. Joag, and °†Yahia Chebloune

°Departments of Microbiology and Molecular Genetics and †Immunology, University of Kansas Medical Center, Kansas City, Kansas 66160; and †Laboratoire des lentivirus des petits ruminants, Institut National de la Recherche Agronomigue, Ecole Vétèrincure de Lyon, Marcy l'Etoile 69630, France

Human immunodeficiency virus types 1 and 2 (HIV-1 and HIV-2) are best known as the causative agents of acquired immunodeficiency syndrome (AIDS) that mechanistically involve the infection and gradual elimination of CD4+ T-lymphocytes (CD4+ counts) by the virus (4). This is accompanied by progressive loss of immunological competence, which in turn creates a fertile environment for development of tumors and uncontrolled replication of opportunistic pathogens. Neurological disease is a major systemic complication of HIV infection (41,61) and was originally attributed to concurrent disease caused by diverse agents including neoplasms (B cell lymphoma) and opportunistic agents such as cytomegalovirus, *Toxoplasma gondii*, papovavirus (the cause of progressive multifocal leukoencephalopathy), and so forth. However, subsequent studies showed that in addition to potentiating these syndromes, HIV itself caused infection and lesions in the central nervous system (CNS), and this correlated with wide-ranging symptomatology affecting mood and cognitive and motor functions with different degrees of severity (9,25,75,76,79,87). Examination of brain tissue from infected people dying accidentally or from AIDS showed either no lesions or variable changes extending from mild focal meningitis to severe inflammation and degenerative changes (8,40,87). CNS lesions are most severe in infants and children dying from AIDS (6,26), and examination of brain tissue from such cases showed that the encephalopathy was associated with productive HIV replication almost exclusively in the macrophage population in the brain (7,55,89) and was accompanied by loss of neurons and proliferation and intense activation of astrocytes and macrophages (27,28).

GENERAL PARAMETERS OF VIRAL ENCEPHALITIS

In general, mechanisms of pathogenesis of neurovirulent viruses follow a few basic pathways with regard to neuroinvasion, neurotropism, and neurovirulence. Neuroinvasion refers to the mechanism by which virus gains access into the CNS from other tissues; neurotropism refers to the ability of the virus to replicate in cells in the neuropil; and neurovirulence refers to the ability of the virus to cause clinical neurologic disease. In experimental animals, neuropathological changes associated with virus replication in brain are considered correlates of neurovirulence, although recently, evaluation of cognition also has been used to assess the neurovirulence of simian immunodeficiency virus in macaques (SIV$_{mac}$) (68). Usually, neurovirulent viruses invade the brain during the acute phase of infection in the host, entering the brain by different mechanisms, specific for each agent. These include direct axoplasmic transport mechanisms (e.g., rabies virus [84] and borna disease virus [10]), replication in vascular endothelium of the brain (e.g., Japanese B encephalitis [42]), replication in the ependyma or cells of the choroid plexus (e.g., mumps virus [100]), or transport across the blood–brain barrier in leukocytes (e.g., canine distemper virus [99]). Although certain agents cause mainly meningitis (e.g., vaccinia [38]) and ependymitis/choroiditis (e.g., mumps virus [48,100]), others continue their replication in the neuropil, targeting cells of neuroectodermal origin (neurons, astrocytes, or oligodendroglia) and/or microglia, which are of mesodermal origin.

Usually, repeated passage of virus brain-to-brain (neuroadaptation process) increases the neurotropism of the agent. Most successful viral adaptations have been accomplished with RNA rather than DNA viruses, presumably because the former are more prone to mutation and appropriate mutants are selected by neuroectodermal cells. First introduced by Pasteur during studies on fixation of rabies virus, neuroadaptation reached its zenith by manipulation of alpha and flavi members of the togavirus family. Neuroadaptation of these viruses not only increased the neurotropism of the viruses that were already neurotropic but also resulted in selection of neurotropic mutants from original virus stock that lacked such tropism (e.g., neuroadaptation of dengue virus [85]). Intracranial inoculation of neurovirulent viruses usually results in exponential replication of the agents in the brain during the next few days. After reaching peak replication virus titers (detectable in cell-free homogenates of brain), the host either dies from encephalitis or immune mechanisms clear the virus from the CNS, often leaving neurological deficits as seen in survivors of poliomyelitis. When neuro-adapted viruses are mainly neuronotropic, such as mouse-adapted Lansing type II poliovirus, replication is confined to the CNS (51). An inability to fix neurovirulence appears to characterize lentiviruses as discussed below and represents one of the major differences between lentiviruses and other neurovirulent viruses.

The neurological disease syndrome caused directly by HIV has several unique features when considered from the perspective of other human viral infections in the nervous system. HIV-induced neurological disease varies from these in two important respects. First, whereas most human viral encephalitides are acute syndromes, the HIV syndrome is a chronic, slowly progressive disease with a long preclinical phase of infection (50). Second, whereas all known viral encephalitides result from infection in neuroectodermal cells, especially neurons (49), HIV replication occurs in cells of mesodermal origin, the macrophages of the brain (33,55). These are the bases of the uniqueness of the disease. However, HIV does not cause disease in host species other than humans; therefore, there are no mechanisms for studies on the pathogenesis of this infection in the brain. Attempts to understand mechanisms of the disease have been made by examining the pathogenesis of neurological disease caused by animal viruses of the same taxonomic group (lentiviruses) to which HIV belongs. These viruses include visna/maedi and caprine arthritis encephalitis viruses of sheep and goats, feline immunodeficiency virus (FIV), and SIV_{mac}.

OVINE–CAPRINE ENCEPHALITIS

The concepts of an apparently unique viral neuropathogenesis that were discovered in HIV infections during the 1980s had begun to unfold more than 30 years earlier during studies in Iceland on a new disease in sheep, visna/maedi, which broke out explosively after introduction of infected rams from Europe into local flocks (94). Clinically, visna was characterized by a gradual onset of ataxia, which progressed during a course of several weeks to paralysis. The syndrome was afebrile, and animals maintained normal appetites. However, they developed severe cachexia along with paralysis. Histologically, lesions appeared as severe meningoencephalomyelitis with dense infiltration of mononuclear cells around blood vessels in Virchow-Robin spaces as well as in the neuropil. Both gray and white matter were involved, but lesions in the white matter were more severe (35) and were frequently diffusely malacic (95). These areas were characterized by destruction of myelinated fibers and the presence of large numbers of debris-laden macrophages (gitter cells) (Fig. 1). Interestingly, cell bodies of neurons in contiguous, relatively unaffected areas appeared normal (Fig. 2). In some animals, this destructive type of lesion was also seen in the dorso (posterior)-lateral columns of the spinal cord (14). In less severely affected areas of the brain and spinal cord where only mononuclear inflammatory cells were present, there was an accompanying activation and proliferation of astrocytes and microglia. The latter cells frequently occurred in nodular arrangements. Interestingly, although visna virus caused multinucleated giant cell formation in cell cultures, giant cells were only rarely seen in the pathologically affected brains.

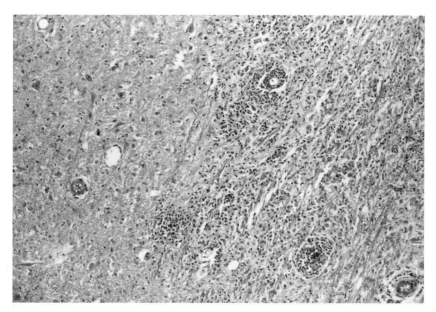

FIG. 1. Diffuse necrotizing encephalitis in the white matter track in the brain stem of a sheep with visna. Note intense perivascular inflammatory response. Hematoxylin and eosin (HE) stain, original magnification ×100.

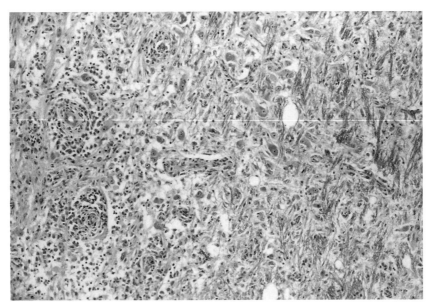

FIG. 2. Necrotizing lesion in brain stem of the same sheep showing destruction of myelinated tracts, presence of inflammatory cells and macrophages around blood vessels and in the neuropil, and relative sparing of neurons. HE stain, original magnification ×100.

Pioneering experiments by Sigurdsson et al. in Iceland, using homogenates of affected brain tissue to inoculate intracerebrally (IC) into new sheep, not only established the infectious nature of visna disease, but also showed that the disease had a remarkably long incubation period that preceded the insidious onset and slow progression of the syndrome. Sigurdsson defined the syndrome as ''slow infection'' in clear distinction from acute disease syndromes caused by other agents (94). This new concept of slow infection constituted one of the main taxonomic criteria for what would be a new virus group—the lentiviruses—which would include the prototypic visna/maedi virus and the newly described HIV. Sigurdsson et al. established that the visna/maedi virus replicated cytopathically in sheep cell cultures causing multinucleated giant cell formation (96), Lin and Thormar discovered that the agent was a retrovirus (62), and later Sonigo et al. showed that the virus had a genetic structure similar to that of HIV (97). Using cell culture–derived visna virus to inoculate sheep in Iceland, Petursson et al. (80) established that visna virus caused a persistent infection in the animals with localization of the agent to mononuclear cells in lymphoid tissues, but the animals did not develop viremia. Furthermore, the IC-inoculated animals developed an acute encephalitic response within 2 weeks of inoculation, but these lesions progressed along the same typical slow tempo reported earlier by Sigurdsson (94). Tissues lacked cell-free virus. Virus was recovered either by cocultivation of mononuclear cells with indicator cultures (80) or by cultivation of macrophages from tissues, a phenomenon that led to induction of virus replication and production of cell-free virus (31,32,70). Using this model, Nathanson et al. showed that development of the acute lesion could be prevented by treatment of the animals with antilymphocyte serum (74), thus establishing that the lesion was immunopathological in character. Further studies by this group showed that the visna lesion was basically similar in character to those of experimental allergic encephalo-myelitis (78).

Identification of visna/maedi virus in Iceland was followed by identification of similar viruses in sheep and goats in the United States. However, the main pathologi-cal responses of infection in sheep in the United States were dyspnea, characterized histologically by severe interstitial pneumonia (19,59,64); synovitis/arthritis, less frequently (39,77); and paralysis and encephalomyelitis of the type reported in Ice-land, only rarely (77,92). All of these diseases followed along the same slow tempo as visna in Icelandic sheep. The disease in goats was characterized by paralysis and leukoencephalomyelitis in young goats (13,14) and by synovitis-arthritis among adult animals (17). Whereas the development of the arthritic syndrome followed along the slow progressive course of visna in sheep, the neurological disease in kids developed frequently within a few weeks of birth. The mothers of affected kids were clinically normal but were infected with caprine arthritis encephalitis virus (CAEV) (1,16). IC inoculation of CAEV into newborn goats resulted in acute inflammatory lesions in the brain, but these animals did not develop paralysis as seen in field cases of the disease (15). Nevertheless, the subacute nature of the natural disease established the concept that young animals are much more susceptible to disease than are adults.

Studies on the cell biology of the ovine/caprine viruses also provided another classical dimension of the lentivirus taxonomic group: the ability to replicate in cells of the monocyte-macrophage lineage. Preliminary studies had shown that inoculation of visna/maedi or CAE viruses into activated lymphocytes did not result in virus production (39). The same study showed that cultivation of mitogen-treated mononu-clear cells from blood or lymphoid tissues from infected animals also failed to yield infectious virus. In contrast, cultivation of similar types of cell suspensions in medium that fostered differentiation of monocytes from the blood into macrophages led to productive virus replication in the cultivated macrophages (31,32,70).

Comparison between primary sheep macrophages and sheep choroid plexus (SCP) fibroblasts, the same type of cell culture used originally by Sigurdsson et al. (96) as host cells for virus replication, showed that in the macrophages, the virus budded into cytoplasmic vesicles where the particles accumulated until lysis of the cells (72). In contrast, virus maturation occurred at the cell plasma membrane of SCP cells (23). The morphogenesis of HIV follows along a similar dual pathway, accumulating intracellularly in macrophages (33) and budding from the plasma membrane of in-fected T-lymphocytes (4).

Studies on the molecular mechanism regulating visna/maedi virus replication showed that the enhancer region of visna/maedi viral LTR contains AP-1 and AP-4 sites that bind inducible transcription factors Fos and Jun (30,93). These nuclear-binding proteins participate in the differentiation of monocytes to macrophages and, during this process, activate transcription of viral RNA. However, regulation of virus replication by transcription factors is probably only one of several mechanisms restricting virus replication in infected animals. In some animals studied longitudi-nally in the field, only unexpressed viral DNA was found in blood-derived macro-phages, and virus replication was not induced when the macrophages had become fully differentiated (Chebloune, submitted for publication). In other animals in the same study, viral RNA but not virus production was found, whereas in still others, viral proteins were identified in cultured macrophages, but no assembly of infectious virus particles occurred. However, the onset of clinical disease correlated with local cell-free virus production in macrophages in the affected tissues. The enigma was that only the macrophages in the pathologically affected tissues were in a virus-productive phase. Macrophages from other tissues expressed variable levels of virus RNA, but these showed minimal evidence of virus production. Although bone marrow cells were high producers, Kupffer macrophages in liver were relatively poor producers of viral RNA (32).

In addition to factors that influenced virus production in macrophages, T-lymphocytes interacting with infected macrophages produced virus-specific cytokines, including a cytokinelike substance that caused activation of macrophages and enhanced expression of major histocompatibility complex (MHC) II antigen (52,71). This activity was also found in synovial fluid of arthritic joints in CAEV-infected goats (53) and in supernatant fluids of lymphocytes cultivated from lungs with progressive pneumonia lesions (58). Whether production of this cytokine was an epiphenomenon or had a role in the pathogenesis of the lesion is not known. However, production of this cytokine may explain activation of macrophages in the lesions, as well as the occurrence of free virus in the inflamed tissues. Cultivation of lymphocytes from these lesions failed to produce virus, whereas macrophages cultivated from the infected tissues produced cell-free virus for several days in culture. Thus, lesions *in vivo* were associated exclusively with productive virus replication in local tissue macrophages, the encephalitic lesions being associated with virus production in microglia, pneumonia with virus production in alveolar macrophages, and arthritis with virus production in synovial macrophages.

Another characteristic of visna/maedi and other lentiviral syndromes in sheep and goats was the presence of high levels of antibodies against the viral glycoproteins at the site of the lentiviral lesion. Such antibodies were present in synovial fluid of arthritic joints of CAEV-infected goats (46,47). Large numbers of plasma cells were also found in lesions of visna (34) and progressive pneumonia (36), suggesting that immunoglobulins were produced locally at these sites also. A suggestion that these antibodies may be important in the pathogenesis of the lesions came from two studies showing that immunization of infected sheep and goats with viral antigens caused increased severity of lesions (65,73). Thus, the local tissue lesions consisted of productive virus replication in the macrophages, activation of the macrophages, production of novel cytokines including a gamma interferon–like substance, and large amounts of antiviral antibodies. All of these factors are also present in HIV-induced encephalitis and may therefore be generic to lesions caused by lentiviruses.

Reexamination of the pathogenesis of visna from the new perspective of macrophage tropism of the virus showed that after IC inoculation of sheep with this agent, macrophages in the brain became infected but these cells did not produce virus and animals did not develop progressive lesions of visna over the course of 3 years. The virus life cycle was limited to a minimal level of virus gene expression. In addition to this restricted type of virus replication in brain macrophages, a similar type of infection had also developed in macrophage precursors in the bone marrow, macrophages in the spleen, and monocytes in peripheral blood. Cultivation of macrophages from these tissues at any time during the infection resulted in productive virus replication. Factors restricting virus replication *in vivo* are not known. In contrast to the ''latent'' infection in subclinically infected animals, fulminant virus replication had occurred in macrophages in pathologically affected tissues during natural disease, irrespective of whether the tissue was the brain, lung, or joint. However, in these animals with clinical disease, virus replication remained at the typical restricted level of expression in macrophages in other nonaffected tissues. Factors responsible for this selectivity of tissues for virus replication or factors responsible for the induction of virus replication in any particular tissue are not known.

The main relationship between the ovine–caprine model of lentiviral disease to HIV-induced neurological disease is the intriguing role that monocyte-macrophages play in the development of disease and the general framework of slow pathogenesis of the disease syndrome. This somehow must be linked to factors restricting virus replication in macrophages during subclinical infection and the release from such restriction during clinical disease. However, the type of lesion in sheep and goats with disease is much more inflammatory and degenerative than that seen in humans with HIV encephalitis. Furthermore, the lack of virus replication in lymphocytes in sheep and goats, together with the failure of these animals to develop AIDS, limits the usefulness of this model system. One possible reason for the less fulminant inflammatory nature of the disease in humans is that HIV-induced neurological disease develops in people who become severely immunosuppressed and are thus incapable of mounting intense cellular immune responses.

THE FIV MODEL

FIV infection in cats provided another aspect of neurological disease caused by lentiviruses. The first report showing that FIV could induce neurologic disease in cats was by Dow et al. (22). These investigators showed that antibodies directed against FIV could be detected in the cerebrospinal fluid (CSF) in nine of 10 naturally infected animals. FIV was isolated from the CSF in five of nine animals examined, as well as from primary cultures of brain tissue derived from the cerebral cortex, caudate nucleus, midbrain, and caudal brain stem. Histological changes in the CNS included perivascular mononuclear infiltrates, diffuse gliosis, and glial nodules in the midbrain. FIV was shown to infect and cause syncytial cytopathology in primary cultures of feline astrocytes. In addition, the virus caused infection in feline microglia cultures but without any cytopathological affects. Other investigators have confirmed the isolation of FIV from the CNS and have shown neurological abnormalities of FIV-infected cats that include abnormal stereotypic behavior, persistent abnormal electroencephalographic recordings, anisocoria, and alterations in sleep patterns (81,82).

THE HIV-2 MODEL

HIV-2 infects several nonhuman primates, including macaques (29) and baboons and causes AIDS in baboons (3). However, no neurological disease has been described in any of these models.

THE SIV$_{MAC}$ MODEL

SIV$_{mac}$ infection provides the best model of the HIV disease complex. SIV$_{mac}$ infects macaque CD4+ counts and monocyte-macrophages and causes AIDS and encephalitis in macaques, following similar mechanisms as those identified in HIV-potentiated AIDS and HIV-induced neurological disease (20,60). SIV$_{mac}$251 and

SIV$_{mac}$B670 are two strains of virus that had been obtained from animals with AIDS after inoculation with tissue material (20,60,67). These biologically purified (but not molecularly cloned) viruses caused typical infection in CD4+ T cells and macrophages and *in vivo* caused productive infection in CD4+ T cells, hyperplastic changes in lymphoid tissues, followed by virus invasion and replication in the brain. Current data suggest that neuroinvasion occurs mainly by transport of infected mononuclear cells across the vascular endothelium of the blood–brain barrier. Studies by Gilles et al. (37) have shown that virus expression in macrophages becomes amplified after contact between these cells and cells of the vascular endothelium. In support of this, Sasseville et al. (86) showed that monocytic cell lines bound preferentially to vascular endothelial cells from brains of macaques with SIV encephalitis via VLA-4 molecules on the monocytic cells and VCAM-1 molecules expressed on the vascular endothelium. Expression of the latter molecule was enhanced in brains with SIV encephalitis (86). More recent data suggest that macrophage-tropic SIV can bind directly and fuse with vascular endothelial cells derived from brain, thus allowing entry of the virus into the vascular endothelium cells (63). It is not known how important this last mechanism is because the bulk of the evidence points to infected cells rather than free virus particles as the source of virus that interacts with the blood–brain barrier. Furthermore, fusion among the vascular endothelial cells of the brain has not been reported in lentiviral encephalitis. Some animals infected with SIV$_{mac}$251 developed infection and encephalitis within 2 weeks of inoculation with virus (11). Lesions in the brain caused by the virus consisted of giant cell encephalitis, perivascular infiltration of mononuclear cells, and activation and proliferation of microglia and astrocytes (11,18,56,57). Similar lesions had been described for animals infected with SIV$_{mac}$B670 (5,88). Thus, these two viruses proved to be highly neurovirulent.

Juvenile rhesus macaques inoculated with SIV$_{mac}$B670 were assessed for development of neurobehavioral changes, and initial experiments showed that both cognitive and motor functions were affected during virus infection (68,83). Many of these symptoms correlated with virus infection in cells of the basal ganglia (83). Virus invasion of the CNS correlated with elevated levels of quinolinic acid in the CSF, and this with impairment of motor skills in the animals (83). Whether infection in the neuropil was essential for causing these symptoms is not known. Interestingly, reactive astrocytosis with diffuse increase in expression of glial fibrillary acid protein (GFAP) was the best predictor of neuropsychological impairment, irrespective of productive virus replication in the brain. Thus, the mere presence of virus-infected cells in the CSF and accompanying meningitis may have been enough to induce neuropsychological changes in the animal. Sequential examination of animals infected with SIV$_{mac}$251 showed that meningitis was a frequent and the earliest lesion in the CNS and this was followed in some of the animals by development of encephalitic changes (18,56,57). Further data in the study by Dean et al. (18) showed that meningitis correlated with hypergammaglobulinemia and probably follicular hyperplasia in the lymphoid tissues (activation of the immune system). In contrast, in the few animals developing encephalitis, these lesions correlated with hypoglobulinemia and presumably involution of the lymphoid tissues (immunosuppression).

As mentioned above, SIV$_{mac}$251 and SIV$_{mac}$ are biologically purified viruses that replicate efficiently in CD4+ T cells and macrophage cell cultures. Whether the dual tropism of these agents are the effects of a single viral phenotype or more than one phenotype is not known. $SIV_{mac}239$ was chosen to evaluate pathogenesis because it is an infectious molecular clone derived from $SIV_{mac}251$ and is pathogenic in macaques (54,69). This provided the potential for determining the viral genetic basis of disease and possibly neuropathogenesis. $SIV_{mac}239$ is mainly a T-lymphocyte–tropic (L-tropic) virus. It replicates productively in human T cell lines and in primary macaque peripheral blood mononuclear cells (PBMCs) previously activated with mitogens and causes multinucleated giant cell formation (syncytia) (2,90). This virus also infects macrophages, causing a persistent, minimally productive type of infection (66). Infected macrophage cultures remain morphologically normal for several days in culture, and virus spread is minimal at best, as evidenced by the rare appearance of syncytial cytopathology. The precursor proteins of the viral envelope (glycoprotein [gp]160) and core (p55) are not processed efficiently, and only minimal assembly of infectious particles occurs (98).

Inoculation of $SIV_{mac}239$ into macaques resulted in dramatic effects that became apparent within the first 2 weeks after inoculation (43). First, the virus caused massive infection in T-lymphocytes, detectable by infectious center assays (43). Second, infected cells became activated and produced large amounts of cell-free virus, which coincided with the onset of viremia (90). During this phase the virus was recovered from PBMCs that had been cultured in medium containing only interleukin (IL)-2 (but no mitogens) (43). This confirmed that the infected T cells had been activated *in vivo* and therefore had no need for further activation by mitogens *in vitro* in order to produce virus. Third, this highly productive phase of virus replication coincided with massive hyperplasia in the lymphoid tissues, as evidenced by prominent increase in lymph node size and by splenomegaly. Fourth, the activated infected T cells crossed the blood–brain barrier and appeared in the CSF (43) within 2 weeks of inoculation. The animals developed lentiviral meningitis, as evidenced by histopathological and *in situ* hybridization procedures (18,56,57). However, these effects were transient, and lesions disappeared from the brains after the phase of activated T cells in the peripheral blood had ended (43,44) (Table 1). Cultivation of macrophages from the virus-producing spleen or lymph nodes or from brain did not yield cytopathic virus. However, cultivation of lymphocytes from the lymphoid tissues produced cytopathic virus (90). These results were in agreement with the inability of macrophages and the permissiveness of lymphocytes to produce virus when inoculated in culture. Notwithstanding the failure to recover infectious virus from brain or brain macrophages, or the lack of neuropathological changes, newer data obtained via polymerase chain reaction (PCR) have shown that the SIV genome was present in CNS tissue in seven of seven animals up to 2 years after inoculation with $SIV_{mac}239$ (Stephens, unpublished observations). Furthermore, homogenates of portions of brain from these animals also had small amounts of the viral core protein p27 (Joag,

TABLE 1. *Neuropathogenesis of SEV_{mac} infection in rhesus macaques*

Virus	No. of animals	Encephalitis	Antiviral immune reponses	Virus replication in brain
SIV_{mac} 239 (L-tropic)	15	0	15	Persistent, minimally productive
Infectious brain	15	3	0	Highly productive
homogenate (MΦtropic)		12	12	Persistent, minimally productive
Chimera (MΦtropic)	4	0	4	Persistent, minimally productive

unpublished observations). Presumably, the virus in brain was not actively replicating, the type of virus replication being similar to that produced in cultured macrophages infected with this virus (98). It is possible that this prolonged, minimally productive state of virus replication in brain, without any accompanying neuropathological changes, was sufficient to cause neuropsychological impairment. This concept may be relevant to HIV neurological disease because many individuals diagnosed with dementia had minimal neuropathological changes in the brain (75,76).

Macaques infected with $SIV_{mac}239$ developed strong humoral and cellular immune responses to the virus but nevertheless gradually lost CD4 + counts during the following 2 years. During this period, the animals also lost immunological competence with different degrees of severity, and most developed opportunistic infections; one animal developed lymphoma in the kidneys with metastasis to the brain but no viral encephalitis (101). Of 15 animals infected with this virus in different experiments, none developed virus encephalitis (Table 1), but as already mentioned, seven of these animals had evidence of persistent low level of virus replication in the brain. In an earlier study on macaques infected with $SIV_{mac}239$ (21), Desrosiers et al. showed that two animals developed encephalitis 2 years after inoculation, and the brains had classical lentiviral neuropathological lesions. Virus in the brains of the two animals was macrophage tropic. Because the animals had been inoculated with molecularly cloned, lymphocyte-tropic $SIV_{mac}239$, the origin of the neurovirulent virus must have been the result of mutation of virus 239 into a macrophage-tropic variant, followed by replication of the virus in the brain.

In hopes of deriving a predictably neurovirulent mutant of $SIV_{mac}239$, we performed two animal-to-animal passages using virus-infected bone marrow cells for IC inoculation and into the bone marrow of new animals. The rationale for this was that (a) it is well established that lentiviruses exist as a swarm of different genotypes; and (b) the bone marrow contains the largest number of different mononuclear cell types and, by inference, the largest number of different potential cells that can select and amplify different clones of virus from the virus swarm. The animal receiving the first bone marrow transplant developed interstitial pneumonia (91) similar to the disease seen in sheep with progressive pneumonia (maedi). The second recipient of the bone marrow cells developed both encephalitis and pneumonia, the macaque equivalent of visna/maedi disease. Cultivation of fragments of brain and lung in macrophage-inducing medium yielded macrophages that produced virus. Cell-free homogenates of both tissues also had infectious macrophage-tropic virus. However, cultivation of spleen cells in macrophage-promoting medium did not result in virus production, although cultivation of lymphocytes from the tissue yielded virus. Thus, these animals had two types of virus: the spleen had predominantly lymphocyte-tropic virus, whereas the brain contained predominantly macrophage-tropic virus. A similar dichotomy in viruses had been observed in spleen and brain from children dying from AIDS (24).

The brain from the animal that developed neurological disease, characterized by ataxia and weakness, had classical lesions of SIV encephalitis. Macrophages and astrocytes were activated, multinucleated giant cells and accumulations of microglia (glial nodules) were present in the neuropil, and cuffs of mononuclear cells were present around many of the blood vessels in the brain (Figs. 3–5). SIV infection was confirmed in brain sections using immunocytochemistry and *in situ* hybridization procedures, and a cell-free homogenate of a portion of the brain had infectious virus.

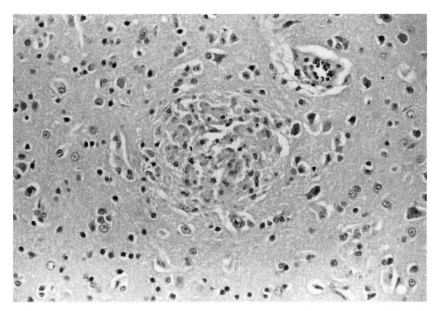

FIG. 3. Glial nodule in the brain of a macaque dying with SIVmac encephalitis. HE stain, original magnification ×150.

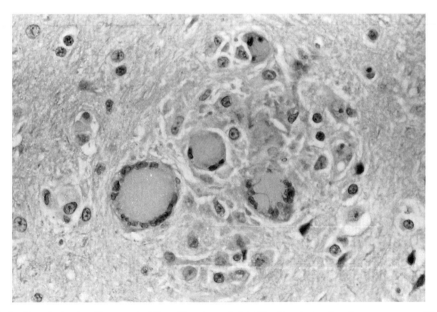

FIG. 4. Focal giant cell encephalitis with microglial infiltration in brain of a macaque with SIV encephalitis. HE stain, original magnification ×150.

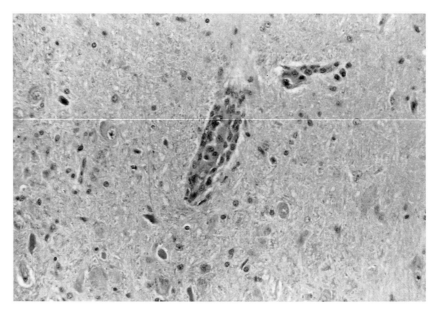

FIG. 5. Focal perivascular accumulation of inflammatory mononuclear cells in the brain of a macaque with SIV encephalitis. HE stain, original magnification ×150.

These results were thus similar to those caused by uncloned $SIV_{mac}251$ and B670. The fact that two types of infection (a lymphocyte-tropic virus infection in lymphoid tissues and a macrophage-tropic virus infection in the brain) were interacting in our animals that developed encephalitis raised a question about the presence of viral multiple genotypes in the stocks of $SIV_{mac}251$ and B670.

Brain homogenate containing infectious virus had been inoculated into 15 macaques (Table 1). Three of these animals developed classical encephalitis 2–6 months after inoculation, and all three had become severely immunosuppressed before the onset of encephalitis. None of these animals had antibodies against the virus as determined by immunoprecipitation, nor did they develop antiviral CD8+ T cells (45). Paradoxically, in the presence of the subtotal collapse of the immune system in lymphoid tissues, brain sections of all three animals with encephalitis had classical hallmarks of intense immunological activation. Microglia were enlarged and had multiple processes and expressed MHC II antigen, and this was accompanied by widespread astrocytosis. These cells expressed GFAP exuberantly. In contrast, the 12 other animals developed antiviral antibodies and antiviral CD8+ T cells. These animals had only latent infection in macrophages in their brains. Productive virus replication did not occur in the brain, and the animals did not develop encephalitis (45). Three of the 12 animals inoculated with infectious brain homogenate were treated with cytokines to determine whether virus replication in the brain would become activated (44). The animals were outfitted with Alzet pumps containing tissue culture fluids with 16 U/ml tumor necrosis factor-alpha and 100 U/ml IL-6. This material was delivered into the brain by a catheter at a rate of 70 mm^3/day for 4 weeks, and all three animals developed transient viremia during the next 2 weeks. All three produced antiviral antibodies. The animals were killed 4–6 weeks later and brains examined for virus content and lesions. There was only minimal evidence of virus replication, and similar to several animals already mentioned, only latent infection was found in the brain. This was evident because macrophages in explants of brain tissue produced virus in culture. Cytokines did not alter this pattern. Thus, it appeared that the encephalitis in macaques could be reproduced with SIV_{mac} that had macrophage tropism, but this was possible only in animals that had become severely immunosuppressed, and only three of 15 animals fell into this category. Moreover, the fact that the animals that developed encephalitis died within 6 months, whereas the others developed only a minimally productive infection irrespective of time, showed that the encephalitic process did not follow a course of gradual increment in severity with time. Rather, the data suggest a precipitous onset of disease. This is in keeping with beliefs on the pathogenesis of the disease in people.

Because the infectious viruses in the brain homogenate undoubtedly contained a virus swarm consisting of many genotypes or quasispecies, we attempted to determine whether a single infectious, molecularly cloned virus whose *env* gene was obtained from brain with encephalitis could cause encephalitis. We used PCR to amplify the *env* gene of the virus from DNA of brain from an animal with encephalitis, cloned the gene using molecular genetic techniques, and substituted this *env* gene for the corresponding *env* gene of infectious $SIV_{mac}239$ DNA (2). The rationale for this approach was that sequences in the *env* gene are the major determinant for cell and tissue tropism of the virus (12). Examination of the replication potential of this chimeric virus showed that it replicated productively in macaque macrophages, killing the cells within 1 week (2,98). We then tested the ability of this chimeric virus to cause encephalitis. To ensure that the viral genome did not undergo variation by passage in cell culture, we transfected bone marrow cells of four macaques with viral DNA, after which the cells were reinfused back into the respective animals (45). All four macaques became infected as determined by PCR evaluation of PBMC DNA and by rescue of infectious virus by cocultivation of mitogen-treated PBMCs with CEMx174 (proving infection in lymphocytes) and in cultures of blood-derived macrophages (proving infection in macrophage lineage cells). None of the animals developed infected activated T cells in peripheral blood, plasma viremia, lymphoid hyperplasia, or infected cells in the CSF. Examination of sections of brain tissue obtained via biopsy from the four animals showed that there were no viral antigens as determined by immunocytochemistry, and no encephalitic lesions were found. All four animals had developed potent antiviral immune responses. Thus, despite the tropism of the virus for macrophages and the fact that the *env* gene of the virus was derived from encephalitic brain, this agent, which seemed to have the ideal genotypic credentials for causing encephalitis, failed to cause this syndrome.

Our present data suggest that lentiviral encephalitis cannot be reproduced predictably using neuroadaptation procedures that have been applied successfully to other RNA viruses. Lentiviruses that cause encephalitis must be macrophage tropic, but their encephalitic potential seems to require a combination of different factors, two of which are (a) the ability to replicate productively in macrophages and (b) the ability to cause suppression of the immune system by elimination of CD4 + T cells. $SIV_{mac}251$ and B670 have both potentials. Their T cell tropism endowed them with potential for causing activation and infection in T cells, which gave rise to viremia, lymphoid hyperplasia, hypergammaglobulinemia, and meningitis. The latter lesion may have been enough to cause neuropsychological problems. AIDS was the end result of infection. Their macrophage tropism endowed them with the potential for causing encephalitis, but only some developed this complication. $SIV_{mac}239$, with its tropism for T cells, caused all of the effects ascribed to the T cell tropism aspect of $SIV_{mac}251$ and B670, but it is not macrophage tropic; hence, it could not cause encephalitis. In contrast, infectious virus in brain homogenates and bone marrow contained both potential factors and caused encephalitis in some, but not all, animals. This two-virus effect was similar to that of viruses 251 and B670. The chimeric virus had the appropriate cell tropism but failed to cause encephalitis, presumably because it failed to cause immunosuppression outright. Our data suggest that, mechanistically, lentiviral, and by inference, HIV-encephalitis is a two-step process. First, immunosuppression, possibly caused by lymphocyte-tropic virus, and second, replication of a macrophage-tropic virus in the brain. Because the replication of the macrophage-tropic virus in brain seemed to be predicated on suppression of the immune system, this encephalitic syndrome could be classified as another of the AIDS syndromes.

ACKNOWLEDGMENT

This work was supported by Public Health Service Grants NS-12127, NS-32203, and RR-06753 from the National Institutes of Health. We thank Jean Pemberton for typing the manuscript, Istvan Adany for preparation of the tables, and David Pinson for preparation of the photomicrographs.

REFERENCES

1. Adams DS, Oliver RE, Ameghino E, et al. Global survey of serologic evidence of caprine arthritis-encephalitis virus infections. *Vet Rec* 1984;115:493–495.
2. Anderson MG, Hauer D, Sharma DP, et al. Analysis of envelope changes acquired by $SIV_{mac}239$ during neuroadaptation in rhesus macaques. *Virology* 1993;195:616–626.
3. Barnett SW, Murthy KK, Herndier BG, Levy JA. An AIDS-like condition induced in baboons by HIV-2. *Science* 1994;266:642–646.
4. Barre-Sinoussi F, Chermann JC, Rey F, et al. Isolation of a T-lymphotropic retrovirus from a patient at risk for acquired immune deficiency syndrome. *Science* 1983;220:868–871.
5. Baskin GB, Murphey-Corb M, Roberts ED, Didier PJ, Martin LN. Correlates of SIV encephalitis in rhesus monkeys. *J Med Primatol* 1992;21:59–63.
6. Belman AL, Lantos G, Horoupian DS, et al. AIDS: calcification of the basal ganglia in infants and children. *Neurology* 1986;36:1192–1199.
7. Brinkmann R, Schwinn A, Narayan O, et al. Human immunodeficiency virus infection in microglia: correlation between cells infected in the brain and cells cultured from infectious brain tissue. *Ann Neurol* 1992;31:361–365.
8. Budka H. Multinucleated giant cells in brain: a hallmark of the acquired immune deficiency syndrome (AIDS). *Acta Neuropathol (Berl)* 1986;69:253–258.
9. Budka H, Costanzi G, Cristina S, et al. Brain pathology induced by infection with the human immunodeficiency virus (HIV). A histological, immunocytochemical, and electron microscopical study of 100 autopsy cases. *Acta Neuropathol (Berl)* 1987;75:185–198.
10. Carbone KM, Duchala CS, Griffin JW, Kincaid AL, Narayan O. Pathogenesis of Borna disease in rats: evidence that intra-axonal spread is the major route for virus dissemination and the determinant for disease incubation. *J Virol* 1987;61:3431–3440.
11. Chakrabarti L, Guyader M, Alizon M, et al. Sequence of simian immunodeficiency virus from macaque and its relationship to other human and simian retroviruses. *Nature* 1987;328:543–547.
12. Cordonnier A, Montagnier L, Emerman M. Single amino-acid changes in HIV envelope affect viral tropism and receptor binding. *Nature* 1989;340:571–574.
13. Cork LC, Hadlow WJ, Crawford TB, Gorham JR, Pyper RC. Infectious leukoencephalomyelitis of goats (CAEV). *J. Infect. Diseases* 1974;129:134–141.
14. Cork LC, Hadlow WJ, Gorham JR, Piper RC, Crawford TB. Pathology of viral leukoencephalomyelitis of goats. *Acta Neuropathol (Berl)* 1974;29:281–292.
15. Cork LC, Narayan O. The pathogenesis of viral leukoencephalomyelitis-arthritis of goats I. Persistent viral infection with progressive pathologic changes. *Lab Invest* 1980;42:596–602.

16. Crawford TB, Adams DS. Caprine arthritis-encephalitis: clinical features and presence of antibody in selected goat populations. *J Am Vet Med Assoc* 1981;178:713–719.

17. Crawford TB, Adams DS, Cheevers WP, Cork LC. Chronic arthritis in goats caused by a retrovirus. *Science* 1980;207:997–999.

18. Dean AF, Montgomery M, Baskerville A, et al. Different patterns of neuropathological disease in rhesus monkeys infected by simian immunodeficiency virus, and their relation to the humoral immune response. *Neuropathol Appl Neurobiol* 1993;19:336–345.

19. DeMartini JC, Brodie SJ, de la Concha Bermejillo A, Ellis JA, Lairmore MD. Pathogenesis of lymphoid interstitial pneumonia in natural and experimental ovine lentivirus infection. *Clin Infect Dis* 1993;17(suppl 1):236–242.

20. Desrosiers RC. Simian immunodeficiency viruses. *Annu Rev Microbiol* 1988;42:607–625.

21. Desrosiers RC, Hansen Moosa A, Mori K, et al. Macrophage-tropic variants of SIV are associated with specific AIDS-related lesions but are not essential for the development of AIDS. *Am J Pathol* 1991;139:29–35.

22. Dow SW, Poss ML, Hoover EA. Feline immunodeficiency virus: a neurotropic lentivirus. *J AIDS* 1990;3:658–668.

23. Dubois-Dalcq M, Reese TS, Narayan O. Membrane changes associated with assembly of visna virus. *Virology* 1976;74:520–530.

24. Epstein LG, Kuiken C, Blumberg BM, et al. HIV-1 V3 domain variation in brain and spleen of children with AIDS: tissue-specific evolution within host-determined quasispecies. *Virology* 1991; 180:583–590.

25. Epstein LG, Sharer LR, Gajdusek DC. Hypothesis: AIDS encephalopathy is due to primary and persistent infection of the brain with a human retrovirus of the lentivirus subfamily. *Med Hypotheses* 1986;21:87–96.

26. Epstein LG, Sharer LR, Joshi VV, Fojas MM, Koenigsberger MR, Oleske JM. Progressive encephalopathy in children with acquired immune deficiency syndrome. *Ann Neurol* 1985;17:488–496.

27. Everall I, Glass J, McArthur J, Spargo E, Lantos P. Neuronal loss in the superior frontal gyrus correlates with HIV associated dementia. *Clin Neuropathol* 1993;12(suppl):10.

28. Everall IP, Luthert PJ, Lantos PL. Neuronal loss in the frontal cortex in HIV infection. *Lancet* 1991; 337:1119–1121.

29. Franchini G, Markham P, Gard E, et al. Persistent infection of rhesus macaques with a molecular clone of human immunodeficiency virus type 2: evidence of minimal genetic drift and low pathogenetic effects. *J Virol* 1990;64:4462–4467.

30. Gabuzda DH, Hess JL, Small JA, Clements JE. Regulation of the visna virus long terminal repeat in macrophages involves cellular factors that bind sequences containing AP-1 sites. *Mol Cell Biol* 1989;9:2728–2733.

31. Gendelman HE, Narayan O, Kennedy-Stoskopf S, et al. Tropism of sheep lentiviruses for monocytes: susceptibility to infection and virus gene expression increase during maturation of monocytes to macrophages. *J Virol* 1986;58:67–74.

32. Gendelman HE, Narayan O, Molineaux S, Clements JE, Ghotbi Z. Slow, persistent replication of lentiviruses: role of tissue macrophages and macrophage precursors in bone marrow. *Proc Natl Acad Sci U S A* 1985;82:7086–7090.

33. Gendelman HE, Orenstein JM, Baca LM, et al. The macrophage in the persistence and pathogenesis of HIV infection. *AIDS* 1989;3:475–495.

34. Georgsson G, Houwers DJ, Palsson P, Petursson G. Expression of viral antigens in the central nervous system of visna-infected sheep: an immunohistochemical study on experimental visna induced by virus strains of increased neurovirulence. *Acta Neuropathol* 1989;77:299–306.

35. Georgsson G, Martin JR, Klein J, Palsson PA, Nathanson N, Petursson G. Primary demyelination in visna. An ultrastructural study of Icelandic sheep with clinical signs following experimental infection. *Acta Neuropathol* 1982;57:171–178.

36. Georgsson G, Palsson PA. The histopathology of maedi, a slow viral pneumonia of sheep. *Vet Pathol* 1971;8:63–80.

37. Gilles PN, Lathey JL, Spector SA. Replication of macrophage-tropic and T cell–tropic strains of human immunodeficiency virus type-1 is augmented by macrophage/endothelial cell contact. *J Virol* 1995;69:2133–2139.

38. Ginsberg AH, Johnson KP. Vaccinia virus meningitis in mice after intracerebral inoculation. *Infect Immun* 1976;13:1221–1227.

39. Gorrell MD, Brandon MR, Sheffer D, Adams RJ, Narayan O. Ovine lentivirus is macrophage-tropic and does not replicate productively in T lymphocytes. *J Virol* 1992;66:2679–2688.

40. Gray FM, Lescs C, Keohane C, et al. Early brain changes in HIV infection: neuropathological study of 11 HIV seropositive, non-AIDS cases. *J Neuropathol Exp Neurol* 1992;51:177–185.

41. Horowitz SL, Benson DF, Gottlieb MS. Neurological complications of gay-related immunodeficiency disorder. *Ann Neurol* 1982;12:80.

42. Huang CH, Wong C. Relation of peripheral multipilication of Japanese B encephalitis virus to the pathogenesis of infection in mice. *Acta* 1963;7:322–330.

43. Joag SV, Adams RJ, Foresman L, et al. Early activation of PBMC and appearance of antiviral CD8$^+$ cells influence the prognosis of SIV-induced disease in rhesus macaques. *J Med Primatol* 1994;23:108–116.

44. Joag SV, Adams RJ, Pinson DM, Adany I, Narayan O. Intracerebral infusion of TNF-α and IL-6 failed to activate latent SIV infection in the brains of macaques inoculated with macrophage-tropic neuroadapted SIV$_{mac}$. *J Leukoc Biol* 1994;56:353–357.

45. Joag SV, Stephens EB, Galbreath D, et al. SIVmac chimeric virus whose env gene was derived from SIV-encephalitic brain is macrophage-tropic but not neurovirulent. *J Virol* 1995 (in press).

46. Johnson GC, Adams DS, McGuire TC. Pronounced production of polyclonal immunoglobulin G1 in the synovial fluid of goats with caprine arthritis encephalitis virus infection. *Infect Immun* 1983; 41:805–815.

47. Johnson GC, Barbet AF, Klevjer-Anderson P, McGuire TC. Preferential immune response to vision surface glycoproteins by caprine arthritis encephalitis virus infected goats. *Infect Immun* 1983;41: 657–665.

48. Johnson RT. Mumps virus. In: Johnson RT, ed. *Viral Infections of the Nervous System.* New York: Raven, 1982:98–100.

49. Johnson RT. Viral infections of the nervous system. New York: Raven, 1982.

50. Johnson RT, McArthur JC, Narayan O. The neurobiology of human immunodeficiency virus infections. *FASEB J* 1988;2:2970–2981.

51. Jubelt B, Narayan O, Johnson RT. Pathogenesis of human poliovirus infection in mice. II. Age-dependency of paralysis. *J Neuropathol Exp Neurol* 1980;39:149–159.

52. Kennedy PGE, Narayan O, Ghotbi Z, Hopkins J, Gendelman HE, Clements JE. Persistent expression of Ia antigen and viral genome in visna-maedi virus-induced inflammatory cells: possible role of lentivirus-induced interferon. *J Exp Med* 1985;162:1970–1982.

53. Kennedy-Stoskopf S, Zink C, Narayan O. Pathogenesis of ovine lentivirus-induced arthritis: phenotypic evaluation of T lymphocytes in synovial fluid, synovium, and peripheral circulation. *Clin Immunol Immunopathol* 1989;52:323–330.

54. Kestler H, Kodama T, Ringler D, et al. Induction of AIDS in rhesus monkeys by molecularly cloned simian immunodeficiency virus. *Science* 1990;248:1109–1112.

55. Koenig S, Gendelman HE, Orenstein JM, et al. Detection of AIDS virus in macrophages in brain tissue from AIDS patients with encephalopathy. *Science* 1986;233:1089–1093.

56. Lackner AA, Smith MO, Munn RJ, et al. Localization of simian immunodeficiency virus in the central nervous system of rhesus monkeys. *Am J Pathol* 1991;139:609–621.

57. Lackner AA, Vogel P, Ramos RA, Kluge JD, Marthas M. Early events in tissues during infection with pathogenic (SIV$_{mac}$239) and nonpathogenic (SIV$_{mac}$1A11) molecular clones of simian immunodeficiency virus. *Am J Pathol* 1994;145:428–439.

58. Lairmore MD, Butera ST, Callahan GN, DeMartini JC. Spontaneous interferon production by pulmonary leukocytes is associated with lentivirus-induced lymphoid interstitial pneumonia. *J Immunol* 1988;140:779–785.

59. Lairmore MD, Poulson JM, Adduci TA, DeMartini JC. Lentivirus-induced lymphoproliferative disease: comparative pathogenicity of phenotypically distinct ovine lentivirus strains. *Am J Pathol* 1988;130:80–90.

60. Letvin NL, Daniel MD, Sehgal PK, et al. Induction of AIDS-like disease in macaque monkeys with T cell tropic retrovirus STLV-III. *Science* 1985;230:71–73.

61. Levy RM, Bredesen DE, Rosenblum ML. Neurological manifestations of the acquired immunodeficiency syndrome: experience at UCSF and review of the literature. *J Neurosurg* 1985;62:475–495.

62. Lin FH, Thormar H. Characterization of ribonucleic acid from visna virus. *J Virol* 1971;7:582–587.

63. Mankowski JL, Spelman JP, Ressetar HG, et al. Neurovirulent simian immunodeficiency virus replicates productively in endothelial cells of the central nervous system *in vivo* and *in vitro. J Virol* 1994;68:8202–8208.

64. Marsh H. Progressive pneumonia in sheep. *J Am Vet Med Assoc* 1923;62:458–473.

65. McGuire TC, Adams DS, Johnson GC, Klevjer-Anderson P, Barbee DE, Gorham JR. Retrovirus challenge of vaccinated on persistently infected goats causes acute arthritis. *Am J Vet Res* 1986;47: 537–540.

66. Mori K, Ringler DJ, Desrosiers RC. Restricted replication of simian immunodeficiency virus strain 239 in macrophages is determined by env but is not due to restricted entry. *J Virol* 1993;67: 2807–2814.

67. Murphey-Corb M, Martin LN, Rangan SRS, et al. Isolation of an HTLV-III related retrovirus from macaques with simian AIDS and its possible origin in asymptomatic mangabeys. *Nature* 1986;321: 435–437.

68. Murray EA, Rausch DM, Lendvay J, Sharer LR, Eiden LE. Cognitive and motor impairments associated with SIV infection in rhesus monkeys. *Science* 1992;255:1246–1249.

69. Naidu YM, Kestler HW, Li Y, et al. Characterization of infectious molecular clones of simian immunodeficiency virus (SIV$_{mac}$) and human immunodeficiency virus type 2: persistent infection of rhesus monkeys with molecularly cloned SIV$_{mac}$. *J Virol* 1988;62:4691–4696.

70. Narayan O, Kennedy-Stoskopf S, Sheffer D, Griffin DE, Clements JE. Activation of caprine arthritis-encephalitis virus expression during maturation of monocytes to macrophages. *Infect Immun* 1983; 41:67–73.

71. Narayan O, Sheffer D, Clements JE, Tennekoon G. Restricted replication of lentiviruses: visna viruses induce a unique interferon during interaction between lymphocytes and infected macrophages. *J Exp Med* 1985;162:1954–1969.

72. Narayan O, Wolinsky JS, Clements JE, Strandberg JD, Griffin DE, Cork LC. Slow virus replication: the role of macrophages in the persistence and expression of visna viruses of sheep and goats. *J Gen Virol* 1982;59:345–356.

73. Nathanson N, Martin JR, Georgsson G, Palsson PA, Lutley RE, Petursson G. The effect of post-infection immunization on the severity of experimental visna. *J Comp Pathol* 1981;91:185–191.

74. Nathanson N, Panitch H, Palsson PA, Petursson G, Georgsson G. Pathogenesis of visna II. Effect of immunosuppression upon the central nervous system lesions. *Lab Invest* 1976;35:444–451.

75. Navia BA, Cho ES, Petito CK, Price RW. The AIDS dementia complex: II. Neuropathology. Ann. Neurol. 1986;19:525–535.

76. Navia BA, Jordan BD, Price RW. The AIDS dementia complex: I. Clinical features. Ann Neurol 1986;19:517–524.

77. Oliver RE, Gorham JR, Parish SF, Hadlow WJ, Narayan O. Ovine progressive pneumonia: pathologic and virologic studies on the naturally occurring disease. *Am J Vet Res* 1981;42:1554–1559.

78. Panitch H, Petursson G, Georgsson G, Palsson PA, Nathanson N. Pathogenesis of Visna. III. Immune responses to central nervous system antigens in experimental allergic encephalomyelitis and visna. *Lab Invest* 1976;35:452–460.

79. Petito CK, Cho ES, Lemann W, Navia BA, Price RW. Neuropathology of acquired immunodeficiency syndrome (AIDS): an autopsy review. *Acta Neuropathol* 1987;75:185–198.

80. Petursson G, Nathanson N, Georgsson G, Panitch H, Palsson PA. Pathogenesis of visna 1. Sequential virologic, serologic and pathologic studies. *Lab Invest* 1976;35:402–412.

81. Phillips TR, Prospero-Garcia O, Puaoi DL, et al. Neurological abnormalities associated with feline immunodeficiency virus infection. *J Gen Virol* 1994;75:979–987.

82. Podell M, Oglesbee M, Mathes L, Krakowka S, Olmstead R, Lafrado L. AIDS-associated encephalopathy with experimental feline immunodeficiency virus infection. *J AIDS* 1993;6:758–771.

83. Rausch DM, Heyes MP, Murray EA, et al. Cytopathologic and neurochemical correlates of progression to motor/cognitive impairment in SIV-infected rhesus monkeys. *J Neuropathol Exp Neurol* 1994;53:165–175.

84. Sabin AB. The nature and rate of centripetal progression of certain neurotropic viruses along peripheral nerves. *Am J Pathol* 1937;13:615–617.

85. Sabin AB, Schlesinger RW. Production of immunity to dengue with virus modified by propagation in mice. *Science* 1945;101:640–642.

86. Sasseville VG, Newman W, Brodie SJ, Hesterberg P, Pauley D, Ringler DJ. Monocyte adhesion to endothelium in simian immunodeficiency virus-induced AIDS encephalitis is mediated by vascular cell adhesion molecule-1/alpha 4 beta 1 integrin interactions. *Am J Pathol* 1994;144:27–40.

87. Sharer LR. Pathology of HIV-1 infection of the central nervous system. A review. *J Neuropathol Exp Neurol* 1992;51:3–11.

88. Sharer LR. Neuropathology and pathogenesis of SIV infection of the central nervous system. In: Price RW, Perry SW, eds. *HIV, AIDS and the Brain.* New York: Raven, 1994:133–145.

89. Sharer LR, Epstein LG, Cho ES, et al. Pathologic features of AIDS encephalopathy in children: evidence for LAV/HTLV-III infection of brain. *Hum Pathol* 1986;17:271–284.

90. Sharma DP, Anderson M, Zink MC, et al. Pathogenesis of acute infection in rhesus macaques with a lymphocyte-tropic strain of simian immunodeficiency virus. *J Infect Dis* 1992;166:738–746.

91. Sharma DP, Zink MC, Anderson M, et al. Derivation of neurotropic simian immunodeficiency virus from exclusively lymphocytetropic parental virus: pathogenesis of infection in macaques. *J Virol* 1992;66:3550–3556.

92. Sheffield WD, Narayan O, Strandberg JD, Adams RJ. Visna-maedi-like disease associated with an ovine retrovirus infection in a Corriedale sheep. *Vet Pathol* 1980;17:544–552.

93. Shih DS, Carruth LM, Anderson M, Clements JE. Involvement of FOS and JUN in the activation of visna virus gene expression in macrophages through an AP-1 site in the viral LTR. *Virology* 1992;190:84–91.

94. Sigurdsson B. Observations on three slow infections of sheep: Maedi, paratuberculosis, rida, a slow encephalitis of sheep with general remarks on infections which develop slowly, and some of their special characteristics. *Br Vet J* 1954;110:255–270.

95. Sigurdsson B, Palsson PA, Grissom H. Visna, a demyelinating transmissable disease of sheep. *J Neuropathol Exp Neurol* 1957;16:389–403.

96. Sigurdsson B, Thormar H, Palsson PA. Cultivation of visna virus in tissue culture. *Arch Virusforsch* 1960;10:368–381.

97. Sonigo P, Alizon M, Staskus K, et al. Nucleotide sequence of visna lentivirus: relationship to the AIDS virus. *Cell* 1985;42:369–382.

98. Stephens EB, McClure HM, Narayan O. The proteins of lymphocyte and macrophage-tropic strains of SIV are processed differently in macrophages. *Virology* 1995;206(1):535–544.
99. Summers BA, Griesen HA, Appel MG. Possible initiation of viral encephalomyelitis in dogs by migrating lymphocytes infected with distemper. *Lancet* 1978;1:187–189.
100. Wolinsky JS, Klassen T, Baringer JR. Persistence of neuroadapted mumps virus in brains of newborn hamsters after intraperitoneal inoculation. *J Infect Dis* 1976;133:260–267.
101. Zhu GW, Liu ZQ, Joag SV, et al. Pathogenesis of lymphocyte-tropic and macrophage-tropic SIVmac infection in the brain. *J Neurovirol* 1995;1:78–91.

AIDS and the Nervous System, Second Edition,
edited by J. R. Berger and R. M. Levy.
Lippincott-Raven Publishers, Philadelphia © 1997.

7

Neurological Symptoms in Human Immunodeficiency Virus Infection

*Gerald J. Dal Pan, °Justin C. McArthur, and
†Michael J.G. Harrison

°Department of Neurology, The Johns Hopkins University School of Medicine,
Baltimore, Maryland 21287-7609, U.S.A., and †University College London
Medical School, Reta Lila Weston Institute of Neurological Studies,
London W1N 8AA, England

A wide variety of nervous system manifestations can complicate HIV infection. This broad spectrum of neurological disease reflects not only the diversity of pathogens capable of causing neurologic dysfunction in the HIV-infected patient, but also the multiple levels of both the central and peripheral nervous system that can be involved. Almost any neurological symptom can thus be seen in an HIV-infected patient.

Despite the wide number of neurological syndromes in HIV infection, a systematic approach to the patient with neurological symptoms can usually narrow the differential diagnosis to two or three specific illnesses before any neurodiagnostic tests are conducted. A few principles should be applied when evaluating neurological symptoms:

1. Specific neurological syndromes are usually restricted to a given stage of HIV disease or to a given range of CD4+ T-lymphocytes (CD4+ counts). For example, cytomegalovirus (CMV) encephalitis generally occurs in the late stage of HIV infection, usually when the CD4+ count is <50 cell/mm^3. On the other hand, acute inflammatory demyelinating polyneuropathy generally occurs during the ''asymptomatic'' period of HIV disease. Knowledge of the patient's CD4+ count is thus crucial in evaluating neurological complaints. Of note, coinfection with human T-lymphotropic virus-1 (HTLV-I) can increase the CD4+ count.

2. Neurological symptoms in HIV-infected patients may be due not only to nervous system involvement by HIV or an opportunistic pathogen, but also to the effects of systemic illness or medications. For example, an acute change in mental status may represent cryptococcal meningitis, or it may represent the effects of hypoxemia caused by *Pneumocystis carinii* pneumonia. A predominantly sensory neuropathy (PSN) may be due to HIV infection, or it may be a toxic sensory neuropathy induced by dideoxyinosine (ddI) or dideoxycytidine (ddC). Knowledge of a patient's medications is essential, and a search for systemic illness may be warranted.

3. Patients may have multiple neurological symptoms. In some cases, these may be due to a single process, whereas in others two or more processes may be at

This work was supported by NS 26643, AI35042, RR00722. Portions of this chapter were modified from Harrison MJG, McArthur JC: *AIDS and Neurology*. New York: Churchill Livingstone, 1995.

work. For example, a patient with cryptococcal meningitis may have not only headache, stiff neck, and fevers, but also may have a unilateral lower motor neuron facial nerve palsy. On the other hand, a patient with painful, numb feet and a spastic gait disorder may have both a PSN as well as an HIV-associated vacuolar myelopathy (VM). Examination of both the peripheral and central nervous systems is essential in evaluating a neurological complaint in an HIV-infected person.

MENTAL STATUS CHANGES

Encephalopathy or altered mentation is one of the most common neurological syndromes encountered during HIV infection. Although altered mentation may indicate central nervous system (CNS) infection either with an opportunistic organism or with HIV, more commonly altered mentation results from metabolic disturbance or intoxication or as an adverse effect of medication. The development of encephalopathy in an HIV-infected person must prompt consideration of a CNS opportunistic process; however, it is rare for these to develop with a CD4+ count of >200 mm^3. In the uncommon situation of dual infection with HIV-1 and HTLV-I, the CD4+ count may be difficult to interpret because HTLV-I may elevate the CD4+ count even though there is a degree of underlying cellular immunodeficiency. Table 1 provides a useful guide to differential diagnosis when a recent CD4+ count is available. In an encephalopathic patient with risk behaviors for HIV infection in whom HIV seropositivity has not been documented, HIV serology should be confirmed. Psychomotor slowing is a hallmark of HIV-associated cognitive disorder. A number of brief cognitive tests have been developed for measurement of cognitive impairment in HIV infection. The Minimental State Examination (MMSE) is relatively insensitive for the detection of HIV dementia because it does not include any timed measures. We have developed a short screening instrument that is superior to the MMSE for detecting dementia: the HIV Dementia Scale (76). This instrument (Fig. 1) combines measures of frontal, memory, and psychomotor speed and requires no equipment or special training. It is particularly useful as a brief screen in an outpatient setting and probably most helpful when it is preformed as a baseline test and then followed at successive visits.

Altered Mentation with a CD4+ Count of >200

There are several important infectious causes of altered mentation that may occur in HIV-infected persons with CD4+ counts of >200. Acute encephalopathy in an

TABLE 1. *Differential diagnosis of mental status changes in HIV infection*

CD4+ >200 cells/mm³	CD4+ <200 cells/mm³
Primary HIV infection with meningoencephalitis	Any causes with CD4+ <200 cells/mm³, except for primary infection
Herpes simplex virus encephalitis	
Tuberculous meningitis	Sepsis
Neurosyphilis	Systemic infections
Substance abuse	Medications (see Table 2)
Cranial trauma	Opportunistic CNS infections (see Tables 3 and 8)
Seizures	
Nutritional deficiency	
Bacterial meningitis	

HIV DEMENTIA SCALE

Max   Score
Score

MEMORY - REGISTRATION

Give four words to recall (dog, hat, green, peach) -
1 second to say each. Then ask the patient all 4
after you have said them.

4   ( )   **ATTENTION**

Anti-saccadic   eye   movements: 20   (twenty)
commands.

_____errors of 20 trials

≤3 errors = 4; 4 errors = 3; 5 errors = 2; 6 errors = 1; >6
errors = 0

6   ( )   **PSYCHOMOTOR SPEED**

Ask patient to write the alphabet in upper case letters
horizontally across the page (use back of this form)
and record time: _____ seconds.

≤21 sec = 6; 21.1 - 24 sec = 5; 24.1 - 27 sec = 4; 27.1 - 30
sec = 3; 30.1 - 33 sec = 2; 33.1 - 36 sec = 1; >36 sec = 0

4   ( )   **MEMORY - RECALL**

Ask for 4 words from Registration above. Give 1
point for each correct. For words not recalled,
prompt with a "semantic" clue, as follows: animal
(dog); piece of clothing (hat), color (green), fruit
(peach). Give 1/2 point for each correct after
prompting.

2   ( )   **CONSTRUCTION**

Copy the cube below; record time: ____ seconds.

< 25 sec = 2; 25 - 35 sec = 1; >35 sec = 0

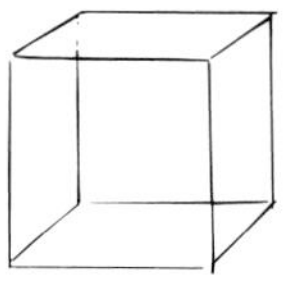

TOTAL SCORE: _____ /16

Department of Neurology

FIG. 1. The HIV Dementia Scale. (From Power C, Selnes OA, Grim JA, McArthur JC. The HIV Dementia Scale: a rapid screening test. *J AIDS* 1995;8:273–278; with permission).

HIV-seronegative individual with risk factors for HIV infection may represent primary HIV infection with seroconversion illness and HIV meningoencephalitis. In this setting, altered mentation is accompanied by fever, macular papular rash, lymphadenopathy, meningismus, and atypical lymphocytosis with serologic conversion within days to weeks. Another cause of viral encephalitis with altered mentation, fever, and seizures is herpes simplex encephalitis. Although there have been several case reports of herpes simplex encephalitis during HIV infection, overall, it is a relatively unusual cause of encephalitis and altered mentation. Its clinical features during HIV infection mirror those of sporadic herpes simplex virus encephalitis with abrupt onset of personality change, altered mentation, seizures, frontotemporal abnormalities on imaging and electroencephalography (EEG), and cerebrospinal fluid (CSF) pleocytosis. Brain biopsy may be required for diagnosis, and treatment with intravenous acyclovir is usually effective.

Apart from CMV and progressive multifocal leukoencephalopathy (PML), which are both rare when the CD4+ count is >200 cells/mm^3, other forms of CNS infection, both viral and bacterial, may develop in the HIV-infected individual, but do not appear to be increased in frequency. The only two exceptions to this are tuberculous (TB) meningitis and neurosyphilis. Worldwide, tuberculosis is the most common opportunistic infection accompanying HIV infection, and TB meningitis has become an important cause of encephalopathy and altered mentation, particularly in developing countries. In contrast to other CNS opportunistic infections, TB meningitis can develop with a CD4+ count of >200. Important clues to the presence of TB meningitis are pulmonary or extrapulmonary tuberculosis, fever, and abnormal CSF profile with hypoglycorrhachia and elevated protein. TB meningitis is usually preceded by a period of malaise, fatigue, and headache. Most patient have confusion and/or headache (20,84). Less than half have meningismus, but one quarter may have focal signs such as hemiparesis or cranial nerve deficits. A predominantly lymphocytic pleocytosis, with up to 1,000 white blood cells (WBC)/mm^3 is the rule with protein content elevated up to 1,000 mg/dl and positive CSF cultures. Imaging studies may show meningeal enhancement or focal lesions representing tuberculomas in about half of patients. Because of the frequency of cutaneous anergy in HIV infection, standard tuberculin skin reactivity is notoriously unreliable for the detection of active tuberculous infection (2).

Neurosyphilis is another infectious process that may be more frequent or its features more florid in the setting of concomitant HIV infection. Several series have suggested that the natural history of syphilis is accelerated with coexisting HIV-induced cellular immunodeficiency. In fact, general paresis is rare as a manifestation of syphilis during HIV infection (39,68). More common is for altered mentation to develop with syphilitic meningitis or meningovascular syphilis. Musher et al. (68) reported signs and symptoms of meningitis, including confusion, in nine of 23 HIV-infected individuals with acute syphilitic meningitis. Important clues to neurosyphilis include history of untreated (or inadequately treated) syphilis, increasing reactive plasma reagin (RPR) titers on serial blood samples, or lymphocytic CSF pleocytosis with or without a positive CSF VDRL. The CSF VDRL test is relatively insensitive and may have a false-negative result rate of 30–40% during this phase of syphilis (86).

Probably the most common cause of altered mentation at this early stage of HIV infection is substance abuse. Alcohol intoxication, alcohol or benzodiazepine withdrawal, and use of sedatives, barbiturates, cocaine, phencyclidine, marijuana, or injection drugs can all induce encephalopathy. Each agent can induce specific clinical features, which facilitate identification. For example, alcohol withdrawal may be associated with delirium tremens, seizures, and sympathetic overactivity; phencyclidine use may be associated with hyperagitation and violent outbursts; use of narcotics may be suspected when recognizing pinpoint pupils or recent needle tracks. History and toxicological screening are important to identify the offending substance. Flumazenil and naloxone may be useful as specific reversal agents for benzodiazepines and opiates, respectively. Additional information on the recognition and treatment of specific intoxication syndromes can be found in the text by Brust (8).

Other causes of altered mentation include cranial trauma, which may result from assaults or falls or may be related indirectly to substance abuse. External signs of cranial trauma, including laceration, bruises, and contusions, are important clues. Cerebral contusion, intraparenchymal hemorrhages, subdural hematomas, and subarachnoid hemorrhage can be readily identified via computed tomography (CT) or magnetic resonance imaging (MRI). Seizures may induce altered mentation, either as a postictal phenomenon or, less commonly, during nonconvulsive status epilepticus. In HIV-infected individuals with normal CD4+ counts, seizures are usually not the result either of HIV infection or opportunistic processes, and usually develop either as a consequence of substance abuse or withdrawal or result secondarily from trauma. History and EEG should identify most patients with epileptiform activity. Finally, nutritional deficiencies, including Wernicke's encephalopathy, may contribute to altered mentation in HIV infection. Although not a direct consequence of HIV infection, cooccurrence of two illnesses, chronic alcoholism and HIV infection, has produced a recent resurgence in cases of Wernicke's encephalopathy. Specific clues for Wernicke's encephalopathy include ophthalmoparesis or ophthalmoplegia, gait ataxia, confabulation, and, in its chronic forms, Korsakoff's psychosis. It is reasonable to treat any HIV-infected patient with altered mentation with additional thiamine, particularly before a glucose load, which may precipitate Wernicke's encephalopathy with thiamine deficiency.

Altered Mentation with a CD4+ Count of <200

Any of the causes of altered mentation described above for the immunocompetent HIV-infected individual can develop with CD4+ counts of <200. However, development of encephalopathy at this stage of HIV infection has much more serious consequences and usually reflects the development of an opportunistic process affecting the central nervous system. For the patient with advanced HIV infection, bacteremia—either from bacterial sepsis or disseminated *Mycobacterium avium-intracellulare*—may produce fevers and altered mentation as a result of a septic/toxic encephalopathy. A common example would be development of transient delirium during *Staphylococcus aureus* bacteremia from an infected central catheter. In this situation, treatment of the underlying infection with antibiotics usually allows normalization of mental status within 24–48 hours. Prolonged, persistent encephalopathy should prompt a search for other causes. Although some substances can and do cause encephalopathy during advanced HIV infection, generally the frequency of illicit drug use declines during this stage of HIV infection. A number of prescribed medications, either singly or in combination, can contribute to the development of altered mentation in a patient with AIDS. Drug interactions or accumulation of active metabolites as a result of hepatic dysfunction or impaired renal clearance may contribute to the adverse effects of medications commonly used during HIV infection. Table 2 lists some of the commonly used medications associated with altered mentation. Patients with preexisting HIV-associated dementia (AIDS dementia complex) are particularly prone to the psychoactive effects of medications. One commonly encountered situation is the mildly demented patient who is treated with tricyclic antidepressants at full dose and develops a "decompensated" dementia with delirium. With discontinuation of the offending medication, the delirium usually clears within a few days. Similarly, other cerebral insults from the effects of sepsis, infection, or metabolic derangements may precipitate altered mentation and delirium in demented individuals.

A range of opportunistic processes can lead to altered mentation. The tempo of onset of encephalopathy and associated clinical features are probably most helpful in recognizing and identifying the causative agent (Table 3). Fungal meningitides, including cryptococcal meningitis, coccidioidomycosis, and histoplasmosis, can all cause acute change in mental status, usually with fever, headache, and varying degrees of meningismus. Focal neurological deficits are uncommon, occurring in cryptococcal meningitis in only 15% of patients in one large series (10). Perhaps surprisingly, in the same series meningismus was detected in just over one quarter of the patients. Cryptococcal meningitis is the first AIDS-defining illness for almost half the patients with cryptococcosis., Many patients may have had undocumented HIV infection before their acute presentation with meningitis and altered mentation. There are important regional differences for the different forms of fungal meningitis. Although cryptococcal meningitis is ubiquitous with worldwide distribution, histoplasmosis is found most commonly in the midwest and coccidioidomycosis in the southwest. Cerebral toxoplasmosis is associated with altered mentation in almost two thirds of patients, many of whom also have fever and headache. An important differentiating point from the fungal meningitides is that ~90% of patients with toxoplasmosis have focal neurological deficits, usually hemiparesis, aphasia, or hemiataxia. The onset of neurological symptoms in toxoplasmosis is usually subacute, developing over 1–2 weeks. Toxoplasmosis develops as a reactivated infection in HIV-infected individuals, rather than as a true opportunistic pathogen. Thus, measurement of toxoplasma serology in neurologically asymptomatic HIV-infected individuals is useful, both to identify individuals at risk for the subsequent development of toxoplasmosis and to initiate anti-toxoplasma prophylaxis with trimethoprim/sulfamethoxazole, pyrimethamine, or dapsone at CD4 + counts of <200 (66,80). Although primary CNS lymphoma, like toxoplasmosis, also can produce altered mentation and may have identical radiological characteristics (see Chapter 13), in general the development of altered mentation is slower with primary CNS lymphoma. Patients first develop personality or behavioral changes that only over a few weeks lead to altered mentation with disorientation, language disturbance, and impairment of cognitive functions. Although both processes may produce multiple ring-enhancing mass lesions, in general, those of cerebral toxoplasmosis tend to be smaller, more numerous, and associated with relatively little edema, whereas primary CNS lymphoma lesions may be single, large (>4 cm), and accompanied by significant edema and mass effect. Recently, thallium SPECT scans have been used to differentiate lymphoma (positive uptake) from toxoplasma abscesses, which fail to take up the radioisotope and appear as "cold" lesions (73).

CMV encephalitis has become a relatively common cause of altered mentation, particularly in very advanced HIV infection with CD4 + counts of <100. In a recent

TABLE 2. *Drugs that cause psychiatric symptoms in HIV infection*

Drug	Reactions	Comments
Acyclovir	Hallucinations, delirium, insomnia, depression	At high doses, particularly with renal impairment
Amphetaminelike drugs	Bizarre behavior, hallucinations, paranoia, agitation, manic symptoms	Usually with overdose or abuse; depression can occur on withdrawal
Amphotericin B	Delirium	With intravenous or intrathecal use
Anabolic steroids	Agression, mania, depression, psychosis	
Anticonvulsants	Agitation, confusion, delirium, depression	Usually with high doses or high plasma concentrations
Antidepressants, tricyclic	Delirium, confusion, hallucinations, mania	Mania or hypomania in ~10% of patients also after withdrawal
Benzodiazepines	Rage, hostility, paranoia, hallucinations, delirium, depression, anterograde, amnesia	During treatment or on withdrawal
Corticosteroids	Mania, depression, confusion, paranoia, hallucinations, catatonia	Especially with high doses; can occur on withdrawal
Dapsone	Insomnia, agitation, hallucinations, mania, depression	Several reports; may occur even with low doses
Dronabinol	Anxiety, disorientation, psychosis	More common in elderly
Fluoxetine	Mania, hypomania, depersonalization	Tremor and myoclonus can occur
Ganciclovir	Hallucinations, delirium, confusion, agitation	With renal dysfunction
Histamine H_2-receptor	Hallucinations, bizarre behavior, delirium, depression	Usually with high doses; more common in elderly or with renal impairment
Interferon alpha	Delirium, depression, suicidal thoughts, anxiety	Occurs in up to 20%; depression treatable with fluoxetine
Iohexol/iopamidol	Confusion, disorientation	Infrequent
Isoniazid	Depression, agitation, hallucinations	Several reports
Ketoconazole	Hallucinations	Single case report
Loperamide	Delirium	Single case report
Methylphenidate	Hallucinations, paranoia	Several reports
Metoclopramide	Mania, depression, delirium	Several reports
Metronidazole	Depresssion, agitation, uncontrollable crying, disorientation, hallucinations	Several case reports, particularly with intravenous use
Narcotics	Nightmares, anxiety, agitation, euphoria, dysphoria, depression, paranoia, hallucinations	Usually with high doses
Nonsteroidal anti-inflammatory drugs	Paranoia, depression, anxiety, disorientation, hallucinations	Uncommon; frequency varies among the NSAIDs
Procaine derivatives	Confusion, "doom" anxiety, psychosis, agitation, bizarre behavior	Many reports, especially with penicillin G procaine
Pseudoephedrine	Hallucinations, paranoia	Reported with overuse in adults
Salicylates	Agitation, confusion, hallucinations, paranoia	Chronic intoxication
Sulfonamides	Confusion, disorientation, euphoria	Several reports
Trimethoprim-sulfamethoxazole	Psychosis, depression, disorientation, hallucinations, delusions	Several reports
Zidovudine	Mania, paranoia, hallucinations	Infrequent, reported in two patients

Modified from *The Medical Letter*, 1993:35; with permission.

TABLE 3. *Common neurological diseases complicating HIV infection: clinical differentiation*

Cause	Neurological syndrome	Gait	Symptoms
Intracranial mass lesion	Focal CNS signs, hemiparesis, truncal ataxia	Hemiparetic	Weakness on one side: arm and leg, drunken gait, wide-based, staggering
Myelopathy	Spastic paraparesis	Spastic	Legs stiff, toes scuff and catch, stumbling when walking or going up steps
CMV radiculitis	Lumbar radiculopathy	Asymmetric weakness	Progressive asymmetric leg weakness; variable sensory loss, bladder/bowel loss, and back pain
Myopathy	Proximal weakness	Waddling	Difficulty rising from chair, knee bend, or climbing stairs; difficulty brushing hair, shampooing; muscle aching
Sensory neuropathy	Distal sensory loss; minimal weakness	Antalgic	Numb, "frost-bitten" or painful feet

series, Holland et al. (30) reviewed the clinical features of pathologically proven CMV encephalitis and contrasted them to the clinical features of HIV-associated dementia. Over 90% of those patients with CMV encephalitis had altered mentation, which typically developed over 1–4 weeks as disorientation, delirium, mental slowing, and apathy. Cranial nerve deficits indicating brain stem involvement were relatively frequent, occurring in three of 14 patients. An important laboratory clue was the presence of hyponatremia, probably reflecting CMV adrenalitis and either an Addisonian state or dilutional hyponatremia. CMV blood cultures were positive in two thirds of patients in this series. Periventricular infection may be recognized on contrast CT or MRI as an irregular enhancement in the subependymal regions.

Management of Altered Mentation

The first step to management is the accurate identification of trigger or cause of the encephalopathy and the exclusion of evolving opportunistic infections, which might need a specific treatment. Metabolic or toxic encephalopathies usually respond quickly to treatment of the underlying infection or correction of metabolic derangements. An agitated or combative patient may require sedation and small doses of haloperidol 0.5 to 1 mg orally or intramuscularly probably provide the best control.

COGNITIVE DISTURBANCE

The American Academy of Neurology introduced the term HIV-associated minor cognitive/motor disorder in 1991 (Table 4). Because of the ill-defined nature of this entity, reliable estimates of its incidence and prevalence are not available, nor has its natural history been characterized. Our clinical experience suggests that it may be even more common than HIV dementia, occurring in perhaps 25–40% of patients with advanced AIDS, although the precise relationship of these cognitive disorders is not understood. Specifically, we do not know that minor cognitive symptoms are caused directly by HIV infection, nor that they inevitably progress to HIV dementia. Use of a screening instrument as already

TABLE 4. *Simplified version of 1991 American Academy of Neurology definitional criteria for HIV neurological CNS disorders*

HIV-1-associated dementia complex
Probable (must have each of the following)
1. Acquired abnormality in two or more cognitive domains, present for at least 1 month and cognitive dysfunction impairing work or activities of daily living, not solely attributable to systemic illness.
2. Acquired abnormality in motor function or performance, verified by clinical examination and/or neuropsychological tests and/or decline in motivation, emotional control, or change in social behavior.
3. Absence of clouding of consciousness, for a period of time sufficient to establish criterion 1.
4. No other etiology present (e.g., medical, psychiatric, substance abuse, CNS infection or neoplasm).
Possible (must have one of the following):
1. Criteria 1, 2, and 3 above are present, but an alternative etiology is present and the cause of criterion 1 is not certain.
2. Criteria 1, 2, and 3 above are present, but the etiology is not certain due to an incomplete evaluation.
HIV-1-associated minor cognitive/motor disorder
Probable (must have each of the following):
1. Acquired cognitive/motor/behavioral abnormalities, verified by both a reliable history and neurological/neuropsychological tests.
2. Mild impairment of work or activities of daily living.
3. Does not meet criteria for HIV dementia or HIV myelopathy.
4. No other etiology present.
Possible:
1. Criteria 1, 2, and 3 above are present, but an alternative etiology is present and the cause of criterion 1 is not certain.
2. Criteria 1, 2, and 3 above are present, but the etiology of criterion 1 cannot be determined due to incomplete evaluation.
Levels of cognitive dysfunction:
Mild: Decline in work and home activities noticeable to others, but person not totally dependent on others. Incapable of more complicated daily tasks. Self-care intact.
Moderate: Unable to work, including in the home. Requires assistance in activities of daily living.
Severe: Unable to perform any activities of daily living without assistance. Requires continual supervision.
Levels of myelopathic dysfunction
Mild: Ambulatory, but requires constant unilateral support.
Moderate: Requires constant bilateral support walking.
Severe: Unable to walk even with assistance.

From Janssen et al. 1991; with permission.

discussed can be particularly useful to detect further decline. However, its detection and presence may have prognostic importance. Mayeux et al. (56) have found that minor cognitive impairment is a marker of reduced survival. A number of observations within prospective studies indicate that minor cognitive/motor disorder may remain stable for many months or years, even without antiretroviral therapy. Several groups have described high rates of neuropsychological test abnormalities in healthy HIV-1–infected homosexual men (27,36) and in injecting drug users (85). The clinical significance of these findings is uncertain because the reported neuropsychological abnormalities do not necessarily progress and so may reflect the effects of low education, age, and alcohol and drug use rather than incipient HIV-1 dementia. By contrast, among several hundred HIV-1–seropositive men without AIDS or constitutional symptoms in the Multicenter AIDS Cohort Study (MACS), the prevalence of HIV dementia was <1% and overall the frequency of neuropsychological impairment was not significantly higher in medically healthy HIV-seropositive individuals than in HIV-1–seronegative controls (59). Similar results have been described in injecting drug users (79) and hemophiliacs (44). From longitudinal neuropsychological evaluation in the MACS and among injecting drug users, no evidence for cognitive decline was found during the asymptomatic phase of infection (82,83), suggesting that cognitive disturbance is uncommon during this phase. Reports of frequent neuropsychological abnormalities may reflect other confounding factors rather than the effects of HIV infection.

MENINGISMUS

Most of the causes of neck stiffness in individuals with HIV infection are infectious, either reflecting bacterial or viral meningitis in an immunocompetent person, or development of a CNS opportunistic infection. Most of these have been reviewed already in the section on altered mentation. Noninfectious causes of meningeal irritation with meningismus include ibuprofen-induced chemical meningitis and chemotherapy-induced meningeal irritation, for example, after intrathecal administration of cytosine arabinoside (Ara-C) for treatment of PML. Systemic lymphoma involves the meninges in up to 40% of cases (38), but meningeal irritation and meningismus are uncommon.

HEADACHE

Headache is an extremely common symptom in HIV infection because of the frequency of intracranial infections and mass lesions, and of pyrexial systemic disorders related to immunosuppression. As with mentation change, the degree of immunodeficiency is a critical factor in the differential diagnosis. As Fig. 2 indicates, with a CD4+ count in the normal range (e.g., >500), opportunistic infections occur only rarely and other causes of headaches predominate. Below 500, the development of headache, particularly if new in onset and accompanied

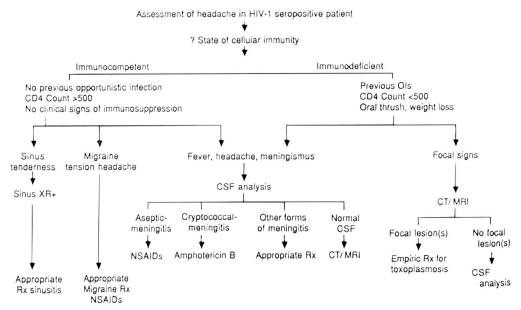

FIG. 2. Evaluation of headache in the HIV-seropositive patient. NSAIDs, nonsteroidal antiinflammatory drugs; OIs, opportunistic infections.

by fever, meningismus, or neurological symptoms should prompt an urgent search for intracranial infection.

Headache in the Immunocompetent HIV-Seropositive Patient

As discussed above, during this phase of HIV infection, opportunistic processes are unlikely to develop. The most common causes of headaches are chronic "tension" headaches, chronic HIV meningitis, and sinusitis. Chronic tension headaches may be recognized by their chronicity and the descriptions of a bandlike, vertex pressure occurring daily. Typically, the headaches worsen as the day progresses, are not accompanied by neurological symptoms or visual phenomena, and worsen during periods of anxiety or stress. As discussed later in this book, HIV is commonly associated with a CSF pleocytosis, particularly in the first few years after infection. In the majority of individuals, this "meningitis" is silent and not accompanied by meningismus. In a small proportion of patients, usually very early in HIV infection, an acute aseptic meningitis develops. This often occurs as part of the so-called sero-conversion illness (13). Far more common is a chronic low-grade meningitis from HIV (32), and it is often difficult to ascertain whether a patient's headache results from a low-grade meningitis. It may be impossible to separate the headache of chronic HIV meningitis from tension headache, and indeed the two may overlap. A persistent CSF pleocytosis with >20 WBC/mm^3 favors HIV chronic meningitis as the cause, and the headache may result from the intrathecal release of cytokines such as tumor necrosis factor-alpha. Sinus disease and sinusitis are a common cause of headache, usually frontal and aching in character and associated with nasal symptoms. MRI studies have shown a high frequency of sinus congestion and mucosal thickening in HIV-seropositive individuals (1). Finally, migraine is an extremely common cause of headache and has been estimated to affect 8–15% of the general population. Episodic headache with nausea, vomiting, and migrainous visual phenomena, such as scintillating scotoma or fortification spectra, are usually easily diagnosable as migrainous. Although it has been suggested that there is an increased frequency of migraine in HIV infection, this has not been confirmed by rigorous surveys. The initiation of zidovudine is frequently accompanied by transient headaches lasting 2–4 weeks after drug initiation. In a migraineur, zidovudine can induce a flurry of migraine attacks. Usually these subside within a few weeks of initiation.

Headaches in the Immunodeficient HIV-Positive Patient

In the setting of immunodeficiency with a CD4+ count of <500, the development of new headache has to be considered a marker of possible intracranial pathology, particularly if accompanied by meningismus, localizing neurological symptoms and signs, or altered mentation. The exception is if the patient is obviously diffusely encephalopathic with a systemic infection such as pneumonia and a pyrexial headache. The most common cause of new headache in an immunodeficient HIV-seropositive patient is cryptococcal meningitis. Forty-five percent of patients developing cryptococcal meningitis have had no previous AIDS-defining illness (10), and in the United States it is not uncommon for an injecting drug user to present for medical attention the first time with fulminant cryptococcal meningitis. The headache is usually severe and frontotemporal and accompanied by fever, nausea, and stiff neck. Visual blurring from papilledema occurs in ~10% of cases, but lateralizing neurologic symptoms are rare. The average duration of headache before diagnosis is ~7 days. Because of the frequency of cryptococcal meningitis and the impracticality of performing lumbar puncture on every HIV-seropositive patient with low CD4 + count and headache, the measurement of serum cryptococcal antigen has come into widespread use for screening. Chuck and Sande (10) reviewed 106 cases of cryptococcal meningitis and found a positive serum cryptococcal antigen in 70 of 71. Only one proved to be falsely negative. Serum cryptococcal antigen is thus a reasonable screening test in an immunodeficient patient with headache.

Other opportunistic processes, including cerebral toxoplasmosis and primary CNS lymphoma, are less common causes of head pain. Headache is described in ~60% of patients with toxoplasmosis (72) and 40% of patients with lymphoma (49). In toxoplasmosis, headache is usually associated with nausea, vomiting, hemiparesis, language dysfunction, behavioral or personality change, or altered mentation. It may be frontal, nuchal, generalized, or unilateral and may be increased by head jolt, coughing, stooping, and straining.

SEIZURES

Both focal and generalized seizures are common in HIV infection, affecting 10–20% of patients with AIDS. Seizures may be the initial presenting symptom, indicating an underlying CNS opportunistic process, or may signal systemic illness, or the effects of drug or alcohol abuse. The most common drugs of abuse associated with seizures are cocaine and "crack," as well as in withdrawal from benzodiazepines and alcohol. In two series studying the cause of seizures in HIV clinics in New York and San Francisco (33,96), half had no obvious explanation in terms of structural deficits, metabolic causes, or intoxication. The implication was that in these cases, seizures might result directly from brain infection with HIV. In our series of 268 demented patients, only 15 had seizures. Thus, the effect of HIV on the seizure threshold must be modest. Long-term follow-up studies will show whether this interpretation is correct.

Among the more clearly defined causes for seizures in AIDS are focal intracranial lesions such as abscesses and lymphomas, meningitis, metabolic problems, and strokes (Table 5). Rarer causes include viral encephalitides related to herpes simplex, herpes zoster, CMV, and JC virus. In the immunocompetent HIV-infected patient, CNS opportunistic processes are unlikely, and particularly careful questioning for alcohol abuse or illicit drug use should be made with appropriate toxicological confir-

TABLE 5. *Causes of seizures*

Cause	San Francisco (Wong)	Cornell (Holtzman)	Total (%)
Toxoplasma	28	11	39 (23)
Lymphoma	4	8	12 (7)
Meningitis	16	7	23 (14)
Cerebrovascular	3	4	7 (4)
Metabolic	3	8	11 (6)
Uncertain HIV encephalitis	46	32	78 (46)
Total	100	70	170

mation. The presence of focal neurological signs is strongly predictive of an underlying structural cause. Thus, in Holzman's study, 53 of 76 patients with neurological signs had a detectable cause, whereas only two of 24 patients with normal neurological examination results had a mass lesion or meningitis (33). Focal seizures more frequently indicate underlying structural lesions.

The investigation of seizures in this setting should include contrast imaging for mass lesions and CSF examination for meningitis. EEG recordings add little to the diagnostic work-up, except when the patient remains confused or encephalopathic. Here, EEG is useful to exclude frequent epileptiform discharges or nonconvulsive status, to search for the characteristic periodic lateralizing epileptiform discharges of herpes simplex encephalitis, or to observe other localizing phenomena. If neurodiagnostic studies and the results of the neurologic examination are normal, the patient can usually be reassured that the seizure has no sinister implications. Advice about driving restrictions (variable from state to state) should be given and secondary prophylaxis considered.

Use of Anticonvulsants

If the seizure can be linked to drug or alcohol use, prophylactic anticonvulsants are generally not advisable. If neuroimaging or CSF examination is abnormal, medication should probably be started even after a single seizure. However, anticonvulsant intolerance is high, and rashes and granulocytopenia are common both with phenytoin and carbamazepine. Phenobarbital can be used as a second line agent, although its sedating properties can pose a major disadvantage. For patients presenting with seizures who have identified mass lesions, there is an immediate risk of further seizures or status epilepticus, and intravenous loading with phenytoin is appropriate.

DIZZINESS AND LIGHTHEADEDNESS

Dizziness and lightheadedness are common symptoms in patients with advanced HIV disease, and their presence usually reflects the effects of systemic illness. Perhaps the most common complaint is that of postural dizziness due to anemia- or hypovolemia-induced orthostatic hypotension. Anemia is common in HIV infections and can be the result of either disease (e.g., disseminated *Mycobacterium avium* complex infection) or therapy (e.g., zidovudine). Correction of the anemia with erythropoietin or treatment with blood transfusions usually improves symptoms. Hypovolemia may result from diarrheal illness (e.g., cryptosporidiosis) or from inability to ingest sufficient food and liquid (e.g., candida esophagitis). Treatment with intravenous fluids and/or parenteral nutrition often alleviates symptoms. Medications are also common causes of dizziness in HIV infection. Tricyclic antidepressants, phosphonoformates, amphotericin B, and narcotics are commonly prescribed agents that often produce these symptoms, even in normal doses. Several studies have suggested that an autonomic neuropathy may develop in advanced HIV infection (23), with a high frequency of abnormal autonomic function tests. It remains unclear whether HIV can cause autonomic dysfunction or whether these abnormalities most likely reflect advanced systemic disease and can contribute to dizziness and lightheadedness. Cardiomyopathies can occur in all stages of HIV infection; the associated hypoxemia and arrhythmias can produce dizziness.

TABLE 6. *Causes of visual symptoms*

Problem	Location	Diagnosis
Field defect	Optic tract	Toxoplasmosis
	Radiation ?	Lymphoma
	Visual cortex	PML, infarct/hemorrhage
Diplopia	Cranial nerve	Lymphomatous meningitis, neurosyphilis, cryptococcal meningitis, elevated intracranial pressure
	Brain stem	PML, lymphoma, toxoplasmosis, infarct, Wernicke's, intoxication
Visual loss	Retina	CMV retinitis, toxoplasmosis, histoplasmosis
	Optic nerve	Syphilis, cryptococcosis, optic neuritis, elevated ICP

VISUAL CHANGES

Several discrete causes of visual disturbance can occur in AIDS. These include visual field deficits, diplopia from oculomotor pareses, optic nerve involvement, retinal damage, and uveitis. Each site of involvement may be associated with different visual complaints, and Table 6 indicates the common organisms or causes of the specific symptoms.

Visual Field Deficits

These usually occur late in HIV infection and are produced by opportunistic processes involving either the visual cortex, optic tracts, or optic radiations. Depending on the specific entity, the onset of visual field deficits may be slow and unnoticed by the patient. This contrasts to retinal or oculomotor dysfunction, in which symptoms are frequently early and obvious. For example, PML commonly produces visual field dysfunction with a slow progression of deficits over several weeks to months.

Oculomotor Palsies

These include direct involvement of the IIIrd, IVth, or VIth cranial nerves with development of diplopia or the false localizing sign of bilateral VIth nerve palsies from elevated intracranial pressure. Relatively common causes (41) of direct cranial nerve involvement include lymphomatous meningitis with infiltration of the cranial nerves as they traverse the subarachnoid space or within the cavernous sinus. Cryptococcal infiltration of the cranial nerves (55) or chronic arachnoiditis (53) can cause optic nerve or oculomotor nerve dysfunction and usually portends poor response to treatment. Cranial nerve involvement with neurosyphilis has been recognized frequently in HIV-seropositive individuals. In one series of 40 HIV-seropositive individuals with neurosyphilis, nine had syphilitic meningitis and 13 developed cranial nerve dysfunction. Involvement of the IInd cranial nerve was most frequent, followed by the VIIIth (69). Cranial nerve lesions are also seen in TB meningitis and CMV ventriculoencephalitis. In three of 14 patient recently reported by Holland (30) with CMV encephalitis, cranial nerve deficits were obvious, reflecting brain stem involvement. Wernicke's encephalopathy is an uncommon but treatable cause of nystagmus and ophthalmoparesis.

Change in Visual Acuity

Visual blurring, the development of scotoma, or blindness are frequent manifestations of CMV retinitis (see Chapter 14). Although peripheral retinal involvement may be visually silent, when CMV retinitis affects central vision, patients describe painless onset of visual blurring with blurring (inflammatory cells in vitreous), black spots, or field deficits. The fundoscopic appearance of CMV retinitis is characteristic, with hemorrhagic exudates tracking along blood vessels. Many patients, particularly when at high risk for CMV infection (CD4+ count <100), perform regular self-checks of vision using an Amsler grid to detect early CMV lesions. Direct ophthalmoscopy is of limited use to screen for CMV retinitis because it only permits visualization of the central retina. Pupillary dilatation and indirect ophthalmoscopy are essential for adequate screening. Less common causes of visual loss include toxoplasmic or histoplasma retinitis, papilledema from elevated intracranial pressure associated with cryptococcal meningitis, or syphilitic optic neuritis (95). The latter is often accompanied by recognizable inflammation of the anterior chamber with uveitis and iritis. A rarer cause of visual loss is optic nerve CMV infection.

Cotton wool spots are common in HIV infection, occurring in 5–10% of asymptomatic seropositives and up to 80% of people with AIDS (24). Thought to represent axonal stasis from retinal ischemia, these lesions were thought not to affect vision. However, a reduction in nerve fibers in the optic nerve has been shown (92), suggesting that cotton wool spots may lead to this loss.

As tuberculosis infection, and its treatment, becomes more frequent, we will probably see more cases of antimicrobial-induced retinal damage. Ethambutol is the major culprit of toxic retinopathy.

CRANIAL NEUROPATHIES

Cranial neuropathies are encountered frequently in HIV infection (Table 7), although no distinctive syndrome specifically caused by HIV has been identified. Facial palsies may be seen with HIV seroconversion. More typically, cranial neuropathies may occur as sequelae to any of the CNS or peripheral nervous system opportunistic processes that can complicate HIV infection. In a review of the neurological manifestations of HIV infection in 2,370 patients, Lewis et al. (50) identified cranial neuropathies in 98 (4.1%). One third of those with cranial neuropathies had multiple cranial nerves involved. The facial nerve was most common (77 cases), followed by the abducens nerve (13 cases), the oculomotor nerve (13 cases), the hypoglossal nerve (10 cases), the trigeminal nerve (nine cases), the vestibulocochlear nerve (eight cases), the optic nerve (three cases), the trochlear nerve (two cases), the glossopharyngeal nerve (two cases), and the vagus nerve (two cases). Cerebral toxoplasmosis was overrepresented in the group of patients with facial palsies, largely because of the upper motor neuron weakness frequently associated with it. Primary CNS lymphoma and cryptococcal meningitis were commonly associated with these cranial neuropathies. Other etiologies included PML, aseptic meningitis, CMV encephalitis, non-Hodgkin's lymphoma, bacterial meningitis, brain stem glioma, and cerebrovascular accident (CVA). About 15% of patients with cranial neuropathies had a coexistent neuropathy, and no CNS process was identified in 15%.

TABLE 7. *Cranial neuropathies in HIV infection*

Condition	Commonly affected CNs	Other associated features	Imaging	CSF
Aseptic meningitis	V, VII, VII	Headache, fever meningismus	Unremarkable cranial imaging	Mild-moderate CSF pleocytosis
Cryptococcal meningitis	II, III, VI, VI, VII	± meningismus fever, progressive cranial neuropathy	May be normal or may show enhancement of cranial nerve	Acellular CSF in about 20% of cases; cryptococcal antigen positive >95% of cases
TB	VI, VII, VII	Aggressive clinical course		Low CSF glucose
CIDP	V, VII	Occurs before other AIDS illnesses	Normal cranial imaging	Elevated protein, mononuclear pleocytosis
GBS	V, VII,	Occurs before other AIDS illnesses	Normal cranial imaging	Elevated protein, mononuclear pleocytosis
Lymphoma	II, V, VI, VII	Systemic lymphoma identifiable; upper motor neuron VIIth nerve lesion may be seen with primary CNS lymphoma	May see enhancing basal meninges	High protein, lymphomatous cells in CSF
Toxoplasmosis	Upper motor neuron VII	Hemiparesis frequent	Solitary or multiple ring-enhancing lesions	Elevated protein
Mononeuritis multiplex	V, VII	Abrupt onset multifocal mononeuropathies	Normal cranial imaging	Elevated protein

The approach to the patient with cranial neuropathies includes identification of neurological deficits at other levels of the neuraxis and a search for the underlying cause. Cranial MRI, CSF analysis, and serologic studies are often useful. Certain patterns of cranial neuropathies are seen with specific underlying causes (64). For example, optic neuropathy is frequently encountered in cases of lymphomatous or cryptococcal meningitis, or rarely with CMV, but is almost never encountered with other diseases. Figure 3 presents an algorithm for the evaluation of cranial neuropathies in HIV infection.

Oculomotor nerve palsy may be due to elevated intracranial pressure resulting from either a mass lesion or meningitis. Opportunistic processes that can directly

FIG. 3. Evaluation of cranial neuropathies in the HIV-seropositive patient. (From Rosenblum ML, Bredensen DE, Levy RM. Algorithms for treatment of AIDS patients with neurological diseases. In: Rosenblum ML, Levy RM, Bredensen DE, eds. AIDS and the Nervous System. New York: Raven Press, 1988;389–395.) et al. 1988; with permission. **A:** Acyclovir is recommended because of the high incidence of herpes zoster infections in patients with HIV infection. DHPG (ganciclovir) is currently used for CMV retinitis; efficacy has been shown for progressive polyradiculopathy due to CMV infection. **B:** Culture of HIV from the CSF does not rule out other causes of HIV-related cranial nerve dysfunction. MM, mononeuropathy multiplex; VZV, varicella zoster virus.

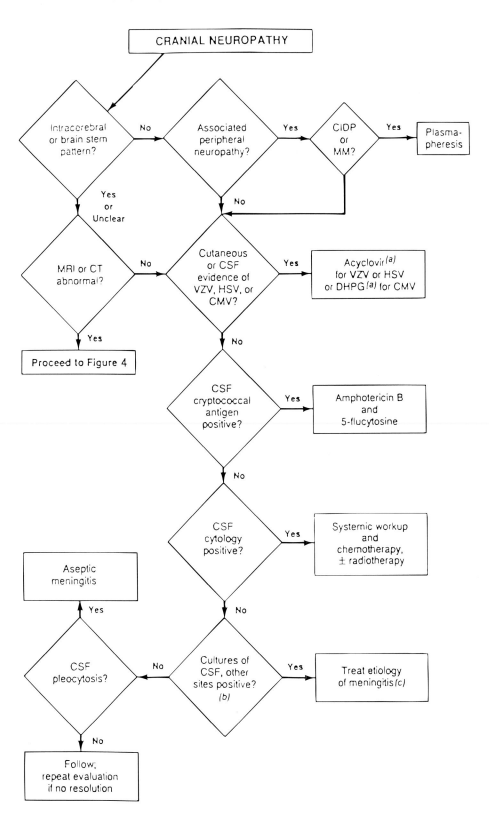

affect the oculomotor nerve include lymphoma (5), herpes family virus infection, cryptococcal meningitis or, rarely, TB meningitis. The trochlear and abducens nerves also can be affected by any of these processes.

The trigeminal nerve can be involved by mononeuritis multiplex (52), chronic inflammatory demyelinating polyradiculopathy (CIDP) (15), lymphoma, or the aseptic meningitis that can occur at the time of seroconversion. Another important cause of trigeminal neuropathy is varicella zoster virus (VZV) infection, which has a predilection for the first division (herpes zoster ophthalmicus). In severe cases, motor as well as sensory roots may be affected (28,67,78)

The facial nerve is one of the most commonly affected cranial nerves in HIV infection. An acute lower motor nerve facial palsy occurs frequently, especially in HIV-seropositive individuals who are otherwise healthy or who have only constitutional symptoms, such as weight loss, fever, fatigue, or thrush. Although recovery may be good, recurrence may occur. Facial palsy also may occur during acute aseptic meningitis (57). Intraaxial processes such as CNS toxoplasmosis, primary CNS lymphoma, and cryptococcomas can result in upper motor neuron facial nerve palsy, whereas extraaxial processes, including meningitides due to syphilis, cryptococcus, tuberculosis, lymphoma (90), or herpes family viruses may produce a lower motor neuron facial palsy. Mononeuritis multiplex (52) and chronic inflammatory demyelinating polyneuropathy (15) may each have facial nerve involvement.

The eighth cranial nerve may be involved in cases of aseptic, cryptococcal (45), syphilitic (51), or TB meningitis.

The lower cranial nerves are less frequently involved, although some cases have been reported of involvement of the laryngeal nerve presenting as hoarseness (89).

HEMIPARESIS

Several of the opportunistic processes can produce hemiparesis. Table 8 summarizes the different neurological syndrome, onset, course, and diagnoses. Two

TABLE 8. *Causes of hemiparesis in HIV infection*

Cause	Neurological syndrome	Onset/course	Diagnosis
Progressive multifocal leukoencephalopathy	Spastic hemiparesis, mentation normal	Unifocal initially, progressing over few weeks to multifocal	Cranial MRI: subcortical white matter lesions (no edema, no enhancement)
Toxoplasmosis	Hemiparesis flaccid → spastic, focal seizures, headache, fever, altered mentation	Subacute onset (days)	Cranial MRI: ring-enhancing lesions (1–3) cm, little mass effect), thallium SPECT negative
Primary CNS lymphoma	Spastic paraparesis, altered behavior, personality and mentation	Develops over weeks	Cranial MRI: ring/homogenous enhancement, large mass lesions (>3 cm); thallium SPECT positive
Cerebrovascular accident	Flaccid → spastic hemiparesis, aphasia, headache	Abrupt, acute	CT scan, MRI, echocardiogram, syphilis and anticardiolipin serologies, carotid duplex (dissection)

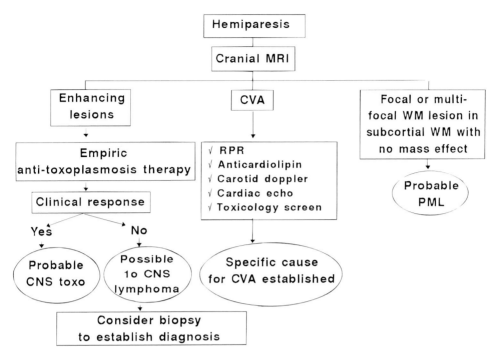

FIG. 4. Evaluation of hemiparesis in the HIV-seropositive patient. CVA, cerebrovascular accident; WM, white matter.

causes—cerebral toxoplasmosis and CVA—have a relatively abrupt to subacute onset, usually presenting first with a flaccid hemiparesis that later becomes spastic (see Chapter 24). CVAs occur reasonably frequently in people with HIV infection; however, it seems unlikely that HIV itself changes the predilection for stroke, but rather that stroke risk is related to the risk behaviors for HIV infection. Thus, an injection drug user with valvular vegetation and endocarditis is at high risk for septic emboli and subsequent stroke. Similarly, with advancing HIV infection, the frequency of anticardiolipin antibodies with thrombotic episodes may increase (6). Finally, meningovascular syphilis is an important and treatable cause of stroke. Carotid or vertebral artery dissection resulting from autoerotic practices such as near asphyxiation during sex are an unusual cause of CVAs in homosexual men. Figure 4 presents an algorithm for the evaluation of the patient with hemiparesis.

PML and primary CNS lymphoma can both cause spastic hemiparesis that develops over several weeks. These conditions can be differentiated by their appearance on cranial MRI.

QUADRIPARESIS

Four-limb hyperreflexia with some spasticity is frequently encountered in HIV dementia, where it is associated with the typical cognitive deficits of dementia, with pathological reflexes above the foramen magnum, such as the jaw jerk and snout reflexes, being present. A spastic quadriparesis without signs or symptoms of dementia suggests a cervical spinal cord process. Although rare, myelopathies in this region have been reported (16). Dal Pan et al. reported three cases of cervical myelopathies in HIV infection. All presented with slowly progressive spastic quadripareses with sensory loss and hyperreflexia. All had cervical cord enlargement, and two had enhancing lesions in the cervical cord. Spinal cord biopsy in each case failed to show an infectious or neoplastic etiology, and no typical features of VM were present. A case of toxoplasmosis in the cervical cord also has been reported (62).

In children, a progressive spastic quadriparesis may be a manifestation of HIV encephalopathy. A flaccid quadriparesis can be seen with the Guillain-Barré syndrome or CIDP, although facial involvement also may be present in either condition.

PARAPARESIS

Myelopathies

Common early symptoms of myelopathy include leg stiffness with resultant tripping, falling, and slowness of gait. Symptoms of a more advanced myelopathy include leg weakness, sexual dysfunction, and bowel and/or bladder incontinence. Sensory symptoms may occur either early or late in the course, and a discrete sensory level may be present in the severe forms of myelopathy. HIV-associated VM, opportunistic infectious and neoplastic myelopathies, HTLV-I associated myelopathy, and cervical spondylitic myelopathy are the principal forms of myelopathy that can occur in HIV-infected patients.

The most frequently encountered is HIV-associated VM. Although most of the reported cases have been in individuals with previous AIDS-defining illnesses (17,75), there have been reports of vacuolar myelopathy occurring before the development of other AIDS-defining illnesses (57) and at the time of seroconversion (19). The clinical features of HIV-1–related VM have been systematically studied (17). Mild to moderate limb weakness is usually present, with severe weakness limited to only the most advanced cases. Knee hyperreflexia, lower limb spasticity, gait spasticity, and vibration and position sense loss are other common features. A sensory ataxia or a coexistent distal sensory neuropathy also can be seen. A discrete thoracic sensory level and bowel and bladder dysfunction are not common in mild cases. The development of symptoms is usually slowly progressive. Standard thoracic spine imaging is generally normal. CSF analysis in cases of VM may show no pleocytosis or a mild pleocytosis (5–10 cells/mm^3) (17). A CSF WBC count of >20 cells/mm^3 is rare. A mild elevation in CSF protein content is seen in most cases (17,58). HIV dementia may be present in some patients with VM (17,34,57,75), although several cases of VM without dementia have been reported (17).

In addition to VM, infectious and neoplastic myelopathies can complicate HIV infection. Myelopathies may be due to syphilis (4), herpes group viruses (7,93), mycobacterial infection (26,97), toxoplasmosis (29), and lymphoma (43). Although myelopathies due to infectious or neoplastic causes can present with a spastic paraparesis, their course is usually more fulminant than that of VM (Table 9). Features suggestive of an infectious or neoplastic cause include an acute (hours to days) onset, a discrete sensory level, localization to the upper thoracic or cervical spine, a CSF pleocytosis (>20 cells/mm^3) (93,94,97), early bladder involvement, and back pain. In those cases, emergent spine imaging by CSF analysis is mandatory.

HTLV-I–associated myelopathy may present with a slowly progressive spastic paraparesis similar to VM, although the course may be more protracted than that of

TABLE 9. *Features distinguishing vacuolar myelopathy from infectious/neoplastic myelopathies*

Clincal feature	Vacuolar myelopathy	Infectious/neoplastic myelopathy
Back pain	Rare	Frequent
Course	Subacute–chronic	Acute–subacute
Bladder/bowel involvement	Usually urgency	Occurs early; usually retention
CSF	Mild–moderate protein elevation, 0–10 WBC/mm^3 in most cases	>20 WBC/mm^3 in many cases
Spinal imaging	Normal in most cases	Cord enhancement and/or mass lesion may be identified

VM (60). Like VM, a discrete sensory level may not be present, and bowel and bladder involvement in rare in all but the most advanced cases. If a diagnosis of HTLV-I–associated myelopathy is being considered, then serology for HTLV-I should be obtained. The similarities between these two myelopathies present a diagnostic challenge for the clinician evaluating a myelopathic patient dually infected with HIV and HTLV-I. A low CD4+ count suggests VM, although a high CD4+ count does not reliably distinguish between VM and HTLV-I–associated myelopathy because HTLV-I can elevate the CD4+ count in an individual who is functionally immunosuppressed. CSF analysis is helpful in these cases because intrathecal synthesis of anti–HTLV-I antibodies strongly suggests HTLV-I myelopathy.

Cervical spondylitic myelopathy also may occur in HIV-infected individuals. This diagnosis should be suspected in individuals with neck pain, as well as in individuals with higher (>300 cells/mm^3) CD4+ counts. Cervical spine MRI can establish the diagnosis.

Figure 5 presents an algorithm for the evaluation of the patient with paraparesis.

RADICULOPATHIES

Monoradiculopathy

The typical features of a monoradiculopathy—pain and paresthesia in a dermatomal distribution, with weakness and diminished reflexes referable to that nerve root—are occasionally seen in HIV-infected patients. In patients with high CD4+ counts (>300 cells/mm^3) and signs and symptoms clearly limited to one root, the most likely cause will be degenerative disk disease. Imaging studies may show a herniated disk. In patients with CD4+ counts of <300/mm^3, concern over an inflammatory or neoplastic process is greater, and imaging studies should be undertaken in all cases to exclude structural lesions. If imaging studies are inconclusive, then CSF analysis should be undertaken. The differential diagnosis of monoradiculopathy is similar to that of polyradiculopathy (see below).

Polyradiculopathy

A distinctive syndrome of acute lumbosacral polyradiculopathy has been recognized in HIV infection (3,18,22,25,37,54,65,91). Multiple lumbosacral roots are al-

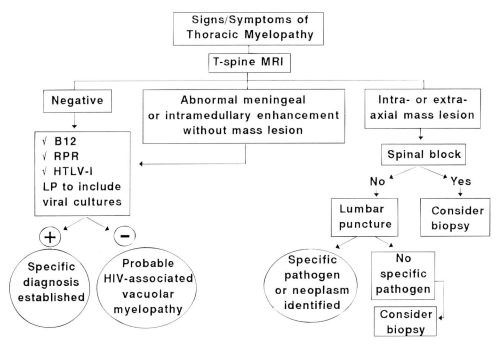

FIG. 5. Evaluation of paraparesis in the HIV-seropositive patient. T-spine MRI, thoracic spine MRI; B12, vitamin B12; LP, lumbar puncture.

most always involved, with progression to adjacent roots. In the series of So and Olney (91), the clinical picture was characterized by rapidly progressive flaccid lower limb paralysis with areflexia in all cases. Lower limb sensory loss occurs in at least three quarters of cases, and perianal anesthesia is seen in about one half of cases. Loss of bowel and bladder control are distinctive early features of this syndrome and occur in about one half of cases.

CMV has been implicated in many cases of acute progressive polyradiculopathy, although other etiologies also have been identified. So and Olney (91) studied 23 cases of acute polyradiculopathy in patients with AIDS and identified CMV as the causative agent in 15 cases. Two other patients had lymphomatous polyradiculopathy from a systemic primary, and the other six had a more benign course with no pathogen identified. Six others had no identifiable etiology. This latter group also tended to have a more benign clinical course, with spontaneous improvement seen in some cases. The majority of patients with CMV polyradiculitis have a prominent pleocytosis (60 to >1,000 cells/mm^3) with a polymorphonuclear predominance, elevated CSF protein content, and low to normal CSF glucose content. CMV is cultured form the CSF in about one half of cases.

Other etiologies of polyradiculitis include toxoplasmosis (40), syphilis (47), and primary CNS lymphoma (43,48).

Nerve conduction studies may be normal early in the course of disease, but the electromyogram (EMG) will show reduced recruitment in weak muscles. With time, the nerve conduction velocity study results will show a reduced compound muscle action potential and fibrillations.

The evaluation of an HIV-seropositive patient with a suspected acute polyradiculo-pathy should include an emergent lumbar puncture. MRI may identify structural problems or infiltrating tumor, although the yield is low (91).

Untreated lumbosacral polyradiculopathy with features of CMV polyradiculitis inevitably leads to progressive neurological deterioration in all cases. Several reports have documented clinical stabilization with ganciclovir treatment, although deterioration during the first 2 weeks of treatment is common (11,18,25,65,91). A failure to respond usually indicates a ganciclovir-resistant CMV strain (11).

NEUROPATHIC SYMPTOMS

A wide variety of syndromes can produce sensory and/or motor disturbances in HIV infection. Many of these entities predominantly affect the lower extremities early in their course and are summarized in Table 10.

The most common neuropathic symptoms in HIV infection are due to a PSN. A variety of sensory complaints can be elicited, including burning, tingling, shooting pain, numbness, throbbing, aching, "frostbite," and a feeling of "walking on a bed of coals." Some patients develop contact hyperalgesia, resulting in exquisite tenderness of the skin when touched. In some instances, walking is limited due to pain. Patients may complain of mild muscle weakness, but this is not a distinct feature. Bowel and/or bladder disturbances are not seen in HIV-associated sensory neuropathies; their presence should prompt a search for other etiologies.

The diagnosis of a sensory neuropathy requires a history compatible with predominantly sensory dysfunction and a physical examination notable for abnormal sensory findings in the feet with reduced or absent ankle jerks. Nerve conduction velocity studies and EMG show a length-dependent axonal degeneration. These studies are generally of little value in the management of patients with the typical features of a PSN, but may be helpful in patients with other neuromuscular manifestations of HIV infection. Nerve biopsy is only rarely indicated in PSN and is usually reserved for those patients for whom a diagnosis is not certain, for example, in cases in which vasculitis in a concern.

The differential diagnosis of a sensory neuropathy (Fig. 6) includes HIV-associated PSN, toxic neuropathies (usually due to antiretroviral medications), nutritional deficiency neuropathies, and tarsal tunnel syndrome. All patients should be asked about a history of diabetes and excessive alcohol consumption, which are other common causes of peripheral neuropathies, and may predispose patients with HIV to develop a sensory neuropathy.

By far the most common peripheral sensory neuropathy that occurs in the later stages of HIV disease, usually after other AIDS-defining illnesses have occurred, is HIV-associated PSN (14). This disorder occurs in >30% of individuals with AIDS.

A variety of neurotoxic medications (Table 11) can cause symptoms similar to those seen with PSN. Three common causes of toxic neuropathies are the antiretroviral agents ddI (didanosine), ddC (zalcitibine), and d4T (stavudine). These agents can result in a dose-dependent toxic neuropathy, with clinical features similar to those of HIV-associated PSN (12,21,42,46,63,74,81,88,98). Whether this is the result of direct neurotoxicity or whether it represents an "unmasking" of a "silent" or latent PSN remains unclear. Frequently, individuals with mild neuropathic symptoms before the initiation of ddI, ddC, or d4T will have an intensification of symptoms

TABLE 10. *Differential diagnosis of lower extremity symptoms in HIV infection*

Syndrome	Symptoms	Clinical features	Ancillary studies/treatment
Predominantly sensory neuropathy	Pain and numbness in toes and feet, involves ankles, calves, and fingers in more advanced cases	Reduced pin/vibratory sensation; reduced or absent ankle jerks; contact hypersensitivity present in some cases	EMG/NCVs show a predominantly axonal neuropathy; see flow sheet for treatment
Toxic neuropathy	Same as PSN (above) but symptoms occur after initiation of ddI/ddC/D4T	Same as PSN (above)	EMG/NCVs show a predominantly axonal neuropathy; discontinuation of presumed neurotoxic medication. Symptoms may worsen for a few weeks ("coasting") before improving; see flow sheet for treatment.
Tarsal tunnel syndrome	Pain and numbness predominantly in anterior portion of soles of feet	Reduced sensation over soles of feet; positive Tinel's sign at tarsal tunnel	Infiltration of local anesthestic into tarsal tunnel may provide symptomatic relief
HIV-associated myopathy/ AZT myopathy	Pain and aching in muscles, usually in thighs and shoulders; weakness, with difficulty arising from a chair or reaching above shoulders	Mild/moderate muscle tenderness; weakness predominantly in proximal muscles (i.e., deltoids, hip flexors); normal sensory examination/normal reflexes	CPK usually elevated; EMG/NCVs show evidence of an irritable myopathy If patient is on AZT, discontinue AZT and follow every 2 weeks. Symptoms/signs/ CPK should improve within 1 month.
Polyradiculitis	Rapidly evolving weakness and numbness in legs (both proximally and distally), with bowel/ bladder incontinence	Diffuse weakness in legs; diffuse sensory abnormalities in legs and buttocks; reduced/ absent reflexes at knees and ankles	EMG/NCV shows multilevel nerve root involvement; spinal fluid helpful in determining etiology (CMV or HSV infections, lymphomatous infiltration); ganciclovir helpful in CMV polyradiculopathy
Vacuolar myelopathy	Stiffness and weakness in legs with leg numbness; bowel/bladder incontinence in advanced cases	Weakness and spasticity mainly in hip flexors, knee flexors, ankle dorsiflexor; brisk knee jerks, upgoing toes (Babinski signs). If sensory neuropathy coexists, then distal sensory loss and reduced/absent ankle jerks will also be seen.	Spinal fluid may show elevated protein, mild ($5–10$ cells/mm^3) or no pleocytosis; thoracic spinal imaging normal; no specific therapy; physical therapy often helpful
Inflammatory demyelinating polyneuropathies	Predominantly weakness in arms and legs, with minor sensory symptoms	Diffuse weakness including facial musculature, asymmetric in early cases, with diffusely absent reflexes; minor sensory signs	EMG/NCVs show a demyelinating polyneuropathy; spinal fluid shows very high protein, with mild–moderate lymphocytic pleocytosis, but all cultures are negative

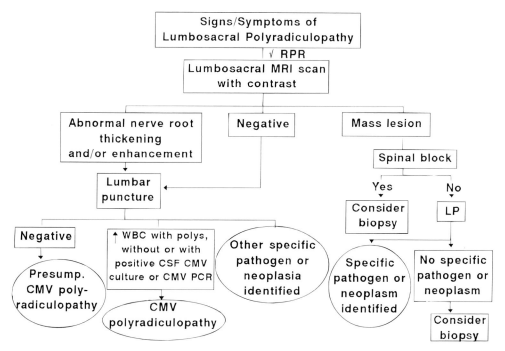

FIG. 6. Evaluation of polyradiculopathy in the HIV-seropositive patient. PCR, polymerase chain reaction.

once the antiretroviral agent has been started. The onset of symptoms can occur at any time after the agent has been started, but typically occurs after several weeks. Symptoms also may worsen for a period of up to 4 weeks after the agent has been discontinued, a phenomenon known as "coasting." If the symptoms persist for several months after the antiretroviral agent has been stopped, then a coexistent HIV-associated PSN is likely to be present. The same logic holds true for other potentially neurotoxic medications.

In individuals with sensory symptoms that spare the top of the foot and are limited to the anterior portion of the sole of the foot, tarsal tunnel syndrome may be present. This disorder is caused by entrapment of the tarsal nerve as it passes through the tarsal tunnel in the ankle, just below the medial malleolus. Lightly tapping the area just beneath the medial malleolus should give rise to shooting pains into the sole of the foot (i.e., a positive Tinel's sign).

In diabetics with AIDS, it is virtually impossible to separate the component of the neuropathy due to diabetes and that due to HIV-associated PSN, although prominent motor signs are more likely the result of diabetes. In HIV-infected diabetics without advanced immunodeficiency (CD4+ count >300 cells/mm^3), peripheral neuropathy should be attributed to the diabetes and not to HIV-associated PSN.

TABLE 11. *Common neurotoxic medications used in HIV infection*

Didanosine (ddI)	Metronidazole	Vincristine
Zalcitabine (ddC)	Isoniazid	Dapsone
Stavudine (d4T)	Pyridoxine (vitamin B6)	Chloramphenicol

Vitamin B12 levels, thyroid function tests, and a glucose level should be obtained as a screen for potentially reversible neuropathies.

INVOLUNTARY MOVEMENTS

The spectrum of abnormal involuntary movements is wide and includes tremor, dystonia, akathisia, and myoclonus. Symmetric tremor may represent the exaggeration of physiological tremor or benign essential tremor in the setting of systemic infection or may be related to medication. Medications that commonly induce tremor include phosphonoformate (Foscarnet), neuroleptics including phenothiazines and metaclopramide, pyrimethamine, and the experimental N-methyl-D-aspartate antagonist memantine. Tremor may be a part of a parkinsonian syndrome from medications. Productive HIV infection has a predilection for the basal ganglia and brain stem, and direct damage or the release of cytokines may trigger tremor and other movement disorders. Reyes et al. (77) demonstrated loss of neurons in the substantia nigra in patients with AIDS, which may explain the higher risk of extrapyramidal symptoms in patients with AIDS, especially those prescribed neuroleptics for agitation, delirium, or frank psychosis (31,35). Hriso reported that the risk was more than doubled. On less than the equivalent of 4 mg/kg/day of chlorpromazine, 50% of the patients with AIDS developed extrapyramidal problems. Over that dose, the rate increased to 78%. One patient with writing tremor had a coincidental old focal lesion due to meningovascular syphilis that preceded his HIV infection.

In addition to tremor and parkinsonismvariety of involuntary movements have been described in patients with AIDS (71). These have included hemidystonia (71), hemichorea (72), hemiballismus (70), and unilateral akathisia (9). Almost all have been related to toxoplasma abscesses in the basal ganglia. Rarer causes have included lymphoma, PML, and zoster vasculitis. The precise localization has varied between the head of the caudate, putamen, thalamus, and subthalamic nucleus. Management of involuntary movement disorders depends on treatment of the underlying structural lesion, e.g., toxoplasmosis, or dose reduction of the provoking medication.

GAIT DISTURBANCE

Gait disturbance is a common, yet nonspecific, symptom in HIV infection and represents a common reason for neurological consultation. Obviously, in patients with very advanced HIV infection with cachexia and wasting syndrome, a general loss of muscle bulk can lead to diffuse weakness that affects gait. Most of the specific neurological disorders that affect gait occur after AIDS with CD4 + counts of <200. Two exceptions to this are the development of inflammatory demyelinating polyneuropathy and HIV-associated polymyositis. These conditions can occur relatively early in HIV infection before other medical symptoms or immunodeficiency have appeared. Inflammatory demyelinating polyneuropathy may present either as Guillain-Barré syndrome or CIDP, depending on the tempo with which neuropathic symptoms develop. The condition is generally easily recognized by the combination of motor and sensory peripheral deficits, areflexia, and electrodiagnostic features of demyelination, including conduction block (15). HIV-associated polymyositis can occur at almost any stage of HIV infection and presents in a similar way to sporadic polymyositis with proximal weakness, myalgias, and elevated creatine phosphokinase (CPK).

Patients may have less severe myalgias than with toxic myopathies, although this is not always a reliable differentiating point. Functional limitations reflect the proximal weakness, including difficulty lifting grocery bags, brushing or shampooing hair, rising from a low chair or low commode, and climbing steps. In addition to persistently elevated serum CPKs, EMG demonstrates myopathic features with short unit potentials. Muscle biopsy may be useful in individuals with severe weakness who require immunomodulatory therapy and usually shows prominent inflammation with myofiber necrosis (87).

In patients with more advanced HIV infection, the development of gait difficulties encompasses a more lengthy differential diagnosis (Table 12). Important historical points include history of weight loss, chronic diarrhea, vegetarianism, or nutritional deficiency (which might indicate vitamin B12 deficiency), present or past syphilis (particularly if inadequately treated), and risk behaviors associated with HTLV-I infection (blood transfusion, injection drug use, and residence/travel to endemic areas). Associated symptoms, for example, painful paresthesia or dysesthesias, cognitive dysfunction, or headache and seizures, should point to neuropathy, dementia, or intracranial mass lesions, respectively. Careful neurological examination should include observation of walking, squatting, and, in subtle cases, running. Testing tandem and Romberg maneuver and assessing rapid foot tapping is useful to elicit cerebellar, posterior column, and corticospinal tract dysfunction.

TABLE 12. *Casuses of gait disturbance in HIV infection*

Cause	Neurological syndrome	Gait	Symptoms	Diagnosis
Intracranial mass lesion	Focal CNS signs, hemiparesis, truncal ataxia	Hemiparetic	Weakness on one side: arm and leg, drunken gait, wide-based, staggering	MRI
Myelopathy	Spastic paraparesis	Spastic	Legs stiff, toes scuff and catch, stumbling when walking or going up steps	Spinal MRI, CSF VDRL, vitamin B12, HTLV-I serology
CMV radiculitis	Lumbar radiculopathy	Asymmetric weakness	Progressive asymmetric leg weakness; variable sensory loss, bladder/bowel loss and back pain	CSF: polymorphonuclear pleocytosis, +culture MRI: enhancing nerve roots EMG: radiculopathy
Myopathy	Proximal weakness	Waddling	Difficulty rising from chair, knee bending, or climbing stairs; difficulty brushing hair, shampooing; muscle aching	Elevated serum CK EMG: myopathic potentials Muscle bx: inflammation, myofiber necrosis
Sensory neuropathy	Distal sensory loss; minimal weakness	Antalgic	Numb, "frost-bitten" or painful feet.	Toxic exposure history, vitamin B_1, B_{12} levels NCV's: axonal length–dependent neuropathy
HIV dementia	Nonspecific clumsiness or association with myelopathy	Clumsy	Mental slowing and memory impairment	Cranial MRI: severe atrophy, white matter hyperintensities, neurocognitive testing

Modified from Harrison MJG, McArthur JC. *AIDS and Neurology*, Churchill-Livingstone, 1995; with permission.

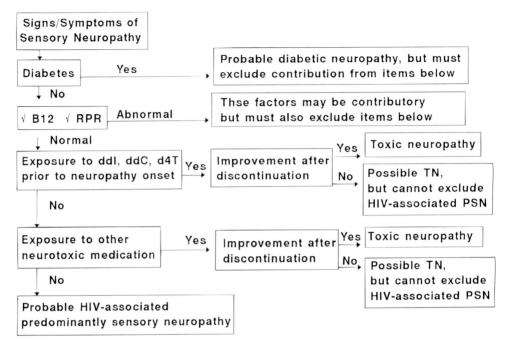

FIG. 7. Evaluation of sensory neuropathy in the HIV-seropositive patient. TN, toxic neuropathy.

Table 12 lists the most common causes of gait disturbance, their symptoms, and helpful diagnostic procedures. Figure 7 presents an algorithm for the evaluation of the patient with gait disturbance. For many of these conditions, history and examination alone are sufficient to localize the cause of the gait disturbance. The tempo of the evolution of the gait disturbance also may be helpful. For example, a slowly progressive myelopathy with spastic paraparesis over 5–10 years would be much more consistent with HTLV-I–associated myelopathy than with the rapidly developing ascending myelopathy associated with herpes group infections. Other causes of myelopathy are discussed more fully in Chapter 8. As the HIV epidemic broadens its reach and affects older individuals, one should not overlook cervical spondylitic myelopathy as a cause of progressive gait disturbance in an HIV-infected person. HIV-associated myelopathy (which induces vacuolar changes in the posterior columns and corticospinal tracts typically in the thoracic area) occurs in ~10% of patients, usually with advanced HIV infection. Rarely is it one of the presenting neurological illnesses or an AIDS-defining illness. Many, but not all, patients with HIV-associated VM develop concurrent HIV dementia. HIV-associated dementia as a cause of gait disturbance is probably under-recognized. In a recent series of 268 patients with HIV dementia evaluated at Johns Hopkins Hospital, 45% had gait dysfunction as one of the presenting symptoms (61). The gait complaints of HIV dementia are nonspecific and usually include mild gait instability or incoordination of leg movements, noticed, for example, while driving, dancing, or using foot pedals. In some patients, the gait instability reflects an evolving concomitant HIV-associated myelopathy. In others, the signs seem predominantly cerebral.

CMV radiculitis is a relatively uncommon but dramatic cause of acute gait disturbance and lower extremity weakness. As with CMV encephalitis, it usually develops in patients with very advanced HIV infection with CD4+ counts of <100. Most patients develop leg weakness with sensory deficits and bowel or bladder dysfunction that evolve rapidly over 1–3 weeks. The CSF profile is particularly helpful, showing a polymorphonuclear pleocytosis in the majority of cases, with positive CMV culture of polymerase chain reaction in 50–60% (65). A less common cause of gait instability may be seen in patients who have recovered from cryptococcal meningitis. They may have a vestibular dysfunction from inner ear involvement or may have a degree of communicating hydrocephalus with dysfunction of the descending leg fibers.

CONCLUSION

The HIV-infected patient is vulnerable to a wide variety of central and peripheral nervous system complications. These may be due to specific opportunistic pathogens or neoplasms, HIV itself, the effects of medications, or the neurological complications of systemic illness. A careful clinical evaluation, together with knowledge of a patient's CD4+ count, coexistent medical problems, and medications, can usually narrow the differential diagnosis. Appropriate neurodiagnostic tests can then establish the specific diagnosis.

REFERENCES

1. Armstrong M, McArthur JC, Zinreich SJ. Radiographic imaging of sinusitis in HIV infection. *Otolargyngol Head Neck Surg* 1993;108:36–43.
2. Barnes PF, Bloch AB, Davidson PT, Snider DE. Tuberculosis in patients with acquired immunodeficiency virus infection. *N Engl J Med* 1991;324:1644–1650.
3. Behar R, Wiley C, McCutchan JA. Cytomegalovirus polyradiculoneuropathy in acquired immune deficiency syndrome. *Neurology* 1987;37:557–561.
4. Berger JR. Spinal cord syphilis associated with human immunodeficiency virus infection: a treatable myelopathy. *Am J Med* 1992;92:101–103.
5. Berger JR, Flaster M, Schatz N, et al. Cranial neuropathy heralding otherwise occult AIDS-related large cell lymphoma. *J Clin Neuro Ophthalmol* 1993;13:113–118.
6. Brey RL, Hart RG, Sherman DG, Tegeler CH. Antiphospholipid antibodies and cerebral ischemia in young people. *Neurology* 1990;40:1190–1196.
7. Britton CB, Mesa-Tejada R, Fenoglio CM, Hays AP, Garvey GG, Miller JR. A new complication of AIDS: thoracic myelitis caused by herpes simplex virus. *Neurology* 1985;35:1071–1074.
8. Brust JCM. *Neurological Aspects of Substance Abuse*. Boston: Butterworth-Heinemann, 1993.
9. Carrazone EJ, Rossitch E, Martinez J. Unilateral "akathisia" in a patient with AIDS and a toxoplasma subthalamic abscess. *Neurology* 1989;39:449–450.
10. Chuck SL, Sande MA. Infections with *Cryptococcus neoformans* in acquired immunodeficiency syndrome. *N Engl J Med* 1989;321:794–799.
11. Cohen BA, McArthur JC, Grohman S, Patterson B, Glass JD. Neurologic prognosis in CMV polyradiculomyelopathy in AIDS. *Neurology* 1993;43:493–499.
12. Cooley TP, Kunches LM, Saunders CA, et al. Once-daily administration of 2′,3′-dideoxyinosine (ddI) in patients with the acquired immunodeficiency syndrome or AIDS-related complex. *N Engl J Med* 1990;322:1340–1345.
13. Cooper DA, Gold J, Maclean P, et al. Acute AIDS retrovirus infection: definition of a clinical illness associated with seroconversion. *Lancet* 1985;1:537–540.
14. Cornblath DR, McArthur JC. Predominantly sensory neuropathy in patients with AIDS and AIDS-related complex. *Neurology* 1988;38:794–796.
15. Cornblath DR, McArthur JC, Kennedy PG, Witte AS, Griffin JW. Inflammatory demyelinating peripheral neuropathies associated with human T cell lymphotropic virus type III infection. *Ann Neurol* 1987;21:32–40.
16. Dal Pan GJ, Glass J, Zeidman S, McArthur J. Atypical HIV-associated myelopathy: diagnosis by cord biopsy [Abstract]. *Neurology* 1992;42:257.
17. Dal Pan GJ, Glass JD, and McArthur JC. Clinicopathological correlations of HIV-1–associated vacuolar myelopathy: an autopsy-based case-control study. *Neurology* 1994;44:2159–2164.

18. de Gans J, Tiessens G, Portegies P, Tutuarima JA, Troost D. Predominance of polymorphonuclear leukocytes in cerebrospinal fluid of AIDS patients with cytomegalovirus polyradiculomyelitis. *J AIDS* 1990;3:1155–1158.

19. Denning DW, Anderson J, Rudge P, Smith H. Acute myelopathy associated with primary infection with human immunodeficiency virus. *Br Med J* 1987;294:143–144.

20. Dube MP, Holtom PD, Larsen RA. Tuberculous meningitis in patients with and without human immunodeficiency virus infection. *Am J Med* 1992;93:520–524.

21. Dubinsky RM, Yarchoan R, Dalakas M, Broder S. Reversible axonal neuropathy from the treatment of AIDS and related disorders with 2′,3′-dideoxycytidine (ddC). *Muscle Nerve* 1989;12:856–860.

22. Eidelberg D, Sotrel A, Vogel H, Walker P, Kleefield J, Crumpacker CS III. Progressive polyradiculopathy in acquired immune deficiency syndrome. *Neurology* 1986;36:912–916.

23. Freeman R, Roberts MS, Friedman LS, Broadbridge C. Autonomic function and human immunodeficiency virus infection. *Neurology* 1990;40:575–580.

24. Freeman WR, Lerner CW, Mines JA, et al. A prospective study of the ophthalmologic findings in the acquired immune deficiency syndrome. *Am J Ophthalmol* 1984;97:133–142.

25. Fuller GN, Gill SK, Guiloff RJ, et al. Ganciclovir for lumbosacral polyradiculopathy in AIDS [Letter]. *Lancet* 1990;335:48–49.

26. Gallant JE, Mueller PS, McArthur JC, Chaisson RE. Intramedullary tuberculoma in a patient with HIV infection [Letter]. *AIDS* 1992;6:889–891.

27. Grant I, Atkinson JH, Hesselink JR, et al. Evidence for early central nervous system involvement in the acquired immunodeficiency syndrome (AIDS) and other human immunodeficiency virus (HIV) infections. Studies with neuropsychologic testing and magnetic resonance imaging [erratum in *Ann Intern Med* 1988;108:496]. *Ann Intern Med* 1987;107:828–836.

28. Harrison MJG, McAllister RH. Neurologic complications of HIV infection. In: Lambert H, ed. *Infections of the Nervous System*. Philadelphia: BC Decker, 1991.

29. Herskovitz S, Siegel SE, Schneider AT, Nelson SJ, Goodrich JT, Lantos G. Spinal cord toxoplasmosis in AIDS. *Neurology* 1989;39:1552–1553.

30. Holland NR, Power C, Mathews VP, Glass JD, Forman M, McArthur JC. CMV encephalitis in acquired immunodeficiency syndrome (AIDS). *Neurology* 1994;44:507–514.

31. Hollander H, Golden J, Mendelson T, Cortland D. Extrapyramidal symptoms in AIDS patients given low-dose metoclopramide or chlorpromazine [Letter]. *Lancet* 1985;2:1186.

32. Hollander H, Stringari S. Human immunodeficiency virus–associated meningitis. Clinical course and correlations. *Am J Med* 1987;83:813–816.

33. Holtzman DM, Kaku DA, So YT. New-onset seizures associated with human immunodeficiency virus infection: causation and clinical features in 100 cases. *Am J Med* 1989;87:173–177.

34. Horoupian DS, Pick P, Spigland I, et al. Acquired immune deficiency syndrome and multiple tract degeneration in a homosexual man. *Ann Neurol* 1984;15:502–505.

35. Hriso E, Kuhn T, Masdeu JC, Grundman M. Extrapyramidal symptoms due to dopamine-blocking agents in patients with AIDS encephalopathy. *Am J Psychiatry* 1991;148:1558–1561.

36. Janssen RS, Saykin AJ, Kaplan JE, et al. Neurological complications of human immunodeficiency virus infection in patients with lymphadenopathy syndrome. *Ann Neurol* 1988;23:49–55.

37. Jeantils V, Lemaitre MO, Robert J, Gaudouen Y, Krivitzky A, Delzant G. Subacute polyneuropathy with encephalopathy in AIDS with human cytomegalovirus pathogenicity? [Letter]. *Lancet* 1986;2:1039.

38. Kaplan LD, McGrath MS. AIDS-associated non-Hodgkin's lymphoma. *AIDS Update* 1991;2:1–11.

39. Katz DA, Berger JR, Duncan RC. Neurosyphilis—a comparative study of the effects of infection with human immunodeficiency virus. *Arch Neurol* 1993;50:243–249.

40. Kayser C, Campbell R, Sartorious C, Bartlett M. Toxoplasmosis of the conus medullaris in a patient with hemophilia A–associated AIDS. Case report. *J Neurosurg* 1990;73:951–953.

41. Keane JR. Neuro-ophthalmologic signs of AIDS: 50 patients. *Neurology* 1991;41:841–845.

42. Kieburtz KD, Seidlin M, Lambert JS, Dolin R, Reichman R, Valentine F. Extended follow-up of peripheral neuropathy in patients with AIDS and AIDS-related complex treated with dideoxyinosine. *J AIDS* 1992;5:60–64.

43. Klein P, Zientek G, VandenBerg SR, Lothman E. Primary CNS lymphoma: lymphomatous meningitis presenting as a cauda equina lesion in an AIDS patient. *Can J Neurol Sci* 1990;17:329–331.

44. Kokkevi A, Hatzakis A, Maillis A, et al. Neuropsychological assessment of HIV-seropositive haemophiliacs. *AIDS* 1991;5:1223–1229.

45. Kwarteler JA, Linthicum FH, Jahn AF, Hawke M. Sudden hearing loss due to AIDS-related cryptococcal meningitis—a temporal bone study. *Otolargyngol Head Neck Surg* 1991;104:265–269.

46. Lambert JS, Seidlin M, Reichman RC, et al. 2′,3′-dideoxyinosine (ddI) in patients with the acquired immunodeficiency syndrome or AIDS-related complex. A phase I trial. *N Engl J Med* 1990;322:1333–1340.

47. Lanska MJ, Lanska DJ, Schmidley JW. Syphilitic polyradiculopathy in an HIV-positive man. *Neurology* 1988;38:1297–1301.

48. Leger JM, Henin D, Belec L, Mercier B, et al. Lymphoma-induced polyradicuolapthy in AIDS: two cases. *J Neurol* 1992;239:132–134.
49. Levy RM, Bredesen DE. Central nervous system dysfunction in acquired immunodeficiency syndrome. *J AIDS* 1988;1:41–64.
50. Lewis EM, Mahawar S, Wesley AM, Bredesen DE. Cranial neuropathies in AIDS patients. *International Conference on AIDS.* 1989;5:450.
51. Linstrom CJ, Pincus RL, Leavitt EB, Urbina MC. Otologic neurotologic manifestations of HIV-related disease. *Otolargyngol Head Neck Surg* 1993;108:680–687.
52. Lipkin WI, Parry G, Kiprov D, Abrams D. Inflammatory neuropathy in homosexual men with lymphadenopathy. *Neurology* 1985;35:1479–1483.
53. Lipson BK, Freeman WR, Beniz J, et al. Optic neuropathy associated with cryptococcal arachnoiditis in AIDS patients. *Am J Ophthalmol* 1989;107:523–527.
54. Mahieux F, Gray F, Fenelon G, et al. Acute myeloradiculitis due to cytomegalovirus as the initial manifestation of AIDS. *J Neurol Neurosurg Psychiatry* 1989;52:270–274.
55. Mathews VP, Alo PL, Glass JD, Kumar AJ, McArthur JC. AIDS-related CNS cryptococcosis—radiologic-pathologic correlation. *AJNR* 1992;13:1477–1486.
56. Mayeux R, Stern Y, Tang MX, et al. Mortality risks in gay men with human immunodeficiency virus infection and cognitive impairment. *Neurology* 1993;43:176–182.
57. McArthur JC. Neurologic manifestations of AIDS. *Medicine (Baltimore)* 1987;66:407–437.
58. McArthur JC, Cohen BA, Farzedegan H, et al. Cerebrospinal fluid abnormalities in homosexual men with and without neuropsychiatric findings. *Ann Neurol* 1988;23(suppl):34–37.
59. McArthur JC, Cohen BA, Selnes OA, et al. Low prevalence of neurological and neuropsychological abnormalities in otherwise healthy HIV-1–infected individuals: results from the multicenter AIDS Cohort Study. *Ann Neurol* 1989;26:601–611.
60. McArthur JC, Griffin JW, Cornblath DR, et al. Steroid-responsive myeloneuropathy in a man dually infected with HIV-1 and HTLV-I. *Neurology* 1990;40:938–944.
61. McArthur JC, Harrison MJG. HIV-associated dementia. In: Appel S, ed. *Current Neurology.* Chicago: Mosby-Year Book, 1994.
62. Mehren M, Burnes PJ, Mamani F, Levy CS, Laureno R. Toxoplasma myelitis mimicking intramedullary spinal cord tumor. *Neurology* 1988;38:1648–1650.
63. Merigan TC, Skowron G, Bozzette SA, et al. Circulating p24 antigen levels and responses to dideoxycytidine in human immunodeficiency virus (HIV) infections: a phase I and II study. *Ann Intern Med* 1989;110:189–195.
64. Miller RG, Kiprov DD, Parry G, Bredesen DE. Peripheral nervous system dysfunction in acquired immunodeficiency syndrome. In: Rosenblum ML, Levy RM, Bredesen DE, eds. *AIDS and the Nervous System.* New York: Raven, 1987:65–78.
65. Miller RG, Storey JR, Greco CM. Ganciclovir in the treatment of progressive AIDS-related polyradiculopathy. *Neurology* 1990;40:569–574.
66. Morlat P, Chene G, Leport C, et al. Primary prophylaxis of cerebral toxoplasmosis in the HIV patient—results of a double-blind randomized trial (pyrimethamine versus placebo). *Rev Med Intern* 1993;14:1002.
67. Moskow BS, Hernandez G. Aggressive periodontal destruction and herpes zoster in a suspected AIDS patient. *J Paradontol* 1991;10:359–369.
68. Musher DM. Syphilis, neurosyphilis, penicillin, and AIDS. *J Infect Dis* 1991;163:1201–1206.
69. Musher DM, Hamill RJ, Baughn RD. Effect of human immunodeficiency virus (HIV) infection on the course of syphilis and on the response to treatment. *Ann Intern Med* 1990;113:872–881.
70. Namer IJ, Tan E, Akalim E. Un cas d'hemiballisme au cours d'une meningite a cryptococque. *Rev Neurol* 1990;146:153–154.
71. Nath A, Jankovic J, Pettigrew LC. Movement disorders and AIDS. *Neurology* 1987;37:37–41.
72. Navia BA, Petito CK, Gold JW, Cho ES, Jordan BD, Price RW. Cerebral toxoplasmosis complicating the acquired immune deficiency syndrome: clinical and neuropathological findings in 27 patients. *Ann Neurol* 1986;19:224–238.
73. O'Malley JP, Ziessman HA, Pierce PF, Kumar PN. Tl-201 SPECT diagnosis of intracranial lymphoma in AIDS patients [Abstract]. *Radiology* 1992;185(P):233.
74. Parry GJ. Peripheral neuropathies associated with human immunodeficiency virus infection. *Ann Neurol* 1988;23(suppl):49–53.
75. Petito CK, Navia BA, Cho ES, Jordan BD, George DC, Price RW. Vacuolar myelopathy pathologically resembling subacute combined degeneration in patients with the acquired immunodeficiency syndrome. *N Engl J Med* 1985;312:874–879.
76. Power C, Selnes OA, Grim JA, McArthur JC. The HIV Dementia Scale: a rapid screening test. *J AIDS* 1994 (in press).
77. Reyes MG, Faraldi F, Senseng CS, Flowers C, Fariello R. Nigral degeneration in acquired immune deficiency syndrome (AIDS). *Acta Neuropathol (Berl)* 1991;82:39–44.
78. Rosenblum MK. Bulbar encephalitis complicating trigeminal zoster in the acquired immune deficiency syndrome. *Hum Pathol* 1989;20:292–295.

79. Royal W, Updike M, Selnes OA, et al. HIV-1 infection and nervous system abnormalities among a cohort of intravenous drug users. *Neurology* 1991;41:1905–1910.
80. Ruf B, Schurmann D, Bergmann F, et al. Efficacy of pyrimethamine sulfadoxine in the prevention of toxoplasmic encephalitis relapses and *Pneumocystis carinii* pneumonia in HIV-infected patients. *Eur J Clin Microbiol Infect Dis* 1993;12:325–329.
81. Schaumburg HH, Arezzo J, Berger A, Skowron G, Bozzette SA, Soo W. Dideoxycytidine (ddC) neuropathy in human immunodeficiency virus infection: a report of 52 patients [Abstract]. *Neurology* 1990;40(suppl):248.
82. Selnes OA, McArthur JC, Royal W, et al. HIV-1 infection and intravenous drug use: longitudinal neuropsychological evaluation of asymptomatic subjects. *Neurology* 1992;42:1924–1930.
83. Selnes OA, Miller E, McArthur JC, et al. HIV-1 infection: no evidence of cognitive decline during the asymptomatic stages. *Neurology* 1990;40:204–208.
84. Shafer RW, Kim DS, Weiss JP, Quale JM. Extrapulmonary tuberculosis in patients with human immunodeficiency virus infection. *Medicine (Balt)* 1991;70:384–397.
85. Silberstein CH, McKegney FP, O'Dowd MA, et al. A prospective longitudinal study of neuropsychological and psychosocial factors in asymptomatic individuals at risk of HTLV-III/LAV infection in a methadone program: preliminary findings. *Int J Neurosci* 1987;32:669–676.
86. Simon RP. Neurosyphilis. *Arch Neurol* 1985;42:606–616.
87. Simpson DM, Citak KA, Godfrey E, Godbold J, Wolfe DE. Myopathies associated with human immunodeficiency virus and zidovudine—can their effects be distinguished. *Neurology* 1993;43:971–976.
88. Simpson DM, Wolfe DE. Neuromuscular complications of HIV infection and its treatment. *AIDS* 1991;5:917–926.
89. Small PM, McPhaul LW, Sooy CD, Wofsy CB, Jacobson MA. Cytomegalovirus infection of the laryngeal nerve presenting as hoarseness in patients with acquired immunodeficiency syndrome. *Am J Med* 1989;86:108–110.
90. Snider WD, Simpson DM, Nielsen S, Gold JW, Metroka CE, Posner JB. Neurological complications of acquired immune deficiency syndrome: analysis of 50 patients. *Ann Neurol* 1983;14:403–418.
91. So YT, Olney RK. Acute lumbosacral polyradiculopathy in acquired immunodeficiency syndrome: experience in 23 patients. *Ann Neurol* 1994;35:53–58.
92. Tenhula WN, Xu SZ, Madigan MC, Heller K, Freeman WR, Sadun AA. Morphometric comparisons of optic nerve axon loss in acquired immunodeficiency syndrome. *Am J Ophthalmol* 1925;113:14–20.
93. Tucker T, Dix RD, Katzen C, Davis RL, Schmidley JW. Cytomegalovirus and herpes simplex virus ascending myelitis in a patient with acquired immune deficiency syndrome. *Ann Neurol* 1985;18:74–79.
94. Watkins BA, Dorn HH, Kelly WB, et al. Specific tropism of HIV-1 for microglial cells in primary human brain cultures. *Science* 1990;249:549–553.
95. Winward KE, Hamed LM, Glaser JS. The spectrum of optic nerve disease in human immunodeficiency virus infection. *Am J Ophthalmol* 1989;107:373–380.
96. Wong MC, Suite NDA, Labar DR. Seizures in human immunodeficiency virus infection. *Arch Neurol* 1990;47:640–642.
97. Woolsey RM, Chambers TJ, Chung HD, McGarry JD. Mycobacterial meningomyelitis associated with human immunodeficiency virus infection. *Arch Neurol* 1988;45:691–693.
98. Yarchoan R, Pluda JM, Thomas RV, et al. Long-term toxicity/activity profile of 2',3'-dideoxyinosine in AIDS and AIDS-related complex. *Lancet* 1990;336:526–529.

AIDS and the Nervous System, Second Edition,
edited by J. R. Berger and R. M. Levy.
Lippincott-Raven Publishers, Philadelphia © 1997.

8

Spinal Cord Disease in Human Immunodeficiency Virus Infection

*Gerald J. Dal Pan and †Joseph R. Berger

*Department of Neurology, Johns Hopkins University School of Medicine,
Baltimore, Maryland 21287-7609; and †Department of Neurology, University of
Kentucky Medical Center, Lexington, Kentucky 40536

The neurological complications of human immunodeficiency virus (HIV) infection can involve any part of the central or peripheral nervous systems. The spinal cord is no exception. Because both peripheral neuropathy and dementia are so frequent in HIV infection, the clinical manifestations of spinal cord involvement may be overlooked. Nonetheless, specific spinal cord syndromes, both those due to HIV itself and those resulting from opportunistic processes, have been well characterized (Table 1).

HIV-ASSOCIATED VACUOLAR MYELOPATHY

The most common spinal cord disease complicating HIV infection is HIV-associated vacuolar myelopathy (VM). This pathologically defined entity was first described in a case report by Goldstick et al.(35), whose patient, a 36-year-old homosexual man with acquired immunodeficiency syndrome (AIDS), developed a progressive symmetric paraparesis with muscle wasting, loss of vibratory and position sensation in the lower limbs, and bowel and bladder incontinence. Autopsy examination of the spinal cord showed a relatively symmetric spongy degeneration of the lateral and anterior pyramidal tracts, as well as of the posterior columns. The etiology of this spinal cord degeneration was not known, and a search for infectious and nutritional causes was inconclusive.

After this initial case report, Petito et al. (68) reported a high incidence of myelopathy in patients with AIDS. In 20 of 89 consecutive autopsies of patients with AIDS, a myelopathy resembling the myelopathy of subacute combined degeneration was identified. This was most severe in the posterior and lateral columns of the thoracic cord. Clinically, all 20 of these patients had shown evidence of myelopathy of varying degrees of clinical and pathological severity. In those with pathologically moderate or severe myelopathy, leg weakness, ataxia, and incontinence were common. Motor signs were rare in those with pathologically mild spinal cord degeneration. Progressive dementia occurred in 14 of these 20 patients. The 20 patients with myelopathy were comparable with the remainder of patients with AIDS studied with respect to opportunistic infection, neoplasm, medications, or clinical laboratory findings. There

TABLE 1. *Diseases of the spinal cord associated with HIV-1 infection*

Infectious	Fungal
HIV-associated	*Nocardia*
Vacuolar myelopathy	*Cryptococcus*
Acute transient myelopathy	*Aspergillus*
Relapsing and remitting myelitis	Other
Spinal myoclonus	Parasitic
Other Viral	*Toxoplasma gondii*
Cytomegalovirus	**Neoplastic**
Herpes simplex types 1 and 2	Primary CNS lymphoma
Varicella zoster	Metastatic lymphomas
HTLV-1	Astrocytoma/glioma
Measles	Plasmacytoma
Progressive multifocal leukoencephalopathy	**Vascular**
Bacterial	Necrotizing vasculitis
M. tuberculosis	Disseminated intravascular coagulation
Pseudomonas cepacia	**Metabolic**
Syphilitic meningomyelitis	Vitamin B12 deficiency

was no evidence of spinal cord compression or other structural lesions, nor was there evidence of an infectious process within the spinal cord. They termed this entity VM.

Although most studies of HIV-1–associated myelopathy have been of adults, children also may be similarly affected (79). Histological examination by Sharer et al. found inflammatory cell infiltrates in nine and multinucleated giant cells in six of 16 spinal cords of children (79). Only two children exhibited VM (79). Dickson et al. detected significant changes in corticospinal tract degeneration in 15 of 20 spinal cords studied from children dying with AIDS (26). Pathological changes in the corticospinal tract included axonal loss and diminished myelin, but vacuolar changes were not observed in this series of children (25). Therefore, the frequency of certain pathological abnormalities of the spinal cord may not be the same in children as in adults. Parenthetically, the pathology of the spinal cord in adults need not always be that of vacuolar change; other abnormalities that may occur in the absence of vacuolar change include HIV myelitis, microglial nodules, and pallor of the gracile tracts (77).

The frequency of VM in autopsy series has varied. Petito et al. (68) observed a frequency of 22%. In a study of 40 patients dying of AIDS, Artigas et al. (83) reported a prevalence of 55%. In a series of 215 consecutive AIDS autopsies in which the spinal cord was examined, Dal Pan et al. (22) identified VM in 46%.

The neuropathologic features of VM are covered in detail in Chapter 17. However, because this entity is pathologically defined, the salient histopathologic features are reviewed here. Patchy vacuolization, most prominent in the thoracic spinal cord, is the pathological hallmark of HIV-1 VM (68). Petito et al. (68) required the presence of lipid-laden macrophages within the vacuoles to avoid confusion with postmortem artifact. Although they are distributed throughout the spinal white matter, the vacuoles are more numerous in the middle and lower thoracic spinal cord. The cervical cord is also frequently involved, whereas involvement of the lumbar cord is rare (3,68). The lateral columns are more frequently involved than the posterior columns, and the anterolateral and anterior columns are least often involved. In mild cases, the distribution of vacuoles is symmetric, but it is often asymmetric in more advanced cases. On the basis of these findings, Petito et al. have developed a grading system:

Grade I: no more than 15 vacuoles per transverse section
Grade II: numerous but nonconfluent vacuoles
Grade III: areas of confluent vacuolization

Vacuoles are surrounded by a thin myelin sheath. The vacuoles themselves may be the result of intramyelinic edema, which causes enlargement of the periaxonal space and splitting of the myelin lamellae. Macrophages may be found either within the vacuole or within the myelin sheath. Artigas et al. (3), using electron microscopic techniques, have argued, however, that the vacuole arises between the axolemma and the myelin sheath.

In areas of mild or moderate vacuolization, the axons generally appear normal. Only in areas of advanced vacuolization is there axonal disruption. Although multinucleated giant cells are only occasionally seen (15,58), florid infiltration may be observed (33). Typically, lymphocytic infiltrates are not seen. Microglial nodules also are seen (35,68). Similar pathological changes have been noted in the brain (23,78), but not invariably (33).

Becker et al. (6) have applied electromicrographic techniques to further elucidate the pathology of VM. They found that within the same spinal cord there were differences in the stage and severity of individual lesions. Even in early lesions with only a small number of fibers undergoing vacuolization, intramyelinic macrophages could be identified. These lesions often progressed to complete demyelination, with the demyelinated axons surrounded by interdigitated fibrillary astrocytic processes. Some of the lesions were subsequently remyelinated by oligodendrocytes, appearing as thinly myelinated fibers in a field of astrocytic gliosis. Other lesions progressed to necrosis, with initial replacement of most tissue elements by foamy macrophages and later by a matrix of fibrillary astrocytic processes. These observations have suggested that the individual lesions have variable time course and outcome.

The clinical features of HIV-1–related VM have been systematically studied. In an autopsy-based clinicopathological correlation, Dal Pan et al. (22) found that 15 of 56 patients with pathologically confirmed VM had had clinical evidence of myelopathy. Mild to moderate limb weakness was present in all cases, with severe weakness limited to only the most advanced cases. Knee hyperreflexia was common (14 of 15, 93%), as were lower limb spasticity (eight of 15, 53%) and gait spasticity (60%). A sensory ataxia was seen in 20% of cases. A coexistent distal sensory neuropathy with ankle areflexia or hyporeflexia was also common (eight of 15, 53%). A discrete thoracic sensory level was seen in two of 15 of cases (13%). Vibration and position sense loss were common. Bowel and bladder dysfunction were seen in only one case. In all cases, the development of symptoms was slowly progressive, with onset of symptoms ranging from 3 to 16 weeks before the diagnosis of myelopathy. The development of symptomatic myelopathy is more frequent in patients with pathologically more severe VM. For example, Dal Pan et al. (22) found that none of 17 patients with grade I VM had signs or symptoms of myelopathy, whereas five of 26 with grade II VM and 10 of 13 with grade III VM were clinically affected.

Most studies examining the onset of VM in relation to the degree of immunosuppression have concluded that it is a manifestation of advanced HIV disease. Most of the reported cases have occurred in individuals with previous AIDS-defining illnesses (22,35,44,59,68,80). However, there have been reports of VM occurring before the development of other AIDS-defining illnesses (22,59) and at the time of seroconversion (30). Cerebrospinal fluid (CSF) analysis in cases of VM shows only nonspecific abnormalities. Most cases show no pleocytosis or a mild pleocytosis (5–10 cells/mm^3). A CSF white blood cell (WBC) count of >20 cells/mm^3 is rare (22). A mild elevation in CSF protein content is seen in most cases (22,60). These findings contrast with those from cases of infectious myelopathies in AIDS, in which a prominent CSF pleocytosis (>30 WBC/mm^3) can be found (67,86,93). Standard thoracic spine imaging is generally normal. Despite reports of high-intensity signal abnormalities on T2-weighted magnetic resonance images (MRI) of the spinal cord in a rare patient with AIDS myelopathy (4), the presence of this abnormality should suggest another etiology.

Many case series have reported a high frequency of HIV dementia in cases of VM (36,44,59,68). In a case-control study, however, no association was found between HIV dementia (clinically defined) and VM (both clinically and pathologically defined) (22).

Subclinical myelopathy has also been recognized. Jakobsen et al. (45) evaluated the frequency of subclinical neuropathy and myelopathy in a group of 12 HIV-1–infected homosexual men using serial somatosensory evoked potentials. After a 2-year follow-up period, they found a 32% prolongation of the latency from the gluteal crease to the 12th thoracic vertebra after tibial nerve stimulation at the ankle. Tibial nerve conduction time was not significantly increased. The relative delay in conduction from the gluteal crease to T12 exceeded that in the median nerves and from Erb's point to C7. They found no relationship between the degree of abnormality in the somatosensory evoked potential and the clinical stage of HIV infection, the duration of HIV infection, and the CD4+ T-lymphocyte count (CD4+ count). They suggested that subclinical myelopathy is a frequent accompaniment of HIV-1 infection and is probably not related to an opportunistic infection. However, this finding also could be explained by subclinical lumbar root disease and not by thoracic cord disease.

The diagnosis of VM is one of exclusion. Myelopathies due to infectious or neoplastic causes can present with a spastic paraparesis. Features suggestive of an infectious or neoplastic cause include an acute (hours to days) onset, a discrete sensory level, localization to the upper thoracic or cervical spine, a CSF pleocytosis (<20 cells/mm^3), early bladder involvement, and back pain. In those cases, emergent spine imaging followed by CSF analysis is mandatory.

No specific treatment for VM is available. One report showed no benefit of antiretroviral therapy (94), whereas another (66) reported a beneficial response to once-daily high-dose zidovudine (ZDV) (10 mg/kg). The use of corticosteroids, intravenous immunoglobulin, or high-dose, parenteral vitamin B12 has not been effective either (J Berger, personal observations).

Other types of myelopathy attributed directly to HIV-1 have been observed. An acute myelopathy occurring at the time of primary infection with HIV-1 has been reported by Denning et al. (24). Fatigue, sore throat, fever, rash, lymphadenopathy, and conjunctivitis were associated with the acute onset of paraparesis. The patient demonstrated "spasms of the uncontrolled shaking of the lower extremities" and complained of severe, episodic, lancinating, electriclike shocks in his back. Upper extremity hyperreflexia was also noted. HIV-1 was isolated from the peripheral blood and CSF during acute illness. Over several months, the neurological symptoms improved.

A relapsing and remitting myelopathy may accompany optic neuritis in patients with HIV-1 infection. The illness appears to be indistinguishable from multiple sclerosis (10) and is frequently observed in the early stages of HIV-1 infection. A leukoencephalopathy possibly related to this disorder may be monophasic and more aggressive (12). Cranial and spinal MRI shows discrete white matter lesions that may enhance with gadolinium. CSF findings generally reflect those observed with HIV-1 infection, but oligoclonal bands are noted with greater frequency, and myelin basic protein may be elevated. Evoked potentials demonstrate increased latency. In one patient, electron microscopy showed HIV-1 in an affected area of the brain (10). The myelopathy typically responds to corticosteroid administration.

Another curious spinal abnormality associated with HIV-1 infection is spinal myoclonus (8). An increased intrablood–brain barrier synthesis of antibody to HIV-1 was demonstrated in an otherwise asymptomatic man with rhythmic (40–70 contractions per minute) ''beating'' of the abdomen just below the segmental level of T10. The neurological examination was normal apart from the inability to elicit superficial abdominal reflexes. Within 2 months, the myoclonus resolved spontaneously in the absence of medical therapy. Similarly, a 28-year-old HIV-seropositive patient was observed with axial myoclonus affecting the trunk, neck, left shoulder, hips, and knees without other explanation (56). HIV-specific antibodies were detected in the CSF (56). Segmental myoclonus has also been observed preceding herpes zoster radiculitis in a patient with AIDS (54).

Cervical myelopathies are not frequent in HIV infection. Dal Pan et al. reported three cases of cervical myelopathies in HIV infection. All presented with slowly progress spastic quadripareses with sensory loss and hyperreflexia. All had cervical cord enlargement, and two had enhancing lesions in the cervical cord. Spinal cord biopsy in each case failed to show an infectious or neoplastic etiology, nor were the typical features of VM present (21).

The pathogenesis of HIV-1–related VM remains obscure to date. Current hypotheses have centered around a role for the HIV-1 virus (either direct or indirect). A disorder of vitamin B12 has also been considered.

ROLE OF HIV-1 INFECTION

Shortly after the description of VM by Petito et al. (68), Ho et al. (42) reported the isolation of HIV-1 from the CSF and neural tissues from 24 of 33 patients with AIDS-related neurologic syndromes. HIV was isolated from the spinal cord of one of two patients with VM and from the CSF of each of these two patients. They speculated that VM may be a direct neurologic sequel of HIV infection.

In 1988, Budka et al. (15,27) reported that, using monoclonal antibodies against HIV-1 p24 and p17, they had identified HIV-1 antigens in mono- or multinucleated giant cells in the cerebral white matter of a 43-year-old man who had died with AIDS-related VM. In the spinal cord, they noted that HIV antigens were limited to areas with vacuolar damage, where cells with features of macrophages were immunostained. This finding linked productive HIV-1 infection to VM.

Using immunohistochemistry, *in situ* hybridization, and culture of tissue homogenates, Rosenblum et al. (74) found that neither the presence nor the severity of VM correlated with the presence of HIV-1 in the spinal cord. Rather, they found that detection of viral p24 and of HIV-1 messenger RNA correlated with the histopathologic findings of cellular infiltrates: multinucleated giant cells, macrophages, and microglia. HIV-1 infection was detected in the brain of several of these patients, although there was no correlation between brain infection and VM. They concluded that VM is independent of productive spinal cord or brain HIV-1 infection.

On the other hand, Rhodes et al. (71), using immunohistochemical techniques, found a high correlation of immunolocalization of HIV-1 in the spinal cord with clinical signs and symptoms. Such immunoreactivity was localized to macrophages, multinucleated giant cells, microglial nodules, glial cells, and vascular endothelial cells. They postulated that HIV-1 could enter the spinal cord via infected endothelial cells and that a vasculitis could lead to the myelitis.

Using *in situ* hybridization techniques, Weiser et al. (91) detected HIV-1 RNA in the spinal cords of 10 of 10 patients with clinical and histopathological evidence of VM. HIV-1 RNA was detected in none of 10 spinal cords from HIV-1–infected patients without myelopathy, nor was it detected from the spinal cords of HIV-1–seronegative controls. In their study group, five of six subjects with severe VM had coexistent HIV-1 encephalitis, whereas only one of the HIV-1–infected individuals without VM had HIV-1 encephalitis.

Combining the techniques of *in situ* hybridization and immunohistochemistry, Eilbott et al. (29) demonstrated that HIV-1 was expressed in the cells of the monocyte/macrophage lineage, primarily in the areas of myelopathy in the white matter of the spinal cord. Electron microscopy showed retroviral particles associated with and budding from macrophages. Myelin was identified within macrophages as well. In two of the three cords examined, the number of macrophages and viral particles paralleled the degree of pathologic change.

What is the role of the HIV-1 virus in the pathogenesis of VM? The above studies suggest that the virus is present in the spinal cord of patients with VM, although these findings do not confirm a direct role for the virus in the development of the myelopathy.

Tyor et al. (87) have studied cytokine expression of macrophages in HIV-associated VM. They found that the predominant mononuclear cells present in spinal cord specimens from HIV-seropositive individuals were macrophages and that both macrophages and microglia were more frequent in the cords of HIV-seropositive compared with seronegative individuals. Macrophages were located primarily in the posterior and lateral funiculi in the cords of all the HIV-seropositive cases, including those in which no vacuolar changes were evident. These macrophages stained for class I and class II major histocompatibility antigens, interleukin-1 (IL-1), and tumor necrosis factor-alpha (TNF-α). The finding of activated macrophages in the posterior and lateral columns of spinal cords form AIDS autopsies with and without VM suggests that they are present before the development of the vacuoles and that cytokines, such as TNF-α, may be toxic for myelin or oligodendrocytes. The resultant myelin damage may then be followed by removal by macrophages and vacuole formation.

The occurrence of a clinically and pathologically indistinguishable myelopathy occurring in patients with underlying illnesses other than AIDS, including leukemia, lymphoma, systemic lupus erythematosus, chronic lung disease, renal transplantation, cirrhosis, diabetes, hemophagocytic syndrome, and viral encephalitis (48), suggests an etiology other than HIV-1. Kamin and Petito, who observed this VM in 21 patients who did not have AIDS, speculated that another opportunistic viral infection may be responsible for the disorder. However, another possibility is a nutritional deficiency.

VITAMIN B12 DEFICIENCY AND VM

VM has certain clinical and pathological characteristics suggestive of vitamin B12 deficiency. The micovacuolation observed is similar in both conditions; however, the lesions tend to predominate in the cervical region in association with B12 deficiency. Gait abnormalities, hyperreflexia and concomitant peripheral neuropathy are common to both conditions. Retrospective analysis of vitamin B12 levels in pathological series has failed to show an association (68). However, in a preliminary study performed as a substudy within a prospective, longitudinal study of the neurological complications of HIV infection, four of six HIV-1 patients with an unexplained myelopathy clinically indistinguishable from VM had a low B12 level of ~250 pg/ml in contrast to none of seven patients with identifiable etiologies for their myelopathy (J. Berger, personal observation).

None of 12 patients in the study by Petito et al. (68) had a low serum vitamin B12 level. Harriman et al. (37) have examined the prevalence of B12 deficiency in various groups of HIV-1–infected individuals. They found that 15% of an unselected population of patients with AIDS had low serum B12 levels, wheres 7% of asymptomatic HIV seropositives had low serum vitamin B12 levels. Other groups (5,16,40,69) have demonstrated an even higher prevalence of vitamin B12 deficiency (up to one third of patients with AIDS) and have attributed this in part to impaired ileal absorption.

One study reported a high prevalence of abnormally low serum cobalamin levels and/or an abnormal Schilling test result in HIV-1–infected patients with myelopathy and neuropathy (52). CSF studies have suggested inhibition of brain methyltransferase activity in patients with various stages of HIV-1 infection and with various degrees of neurologic dysfunction, but no specific correlation was made with VM (51). Other studies, in children, have suggested that elevation of CSF neopterin leads to inhibition of folate-dependent methylation reactions, thus resulting in demyelination (81,85).

Studies of the potential role of altered cobalamin-dependent or folate-dependent metabolism in the pathogenesis of VM are confounded by the high frequency of nutritional deficiency in the advanced stages of HIV-1 infection and the association of VM with the later stages of HIV-1 infection. Furthermore, because serum cobalamin and folate levels are not the most sensitive indicators of the integrity of cobalamin- and folate-dependent methylation reactions, a normal cobalamin or folate level may be seen even in the presence of abnormal methylation reactions. In a case-control study, Dal Pan et al. (20) measured cobalamin, folate, and several intermediary metabolites involved in methylation reactions, including methylmalonic acid, 2-methylcitric acid homocysteine, and cystathionine in stored sera of individuals who died with HIV-1 infection, some with autopsy-proven VM, others with no autopsy evidence of VM. No differences in cobalamin, folate, or the other metabolites was found between the two groups. In addition, the vast majority of patients in both groups had values of all metabolites that were not suggestive of cobalamin or folate deficiency.

INFECTIOUS MYELOPATHIES

Though the noninflammatory VM is the most common cause of spinal cord disease in HIV-1 infection, there have been several case reports of myelopathy attributed to other infectious agents.

HTLV-I Infection

The human T-lymphotropic virus type 1 (HTLV-I) is a human retrovirus that has been associated with both adult T cell leukemia/lymphoma and myelopathies in both tropical (34,46,72,73,88) and nontropical regions. HTLV-I–associated myelopathy (HAM), also called tropical spastic paraparesis, is a slowly progressive spastic paraparesis. Only rarely does HAM involve the upper extremities, although brisk upper extremity reflexes and positive Hoffman's sign are the rule rather than the exception. A mild sensory neuropathy with pedal paraesthesias may be present, but other sensory symptoms are usually absent. Unlike HIV-1–related VM, a discrete sensory level may be present, but it is exceptional. Bowel and bladder involvement may occur with advanced disease. A CSF pleocytosis (20–100 WBC/mm^3) can occur in 40–60% of cases. Pathologically, there is an inflammatory myelitis with leptomeningitis affecting the thoracic cord, and in chronic cases, spongiform changes may be seen. Diagnosis rests upon isolation of HTLV-I within the CSF or measurement of intrathecal synthesis of anti–HTLV-I immunoglobulin G (IgG). Unlike HIV-1–related VM, there are no associated dementia or cranial nerve abnormalities (1,9,75).

Because of the similarities of HAM and HIV-1–related VM, several groups have attempted to isolate HTLV-I from patients with VM. Brew et al. (13) examined sera from 28 patients with AIDS: 23 with pathologically confirmed VM, four with clinically diagnosed VM, and one with an atypical myelopathy, which had its onset several years before the AIDS epidemic. None of the 27 patients with VM had serological evidence of HTLV-I. The patient with the atypical myelopathy, however, was seropositive for both HTLV-I and HIV-1.

Although HTLV-I is not the etiologic agent of myelopathy in VM, coinfection with both HIV-1 and HTLV-I may occasionally occur. McArthur et al. (61) reported the unusual case of a 28-year-old American bisexual man dually infected with HIV-1 and HTLV-I who developed a myeloneuropathy. His blood CD4+ count was persistently in the normal range. MRI of the brain was normal; spinal MRI showed atrophy from T3 to T10. CSF analysis was notable for a lymphocytic pleocytosis, elevated protein and IgG, oligoclonal bands, and elevated intrathecal synthesis of anti–HTLV-I IgG. Soluble IL-2 receptor and soluble CD8 were elevated in both blood and CSF when compared with patients with VM and with those with other causes of myelopathy. Nerve biopsy showed a CD8+ lymphocytic infiltration. The patient responded to a 6-week course of prednisone. Based on these features, the authors concluded that the myelopathy was caused by HTLV-I.

Berger et al. (11) described a 34-year-old parenteral drug abuser with a myelopathy clinically indistinguishable from HAM who was coinfected with HIV-1 and HTLV-II. A mixed axonal and demyelinative peripheral neuropathy coexisted. Although unresponsive to 10 months of zidovudine therapy over the course of 2 years, the neurological symptoms abated dramatically in the absence of specific therapy.

Toxoplasma gondii

Toxoplasma gondii is an obligate intracellular protozoan parasite that causes symptomatic cerebral infection in individuals with impaired cellular immunity. In HIV-infected patients, it most commonly presents as multiple ring-enhancing lesions in the cerebrum (65). An encephalitic form, clinically similar to a viral encephalitis, also has been reported (2,17).

Although it is one of the most common forms of intracerebral mass lesions in AIDS, toxoplasmosis of the spinal cord is rare. Mehren et al. (62) reported the case of a 63-year-old man with AIDS who developed weakness and numbness of the left arm. Neurological examination was notable for weakness of the left arm and leg, a left hemisensory deficit to vibration up to C3, diminished pinprick and temperature sensation on the right side of the body to a similar level, and a left Babinski sign. Cervical spine MRI showed a variable signal intensity at the C2–4 level and thickening of the spinal cord at that level, suggestive of an intramedullary lesion. A serum toxoplasma titer (IgG) was 1 : 16. Empiric treatment of lymphoma with radiation and steroid therapy resulted in only transient improvement. Autopsy showed multiple circumscribed lesions in the brain and softening in the brain stem and upper cervical spinal cord. The necrotic lesions contained multiple cysts filled with toxoplasma trophozoites.

A second case of intramedullary spinal cord toxoplasmosis was reported by Herskovitz et al. (41). Their patient presented with 3 months of upper thoracic back pain, 1 month of urinary hesitancy, and 2 weeks of urinary and fecal incontinence accompanied by progressive bilateral leg weakness. Examination was notable for a flaccid paraparesis and a T2 sensory level bilaterally. He underwent spinal cord biopsy with decompressive laminectomy. Neuropathologic examination of the posterior column biopsy showed a pseudocyst containing *T. gondii*. Despite antitoxoplasma therapy, there was no improvement.

Toxoplasma gondii also has been the etiologic agent of a conus medullaris syndrome in a 32-year-old hemophilic man with AIDS who developed the acute onset of fever, bilateral leg weakness, urinary retention, and decreased anal sphincter tone (38,50,67). The CSF was suggestive of an infection (30 WBC/mm^3; 35% polys, 38% lymphocytes, and 25% monocytes, protein 220 mg/dl, and glucose 43 mg/dl). A fine-needle aspiration biopsy was nondiagnostic. Open surgical biopsy was performed, and staining of the lesion was positive for *T. gondii*. The patient improved with antitoxoplasma therapy.

Other cases of *T. gondii* of the spinal cord include that described by Fairley (31) and that of Resnick et al. (70). These cases resulted from an intramedullary lesion of the spinal cord due to *T. gondi* that resulted in progressive paraparesis. An antemortem diagnosis was possible.

Treponemal Infection

Though infection with the spirochete *Treponema pallidum*, the etiologic agent of syphilis, is common in HIV-1 infection, the incidence of neurosyphilis in HIV-1 infection has never been firmly established, in part because of the lack of sensitivity of commonly used tests to detect the presence of antitreponemal antibodies in the setting of HIV-1 infection. Katz and Berger (49) have conservatively estimated that 1.5% of all hospitalized patients with AIDS have neurosyphilis. In the majority of cases, the neurological manifestations have been an altered mental status and hemiparesis. Eye disease is also common. Apart from meningitis, spinal cord disease attributable to *T. pallidum* is apparently not very common. Berger (7) described three patients with a syphilitic myelopathy, confirmed at autopsy in two cases. One patient demonstrated a dramatic response within 2 weeks of receiving high-dose intravenous penicillin therapy. In that patient, serum and CSF FTA-ABS were positive, as was serum VDRL. An elevated CSF protein and lymphocytic pleocytosis were also noted. Strom and Schneck reported on a 28-year-old patient with secondary syphilis who was not immunocompromised and developed spastic paraparesis secondary to syphilitic meningomyelitis with other hallmarks of secondary syphilis (84).

Herpes Group Myelitides

The herpes viruses include herpes simplex types I and II (HSV I and II), cytomegalovirus (CMV), varicella zoster virus (VZV), and Epstein-Barr virus (EBV). In non–HIV-1–infected individuals, these viruses may cause a variety of neurologic syndromes at any level of the neuraxis. In HIV-1 infection, CMV has been well recognized as the etiologic agent of both an encephalitis (39,43,47,55,64,82,90) and a polyradiculitis (19,57,63). Although it typically occurs with advanced degrees of immunosuppression, on rare occasion CMV myelopathy may be the initial manifestation of AIDS (57).

Britton et al. (14) reported on a 24-year-old intravenous drug user coinfected with CMV and HSV who developed CMV colitis and chorioretinitis, as well as a progressive thoracic myelopathy, resulting in weakness and diminished vibration in the right leg, a left T8 sensory level to pin, and a right Babinski sign. The CSF was acellular with normal glucose and protein and negative viral, fungal, and bacterial cultures. At autopsy, there was a necrotizing arteritis of the anterior spinal artery and old cystic myelomalacia involving the ventral gray and much of the lateral column on the right side. The cavity contained macrophages, cellular debris, blood vessels with reactive changes, and many cells with Cowdry type A intranuclear inclusions. Immunostaining in spinal cord sections from the T7 to T8 levels showed that most cells in that region stained heavily with monoclonal antiserum to HSV-2 antigen, but only a small focus on CMV antigen-positive cells were seen and were felt to represent a superinfection. They concluded that the patient had a herpes simplex type 2 thoracic myelitis.

Tucker et al. (86) reported the case of a 26-year-old man whose presenting feature of AIDS was a progressive ascending myelitis, causing right leg weakness, leg areflexia, and a T10 sensory level. CSF analysis showed xanthochromia (14,000 red blood cells [RBC]/mm^3), a polymorphonuclear pleocytosis (1,200 WBC/mm^3), elevated protein (295 mg/dl), and hypoglychoracchia (28 mg/dl). His symptoms progressed, and he soon developed Kaposi's sarcoma and *Pneumocystis carinii* pneumonia. At autopsy, both CMV and HSV-2 were recovered from the nervous system. CMV also was recovered from the liver, gastrointestinal tract, adrenal, and lungs. The only extraneural site from which HSV-2 was recovered, however, was the anus. Which of the two viruses—CMV or HSV-2—was responsible for the myelitis remains unknown; however, the widespread recovery of CMV suggests that its presence in the CNS may have been due to hematogenous spread and that its presence was incidental to the HSV-2–caused myelitis.

Herpes zoster also has been observed as a cause of severe meningomyeloradiculitis (18). In a 30-year-old man without cutaneous eruption, a rapidly progressive paraplegia was demonstrated to be the result of HZV by immunocytochemistry studies (18). A similar fulminant ascending myeloradiculitis affected a 40-year-old patient with

AIDS (18). In both a necrotizing vasculitis involved the spinal cord and spinal roots (18).

Progressive myelopathy has been observed (J. Berger, personal communication) in rare patients with very advanced immunosuppression having either HSV-1 or HSV-2 isolated from their CSF. A lymphocytic pleocytosis (<200 cells/mm^3) and increased protein were present in these individuals. Abnormal hyperintense signals in the thoracic spinal cord on T2-weighted MRI were seen. Pathological confirmation of a herpes myelitis was not available. A discussion of CMV disease can be found in Chapter 23.

Mycobacterial Infection

Infection with *Mycobacterium tuberculosis* is a cause of substantial morbidity and mortality in HIV-1-infection. Tuberculous meningitis and intracerebral tuberculomas have been seen in HIV-1–infected individuals. Woolsey et al. (93) reported a case of an intramedullary tuberculoma. Their patient, a 44-year-old homosexual man, developed moderately severe low back pain, extending to his right hip and thigh. He developed weakness in his legs, more in the right than in the left, as well as decreased sensation below both knees. Spinal fluid analysis showed 120 RBC/mm^3, 40 WBC/mm^3 (93% lymphocytes), protein 105 mg/dl, glucose 43 mg/dl, negative VDRL, negative cryptococcal antigen, and no oligoclonal bands. Cultures were negative. His neurologic deficits progressed, and he became anesthetic below the T10 dermatome. Two months after his initial presentation, he underwent a T11–12 laminectomy with spinal cord biopsy. Microscopic examination of the biopsy specimen showed an intramedullary noncaseating granuloma with numerous acid-fast organisms in the epithelioid cells of the granuloma. He was treated with isoniazid, rifampin, pyrazinamide, and ethambutol, with no change in his neurological status.

Rare Infectious Myelopathies

Sharer et al. observed only one child of 18 HIV-infected children coming to autopsy with spinal cord disease who had an opportunistic infection (79). Myelitis occurring as a consequence of opportunistic infection appears to be less common in children than in adults. Their one case of myelitis due to opportunistic infection was in a 30-month-old child with VM and concomitant measles (rubeola) infection of the spinal cord (79). A myeloradiculitis due to *Cryptococcus curvatus* was reported by French investigators (28). This patient presented with numbness of the hands and feet, bilateral paresthesias of the legs, pyramidal tract findings in the arms and legs, and a gait disorder. *Aspergillus fumigatus* of the spinal cord also has been reported (92). To date, no intramedullary bacterial spinal cord abscesses have been reported in HIV infection. On rare occasions, the demyelinative lesions of progressive multifocal leukoencephalopathy may affect the spinal cord as well as the brain.

NEOPLASTIC CAUSES OF MYELOPATHY

Lymphoma

Primary central nervous system lymphoma occurs in ~2% of patients with AIDS (76). It presents almost exclusively in the cerebrum and only rarely in the brain stem.

Klein et al. (53) have reported a single case of a spinal mass lesion and lymphomatous meningitis in a patient with AIDS. Their patient had two bouts of *P. carinii* pneumonia as well as herpes simplex dorsal radiculitis and a distal sensory neuropathy. She then developed acute low back pain radiating to her thighs and calves, as well as weakness of the left leg and urinary hesitancy. CSF protein was elevated (188 mg/dl), glucose was reduced (13 mg/dl), and there were 20 WBCs in the CSF (75% neutrophils, 15% monocytes, and 9% lymphocytes). Cytological examination showed atypical lymphocytes but no malignant cells. *Mycobacterium avium-intracellulare* was isolated from the CSF. MRI of the spinal cord showed an expansive lesion at the cauda equina at the L1 level and a thickening of the nerve roots at the L1–2 level. CT myelography showed an intradural lesion at that level with thickening of multiple nerve roots below the L1 level. Biopsy showed diffuse infiltration of the nerve roots by a large cell lymphoma. Within 5 weeks, the lymphomatous meningitis had spread rostrally to involve multiple cranial nerves and finally the brain. At autopsy, there was diffuse lymphomatous leptomeningitis throughout the neuraxis, but no evidence of lymphoma outside of the CNS.

Other Neoplasms

Myelopathy also has been observed occurring in association with spinal cord astrocytomas. Other neoplasms such as Kaposi's sarcoma have not been reported as causes of myelopathy in HIV-1 infection, but they are anticipated. One patient with AIDS developed a rapidly progressive myelopathy secondary to thoracic cord involvement by a plasmacytoma (Berger, personal observation).

Vascular Myelopathies

Fenelon et al. (32) described a 39-year-old man with AIDS who lost vision in his left eye and then developed lower extremity numbness. A rapidly progressive myelopathy with partial Brown-Sequard syndrome ensued, and he died within 9 weeks of onset. Neuropathological examination showed multiple, hemorrhagic infarcts and fibrin thrombi of the penetrating vessels of the brain and spinal cord characteristic of disseminated intravascular coagulation. No etiology was defined.

Another form of vascular injury to the cord was described by Vinters et al (89). This patient developed an ascending myelopathy and died within 48 hours of onset. A severe necrotizing vasculitis was observed at autopsy.

ACKNOWLEDGMENT

This work was supported by NS 26643, RR00722.

REFERENCES

1. Aboulafia DM, Sexton EH, Koga H, Diagne A, Rosenblatt JD. A pateint with progressive myelopathy and antibodies to human T cell leukemia virus type I and human immunodeficieny virus type I in serum and CSF. *Arch Neurol* 1990;47:477–479.
2. Arendt G, Hefter H, Figge C, et al. Two cases of cerebral toxoplasmosis in AIDS patients mimicking HIV-related dementia. *J Neurol* 1991;238:439–442.

3. Artigas J, Grosse G, Niedobitek F. Vacuolar myelopathy in AIDS. A morphological analysis. *Pathol Res Pract* 1990;186:228–237.
4. Barakos JA, Mark AS, Dillon WP, Norman D. MR imaging of acute transverse myelitis and AIDS myelopathy. *J Comput Assist Tomogr* 1990;14:45–50.
5. Beach RS, Mantero-Atienza E, Shor-Posner G, et al. Specific nutrient abnormalities in asymptomatic HIV-1 infection. *AIDS* 1992;6:701–708.
6. Becker PS, Griffin JW, McArthur JC, Price DL, Johnson RT. Vacuolar myelopathy in human immunodeficiency virus (HIV) infection: central remyelination. *J Neuropathol Exp Neurol* 1989;48:383.
7. Berger JR. Spinal cord syphilis associated with human immunodeficiency virus infection: a treatable myelopathy. *Am J Med* 1992;92:101–103.
8. Berger JR, Bender A, Resnick L, Perlmutter D. Spinal myoclonus associated with HTLV III/LAV infection. *Arch Neurol* 1986;43:1203–1204.
9. Berger JR, Raffanti S, Svenningison A, McCarthy M, Snodgrass S, Resnick L. The role of HTLV in HIV-associated neurologic disease. *Neurology* 1991;41:197–202.
10. Berger JR, Sheremata WA, Resnick L, Atherton S, Fletcher MA, Norenberg M. Multiple sclerosis–like illness occurring with human immunodeficiency virus infection. *Neurology* 1989;39:324–329.
11. Berger JR, Svenningsson A, Rafanti S, Resnick L. Tropical spastic paraparesis-like illness occurring in a patient dually infected with HIV-I and HTLV-II. *Neurology* 1991;41:85–87.
12. Berger JR, Tornatore C, Major EO, Bruce J, et al. Relapsing and remitting human immunodeficinecy virus–associated leukoencephalomyelopathy. *Ann Neurol* 1992;31:34–38.
13. Brew BJ, Hardy W, Zuckerman E, et al. AIDS-related vacuolar myelopathy is not associated with coinfection by human T-lymphotropic virus type I. *Ann Neurol* 1989;26:679–681.
14. Britton CB, Mesa-Tejada R, Fenoglio CM, Hays AP, Garvey GG, Miller JR. A new complication of AIDS: thoracic myelitis caused by herpes simplex virus. *Neurology* 1985;35:1071–1074.
15. Budka H, Maier H, Pohl P. Human immunodeficiency virus in vacuolar myelopathy of the acquired immunodeficiency syndrome [letter]. *N Engl J Med* 1988;319:1667–1668.
16. Burkes RL, Cohen H, Krailo M, Sinow RM, Carmel R. Low serum cobalamin levels occur frequently in the acquired immune deficiency syndrome and related disorders. *Eur J Haematol* 1987;38:141–147.
17. Carrazana EJ, Rossitch E Jr, Schachter S. Cerebral toxoplasmosis masquerading as herpes encephalitis in a patient with the acquired immunodeficiency syndrome. *Am J Med* 1989;86:730–732.
18. Chretien F, Gray F, Lescs MC, et al. Acute varicella zoster virus ventriculitis and meningo-myelo-radiculitis in acquired immunodeficiency syndrome. *Acta Neuropathol (Berl)* 1993;86:659–665.
19. Cohen BA, McArthur JC, Grohman S, et al. Neurologic prognosis in CMV polyradiculomyelopathy in AIDS. *Neurology* 1993;43:493–499.
20. Dal Pan GJ, Allen RH, Glass JD, et al. Cobalamin (vitamin B12) dependent metabolism is not specifically altered in HIV-1–associated vacuolar myelopathy [Abstract]. *Ann Neurol* 1993;34:281.
21. Dal Pan GJ, Glass J, Zeidman S, McArthur J. Atypical HIV-associated myelopathy: diagnosis by cord biopsy. *Neurology* 1992;42(suppl 3):257.
22. Dal Pan GJ, Glass JD, McArthur JC. Clinicopathologic correlations of HIV-associated vacuolar myelopathy: an autopsy-based case-control study. *Neurology* 1994;44:2159–2164.
23. de la Monte SM, Moore T, Hedley-Whyte ET. Vacuolar encephalopathy of AIDS [Letter]. *N Engl Med* 1986;315:1549–1550.
24. Denning DW, Anderson J, Rudge P, Smith H. Acute myelopathy associated with primary infection with human immunodeficiency virus. *Br Med J [Clin Res]* 1987;294:143–144.
25. Dickson DW, Belman AL, Kim TS, Horoupian DS, Rubinstein A. Spinal cord pathology in pediatric acquired immunodeficiency syndrome. *Neurology* 1989;39:227–235.
26. Dickson DW, Belman AL, Park YD, et al. Central nervous system pathology in pediatric AIDS: an autopsy study. *APMIS Suppl* 1989;8:40–57.
27. Dilley JW, Ochitill HN, Perl M, Volberding P. Findings in psychiatric consultations with patients with acquired immune deficiency sydrome. *Am J Psychiatry* 1985;142:82–86.
28. Dromer F, Moulignier A, Dupont B, et al. A myeloradiculitis due to *Cryptococcus curvatus* in AIDS. *AIDS* 1995;9:395–396.
29. Eilbott DJ, Peress N, Burger H, et al. Human immunodeficiency virus type 1 in spinal cords of acquired immunodeficiency syndrome patients with myelopathy: expression and replication in macrophages. *Proc Natl Acad Sci U S A* 1989;86:3337–3341.
30. Epstein LG, Sharer LR, Oleske JM, et al. Neurologic manifestations of human immunodeficiency virus infection in children. *Pediatrics* 1986;78:678–687.
31. Fairley CK, Wodak J, Benson E. Spinal cord toxoplasmosis in a pateint with human immunodeficiency virus infection. *J STD AIDS* 1992;3:366–368.
32. Fenelon G, Gray F, Scaravilli F, et al. Ischemic myelopathy secondary to disseminated intravascular coagulation in AIDS. *J Neurol* 1991;238:51–54.
33. Geny C, Gherardi R, Boudes P, Lionet F, et al. Multifocal multinucleated giant cell amyelitis in an AIDS patient. *Neuropathol Appl Neurobiol* 1991;17:157–162.
34. Gessain A, Barin F, Vernant JC, et al. Antibodies to human T-lymphotropic virus type-I in patients with tropical spastic paraparesis. *Lancet* 1985;2:407–410.

35. Goldstick L, Mandybur TI, Bode R. Spinal cord degeneration in AIDS. *Neurology* 1985;35:103–106.
36. Griffin JW, McArthur JC, Cornblath DR. Peripheral nerve and spinal cord disease in human retroviral infections. *Curr Opin Neurol Neurosurg* 1990;3.
37. Harriman GR, Smith PD, Horne MK, et al. Vitamin B12 malabsorption in patients with acquired immunodeficiency syndrome. *Arch Intern Med* 1989;149:2039–2041.
38. Harris TM, Smith RR, Bognanno JR, Edwards MK. Toxplasmic myelitis in AIDS: gadolinium-enhanced MR. *J Comput Assist Tomogr* 1990;14:809–811.
39. Hawley DA, Schaefer JF, Schulz DM, Muller J. Cytomegalovirus encephalitis in acquired immunodeficiency syndrome. *Am J Clin Pathol* 1983;80:874–877.
40. Herbert V. B12 deficiency in AIDS. *JAMA* 1988;260:2837.
41. Herskovitz S, Siegel SE, Schneider AT, Nelson SJ, Goodrich JT, Lantos G. Spinal cord toxoplasmosis in AIDS. *Neurology* 1989;39:1552–1553.
42. Ho DD, Rota TR, Schooley RT, et al. Isolation of HTLV-III from cerebrospinal fluid and neural tissues of patients with neurologic syndromes related to the acquired immunodeficiency syndrome. *N Engl J Med* 1985;313:1493–1497.
43. Holland NR, Power C, Matthews VP, et al. CMV encephalitis in acquired immunodeficiency syndrome (AIDS). *Neurology* 1994;44:507–514.
44. Horoupian DS, Pick P, Spigland I, et al. Acquired immune deficiency syndrome and multiple tract degeneration in a homosexual man. *Ann Neurol* 1984;15:502–505.
45. Jakobsen J, Smith T, Gaub J, Helweg-Larsen S, Trojaborg W. Progressive neurological dysfunction during latent HIV infection. *Br Med J* 1989;299:225–228.
46. Johnson RT, Griffin DE, Arregui A, et al. Spastic paraparesis and HTLV-I infection in Peru. *Ann Neurol* 1988;23(suppl):151–155.
47. Kalayjian RC, Cohen ML, Bonomo RA, Flanigan TP. Cytomegalovirus ventriculoencephalitis in AIDS. *Medicine* 1993;72:67–77.
48. Kamin SS, Petito CK. Idiopathic myelopathies with white matter vacuolation in non-acquired immunodeficiency syndrome patients. *Hum Pathol* 1991;22:816–824.
49. Katz DA, Berger JR. Neurosyphilis in acquired immunodeficiency syndrome. *Arch Neurol* 1989;46:895–898.
50. Kayser C, Campbell R, Sartorious C, Bartlett M. Toxoplasmosis of the conus medullaris in a patient with hemophilia A–associated AIDS. *J Neurosurg* 1990;73:951–953.
51. Keating JN, Trimble KC, Mulcahy F, Scott JM, Weir DG. Evidence of brain methyltransferase inhibition and early brain involvement in HIV-positive patients. *Lancet* 1991;337:935–939.
52. Kieburtz KD, Giang DW, Schiffer RB, Vakil M. Abnormal vitamin B12 metabolism in human immunodeficiency infection. Association with neurologic dysfunction. *Arch Neurol* 1991;48:312–314.
53. Klein P, Zientek G, VandenBerg SR, Lothman E. Primary CNS lymphoma: lymphomatous meningitis presenting as a cauda equina lesion in an AIDS patient. *Can J Neurol Sci* 1990;17:329–331.
54. Koppel BS, Daras M. Segmental myoclonus preceding herpes zoster radiculitis. *Eur Neurol* 1992;32:264–266.
55. Levy RM, Bredesen DE, Rosenblum ML. Neurological manifestations of the acquired immunodeficiency syndrome (AIDS): experience at UCSF and review of the literature. *J Neurosurg* 1985;62:475–495.
56. Lubetzki C, Vidailhet M, Jednyak CP, Thibault S, et al. Propriospinal myoclonus in an HIV seropostive pateint. *Rev Neurol* 1994;150:70–72.
57. Mahieux F, Gray F, Fenelon G, et al. Acute myeloradiculitis due to cytomegalovirus as the initial manifestation of AIDS. *J Neurol Neurosurg Psychiatry* 1989;52:270–274.
58. Maier H, Budka H, Lassmann H, Pohl P. Vacuolar myelopathy with multinucleated giant cells in the acquired immune deficiency syndrome (AIDS). Light and electron microscopic distribution of human immunodeficiency virus (HIV) antigens. *Acta Neuropathol (Berl)* 1989;78:497–503.
59. McArthur JC. Neurologic manifestations of AIDS. *Medicine (Balt)* 1987;66:407–437.
60. McArthur JC, Cohen BA, Farzedegan H, et al. Cerebrospinal fluid abnormalities in homosexual men with and without neuropsychiatric findings. *Ann Neurol* 1988;23(suppl):34–37.
61. McArthur JC, Griffin JW, Cornblath DR, et al. Steroid-responsive myeloneuropathy in a man dually infected with HIV-1 and HTLV-I. *Neurology* 1990;40:938–944.
62. Mehren M, Burns PJ, Mamani F, Levy CS, Laureno R. Toxoplasmic myelitis mimicking intramedullary spinal cord tumor. *Neurology* 1988;38:1648–1650.
63. Miller RG, Storey JR, Greco CM. Ganciclovir in the treatment of progressive AIDS-related polyradiculopathy. *Neurology* 1990;40:569–574.
64. Moskowitz LB, Gregorios JB, Hensley GT, Berger JR. Cytomegalovirus. Induced demyelination associated with acquired immune deficiency syndrome. *Arch Pathol Lab Med* 1984;108:873–877.
65. Navia BA, Petito CK, Gold JW, Cho ES, Jordan BD, Price RW. Cerebral toxoplasmosis complicating the acquired immune deficiency syndrome: clinical and neuropathological findings in 27 patients. *Ann Neurol* 1986;19:224–238.

66. Oksenhendler E, Ferchal F, Cadranel J, Sauvageon-Martre H, Clauvel J. Zidovudine for HIV-related myelopathy. *Am J Med* 1990;88:5-65N–5-66N.
67. Overhage JM, Greist A, Brown DR. Conus medullaris syndrome resulting from *Toxoplasma gondii* infection in a patient with the acquired immunodeficiency syndrome. *Am J Med* 1990;89:814–815.
68. Petito CK, Navia BA, Cho ES, Jordan BD, George DC, Price RW. Vacuolar myelopathy pathologically resembling subacute combined degeneration in patients with the acquired immunodeficiency syndrome. *N Engl J Med* 1985;312:874–879.
69. Remacha AF, Riera A, Cadafalch J, Gimferrer E. Vitamin B-12 abnormalities in HIV-infected patients. *Eur J Haematol* 1991;47:60–64.
70. Resnick L, Comey CH, Welch WC, Martinez AJ, et al. Isolated toxoplasmosis of the thoracic spinal cord in a patient with acquired immunodeficiency syndrome. *J Neurosurg* 1995;82:493–496.
71. Rhodes RH, Ward JM, Cowan RP, Moore PT. Immunohistochemical localization of human immunodeficiency viral antigens in formalin-fixed spinal cords with AIDS myelopathy. *Clin Neuropathol* 1989;8:22–27.
72. Rodgers-Johnson P, Gajdusek DC, Morgan OS, Zaninovic V, Sarin PS, Graham DS. HTLV-I and HTLV-III antibodies and tropical spastic paraparesis [Letter]. *Lancet* 1985;2:1247–1248.
73. Roman GC. Retrovirus-associated myelopathies. *Arch Neurol* 1987;44:659–665.
74. Rosenblum M, Scheck AC, Cronin K, et al. Dissociation of AIDS-related vacuolar myelopathy and productive HIV-1 infection of the spinal cord. *Neurology* 1989;39:892–896.
75. Rosenblum MK, Brew BJ, Hahn B, et al. Human T-lymphotropic virus type I–associated myelopathy in patients with the acquired immunodeficiency syndrome. *Hum Pathol* 1992;23:513–519.
76. Rosenblum ML, Levy RM, Bredesen DE, So YT, Wara W, Ziegler JL. Primary central nervous system lymphomas in patients with AIDS. *Ann Neurol* 1988;23(suppl):13–16.
77. Scaravilli F, Sinclair E, Arango J-C, Manji H, Lucas S, Harrison MJG. The pathology of the posterior root ganglia in AIDS and its relationship to the pallor of the gracile tract. *Acta Neuropathol (Berl)* 1992;84:163–170.
78. Schmidbauer M, Budka H, Okeda R, Cristina S, Lechi A, Trabattoni GR. Multifocal vacuolar leucoencephalopathy: a distinct HIV-associated lesion of the brain. *Neuropathol Appl Neurobiol* 1990; 16:437–443.
79. Sharer LR, Dowling PC, Michaels J, Cook SD, et al. Spinal cord disease in children with HIV-1 infection: a combined molecular biological and neuropathological study. *Neuropathol Appl Neurobiol* 1990;16:317–331.
80. Singh BM, Levine S, Yarrish RL, Hyland MJ, Jeanty D, Wormser GP. Spinal cord syndromes in the acquired immune deficiency syndrome. *Acta Neurol Scand* 1986;73:590–598.
81. Smith I, Howells DW, Kendall B, Levinsky R, Hyland K. Folate deficiency and demyelination in AIDS [Letter]. *Lancet* 1987;2:215.
82. Snider WD, Simpson DM, Nielsen S, Gold JW, Metroka CE, Posner JB. Neurological complications of acquired immune deficiency syndrome: analysis of 50 patients. *Ann Neurol* 1983;14:403–418.
83. Stabler SP, Lindenbaum J, Savage DG, Allen RH. Elevation of serum cystathione levels in patients with cobalamin and folate deficiency. *Blood* 1993;81:3404–3413.
84. Strom T, Schneck SA. Syphilitic meningomyelitis. *Neurology* 1991;41:325–326.
85. Surtees R, Hyland K, Smith I. Central nervous system methyl-group metabolism in children with neurological complications of HIV infection. *Lancet* 1990;335:619–621.
86. Tucker T, Dix RD, Katzen C, Davis RL, Schmidley JW. Cytomegalovirus and herpes simplex virus ascending myelitis in a patient with acquired immune deficiency syndrome. *Ann Neurol* 1985;18:74–79.
87. Tyor WR, Glass JD, Baumrind N, et al. Cytokine expression of macrophages in HIV-1–associated vacuolar myelopathy. *Neurology* 1993;43:1002–1009.
88. Vernant JC, Maurs L, Gessain A, et al. Endemic tropical spastic paraparesis associated with human T-lymphotropic virus type I: a clinical and seroepidemiological study of 25 cases. *Ann Neurol* 1987; 21:123–130.
89. Vinters HV, Guerra WF, Eppolito L, Keith PE III. Necrotizing vasculitis of the nervous system in a patient with AIDS-related complex. *Neuropathol Appl Neurobiol* 1988;14:417–424.
90. Vinters HV, Kwok MK, Ho HW, et al. Cytomegalovirus in the nervous system of patients with the acquired immune deficiency syndrome. *Brain* 1989;112:245–268.
91. Weiser B, Peress N, LaNeve D, Eilbott DJ, Seidman R, Burger H. Human immunodeficiency virus type 1 expression in the central nervous system correlates directly with extent of disease. *Proc Natl Acad Sci U S A* 1990;3997:4001.
92. Woods GL, Goldsmith JC. Aspergillus infection of the central nervous system in patients with acquired immunodeficiency syndrome. *Arch Neurol* 1990;47:181–184.
93. Woolsey RM, Chambers TJ, Chung HD, McGarry JD. Mycobacterial meningomyelitis associated with human immunodeficiency virus infection. *Arch Neurol* 1988;45:691–693.
94. Yarchoan R, Berg G, Brouwers P, et al. Response of human immunodeficiency virus–associated neurological disease to 3′-azido-3′-deoxythymidine. *Lancet* 1987;1:132–135.

AIDS and the Nervous System, Second Edition,
edited by J. R. Berger and R. M. Levy.
Lippincott-Raven Publishers, Philadelphia © 1997.

9

Neuromuscular Syndromes in Human Immunodeficiency Virus Disease

David M. Simpson and Michele Tagliati

*Department of Neurology, Clinical Neurophysiology Laboratories, The Mount
Sinai Medical Center, New York, New York 10029*

The nervous system may be affected at virtually every level in individuals infected with human immunodeficiency virus-1 (HIV-1) infection (107,119,160,167), and multiple pathologies may coexist in the same patient. Although neuromuscular disorders are often the presenting symptom of HIV disease, they may be masked by coexistent central nervous system disorders such as dementia, focal brain lesions, or myelopathy. Furthermore, the insidious progression of peripheral neuropathy or myopathy may be overlooked in advanced acquired immunodeficiency syndrome (AIDS), when the clinician may concentrate on other life-threatening complications. However, prompt recognition and therapy of neuromuscular disease may dramatically improve the patient's quality of life.

The prevalence of neurological complications is likely to increase as more effective therapies for HIV and its associated opportunistic infections lengthen survival. A variety of peripheral neuropathies and myopathies have been described in association with HIV infection (Table 1). Although the incidence of certain forms of neuromuscular disease are clearly increased in HIV infection, in other cases the association may be fortuitous.

Myopathy may occur at any time in the course of HIV disease and is not associated with any particular stage of immunosuppression. However, different forms of peripheral neuropathy occur with increased frequency at particular stages of HIV disease. For example, inflammatory demyelinating neuropathy (IDP) is often the first manifestation of HIV disease, when CD4+ T-lymphocyte counts (CD4+ counts) are relatively high (36). As immunosuppression progresses, the prevalence of distal symmetrical polyneuropathy (DSP) increases (7,163). In advanced stages of HIV disease (CD4+ count <50 cells/mm^3) patients may develop opportunistic cytomegalovirus (CMV) nerve infections, which can present as progressive polyradiculopathy (PP) (170) or mononeuritis multiplex (MM) (146). In addition to the neuromuscular disorders caused by HIV and its concomitant immunosuppression, the use of antiretroviral drugs and other therapeutic agents in HIV disease is frequently limited by neuromuscular side effects.

This chapter reviews the spectrum of neuromuscular disorders that occur in association with HIV infection and nucleoside analogue therapy. We describe the clinical, electrophysiologic, and pathologic features of these disorders and discuss theories of pathogenesis and results of treatment to date.

TABLE 1. *Neuromuscular syndromes in HIV disease*

Peripheral neuropathies	Progressive polyradiculopathy
Distal symmetrical polyneuropathy	CMV
HIV-related	Lymphoma
Neurotoxic drugs	Autonomic neuropathy
Vitamin B$_{12}$ deficiency	Motor neuron disease (?)
Inflammatory demyelinating polyneuropathy	Sensory neuronopathy (?)
Autoimmune	**Myopathies**
CMV	HIV-associated myopathy
Mononeuropathy multiplex	Zidovudine myopathy
Autoimmune	Wasting syndrome
Vasculitic	**Neuromuscular junction disorders**
CMV	Myasthenia gravis (?)

INFLAMMATORY DEMYELINATING POLYNEUROPATHY

Acute IDP (AIDP) and chronic IDP (CIDP) are most common in patients who are HIV seropositive and otherwise asymptomatic (36,69,125). AIDP may occur at the time of HIV seroconversion (80, 138,181). An increased incidence of HIV seropositivity in patients with IDP has been reported in several studies (14,36,178). The prevalence of IDP in HIV infection is unknown, with a wide range reported in different series. Several investigators have reported IDP in up to one third of HIV-infected patients referred for evaluation of peripheral neuropathy (36,69,101,125), whereas others have found a much lower incidence (64,190). At present, it appears that IDP is a relatively infrequent neuropathic complication of HIV infection (D. Simpson, unpublished observations).

Clinical Features

The clinical features of IDP are similar in patients with and without HIV infection (2,36,125). AIDP is characterized by rapidly progressive weakness in distal and proximal muscles of two or more limbs associated with generalized areflexia. Occasionally, bilateral facial weakness may be the presenting symptom (14). The clinical progression of AIDP is usually rapid and reaches its peak within the first 4 weeks of neurologic illness (14,36), with involvement of respiratory muscles in the most severe cases (36). Although sensory symptoms may precede the onset of weakness, sensory signs generally remain mild even in patients with severe motor impairment. CIDP is distinguished by a more slowly progressive clinical course, that may be monophasic or relapsing over several months (36,69),

Electrodiagnostic Features

Electrophysiologic signs of acquired demyelination are usually more prominent in patients with CIDP than with AIDP. Motor nerve conduction studies (NCS) in patients with AIDP or CIDP may show one or more of the following findings: (a) reduced conduction velocity in two or more nerves; (b) evidence of conduction block between proximal and distal nerve stimulation sites; (c) prolonged distal latencies in two or more nerves; (d) prolonged or absent late responses; and (e) reduced compound muscle action potential (CMAP) amplitudes as a result of axonal degeneration or distal conduction block (2). In HIV-infected patients with CIDP, nerve conduction velocities (NCVs) are typically slow, with delayed F-wave latencies in two or more nerves, and in a range consistent with the diagnosis of primary demyelination (36,125). Electrophysiologic signs of conduction block are often prominent. Sensory nerve action potential (SNAP) amplitudes may be small, and sensory conduction velocities are slow. Needle electromyography (EMG) shows reduced motor unit recruitment proportional to the degree of weakness, although denervation potentials may be minimal because weakness may be a result of conduction block without associated axonal degeneration (36,125). In patients with early AIDP, electrophysiological signs of demyelination are often less pronounced, with minor slowing of motor NCV and mildly prolonged F-wave latencies (36).

Other Laboratory Results

The analysis of cerebrospinal fluid (CSF) in IDP associated with HIV infection yields important findings. A lymphocytic pleocytosis of 10–50 cells/mm^3 is present in a majority of HIV-infected patients (36), which serves to distinguish them from HIV-negative subjects with typically acellular CSF. Thus, the finding of CSF pleocytosis in a patient with IDP not previously known to be infected with HIV mandates HIV antibody testing. CSF protein levels are elevated (50–250 mg/dl), as in seronegative patients.

Pathologic Features

Sural nerve biopsy specimens of HIV-infected patients with IDP show subperineurial edema with endoneurial and perivascular mononuclear cell infiltrates and macrophage-mediated segmental demyelination (36). In addition to signs of primary demyelination, axonal degeneration may be present to a variable degree. In two cases of demyelinative neuropathy associated with AIDS, CMV inclusions in the Schwann cells have been described, implicating a direct role of this virus (Fig. 1) (18,128),

Etiology

The etiology of IDP associated with early HIV infection is thought to be autoimmune, with mechanisms similar to those proposed in HIV-seronegative patients (36,135,164). Other autoimmune disorders such as thrombocytopenic purpura (186) may occur in association with early HIV infection. Furthermore, abnormal immune activation in IDP is supported by increased CSF levels of soluble CD8 and neopterin (76,77). Antiperipheral nerve myelin antibodies have been found in HIV-seropositive patients with AIDP, with titers that parallel the course of illness (127). In the late stages of HIV disease, primary CMV infection of peripheral nerve may cause IDP (128), as discussed above.

Treatment

In the absence of large series and controlled treatment trials, definitive statements concerning the natural history and therapy of HIV-associated IDP cannot be made.

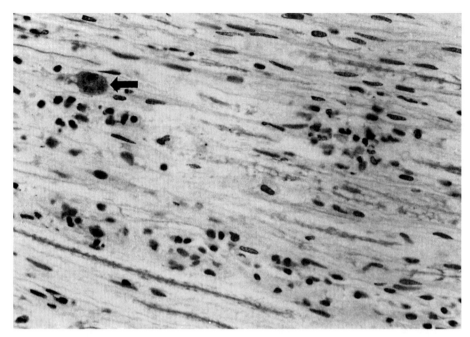

FIG. 1. Photomicrograph of right brachial nerve from HIV patient with IDP showing endoneurial cell with CMV inclusion *(arrow)* and scattered mild inflammatory infiltrates. Hematoxylin and eosin stain (HE), original magnification ×100. (From Morgello S, Simpson D. Multifocal cytomegalovirus demyelinating polyneuropathy associated with AIDS. *Muscle Nerve* 1994; 17:176–182, with permission.)

The clinical course and response to treatment in HIV-infected patients with AIDP or CIDP appear to be similar to those of seronegative patients. Prednisone (34,36,69) or plasmapheresis (34,36,125) has been reported to be effective in several patients. Cornblath et al. (36) found that HIV-positive patients with AIDP had a relatively poor prognosis despite immunomodulating treatment. However, Berger et al. (14) reported several patients with IDP with an excellent recovery in 1–6 months, even without specific therapy. Patients with CIDP may improve during treatment with prednisone or plasmapheresis and often relapse when therapy is stopped (34,36,104,125). These and other interventions such as intravenous immunoglobulin (Ig) (69,114) await evaluation in controlled trials of HIV-seropositive patients with acute or chronic IDP. A treatment algorithm for HIV-associated neuropathies is shown in Fig. 2.

--→

FIG. 2. Diagnostic treatment algorithm for patients with peripheral neuropathies associated with HIV infection. NCS, nerve conduction studies; EMG, electromyography; DSP, distal symmetrical polyneuropathy; IDP, inflammatory demyelinating polyneuropathy; MM, mononeuropathy multiplex; LP, lumbar puncture; CMV, cytomegalovirus; IVIG, intravenous immunoglobulin; bx, biopsy; PMN, polymorphonuclear cells; Mono, Mononuclear cells; RT, radiation therapy. (Adapted from Simpson D, Olney R. Peripheral neuropathies associated with human immunodeficiency virus infection. In: Dyck PJ, ed. *Peripheral Neuropathies: New Concepts and Treatments.* Philadephia: WB Saunders, 1992:685–711, with permission.)

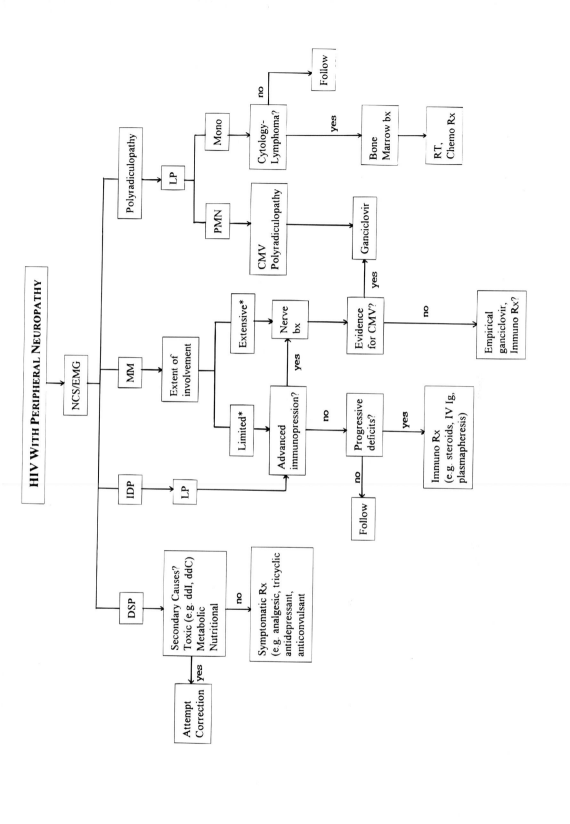

HIV WITH PERIPHERAL NEUROPATHY

NCS/EMG

DSP

Secondary Causes?
Toxic (e.g. ddI, ddC)
Metabolic
Nutritional

→ yes → Attempt Correction

→ no → Symptomatic Rx
(e.g. analgesic, tricyclic antidepressant, anticonvulsant)

IDP

LP

→ Advanced immunopression?

→ no → Progressive deficits?
→ no → Follow
→ yes → Immuno Rx (e.g. steroids, IV Ig, plasmapheresis)

→ yes → Nerve bx

MM

Extent of involvement

Limited* → Advanced immunopression?

Extensive* → Nerve bx

Nerve bx → Evidence for CMV?
→ yes → Ganciclovir
→ no → Empirical ganciclovir, Immuno Rx?

Polyradiculopathy

LP

PMN → CMV Polyradiculopathy → Ganciclovir

Mono → Cytology-Lymphoma?
→ no → Follow
→ yes → Bone Marrow bx → RT, Chemo Rx

DISTAL SYMMETRICAL POLYNEUROPATHY

DSP was initially described in patients with AIDS by Snider et al. (167), and its clinical and pathological features have been further characterized by numerous investigators (6,35,46,56,92,101,104, 107,112,172). Recent data from the Multicenter AIDS Cohort Study indicate that in the interval between 1988 and 1992 DSP had the highest yearly rate of increase in incidence among the neurological complications of HIV infection and reached a peak incidence of 2.81% in 1992 (5). DSP may be diagnosed in >30% of patients with AIDS, after other recognized causes for polyneuropathy are excluded (56,92,172). DSP is usually associated with late stages of HIV disease, as indicated by the presence of opportunistic infections and significant wasting in the majority of patients with DSP (101,104,172). Emerging data from several clinical trials indicate that the prevalence of DSP increases in the strata of patients with low CD4+ counts (7,163).

Clinical Features

The major presenting symptoms of DSP are numbness, distal paresthesias, and dysesthesias, usually beginning in the lower extremities. A complaint of "burning feet" is reported by 23–100% of patients with AIDS evaluated for DSP in different series (6,35,101,172). These patients may alter their gait to avoid pressure on their soles and often report that even the lightest contact (i.e., socks, bed sheets) increases their pain (35). The upper extremities may be affected in a distal and symmetrical fashion later in the course of DSP. Muscle weakness is not a prominent symptom of DSP and generally occurs only late in disease (35).

The most common signs of DSP in AIDS are depressed or absent reflexes at the ankles relative to the knees (5,35,101,172). The presence of hyperactive knee reflexes and depressed ankle reflexes may indicate concurrent myelopathy and neuropathy, which is a common association in HIV-infected individuals (44). Vibratory thresholds are increased, and pinprick and temperature are reduced in a stocking and glove distribution, whereas joint position sensation is relatively normal (104). Weakness is generally restricted to intrinsic foot muscles (35,172), unless DSP is very advanced, or other neurologic disorders are also present.

Electrodiagnostic Features

Several studies have demonstrated that mean sural nerve conduction velocity or amplitude is significantly reduced in HIV-seropositive patients as compared with controls (25,62,91,133,163). The electrodiagnostic features of DSP in AIDS are indicative of distal and symmetrical degeneration of sensory and motor axons in a pattern similar to other forms of DSP. Small or absent sural nerve action potentials are the most common abnormalities in patients with DSP (35,154,163,167), although occasional patients with DSP and normal sural responses have been reported (35,101,104,167). Less commonly, reduced sensory or motor amplitudes of the median or ulnar nerves are found (35,167). Sensory and motor NCV are normal or only mildly reduced in proportion to the reduction in amplitude (35,154,167). Late responses are also delayed in a pattern consistent with axonal neuropathy (6,101,163).

Needle EMG may demonstrate signs of active or chronic partial denervation with reinnervation in distal leg muscles (6,35,101,104).

Other Laboratory Results

The results of other laboratory studies are usually normal in patients with AIDS and DSP. Serum vitamin B12 levels, folate, erythrocyte sedimentation rate, antinuclear antibodies, fasting blood glucose, liver enzymes, creatinine, thyroid function tests, and serum protein electrophoresis have been normal in most of these subjects (6,34,167,172). Data from our longitudinal cohort study indicate that serum albumin, hemoglobin levels, and weight loss are significantly correlated with reduced NCS values in HIV-infected patients (162). In patients with DSP and HIV infection, CSF often shows mild, nonspecific abnormalities in white blood cell count and protein, similar to those commonly present in neurologically asymptomatic patients with HIV infection (87,88,120,121).

Pathologic Features

Pathologically, evidence of axonal neuropathy is present in nearly all patients dying with AIDS (78). The most common nerve biopsy finding in patients with DSP is degeneration of myelinated and unmyelinated axons (6,46,78,112). Mild epineural and endoneurial perivascular mononuclear inflammation may be observed in up to two thirds of specimens (46,78,109,112). De la Monte et al. (46) characterized these inflammatory cells as T-lymphocytes and activated macrophages, with suppressor/cytotoxic cells (CD8) predominating over helper/inducer cells (CD4) endoneurially and a more equal ratio seen epineurally and perineurally. These investigators were unable to detect deposition of Ig, complement, or fibrin by direct immunofluorescence. Several investigators have observed associated demyelination (6,46), but this does not appear to be either macrophage mediated or segmental (6,112).

Distal axonal degeneration may affect both central and peripheral projections of dorsal root ganglion cells. Rance et al. (141) observed gracile tract degeneration selective for upper thoracic and cervical segments in four of 27 patients with DSP. Loss of dorsal root ganglion cells and mononuclear infiltration is usually mild in comparison with the degree of axonal degeneration and inflammation noted in distal nerves (46,73,78,141).

Etiology

Although the specific etiology for most cases of DSP in AIDS is obscure, several mechanisms have been proposed.

Direct HIV infection

Several investigators have reported that HIV infection of peripheral nerve or dorsal root ganglion cells may cause DSP. Ho et al. (84) cultured HIV from sural nerve homogenates in two patients and from CSF in these two and one additional patient. Bailey et al. (6) reported electron microscopic evidence of retroviral-like inclusions in myelinated nerve fibers of the sural nerve in one of six patients with DSP. Based on this evidence and the type of mononuclear infiltration suggesting a cell-mediated immune response, de la Monte et al. (46) proposed that peripheral neuropathy in AIDS results from direct HIV infection of peripheral nerve. However, this interpretation is open to question. Neither of the patients in whom HIV was cultured from sural nerve appears to have had DSP. The first subject had disseminated CMV infection and presented with a peripheral neuropathy characterized by subacute progression to paraplegia and incontinence (patient 10 of Ho et al. [84]). This syndrome is now recognized as PP and is usually caused by CMV infection. The second patient was later described as having CIDP that was responsive to both plasmapheresis and prednisone (patient 26 of Ho et al. [84] and patient 4 of Cornblath et al. [36]). Several pathological studies have failed to identify retroviral-like particles or HIV antigens in dorsal root ganglion cells, nerve roots, or peripheral nerves (46,73,112,141), making direct HIV infection of peripheral nerve an unlikely cause of DSP. However, a role for the glycoprotein (gp)120 subunit of HIV has been proposed as a cofactor in the pathogenesis of DSP (3).

Cytokines

Because HIV may not be the principal pathogenetic agent in DSP, recent research has focused on indirect mechanisms, such as the action of cytokines. Tumor necrosis factor-alpha, interleukin-1, and other cytokines have been identified in peripheral nerves (79,189) and dorsal root ganglia (194) of HIV-infected patients. Griffin et al. (79) have suggested that cytokines may interact with nerve growth factors. Further studies are needed to clarify the role of these agents in the pathogenesis of DSP in AIDS.

CMV Infection

Several authors have described CMV inclusions or antigens in peripheral nerve specimens, nerve roots, or dorsal root ganglion cells in some patients with AIDS with DSP (46,73,112,141). Fuller et al. (61) reported a series of 12 patients with painful neuropathy, of whom nine had concurrent active systemic CMV infection. Only 11 of 30 patients without DSP had evidence of CMV infection. However, there is no compelling evidence at this time that direct CMV infection causes DSP.

Vitamin B12 Deficiency

Kieburtz et al. (95) reported low serum B12 levels or impaired absorption of vitamin B12 in 16% of 64 HIV-infected patients that were referred for neurologic evaluation. Ten of 34 patients (29%) with DSP and six of nine patients (67%) with the combination of DSP and myelopathy had B12 abnormalities. The clinical presentation of DSP was comparable in patients with and without B12 deficiency. Patients in both groups complained of pain, burning, or tingling in their feet. Objective signs included reduced sensation distally in the lower extremities and depressed or absent ankle reflexes, with only minor motor impairment. These investigators reported that 60% of B12 abnormalities were detected by low serum levels and 40% by impaired absorption. NCS and nerve biopsy results were not reported. Five of eight patients had improvement of their neuropathic symptoms within 1 week after parenteral vitamin B12 administration. However, other investigators, as well as our longitudinal cohort study (162), have not detected abnormal vitamin B12 levels in the majority of HIV-infected patients with DSP (6,144,167). Although it is prudent to screen B12 levels in all neurologically affected patients with AIDS, the prevalence of vitamin B12 abnormalities appears to be low.

Wasting

Malnutrition and weight loss are common among patients with AIDS who develop DSP (35,167,172,190), leading some investigators to compare AIDS-related DSP to the peripheral neuropathy reported in other chronic diseases (190). Although wasting syndrome may be more prominent in patients with than without DSP (162,172), weight loss and nutritional disorders are also commonly described in advanced patients with AIDS without DSP. Thus, the direct role of malnutrition and wasting in the production of DSP is unclear.

Neurotoxins

Several drugs used in the treatment of HIV-related complications may cause DSP. A majority of patients with lymphoma or Kaposi's sarcoma that are treated with chemotherapeutic regimens including vincristine develop symptoms and signs of DSP (70). Peripheral neuropathy may develop in patients treated with isoniazid (INH) for tuberculosis, particularly when pyridoxine is not supplemented (57). Thalidomide, which is under investigation in the treatment of HIV-associated aphthous ulcers, also may cause DSP (63,132). The nucleoside analogue antiretroviral agents have several dose-limiting toxicities. Although zidovudine (ZDV) is limited by hematologic toxicity, there is no evidence that ZDV causes DSP (157). The dideoxynucleotide analogues didanosine (ddI), zalcitabine (ddC), and stavudine (d4T) have well-recognized neurotoxicity (161). Unexpected peripheral neuropathy was first described in patients receiving ddC (49,122,193). The neuropathy associated with ddC is clinically and electrophysiologically similar to HIV-related DSP. The most common early symptoms are burning, paresthesias, or aching in the distal lower extremities. Reduced pinprick, temperature, light touch; vibratory sensation in the lower extremities; and absent ankle reflexes are typical in these patients. Electrophysiologic abnormalities in toxic neuropathy are similar to those in HIV-associated DSP and indicate distal axonopathy. The acute onset and rapid progression of nucleoside-related DSP, and particularly the effect of drug withdrawal, serve to distinguish HIV-associated DSP from nucleoside toxicity (13,49).

The occurrence of toxic neuropathy is dose dependent. In a series of 52 patients receiving four ddC dose regimens, all who received high-dose (0.12–0.24 mg/kg/day) and 80% who received intermediate dose (0.04 mg/kg/day) developed DSP. Only two of six patients receiving low-dose ddC (0.02 mg/kg/day) complained of neuropathic symptoms (13). Furthermore, the onset and clinical characteristics of DSP were substantially different in the three groups. When ddC was withdrawn, patients in the high-dose group experienced a period of "coasting," during which the symptoms of neuropathy intensified for several weeks before improving (13).

The toxic effects of ddC may be reduced by alternating therapy with ZDV (166), although larger studies are needed to confirm this observation.

Painful DSP also is a common, dose-limiting effect of ddI therapy (33,96,99). The varying incidence of neuropathy in different studies may result from different ddI doses and schedules (33,99). Reversible ddI-related neuropathy was reported in 10 of 44 (23%) patients followed for at least 10 months. These patients were taking higher daily doses (27.2 mg/kg) and had higher cumulative doses (2.6 g/kg) of ddI than did patients who remained asymptomatic (13.9 mg/kg/day and 1.75 g/kg). Once the symptoms of peripheral neuropathy had resolved, most patients tolerated rechallenge with ddI at half-dose (96). A maximum ddI dosage of 12.5 mg/kg/day has been recommended by several investigators to avoid the development of neuropathy (1,33,96,99,129, 193). However, in patients with a low CD4+ count, ddI-related neuropathy may develop at lower cumulative doses (142). Furthermore, patients with a previous history of clinical or subclinical neuropathy are more prone to develop ddI-associated DSP (139).

Stavudine (d4T) is a later generation nucleoside analogue that may also cause DSP (161). In a study of 36 patients taking a maximum d4T dose of 2 mg/kg/day, 20 (55%) developed dose-limiting peripheral neuropathy, similar to ddC and ddI-induced DSP (19). Dose-dependent neuropathic effects of d4T have been better defined in a recent randomized trial comparing doses of 0.5, 1.0, and 2.0 mg/kg/day in 152 patients (median CD4+ count = 246 cells/mm^3). DSP was observed in 6%, 15%, and 31% of patients, respectively, with an onset within 8–16 weeks of therapy (Bristol-Myers-Squibb, data on file). In another large (N = 10,348), blinded randomized study in patients with advanced HIV disease (median CD4+ count = 41 cells/mm^3), DSP was reported in 21% of patients receiving 40 mg twice per day (~1.0 mg/kg/day) and in 15% of those receiving 20 mg twice per day (~0.5 mg/kg/day). Patients with a history of neuropathy, low CD4+ count, Karnofsky score <80, or hemoglobin level <110 g/dl were at increased risk of developing DSP during d4T treatment.

The pathogenetic mechanism of toxic neuropathy related to dideoxynucleotide derivatives is unknown. Chen et al. (26) reported delayed cytotoxicity of ddC on human T-lymphoblasts *in vitro*, associated with decreased cellular content of mitochondrial DNA. This mitochondrial toxicity has been attributed to the reversible inhibition of DNA gamma-polymerase by the drug (26). However, studies of ddC effects on DNA gamma-polymerase in animals documented relatively low levels of enzyme inhibition (94). Species-specific toxicity may account for different outcomes in animal models of ddC-related neuropathy (110).

Treatment

When a patient with DSP is receiving a known neurotoxin, it should be reduced in dosage or discontinued if possible. Although there have been anecdotal reports of DSP improvement with ZDV treatment (193), most investigators have not found that antiretroviral therapy improves symptoms of DSP (35). Plasmapheresis has not been effective in several patients (109,124), although tricyclic antidepressants, carbamazepine, or topical capsaicin have been reported to improve symptoms in uncontrolled series of patients with DSP (164). In a blinded, placebo-controlled study of 81 patients with DSP, peptide T was ineffective in relieving pain and did not produce clinical or electrophysiologic improvement of DSP (158). Controlled studies of amitriptyline, mexiletine, acupuncture, and nerve growth factor are underway in development for the treatment of AIDS-associated DSP (35).

MONONEUROPATHY MULTIPLEX

In 1985, Lipkin et al. (109) first described the occurrence of inflammatory neuropathy in 12 homosexual patients with lymphadenopathy syndrome, of whom nine presented with multiple, asymmetrical nerve involvement. Electrophysiologic and pathologic features of mononeuropathy multiplex (MM) may overlap with IDP and DSP (109,125). However, the clinical features, electrophysiologic findings, pathogenesis, and treatment of this neuropathy warrant its separate classification.

Clinical Features

MM is most easily distinguished from IDP and DSP by its clinical characteristics. Patients with MM have asymmetric or proximal involvement of peripheral nerves and preservation of tendon reflexes in asymptomatic distributions. The typical neurologic presentation includes multifocal sensory and motor abnormalities in the distribution of cutaneous nerves, mixed nerves, and nerve roots (109). Cranial neuropathies are also a frequent feature of MM (101,109,125).

MM may be divided into separate syndromes based on its natural history in HIV-infected patients. Early in the course of HIV infection, usually in association with CD4+ counts of >200/mm^3, patients usually present with a limited distribution of MM, characterized by the acute onset of sensory or motor deficits limited to one or two peripheral or cranial nerves. Deficits commonly resolve within several months spontaneously or with immunomodulating therapy (109,169). In advanced HIV disease, especially when CD4+ counts fall below 50/mm^3, patients develop a more extensive form of MM, involving numerous nerves in two or more limbs or multiple cranial nerves (101,125,169). This neuropathy may rapidly progress and can simulate IDP or PP.

Electrodiagnostic Features

Electrophysiologic studies in patients with MM generally show asymmetric reduction in amplitudes of CMAP and SNAP, with mild reduction in NCV. EMG shows evidence for denervation and neuropathic motor unit recruitment patterns, consistent with axonal degeneration. Electrodiagnostic features of MM may overlap with those of DSP or IDP. Although signs of focal or asymmetrical multifocal axonal lesions are most typical in MM (101), electrodiagnostic abnormalities may be diffuse and symmetrical, similar to DSP (68,109), or may indicate primary demyelination, with slowing of NCV and conduction block (109,140,145).

Other Laboratory Results

CSF results are usually abnormal in most patients with HIV-associated MM (109). However, elevated protein and mild mononuclear pleocytosis are nonspecific findings in HIV-infected patients because they are frequently present in asymptomatic HIV infection (87,88,120,121). Polymerase chain reaction (PCR) for CMV DNA in the CSF may provide more specific diagnostic data in patients with advanced immuno-suppression and MM (145).

Pathologic Features

Several distinctive patterns of nerve biopsy abnormalities have been described in HIV-associated MM. Early in the course of HIV infection, axonal degeneration is generally present, usually accompanied by epineural and endoneural perivascular inflammatory infiltrates. In patients with advanced AIDS and MM, nerve biopsies show more numerous polymorphonuclear infiltrates, with mixed axonal and demyelinative lesions (145). Additionally, cytomegalic inclusion bodies have been identified within some of these nerve lesions (145). Electron microscopy (EM) has shown CMV virions in cells of the monocyte/macrophage lineage, endoneurial fibroblasts, and endothelial cells (146). A less common pathological alteration described in HIV-related MM is necrotizing arteritis (Fig. 3). Said et al. (148) has reported pathological evidence of vasculitis in 10% of HIV-infected patients with peripheral neuropathy.

Etiology

Several pathogenetic mechanisms may underlie HIV-associated MM, in part related to the patient's stage of immunosuppression (146,169). An autoimmune mecha-

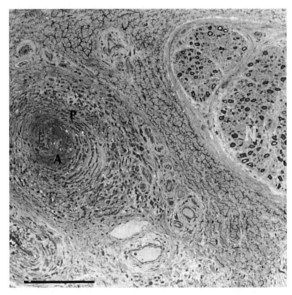

FIG. 3. Sural nerve biopsy from a patient with mononeuropathy multiplex. An occluded small artery *(A)* displays fibrinoid necrosis and transmural and periarterial acute and chronic inflammatory infiltrate *(P)* nerve fascicles *(N)*. Toluidine blue–stained semithin plastic section from gluteraldehyde–fixed postosmicated nerve biopsy. Bar = 200 µm. (From Simpson D, Wolfe D. Neuromuscular complications of HIV infection and its treatment. *AIDS* 1991;5:917–926, with permission.)

nism has been proposed for the type of MM seen early in HIV infection because of its similarities to IDP, response to immunosuppressive therapy, and relatively good prognosis (109,169). The progressive form of MM that develops late in HIV infection may result from identifiable infectious or neoplastic causes. In patients with multiple cranial neuropathies, specific etiologies, including lymphoma (15), cryoglobulinemia (176), cryptococcal meningitis, toxoplasmosis, and herpes zoster have been found in some cases (53). Most importantly, CMV should be considered as a potential pathogen in late-onset MM (145). Patients with systemic CMV infection, such as retinitis or gastroenteritis, are at particular risk for neurologic involvement (145). Nerve biopsy may provide confirmatory evidence of CMV neuropathy in some cases (145).

Although HIV has only rarely been identified as a primary pathogen in peripheral nerve (36,135,164), Gherardi et al. (68) reported *in situ* hybridization evidence for HIV replication in nerve biopsies of two patients with vasculitic neuropathy. The infected cells were located in the epineurium in one patient and in the epineurium, perineurium, and endoneurium in the other. EM showed HIV-like particles in the perivascular cells in one biopsy specimen.

Treatment

The peripheral nerve lesions of early or limited MM usually remit spontaneously within several months (109,169). In some patients with delayed or incomplete recovery, immunomodulating therapy, such as corticosteroids, plasmapheresis, or high-dose intravenous Ig, may be warranted (125). Despite the poor response to immunosuppressive therapy that Lipkin et al. (109) observed in a small number of patients with MM, other investigators have reported good results in uncontrolled series (53). Said et al. (147) reported that three of six patients with multifocal neuropathy and pathologic evidence of CMV on nerve biopsy improved with ganciclovir therapy. In the series of Roullet et al. (145), 14 of 15 patients with MM who were treated with ganciclovir or foscarnet improved within 1–4 weeks. However, neuropathy relapsed in three patients during maintenance therapy. These results suggest that even in the absence of specific evidence of CMV infection, empirical therapy for CMV should be considered in severely immunosuppressed patients with MM.

PROGRESSIVE POLYRADICULOPATHY

Since PP was first reported by Eidelberg et al. in 1986 (51), it has been increasingly recognized as an alarming complication of AIDS (10,45,126). Its rapidly progressive course and potentially good response to early therapy (60,75,126) demand prompt diagnosis and treatment. PP generally occurs late in the course of HIV disease, when CD4 + counts are extremely low and other AIDS-defining opportunistic infections have occurred (45,126). PP is rarely the initial manifestation of AIDS (45,113). It is significant that a large number of patients with polyradiculopathy have coexistent systemic CMV infections, including retinitis, pneumonia, and gastroenteritis (45,51,97,126).

Clinical Features

The clinical presentation of PP is characterized by radiating pain and paresthesias in the cauda equina distribution, followed by rapidly progressive flaccid paraparesis, lower extremity areflexia, mild sensory loss, and sphincter dysfunction. A thoracic sensory level has occasionally been demonstrated, leading some investigators to term this disorder polyradiculomyelitis (45). However, other signs of myelopathy are usually absent. Urinary retention occurs in over two thirds of patients (97). Extraocular movement deficits indicating multiple cranial nerve involvement have been reported in one patient with PP (10). In some cases clinical features of PP and MM may overlap (147). The upper extremities may be involved late in the course of polyradiculopathy (147). In most cases PP has a poor prognosis if untreated, with a mortality rate of nearly 100% and a mean duration of illness from onset of neurologic symptoms to death ranging from 2 to 30 days (10,51,113,147,180). So et al. (173) have reported that a minority of patients may have a more benign form of polyradiculopathy, with a slower evolution and better prognosis.

Electrodiagnostic Features

The most prominent electrophysiologic abnormalities in PP are widespread denervation in lower extremity and lumbar paraspinal muscles, accompanied by abnormal late responses in affected distributions (126,169). NCV results are only mildly affected (10,51,126,147). CMAP amplitudes decline as the disease progresses. These electrodiagnostic findings, indicating severe and widespread proximal axonal pathology in lumbar nerve root segments, are particularly helpful in differentiating PP from IDP or MM, which may have overlapping clinical findings (36). Sural nerve sensory responses may be abnormal in patients with concurrent evidence of DSP (171).

Laboratory Features

The CSF findings in most patients with progressive CMV polyradiculopathy are characterized by marked polymorphonuclear pleocytosis, elevated protein, and hypoglycorrhachia. The CSF white cell count has ranged from 17 to >2,000 cells/mm^3 in different series, with a predominant percentage of polymorphonuclear leukocytes. Protein values can be as high as 920 mg/dl (45), whereas glucose is often <40 mg/dl (97). When CSF analysis shows a mononuclear pleocytosis with a total white cell count of <200/mm^3, other causes of PP should be considered, such as lymphomatous meningitis (105) or a more benign, nonprogressive polyradiculopathy (173). Cytologic examination of CSF by means of immunohistochemistry and in situ hybridization may show CMV-positive cytomegalic cells (45). CSF cultures are positive for CMV in about half of HIV-infected patients with PP (45,97,126), although cultures may remain negative even in autopsy-proven cases of CMV polyradiculopathy (D. Simpson, unpublished observations). Blood and urine cultures also may grow CMV in a smaller percentage of cases (51,90,93,126). PCR for CMV DNA in CSF may prove diagnostically valuable (29), although this assay has not yet been validated in large series.

Radiologic studies may be performed to exclude focal compressive lesions of the spinal cord or cauda equina. Myelography has shown adhesive arachnoiditis in some patients with PP (45,75,93) and magnetic resonance imaging (MRI) studies demonstrated enhancement of the lumbar thecal sac (9) or leptomeninges from the conus medullaris to the cauda equina (97).

Pathologic Features

The predominant pathologic findings in patients with HIV-associated PP are marked inflammation and extensive necrosis of ventral and dorsal nerve roots (45,51,126). Vascular congestion, edema, and infiltrates of polymorphonuclear and mononuclear cells have been observed in areas of severe necrosis (10,51,126). A mild, focal myelitis may be observed in proximity to the inflamed nerve roots (126). Although the inflammatory lesions are most severe in the lumbar region (126), proximal cranial nerves may be similarly affected (10).

In almost all reported autopsied patients with PP, signs of CMV infection have been demonstrated. Nuclear and cytoplasmic cytomegalic inclusions have been observed within endothelial, Schwann, and ependymal cells, particularly in regions of intense inflammation (Fig. 4) (45,51,126). These cellular inclusions stain positively for CMV with immunocytochemical and *in situ* hybridization techniques (51). Evidence of CMV encephalitis has been reported in some patients with PP (126).

Etiology

Considerable evidence indicates that PP in AIDS is usually a direct result of CMV infection. Although the presence of virus in a tissue does not necessarily imply a pathogenetic role, CMV has been isolated from CSF or pathologically identified in the affected nerve roots in most reported patients (45,51,97,126). The extensive presence of CMV in areas of massive inflammation and necrosis and the positive therapeutic response to ganciclovir therapy further suggest a causal link of CMV

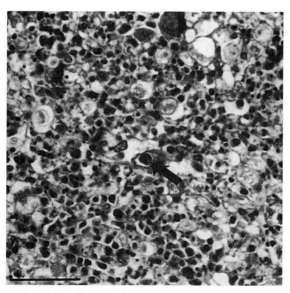

FIG. 4. Acute necrotizing inflammatory infiltrate in lumbar dorsal root of patient with CMV polyradiculopathy. CMV intranuclear inclusions *(arrow)* are evident; axons in cross-section. HE-stained paraffin section, autopsy specimen. Bar = 20 μm. (From Simpson D, Wolfe D. Neuromuscular complications of HIV infection and its treatment. *AIDS* 1991;5:917–926, with permission.)

with PP. Less commonly, AIDS-associated PP has been attributed to other conditions. Neurosyphilis has been diagnosed in one patient with polyradiculopathy who had positive serum and CSF Venereal Disease Research Laboratory (VDRL) tests and rapidly improved with intravenous penicillin therapy (102). Lymphomatous meningitis was diagnosed by abnormal CSF cytology and bone marrow biopsy in several patients with AIDS who also had polyradiculopathy (105,173).

Treatment

Ganciclovir, a nucleoside analogue initially used in the treatment of CMV retinitis and gastroenteritis (103) and capable of penetration of the blood–brain barrier, has been shown to be effective in several series of patients with AIDS-associated PP (45,56,60,75,97,126). Stabilization or improvement of neurologic symptoms has been reported in ~50% of patients with PP treated with ganciclovir (97). Although clinical improvement may be seen within the first 2–4 weeks of treatment (30,60,126), patients may require several months of therapy before recovery (56,75,97). Therefore, ganciclovir therapy must be initiated early, before irreversible nerve root necrosis occurs, and continued indefinitely thereafter even in the absence of immediate benefits (97). Most investigators have suggested that empirical therapy for CMV should be initiated in patients with AIDS with PP even in the absence of positive CSF cultures (45,126). This is particularly true when CSF shows the marked polymorphonuclear pleocytosis distinctive of CMV polyradiculopathy (173). In patients who continue to deteriorate after early therapy, ganciclovir resistance may be responsible (50). Factors predictive of ganciclovir resistance include persistent CSF polymorphonuclear pleocytosis and hypoglycorrhachia, as well as positive CMV cultures of CSF or blood after induction therapy (30). In these cases, an alternate antiviral agent such as foscarnet may be warranted (30,45,60,90,116). Several investigators recommend the initiation of combination therapy with ganciclovir and foscarnet in patients with AIDS and CMV neurologic disease (D. Clifford, personal communication).

AUTONOMIC NEUROPATHY

A number of early reports drew attention to the abnormalities of autonomic function that may occur in HIV-infected patients (55,108). Although the prevalence of autonomic dysfunction in HIV disease is not known, orthostatic hypotension was reported in three of 25 (12%) patients in one series (55). Signs of subclinical autonomic nervous system involvement were described in 30–60% of otherwise neurologically asymptomatic patients (130,183). The highest risk for autonomic abnormalities seems to occur late in HIV disease, particularly when other neurologic deficits are present (31,59).

Clinical Features

Both parasympathetic and sympathetic autonomic dysfunction may occur in HIV-infected patients (31). Parasympathetic abnormalities include resting tachycardia (59,150), impotence, and urinary dysfunction. Failure of sympathetic mechanisms may account for orthostatic hypotension, syncope, diarrhea, and anhidrosis. Cardiac conduction abnormalities are particularly worrisome because they may lead to cardio-respiratory arrest (37).

Laboratory Features

Several tests are helpful in the diagnostic evaluation of autonomic neuropathy. Plasma catecholamine levels may be inappropriately low, suggesting a peripheral postganglionic lesion (55,108). A battery of tests may be used in standardized autonomic nervous system evaluation, including orthostatic blood pressure measures, heart rate responses to provocative tests (Valsalva maneuver, deep breathing, standing up, tilt table), cold pressor test, and quantitative sudomotor axon reflex test responses. Tests of heart rate variability have been used to detect early autonomic dysfunction (31,59,111,130,183). Villa et al. (183) found abnormal RR interval variation on electrocardiographic studies in eight of 37 HIV-positive subjects (22%) without clinical evidence of autonomic dysfunction (183). Mulhall et al. (130) observed cardiac conduction abnormalities in six of 20 patients (20%).

Etiology

A variety of factors may contribute to the symptoms of autonomic dysfunction in HIV-infected patients. Several drugs used in the treatment of HIV-associated complications may cause orthostatic hypotension, including tricyclic antidepressants with anticholinergic activity, vincristine (20), and pentamidine (81). There is no evidence that HIV has a direct role in the pathogenesis of autonomic dysfunction. In later stages of disease, malnutrition and dehydration may be contributory factors (59).

Both central and peripheral nervous system abnormalities may cause autonomic impairment (31). Some patients with autonomic dysfunction have coexistent signs of dementia, myelopathy, and peripheral neuropathy (183). Pathologic studies have suggested several possible sites of the autonomic lesion in AIDS. Chimelli et al. (27) found abnormalities of the cervical sympathetic ganglia in six patients with AIDS. T-lymphocyte inflammatory infiltrates, ganglion nerve cell loss, and increased numbers of macrophages were identified in the sympathetic ganglia at autopsy. Batman et al. (8) demonstrated that autonomic nerves in the jejunal mucosa may be abnormal in AIDS, with severe axonal loss in the mucosal villae. Purba et al. (140) described a decreased number of oxytocin neurons in the paraventricular nucleus, suggesting a possible hypothalamic origin for the dysautonomic symptoms in AIDS.

Treatment

The recognition of symptoms of autonomic dysfunction in the course of HIV infection has important implications in the care of these patients. Life-threatening cardiac arrhythmias may be prevented, and syncope or sphincter abnormalities may be effectively treated. Simple measures include discontinuation of offending drugs and management of fluid and electrolyte imbalance in hypovolemic patients. In subjects with advanced autonomic symptoms, fludrocortisone and antiarrhythmic agents may be necessary.

MYOPATHY

After our description of a patient with AIDS and polymyositis in 1983 (167), numerous cases of HIV-associated myopathy were reported by several groups (41,71,115,151,175). The incidence of myopathy in HIV infection has not been established in prospective studies. This problem is compounded by the fact that different investigators have used variable criteria for the diagnosis of myopathy. We performed a retrospective analysis of a large primary antiretroviral protocol (AIDS Clinical Trials Group 016), comparing the efficacy of ZDV (n = 360) to placebo (n = 351). The incidence of a composite diagnosis of myopathy established from the primary data available in the study was 3% in the ZDV-treated group and 0.4% in the placebo group (159). Over 20% of the HIV-infected patients diagnosed at Mount Sinai Medical Center with a neuromuscular disorder have myopathy as a primary or secondary diagnosis (177). HIV-associated myopathy may develop in patients at all stages of HIV infection (101,151).

Clinical Features

The predominant presenting symptom of myopathy is slowly progressive muscle weakness, typically characterized by difficulty in rising from a chair or climbing stairs (151). Myalgia is present in 25–50% of affected patients (101,151,153). However, myalgia is a nonspecific symptom in HIV-infected individuals (124) and is insufficient for the diagnosis of myopathy, even in the presence of elevated creatine kinase (CK) levels. Neurological examination shows symmetrical weakness of proximal muscle groups, with prominent involvement of neck and hip flexors. The presence of limb weakness, with CK elevation and supportive electrophysiologic and pathologic data, is necessary for a definitive diagnosis of myopathy, particularly when other concurrent neurological disorders complicate the clinical picture. If only some elements of the diagnostic battery are positive, the diagnosis of myopathy may be considered probable (3/4 criteria) or possible (2/4 criteria) in accordance with classical diagnostic standards for polymyositis (17,118).

Myopathy can cause a wasting syndrome in HIV-infected patients, characterized by involuntary weight loss and chronic muscle weakness (152). When systemic or nutritional factors are excluded as the cause of wasting, myopathy may occasionally be diagnosed with rigorous criteria. The importance of determining a specific diagnosis of myopathy in patients with wasting syndrome is evidenced by some patients' improvement after prednisone therapy (152).

HIV-infected individuals may present with acute rhabdomyolysis characterized by a myopathic syndrome (myalgia, muscle weakness) associated with serum CK levels of >1,500 IU/L (24). The cause of acute rhabdomyolysis in HIV disease is unknown, although investigators have suggested several etiologies, including HIV itself, drug toxicity (e.g., ddI, sulfadiazine, pentamidine), and opportunistic infections (24).

Electrodiagnostic Features

EMG is a sensitive diagnostic test in HIV myopathy (153). In our series of 50 patients with HIV myopathy, 94% had myopathic EMG results characterized by small, brief, and polyphasic motor unit potentials that recruit with full interference patterns (153). Abnormal irritative activity (i.e., fibrillation potentials) was also present in 79% of these cases. In ~50% of our patients with HIV myopathy, NCS abnormalities indicated concurrent DSP (151).

Laboratory Studies

The most sensitive serological test for HIV myopathy, as in other primary muscle disorders, is serum CK level. CK was elevated in 92% of patients with HIV myopathy in our retrospective series (153). CK elevation is one of the four classical criteria (clinical, laboratory, EMG, and biopsy) required to establish the diagnosis of HIV-negative polymyositis (118). In HIV myopathy CK levels are usually elevated to a moderate degree, with a median level of ~500 IU/L (153). The CK elevation parallels the degree of myonecrosis observed in coincident muscle biopsies but does not correlate with weakness (164). CK elevation is not a specific marker of HIV myopathy. In the AIDS Clinical Trials Group Protocol 016 analysis, the majority of patients with elevated CK did not have limb weakness or other evidence of myopathy (159).

Pathology

Wrzolek et al. (191) described primary myopathic changes in 24% of 92 autopsies of patients with AIDS. A wide spectrum of histopathological findings has been described in HIV-associated myopathy, including inflammatory infiltrates (Fig. 5A) (41,101,151,191), noninflammatory degeneration (Fig. 5B) (151,175,191), nemaline rod bodies (40,71,151), cytoplasmic bodies (Fig. 5C), and mitochondrial abnormalities (Fig. 5D). The clinical significance of these variable pathological findings is unknown. In our experience, the most common finding on muscle biopsy in HIV-associated myopathy is scattered myofiber degeneration, with occasional associated inflammatory infiltrates. The extent of inflammation is generally less than that observed in HIV-negative polymyositis (164).

Etiology

The pathogenesis of HIV-associated myopathy is unknown. A number of mechanisms have been suggested to contribute to this myopathy.

Direct HIV Infection

HIV may infect infiltrating cells of the monocyte/macrophage lineage (21); however, myofibers remain uninfected (40,89,151). Although more sophisticated assays to detect HIV in tissue, perhaps at a subgenomic level, may yield other information, there is no compelling evidence at this time that HIV infection has a direct role in myopathy.

Immune Mechanisms

Immune mechanisms have been proposed in HIV myopathy (89,153), as in other forms of polymyositis (17,47). HIV antigens have been localized in macrophages

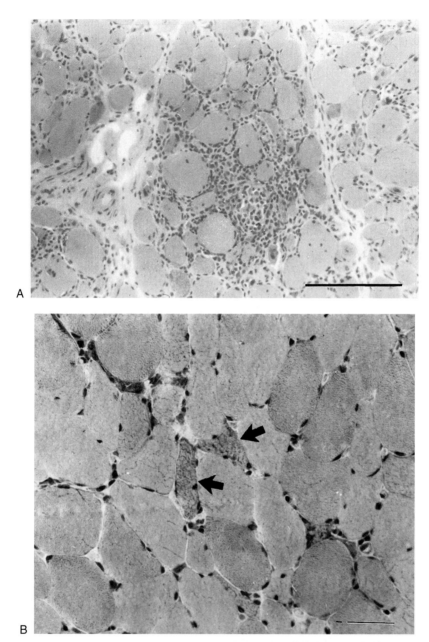

FIG. 5. HIV-associated myopathy. **A:** Focal lymphohistiocytic infiltrate in mild HIV-associated myopathy. Degenerating myofibers, non-necrotic myofibers undergoing circumferential attack, and myophagic figures are present. Modified trichrome-stained cryostat section, quadriceps, original magnification ×33. Bar = 80 μm. **B:** Three moderately atrophic, non-necrotic, degenerating myofibers *(arrows)* not associated with inflammatory infiltrates. Modified trichrome-stained cryostat section, quadriceps, original magnification ×33. Bar = 80 μm.

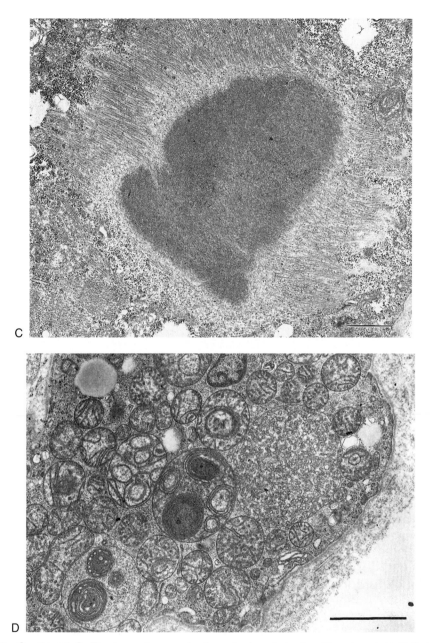

FIG. 5. *Continued.* **C:** Electron micrograph of a cytoplasmic body with a dense central mesh-work and radiating corona of fine filaments. Quadriceps biopsy, original magnification ×3,300. Bar = 2 μm. **D:** Mitochondrial abnormalities seen in non-necrotic degenerating myofibers in HIV-associated myopathy, regardless of ZDV status, include double membrane-bounded profiles containing tubular, circinate, and otherwise convoluted cristae and amorphous dense inclusions. Quadriceps biopsy. Original magnification ×16,000. Bar = 1 μm.

invading muscle (21,89), suggesting a role for virus-infected inflammatory cells in muscle degeneration. It is possible that toxic factors secreted by macrophages mediate myofiber damage. Tumor necrosis factor (cachectin), a cytokine produced largely by monocytes, causes anorexia and cachexia when injected into laboratory animals (12). Wasted patients with congestive heart failure have increased serum cachectin levels (106). Lahdervirta et al. (98) reported that cachectin levels were elevated in patients with AIDS, whereas cachectin levels were normal in HIV-seropositive individuals. The cytokine hypothesis of HIV myopathy has been supported recently by evidence showing interleukin-1 alpha accumulation in muscle fibers of HIV-infected patients, most of whom were treated with ZDV (67).

Other Opportunistic Infections

Several opportunistic agents have been detected in muscles of patients with AIDS, including *Toxoplasma gondii* (66), CMV (85), *Microsporidia* (28), *Cryptococcus neoformans* (191), *Mycobacterium avium-intracellulare* (191), and *Staphylococcus aureus* (11). However, these infections do not play a role in the majority of patients with HIV myopathy.

Zidovudine (ZDV)

In 1987, ZDV began receiving widespread use in HIV infection after the results of several large clinical trials demonstrated clinical efficacy (185,193). In 1988, Bessen et al. (16) first reported polymyositis in four ZDV-treated patients, three of whom improved after ZDV withdrawal (one with concomitant corticosteroid therapy). The investigators attributed this myopathy to ZDV because they had not observed this syndrome in AIDS before the use of ZDV. There are no solid epidemiologic data indicating the incidence of myopathy associated with ZDV therapy. None of the large antiretroviral therapy studies (185,193) were designed to prospectively establish the diagnosis of myopathy, limiting the utility of retrospective data. In a prospective series of 118 patients (136), the incidence of myopathy in the ZDV-treated group was 8% (seven of 88), although the small size of the control group and brief time of follow-up limited the significance of this data.

ZDV has been shown to be an inhibitor of gamma-polymerase of the mitochondrial matrix *in vitro* (165). After Dalakas et al. (42) described a mitochondrial myopathy in patients treated with ZDV, investigators from this group provided evidence of both *in vitro* mitochondrial abnormalities of human and animal muscle cells exposed to ZDV (100) and *in vivo* impairment of muscle energy metabolism in ZDV-treated patients (174). Dalakas et al. also reported depletion of carnitine (43) and muscle mitochondrial DNA in muscle fibers of ZDV-treated patients with molecular and immunocytochemical techniques (4,137). Other groups have described defects of mitochondrial enzymes, such as cytochrome C oxidase and reductase in ZDV-treated patients (23,123), accumulation of cytokines in muscle fiber mitochondria (67), and mitochondrial oxidative dysfunction based on data obtained via ^{31}P MR spectroscopy (187).

However, some of these results could not be replicated in studies using similar techniques. This has contributed to some controversy concerning the role of ZDV in HIV myopathy (83). For example, in an MR spectroscopy study of patients with

AIDS with fatigue and myalgia, Miller et al. (124) were not able to support the hypothesis that ZDV causes a mitochondrial myopathy or to provide "evidence of the metabolic pattern that is commonly associated with mitochondrial myopathy," irrespective of ZDV exposure history or the presence of mitochondrial abnormalities in muscle biopsy. Similarly, Herzberg et al. (82) could not reproduce the results demonstrating abnormalities in cytochrome C oxidase (123) and mitochondrial DNA (4) from ZDV exposure. Finally, Reyes et al. (143) did not observe ragged-red fibers (RRFs) in hamsters treated with intraperitoneal ZDV, none of which developed weakness.

Whether there are distinguishing pathological features between HIV- and ZDV-associated myopathies has been the subject of debate (83,115,153). In 1990, Panegyres et al. (134) first reported ultrastructural abnormalities in muscles of several ZDV-treated subjects with myopathy. The ZDV myopathy described by Dalakas et al. (42) was distinguished by " . . . numerous RRF, indicative of mitochondria with paracrystalline inclusions." Similar findings were reported by Mhiri et al. (123) in a muscle biopsy series. However, mitochondrial abnormalities described in ZDV-exposed biopsies (40) may also be found in ZDV-naive HIV-infected patients with myopathy (115,153). Grau et al. (74) suggested that the pathologic characteristics of degenerate myofibers in ZDV myopathy are sufficiently different from classical RRFs that their name be changed to ZDV fibers. Manji et al. (115) were not able to distinguish the biopsy findings in ZDV-treated and ZDV-naive HIV-infected patients with myopathy.

The clinical significance of RRFs or other laboratory evidence of mitochondrial dysfunction in ZDV-treated patients is unclear. The majority of ZDV-treated patients with RRFs in Grau's series (74) were asymptomatic. Furthermore, the percentage of RRFs did not differ in symptomatic and asymptomatic patients. In Dalakas' series (42), the percentage of RRFs was nearly the same in subjects that improved with ZDV withdrawal (mean = 17.3%) and in those that did not (mean = 15.1%). Manji et al. (115) reported that in the majority of their patients, myopathic symptoms and signs did not improve after ZDV withdrawal. Our experience has been similar (155). This is not surprising because even those investigators who reported a specific ZDV myopathy also noted the coexistence of inflammatory changes identical to HIV polymyositis (42,137). Furthermore, investigators from this group noted that in patients with ZDV myopathy, ZDV may be continued for at least 6 months without clinical or myopathological deterioration (38).

In our experience and that of others, no clinical features have been established to differentiate HIV from ZDV myopathy (54,115,153). Although some patients with HIV myopathy may improve with ZDV withdrawal (16,42,72,134), others do not (54,115,153,179). Furthermore, ZDV rechallenge in some patients has not reproduced their myopathic symptoms (58,65,134). However, all patients on ZDV presenting with a myopathy should have the ZDV withdrawn as initial therapy.

Therapy

Although corticosteroids should be used cautiously in HIV-infected patients because of the risk of further immunosuppression, there is evidence that they provide benefit, with tolerable adverse efforts in other HIV-associated diseases such as *Pneumocystis* pneumonia (32). Numerous investigators have found corticosteroids to be effective in uncontrolled series of patients with HIV-associated myopathy (22,42,115,123). Preliminary data from our randomized, placebo-controlled study of prednisone in HIV-associated myopathy supports these observations (155). Because it may be difficult to prospectively identify patients with ZDV myotoxicity, the initial management of patients with significant limb weakness and objective evidence of myopathy includes ZDV withdrawal. The percentage of ZDV-treated patients that show objective improvement in muscle strength after ZDV withdrawal has varied from 18% to 100% in different series (16,22,42,74,115). In our retrospective series, four of 15 patients with myopathy (26%) improved in strength after ZDV was discontinued (153). We are currently conducting placebo-controlled studies of ZDV withdrawal, prednisone, and anabolic steroid therapy in patients with HIV-associated myopathy. A management algorithm for HIV-associated myopathies is shown in Fig. 6.

OTHER NEUROMUSCULAR DISEASES

Motor Neuron Disease

There are several reports of motor neuron disease (MND) in the course of HIV infection (86,157,182), although this association may be fortuitous. Hoffman et al. (86) reported a 29-year-old homosexual man with progressive weakness and fasciculations in the limbs and bulbar muscles. EMG and muscle biopsy showed signs of widespread denervation and neurogenic atrophy. This patient later tested positive for HIV, but autopsy was not performed, and the association between MND and HIV infection remained speculative.

In 1990, Verma et al. (182) described a 32-year-old HIV-positive man with progressive weakness, widespread fasciculations, and normal tendon reflexes and sensory examination. EMG showed widespread denervation, suggesting the diagnosis of MND or polyradicular syndrome. The neurologic symptoms improved over several months, and the patient later died with progressive AIDS. At autopsy, no significant abnormalities of the anterior horn cells were noted. Other myelopathic changes, including scarring of the ventral nerve roots, moderate loss of myelinated nerve fibers in the peripheral nerves, and mixed features of neurogenic and myopathic atrophy, led to the all-encompassing diagnosis of myeloradiculoneuropathy and myopathy. This case illustrates how multiple neuroanatomic lesions may superimpose in an individual patient. Furthermore, it is not always possible to correlate pathologic abnormalities at autopsy with the antemortem neurologic diagnosis.

We have treated a patient with MND and HIV infection in whom a combination of interesting immunologic abnormalities coexisted (156). A 40-year-old otherwise asymptomatic HIV-positive man developed progressive weakness, hyperreflexia, and extensor plantar responses but had normal sensory and sphincter functions. Results of nerve conduction studies were normal, and EMG showed evidence of widespread active denervation and neurogenic motor unit recruitment patterns. Muscle biopsy showed widespread acute and chronic denervation with mild myopathic changes. Serum immunoelectrophoresis showed mildly elevated total IgM (535 mg/dl) and a monoclonal IgM kappa spike. IgM antibody assays were positive for anti-asialo GM1 (1:3,200), and immunohistochemical studies showed endoneurial staining of IgM and other Ig subtypes.

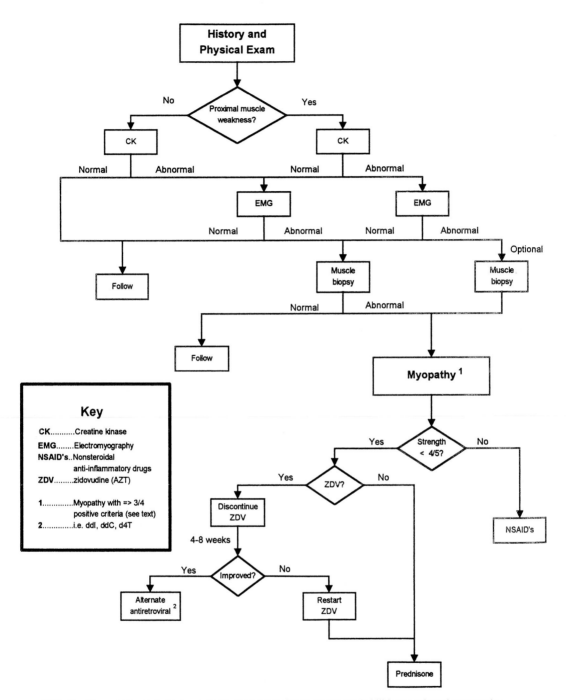

FIG. 6. Diagnosis and management algorithm for patients with HIV-associated myopathy.

Treatment with ZDV and prednisone resulted in no clinical improvement, whereas high-dose intravenous Ig resulted in transient stabilization of his weakness, followed by continued progression. Autopsy showed marked bulbar and spinal motor neuronal loss, associated with pallor in the lateral and anterior funiculi, as well as perivascular aggregates of macrophages and lymphocytes. This case is interesting in light of speculation that some forms of MND may be immunologically mediated (48,149).

Myasthenia Gravis

Myasthenia gravis (MG) has been reported in five HIV-infected patients, although the association may be coincidental (131,188). Wessel and Zitelli (188) described a 15-year-old HIV-positive, hemophiliac boy with progressive proximal weakness subsequently involving facial, bulbar, and extraocular muscles. Symptoms worsened after muscle activity and improved with rest. The tensilon test results were positive, and repetitive stimulation studies showed a decremental response. Antibodies to acetylcholine receptor were absent. The neurologic symptoms improved with anti-cholinesterase drugs.

Nath et al. (131) described a 36-year-old patient with bilateral ptosis and generalized proximal muscle weakness that worsened with exercise. Electrophysiologic and immunologic tests for MG were positive, and the patient responded to high doses of pyridostigmine. Subsequently, the neuromuscular transmission disorder gradually improved in association with progressive decline of the CD4+ count that paralleled the decrease in antiacetylcholine receptor (AchR) antibodies. A similar clinical course was reported by Vittecoq et al. (184) in a myasthenic patient whose recovery was temporally related to HIV infection. Three other cases of patients developing a myasthenic syndrome during HIV disease have been described (117,182a,192). One patient was dually infected with HIV-1 abnd HTLV-I (182a).

In these cases, the investigators speculated that the causal association between HIV infection and MG was based on the ability of the virus to modulate T cell function or to trigger an autoimmune response. Cupler et al. (39) reported three cases of HIV-infected patients with elevated anti-AchR antibodies without clinical or electrophysiological evidence of MG. These investigators concluded that the anti-AchR antibodies may represent a nonspecific effect of B cell stimulation in HIV disease.

Sensory Neuronopathy

Primary sensory ataxia has been described in four HIV-infected patients at different stages of HIV disease (52,171). Because of the infrequency of this syndrome, it is not clearly related to HIV infection.

CONCLUSIONS

Neuromuscular disorders are common complications of AIDS, although their diagnosis is often delayed. Prompt recognition and early treatment of these disorders are crucial because appropriate therapy may dramatically alter the quality of life and length of survival. Basic research advances in the neurobiology of HIV will further elucidate pathogenetic mechanisms of these diseases and should provide a foundation for controlled clinical trials of new therapeutic agents.

ACKNOWLEDGMENT

This work was supported in part by grants from the National Institute of Neurological Disorders and Stroke (RO1-NS28630), National Institute of Allergy and Infectious Disease (UO1-Al-27667), and National Center for Research Resources (5M01 RR00071). We thank Jessica Moise, Arlene Rivera, the Mount Sinai Medical Center Neuromuscular Fellows, and Neuro-AIDS Research Center staff for their dedicated efforts. Drs. David Wolfe and Susan Morgello provided pathological analysis.

REFERENCES

1. Allan JD, Connolly KJ, Fitch H, et al. Long-term follow-up of didanosine administered orally twice daily to patients with advanced human immunodeficiency virus infection and hematologic intolerance of zidovudine. *Clin Infect Dis* 1993;16(suppl 1):46–51.
2. American Academy of Neurology. Criteria for diagnosis of chronic inflammatory demyelinating polyneuropathy. *Neurology* 1991;41:617–618.
3. Apostolski S, McAlarney T, Quattrini A, et al. The gp120 glycoprotein of human immunodeficiency virus type 1 binds to sensory ganglion neurons. *Ann Neurol* 1993;34:855–863.
4. Arnaudo E, Dalakas M, Shanske S, et al. Depletion of muscle mitochondrial DNA in AIDS patients with zidovudine-induced myopathy. *Lancet* 1991;337:508–510.
5. Bacellar H, Munoz A, Miller EN, et al. Temporal trends in the incidence of HIV-1–related neurologic diseases: Multicenter AIDS Cohort Study, 1985–1992. *Neurology* 1994;44:1892–1900.
6. Bailey RO, Baltch AL, Benkatesh R, et al. Sensory motor neuropathy associated with AIDS. *Neurology* 1988;38:886–891.
7. Barohn RJ, Gronseth GS, LeForce BR, et al. Peripheral nervous system involvement in a large cohort of human immunodeficiency virus–infected individuals. *Arch Neurol* 1993;50:167–171.
8. Batman PA, Miller ARO, Sedgwick PM, Griffin GE. Autonomic denervation in jejunal mucosa of homosexual men infected with HIV. *AIDS* 1991;5:1247–1252.
9. Bazan C 111, Jackson C, Jinkins JR, Barohn RJ. Gadolinium enhanced MRI in a case of cytomegalovirus polyradiculopathy. *Neurology* 1991;41:1522–1523.
10. Behar R, Wiley C, McCutchan JR. Cytomegalovirus polyradiculopathy in AIDS. *Neurology* 1987; 37:557–561.
11. Belec L, Di Costanzo B, Georges AJ, Gherardi R. HIV infection in African patients with tropical pyomyositis. *AIDS* 1991;5:234.
12. Bentler B, Cerami A. Cachectin: more than a tumor necrosis factor. *N Engl J Med* 1987;316: 479–485.
13. Berger AR, Arezzo JC, Schaumburg HH, et al. 2′,3′-Dideoxycytidine (ddC) toxic neuropathy: a study of 52 patients. *Neurology* 1993;43:358–362.
14. Berger JR, Difini JA, Swerdloff MA, Ayyar RD. HIV seropositivity in Guillain-Barré syndrome [Letter]. *Ann Neurol* 1987;22:393–394.
15. Berger JR, Flaster M, Schatz N, et al. Cranial neuropathy heralding otherwise occult AIDS-related large cell Iymphoma. *J Clin Neurophysiol* 1993;13:113–118.
16. Bessen LJ, Greene JB, Louie E, et al. Severe polymyositis-like syndrome associated with zidovudine therapy of AIDS and ARC. *N Engl J Med* 1988;318:708.
17. Bohan A, Peters JB. Polymyositis and dermatomyositis. Part I. *N Engl J Med* 1975;292:344–347.
18. Budzilovich G, Avitabile A, Niedt G, et al. Polyradiculopathy and sensory ganglionitis due to cytomegalovirus in acquired immune deficiency syndrome (AIDS). *Prog AIDS Pathol* 1989;1: 143–157.
19. Browne MJ, Mayer KH, Chafee SB, et al. 2′,3′-didehydro-3′-deoxythymidine (d4T) in patients with AIDS or AIDS-related complex: a phase I trial. *J Infect Dis* 1993;167:21–29.
20. Carmichael SM, Engleton L, Ayers CR, et al. Orthostatic hypotension during vincristine therapy. *Arch Intern Med* 1970;126:290–293.
21. Chad DA, Smith TW, Blumenfeld DA, Fairchild PG, DeGirolami U. HIV-associated myopathy: immunocytochemical identification of an HIV antigen (gp 41) in muscle macrophages. *Ann Neurol* 1990;28:579–582.
22. Chalmers AC, Greco CM, Miller RG. Prognosis in AZT myopathy. *Neurology* 1991;41:1181–1184.
23. Chariot P, Monnet I, Gherardi R. Cytochrome C reaction improves histopathological assessment of zidovudine myopathy. *Ann Neurol* 1993;34:561–565.
24. Chariot P, Ruet E, Authier FJ, Levy Y, Gherardi R. Acute rhabdomyolysis in patients infected by human immunodeficiency virus. *Neurology* 1994;44:1692–1696.

25. Chavanet P, Solary E, Giroud M, et al. Infraclinical neuropathies related to immunodeficiency virus infection associated with higher T-helper cell count. *J AIDS* 1989;2:564–569.

26. Chen C-H and Chen Y-C. Delayed cytotoxicity and selective loss of mitochondrial DNA in cells treated with the anti-human immunodeficiency virus compound 2'-3'-dideoxycytidine. *J Biol Chem* 1989;264:11934–11937.

27. Chimelli L, Scaravilli F. Morphological changes in the autonomic nervous system of patients with AIDS. In: *Proceedings of the Seventh International Conference on Neuroscience of HIV Infection.* Padova, Italy, 1991:89.

28. Chupp GL, Alroy J, Adelman iS, Breen JC, Skolnik PR. Myositis due to *Pleistosphora (Microsporidia)* in a patient with AIDS. *Clin Infect Dis* 1993;16:15–21.

29. Clifford DB, Buller RS, Mohammed S, Robison L, Storch GA. Use of polymerase chain reaction to demonstrate cytomegalovirus DNA in CSF of patients with human immunodeficiency virus infection. *Neurology* 1993;43:75–79.

30. Cohen BA, McArthur JC, Grohman S, Patterson B, Glass JD. Neurologic prognosis of cytomegalovirus polyradiculomyelopathy in AIDS. *Neurology* 1993;43:493–499.

31. Cohen JR, Laudenslager M. Autonomic nervous system involvement in patients with human immunodeficiency virus infection. *Neurology* 1989;39:1111–1112.

32. Consensus statement on the use of corticosteroids as adjunctive therapy for pneumocystis pneumonia in the acquired immunodeficiency syndrome. *N Engl J Med* 1990;323:1500–1504.

33. Cooley TP, Kunches LM, Saunders CA, et al. Once-daily administration of 2',3'-dideoxyinosine (ddI) in patients with the acquired immunodeficiency syndrome or AIDS-related complex. *N Engl J Med* 1990;322:1340–1345.

34. Cornblath DR. Treatment of the neuromuscular complications of human immunodeficiency virus infection. *Ann Neurol* 1988;23(suppl):88–91.

35. Cornblath DR, McArthur JC. Predominantly sensory neuropathy in patients with AIDS and AIDS-related complex. *Neurology* 1988;38:794–796.

36. Cornblath DR, McArthur JC, Kennedy PGE, et al. Inflammatory demyelinating peripheral neuropathies associated with human T cell lymphotropic virus type 111 infection. *Ann Neurol* 1987;21:32–40.

37. Craddock C, Pasvol G, Bull R, et al. Cardiorespiratory arrest and autonomic neuropathy in acquired immunodeficiency syndrome. *Lancet* 1987;2:16–18.

38. Cupler EJ, Hench K, Jay CA, et al. The natural history of zidovudine (AZT)-induced mitochondrial myopathy (ZIMM) [Abstract]. *Neurology* 1994;44:132.

39. Cupler EJ, Otero C, Hench K, Dalakas MC. Fatigue related to acetylcholine receptor antibodies in HIV-infected individuals [Abstract]. In: *Proceedings of the InternationalConference on Neuroscience of HIV Infection.* Vancouver, Canada, August 2–5, 1994.

40. Dalakas MC, Pezeshkpour GH. Neuromuscular diseases associated with human immunodeficiency virus infection. *Ann Neurol* 1988;23(suppl):38–48.

41. Dalakas MC, Pezeshkpour GH, Gravell M, Sever JL. Polymyositis associated with AIDS retrovirus. *JAMA* 1986;256:2381–2383.

42. Dalakas MC, Illa I, Pezeshkpour GH, et al. Mitochondrial myopathy caused by long-term zidovudine therapy. *N Engl J Med* 1990;322:1098–1105.

43. Dalakas MC, Leon-Monzon ME, Bernardini I, Gahl WA, Jay CA. Zidovudine-induced mitochondrial myopathy is associated with muscle carnitine deficiency and lipid storage. *Ann Neurol* 1994;35:482–487.

44. Dal Pan GJ, Glass JD, McArthur JC. Clinicopathologic correlations of HIV-I associated vacuolar myelopathy: an autopsy based case-control study. *Neurology* 1994;44:2159–2164.

45. de Gans J, Portegies P, Tiessens G, et al. Therapy for cytomegalovirus polyradiculopathy in patients with AIDS. Treatment with ganciclovir. *AIDS* 1990;4:421–425.

46. de la Monte SM, Gabuzda DH, Ho DD, et al. Peripheral neuropathy in the acquired immunodeficiency syndrome. *Ann Neurol* 1988;23:485–492.

47. DeVere R, Bradley WG. Polymyositis: presentation, morbidity and mortality. *Brain* 1975;98:637–666.

48. Drachman DE, Kuncl RW. Amyotrophic lateral sclerosis: an unconventional autoimmune disease? *Ann Neurol* 1989;26:269–274.

49. Dubinsky RM, Yarchoan R, Dalakas M, et al. Reversible axonal neuropathy from the treatment of AIDS and related disorders with 2',3'-dideoxycytidine (ddC). *Muscle Nerve* 1989;12:856–860.

50. Ebright JR, Crane LR. Ganciclovir-resistant cytomegalovirus [Letter]. *AIDS* 1991;5:604.

51. Eidelberg D, Sotrel A, Vogel H, et al. Progressive polyradiculopathy in acquired immune deficiency syndrome. *Neurology* 1986;36:912–916.

52. Elder G, Dalakas M, Pezeshkpour G, et al. Ataxia neuropathy due to ganglioneuritis after probable acute human immunodeficiency virus infection. *Lancet* 1986;11:1275–1276.

53. Engstrom JW, Lewis E, McGuire D. Cranial neuropathy and the acquired immunodeficiency syndrome. *Neurology* 1991;41(suppl 1):374.

54. Espinoza LR, Aguilar JL, Espinoza CG, et al. Characteristics and pathogenesis of myositis in human

immunodeficiency virus infection. Distinction from azidothymidine-induced myopathy. *Rheum Dis Clin North Am* 1991;17:117–129.

55. Evenhouse M, Hans E, Snell E, et al. Hypotension in infection with the human immune-deficiency virus [Letter]. *Ann Intern Med* 1987;107:598–599.
56. Fiala M, Cone LA, Cohen L, et al. Responses of neurologic complications of AIDS to 3'-azido-2'3'-dideoxythymidine and 9-(1,3-dihydroxy-2-propoxymethyl) guanine I. Clinical features. *Rev Infect Dis* 1988;10:250–256.
57. Figg WD. Peripheral neuropathy in HIV patient after isoniazid therapy initiated. *DICP* 1991;25:100–101.
58. Fischl M, Gagnon S, Uttamchandani R, et al. Myopathy associated with long-term zidovudine therapy. *Final program and abstracts, 5th International Conference on AIDS*. Montreal, 1989:MBP 329.
59. Freeman R, Roberts M, Friedman L, et al. Autonomic function and human immunodeficiency virus infection. *Neurology* 1990;40:575–580.
60. Fuller GN, Gill SK, Guiloff RJ, et al. Ganciclovir for lumbosacral polyradiculopathy in AIDS [Letter]. *Lancet* 1990;335:48–49.
61. Fuller GN, Jacobs JM, Guiloff RJ. Association of painful peripheral neuropathy in AIDS with cytomegalovirus infection. *Lancet* 1989;11:937–941.
62. Fuller GN, Jacobs JM, Guiloff RJ. Subclinical peripheral nerve involvement in AIDS: an electrophysiological and pathological study. *J Neurol Neurosurg Psychiatry* 1991;54:318–324.
63. Fuller GN, Jacobs JM, Guiloff RJ. Thalidomide, peripheral neuropathy and AIDS. *Int J STD AIDS* 1991;2:369–370.
64. Fuller GN, Jacobs JM, Guiloff RJ. Nature and incidence of peripheral nerve syndromesin HIV infection. *J Neurol Neurosurg Psychiatry* 1993;56:372–381.
65. Gertner E, Thurn JR, Williams DN, et al. Zidovudine-associated myopathy. *Am J Med* 1989;6:814–818.
66. Gherardi R, Baudrimont M, Lionnet F, et al. Skeletal muscle toxoplasmosis in patients with acquired immunodeficiency syndrome: a clinical and pathological study. *Ann Neurol* 1992;32:535–542.
67. Gherardi R, Florea-Strat A, Fromont G, Poron F, Sabourin J-C, Authier J. Cytokine expression in the muscle of HIV-infected patients: evidence for interleukin-1alpha accumulation in mitochondria of AZT fibers. *Ann Neurol* 1994;36:752–758.
68. Gherardi R, Lebargy F, Gaulard P, et al. Necrotizing vasculitis and HIV replication in peripheral nerves [Letter]. *N Engl J Med* 1989;321:685–686.
69. Ghika-Schmid F, Kuntzer T, Chave JP, Miklossy J, Regli F. Diversite de l'atteinte neuromusculaire de 47 patients infectes par le virus de l'immunodeficience humaine. *Schweiz Med Wochenschr* 1994;124:791–800.
70. Gill P, Rarick M, Bernstein-Singer M, et al. Treatment of advanced Kaposi's sarcoma using a combination of bleomycin and vincristine. *Am J Clin Oncol* 1990;13:315–319.
71. Gonzales MF, Olney RK, So YT, et al. Subacute structural myopathy associated with human immunodeficiency virus infection. *Arch Neurol* 1988;45:585–587.
72. Gorard DA, Henry K, Guiloff RJ. Necrotizing myopathy and zidovudine. *Lancet* 1988;1:1050–1051.
73. Grafe MR, Wiley CA. Spinal cord and peripheral nerve pathology in AIDS: the roles of cytomegalovirus and human immunodeficiency virus. *Ann Neurol* 1989;25:561–566.
74. Grau JM, Masanes F, Pedro E, et al. Human immunodeficiency virus type 1 infection and myopathy: clinical relevance of zidovudine therapy. *Ann Neurol* 1993;34:206–211.
75. Graveleau P, Perol R, Chapman A. Regression of cauda equina syndrome in AIDS patient being treated with ganciclovir [Letter]. *Lancet* 1989;11:511–512.
76. Griffin DE, McArthur JC, Cornblath DR. Soluble interleuken-2 receptor and soluble CD8 in serum and cerebrospinal fluid during human immunodeficiency virus–associated neurologic disease. *J Neuroimmunol* 1990;28:97–109.
77. Griffin DE, McArthur JC, Cornblath DR. Neopterin and interferon gamma in serum and cerebrospinal fluid of patients with HIV-associated neurologic disease. *Neurology* 1991;41:69–74.
78. Griffin JW, Crawford TO, Tyor WR, et al. Sensory neuropathy in AIDS. I. Neuropathology. *Brain* (in press).
79. Griffin JW, Wesselingh S, Oaklander AL, Kuncl RW, Griffin DE. mRNA fingerprinting of cytokines and growth factors: a new means of characterizing nerve biopsies [Abstract]. *Neurology* 1993; 43(suppl 2):232.
80. Hagberg L, Malmvall BE, Svennerholm L, et al. Guillain-Barre syndrome as an early manifestation of HIV central nervous system infection. *Scand J Infect Dis* 1986; 18:591–592.
81. Helmich CG, Green JK. Pentamidine-associated hypotension and route of administration. *Ann Intern Med* 1985;103:480.
82. Herzberg NH, Zorn I, Zwart R, Portegies P, Bolhuis P. Major growth reduction and minor decrease in mitochondrial enzyme activity in culture human muscle cells after exposure to zidovudine. *Muscle Nerve* 1992;15:706–710.
83. HIV or zidovudine myopathy? [Correspondence]. *Neurology* 1994;44:360–364.

84. Ho DD, Rota TR, Schooley RT, et al. Isolation of HTLV-III from cerebrospinal fluid and neural tissues of patients with neurologic syndromes related to the acquired immunodeficiency syndrome. *N Engl J Med* 1985;313:1493–1497.

85. Ho HW, Bayley R, Rhee JM, Vinters HV. Neuromuscular pathology in patients with acquired immune deficiency syndrome (AIDS): an autopsy study. *J Neuropathol Exp Neurol* 1989;48:382.

86. Hoffman PM, Festaff BW, Giron CT, et al. Isolation of LAV/HTLV-3 from a patient with amyotrophic lateral sclerosis [Letter]. *N Engl J Med* 1985;313:324–325.

87. Hollander H. Cerebrospinal fluid normalities and abnormalities in individuals infected with human immunodeficiency virus. *J Infec Dis* 1988;158:855–858.

88. Hollander H, Stringari S. Human immunodeficiency virus–associated meningitis: clinical course and correlations. *Am J Med* 1987;83:813–816.

89. Illa I, Nath A, Dalakas M. Immunocytochemical and virological characteristics of HIV-associated inflammatory myopathies: similarities with seronegative patients. *Ann Neurol* 1991;29:474–481.

90. Jacobson MA, Mills J, Rush J, et al. Failure of antiviral therapy for acquired immunodeficiency syndrome–related cytomegalovirus myelitis. *Arch Neurol* 1988;45:1019–1092.

91. Jakobsen J, Smith T, Gaub J, et al. Progressive neurological dysfunction during latent HIV infection. *Br Med J* 1989;299:225–228.

92. Janssen R, Saykin A, Kaplan J, et al. Neurologic complications of human immunodeficiency virus infection in patients with lymphadenopathy syndrome. *Ann Neurol* 1988;23:49–55.

93. Jeantils V, Lemaitre MO, Robert J, et al. Subacute polyneuropathy with encephalopathy in AIDS with human cytomegalovirus pathogenicity? [Letter]. *Lancet* 1986;11:1039.

94. Keilbaugh SA, Moschella JA, Chin CD, et al. Role of mtDNA replication in the toxicity of 3'-azido-3'-deoxythymidine (AZT) in AIDS therapy and studies on other anti–HIV-1 dideoxynucleotides. In: Ouagliarello E, Papa S, Palmieri F, Saccone C, eds. *Structure, Function and Biogenesis of Energy-Transfer Systems.* New York: Elsevier Science, 1990:159–162.

95. Kieburtz KD, Ciang DW, Schiffer RB, et al. Abnormal vitamin B_{12} metabolism in human immunodeficiency virus infection: association with neurological dysfunction. *Arch Neurol* 1991;48:312–314.

96. Kieburtz KD, Seidlin M, Lambert JS, et al. Extended follow-up of peripheral neuropathy in patients with AIDS and AIDS-related complex treated with dideoxyinosine. *J AIDS* 1992;5:60–64.

97. Kim YS, Hollander H. Polyradiculopathy due to cytomegalovirus: report of two cases in which improvement occurred after prolonged therapy and review of the literature. *Clin Infect Dis* 1993;17:32–37.

98. Lahdevirta J, Maury C, Teppo A-M, Repo H. Elevated levels of circulating cachectin-tumor necrosis factor in patients with AIDS. *Am J Med* 1988;85:289–291.

99. Lambert JS, Seidlin M, Reichman RC, et al. 2',3'-dideoxyinosine (ddI) in patients with the acquired immunodeficiency syndrome or AIDS-related complex: results of a phase 1 trial. *N Engl J Med* 1990;322:1333–1340.

100. Lamperth L, Dalakas MC, Dagani F, et al. Abnormal skeletal and cardiac muscle mitochondria induced by zidovudine (AZT) in human muscle *in vitro* and in an animal model. *Lab Invest* 1991;65:742–751.

101. Lange DJ, Britton CB, Younger DS, et al. The neuromuscular manifestations of human immunodeficiency virus infections. *Arch Neurol* 1988;45:1084–1088.

102. Lanska MJ, Lanska DJ, Shmidley JW. Syphilitic polyradiculopathy in an HIV-positive man. *Neurology* 1988;38:1297–1301

103. Laskin OL. Use of ganciclovir to treat serious cytomegalovirus infections in patients with AIDS. *J Infect Dis* 1987;155:323–328.

104. Leger JM, Bouche P, Bolgert F, et al. The spectrum of polyneuropathies in patients infected with HIV. *J Neurol Neurosurg Psychiatry* 1989;52:1369–1374.

105. Leger JM, Henin D, Belic L, et al. Lymphoma-induced polyradiculopathy in AIDS: two cases. *J Neurol* 1992;239:132–134.

106. Levine E, Kalman J, Mayor L, et al. Elevated circulating levels of tumor necrosis factor in severe chronic heart failure. *N Engl J Med* 1990;323:236–241.

107. Levy RM, Bredesen DE, Rosenblum ML. Neurological manifestations of the acquired immunodeficiency syndrome (AIDS): experience at UCSF and review of the literature. *J Neurosurg* 1985;62:475–495.

108. Lin-Greenberg A, Taneja-Uppal N. Dysautonomia and infection with the human immuno-deficiency virus [Letter]. *Ann Intern Med* 1987;106:167.

109. Lipkin WI, Parry G, Kiprov D, et al. Inflammatory neuropathy in homosexual men with lymphadenopathy. *Neurology* 1985;35:1479–1483.

110. Lipman JM, Reichert JA, Davidovich A, Anderson TD. Species differences in nucleotide pool levels of 2'-3'-dideoxycytidine: a possible explanation for species-specific toxicity. *Toxicol Appl Pharmacol* 1993;123:137–143.

111. Lohmuller G, Matuschke A, Goebl FD. Testing for neurological involvement in HIV infection [Letter]. *Lancet* 1987;11:1532.

112. Mah V, Vartavarian LM, Akers MA, et al. Abnormalities of peripheral nerve in patients with human immunodeficiency virus infection. *Ann Neurol* 1988;24:713–717

113. Mahieux F, Gray F, Fenelon G, et al. Acute myeloradiculitis due to cytomegalovirus as the initial manifestation of AIDS. *J Neurol Neurosurg Psychiatry* 1989;52:270–274.

114. Malamut RI, Leopold N, Parry GL. The treatment of HIV-associated chronic inflammatory demyelinating polyneuropathy (HIV-CIDP) with intravenous immunoglobulin (IVIG). *Neurology* 1992; 42(suppl 3):335.

115. Manji H, Harrison MJG, Round JM, et al. Muscle disease, HIV and zidovudine: the spectrum of muscle disease in HIV-infected individuals treated with zidovudine. *J Neurol* 1993;240:479–488.

116. Manji H, Malin A, Connolly S. CMV polyradiculopathy in AIDS—suggestion for new strategies in treatment [Letter]. *Genitourin Med* 1992;68:192.

117. Martini L, Vion P, LeGangneux E, Grandpierre G, Becquet D. SIDA et myasthenie: une association exceptionelle. *Rev Neurol* 1991;147:395–397.

118. Mastaglia FL, Ojeda VJ. Inflammatory myopathies: Part 2. *Ann Neurol* 1985;17:317–323.

119. McArthur JC. Neurologic manifestation of AIDS. *Medicine* 1987;66:407–437.

120. McArthur JC, Cohen BA, Farzedegan H, et al. Cerebrospinal fluid abnormalities in homosexual men with and without neuropsychiatric findings. *Ann Neurol* 1988;23(suppl):34–37.

121. McArthur JC, Sipos E, Cornblath DR, et al. Identification of mononuclear cells in CSF of patients with HIV infection. *Neurology* 1989;39:66–70.

122. Merigan TC, Skowron G, Bozzette SA, et al. Circulating p24 antigen levels and responses to dideoxy-cytidine in human immunodeficiency virus (HIV) infections. *Ann Intern Med* 1989;110:189–194.

123. Mhiri C, Baudrimont M, Bonne G, et al. Zidovudine myopathy: a distinctive disorder associated with mitochondrial dysfunction. *Ann Neurol* 1991;29:606–614.

124. Miller RG, Carson PJ, Moussavi RS, et al. Fatigue and myalgia in AIDS patients. *Neurology* 1991; 41:1603–1607.

125. Miller RG, Parry CJ, Pfae MW, et al. The spectrum of peripheral neuropathy associated with ARC and AIDS. *Muscle Nerve* 1988;11:857–863.

126. Miller RG, Storey JR, Greco CM. Ganciclovir in the treatment of progressive AIDS-related polyradiculopathy. *Neurology* 1990;40:569–574.

127. Misha BE, Sommers W, Koski CL, et al. Acute inflammatory demyelinating polyneuropathy in the acquired immune deficiency syndrome. *Ann Neurol* 1985;18:131–132.

128. Morgello S, Simpson DM. Multifocal cytomegalovirus demyelinative polyneuropathy associated with AIDS. *Muscle Nerve* 1994;17:176–182.

129. Moyle GJ, Nelson MR, Hawkins D, Gazzard BG. The use and toxicity of didanosine (ddI) in HIV antibody-positive individuals intolerant to zidovudine (AZT). *Q J Med* 1993;86:155–163.

130. Mulhall BP, Jennens I. Testing for neurological involvement in human immunodeficiency virus infection [Letter]. *Lancet* 1987;11:1531–1532.

131. Nath A, Kerman RH, Novak IS, Wolinsky JS. Immune studies in human immunodeficiency virus infection with myasthenia gravis: a case report. *Neurology* 1990;40:581–583.

132. Ochonisky S, Verroust J, Bastuji-Garin S, Gherardi R, Revuz J. Thalidomide neuropathy incidence and clinicoelectrophysiologic findings in 42 patients. *Arch Dermatol* 1994;130:66–69.

133. Olney RK, So YT, Hollander H. Electrodiagnostic results in different stages of HIV infection [Abstract]. *Muscle Nerve* 1990;13:854–855.

134. Panegyres PK, Tan M, Kakulas BA, et al. Necrotising myopathy and zidovudine. *Lancet* 1988;1: 1050–1051.

135. Parry GJ. Peripheral neuropathies associated with human immunodeficiency virus infection. *Ann Neurol* 1988;23(suppl):49–53.

136. Peters BS, Winer J, Landon DN, et al. Mitochondrial myopathy associated with chronic zidovudine therapy in AIDS. *Q J Med* 1993;86:5–15.

137. Pezeshkpour GH, Illa I, Dalakas MC. Ultrastructural characteristics and DNA immunochemistry in HIV and AZT-associated myopathies. *Hum Pathol* 1991;22:1281–1288.

138. Piette AM, Tusseau F, Vignon D, et al. Acute neuropathy coincident with seroconversion for anti-LAV/HTLV-III. *Lancet* 1986;1:852.

139. Pike IM, Nicaise C. The didanosine expanded access program: safety analysis. *Clin Infect Dis* 1993; 16(suppl 1):63–68.

140. Purba JS, Hofman MA, Portegies P, et al. Decreased number of oxytoxin neurons in the paraventricular nucleus of the human hypothalamus in AIDS. *Brain* 1993;116:795–805.

141. Rance NE, McArthur JC, Cornblath D, et al. Gracile tract degeneration in patients with sensory neuropathy and AIDS. *Neurology* 1988;38:265–271.

142. Rathbun RC, Martin ES 111. Didanosine therapy in patients intolerant of or failing zidovudine therapy. *Ann Pharmacother* 1992;26:1347–1351.

143. Reyes MG, Casanova J, Varricchio F, et al. Zidovudine myopathy [Letter]. *Neurology* 1992;42: 1252.

144. Robertson KR, Stern RA, Hall CD, et al. Vitamin B_{12} deficiency and the nervous system in HIV infection. *Arch Neurol* 1993;50:807–811.

145. Roullet E, Assuerus V, Gozlan J, et al. Cytomegalovirus multifocal neuropathy in AIDS: analysis of 15 consecutive patients. *Neurology* 1994;44:2174–2182.
146. Said C. Multifocal neuropathy in HIV infection. In *Proceedings of the Seventh International Conference of HIV Infection*. Padova, Italy, 1991:89.
147. Said G, Lacroix C, Chemouilli P, et al. Cytomegalovirus neuropathy in acquired immunodeficiency syndrome: a clinical and pathological study. *Ann Neurol* 1991;29:139–146.
148. Said G, Lacroix-Ciando C, Fujimura H, et al. The peripheral neuropathy of necrotizing arteritis: a clinicopathological study. *Ann Neurol* 1988;23:461–465.
149. Savery F, Hang LM. Immunodeficiency associated with motor neuron disease treated with intravenous immunoglobulin. *Clin Ther* 1986;8:700–702.
150. Shamanesh M, Bradber CS, Edwards A, Smith SE. Autonomic dysfunction in patients with human immunodeficiency virus infection. *Int J STD AIDS* 1991;2:419–423.
151. Simpson DM, Bender AN. Human immunodeficiency virus–associated myopathy: analysis of 11 patients. *Ann Neurol* 1988;24:79–84.
152. Simpson DM, Bender AN, Farraye J, et al. Human immunodeficiency virus wasting syndrome may represent a treatable myopathy. *Neurology* 1990;40:535–538.
153. Simpson DM, Citak KA, Godfrey E, Godbold J, Wolfe D. Myopathies associated with human immunodeficiency virus and zidovudine: can their effects be distinguished? *Neurology* 1993;43: 971–976.
154. Simpson DM, Cohen JR, Sivak MA, et al. Neuromuscular complications in association with acquired immunodeficiency syndrome. *Ann Neurol* 1985;18:160.
155. Simpson DM, Godbold J, Hassett J, et al. HIV associated myopathy, and the effects of zidovudine and prednisone: preliminary results of placebo-controlled trials [Abstract]. *Clin Neuropathol* 1993; 12(suppl 1):20.
156. Simpson DM, Morgello S, Citak K, Corbo M, Latov N. Motor neuron disease associated with HIV and anti-asialo GM1 antibody [Abstract]. *Muscle Nerve* 1994;17:1091.
157. Simpson DM, Olney RK. Peripheral neuropathies associated with human immunodeficiency virus infection. In: Dyck PJ, ed. *Peripheral Neuropathies: New Concepts and Treatments*. Philadephia: WB Saunders, 1992:685–711.
158. Simpson DM, Olney RK, So YT, et al. A placebo-controlled study of peptide T for painful distal neuropathy associated with AIDS [Abstract]. *Neurology* 1994;44:249.
159. Simpson DM, Slasor P, Dafni U, et al. Analysis of myopathy in a placebo-controlled zidovudine trial. *Muscle Nerve* 1996 (in press).
160. Simpson DM, Tagliati M. Neurological manifestations of HIV infection. *Ann Intern Med* 1994;121: 769–785.
161. Simpson DM, Tagliati M. Nucleoside analogue–associated peripheral neuropathy in human immunodeficiency virus infection. *J AIDS* 1995;9:153–161.
162. Simpson DM, Tagliati M, Grinnell J, Bittner E, Hassett J, Godbold J. Peripheral nerve function in HIV infection: clinical and electrophysiological analysis of 300 subjects [Abstract]. *Neurology* 1995; 45:926.
163. Simpson DM, Tagliati M, Grinnell J, Godbold J. Electrophysiological findings in HIV infection: association with distal symmetrical polyneuropathy and CD4 level [Abstract]. *Muscle Nerve* 1994; 17:1113–1114.
164. Simpson DM, Wolfe DE. Neuromuscular complications of HIV infection and its treatment. *AIDS* 1991;5:917–926.
165. Simpson MV, Chin CD, Keilbough SA, Lin T-S, Prusoff WH. Studies on the inhibition of mitochondrial DNA replication of 3′-azido-3′-deoxythymidine and other deoxynucleoside analog which inhibit HIV-1 replication. *Biochem Pharmacol* 1989;38:1033–1036.
166. Skowron G, Bozzette SA, Lim L, et al. Alternating and intermittent regimens of zidovudine and dideoxycytidine in patients with AIDS or AIDS-related complex. *Ann Int Med* 1993;118:321–330.
167. Snider WD, Simpson DM, Nielsen S, et al. Neurological complications of acquired immune deficiency syndrome: analysis of 50 patients. *Ann Neurol* 1983;14:403–418.
168. So YT, Engstrom JW, Olney RK. The spectrum of electrodiagnostic abnormalities in patients with human immunodeficiency virus infection. *Muscle Nerve* 1990;13:855.
169. So YT, Olney RK. The natural history of mononeuritis multiplex and simplex in HIV infection. *Neurology* 1991;41(suppl 1):375.
170. So YT, Olney RK. Acute lumbosacral polyradiculopathy in acquired immunodeficiency syndrome: experience in 23 patients. *Ann Neurol* 1994;35:53–58.
171. So YT, Holtzman DM, Miller RG. Sensory myeloneuropathy in patients with human immunodeficiency virus (HIV) infection. *Neurology* 1990;40(suppl 1):429.
172. So YT, Holtzman DM, Abrams DJ, et al. Peripheral neuropathy associated with acquired immunodeficiency syndrome: prevalence and clinical features from a population-based survey. *Arch Neurol* 1988;45:945–948.
173. So, YT, Holtzman DM, Olney RK. The spectrum of progressive lumbosacral polyradiculopathy seen in acquired immune deficiency syndrome. *Neurology* 1989;39(suppl 1):382.

174. Soueidan S, Sinnwell T, Jay C, Frank J, McLaughlin A, Dalakas M. Impaired muscle energy metabolism in patients with AZT-myopathy: a blinded comparative study of exercise ^{31}P magnetic resonance spectroscopy (MRS) with muscle biopsy [Abstract]. *Neurology* 1992;42(suppl 3):146.

175. Stern R, Gold J, DiCarlo EF. Myopathy complicating the acquired immunodeficiency syndrome. *Muscle Nerve* 1987;10:318–322.

176. Stricker RB, Sanders KA, Owen WF, et al. Mononeuritis multiplex associated with cryoglobulinemia in HIV infection. *Neurology* 1992;42:2103–2105.

177. Tagliati M, Godbold J, Hassett J, Godfrey E, Grinnell J, Simpson DM. Neuromuscular disorders in HIV infection: cross-sectional cohort analysis of 250 patients [Abstract]. *Neurology* 1994;44(suppl 2):367.

178. Thornton CA, Latif AS, Emmanuel JC. Guillain-Barré syndrome associated with human immunodeficiency virus infection in Zimbabwe. *Neurology* 1991;41:812–815.

179. Till M, MacDonnell KB. Myopathy with human immunodeficiency virus type 1 (HIV-1) infection: HIV-1 or zidovudine. *Ann Intern Med* 1990;113:492–494.

180. Tucker T, Dix RD, Kazten C, Davis RL, Schmidley JW. Cytomegalovirus and herpes simplex virus ascending myelitis in a patient with acquired immune deficiency syndrome. *Ann Neurol* 1985;18: 74–79.

181. Vendrell J, Heredia C, Pujol M, et al. Guillain-Barré syndrome associated with seroconversion for anti–HTLV-III. *Neurology* 1987;37:544.

182. Verma RK, Ziegler DK, Kepes JJ. HIV-related neuromuscular syndrome simulating motor neuron disease. *Neurology* 1990;40:544–546.

182a. Verma A, Berger JR. Myasthenia gravis with dual infection of HIV and HTLV-I. *Muscle and Nerve* 1995;18:1355–1356.

183. Villa A, Foresti V, Confalonieri F. Autonomic nervous system dysfunction associated with HIV infection in intravenous heroin users. *AIDS* 1992;6:85–89.

184. Vittecoq D, Morel C, Eymard B, Bach JF. Recovery from myasthenia gravis of a patient infected with human immunodeficiency virus. *Clin Infect Dis* 1992;15:379–380.

185. Volberding PA, Lagakos SW, Koch MA, et al. Zidovudine in asymptomatic human immunodeficiency virus infection: a controlled trial in persons with fewer than 500 CDV-positive cells per cubic millimeter. *N Engl J Med* 1990;322:941–949

186. Walsh C, Krigel R, Lennett E, et al. Thrombocytopenia in homosexual patients. *Ann Intern Med* 1985;103:542–545.

187. Weissman JD, Constantinitis I, Hudgins P, Wallace DC. [31]P magnetic resonance spectroscopy suggests impaired mitochondrial function in AZT-treated HIV-infected patients. *Neurology* 1992;42: 619–623.

188. Wessel HB, Zitelli BJ. Myasthenia gravis associated with human T cell lymphotropic virus type 111 infection. *Pediatr Neurol* 1987;3:238–239.

189. Wesselingh SL, Power C, Fox R, et al. Cytokine mRNA expression in HIV-associated neurological disease [Abstract]. *Neurology* 1993;43(suppl 2):291.

190. Winer JB. Neuropathies and HIV disease [Editorial]. *J Neurol Neurosurg Psychiatry* 1993;56: 739–741.

191. Wrzolek MA, Sher JH, Kozlowski PB, Rao C. Skeletal muscle pathology in AIDS: an autopsy study. *Muscle Nerve* 1990;13:508–515.

192. Wullenweber M, Schneider U, Hegenah R. Myasthenia gravis bei AIDS und Neurolue. *Nervenarzt* 1993;64:273–277.

193. Yarchoan R, Berg G, Brouwers P, et al. Response of human immunodeficiency virus–associated neurological disease to 21-azido-3′-deoxythymidine. *Lancet* 1987;1:132–135.

194. Yoshioka M, Shapshak P, Srivasta AK, et al. Expression of HIV-1 and interleukin-G in lumbosacral dorsal root ganglia of patients with AIDS. *Neurology* 1994;44:1120–1130.

AIDS and the Nervous System, Second Edition,
edited by J. R. Berger and R. M. Levy.
Lippincott-Raven Publishers, Philadelphia © 1997.

10

Infants, Children, and Adolescents

Anita L. Belman

*Department of Neurology and Pediatrics, School of Medicine, State University of
New York, Stony Brook, New York 11790*

PEDIATRIC HIV-1 INFECTION AND AIDS

The first cases of AIDS in children were described over a decade ago (2, 104, 121). Since then, HIV-1 infection has become one of the leading causes of morbidity and mortality in children worldwide.

Early in the AIDS epidemic it was recognized that HIV-1, a lentivirus, affects the central nervous system (CNS), as well as the immune system (15,62,64,71,75, 76,79,84,101,114,117,128,130,150). Because of this selective tropism, HIV-1 causes a wide spectrum of disease in infants and children (Table 1). The most severe form of the disease results in AIDS. Table 2 lists the current Centers for Disease Control (CDC) classifications for pediatric HIV disease. Neurological disorders associated with HIV-1 are common, add significantly to the morbidity of the disease, and often have devastating complications. This chapter will focus on neurological aspects of HIV-1 infection in children. Epidemiological and clinical features of pediatric HIV-1 infection and AIDS will be reviewed briefly.

Time of Infection

Pediatric HIV-1 infection results from maternal-infant transmission (vertically-acquired; also termed congenital, HIV-1 infection), transfusion with contaminated blood or blood products, or in some adolescent cases, from sexual or IV drug use.

Mother to Child Transmission

Estimates of the rate of mother-to-child transmission range from 13-45% (European Collaborative Study, 14.4%; New York City, 28%; San Francisco, 31%; areas in Kenya, 45%) (66,105,118). It is not clear what percentage of transmission occurs *in utero*, during labor and delivery, and postnatally by breast feeding (99,105). It is also not certain in which trimester of gestation most transmission occurs. Both the risk factors of perinatal transmission and its timing remain under active investigation. Although transmission of HIV-1 to a fetus can occur prior to the 20th week of gestation (82,86,93), current data suggests that at least one half of perinatally acquired infections occur before or during the birth process (22,29,32,46,49,50,57,58,

TABLE 1. *Diagnoses that indicate AIDS: 1993 CDC revised surveillance definition for AIDS*

Multiple or recurrent bacterial infections[a]
Candidiasis of the trachea, bronchi, or lungs[b]
Candidiasis of the esophagus[b,c]
Invasive cervical cancer[d]
Coccidioidomycosis, disseminated or extrapulmonary[a]
Cryptococcosis, extrapulmonary[b]
Cryptosporidiosis, chronic intestinal[b]
CMV disease (other than liver, spleen, nodes) onset at age >1 month[b]
CMV retinitis (with loss of vision)[b,c]
HIV encephalopathy[a]
Chronic herpes simplex ulcer (>1 mo duration) or pneumonitis or esophagitis onset at >1 mo of age[b]
Histoplasmosis, disseminated or extrapulmonary[b]
Isosporiasis, chronic intestinal (>1 month duration)[a]
Kaposi's sarcoma[b,c]
Lymphoid interstitial pneumonitis[b,c]
Lymphoma, primary brain[b]
Lymphoma (Burkitt's or immunoblastic sarcoma)[a]
Mycobacterium avium complex or *M. kansasii*, disseminated or extrapulmonary[b]
M. tuberculosis or acid-fast infection (species not identified), disseminated or extrapulmonary[a] or pulmonary[d]
Pneumonia, recurrent[d]
P. carinii pneumonia[b,c]
Progressive multifocal leukoencephalopathy[b]
Toxoplasmosis of brain, onset of age >1 mo[b,c]
Wasting syndrome caused by HIV[a]

[a] Requires laboratory evidence of HIV infection (1987 addition)
[b] If indicator disease is diagnosed definitively (e.g., biopsy, culture) and there is no other cause of immunodeficiency, laboratory documentation of HIV infection is not required.
[c] Presumptive diagnosis of indicator disease is accepted, if there is laboratory evidence of HIV infection (1987 addition)
[d] Requires laboratory evidence of HIV infection (1993 addition; adults and adolescents).

73,86,99,116,118,120,132). Several maternal factors are reported to be associated with increased risk of maternal-fetal transmission. These include low CD4- counts, high viral titers, advanced HIV-1 disease, placental membrane inflammation, premature rupture of membranes, premature delivery, increased exposure of infant to maternal blood, and low vitamin A (22,34,99,122,125,133,145).

NATURAL HISTORY

The natural history of vertically-acquired HIV-1 infection differs from that of adults. The adverse effects of HIV-1 on the developing immune system and nervous

TABLE 2. *CDC pediatric HIV classification (1994)*

Immunonological categories	Clinical categories			
	No signs/ symptoms (N)	Mild signs/ symptoms (A)	Moderate signs/ symptoms (B)	Severe signs/ symptoms (C)
No evidence of suppression	N1	A1	B1	C1
Evidence of moderate suppression	N2	A2	B2	C2
Severe suppression	N3	A3	B3	C3

From the CDC. 1994 Revised classification system for human immunodeficiency virus infection in children less than 13 years of age. Official authorized addenda—human immunodeficiency virus infection codes and official guidelines for coding and reporting ICD-9-CM. *MMWR* 1994;43(RR-12); with permission.

system often result in more rapid onset of clinical symptoms and progression to death. A bimodal evolution of symptomatic pediatric HIV-1 disease is recognized from clinical and data modeling studies. The first "hump" occurs in infancy, and the second later in childhood (3,21,105,124). There may actually be a trimodal evolution, with the third "hump" (albeit smaller) occurring in the pre- and early adolescent years (26,33,99,105,107). Latency to onset of symptoms, in this group, as in adults, may be 10 years or more.

Among infants diagnosed with AIDS (the first group), CDC AIDS case surveillance reports indicate that 62% had *Pneumocystis carinii* pneumonia (PCP) as an AIDS indicator disease versus only 20% of children diagnosed at >1 year of age (105). These infants often present between 3–8 months of age with symptoms including HIV encephalopathy (see HIV–associated CNS disease syndromes), PCP, cytomegalovirus (CMV), and/or wasting syndrome. The risk that this early and severe form of disease will develop is highest in those infants who as newborns have detectible levels of serum p24 antigen, and to a lesser degree, in those infants in whom virus could be isolated by culture or polymerase chain reaction (PCR) (20,32,118,119).

The children in the second group usually have a more indolent initial course (and did not have detectible serum levels of p24 as neonates as determined by the methodology used in the study). Lymphoid interstitial pneumonitis (LIP) is their most frequent AIDS indicator disease (105). Evidence of other lymphoproliferative processes characteristic of pediatric HIV-1 infection is frequent and includes lymphadenopathy, hepatosplenomegaly, and parotid gland enlargement. LIP carries a much better prognosis for survival.

Multiple or recurrent bacterial infections, (another pediatric AIDS-defining condition), ranging from otitis media, pneumonia, bone and joint infection, to sepsis and meningitis are common in both groups, as is failure to thrive, persistent oral candidiasis, and chronic or recurrent diarrhea.

Data modeling of the CDC's Pediatric Spectrum of Disease Study also supports the clinical impression of two distinct populations of children with different rates of survival. Analysis showed that the difference between the groups was not related to any difference in PCP prophylaxis, specific AIDS-defining conditions, antiviral therapy or birth weight (36,105). Clinical studies do suggest that the stage of maternal HIV-1 illness during pregnancy and delivery (maternal viremia) may be an important factor. The different rates of disease progression may relate to viral load, phenotype of the infecting virus, maternal HIV-1 disease stage, and perhaps timing of perinatal infection (20,32,49,58,105).

EPIDEMIOLOGY

Infants and Children

The worldwide increase in the number of AIDS cases in women of childbearing age is paralleled by an increasing number of children with vertically transmitted HIV-1 infection. Maternal-infant transmission currently accounts for virtually all reported new cases in the United States (105). Over 5,000 children with AIDS (vertically acquired) were reported to the CDC in 1995 (37). It is estimated that between 1989 and 1992, approximately 7,000 HIV-1–infected women have given birth each year. Assuming a 20% transmission rate (15%-30%) of infection from mother to infant, it is estimated that 1,000–2,000 HIV-1–infected infants were born each year.

The true number of HIV-1–infected children is unknown as surveillance systems have relied mostly on identification of children with clinical manifestations of AIDS. Reports based on seroprevalence and AIDS mortality data suggest that there are 15,000-20,000 HIV-1– infected infants and children in the United States. The World Health Organization projects that by the year 2000, 3 million women and children will die from HIV related disease, and 10 million children will be born infected (42,43,99).

Adolescents

Although adolescents (13–19 years of age) comprised ~ 1% of total AIDS cases in the United States, as of March 1993, statistics show that 20% of total AIDS cases are in the 13-29 year age group (70). Given that it may take ~10 years between infection with HIV and the onset of symptoms, it can be assumed that many of these patients were infected as adolescents. In the past, transfusion-acquired HIV-1 infection was the most common cause. Individuals with hemophilia, and other coagulation defects, and recipients of blood or blood product due to other illness, represented the majority of teenage AIDS cases. However, the percentage of all cases that this group represents is declining because of blood screening for HIV-1. Currently the most common risk factors for adolescents include sexual exposure and IV drug use. In fact it is estimated that ~65% of adolescents 13–19 years of age and 90% of individuals 20–24 years of age with AIDS were infected through these means (33,47,105). As already noted, some adolescents have vertically acquired HIV-1 infection. Since the first reported cases of HIV-1 in adolescents there has been a steady increase in the number of new cases (46,105).

PEDIATRIC HIV-1 INFECTION: A CHRONIC DISEASE

Infants and children with HIV-1 infection, including those who have developed an AIDS-defining condition, are currently living longer. In part this is due to more reliable techniques for early diagnosis and thus identification of infants and children when they are still asymptomatic or mildly symptomatic. In part it is due to successful prophylactic therapy for life threatening opportunistic infections, and to more aggressive and successful medical management of serious infections (including Ois), and other HIV-1 related conditions. It is also due to primary antiretroviral and immunomodulating therapies. Pediatric HIV-1 infection can now be thought of as a chronic disease, with multisystem involvement, that had periods of progression and periods of relative stability.

Prevention

The most important and effective strategy for preventing maternal-infant HIV-1 transmission involves prevention of HIV-1 infection in the mother before pregnancy, and indeed in all women of child bearing age.

The second most important strategy is detection of HIV-1 infection in pregnant women. In a study conducted by the AIDS Clinical Trials Group (ACTG 076), it was shown that administration of Zidovudine (ZDV) to a selected group of HIV-1–infected pregnant women and their newborns, reduced the risk for perinatal transmission by approximately two thirds. This trial begun in April 1991, was designed to evaluate the efficacy, safety, and tolerance of ZDV in preventing maternal transmission of HIV-1 to the fetus. Preliminary analyses in February 1994 indicated a substantial reduction in HIV-1 infection among infants born to women and their newborns treated with ZDV. There was a 67% relative reduction in the risk of HIV infection for infants whose mothers had taken ZDV. The rate of perinatal infection in the placebo group was 25.5%, consistent with the expected U.S. transmission rate, and only 8.3 % in the treated group (40). Based on these findings the U.S. Public Health Service provided guidelines and recommendations for treating pregnant HIV-1–infected women after the 14th week of gestation (see ref. 38).

HIV-1 AND THE NERVOUS SYSTEM

In 1983 the clinical and immunological features of pediatric AIDS were described in the literature. The investigators of these landmark reports noted that developmental delays were a common finding; an observation implicating CNS involvement. Shortly thereafter the characteristics of pediatric neuro AIDS were described (15,64). CNS involvement manifested by a progressive encephalopathy was recognized as a major complication (9,15,64,65,140). It was observed that by the time HIV-1 infection had advanced to ''full blown'' AIDS, cognitive and motor impairment of varying duration, progression, and severity were common (9). Neuropathological studies, in the majority of cases, revealed no evidence of CNS opportunistic infections or neoplasms (9,53,65,128). Furthermore, investigations from various clinical and laboratory studies indicated that the CNS was infected by HIV-1. Morphological and genetic similarities were documented between HIV-1 and visna virus, an ovine retrovirus with well known neurotropic properties (15,64,71,75,76,79,84,91,114,117,128,130,150). These studies suggested that the clinical syndromes of progressive encephalopathy (PE) in children and the adult counterpart AIDS-dementia complex (101) (now termed HIV–associated dementia) were directly related to HIV-1.

Neurological and Neurobehavioral Disorders

The neurological and developmental status of HIV-1–infected infants and children may be adversely affected by conditions directly associated with HIV-1 infection. It may also be affected by coexisting, and at times, confounding and compounding conditions that are not themselves HIV-1 related, but that occur with significant frequency in this population.

HIV-1 Related

The CNS in HIV-1–infected children may be affected by: (a) HIV-1, itself. This category includes the clinically recognized syndromes with cognitive, motor and behavioral manifestation that are related to CNS HIV-1 infection and HIV-1–associated CNS disease ; (b) secondary CNS complications. This group of disorders are associated with immunosuppression or with distinct systemic AIDS-related conditions. Infections caused by pathogens, other than HIV-1, neoplasms and strokes are included in this category; (c) metabolic and endocrinological derangements associated with systemic HIV-1 infection and AIDS-related disorders. They are often amenable to medical therapy and therefore may be transient and reversible; and (d) toxic or metabolic complications of antiretroviral, antimicrobial and other therapies. As new, more specific antiretroviral, antimicrobial, immunomodulating agents are developed, and new treatment protocols for HIV-1 infection and AIDS-related diseases are instituted, there is the possibility that the infant or child's nervous system may be adversely affected by toxic or metabolic complications of therapy.

Coexisting Conditions

Antenatal and Perinatal Complications

The developing nervous system in HIV-1–infected infants, as in non-HIV-1–infected infants, may be adversely affected by maternal illnesses and high risk behaviors during gestation (6,7). Some factors are related to maternal AIDS–associated disorders or infections with pathogens other than HIV-1, whereas others are not. Some factors are related to maternal behaviors and conditions such as substance use, inadequate nutrition, and deficient prenatal care.

The developing CNS in HIV-1–infected infants, as in non-HIV-1–infected infants may be adversely affected by CNS complications in the perinatal period. Some of these are interlinked with "high risk" maternal factors and are associated with premature delivery. The prematurely born HIV-1–infected infant, as is true for any premature infant, is at high risk for developing the well described perinatal CNS complications of the preterm infant, that often result in neurological deficits. Some of these conditions include the following (144):

Hypoxic-ischemic encephalopathy
Periventricular leukomalacia
Intracranial hemorrhage (intraventricular, intraparenchymal)
Hydrocephalus
CNS infections caused by common and opportunistic pathogens
CNS "problems" related to systemic conditions e.g. bronchopulmonary dysplasia
     etc

The question of whether *in utero* exposure to HIV-1 has a deleterious effect on the neurological status of the uninfected infant was recently addressed in a prospective longitudinal study. Results suggest that maternal HIV-1 infection during gestation, per se, does not adversely affect the neurological outcome of the infant, if the infant is not infected. The neurological and developmental status of "seroreverters" between ages 3-24 months was found to be no different from their controls (HIV-1 negative infants born to HIV-1 negative women) (12,102). Although some of the infants were found to have neurological and neurodevelopmental abnormalities, these were present in both seroreverters and controls. Not surprisingly they were often associated with "high risk" maternal conditions discussed in this above.

Psychosocial Factors

Infants and Children. Neurobehavioral and neurological function of infants and children with HIV-1 infection may also be affected by coexisting psychosocial stressors that occur with significant frequency in this population and that at times, are both confounding and compounding. Some of these conditions are connected to HIV-1 infection (e.g. death of an HIV-1–infected parent or sibling), whereas others are not. During infancy and early childhood the HIV-1–infected child's development may be adversely affected by a myriad of complex psychosocial stressors, including unstable family units, poverty, maternal illness, death of parents and siblings, changing caretakers, impoverished environments, chronic illnesses, frequent hospitalizations, poor or no school attendance, and painful and unpleasant medical procedures and experiences.

Older Children and Adolescents. Additional psychosocial stressors which may impact upon the older child and teenager (as in children with other chronic illnesses) include, but are not limited to, poor self-esteem and body image, unresolved issues of sexuality, and struggles with issues related to death and dying. Moreover, the child with HIV-1 infection must contend with the societal stigmata associated with HIV-1 infection and AIDS, itself.

Disorders Related to Underlying Illness: Transfusion-Acquired HIV-1 Infection

Children with transfusion-acquired HIV-1 infection may have coexisting nervous system disorders that predate HIV-1 infection, and are related to the underlying disease or, therapies for the disease, that necessitated the transfusion of blood or blood products in the first place (e.g., hemophilia, other blood dyscrasias, cancer, sick neonates) (5,7,146). (Fortunately, since 1985, with the advent of blood and blood product testing, new cases of transfusion acquired HIV-1 are virtually nonexistent in the United States.)

HIV-1–ASSOCIATED CNS DISEASE

Terminology and Definitions

The pediatric AIDS literature contains many terms pertaining to neurological dysfunction associated with HIV-1 infection. At times these terms are used without accompanying descriptors. This has led to much ambiguity because there is a lack of clarity about what deficits, impairments or disabilities the particular child or cohort of children actually had.

A consensus report on nomenclature suggested that the term HIV–associated PE of childhood replace the various terms found in the literature (1). The well described late manifestations were enumerated (Table 3). However, early manifestations, rate of CNS disease progression, and stage of CNS disease were not delineated nor defined.

Initially, a progressive encephalopathy was described, as was more stable neurological impairments. As children were followed longitudinally several patterns of disease were recognized. Based on progression and severity of neurological deficits,

TABLE 3. *HIV-1–associated progressive encephalopathy of childhood*

Probable (must have each of the following):
1. Evidence for systemic HIV-1 infection:
    a. Infants and children <15 months
        i. Virus in blood or tissues, or
        ii. Presence of HIV-1 antibody *and* evidence of cellular and humoral immune deficiency *or* other conditions meeting CDC case definition for AIDS
    b. Children ≥15 months
        i. Antibody or virus in blood or tissues
2. At least one of the following progressive findings present at least 2 months:
    a. Failure to attain or loss of developmental milestones or loss of intellectual ability, verified by standard developmental scale or neuropsychological tests
    b. Impaired brain growth (acquired microcephaly or brain atrophy demonstrated on serial CT or MRI)
    c. Acquired symmetric motor deficits manifested by two or more of the following: paresis, abnormal tone, pathologic reflexes, ataxia, or gait disturbance
3. Evidence of another etiology, including active CNS opportunistic infection or malignancy, must be sought from history, physical examination, and appropriate laboratory and radiologic investigation (e.g., lumbar puncture, neuroimaging). If another potential etiology is present, it is not thought to be the cause of the above cognitive/motor/behavioral/developmental symptoms and signs.
Possible (must have one of the following):
1. Other potential etiology present (must have each of the following):
    a. As above (see *Probable* 1 and 2)
    b. Other potential etiology is present but the cause of 2 is uncertain
2. Incomplete clinical evaluation (must have each of the following):
    a. As above (see *Probable* 1 and 2)
    b. Etiology cannot be determined (appropriate laboratory or radiologic investigations not performed)

From American Academy of Neurology AIDS Task Force. Nomenclature and research case definitions for neurologic manifestations of human immunodeficiency virus type 1. *Neurology* 1991;41:778–785; with permission.

the terms "subacute progressive," "plateau" (with improvement; with deterioration), and "static/stable" were introduced to allow further clinical characterization (9). However during the past several years, continued observations of children in both clinical and research settings suggested that the spectrum and diversity of "HIV-1 encephalopathy" is much wider than previously appreciated. The term HIV-1–associated CNS disease syndromes, as used herein refers to the CNS disorders (including PE) with a constellation of cognitive, motor, and behavioral manifestations currently believed to be related to the CNS effects of HIV-1. It is anticipated that in the future more precise classification and definitions will evolve as clinical features are further delineated and correlated with underlying neuropathophysiological processes.

HIV-1–ASSOCIATED CNS DISEASE SYNDROMES

Clinical Manifestations

The most frequent signs of HIV-1–associated CNS disease are cognitive impairment (developmental delays), poor brain growth, and abnormalities of tone and motor function (9,15,55,65) . Movement disorders (rigidity, opisthotonic posturing) may develop and are usually superimposed upon spasticity. Cerebellar signs also may occur. Symptoms and signs of myelopathy are uncommon (127). Mood and behavioral problems may manifest with progressive disease (9,24,25,100).

Patterns of Disease

Considerable clinical variability is noted with regard to age of onset of clinically apparent disease, domains of function most affected, and rate and pattern of disease progression (6,7,9,13,14).

The rate of neurological deterioration, domains of function most affected, and severity of neurological deficits vary among patient subsets (9,14). Neurological deterioration in some infants and young children will be rapidly progressive. Within a few months they develop severe and progressive CNS dysfunction resulting in quadriparesis and mental deficiency. Others have progressive and disabling motor deficits with relatively stable socially adaptive skills and cognitive function. Other children have more cognitive than motor impairment, whereas still others, will have relatively minor and stable motor and cognitive findings (6,7). Moreover, an individual child may have progressive neurological deterioration that occurs over a period of months followed by a relatively stable period, which then may or may not be followed then by further deterioration (see refs. 7 and 15 and Fig. 1).

Age of Onset and Patterns of Neurological Disease

Because of the considerable clinical diversity we have adapted a classification based on (a) age of onset of clinically apparent disease, (b) domains of function most affected and severity of deficits, and (c) rate and pattern of disease progression (13, 14).

Neonates

The vast majority of congenitally HIV-1–infected neonates are clinically well at birth and are indistinguishable from uninfected newborns. Clinically recognizable neurological features of HIV-1–associated CNS disease are exceedingly rare in newborns. Review of the literature reveals single case reports of neonatal neurological dysfunction ascribed to HIV-1 (131,139).

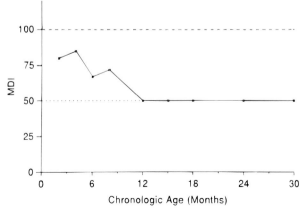

FIG. 1. Psychometric evaluations (Bayley Scales of Infant Development [BSID]) show decline in Mental Developmental Index (MDI) (note scores <50 are not defined on the BSID).

However, some HIV-1–infected neonates do have neurological problems due to comorbid conditions associated with disorders of the pre-term infant, *in utero* exposure to drugs, or congenital, or acquired infections, (see above, Coexisting Conditions: Antenatal/Perinatal complications).

Infants

The most severe and devastating syndrome is HIV-1–associated progressive encephalopathy (PE), severe infantile form. Age of onset is usually in the first year of life (3-8 months of age) but may begin in the second year. Neurological deterioration results in spastic quadriparesis and mental deficiency. Characteristic features are: (a) progressive corticospinal tract (CST) signs with (b) concomitant loss of previously acquired motor milestones, or markedly deviant rate of acquiring motor skills, (c) acquired microcephaly, and (d) marked "delays" in mental development. Opisthotonic posturing and rigidity may develop, and are usually superimposed upon spasticity. Pseudobulbar signs may also develop and feeding difficulties are frequent. The children develop a characteristic "mask-like" facial appearance (8,9). They appear alert and wide-eyed but have a paucity of spontaneous facial expression (manifestations of the basal ganglia and subcortical pathology). Despite these features, there is little facial weakness evidenced by full movement when crying. The child is hypophonic with decreased vocalizations, both spontaneous and responsive. Serial head circumference measurements document poor brain growth (acquired microcephaly).

As the CNS disease progresses, play deteriorates, and previously acquired language skills and/or adaptive skills are lost. The end stage picture is an apathetic, withdrawn quadriparetic child who has markedly impaired higher cortical function (9,15,64,65).

The rate of neurological deterioration in this subacute PE, may be slowly progressive with an insidious decline. Some patients experience rapid deterioration (over weeks), whereas others will have an episodic course. Periods of deterioration interrupted by periods of relative neurological stability (see Fig. 1 and ref. 15).

Psychometric measures document a decline in the composite cognitive score [e.g. Mental Developmental Index (MDI) of the Bayley Scales of Infant Development (BSID)]. The Mental Developmental Age (MDA) may remain stable (no or little gain in "raw" score) (Fig. 2A). With advanced disease it may actually decline (9) (Fig. 2B).

A less severe and more indolent neurological course may also occur in the first two years of life. This had been termed "plateau" (9). Motor involvement is common, but rate of progression and severity of deficits differ among subsets of patients. Some infants and young children are hypotonic and have delays in attaining motor milestones. For example, some children will not be able to sit unsupported until age 12 months and not walk independently until age 24 months (most neurologically normal infants sit by age 6 months and walk by age 12 months). Mental development may also be delayed and concomitant expressive language delays and deficiencies are common (9,13,14,15,45,64,151).

Some of these children will with time develop a diparesis-type syndrome. Other children will have further neurological deterioration and develop a progressive paraparesis-type syndrome (6,7,9). Other children remain stable.

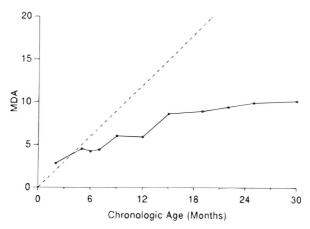

FIG. 2. Serial psychometric evaluations (BSID expressed as equivalent Mental Developmental Age [MDA]) in a child who was born at term to a mother with heterosexually acquired HIV-1 infection. Neurological assessments were normal until age 4 months. At 5 months of age there was mild axial hypotonia. At 6 months of age she had stopped vocalizing, lost head control, and was hypotonic and hyperreflexic. Examination at 1 year of age showed acquired microcephaly and spastic quadriparesis. Note she continues to acquire "skills," but the rate deviates markedly from the norm.

Toddlers and Young Children

In toddlers or young children, early signs of motor involvement include a change of gait. Children begin to toe walk, and develop increased tone and hyperreflexia in the lower extremities (6). Rate of progression and severity of deficits vary. In some children independent ambulation is maintained for years. They have a mildly spastic gait, or hyperreflexia and clumsiness, often associated with impairment of fine motor ability (14). In others, progression is more rapid and they require orthotics to maintain independent ambulation. Severity in some children is more marked and they become wheel chair bound within months. Some children progress to quadriparesis (Fig. 3) (9,14). Poor brain growth can usually be documented in the younger patients by serial head circumference measurements, and some children will develop acquired microcephaly (9,15,64,65).

Cognitive impairment is usual, although degree of impairment may range from "borderline" intelligence, to mild or moderate retardation. Cognitive problems become evident as the rate of mental development declines and deviates from the norm. Over time, although the child gains further cognitive, language, and socially adaptive skills, the rate of acquisition of these new skills deviates from the norm (Fig. 4), and in some cases from the child's previous rate of developmental progress (9). Serial psychometric evaluations show a decline in the composite cognitive score. The MDA, which reflects the "raw" scores, may gradually increase. There is an incremental rise over time, but the slope of the curve clearly deviates from the norm (see Fig. 4) (6). Less commonly, the MDA will remain the same for a period of months. Loss of milestones and previously acquired abilities is not observed.

A subset of these children who had a prolonged stable course will ultimately develop further neurological deterioration: plateau followed by further deterioration. The course then becomes similar to that of subacute PE (9). In contrast, other children

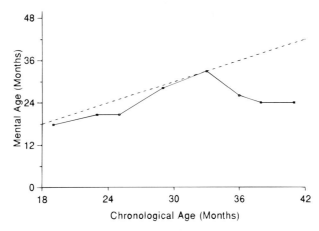

FIG. 3. Serial psychometric evaluation, expressed as mental developmental age, on another child who was born at term (birth weight 7 lb 1 oz) to a mother with transfusion-acquired HIV-1 infection. Neurological examinations during the first year of life showed hypotonia and delayed acquisition of motor skills. She walked independently at 26 months of age. Mental development was normal. At 30 months of age there was a change in gait; by 34 months of age she was no longer ambulating; and by 36 months of age she was quadriplegic and cognitive decline was apparent.

show improvement. They steadily acquire additional developmental skills, and their rate of acquisition of new skills accelerates compared to their previous performance. This course then is stable or static (9).

It is noteworthy that we have now followed some children from birth in our prospective studies who had marked delays in motor and mental development. They did not have *in utero* exposure to drugs or any of the other confounding conditions described above. They continued to acquire milestones and skills although the rate and quality deviated from the norm (10,12,14). This suggests that HIV-1 may com-

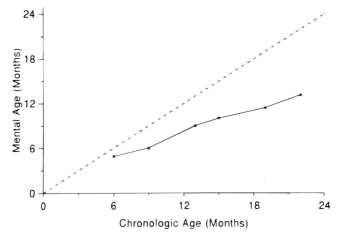

FIG. 4. Psychometric evaluations (expressed as equivalent Mental Developmental Age) of a child born to a mother with heterosexually acquired HIV-1 infection. Note that he steadily acquires new "skills," although the rate (and quality) deviate from the norm.

promise the normal developmental process and result in a stable/static encephalopathy.

School Age Children

Cognitive decline, loss of interest in school performance, social withdrawal, emotional lability, decreased attention and psychomotor slowing are reported as signs of HIV-1–associated PE (6,9,11,24,92). With advancing disease, psychometric tests show a decline in composite IQ score (see ref. 9). Motor involvement of varying severity is common. There is usually hyperreflexia, with or without increased extensor tone in the lower extremities. Clumsy and poor fine motor ability and coordination are often noted. Progressive long tract signs, movement disorders, cerebellar signs, and myelopathy also may develop. In the advanced stages of CNS disease the child has cognitive impairment, and at end stage is apathetic and abulic (11).

The term static encephalopathy was used by our group in the early years of the AIDS epidemic to describe a group youngsters who had (a) varying degrees of cognitive and/or motor impairment, (b) histories of developmental abnormalities (delays in acquisition of language and motor milestones), and (c) no history of loss of milestones or progressive neurological deficits (9,15,62,141). Longitudinal follow-up documented a pattern of continued but impaired development. Developmental and intelligence quotients ranged from low average or borderline to retarded. These scores remained relatively stable during the study period (9,24,88,137,90,141). The children acquired new skills and abilities at a rate fairly consistent with their level of functioning at initial evaluation. Motor dysfunction was also common. The most frequent findings were hyperreflexia, increased tone in the lower extremities, and poor fine motor skills and coordination. Some children had a mildly spastic gait. This pattern was in direct contrast to the deteriorating neurological pattern of PE. It still remains unclear what role, if any, HIV-1 plays in this syndrome. It is possible that abnormalities are related to concurrent or previous effects of HIV-1 CNS disease. However, confounding uncontrolled factors have made interpretation and analysis difficult (24). Continued follow up of children who were enrolled as infants in controlled studies as described earlier should help clarify this question.

Adolescents

It is as yet unknown whether HIV-1–associated CNS disease manifestations in adolescents differs in early signs and progression from that of adults or of children, although it is anticipated that manifestations will be similar to adults.

Neurobehavioral and Cognitive Profiles of HIV-1–Infected Children

The declining pattern of neuropsychological function as assessed by serial psychometric and neurodevelopmental measures in infants and children with HIV-1–associated CNS disease are described earlier. The question of early signs of HIV-1 related neuropsychological impairment and domains affected remains unanswered. Several domains of cognitive function have been reported to be affected in children with symptomatic HIV-1 infection who did not have overt clinical evidence of PE and who functioned in the borderline, low, or average range of cognitive ability (24,45,51,77,136,151). These include relative deficits in attention, perceptual motor function, and expressive language and memory. Mood and affective disorders are noted as well.

Attention

In adults, attentional problems are reported as an early manifestation of HIV-1–associated dementia. The *new* onset of difficulties with attention have also been described in some children who developed PE. Therefore, attentional problems may indeed be an early behavioral manifestation of HIV-1–associated CNS disease. However, the problem that confronts clinicians is that although attention deficit disorders (ADD) and attention deficit hyperactivity disorders (ADHD) occur with significant frequency in children with HIV-1 infection, the prevalence of ADHD is relatively high in the general population, particularly in children with *in utero* exposure to drugs and alcohol, those who are born prematurely, and those who have strong family histories of ADHD (24). Recent well-designed studies of HIV-1–infected children, HIV-1 seroreverters, and controls have shown a high rate of ADHD and other disruptive behavior disorders in all three groups, suggesting to the investigators that genetic and/or background factors common to this high-risk group of children may be important factors (4,78). Thus, it is not yet certain if ADD/ADHD, as such, should be attributed to HIV-1 CNS disease unless it is of recent onset.

Visual-Spatial and Organization Skills

Selective deficits in visual-spatial and organizational skills in HIV-1–infected children with "normal" composite IQ scores are reported from several different studies. Cohen et al. studied a cohort of asymptomatic and mildly symptomatic HIV-1–infected children who acquired infection via blood transfusions as neonates (44). Overall IQ test scores did not differ between the cohort and the HIV-1 seronegative control group. However, the investigators reported small but consistently significant differences in motor speed, visual scanning, and cognitive flexibility. This is in agreement with the earlier studies of Diamond and colleagues, and more recently Tardieu et al., in vertically HIV-1–infected children (51,136,146).

Language

Investigators have also noted problems with language (7,10,24,45). As described earlier, infants with PE often stop vocalizing (6,7,64), and older children who previously spoke in full sentence may regress and only speak in short phrases or single words (24).

Many children who do not have overt clinical manifestations of HIV-1–associated disease are also noted to have delayed language development and impairment of expressive language relative to receptive ability (45,151).

Havens et al. reported preliminary findings from their study of cognitive and language function in HIV-1–infected children (78). The HIV-1–infected children were relatively well and were said to have no evidence of encephalopathy. The HIV-

1–infected cohort showed deficits in short-term memory (Stanford-Binet 4th edition) relative to seroreverters and controls. There was no difference between the groups on language testing or general intelligence.

However Wolters et al. recently studied language ability in a cohort of HIV-1–infected children and their controls (non-HIV-1–infected siblings of the case cohort). The HIV-1–infected children were stratified into two groups: encephalopathic and nonencephalopathic. Expressive language impairment was noted in both groups but not their controls. Severity of language dysfunction was marked in the encephalopathic and included impairment of both expressive and receptive ability, with expressive language more affected than receptive. Correlation of neuroimaging evidence of cerebral atrophy was also noted in the encephalopathic group.

Mood and Affect

Signs and symptoms of neurobehavioral dysfunction in children with HIV-1–associated CNS were mentioned above. These include flattened affect, lack of social responsiveness, withdrawal, and declining interest in the environment. Manifestations may also include depression, mood swings, agitation, extreme impulsiveness, and new onset (or change) of attentional problems (6,7,24).

NEUROEPIDEMIOLOGY

The true incidence of pediatric HIV-1–associated CNS disease is not yet known. Information derived from the published literature is difficult to interpret because of lack of standardized definition (see terminology), differences in study populations, and difference in study design. A 23.8% prevalence is reported by Tovo et al. in their study of 433 HIV-1 perinatally infected P-2 classified children (138). Blanche and colleagues reported a 20% incidence of HIV-1 encephalopathy by 3 years of age in their cohort of patients followed prospectively from birth (20,21). In contrast, studies of children with advanced symptomatic HIV-1 infection and AIDS estimate a frequency of 31–75% (9,63,67,97).

The frequency with which HIV-1–associated PE was reported as the initial AIDS-defining illness has ranged from to 12% to 16% (105,124). This contrasts to the much lower figures reported for adults 0.8%–2.2% (17,80).

Extrapolating from the experiences of many investigators, it appears that in general HIV-1–associated CNS disease parallels progression and severity of immunodeficiency and systemic disease. However, it is also very clear that some patients will develop HIV-1–associated CNS disease as their first AIDS defining illness (6,7,8,26,48,131).

CEREBROSPINAL FLUID FINDINGS

HIV-1 has been recovered from the CSF of children with HIV-1–associated CNS disease as well as neurologically normal children. Detectable levels of HIV-1 antigen, intrathecal production of anti-HIV-1 antibodies, oligoclonal bands, and cytokines may be found in some children with PE, static encephalopathy, or neurologically normal children (21,61,72,89,97). Markers of immune activation are reported to be elevated in children with PE (IL-6, IL-1B) (24,72). The prognostic significance of these findings is unclear, and to date, data is still limited to a few cross sectional studies of small numbers of patients. However these findings indicate that the CNS is infected with HIV-1 and also verify early CNS invasion.

NEUROIMAGING FINDINGS

Computed Tomography

Computed tomographic (CT) examinations of the brain in PE usually show variable degrees of cerebral atrophy and white matter (WM) abnormalities (Figs. 5B, 5C and Table 4) (9,11,15,42,52,62). There may be bilateral symmetrical calcification of the basal ganglia (BG), and less frequently, of the frontal WM. In general, calcification of the BG is more frequently seen in younger children, and those with clinical signs of HIV-1 CNS disease, than in older children (52).

Serial studies often show progressive atrophy and WM changes (rarefaction), and in some cases, progressive calcification of the BG (Fig. 6) (7,9,11,15). However it is noteworthy that in some children serial CT studies show no change, even though poor brain growth is demonstrated by serial head circumference and serial clinical examinations show "plateau" or marked delays in mental function (with or without progressive motor findings) (147). It is also noteworthy that some neurologically normal children may have mild to moderate atrophic findings. Nevertheless, there does appear to be a strong correlation between cerebral atrophy and severity of encephalopathy, cognitive dysfunction, and aberrant behavior (25,27,41,151).

Magnetic Resonance Imaging

Magnetic resonance imaging (MRI) may reveal atrophy on T1 and T2-weighted images. T2 images may show abnormal signal intensity in the WM and deep grey structures (6,7,11,135). Tardieu et al. found MRI abnormalities of WM in 40% of HIV-1–infected children (135). Because this finding was present in both neurologically normal and symptomatic children, the investigators suggested that it may serve as a marker for CNS HIV-1 infection. Leukomalacia and cerebral atrophy were found more frequently in patients with clinical evidence of HIV-1–associated PE than in the neurologically normal cohort.

MRI is more sensitive to image WM abnormalities (Fig. 5A), maturational changes

---

TABLE 4. *Neuroimaging findings*

CT
  Cerebral atrophy: present in majority of patients serial studies often show progressive atrophy
  Basal ganglia calcification, ± frontal white matter: present in a subset of patients serial studies may show progressive 'calcification'
  White matter: white matter changes [hypodensity-rarefaction] serial studies often show progressive changes
MRI
  Cerebral atrophy: present in majority of patients serial studies often show progressive atrophy
  Basal ganglia: may show abnormal high signal [T2-weighted images] [At time when CT is "normal"] may show abnormal low signal [T2-weighted images] [at time when CT shows calcification]
  White matter: may show abnormal high signal [T2-weighted images]

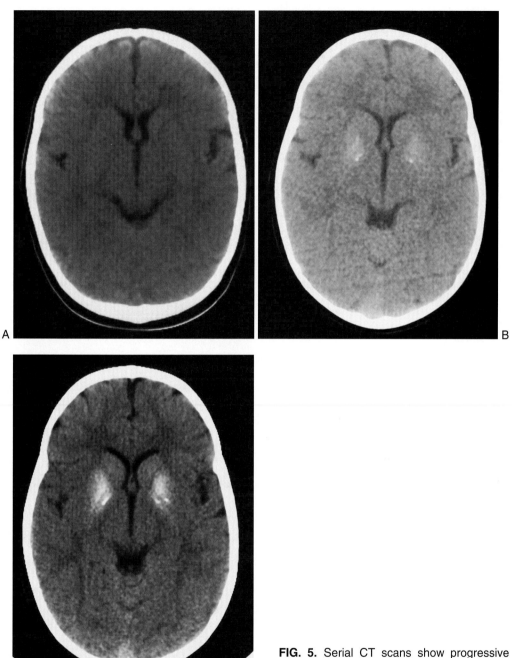

FIG. 5. Serial CT scans show progressive calcification of the BG. **A:** 4 months of age. **B:** 20 months of age. **C:** 41 months of age.

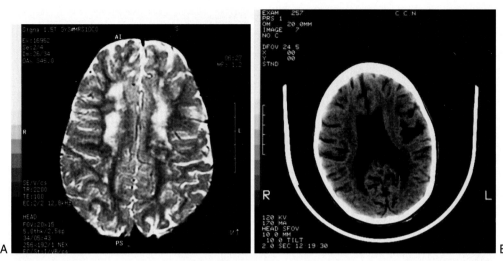

FIG. 6. A: T2-weighted MRI scan of child in Fig. 3 at 40 months of age shows marked WM abnormalities and atrophy. **B:** CT scan of the same child shows marked atrophy and WM abnormalities.

in myelination, and structural abnormalities. CT is more sensitive to detect calcification. Cerebral atrophy is well demonstrated by both techniques.

PET

In a recent study of eight children (neurologically normal:5; PE:3), diffuse hypometabolism and subcortical hypermetabolism was seen in the three children with PE, whereas temporo-occipital cortical hypometabolism was seen in the five neurologically normal children. Interestingly, Pizzo reported ''normalization'' of PET in one child after ZDV.

Magnetic Resonance Spectroscopic

Magnetic resonance spectroscopic (MRS) studies in a limited number of children suggest that there is a lower n-acetylaspartate/creatinine ratio in subcortical structures in children with encephalopathy (108).

NEUROPHYSIOLOGICAL STUDIES

Electroencephalographic studies in children with HIV-1–associated PE may show diffuse mild to moderate slowing of background rhythm. Abnormal evoked potentials including increased central latencies, (prolongation of the 1-V interwave latency) and abnormal responses to increased rate of stimulation have also been demonstrated (7,15,23,69,123,140).

NEUROPATHOLOGICAL FINDINGS

Brain

Gross neuropathological features include variable degrees of cerebral atrophy, ventricular enlargement, widening of sulci, ventricular dilation, and attenuation of deep cerebral WM (9,15,54,63,85).

Histopathological examination may reveal HIV encephalitis (28,55,63,85,143). Although this is one of the most impressive postmortem findings of HIV-1 CNS infection (30), it appears to be more frequent in adults than young children (30,88).

Calcification of the basal ganglia (BG) is the most characteristic and consistent neuropathological finding (54,63,85). In some cases mineralization is also noted in vessels of the centrum semiovale. Although this vasculopathy is frequently seen with HIV encephalitis, the association is not invariable. Many cases have BG calcification without inflammatory disease and with no sign of acute infection. Nevertheless, accompanying WM changes and gliosis are common.

HIV leukoencephalopathy is characterized by diffuse staining pallor of myelin (30). There is damage to the WM, including myelin loss, reactive astrogliosis, presence of macrophages and multinucleated giant cells, but little or no inflammatory infiltrates. This is a common finding in pediatric AIDS.

Diffuse reactive astrogliosis, as demonstrated by glial fibrillary acidic protein (GFAP) immunocytochemical staining is a frequent finding in pediatric AIDS (53,63,147).

TABLE 5. *Neuropathologic findings*

Brain
GROSS
Cerebral atrophy of variable degrees
Ventricular enlargement
Widening of sulci
Attenuation of deep cerebral WM
MICROSCOPIC
HIV-1 encephalitis
Foci of inflammatory cells, microglia, macrophages, MGC
One of the most impressive postmortem findings of CNS HIV-1 infection
More common in adults than infants and young children
HIV-1 leukoencephalopathy
Diffuse staining pallor of myelin; diffuse damage to WM; myelin loss, reactive astrogliosis; ± MGC, macrophages
Calcific vasculopathy
Mineralization walls of small vessels (± large vessels) BG; ^ WM accompanying WM changes and gliosis are common
Frequently seen with HIV encephalitis, but association not invariable. Many cases have BG calcification without inflammatory disease and with no sign of acute infection
Calcific vasculopathy of the BG most characteristic and consistent neuropathological finding in infants and children
Spinal cord
Corticospinal tract "degeneration" striking myelin pallor restricted to the corticospinal tracts
Axonopathy type
Myelinopathy type
Myelitis (more common in adults)
Vacuolar myelopathy (older children)

Spinal Cord

Unlike adults with HIV–associated myelopathy, the most common and striking pathological finding in the spinal cord of young children is myelin pallor restricted to the CST (53,54). In some cases there is both axonal and myelin pathology, suggesting that CST findings are due to axonal injury. In other cases, pathological findings are predominantly related to myelin. Because the CSTs are the last tracts to myelinate, it is hypothesized that HIV-1 in some way, directly or indirectly, affects the developmental–maturational process. Injury may occur to myelinating glial cells, newly formed myelin, or even antenatally to proliferating glial precursor cells.

Vacuolar myelopathy, a common neuropathological feature of adult HIV-1 spinal cord disease, has also been described in pediatric AIDS, but rarely, and only in older children. Myelitis has also been described, but is not a common finding (127).

NEUROPATHOPHYSIOLOGICAL CONSIDERATIONS

Localization

HIV-1 is most frequently localized in cells of bone-marrow lineage (see refs. 55 and 112 for review). These include blood-derived macrophages, intrinsic microglia, (the resident mononuclear phagocytic system of the brain), and multinucleated giant cells, formed by the fusion of these cell types (productive infection). Endothelial cell infection has also been reported, but not consistently. *In vitro* studies show that HIV-1 can infect neuronal and glial cell lines. There is also *in vivo* evidence that glia in children may also be infected (60,137); however, this may be restricted infection.

It is now well accepted that HIV-1–associated CNS disease (PE) is related to HIV-1 CNS infection. Neuropathological findings, however, often reveal little evidence of active infection or inflammation (54,143) ; there is a paucity of infected cells. Even when there is more marked pathological findings, the proportion of infected cells is small and does not always correlate well with the clinical course. These incongruities suggest that other factors besides direct cellular damage by HIV-1 may be important in pathogenesis (reviewed in refs. 60,81,113). Neuropathophysiological mechanisms are the focus of active investigation.

It is unclear whether one or several neuropathophysiological processes underlie the clinical diversity described above. It may be that different pathogenetic mechanisms account, at least in part, for different clinical expressions and patterns of pediatric HIV-1–associated CNS disease syndromes. Distinct clinical CNS syndromes may in some subsets of children reflect a continuum of the disease process, with different stages of disease progression. In others, clinical findings may reflect separate and distinct pathophysiological processes. In still other subsets of patients, these processes may coexist or interlink and may be manifested clinically by overlapping signs and symptoms. In other words, it is currently uncertain if there is one or several causes to account for the clinical diversity of HIV-1–associated CNS disease(s) syndromes (described earlier). However, to this investigator, it seems most likely that different neuropathophysiological mechanisms account, at least in part, for the different clinical expressions of this syndrome complex.

The frequent finding of basal ganglia calcification suggests a hematogenous route consistent with early CNS infection. It also points to the vulnerability of this immature vasculature, and perhaps to selective tropism for the basal ganglia (and other subcortical structures) and its resident microglial (88).

Cerebral atrophy is a common finding in both adults and children. Recent quantitative and morphometric studies in adults have identified loss of neurons with a frontal and temporal predominance, and loss of dendritic arborizations (reviewed in ref. 113) (83,94,148,149). Similar studies have not been performed in pediatric AIDS. However, it is tempting to speculate that comparable abnormalities in some subsets of children result in poor brain growth and development of acquired microcephaly. Interference with synaptogenesis could explain in part developmental ''delays'' and cognitive impairment. Astrogliosis, an extremely common finding in pediatric AIDS, is also noted in the simian immune deficiency virus model. Of note, is a recent report showing the correlation between this pathological finding and functional impairment in juvenile macaques.

Developmental–Maturational Considerations

Issues concerning neuropathophysiological mechanisms and clinicopathological correlations are germane to the understanding of HIV-1–associated CNS disease in adults and children. However, the study of pediatric HIV-1–associated CNS disease syndromes becomes even more complex because developmental–maturational issues must also be considered.

Adult HIV-1 CNS infection and disease occurs in mature, fully developed, and completely myelinated nervous systems. The immune system and CNS elements of the mononuclear phagocyte system (intrinsic microglia) are also fully developed. Vertically transmitted HIV-1 infection occurs in an immature evolving organism. It is believed that HIV-1 invades the CNS early in the course of infection. However, maternal-infant transmission may occur during gestation in some patients, whereas in others, infection may occur during the perinatal period. The time of fetal infection (i.e. perinatal versus during gestation, and which trimester [early, mid, late?] is likely to be an extremely important factor. The developmental stage of the nervous and immune system when exposed to the direct or indirect effects of the virus must be considered. Innumerable dynamic interactions occur between these two systems during development, which will interact in complex ways with HIV-1 variables. The maturational stage of CNS development when exposed to the virus will also vary, and this is likely to manifest as different patterns of HIV-1 CNS disease (7).

Thymic abnormalities in some fetuses of HIV-1–infected women suggest that an interaction between the virus and the developing fetal immune system may account for the early and severe immune deficiency and profound CNS disease observed in 15-25% of congenitally infected HIV-1 infants. The pathophysiological mechanism is as yet unclear; both induction of an immune deficiency *in utero* and a state of immune tolerance have been proposed (55,104).

A large number of peripheral and tissue-based immunocytes are chronically infected with HIV-1 persisting as stationary cell intermediate from which HIV may be induced. HIV-1–infected macrophages are also infected with high frequency in brain, spinal cord, lymphatic tissue, and lung, and it is hypothesized that this may parallel organ-specific manifestations of HIV-1 disease. It is unknown whether overall virus burden in peripheral blood reflects the level of compartmentalization of HIV-1 in tissues and whether differences in relative tissue distribution of the retrovirus may contribute to differences in the clinical outcome. It is possible that the subsequent disease course may be determined in part by tissue distribution, maturity of CD4 cells and bone marrow-derived myelomonocytic cells in the immature host (112). Additional factors including differential timing of infection, strain of virus, and increased sequence diversity along with the high mutation rate of specific HIV-1 genes, may allow the virus to evade immune surveillance and persist within the host. Emergence of genotypic variants with altered biological activity such as increased replication rate and cytopathogenicity may also increase the pathogenicity of the virus (33,46,113,118).

It is also necessary to remember that we are dealing with two different trajectories: (a) the developing brain and (b) a progressive neurological disease. During the designated time period of a particular study or observational period, it is not always clinically apparent (a) if the rate of CNS maturation and development is exceeding the slower rate of the ongoing disease process(es), (b) if the disease process is quiescent, or (c) if the disease process has been abated or arrested by therapeutic interventions. Currently there are few prognostic indicators to predict rapidity and severity of CNS disease.

THERAPY

Clinical trials in progress are investigating various antiretroviral agents, different dosage regimens, combination therapies, and immunomodulating agents. New targets for therapy are in investigation and new protocols are in development. In parallel are rehabilitation programs, including infant stimulation programs, therapeutic nursery schools, and special educational classes, as well as physical and occupational therapy programs and management of pain.

Antiretroviral Therapy

Drugs that treat HIV-1 infection attempt to interfere with the replication of HIV. Targeted points in the growth cycle of the virus include: blockage of viral entry (soluble CD4- preparations); prevention of transcription of RNA to DNA (reverse transcriptase inhibitors); interference with translation (drugs acting on regulatory genes or their proteins); and inhibition of assembly (protease inhibitors) and release of virus (interferon) (reviewed in ref 112).

In this country, clinical trials with antiretroviral agents have been performed largely by the AIDS Clinical Trials Group of the National Institutes of Health and the National Cancer Institute. There is still limited published data concerning antiretroviral therapy of children with HIV-1 infection. In clinical trials, children treated with ZDV had improvement in weight gain and growth, stabilization of CD4 counts, a reduction in serum and CSF p24 antigen levels, decrease in immunoglobulin levels, and improvement or stabilization of cognitive function (21,26,110). At the present time, the number of therapeutic agents available for the treatment HIV-1 infection and its complications is limited. ZDV and dideoxyinosine (DDI) are the only antiretroviral agents approved by the FDA for treatment of HIV infection in children <13 years of age. The optimal time to initiate antiretroviral therapy in children is unknown. Currently antiretroviral therapy is recommended for children who either have evidence of significant immunodeficiency or who have defined HIV–associated symptoms (112). It is recommended that initial therapy should begin with DDI alone or DDI in combination with ZDV (although toxicity of combination therapy may be greater than monotherapy).

Antiretroviral agents clearly offer promising therapeutic interventions (26,35,46,

52,96,109,110). Improvement of cognition and mood, decrease of CT evidence of brain atrophy, improvement of auditory brain stem responses, and immunological parameters have been documented. Both cognitive and behavioral function gains were noted in many children who received ZDV via continuous parenteral infusion. Intermittent orally administered antiretroviral agents have been efficacious in some children (although improvements were less dramatic than with continuous dosing) (25). With each of these agents, on an individual basis, some patients have shown improvement, some have remained stable, while some have continued to decline. Unfortunately, some children after an initial favorable response to antiretroviral agents, relapse and develop progressive clinical and neuroimaging signs of HIV-1–associated CNS disease (97,103).

DIAGNOSIS

The evaluation of the HIV-1–infected child with neurological involvement requires the clinical skills and major diagnostic tools of the neurologist. The approach to the diagnosis of HIV-1–associated CNS disease, including differential diagnosis (secondary complications, comorbid complications), involves a careful medical and developmental history, HIV-1 systemic disease history, current immunological status, neurological examination, psychological assessment, and neuroimaging studies (6,7).

The diagnosis of HIV-1–associated PE is relatively straight forward if the patient has been followed prospectively. Longitudinal assessments of the infant or child will show progressive involvement. The infant may stop vocalizing, lose head control, develop axial hypotonia and upper motor neuron signs. The toddler or older child may have a change in gait, become hyperreflexic, refuse to walk, and over time develop progressive CST signs, or less frequently, ataxia. Concomitant cognitive problems with a relative ''plateau'' or decline in psychometric test scores may also be documented.

The diagnosis is also fairly straight forward if the child, on initial examination, is found to have motor deficits (spasticity, ataxia, weakness, abnormalities of tone, change in gait, etc.), and a careful history can document either the new onset or progression of motor impairment (again, when other causes for progressive motor dysfunction have been excluded). Confirmation of progression can at times be obtained by review of family photographs of the child.

However, diagnostic difficulties arise when an HIV-1–infected youngster, who was not followed from birth or infancy by the examiner, is found at the initial neurological evaluation to have neurological deficits or delays. Because the frequency of neurological and developmental impairment in this population is high, it is often impossible for the clinician to ascribe these findings to HIV-1–associated CNS disease rather than to possible comorbid conditions. A careful history is paramount. If there are no other risk factors, the diagnosis is likely. The child should have a formal psychological assessment and be reevaluated by the neurologist and psychologist in 2–4 months.

Neuroimaging studies are extremely helpful and in fact are critical. If calcification of BG, is present, it is probable that the child has HIV-1–associated CNS disease. If cerebral atrophy is present in the absence of documented perinatal complications, steroid use, or other known causes of atrophy, the diagnosis becomes extremely likely. Follow-up neuroimaging studies should be requested in addition to the above mentioned serial neurological and psychological evaluations.

Head circumference measurements are also helpful. It has been our experience that a careful review of medical records will document at least one or two past head circumference measurements. This allows the examiner to plot serial measurements. The pattern of downward deviation and crossing percentiles makes the diagnosis of HIV-1–associated CNS disease likely. This is especially true if acquired microcephaly is documented. Thus, neuroimaging evidence of atrophy accompanied by acquired microcephaly clearly strengthens the diagnosis.

PERIPHERAL NERVOUS SYSTEM INVOLVEMENT

Although peripheral nervous system (PNS) involvement is well-documented in adult patients with HIV-1 infection, there is little information concerning PNS complications in infants and children other than anecdotal reports (7,115). We and others have followed some infants and young nonverbal children who became marked more irritable and distressed when their lower extremities were lightly touched, increasing the possibility of painful dysethesias of neuropathic origin. We have also followed a few children who developed a mononeuritis multiplex type syndrome that was transient and reminiscent of HIV-1–associated neuropathy described in adults (M. Kaufman, unpublished information).

It remains unclear if HIV-1–associated and/or CMV associated neuropathies are indeed rare in infants and children or if these conditions go undiagnosed because symptoms are not verbalized by these young and often very ill patients. Peripheral nervous system toxicity in association with antiretroviral therapy has also been noted in children.

SECONDARY CNS COMPLICATIONS

The common denominator of HIV-1 infection is the development of profound immunosuppression. The patient becomes susceptible to a variety of infections. Neoplasms (mainly lymphoma) may also develop. Strokes may also complicate the course of HIV-1 infection in infants and children, and in general, are related to infection or other AIDS–associated illnesses. In one longitudinal series, secondary CNS complications occurred in ~18% of patients (9). The infants and children often had more than one complication, and the majority of children had coexisting or subsequently developed HIV-1–associated CNS disease.

Secondary CNS complications must be considered in the differential diagnosis of the child with HIV-1 infection who presents with the new onset of neurological deficits, headache, seizures, or mental status changes.

CNS Infections

Infants and children with HIV-1 infection are at risk for CNS infections caused by the usual childhood pathogens as well as OIs (reviewed in refs. 18 and 113). Congenital CNS infections (toxoplasmosis, CMV) have also been reported in infants with vertically transmitted HIV-1 infection, although not frequently (98,126,134).

Syphilis in women of child bearing age appears to be on the rise, and as such must also be considered in infants. The most frequent OIs reported are CMV encephalitis *Candida albicans* meningitis, and microabscesses (15,19,59,95). Measles encephalitis has also recently been described as a complicator (26).

In adults most CNS OIs are due to reactivation of previously acquired infection (e.g. toxoplasmosis, CMV, herpes simplex virus, and JC virus infection). Therefore, reactivation of latent agents would not be expected in infants and young children; indeed, CNS OI's are uncommon. However, due to more aggressive medical management as well as antiretroviral and immunomodulating therapy, children with HIV-1 infection and AIDS are living longer. Infections common in HIV–infected adults (see CNS infections) can now be anticipated to occur in older children and adolescents. In fact, progressive multifocal leukoencephalopathy, a rare CNS disease in children, has now been reported in three HIV-1–infected children (16,142).

Neoplasms

Primary CNS lymphoma and systemic lymphoma metastatic to the CNS may occur in HIV-1–infected children (9,59,106). Presenting signs of lymphoma include the new onset of focal neurological deficits, seizures, and/or a change in mental status. Neurological deterioration at times may be rapidly progressive and fulminant (48,85,117). Computed tomography characteristics of lymphoma include (a) hyperdense or isodense mass lesions with variable contrast enhancement; (b) diffusely infiltrating contrast enhancing lesions; and (c) periventricular contrasting lesions. Reduction in tumor size has been noted in some patients after radiation therapy; however, long- term survival rates have not been affected (74).

Strokes

Cerebrovascular accidents may also complicate the course of HIV-1 infection in children. Both hemorrhagic and nonhemorrhagic strokes have been described (9,68,74,87,106). Intracerebral hemorrhage usually occurs in the setting of immune-mediated thrombocytopenia. Clinical presentation is variable, reflecting the severity and location of the hemorrhage. Hemorrhage into tumor may also occur. Strokes may be catastrophic and fatal or clinically silent evennts. Nonhemorrhagic infarctions are most often associated with pathological changes of cerebral blood vessels, meningeal infections, or cardiomyopathy.

The clinical presentation of stroke includes the new onset of focal neurological deficits, most commonly hemiparesis, with or without seizures.

SUMMARY

It is now well recognized that HIV-1–associated CNS disease may complicate the course of HIV-1 infection and AIDS in infants and children. Neurological dysfunction in these young patients adds significantly to the morbidity of the disease and is often a devastating complication (7). Neurological complications secondary to immunosuppression or other AIDS-related conditions may also occur, as may complications due to therapy and comorbid conditions.

Vertically transmitted HIV-1 infection occurs in an immature developing organism. The maturational stage of the nervous and immune system when exposed to the direct or indirect affects of the virus is likely to be of utmost importance. Innumerable dynamic interactions occur between these two systems during development, and these undoubtedly interact in complex ways with HIV-1 variables. In order to care for these children and to design rational approaches for treatment and prevention, it is now critical to develop a better understanding of how HIV-1 effects the developing nervous system (7).

REFERENCES

1. American Academy of Neurology AIDS Task Force. Nomenclature and research case definitions for neurological manifestations of human immunodeficiency virus type 1. *Neurology* 1991;41:778–785.
2. Ammann AJ, Cowan M, Wara DW, et al. Acquired immunodeficiency in an infant: possible transmission by means of blood products. *Lancet* 1983;1:956–958.
3. Auger I, Thomas P, De Gruttola V, et al. Incubation periods for paediatric AIDS patients. *Nature* 1988;336:575–577.
4. Aylward EH, Butz AM, Hutton N, et al. Cognitive and motor development in infants at risk for human immunodeficiency virus. *Am J Dis Child* 1992;146:218–222.
5. Bales JF, Constant CF, Garg B, Tilton A, Kaufman DM, Wasiewski. Neurological history and examination results and their relationship to human immunodeficiency virus type I serostatus in hemophilic subjects: result from the hemophilia growth and development study. *Pediatrics* 1993; 91:736–741.
6. Belman AL. AIDS and the child's central nervous system. *Ped Clin of North Am* 1992:39;691–714.
7. Belman AL. AIDS and pediatric neurology. *Neurological Clinics* 1990;8:571–603.
8. Belman AL, Calvelli T, Nozyce M, et al. Neurological and immunological correlates in infants with vertically transmitted HIV infection. *Neurology* 1990;40(1):409.
9. Belman AL, Diamond G, Dickson D, et al. Pediatric AIDS: neurological syndromes. *Am J Dis Child* 1988;142:29–35.
10. Belman AL, Diamond G, Park Y, et al. Perinatal HIV infection: a prospective longitudinal study of the initial CNS signs. *Neurology* 1989;39[suppl] 8–279.
11. Belman AL, Lantos G, Horoupian D, et al. AIDS: calcification of the basal ganglia in infants and children. *Neurology* 1986;36:1192–1199.
12. Belman AL, Marcus J, Muenz L, Durako S, Willoughby A. Neurological status of infants born to HIV-I–infected mothers and their controls: a prospective study from birth to 24 months of age. *Neurology* (Abstract) 1993.
13. Belman AL, Preston T, Milazzo M. HIV-1–associated CNS disease syndromes in infants and children: a proposal for "working" research case definitions according to age. *Journal of Neuro-AIDS* 1994 (in press).
14. Belman AL, Taylor FL, Nachman S, Milazzo M. HIV-1–associated CNS disease syndromes in infants and children. *Neurology* 1994;44[suppl 2]:A168.
15. Belman AL, Ultmann MH, Horoupian D, et al. Neurological complications in infants and children with acquired immune deficiency syndrome. *Ann Neurol* 1985;18:560–566.
16. Berger J, Albrecht J, Belman AL, et al. Progressive multifocal leukoencephalopathy in children with HIV infection. *AIDS* 1992;6:837–841 .
17. Berger JR, Moskowitz L, Fischl M, Kelley RE. Neurological disease as the presenting manifestation of acquired immunodeficiency syndrome. *Southern Medical Journal* 1987;80:683–686.
18. Bernstein LJ, Ochs HD, Wedgewood RJ, Rubinstein A. Defective humoral immunity in pediatric acquired immunodeficiency syndrome. *J Pediatr* 1985;107:352–357.
19. Biggemann B, Voit T, Neuen E, et al. Neurological manifestations in three German children with AIDS. *Hippokrates* 1987;1:99–106.
20. Blanche S, Mayaux MJ, Rouzioux C, et al. Relation of the course of HIV infection in children to the severity of the disease in their mothers at delivery. *N Engl J Med* 1994;330:308–312.
21. Blanche S, Tardieu M, Duliege AM, et al. Longitudinal study of 94 symptomatic infants with materno fetal HIV infection: evidence for a bimodal expression of clinical and biological symptoms. *Am J Dis Child* 1990;144:1210–1215.
22. Boyer PJ, Dillon M, Navaie M, et al. Factors predictive of maternal-fetal transmission of HIV-1: preliminary analysis of zidovudine given during pregnancy and/or delivery. *JAMA* 1994; 271: 1925–1930.
23. Brivio L, Tornaghi R, Musetti L, Marchisio P, Principi N. Improvement of auditory brainstem responses after treatment with zidovudine in a child with AIDS. *Pediatr Neurol* 1991;7(1):53–55.

24. Brouwers E, Belman AL, Epstein L. Central nervous system involvement: manifestations and evaluation. In: Pizzo PA, Wilfert CM, eds. *Pediatric AIDS: The challenge of HIV Infection in Infants, Children and Adolescents*, 2nd Edition. New York: Williams & Wilkins, 1994:433–455.
25. Brouwers P, DeCarli C, Civitello AL. Correlation between CT Brain scan abnormalities and neuropsychological function in children with symptomatic HIV diesease. *Arch Neurol* 1995; 52:39–44.
26. Brouwers P, Moss H, Wolters P, et al. Effect of continuous-infusion zidovudine therapy on neuropsychological functioning in children with symptomatic human immunodeficiency virus infection. *J Peds* 1990;117:980–985.
27. Brouwers P, Tudor-Williams G, DeCarli C, et al. Relationship between stage of disease and neuro behavioral measures in children with symptomatic disease. *AIDS* 1995; 9:713–720.
28. Brustels O, Spiegel H, Leib SL, Finn T, Stein H, Kleihues P, Wiestler. Distribution of HIV in the CNS of children with severe HIV encephalopathy. *Acad Neuropathol* 1992;84:24–31.
29. Bryson YJ, Luzariaga K, Sullivan JL, Wara DW. Proposed definitions for *in utero* versus intrapartum transmission of HIV-1. *N Engl J Med* 1992;327:1246–1247.
30. Budka H. Neuropathology of human immunodeficiency virus infection. *Brain Pathology* 1991;1: 163–175.
31. Budka H, Wiley CA, Kleihues P, et al. HIV-1–associated disease of the nervous system: review of nomenclature and proposal for neuropathology-based terminology. *Brain Pathol* 1991;1:143–152.
32. Burgard M, Mayaux MJ, Blanche S, et al. The use of viral culture and p24 antigen testing to diagnose HIV infection in neonates. *N Engl J Med* 1992;327:1192–1197.
33. Burger H, Belman AL, Grimson R, et al. Long HIV-1 incubation periods and dynamics of transmission within a family. *Lancet* 1990;336:134–136.
34. Burns DN, Landesman S, Muenz LR, et al. Cigarette smoking, premature rupture of membranes, and vertical transmission of HIV-1 among women with low CD4- levels. *J Acquir Immune Defic Syndr* 1994; 7:718–726.
35. Butler KM, Husson RM, Balis J, et al. Dideoxginosine in children with symptomatic human immunodeficiency virus infection. *N Engl J Med* 1990;324:137–144.
36. Byers B, Caldwell B, Oxtoby M. Pediatric spectrum of disease project. Survival of children with perinatal HIV infection: Evidence for two distinct populations (Abstract WS-C10-6). *Ninth International Conference on AIDS*, Berlin, June 1993.
37. CDC. U.S. Public Health Service Recommendations for Human Immunodeficiency Virus Counseling and Voluntary Testing for Pregnant Women. *MMWR* 1995;44:(No. RR-7).
38. CDC. Recommendations of the U.S. Public Health Service Task Force on the Use of Zidovudine to Reduce Perinatal Transmission of Human Immunodeficiency Virus. *MMWR* 1994:43 (No RR-11).
39. CDC. 1994 Revised classification system for human immunodeficiency virus infection in children less than 13 years of age; Official authorized addenda—human immunodeficiency virus infection codes and official guidelines for coding and reporting ICD-9-CM. *MMWR* 1994;43(No. RR-12).
40. CDC. Birth outcomes following zidovudine therapy in pregnant women. *Morbidity & Mortality Weekly Report* 1994;43(22):409,415–416.
41. Chamberlin MC. Pediatric AIDS: a longitudinal comparative MRI and CT brain imaging study. *J Child Neurol* 1993;8(2):175.
42. Chin J. Current and future dimensions of the HIV/AIDS pandemic in women and children. *Lancet* 1990; 336:221–224.
43. Chin J, Mann J. Global surveillance and forecasting of AIDS. *Bull WHO* 1989; 67:1–7.
44. Cohen SL, Mundy T, Kaarassik B, et al. Neuropsychological functioning in children with HIV-1 infection through neonatal blood transfusion. *Pediatrics* 1991;88:58–68.
45. Condini A, Axia G, Cattelan C, D'Urso MR, Lavera AM, Viero F, Zacchello F. Development of language in 18-30 month old HIV-1–infected but not ill children. *AIDS* 1991;5:735–739.
46. Connor EM, Sperling RS, Gelber R, et al. Reduction of maternal-infant transmission of human immunodeficiency virus type 1 with zidovudine treatment. *N Engl J Med* 1994;331:1173–1180.
47. D'Angelo LJ. HIV infection and AIDS in adolescents. In: Pizzo PA, Wilfert CM, eds. *Pediatric AIDS: the challenge of HIV infection in infants, children and adolescents*, 2nd edition. New York: Williams and Wilkins. 1994;71–81.
48. Davis SL, Halsted C, Levy N, Ellis W. Acquired immunodeficiency virus syndrome presenting as progressive infantile encephalopathy. *J Pediatr* 1987; 110:884–888 .
49. Delfraissy JF, Blanche S, Rouzioux C, Mayaux MJ. Perinatal HIV transmission facts and controversies. *Immunodef Rev* 1992;3:305– 327.
50. de Rossi A, Ometto L, Mammoano F, et al. Time course of antigenaemia and seroconvrsion in infants with vertically acquired HIV-1 infection. *AIDS* 1993;7:1528–1529.
51. Diamond GW, Kaufman J, Belman AL, et al. Characterization of cognitive functioning in a subgroup of children with congenital HIV infection. *Archives of Clinical Neuropsychology* 1987;2:1–6.
52. Di Carli C, Civitello AL, Brouwers P, Pizzo PA. The prevalence of computed tomographic abnormalities of the cerebrum in 100 consecutive children symptomatic with the human immune deficiency virus. *Ann Neurol* 1993;34:198–205.

53. Dickson DW, Lee SC, Hatch W, Mattiace LA, Broshan C, Lyman WD. Macrophages and Microglia in HIV-related CNS neuropathology. In: Price RW, Perry S, eds. *HIV, AIDS and the brain*. New York: Raven Press 1993;99–118.

54. Dickson DW, Belman AL, Kim TS, Horoupian D, Rubinstein A. Spinal cord pathology in pediatric acquired immunodeficiency syndrome. *Neurology* 1989;39:227–235.

55. Dickson DW, Belman AL, Park YD, et al. Central nervous system pathology in pediatric AIDS: an autopsy study. *APMIS* 1989;8[suppl]:40–57.

56. Duliege AM, Messiah A, Blanche S, et al. Natural history of HIV-1 infection in children: prognostic value of the laboratory parameters on the bimodal progression of the desease. *Pediatr Infect Dis J* 1992;11:630–635.

57. Ehrnst A, Lindgren S, Belfrage E, et al. Intrauterine and intrapartum transmission of HIV. *Lancet* 1992;339:245–246.

58. Ehrnst A, Lindgren S, Dictor M, et al. HIV in pregnant women and their offspring: evidence for late transmission. *Lancet* 1991;338:203–207.

59. Epstein LG, Dicarlo F, Joshi V, et al. Primary lymphoma of the central nervous system in children with acquired immunodeficiency syndrome. *Pediatrics* 1988;82:355–363.

60. Epstein LG, Gendelman HE. Human immunodeficiency virus type 1 infection of the nervous system: pathogenetic mechanisms. *Ann Neurol* 1993;33:429–436.

61. Epstein LG, Goudsmit J, Paul DA, et al. Expression of human immunodeficiency virus in cerebrospinal fluid of children with progressive encephalopathy. *Ann Neurol* 1987;21:397–401

62. Epstein LG, Sharer LR, Cho S- E, et al. HTLV-III/LAV-like retrovirus particles in the brains of patients with AIDS encephalopathy. *AIDS Res* 1985;1:477–454.

63. Epstein LG, Sharer LR, Goudsmit J. Neurological and neuropathological features of HIV in children. *Ann Neurol* 1988;23[suppl]d9–S23 .

64. Epstein LG, Sharer LR, Joshi VV, et al. Progressive encephalopathy in children with acquired immune deficiency syndrome. *Ann Neurol* 1985;17:488–496.

65. Epstein LG, Sharer LR, Oleske JM, et al. Neurological manifestations of human immunodeficiency virus infection in children. *Pediatrics* 1986;78:678–687.

66. European Collaborative Study: Risk factors for mother-to-child transmission of HIV-1. *Lancet* 1992; 339:1007–1012.

67. European Collaborative Study. Cogo P, Laverda AM, Ades AE, et al. Neurological signs in young children with human immunodeficiency virus infection. *Ped Inf Dis J* 1990;9:402–406.

68. Frank Y, Lim W, Kahn E, et al. Multiple ischemic infarcts in a child with AIDS, varicella zoster infection and cerebral vasculitis. *Pediatr Neurol* 1989;5:64–67.

69. Frank Y, Vishnubhakat SM, Pahwa S. Brainstem auditory evoked responses in infants and children with AIDS. *Pediatr Neurol* 1992;8(4):262–266.

70. Futterman D, Hein K. Medical management of adolescents. In: Pizzo PA, Wilfert CM, eds. *Pediatric AIDS: the challenge of HIV infection in infants, children and adolescents*, 2nd ed. New York: Williams and Wilkins, 1994;546–560.

71. Gabuzda DH, Ho DD, de la Monte, et al. Immunohistochemical identification of HTLV-III antigen in brain of patients with AIDS. *Ann Neurol* 1986;20:289–295.

72. Gallo P, Laverda AM, DeRossi A, et al. Immunological markers in the cerebrospinal fluid of HIV-1–infected children. *ACTA Ped Scandi* 1991;80:659–666.

73. Goedert JJ, Duliege AM, Amos CI, Felton S, Biggar RJ. High risk of HIV-1 infection for first-born twins: the International Registry of HIV-exposed Twins. *Lancet* 1991;338:1471–1475.

74. Goldstein J, Dickson DW, Rubinstein A, Woods W, Miner F, Belman AL, Davis L. Primary CNS lymphoma in a pediatric patient with acquired immunodeficiency syndrome treatment with radiation. *Cancer* 1990;66:2503–2508.

75. Gonda MA, Wong-Stall F, Gallo RC, et al. Sequence homology and morphological similarity of HTLV-III and visna virus, a pathogenic lentivirus. *Science* 1985;227:173–177.

76. Goudsmit J, Wolters EC, Bakker M, et al. Intrathecal synthesis of antibodies to HTLV-III in patients without AIDS or AIDS related complex. *Br Med J* 1986;292:1231–1234.

77. Havens J, Whitaker A, Felman J, Alvarado L, Ehrhardt AA. A controlled study of cognitive and language function in school-aged HIV-infected children. *Ann NY Acad Sci* 1993;693:249–251.

78. Havens J, Whitaker AH, Feldman JF, Ehrhardt AA. Psychiatric morbidity in school-aged children with congenital human immunodeficiency virus infection: a pilot study. *J of Devel and Behav Pediatri* 1994;15(suppl):S18–S25.

79. Ho DD, Rota TR, Schooley RT, et al. Isolation of HTLV-III from CSF and neural tissues of patients with AIDS related neurological syndromes. *N Engl J Med* 1985;313:1493–1497.

80. Jannsen RS, Cornblath DR, Epstein LG, McArthur J, Price R. HIV infection and the nervous system: report from the American Academy of Neurology Task Force. *Neurology* 1989;39:111–122.

81. Johnson RT, McArthur JC, Narayan O. The neurobiology of human immunodeficiency virus infections. *FASEB J* 1988;2:2970–2981.

82. Jovaisas E, Koch MA, Schafer A, et al. LAV/HTLV-III in 20-week fetus (letter). *Lancet* 1985;2: 1129.

83. Ketzlen S, Weiss S, Haug H, Budka H. Loss of neurons in frontal cortex in AIDS brains. *Acta Neuropath (Berl)* 1990; 80:92–94.
84. Koenig S, Gendelman HE, Orenstein JM, et al. Detection of AIDS virus in macrophage in brain tissue from AIDS patients with encephalopathy. *Science* 1986;233:1089–1093.
85. Kozlowski PB, Sher JH, Rao, et al. Central nervous system in pediatric AIDS registry. *Ann NY Acad Sci* 1993;693:295–296.
86. Krivine A, Firtion G, Gao L, Francoual C, et al. HIV replication during the first few weeks of life. *Lancet* 1992;339:1187–1189.
87. Kure K, Park YD, Kim TS, et al. Immunohistochemical localization of an HIV epitope in cerebral aneurysmal arteriopathy in pediatric AIDS. *Pediatr Pathol* 1989;9:655–662.
88. Kure K, Weidenheim KM, Lyman WD, Dickson DW. Morphology and distribution of HIV-1 qp 41 positive microglia in subacute AIDS encephalitis. *ACTA Neuropathol (Ber 1)* 1990;80:393–400.
89. Laverda AM, Gallo P, Tavolato B, et al. Cerebrospinal fluid findings in neurologically symptomatic and asymptomatic HIV-1–infected children. Neuroscience of HIV-1 Infection [Abstract]. *Satellite Conference, VII International Conferenbce on AIDS*, Padova, Italy, 1991:120.
90. Levenson RL, Mellins CA, Zawadzki R, Kairam R, Stein Z. Cognitive assessment of human immunodeficiency virus exposed children. *AJDC* 1992;146:1479–1483.
91. Levy JA, Shimabukuro J, Hollander H, et al. Isolation of AIDS–associated retrovirus from cerebrospinal fluid and brain of patients with neurological symptoms. *Lancet* 1985;2:586–588.
92. Lifschitz M, Hanson C, Wilson G, Shearer WT. Behavioral changes in children with human immunodeficiency virus (HIV) infection. T.B.P.175. *V International Conference on AIDS*, Montreal, June 4-9, 1989.
93. Lyman WD, Kressy Y, Kure K, et al. Detection of HIV in fetal central nervous system tissue. *AIDS* 1990;4:917–920.
94. Masliah E, Achim CL, Ge N, DeTeresa R, Terry RD, Wiley CA. Spectrum of human immunodeficiency virus-associated neocortical damage. *Ann Neurol* 1992; 32:321–329.
95. McAbee GN, Belman AL, Knapik M, Solitare G, Ciminera P, Dickson D. Rapid and fatal neurological deterioration due to CNS candida infection in an HIV-1–infected child. *J Child Neurol* [in press].
96. McKinney RE, Maha MA, Conners EM, et al. A multicenter trial of oral zidovudine in children with advanced HIV disease. *N Engl J Med* 1991;324:1018–1025.
97. Mintz M, Epstein LE. Neurological manifestations, clinical features and therapeutic approaches. *Sem in Neurol* 1992;12:51–56.
98. Mitchell CD, Erlich SS, Mastrucci MT, et al. Congenital toxoplasmosis occurring in infants perinatally infected with HIV-1. *Pediatr Infect Dis J* 1990;9:512–518.
99. Mofenson LM, Wolinsky SM. Current insights regarding vertical transmission. In: Pizzo PA, Wilfert CM, eds. *Pediatric AIDS: the challenge of HIV Infection in infants, children and adolescents*, 2nd edition. Baltimore: Williams and Wilkins, 1994;179–203.
100. Moss H, Brouwers E, Walters P, Weiner L, Hersh S, Pizzo PA. The development of a Q sort behavioral rating procedure for pediatric HIV patients. *J Pediatr Psychol* 1994;19:27–46.
101. Navia BA, Jordon BD, Price RW. The AIDS dementia complex: I. Clinical features. *Ann Neurol* 1986;19:517–524.
102. Nozyce M, Hittleman J, Muenz L, et al. Effect of perinatally acquired human immunodeficiency virus infection on neurodevelopment in children during the first two years of life. *Pediatrics* 1994; 94:883–889.
103. Nozyce M, Hoberman M, Arpade S, et al. The effects of oral AZT on neurodevelopmental, immunological and clinical outcomes in vertically HIV infected children. *Ann NY Acad Sci* 1993;693[Abstract]:1992.
104. Oleske J, Minnefor A, Cooper R, et al. Immune deficiency syndrome in children. *JAMA* 1983;249:2345.
105. Oxtoby MJ. Vertically acquired HIV infection in the United States. In: Pizzo PA, Wilfert CM, eds. *Pediatric AIDS: The challenge of HIV infection in infants, children and adolescents*, 2nd Edition. New York: Williams and Wilkins, 1994;5–20.
106. Park Y, Belman AL, Dickson DW, et al. Stroke in pediatric acquired immunodeficiency syndrome. *Ann Neurol* 1988;24:359.
107. Pavlakis SG, Lu PF, Frank Y, et al. MRS of the basal ganglia: diagnosis of childhood AIDS encephalopathy. *Neurology* 1994;suppl2A:44.
108. Persaud D, Chadwani S, Rigaud M, et al. Delayed recognition of human immunodeficiency virus infection in pre adolescent children. *Pediatrics* 1992;90:688–669.
109. Pizzo PA, Butler K, Balis F, et al. Dideoxycytidine alone and in an alternating schedule with zidovudine in children with symptomatic human immunodeficiency virus infection. *J Peds* 1990; 117:799–808.
110. Pizzo PA, Eddy J, Balis FM, et al. Effect of continuous intravenous infusion of zidovudine (AZT) in children with symptomatic HIV infection. *N Engl J Med* 1988;319:889–896.
111. Pizzo PA, Wilfert CM. Antiretroviral treatment for children with HIV infection. In: Pizzo PA,

Wilfert CM, eds. *Pediatric AIDS: the challenge of HIV infection in infants, children and adolescents*, 2nd edition. New York: Williams and Wilkins, 1994:651–687.

112. Pizzo PA, Wilfert CM, Editors. *Pediatric AIDS: the challenge of HIV infection in infants, children and adolescents*, 2nd Edition. New York: Williams and Wilkins, 1994:651–687.

113. Price RW, Perry S, Eds. *HIV, AIDS and the brain*. New York: Raven Press, 1993.

114. Pumarola–Sune T, Navia BA, Cordon–Cardo D, et al. HIV antigen in the brains of patients with the AIDS dementia complex. *Ann Neurol* 1987;21:490–496.

115. Raphael SA, Price ML, Lischner HW, et al. Inflammatory demyelinating polyneuropathy in a child with symptomatic human immunodeficiency virus infection. *J Pediatrics* 1991;118:242–245.

116. Report of a consensus workshop, Siena, Italy, January 17– 18, 1992: Early diagnosis of HIV infection in infants. *J Acquir Immune Defic Syndr* 1992;5:1169– 1178.

117. Resnick L, DiMarzo–Veronese F, Schupbach J, et al. Intra–blood–brain barrier synthesis of HTLV–III specific IgG in patients with neurological symptoms associated with AIDS or AIDS–related complex. *N Engl J Med* 1985;313:1498–1504.

118. Rogers MF, Ou CY, Rayfield M, et al. Use of polymerase chain reaction for early detection of the proviral sequences of human immunodeficiency virus in infants born to seropositive mothers. *N Eng J Med* 1989;320:1649–1654.

119. Rogers MF, Schochetman G, Hoff R. Advances in diagnosis of HIV infection. In: Pizzo PA, Wilfert CM, eds. *Pediatric AIDS: the challenge of HIV infection in infants, children and adolescents*, 2nd Edition. New York: Williams and Wilkins, 1994:219–240.

120. Rouzioux C, Burgard M, Blanche S, Costagliola D. HIV Infection in Newborns: French Collaborative Study. Estimate of the period of perinatal HIV–1 transmission. *J Cell Biochem* 1993;17E(suppl): 100(Abstract).

121. Rubinstein A. Acquired immunodeficiency syndrome in infants. *Am J Dis Child* 1983;137:825–827.

122. Ryder RW, Nsa W, Hassig SE, et al. Perinatal transmission of the human immunodeficiency virus type 1 to infants of seropositive wormen in Zaire. *N Engl J Med* 1989;320:1637–1642.

123. Schmidt B, Seeger J, Jacobi G. EEG and evoked potentials in HIV–infected children. *Clin Electroencephalogr* 1992;23(3):111–117.

124. Scott G. Survival in children with perinatally acquired human immunodeficiency virus type infection. *N Engl J Med* 1989;3211:1791–1796.

125. Semba RD, Miotti PG, Chiphangwi JD, et al. Maternal vitamin A deficiency and mother–to–child transmission of HIV–1. *Lancet* 1994; 343:1593–1597.

126. Shanks GD, Redfield RR, Fischer GW. Toxoplasma encephalitis in an infant with acquired immuno-deficiency syndrome. *Pediatr Infect Dis* 1987;6:70.

127. Sharer LR, Dowling PC, Michaels J, et al. Spinal cord disease in children with HIV–1 infection: a combined molecular and neuropathological study. *Neuropathol Appl Neurobiol* 1990;16:317–331.

128. Sharer LR, Epstein LG, Cho ES, et al. Pathologic features of AIDS encephalopathy in children: evidence for LAV/HTLV–III infection of the brain. *Hum Pathol* 1986;17:271–284.

129. Sharer LR, Fischer B, Blumberg BM, Epstein LG. CNS measles virus infection in AIDS. *Journal of Neuro–AIDS* 1994 (in press).

130. Shaw GM, Harper ME, Hahn BH, et al. HTLV–III infection in brains of children and adults with AIDS encephalopathy. *Science* 1985;227:177–181.

131. Srugo I, Wittek AE, Israele V, Brunell PA. Meningoencephalitiis in a neonate congenitally infected with human immunodeficiency virus type 1. *J Pediatr* 1992;120:93–95.

132. St. Louis ME, Kalish M, Kamenga M, et al. The timing of perinatal HIV–1 transmission in an African setting [Abstract]. *First national conference on human retroviruses and related infections*, Washington, DC, 1993.

133. St. Louis ME, Kamenga M, Brown C, et al. Risk for perinatal HIV–1 transmission accourding to maternal immunologic, virologic, and placental factors. *JAMA* 1993; 269:2853–2859.

134. Taccone A, Fondelli MP, Ferra G, Marzoli A. An unusual CT presentation of congenital cerebral toxoplasmosis in an 8 month–old boy with AIDS. *Pediatr Radiol* 1992; 22(1):68–69.

135. Tardieu M, Blanche S, Brunelle F. Cerebral magnetic resonance imaging studies in HIV-1–infected children born to seropositive mothers. Neuroscience of HIV-1 infection [Abstract]. *Satellite Conference, VII International Conference on AIDS*, Padova, Italy, 1991:60.

136. Tardieu M, Mayaux M–J, Seibel N, Funck–Brentano I, Straub E, Teglas J–P, Blanche S. Maternally transmitted HIV–1 infection: cognitive assessment of school age children. *J of Pediatr* 1995;126: 375–379.

137. Tornatore C, Meyers K, Atwood W, Conant K. Major E temporal patterns of human immunodeficiency virus type 1; transcripts in human fetal astrocytes. *J Virol* 1994;68:93–102.

138. Tovo PA, Demartino M, Gabiano C, et al. Prognostic factors and survival in children with perinatal HIV–I infection. Italian register for HIV infection in children. *Lancet* 1992;339:1249–1253.

139. Tovo PA, Gabiano C, Favro–Paris S, et al. Brain atrophy with intracranial calcification following congenital HIV infection. *Acta Paediatr Scand* 1988;77:776–779.

140. Ultmann MH, Belman AL, Ruff HA, Novick BE, Cone–Wesson B, Cohen HJ, Rubinstein A.

Developmental abnormalities in infants and children with acquired immune deficiency syndrome (AIDS) and AIDS–related complex. *Dev Med Child Neurol* 1985;27:563–571.

141. Ultmann MH, Diamond G, Ruff HA, Belman AL, et al. Developmental abnormalities in infants and children with acquired immune deficiency syndrome (AIDS): a follow up study. *Intern J Neurosci* 1987;32:661–667.
142. Van der Steenhoven JJ, Dbaibo G, Boyko OB, et al. Progressive multifocal leukoencephalopathy in pediatric acquired immunodeficiency syndrome. *J Neuropathol Exp Neurol* 1990;50:326.
143. Vazeux R, Lacroix–Ciaudo C, Blanche S, et al. Low levels of human immunodeficiency virus replication in the brain tissue of children with severe acquired immunodeficiency syndrome encephalopathy. *Am J Pathol* 1992;140:137–144.
144. Volpe J. *Neurology of the newborn*, 2nd ed. Philadelphia: WB Saunders, 1994.
145. Weisner B, Nachman S, Tropper P, et al. Quantitation of human immunodeficiency virus type 1 during pregnancy: relationship of viral titer to mother–to–child transmission and stability of viral load. *Proc Natl Acad Sci USA* 1994;91:8037–8041.
146. Whitt JK, Hooper SR, Tennison MB, et al. Neuropsychological functioning of human immunodeficiency virus–infected children with hemophilia. *J Pediatr* 1993;122:52–59.
147. Wiley CA, Belman AL, Dickson D, Rubinstein A, Nelson JA. Human immunodeficiency virus within the brains of children with AIDS. *Clin Neuropath* 1990;1:1–6.
148. Wiley CA, Masliah E, Morey, et al. Neocortical Damage during HIV Infection. *Ann Neurol* 1991;29:651–657.
149. Wiley CA, Masliah E, Achim CL. Measurement of CNS HIV burden and its association with neruological damage. *Adv in Neuroimmunol* 1994;4:319–325.
150. Wiley CA, Schrier RD, Nelson AS, et al. Cellular localization of human immunodeficiency virus infection within the brains of acquired immune deficiency syndrome patients. *Proc Natl Acad Sci* 1986;83:7089–7093.
151. Wolters PL, Brouwers P, Moss HA, Pizzo PA. Differential receptive and expressive language functioning of children with symptomatic HIV disease: comparison with the language of sibling controls and CT scan brain abnormalities. *Pediatrics* 1995;1:112–119.

AIDS and the Nervous System, Second Edition,
edited by J. R. Berger and R. M. Levy.
Lippincott-Raven Publishers, Philadelphia © 1997.

11

Neurodiagnostic Testing in Human Immunodeficiency Virus Infection (Cerebrospinal Fluid)

Elyse J. Singer, Karl Syndulko, and Wallace W. Tourtellotte

*Department of Neurology, University of California Los Angeles Medical Center,
Veterans Administration Medical Center West Los Angeles,
Los Angeles, California 90073*

Human immunodeficiency virus (HIV) invades the central nervous system (CNS) early in infection (50,107,181) and is associated with a spectrum of devastating neurological diseases. The consequences of CNS HIV infection were not readily appreciated early in the epidemic. Interest in the CNS was focused on the secondary consequences of immunosuppression, such as opportunistic infections (OIs) and neoplasms (205). Little attention was given to the cerebrospinal fluid (CSF) except as a medium to diagnose CNS OIs, neurosyphilis, and tumors. As the epidemic matured, CSF studies have contributed significantly to our understanding of the natural history and pathophysiology of HIV CNS disease, especially illnesses that occur as a direct consequence of HIV infection alone (primary HIV-associated neurological disease). CSF is a potential source of laboratory markers to follow the progression of CNS HIV infection and its response to therapy. Sophisticated new diagnostic tests have been developed that extend the role of CSF in the diagnosis and management of HIV neurological disease.

This chapter reviews the physiology and composition of the CSF in HIV infection and discusses the use of CSF as a diagnostic tool in specific pathological states.

CEREBROSPINAL FLUID

CSF is produced by the choroid plexus and, to a lesser degree, by brain parenchyma (70). The CSF is contiguous between the interstitial spaces surrounding individual CNS cells and the macroscopic spaces surrounding the brain and spinal cord. Solutes from the CNS extracellular space sink into CSF and become accessible to measurement. The CSF reflects these constituents in a dynamic fashion. In adults, CSF is secreted at ~0.35 ml/min (500 ml/day) (70), resulting in a total volume of ~150 ml, which is turned over about three times per day (47,70). Normal adult CSF pressure is <200/mm in the lateral decubitus position (80) and is maintained by constant resorption of CSF in the arachnoid villi.

The blood–brain barrier (BBB) and blood–CSF barrier surround the CNS and help maintain internal homeostasis by regulating the passage of substances in and out of the brain. They also partially isolate the CNS from the peripheral immune system. HIV infection disrupts these barriers, as reflected by changes in the CSF profile.

The BBB is formed by tight junctions between CNS capillary endothelial cells and is reinforced by the foot processes of astrocytes (70). In health, the tight junctions are open in the choroid plexus and permit the entry of small amounts of albumin and immunoglobulin (Ig)G from blood. The BBB also admits a few white blood cells (WBCs), mostly T-lymphocytes and monocytes (70). These cells transit between the CNS and the periphery and maintain a form of immune surveillance of the CNS.

Evidence suggests that HIV enters the CNS during primary infection (seroconversion) (50,107), possibly within infected macrophages, which can cross the BBB (116,153). HIV infects resident brain macrophages, microglia, and astrocytes (221,233,240). The presence of viral antigens expressed on the surfaces of infected CNS cells, in association with major histocompatibility complex (MHC) molecules, signals T cells that induce an intrathecal immune response, including the release of cytokines, chemotactic factors, adhesion molecules, and other substances that attract immune cells from the periphery (229). The first cells to arrive are usually activated T cells, macrophages, and/or neutrophils, followed by activated antigen-specific B-lymphocytes, which mature into antibody-producing plasma cells within the CNS (115).

This process is reflected in CSF by an initial increase in WBCs, the onset of intrathecal Ig synthesis (as manifested by an elevated IgG synthesis rate), the presence of unique oligoclonal bands (OBs), and an increase in the CSF total protein. The latter occurs both because of damage to the BBB, which allows excessive influx of proteins such as albumin and IgG from blood, and intrathecal antibody synthesis. HIV disease progression is associated with immune dysfunction, allowing for the proliferation of HIV and/or opportunistic organisms within the CNS. Intrathecal replication of HIV is reflected by elevated levels of viral proteins such as p24 antigen and by an increase in viral nucleic acids as measured by quantitative polymerase chain reaction (PCR). HIV progression is also associated with an increase in inflammation, including synthesis of cytokines, neopterin, beta-2-microglobulin (β2M), quinolinic acid, and prostaglandins. CNS infection by opportunistic pathogens is reflected by positive cultures, an increase in serologies, and other organism-specific assays in the CSF and serum. The proliferation of pathogens and inflammatory cells may occlude the arachnoid villi, leading to decreased resorption of CSF, obstruction of CSF flow, increased intracranial pressure, and/or hydrocephalus. Unfortunately, the same barriers that permit HIV entry into the CNS can fully or partially exclude many therapeutic drugs (188). In late disease there may be a decline in CSF WBCs and IgG despite increasing antigenic stimulation (139). This probably reflects an overall decline in the core immune response.

LUMBAR PUNCTURE

Lumbar puncture (LP) is the most commonly used method to collect CSF and to measure intracranial pressure. An LP is contraindicated in several situations, including coagulopathy, thrombocytopenia, presence of infection in the overlying tissues, and presence of a mass lesion associated with increased intracranial pressure and asymmetric pressure gradients. LPs performed under these conditions can result in complications such as spinal epidural hematoma, meningitis, or brain herniation. Less serious but more common problems include nerve root irritation, backache, and post-LP headache. The latter occurs when continued leakage of CSF through the dural tear results in lowered CSF pressure. The incidence of post-LP headache is proportional to the needle gauge used and can be reduced by the use of a small-gauge (no. 26) needle (225). However, small-gauge needles are less accurate to record CSF pressure (70).

CSF PROFILE IN HIV INFECTION

Abnormal laboratory values are found in the CSF of 60–90% of HIV-infected adults without CNS OIs or tumors, including asymptomatic, neurologically normal subjects (55,138,202,203). The rate and type of CSF abnormalities are influenced by factors such as the subject sample, staging criteria used, presence of "confounding" factors, choice of "normal" reference values, method of specimen collection, and type of assay technique used. The most commonly reported abnormalities are CSF pleocytosis, elevation of total protein and albumin, and intrathecal IgG synthesis. At this time there is no single laboratory value, or constellation of values, that can be used to diagnose or predict the onset of primary HIV neurological disease. Many putative CSF markers exist on a continuum and are present in small amounts in HIV-seronegative controls as well as in asymptomatic HIV-seropositive individuals. Large cross-sectional studies and longitudinal studies that measure intraindividual change over time are needed to determine the predictive value of these tests.

CELLS

A CSF WBC count >5 cells/mm^3 is abnormal in adults (70) and has been reported in 18–32% of asymptomatic, neurologically normal HIV-infected persons (36,139,147,203). Most studies report a predominance of lymphocytes; however, monocytes, macrophages, plasma cells, and atypical lymphocytes also have been reported (7,96). The presence of polymorphonuclear leukocytes indicates a secondary infection, such as cytomegalovirus (CMV) (43,52,53). Flow cytometry of the CSF suggests that the percentages of CD8 and CD4 cells are highly correlated with those in peripheral blood (136,149). The proportion of CD4 lymphocytes (CD4 + counts) is significantly decreased in patients with HIV dementia, which parallels the findings in blood (136,149).

Many studies have reported CSF pleocytosis in HIV-infected adults without CNS OIs, neurosyphilis, or tumors. Marshall et al. (139) collected >500 samples of CSF from 424 HIV-infected Air Force personnel characterized by the Walter Reed (WR) criteria (179) and neurological examination. Eighty percent of these subjects were asymptomatic and neurologically normal. Using extremely strict criteria (>10 CSF WBC/mm^3 rather than >5), CSF pleocytosis was found in 15% of WR stage 1 (WR1) subjects, 18% of WR2 subjects, 19% of WR3 subjects, and 22% of WR4 subjects, but only in 11% of WR5 and in no WR6 subjects. The highest CSF WBC count was 75 cells/mm^3. Pleocytosis was not associated with neurological disease; however, few subjects were neurologically abnormal. One hundred twenty-four of these subjects who remained healthy and neurologically normal were followed over a 2-year period with THREE LPs (137). The mean CSF cell count tended to increase over time, regardless of changes in CD4+ count. Collier et al. (44) found CSF pleocytosis (mean WBC of 8 cells/mm^3) in 65% of HIV-infected men without acquired immunodeficiency syndrome (AIDS), constitutional symptoms, or known neurological disease. Pleocytosis was not associated with any other clinical or laboratory findings. Singer et al. reported on two large groups of adults composed of healthy seronegative controls, and HIV-infected subjects in varying stages of systemic disease without CNS OIs, tumors, or neurosyphilis (202,203). The HIV-infected group included both neurologically normal subjects and subjects with primary HIV neurological disease. HIV-seropositive individuals had significantly higher mean CSF WBC counts and a higher incidence of abnormal (>5 cells/mm^3) counts than did seronegative controls; however, there were no significant differences noted in mean WBC or frequency of elevated (>5 WBC/mm^3) between the HIV-infected groups with or without neurological disease. The highest WBC count found was 120/mm^3. CSF WBCs in HIV-infected subjects without OIs is not altered by zidovudine treatment (217).

A few studies have commented on CSF WBCs in specific diseases. CSF pleocytosis characterizes an aseptic meningitis that may accompany primary infection (108). McArthur et al. (146) reported a mean CSF WBC count of 41 cells/mm^3 (range 5–176) in subjects with aseptic meningitis. Pleocytosis (up to 50 cells/mm^3) is commonly found in subjects with HIV-associated inflammatory demyelinating neuropathies (4), in contrast with the HIV-seronegative inflammatory neuropathies. Normal or hypocellular counts have been reported in many patients with HIV dementia (118,146). Although pleocytosis is common in CNS OIs, acellular CSF has been reported in patients with AIDS who also have cryptococcal meningitis (94,121), tuberculous meningitis (123), neurosyphilis (220), and toxoplasmosis (175).

In summary, CSF pleocytosis usually appears early in HIV infection. Most studies have reported modestly elevated CSF WBCs, which may decline with disease progression in the absence of a secondary CNS infection or tumor. However, a normal or hypocellular CSF WBC count does not reliably exclude CNS OIs in an immunosuppressed patient with AIDS.

CSF GLUCOSE

CSF glucose concentrations are usually normal in HIV infection (96,118,129). Marshall et al. (139) reported a tendency for CSF glucose to decrease in a linear fashion across progressive WR stages 1–6, although mean values remained within the normal range. A CSF glucose well below the normal range suggests a CNS OI or neoplasm.

TOTAL PROTEIN AND ALBUMIN

Elevated levels of CSF total protein and two of its components, albumin and Ig, have been reported in all stages of HIV disease (44,61,127,139). CSF total protein levels in healthy adults range from 0.15 to 0.45 g/L depending on the gender and age (20,57) of the control subjects. CSF total protein can be falsely elevated by blood (hemolyzed red blood cells). Likewise, contamination of CSF by >0.2% serum produces a falsely elevated IgG synthesis rate and IgG index (170). A gradient exists for total protein, CSF/serum albumin ratio, and IgG along the neuraxis; concentrations are higher in lumbar than in cisternal or ventricular CSF (19,177). Failure to control for this gradient may increase the variability of CSF analysis.

Marshall et al. (139), using strict criteria for elevated CSF total protein (>0.55 g/L rather than 0.45 g/L), found that the percentage of subjects with elevated total protein increased from 6.1% in WR1 to 33% in WR4 and declined to 0 in WR6. However, few late-stage subjects were included. One hundred twenty-four asymptomatic, neurologically normal subjects from the latter study were followed over 2 years (137). A small decrease in CSF total protein and increase in the CSF/serum albumin index was noted; however, the mean values remained within the normal range. Portegies et al. (173) reported that 55% of 40 HIV dementia patients had elevated CSF total protein. McArthur et al. (148) reported that subjects with mild HIV dementia had significantly higher CSF total protein levels than did nondemented subjects and that there was no relationship between total protein levels and disease duration in the nondemented group. The total protein level in adults reportedly does not change after zidovudine treatment (217).

Because CSF total protein is a relatively nonspecific marker, it is useful to analyze its major components. Elevation of CSF total protein can occur as follows: increased levels of serum protein with a proportionately greater amount crossing a normal BBB; transudation of serum proteins across an abnormally leaky BBB; intrathecal synthesis of Ig by antibody-secreting plasma cells; or a combination of these processes. The major component of CSF protein, albumin, is synthesized in the liver. Normal CSF albumin concentration is determined by serum concentration (180,223,235) and by the natural leakiness of endothelial capillary tight junctions (28). CSF albumin is a useful index of BBB integrity or leakiness to midsize protein molecules (180). Autopsy studies have demonstrated BBB damage and leakage of serum proteins into the brains of individuals with AIDS (171,176,183), which may contribute both to abnormal CSF and the pathogenesis of HIV dementia. The albumin index (the CSF to serum ratio of albumin) (219) and a formula that calculates trans-BBB albumin leakage rate (228) are used to measure BBB damage. The albumin index and trans-BBB albumin leakage rate are tightly correlated ($r = 0.99$) in subjects with multiple sclerosis (216) and HIV (Syndulko and Singer, unpublished data). Normal values for the albumin index range from 6 to 9. Albumin index values vary with age in normal individuals (20) and thus ideally should be matched to the age of the subjects studied.

In Marshall's predominantly asymptomatic cohort (139), only 2% had an elevated albumin index using an extremely strict cut-off value (>9). In other studies, neurologically symptomatic HIV-seropositive subjects were found to have higher albumin index values than neurologically normal HIV-seropositive individuals (61,134). McArthur (148) reported that subjects with mild HIV dementia had significantly higher CSF/serum albumin ratios than did nondemented subjects.

Singer et al. (203) studied 137 subjects without confounding neurological disease. Paired CSF and serum were collected in a standardized fashion that controlled for CSF rostral-caudal gradients. Albumin leakage increased significantly across disease groups (HIV-seronegative controls < neurologically normal HIV-seropositive individuals < neurologically abnormal HIV-seropositive individuals), and was significantly higher in subjects with CD4+ counts of <100/mm^3 than in subjects with CD4+ counts of >100/mm^3. In contrast, Brew et al. (27) found no correlation between CSF/serum albumin ratio and neurological impairment. Van Weilink et al. (232), in a cross-sectional study, observed that elevated (>6) albumin index values were (nonsignificantly) associated with disease duration in asymptomatic HIV-sero-positive individuals. Elovaara et al. (62), using a CSF/serum albumin ratio of >7, found no significant change in albumin indices over three evaluations in 28 subjects.

In summary, albumin leakage, and to a lesser degree total protein levels, tend to be higher in subjects with HIV neurological disease than those without. Further studies are needed to determine if measures of BBB integrity are useful predictive markers or offer insight into disease pathogenesis.

INTRATHECAL ANTIBODY SYNTHESIS

Studies of intrathecal antibody synthesis have played an important role in establishing the natural history of HIV in the CNS. Two types of markers have been used extensively: (a) indices that quantitate the amount of antibodies synthesized in brain, such as the total intrathecal IgG synthesis rate, the IgG index, and the antigen-specific IgG index, and (b) a qualitative measure, CSF oligoconal bands (OBs).

Igs are synthesized by plasma cells, which are not present in the healthy CNS. The small amount of IgG in normal CSF enters from serum by transudation across the BBB. IgG concentration is determined by serum concentration (180) and by the natural permeability of endothelial capillary tight junctions (28). Elevated intrathecal antibody levels occur by one or more of the following mechanisms: increased serum concentration, with proportionately increased passage across the BBB; damage to the BBB, with increased leakage from serum to CSF; or intrathecal antibody synthesis, which occurs when B-lymphocytes are recruited into the CNS and mature there to plasma cells. An excessively leaky BBB can confound the determination of intrathecal IgG synthesis. However, if CSF IgG concentration is corrected for high serum concentration and/or leakage across the BBB and remains elevated, there is evidence for intrathecal IgG synthesis (227). A number of formulas have been used to calculate intrathecal IgG synthesis rate. Four of the most common are (a) the IgG index

$$\frac{CSF}{serum} \; IgG/CSF \; \frac{albumin}{serum \; albumin}$$

(219); (b) the Tourtellotte intrathecal IgG synthesis rate formula (227); (c) IgG (loc) (180); and (d) intrathecal IgG synthesis (190,191). Although there is controversy over which formula is most valid and least affected by BBB damage (126,162,224), the values from all four formulas are highly correlated (216,224,226). The Tourtellotte equation and the IgG index are the most frequently cited in the HIV literature. Studies that used other methods to detect intrathecal IgG synthesis have obtained results similar to those obtained by using the IgG index and Tourtellotte equation (2,18,64,68,134,178). The presence of elevated intrathecal IgG synthesis was first reported in patients with AIDS-related complex (ARC) and AIDS (182). Subsequently, elevated IgG synthesis was reported in systemically asymptomatic, neurologically normal subjects (39,44,61,76,86,96,138,139,181,201,232). This observation was important because it provided evidence of early HIV penetration of the CNS at a time when HIV could not be reliably recovered from CSF by the available techniques. The case for early penetration was further supported by instances in which antibodies appeared in CSF before blood (61,184).

Total intrathecal IgG synthesis has been found to increase during the early stages of HIV disease but may decrease in late infection (61,139). The latter probably results from immunological failure rather than clearance of virus. Studies using Tourtellotte's intrathecal IgG synthesis rate formula have found that intrathecal IgG synthesis is elevated in 22–88% of HIV-1–infected individuals (6,8,17,137–139,181,182, 202,203). Most studies have not found significant differences in the means or frequency of abnormal total intra-BBB IgG synthesis rate between HIV-infected subjects with primary HIV neurological disease versus those without primary HIV neurological disease (25,148,181). Singer et al. (203) studied 139 subjects, including high-risk seronegative controls and HIV-infected subjects with or without primary HIV neurological disease, and found that the total intrathecal IgG synthesis rate (as measured by nephelometry) was significantly different among groups (HIV neurological disease > HIV neurologically normal > seronegative). In another study of 142 HIV-infected subjects without CNS OIs (202), the mean total intra-BBB IgG synthesis rate (measured by Rocket electroimmunodiffusion) was significantly higher in subjects with moderate to severe HIV-related cognitive dysfunction compared with those with no or mild cognitive abnormalities. These two studies used a methodology that corrected for the CSF gradient of IgG.

Elevated total IgG index has been found in 35–80% of HIV-infected individuals in all clinical stages (61,96,138,139,202,203,210) and has been correlated with duration of infection (5,62). In contrast to the total intrathecal IgG synthesis rate, the total (nonspecific) IgG index has not been reported to differ significantly between subjects with or without primary HIV neurological disease in most (5,203) but not all (63) studies.

HIV-specific antibodies comprise only a small portion of total intrathecal antibody synthesis (134,181). Antibodies to CMV and herpes make up another small percentage of the total (134) and usually appear in advanced disease (134,145). Most intrathecal antibodies in HIV infection are of unknown specificity and may be synthesized in response to polyclonal B cell activation rather than a specific antigen.

HIV-specific intrathecal antibody synthesis has been measured by the HIV-specific antibody index (CSF/serum anti-HIV antibody ratio divided by the CSF/serum albumin ratio), using an upper-limit cut-off equal to 1.5 or 2.0 as abnormal. Intrathecal synthesis of anti-HIV antibodies occurs in all stages of disease (145) but has not been found in all HIV-infected persons. The frequency and/or level of HIV-specific antibody synthesis has been reported to increase with disease severity (134,210), duration of infection (62,232), and the presence of HIV neurological disease (18,63). Sönnenberg et al. reported a strong relationship between positive CSF HIV cultures and the mean HIV antibody index (210), suggesting that intrathecal IgG synthesis is a response to persistent antigenic stimulation rather than polyclonal B cell activation (142). The association between HIV recovery and high levels of anti-HIV IgG indicates that these antibodies do not neutralize HIV or clear infection (11,64,210). No significant association between neurological symptoms and the frequency of HIV-specific antibody production was seen in Sönnerborg's study. However, subjects with moderate-severe dementia had higher mean intrathecal anti-HIV IgG production than did those with no or mild dementia.

The detection of antibodies to viral core proteins in CSF has been observed to decline with disease progression (40,59). Antibody profiles in CSF may differ from blood (40,55,59,178), suggesting different antigenic profiles between the two compartments.

OBs are homogenous protein (Ig) bands, which are demonstrated when CSF and/

or serum proteins are separated electrophoretically on a gel and then stained. Each OB is synthesized by a single clone of plasma cells and is directed against a specific organism or its individual proteins. OBs that are found in CSF alone or are more intense (highly concentrated) in CSF than in serum are abnormal and represent the presence and activation of plasma cells within the CNS (81,212). The number of bands detected is technique specific but, within a given study, can provide a quantitative estimate of intrathecal IgG synthesis. A single CSF OB is sometimes observed in normal individuals. Two or more CSF OBs are considered to be abnormal. CSF OBs can be masked by >2% serum contamination (~100,000 red blood cells/mm^3) (170). OBs can consist of any type of Ig, but IgG has been the most frequently reported in the AIDS literature.

Unique CSF OBs have been detected in all stages of HIV-1 infection, regardless of the presence or absence of HIV neurological disease (7,8,32,39,56,76,82,86, 91,96,117,132,133,139,164,204,235). Significant differences have not been reported in the mean number of OBs or the presence of any antigen-specific OB and in the neurological disease status (82,203). However, two investigators reported a decline in certain antigen-specific OBs with HIV progression (91,117). Grimaldi et al. (92) reported that most CSF OBs are not directed against glycoprotein 120 or p24. He suggested that these unidentified OBs were directed against opportunistic organisms or were nonspecific antibodies due to immune dysregulation.

In summary, intrathecal IgG synthesis begins shortly after infection and persists throughout all stages of HIV disease, although levels may decrease in the late stages of AIDS. The presence of intrathecal IgG synthesis is not invariably associated with clinical HIV neurological disease because the frequency of intrathecal IgG synthesis is similar for both neurologically asymptomatic and symptomatic HIV-seropositive individuals. However, quantitative and qualitative differences in CSF antibodies may occur between neurologically normal and abnormal subject groups.

HIV CULTURE

HIV has been isolated from the CSF of patients in all stages of infection (31,37,38,44,48,54,107,109,114,181,206–208,214), including primary infection (108), at rates from 14% (31) to 92% (128). The relationship of clinical disease to rate of CSF culture positivity is controversial. Some investigators have reported rates of virus recovery corresponding to clinical disease stage (40,107,206,208). Conversely, other studies found no correlation between the frequency of HIV isolation from CSF and stage of infection (31,109,207). No association has been reported between neurological status and HIV isolation (31,37,96,109,181,207). The conflicting results of these studies may be due to methodological differences such as the time from specimen collection to culture (recovery of HIV from CSF is reported to decrease sharply after 5 hours) (207) and the fraction of CSF used (cellular versus cell free) (39,40,211). Successful CSF HIV culture has been associated with an elevated CSF WBC count (31,207,211), elevated CSF total protein level (211), multiple CSF samples (211), HIV-specific intrathecal antibody synthesis (207,210), and CSF and serum levels of β2M and neopterin (209). Zidovudine does not influence the rate of HIV recovery from CSF (31,211,217). Quantitative serum HIV cultures have shown an association between HIV titer and disease stage (45,106); however, this technique has not been used in CSF.

HIV strains isolated from blood, CSF, and the brain may have different biological properties (69,122,166,214). Some investigators have speculated that this may be associated with neurotropism (122).

In summary, HIV culture has been used to document CNS penetration and to examine differences in the biological characteristics of HIV. Its usefulness in CSF is limited by the low rate of recovery, lack of accurate quantitative techniques, and other technical problems that have stimulated interest in alternative methods, such as PCR.

HIV P24 ANTIGEN

HIV p24 antigen, a viral core protein, has been used as a serum marker of viral replication and systemic disease progression (3,124,135). Matched samples of serum and CSF from one patient may show p24 antigen in either one or both compartments, indicating that p24 is synthesized independently in the periphery versus CNS (35,174).

The majority of reports indicate that CSF p24 antigen is detected more frequently in symptomatic (35,84) than asymptomatic (139,186) subjects. The relationship between CSF p24 antigen and HIV neurological disease is less clear, in part because of the varying methods used (e.g., using qualitative rather than quantitative assays or using subject samples from heterogenous groups of patients with neurological disease). Additionally, the majority p24 antigen is complexed with anti-p24 antibody and is not detectable by standard assays. For example, in a group of 34 untreated patients with AIDS dementia, only 13 (38%) were p24 antigen positive in CSF (173).

Singer et al. (202) studied a sample of matched serum and CSF collected from HIV-infected subjects without secondary HIV CNS disease. Mean CSF p24 antigen levels (quantitative) were significantly associated with both the presence of any primary HIV neurological disease and the degree of cognitive impairment. No association with systemic disease stage was found. However, only 43% of the neurologically abnormal subjects (vs. 17% of neurologically normal subjects) were CSF p24 positive. Epstein et al. (65), in a qualitative study, detected CSF p24 antigen in eight of 11 children with progressive encephalopathy but in none of 16 children without progressive encephalopathy. Goudsmit et al. (85) found CSF HIV p24 antigen in six of seven patients with HIV dementia, compared with one of 18 systemically symptomatic HIV-infected subjects without dementia. No CSF p24 antigen was detected in any of eight asymptomatic, experimentally infected chimpanzees, supporting the association between CSF p24 antigen and symptomatic HIV disease. Carbonara et al. (35) reported qualitative p24 antigen results in 209 paired CSF and serum samples from 101 HIV-infected subjects classified by the U.S. Centers for Disease Control and Prevention (CDC) stage and neurological evaluation. Serum HIV p24 antigen was detected at all disease stages. In contrast, CSF p24 antigen was detected in only a few subjects with HIV dementia or CNS OIs. Scalzini et al. (186) detected CSF p24 antigen only in subjects with neurological abnormalities, such as HIV dementia, neuropathy, or CNS opportunistic infections (OIs). Portegies et al. (174) studied 85 HIV-infected adults and 58 children. The presence of CSF p24 antigen was strongly associated with neurological impairment in both adults and children. However, only 12 of 24 adults and 19 of 27 children with neurological impairment were CSF p24 positive, compared with eight of 61 neurologically normal adults and two of 31 neurologically normal children. When a subset of these subjects was evaluated longitudinally, CSF p24 was not found to be predictive of neurological decline. CSF p24 antigen levels have been reported to decline with zidovudine therapy; however, decline in p24 levels did not correspond to clinical improvement (51).

In summary, CSF p24 antigen has been used as both a qualitative and quantitative measurement that provides an index of viral replication in the CNS. When present, it may be useful in following the effect of therapy. The association of CSF p24 antigen with CNS disease suggests a relationship between viral load and neurological decline. Like serum p24, it is not uniformly detectable in all HIV-infected persons, probably due to the masking effect of anti-p24 antibodies. CSF p24 antigen values do not appear to be a useful diagnostic marker for HIV dementia, nor do they differentiate between primary and secondary HIV CNS disease. At this time, it does not appear to be a useful predictive marker for neurological decline. A new and more sensitive assay, acid-dissociated p24 antigen, has been used successfully in peripheral blood (130,154) and also may be useful in CSF.

POLYMERASE CHAIN REACTION

PCR is a new technique for the *in vitro* amplification (49) of specific sequences of DNA (218) and, with modification, of RNA (33,49). It is faster and more sensitive than culture techniques, is not masked by antibodies, can be performed on archival material, and is less susceptible to some of the methodological variables of specimen collection. Initially, PCR was used as a qualitative assay; however, there is a burgeoning body of literature on the use of quantitative PCR techniques (215), which have been used to estimate viral load. For these reasons, PCR may solve some of the problems reported with older assays. However, the extreme sensitivity of PCR makes this technique susceptible to false-positive results caused by contamination of the laboratory with minute amounts of post-PCR HIV products (112).

Recent reports support the notion that PCR techniques are useful to estimate viral load in blood (163). Although the levels of HIV in peripheral CD4 cells appear to be variable, overall, HIV load appears to correlate with disease stage, with the highest loads found in subjects with advanced disease (66,152). An association between viral burden and declining CD4+ count also has been reported (163). In one study (187), proviral DNA was detected by PCR in the blood of 83% of 158 HIV-seropositive men. Subjects who were PCR negative tended to have higher CD4+ counts and to progress more slowly than did those who were PCR positive.

Sinclair and Scaravilli (199) used PCR to detect HIV provirus DNA in the cortex and/or white matter of 12 of 18 patients with AIDS, two of eight HIV-seropositive subjects, and none of five HIV-seronegative controls. PCR detected HIV more frequently than did p24 antigen from the same tissue. Boni et al. (22), in a postmortem study, detected HIV provirus DNA in the brains of two thirds of patients with AIDS; the highest levels were found in subjects with a history of HIV dementia. Pang et al. (165) examined the brain tissue of patients with AIDS using a semiquantitative DNA PCR technique. Higher levels of HIV proviral DNA were found in subjects with histopathological evidence of HIV encephalitis than in those without. Additionally, the vast amount of proviral DNA was in an unintegrated form, in contrast to peripheral blood from the same group, in which the ratio of integrated to unintegrated viral DNA varied.

Few studies of CSF PCR are available. In a retrospective study, Shaunak et al. (196) reported detection of HIV provirus sequences in the CSF WBCs of 20 of 31 (64%) HIV-infected subjects. Thirteen subjects had a CNS OI or tumor at the time of evaluation, and neurological data for some subjects were unavailable. However, it appeared that a positive PCR result was more common in neurologically abnormal persons. Subsequently, they reported on four study subjects without clinical or PCR evidence of neurological disease, who were followed for 3 years. All four subjects remained neurologically normal. One neurologically normal PCR-positive subject and one neurologically normal PCR "indeterminate" subject developed dementia ~15 months after evaluation. Sönnerberg et al. (208) performed viral cultures and DNA PCR on the CSF WBCs and cell-free CSF of 29 HIV-infected subjects in all stages of systemic disease. All four neurologically symptomatic subjects and 20 nonsymptomatic subjects (24 of 28 tested, or 86%) were PCR positive in CSF. Sixteen of 29 subjects tested had positive CSF HIV cultures. One subject was culture positive and PCR negative, demonstrating that PCR was significantly better (p < 0.02) at detecting HIV, but not infallible. In a series of 53 HIV-seropositive subjects with paired CSF and serum samples assayed by RNA PCR, Goswami et al. (83) reported that 23 of 24 subjects with neurological disease had HIV RNA detected by PCR, versus eight of nine subjects with transient neurological symptoms and four of 20 asymptomatic subjects. The neurologically abnormal group was heterogenous and included subjects with CNS OIs; consequently, no associations could be made regarding the relationship between HIV PCR and HIV dementia.

Two studies have analyzed the viral load in CSF using PCR. Steuler et al. (213) assayed the number of copies of HIV provirus DNA in CSF cells. HIV DNA was detected in 13 of 15 (86%) of HIV-seropositive individuals and none of the HIV-seronegative individuals. In the 13 PCR-positive cases, HIV provirus DNA was detected at a median value of one copy per 300 CSF cells (or 3.33/1,000 cells) and a mean of one provirus per 570 CSF cells, with a range from 1/20 (50/1,000) to 1/2,400 (0.42/1,000). The viral load in CSF cells did not correlate with CDC disease stage or neurological status. Given that seven of the 13 PCR-positive subjects had CNS OIs, these results may not generalize to primary HIV neurological disease. However, these results do provide evidence that the level of HIV-1 provirus in CSF WBCs may be higher than in peripheral blood (198).

Schmid et al. (189) used DNA PCR to detect HIV in 87 HIV-seropositive subjects without CNS OIs, tumors, or neurosyphilis. All subjects were examined in a standardized, prospective fashion, and 63 had matched CSF and blood samples. HIV provirus was detected in blood in 93% of subjects and in CSF WBCs in 90% of HIV-seropositive subjects' samples. Detection rates in CSF WBCs did not differ significantly among asymptomatic seropositive individuals (85%), those with ARC (97%), and those with AIDS (83%), nor between those with (90%) versus those without (90%) HIV-associated neurological disease. Viral load in blood was significantly related to systemic disease stage. The median viral load in blood was 0.1 copies per 1,000 CD4 cells in asymptomatic seropositive individuals, 1.4 in those with ARC, and 10.7 in those with AIDS (p = 0.028). The viral load in subjects with HIV-related neurological disease was nonsignificantly greater than in those without, median 43.5 copies versus 17.6 copies per 1,000 CD4 cells in CSF (p = 0.06). The median proviral load in subjects in all stages of HIV infection was significantly higher in CSF than in blood, median 25 versus 0.6 copies per 1,000 CD4 cells (p = 0.0001).

PCR technology has been applied to other CNS pathogens, including treponemes

(97), *Toxoplasmosis gondii* (46), *Listeria monocytogenes* (113), *Mycobacterium tuberculosis* (131,194), herpes zoster (197), HTLV-I (119), JC virus (98), CMV (9,42,87), herpes simplex (9), and Epstein-Barr virus (41).

In summary, PCR is a sensitive method to detect and quantify the presence of HIV, with detection rates in CSF ranging from 64% (196) to 90% (189). Because qualitative PCR detects HIV in most seropositive subjects, regardless of neurological status, it may not be a helpful diagnostic test for HIV dementia unless quantitative differences can be demonstrated. Preliminary results suggest an association between CSF viral load and clinical disease. Quantitative CSF HIV PCR awaits study as a tool to follow the effects of therapy and as a marker to predict the progression of HIV neurological disease.

CYTOKINES

Cytokines are soluble peptide mediators synthesized by activated immune cells, such as macrophages, lymphocytes, microglia, and monocytes (10). In some instances, astrocytes (150), oligodendrocytes (151), and endothelial cells (241) also synthesize cytokines. Cytokines serve to mediate and regulate (stimulate and/or suppress) the immune and inflammatory responses (10). Individual cytokines may have multiple functions (mediate more than one event) and overlapping functions (several cytokines can mediate an event). One cytokine may stimulate the synthesis and function of other cytokines, resulting in a cascade effect. The cytokines interleukin (IL)-1 and tumor necrosis factor (TNF) have been found within neurons, implying that they may also function as neuromodulators (23,24).

Cytokines found to be elevated in the CSF and/or brain tissue of HIV-infected individuals and implicated in the pathogenesis of neurological disease (12,234) include gamma interferon (90,229), TNF (72,143,168), IL-1 (77,168,234), IL-6 (222,229,241), macrophage-colony stimulating factor (78), and transforming growth factor-β (234). Expression of a cytokine in brain tissue may not correlate with its level in CSF (1,229). Furthermore, elevated levels of CSF cytokines are not specific for primary HIV neurological disease and, in some instances, are highest in CNS OIs (143). TNF is associated with systemic effects on body temperature, circulation, appetite, coagulation, metabolism, and other functions 16, 141. TNF is associated with autoimmune demyelination (193) and with the upregulation of HIV replication (185), both of which have been implicated in HIV encephalitis. Elevated serum levels of TNF were found in children with progressive encephalopathy (155), but this has not been confirmed in another study (58). Grimaldi et al. (93) reported that TNF was detected more frequently in the CSF and serum of subjects with advanced versus early HIV disease, but found no correlation between TNF levels and dementia or demyelination. Franciotta et al. (72) reported that 19 of 30 CSF samples from HIV-seropositive individuals had detectable TNF, with the highest levels in subjects with neurological disease. However, TNF levels did not distinguish between subjects with primary versus secondary HIV CNS disease. Mastroianni et al. (144) confirmed that CSF levels of TNF were elevated in subjects with advanced HIV disease; the highest levels were found in subjects with CNS OIs rather than HIV dementia. In contrast, two groups (79,195) failed to detect TNF in the CSF of patients with AIDS.

Gamma interferon is produced mostly by T-lymphocytes (120). Macrophages appear to be a major target of gamma interferon activity (160). Among its many functions, gamma interferon induces the enzyme 2,3-indoleamine dioxygenase (172) and the synthesis of neopterin (110). Neopterin activates the kynurenine pathway of tryptophan metabolism, causing the accumulation of the neurotoxic metabolite quinolinic acid (QUIN) (237). QUIN has been implicated in the pathogenesis of HIV dementia (100). CSF gamma interferon levels are significantly higher in HIV-infected subjects than in seronegative controls, but do not differ between HIV-infected subjects with or without various CNS diseases (90).

IL-6, a B cell stimulatory factor, has been detected in the CSF of HIV-infected subjects (77,168,222) and in the dorsal root ganglia of patients with AIDS (241) and may contribute to polyclonal B cell activation and IgG synthesis (231). However, IL-6 is not specific for primary HIV neurological disease.

In summary, various cytokines implicated in the pathogenesis of HIV neurological disease can be assayed in CSF. To date, there is equivocal evidence for quantitative correlation between HIV neurological disease and CSF cytokine levels. Elevated levels of CSF cytokines do not differentiate between primary and secondary HIV CNS disease. However, relatively few studies have addressed this issue, and most appear to be retrospective and nonstandardized, and thus the methods used may have been suboptimal. Levels of cytokines in brain tissue and CSF may not increase in parallel. Because most cytokines act locally and synergistically, measuring the levels of individual cytokines may not prove to be clinically useful. Standardized prospective studies are needed to determine if CSF cytokine assays are worthwhile investigative tools in HIV neurological disease.

β2M AND NEOPTERIN

Both β2M and neopterin are nonspecific indicators of inflammation. Elevated serum levels of β2M and neopterin, along with CD4 + counts, predict HIV disease progression (67,74,158,230) and have been proposed as markers for HIV neurological disease (60). Levels of β2M and neopterin tend to correlate and increase in parallel (95), along with the putative CSF markers QUIN, L-kynurenine, and kynurenine (102). Both β2M and neopterin can be synthesized independently in blood and the CNS (209). Both can be detected in CSF during seroconversion (209); higher levels were noted in subjects who had HIV cultured from their CSF. In 118 subjects classified by the WR staging system, Bogner et al. (21) reported that CSF neopterin and β2M levels increased in an early (WR2) stage of infection, then declined in WR3–4, rising again in WR5–6. Subjects with HIV dementia had significantly higher levels of CSF β2M and nonsignificantly higher levels of CSF neopterin than did asymptomatic HIV-seropositive individuals.

β2M is a peptide that comprises part of the class I MHC structures on the surfaces of nucleated cells (14). Little or no β2M is found in normal CSF. Elevated levels of β2M are associated with activation of the cellular immune system, especially T-lymphocytes and macrophages (15,161), and with increased MHC class I expression. Consequently, β2M, like neopterin, is not specific for HIV and can be used as a reliable marker only if other inflammatory processes are excluded.

Serum and CSF β2M levels were found to be significantly higher in HIV-infected subjects with dementia than in those without (167). In one series (27), CSF β2M concentrations were significantly higher in 78 subjects with HIV dementia than in 11 seronegative controls and correlated with the severity of dementia. Zidovudine-treated subjects had a significant decrease in CSF β2M levels, as reported elsewhere (95). However, β2M levels did not differentiate between the various stages of dementia. Furthermore, some neurologically normal subjects had elevated (>3.1 mg/L) β2M levels, whereas 12% of subjects with mild dementia had levels within the normal range, suggesting that there is a great deal of variability in this parameter. McArthur et al. (148) compared β2M levels in HIV-seropositive subjects with mild to moderate dementia to those without dementia. Demented subjects had significantly higher intrathecal synthesis of β2M than did nondemented subjects. Using a cutoff value of 3.82 mg/L that was derived from their nondemented group (mean $\pm$ 2 SD), rather than the previously published value of 2.2 (60), they found a specificity of 90%, a sensitivity of 44%, a positive predictive value (proportion of subjects with a positive test who were demented) of 88%, and an efficacy (percentage of subjects correctly classified) of 61%. Lucey et al. (133) studied 163 neurologically normal untreated HIV-infected Air Force personnel. Elevated levels of CSF β2M were associated with declining CD4+ counts and declining functional status of T cells. In contrast to other investigators, they reported that CSF β2M levels paralleled CSF IgG levels, IgG index, and IgG synthesis rates.

Neopterin is synthesized by macrophages and, to a lesser degree, by lymphocytes. Gamma interferon induces neopterin synthesis (34,159,160). However, CSF neopterin levels do not appear to correlate with CSF gamma interferon levels (90). CSF neopterin levels parallel soluble IL-2 receptors and soluble CD8 levels in HIV-infected subjects (89), but do not correlate with CSF pleocytosis (90), BBB dysfunction (90,209), or intrathecal IgG synthesis (169).

Elevated levels of CSF neopterin have been associated with systemic disease progression (73,90,111,209) and with the presence (209) and severity of HIV-related neurological disease (26,60,209). Two studies (21,26) reported that CSF neopterin levels were higher in subjects with AIDS-defining CNS infections, lymphomas, or HIV dementia than in neurologically normal HIV-seropositive individuals; however, CSF neopterin levels may be higher in CNS OIs than in HIV dementia (21). Although CSF neopterin levels tend to correlate with the severity of HIV dementia (26), there is substantial overlap between neurologically symptomatic groups. Like β2M, neopterin levels parallel the degree of CNS inflammation and the course of markers such as QUIN (102). CSF neopterin levels decreased nonsignificantly in conjunction with clinical improvement after zidovudine treatment (26,95).

In summary, CSF β2M and neopterin are easily measured, quantitative, nonspecific markers of cell-mediated immunity that parallel the degree of immune activation and disease progression systemically and in the CNS. Both β2M and neopterin levels decline, at least temporarily, with zidovudine therapy. They are useful to assess the course of primary HIV neurological disease only when OIs and tumors have been excluded and reflect the pathophysiology of HIV CNS disease in an indirect rather than a direct fashion.

EXCITOTOXIC METABOLITES

QUIN is a putative marker for HIV neurological disease, which, like β2M and neopterin, reflects the degree of immune activation in blood and brain and correlates with systemic and neurological disease status (99–105). In addition, QUIN appears to be an important participant in the pathogenesis of neuronal damage in AIDS.

QUIN is an intermediate metabolite in the degradation of the amino acid tryptophan and is classified as an excitotoxic metabolite and an agonist at N-methyl-D-aspartate receptors (9,71,100,105,157). In high concentrations, QUIN can act as a convulsant and a neurotoxin (192). During immune activation, particularly when levels of gamma interferon are elevated, induction of the enzyme indoleamine 2,3-dioxygenase occurs. The latter increases the metabolism of tryptophan through the kynurenine pathway, resulting in an accumulation of QUIN (34,75,237) and related metabolites (103). This process can occur in human macrophages and other cells in conjunction with neopterin synthesis (103,105,236).

QUIN levels are significantly elevated in HIV-infected individuals, with the highest values present in those with moderate to severe HIV-1–related neurological disease (30,99–101,104,105). Elevated levels of CSF QUIN also have been associated with declining neuropsychological test performance, especially reaction time (140). Treatment with zidovudine is associated with a decline in CSF QUIN levels (30). Elevated levels of QUIN are not specific to HIV, however, limiting its use as a diagnostic tool (100). As in other putative markers, there is a high degree of variability in CSF QUIN levels. One group failed to find a significant correlation between QUIN levels in the CSF and brain (1,239). Currently, the measurement of QUIN is a complex process that can only be performed in a few research centers.

In summary, CSF QUIN is a promising quantitative marker for HIV dementia when confounding disease has been excluded. It also may play a role in the pathogenesis of HIV dementia. It is currently not available from commercial laboratories, thus limiting its use for research.

MISCELLANEOUS

CSF and serum levels of tryptophan, precursor of the neurotransmitter serotonin and of QUIN (238), are reportedly lower in HIV-infected subjects than in HIV-seronegative subjects (238). Levels of 5-hydroxy-indoleacetic acid (5HIAA), the major metabolite of serotonin, have been found to be decreased in HIV-infected subjects in two of three reports (29,125,156). Singer et al. (200) found that CSF 5HIAA levels were significantly lower in subjects with HIV dementia than in neurologically normal, systemically asymptomatic HIV-seropositive individuals. Berger et al. (13) found that CSF levels of the neurotransmitter dopamine were significantly lower in HIV-infected subjects than in high-risk seronegative controls. Griffin et al. (88) reportedly found elevated levels of CSF prostaglandins in subjects with HIV dementia.

CONCLUSIONS AND SUMMARY

CSF is an important medium for the diagnosis of HIV-associated neurological diseases and provides valuable information that often cannot be obtained from peripheral blood. Advances in molecular biology have expanded the sensitivity of organism-specific assays as well as important quantitative techniques to follow the progression of HIV disease and its response to treatment.

ACKNOWLEDGMENT

We appreciate the assistance of Julie Kim, Rachel Braum, and Bridget Fahy-Chandon in bibliographic research. This work was supported in part by the National

Institutes of Mental Health (Grant RO1 MH 47281) and by the Veterans Health Services and Research Administration, Department of Veteran Affairs.

REFERENCES

1. Achim CL, Heyes MP, Wiley CA. Quantitation of human immunodeficiency virus, immune activation factors, and quinolinic acid in AIDS brains. *J Clin Invest* 1993;91:2769–2775.
2. Ackermann R, Nekic M, Jurgens R. Locally synthesized antibodies in cerebrospinal fluid of patients with AIDS. *J Neurol* 1986;233:140–141.
3. Allain JP, Laurian Y, Paul D. Long term evaluation of HIV antigen and antibodies to p24 and gp41 in patients with hemophilia. *N Engl J Med* 1987;317:1114–1121.
4. American Academy of Neurology. Ad Hoc Subcommittee of the American Academy of Neurology (AAN) AIDS Task Force. Research criteria for diagnosis of chronic inflammatory demyelinating polyneuropathy (CIDP). *Neurology* 1991;41:617–618.
5. Andersson M. Cerebrospinal fluid in HIV infection. *J Neurol Immunol* 1987;16:12.
6. Andersson M, Bergström T, Blomstrand C, Hermodsson S, Häkansson C, Löwhagen GB. Cerebrospinal fluid changes in HIV-1 infection. *Ann N Y Acad Sci* 1988;540:624–627.
7. Andersson MA, Bergstrom TB, Blomstrand C, Hermodsson SH, Hakanssen C, Lowhagen GBE. Increasing intrathecal lymphocytosis and immunoglobulin G production in neurologically asymptomatic HIV infection. *J Neuroimmunol* 1988;19:291–304.
8. Appleman ME, Marshall DW, Brey RL, et al. Cerebrospinal fluid abnormalities in patients without AIDS who are seropositive for the human immunodeficiency virus. *J Infect Dis* 1988;158:193–199.
9. Aurelius E, Johansson B, Sköldenberg B, Staland A, Forsgren M. Rapid diagnosis of herpes simplex encephalitis by nested polymerase chain reaction assay of cerebrospinal fluid. *Lancet* 1991;337:189–192.
10. Balkwill FR, Burke F. The cytokine network. *Immunol Today* 1989;10:299–304.
11. Beilke MA, Minagawa H, Stone G, Leon-Monzon M, Gibbs CJJ. Neutralizing antibody responses in patients with AIDS with neurological complications. *J Lab Clin Med* 1991;118:585–588.
12. Beneveniste E. *Cytokine circuits in brain: implications for AIDS dementia complex.* New York: Raven, 1994.
13. Berger J, Kumar M, Kumar A, Fernandez J, Levin B. Cerebrospinal fluid dopamine in HIV-1 infection. *AIDS* 1994;8:67–71.
14. Berggard I, Bearn A. Isolation of a low molecular weight microglobulin occuring in human biological fluids. *J Biol Chem* 1968;243:4095–5103.
15. Bernier G, Fanger M. Synthesis of Beta-2-microglobulin by stimulated lymphocytes. *J Immunol* 1972;109:407–409.
16. Beutler B, Cerami A. Cachectin: more than a tumor necrosis factor. *N Engl J Med* 1987;316:379–385.
17. Biniek R, Bartholome M, Schultz M, et al. Intrathecal production of HIV antibodies in suspected AIDS encephalopaty. *J Neurol* 1988;235:131–135.
18. Biniek R, Gesemann M, Scheirmmann NH, Llehmann HJ. Human immunodeficiency virus antibodies in cerebrospinal fluid. *J Neuroimmunol* 1988;20:149–150.
19. Blennow K, Fredman P, Wallin A. Protein analysis in cerebrospinal fluid. I. Influence of concentration gradients for proteins on cerebrospinal fluid/serum albumin ratio. *Eur Neurol* 1993;33:126–128.
20. Blennow K, Fredman P, Wallin A, et al. Protein analysis in spinal fluid II. Reference values derived from healthy individuals 18–88 years of age. *Eur Neurol* 1993;33:129–133.
21. Bogner JR, ge-Hulsing B, Kronawitter U, Sadri I, Matuschke A, Goebel FD. Expansion of neopterin and beta 2-microglobulin in cerebrospinal fluid reaches maximum levels early and late in the course of human immunodeficiency virus infection. *Clin Invest* 1992;70:665–669.
22. Boni J, Emmerich BS, Leib SL, Wiestler OD, Schupbach J, Kleihues P. PCR identification of HIV-1 DNA sequences in brain tissue of patients with AIDS encephlopathy. *Neurology* 1993;43:1813–1817.
23. Breder C, Dinarello C, Saper C. Interleukin-1 immunoreactive innervation of the human hypothalamus. *Science* 1988;240:321–324.
24. Breder C, Saper C. TNF immunoreactive innervation in the mouse brain. *Soc Neurosci Abstr* 1988;144:1280.
25. Brew BJ, Bhalla RB, Fleisher M, et al. Cerebrospinal fluid beta 2 microglobulin in patients infected with human immunodeficiency virus. *Neurology* 1989;39:830–834.
26. Brew BJ, Bhalla RB, Paul M, et al. Cerebrospinal fluid neopterin in human immunodeficiency virus type 1 infection. *Ann Neurol* 1990;28:556–560.
27. Brew BJ, Bhalla RB, Paul M, et al. Cerebrospinal fluid beta 2-microglobulin in patients with AIDS dementia complex: an expanded series including response to zidovudine treatment. *AIDS* 1992;6:461–465.

28. Brightman MW. The distribution within the brain of ferritin injected into cerebrospinal fluid compartments. II. Parenchymal distribution. *Am J Anat* 1965;117:193–220.

29. Britton CB, Cote L, Altsteil L. Cerebrospinal fluid biogenic amine metabolites in patients with AIDS. *Neurology* 1989;39(suppl 1):380.

30. Brouwers P, Heyes MP, Moss HA, et al. Quinolinic acid in the cerebrospinal fluid of children with symptomatic human immunodeficiency virus type 1 disease: relationships to clinical status and therapeutic response. *J Infect Dis* 1993;168:1380–1386.

31. Buffet R, Agut H, Chieze F, et al. Virological markers in the cerbrospinal fluid from HIV-1–infected individuals. *AIDS* 1991;5:1419–1424.

32. Bukasa KS, Sindic CJ, Bodeus M, Burtonboy G, Laterre C, Sonnet J. Anti-HIV antibodies in the CSF of AIDS patients: a serological and immunoblotting study. *J Neurol Neurosurg Psychiatry* 1988;51:1063–1068.

33. Byrne B, Li J, Sninsky J, Poiesz B. Detection of HIV-1 RNA sequences by *in vitro* DNA amplification. *Nucleic Acids Res* 1988;16:4165.

34. Byrne GI, Lehmann LK, Kirschbaum JG, Borden EC, Lee CM, Brown RR. Induction of tryptophan degradation *in vitro* and *in vivo:* a gamma-interferon–stimulated activity. *J Interferon Res* 1986;6:389–396.

35. Carbonara S, Angarano G, Zimatore GB, et al. Clinical value of HIV p24 Ag in cerebrospinal fluid of symptomatic or asymptomatic HIV-infected patients. *Acta Neurol* 1990;12:44–48.

36. Chalmers AC, Aprill BS, Shephard H. Cerebrospinal fluid and human immunodeficiency virus. *Arch Intern Med* 1990;150:1538–1540.

37. Chiodi F, Albert J, Olausson E, et al. Isolation frequency of HIV from CSF and blood of patients with varying severity of HIV infection. *AIDS Res Hum Retrovir* 1988;4:351–358.

38. Chiodi F, Åsjö B, Fenyö EM, Norkrans G, Hagber L, Albert J. Isolation of human immunodeficiency virus from cerebrospinal of an antibody positive virus carrier without neurological symptoms. *Lancet* 1986;2:1276–1277.

39. Chiodi F, Norkrans G, Hagberg L, et al. Human immunodeficiency virus infection of the brain. II. Detection of intrathecally synthesized antibodies by enzyme linked immunosorbent assay and imprint immunofixation. *J Neurol Sci* 1988;87:37–48.

40. Chiodi F, Sönnerborg A, Albert J, et al. Human immunodeficiency virus infection of the brain. I. Virus isolation and detection of HIV specific antibodies in the cerebrospinal fluid of patients with varying clinical conditions. *J Neurol Sci* 1988;85:245–257.

41. Cinque P, Brytting M, Vago L, et al. Epstein-Barr virus DNA in cerebrospinal fluid from patients with AIDS-related primary lymphoma of the central nervous system. *Lancet* 1993;342:398–401.

42. Clifford DB, Buller RS, Mohammed S, Robison L, Storch GA. Use of polymerase chain reaction to demonstrate cytomegalovirus DNA in CSF of patients with human immunodeficiency virus infection. *Neurology* 1993;43:75–79.

43. Cohen BA, McArthur JC, Grohman S, Patterson B, Glass JD. Neurological prognosis of cytomegalovirus polyradiculomyelopathy in AIDS. *Neurology* 1993;43:493–499.

44. Collier AC, Marra C, Coombs RW, et al. Central nervous system manifestations in human immunodeficency virus infection without AIDS. *J AIDS* 1992;5:229–241.

45. Coombs RW, Collier AC, Allain JP, et al. Plasma viremia in human immunodeficiency virus infection. *N Engl J Med* 1989;321:1626–1631.

46. Cristina N, Pelloux H, Goulhot C, Brion J, Leclercq P, Ambroise-Thomas P. Detection of toxoplasma gondii in AIDS patients by the polymerase chain reaction. *Infection* 1993;21:150–153.

47. Cutler R, Page L, Galicich J, Watters G. Formation and absorption of cerebrospinal fluid in man. *Brain* 1968;91:707–720.

48. D'Agaro P, Andrian P, Roscioli B, et al. HIV-1 isolation and p24 antigen detection in cerebrospinal fluid of subjects with neurological abnormalities related to AIDS. *Acta Neurol* 1990;12:49–52.

49. Dallman M, Porter A. Semi-quantitative PCR for the analysis of gene expression. In: McPherson M, Quirke P, Taylor G, eds. *PCR: A Practical Approach.* New York: Oxford University Press, 1991:215–224.

50. Davis LE, Hjelle BL, Miller VE, et al. Early viral brain invasion in iatrogenic human immunodeficiency virus infection. *Neurology* 1992;42:1736–1739.

51. de Gans J, Lange JMA, Derix MMA, et al. Decline of HIV antigen levels in cerebrospinal fluid during treatment with low-dose zidovudine. *AIDS* 1988;2:37–40.

52. de Gans J, Portegies P, Tiessens G, Troost D, Danner SA, Lange JM. Therapy for cytomegalovirus polyradiculomyelitis in patients with AIDS: treatment with ganciclovir. *AIDS* 1990;4:421–425.

53. de Gans J, Tiessens G, Portegies P, Tutuarima J, Troost D. Predominance of polymorphonuclear leukocytes in cerebrospinal fluid of AIDS patients with cytomegalovirus polyradiculomyelitis. *J AIDS* 1990;3:1155–1158.

54. DeRossi A, Gallo P, Amadori A, et al Isolation of HTLV-III from cerebrospinal fluid and neural tissues of patients with neurological syndromes related to the acquired immunodeficiency syndrome. *N Engl J Med* 1985;313:1493–1497.

55. Diederich N, Ackermann R, Jürgens R, et al. Early involvement of the nervous system by human immune deficiency virus (HIV). *Eur Neurol* 1988;28:93–103.
56. Dorries R, Kaiser R, Meulen VT. Human immunodeficiency virus infection: Affinity-mediated immunoblot detects intrathecal synthesis of oligoclonal IgG specific for individual viral protein. *AIDS Res Hum Retrovir* 1989;5:303–310.
57. Duquette P, Charest L. Cerebrospinal fluid findings in healthy siblings of multiple sclerosis patients. *Neurology* 1986;36:727–729.
58. Ellaurie M, Rubinstein A. Tumor necrosis factor-alpha in pediatric HIV-1 infection. *AIDS* 1992;6:1265–1268.
59. Elovaara I, Albert PS, Ranki A, Krohn K, Seppälä I. HIV-1 specificity of cerebrospinal fluid and serum IgG, IgM, and IgG1-G4 antibodies in relation to clinical disease. *J Neurol Sci* 1993;117:111–119.
60. Elovaara I, Iivanainen M, Poutiainen E, et al. CSF and serum beta-2-microglobulin in HIV infection related to neurological dysfunction. *Acta Neurol Scand* 1989;79:81–87.
61. Elovaara I, Iivanainen M, Valle SL, Suni J, Tervo T, Lähdevirta J. CSF protein and cellular profiles in various stages of HIV infection related to neurological manifestations. *J Neurol Sci* 1987;78:331–342.
62. Elovaara I, Nykyri E, Poutiainen E, Hokkanen L, Raininko R, Suni J. CSF follow-up in HIV-1 infection: intrathecal production of HIV-specific and unspecific IgG, and beta-2-microglobulin increase with duration of HIV-1 infection. *Acta Neurol Scand* 1993;87:388–396.
63. Elovaara I, Seppälä I, Poutiainen E, Sun J, Valle S-L. Intrathecal humoral immunological response in neurologically symptomatic and asymptomatic patients with human immunodeficiency virus infection. *Neurology* 1988;38:1451–1456.
64. Emskoetter T, Laer D, Veismann S, Ermer M. Human immunodeficiency virus (HIV)-specific antibodies, neutralizing activity and antibody-dependent cellular cytotoxicity (ADCC) in the cerebrospinal fluid of HIV infected patients. *J Neuroimmunol* 1989;24:61–66.
65. Epstein LG, Goudsmit J, Paul DA, et al. Expression of human immunodeficiency virus in cerebrospinal fluid of children with progressive encephalopathy. *Ann Neurol* 1987;21:397–401.
66. Escaich S, Ritter J, Rougier P, et al. Plasma viraemia as a marker of viral replication in HIV-infected individuals. *AIDS* 1991;5:1189–1194.
67. Fahey JL, Taylor JM, Detels R, et al. The prognostic value of cellular and serological markers in infection with HIV-1. *N Engl J Med* 1990;322:166–172.
68. Felgenhauer K, Lüer W, Poser P. Chronic HIV encephalitis. *J Neuroimmunol* 1988;20:141–144.
69. Fiore JR, Angarano G, Fico C, et al. Different biological properties of paired HIV-1 isolates from peripheral blood mononuclear cells and cerebrospinal fluid. *Acta Neurol* 1991;13:31–36.
70. Fishman RA. *Cerebrospinal Fluid in Diseases of the Nervous System.* 2nd ed. Philadelphia: WB Saunders, 1992.
71. Foster AC, Collins JF, Schwarcz R. On the excitotoxic properties of quinolinic acid, 2,3-piperidine dicarboxylic acids and structurally related compounds. *Neuropharmacology* 1983;22:1331–1342.
72. Franciotta DM, Melzi d'Eril GL, Bono G, Brustia R, Ruberto G, Pagani I. Tumor necrosis factor alpha levels in serum and cerebrospinal fluid of patients with AIDS. *Funct Neurol* 1992;7:35–38.
73. Fuchs D, Chiodi F, Albert J, et al. Neopterin concentrations in cerebrospinal fluid and serum of individuals infected with HIV-1. *AIDS* 1989;3:285–288.
74. Fuchs D, Reibnegge G, Wachter H, Jaeger H, Popescu M. Neopterin levels correlating with the Walter Reed staging classification in human immunodeficiency virus (HIV) infection. *Ann Intern Med* 1987;107:784–785.
75. Fuchs D, Shearer GM, Boswell RN, et al. Negative correlation between blood cell counts and serum neopterin concentration in patients with HIV-1 infection. *AIDS* 1991;5:209–212.
76. Gallo P, De Rossi A, Cadrobbi P, Francavilla E, Chieco-Bianchi L, Tavolato B. Intrathecal synthesis of anti-HIV oligoclonal IgG in HIV-seropositive patients having no signs of HIV-induced neurological diseases. *Ann NY Acad Sci* 1988;540:615–618.
77. Gallo P, Frei K, Rordorf C, Lazdins J, Tavolato B, Fontana A. Human immunodeficiency virus type 1 (HIV–1) infection of the central nervous system: an evaluation of cytokines in cerebrospinal fluid. *J Neuroimmunol* 1989;23:109–116.
78. Gallo P, Pagni S, Giometto B, et al. Macrophage-colony stimulating factor (M-CSF) in cerebrospinal fluid. *J Neuroimmunol* 1990;29:105–112.
79. Gallo P, Piccinno MG, Krzalic L, Tavolato B. Tumor necrosis factor alpha (TNF alpha) and neurological diseases. Failure in detecting TNF alpha in the cerebrospinal fluid from patients with multiple sclerosis, AIDS dementia complex, and brain tumours. *J Neuroimmunol* 1989;23:41–44.
80. Gilland O, Tourtellotte W, O'Tauma L, Henderson W. Normal cerebrospinal fluid pressure. *J Neurosurg* 1974;40:587–593.
81. Glynn P, Gilbert H, Newcombe JIA, Cuzner ML. Rapid analysis of immunoglobulin isoelectric focusing patterns with cellulose nitrate sheets immunoperoxidase staining. *J Immunol Methods* 1982;51:251–257.
82. Goswami K, Kaye R, Miller R, McAllister R, Tedder R. Intrathecal IgG synthesis and specifity of

oligoclonal IgG in patients infected with HIV-1 do not correlate with CNS disease. *J Med Virol* 1991;33:106–113.

83. Goswami KK, Miller RF, Harrison MJ, et al. Expression of HIV-1 in the cerebrospinal fluid detected by the polymerase chain reaction and its correlation with central nervous system disease. *AIDS* 1991;5:797–803.

84. Goudsmit J, de Wolf F, Paul DA, et al. Expression of human immunodeficiency antigen (HIV-Ag) in serum and cerebrospinal fluid during acute and chronic infection. *Lancet* 1986;2:177–180.

85. Goudsmit J, Epstein LG, Paul DA, et al. Intra–blood-brain barrier synthesis of humans and chimpanzees. *Proc Natl Acad Sci U S A* 1987;84:3876–3880.

86. Goudsmit J, Wolters EC, Bakker M, et al. Intrathecal synthesis of antibodies to HTLV-III in patients without AIDS or AIDS related complex. *Br Med J* 1986;292:1231–1234.

87. Gozlan J, Salord J, Roullet E, et al. Rapid detection of cytomegalovirus DNA in cerebrospinal fluid of AIDS patients with neurological disorders. *J Infect Dis* 1992;166:1416–1421.

88. Griffin D, Wesselingh S, McArthur J. Elevated central nervous system prostaglandins in human immunodeficiency virus–associated dementia. *Ann Neurol* 1994;35:592–597.

89. Griffin DE, McArthur JC, Cornblath DR. Soluble interleukin-2 receptor and soluble CD8 in serum and cerebrospinal fluid during human immunodeficiency virus–associated neurological disease. *J Neuroimmunol* 1990;28:97–109.

90. Griffin DE, McArthur JC, Cornblath DR. Neopterin and interferon-gamma in serum and cerebrospinal fluid of patients with HIV-associated neurological disease. *Neurology* 1991;41:69–74.

91. Grimaldi LME, Castagna A, Lazzarin A, et al. Oligoclonal IgG bands in cerebrospinal fluid and serum during asymptomatic Immunodeficiency virus infection. *Ann Neurol* 1988;24:277–279.

92. Grimaldi LME, Castagna A, Roos RP, Devare SG, Casey JM, Lazzarin A. An isoelectric focusing HIV p24 and gp120 overlay study of specimens from asymptomatic HIV seropositive individuals. *Ann Neurol* 1988;24:35–36.

93. Grimaldi LME, Martino GV, Franciotta DM, et al. Elevated alpha–tumor necrosis factor levels in spinal fluid from HIV-1–infected patients with central nervous system involvement. *Ann Neurol* 1991;29:21–25.

94. Gudesblatt M, Gerber O, Vaillancourt PD, Bronster D. Quasi-normal cerebrospinal fluid in patients with acquired immunodeficiency syndrome and cryptococcal meningitis [in French]. *Rev Neurol (Paris)* 1987;143:290–293.

95. Gulevich SJ, McCutchan JA, Thal LJ, et al. Effect of antiretroviral therapy on the cerebrospinal fluid of patients seropositive for the human immunodeficiency virus. *J AIDS* 1993;6:1002–1007.

96. Hagberg L, Forsman A, Norkrans G, Rybo E, Svennerholm L. Cytological and immunoglobulin findings in cerebrospinal fluid of symptomatic and asymptomatic human immunodeficiency virus (HIV) seropositive patients. *Infection* 1988;16:13–22.

97. Hay PE, Clarke JR, Taylor-Robinson D, Goldmeier D. Detection of treponemal DNA in the CSF of patients with syphilis and HIV infection using the polymerase chain reaction. *Genitourin Med* 1990;66:428–432.

98. Henson J, Rosenblum M, Armstrong D, Furneaux H. Amplification of JC virus DNA from brain and cerebrospinal fluid of patients with progressive multifocal leukoencephalopathy. *Neurology* 1991;41:1967–1971.

99. Heyes MP, Brew B, Martin A, et al. Increased quinolinic acid and decreased l-tryptophan in cerebrospinal fluid and plasma in AIDS: correlates to AIDS dementia complex. Presented at the meeting of Neurological and Neuropsychological Complications of HIV Infection, Quebec, Canada, May 31–June 3, 1989, 1989:32.

100. Heyes MP, Brew BJ, Martin A, et al. Quinolinic acid in cerebrospinal fluid and serum in HIV 1 infection: relationship to clinical and neurological status. *Ann Neurol* 1991;29:202–209.

101. Heyes MP, Brew BJ, Price RW, Markey SP. Cerebrospinal fluid quinolinic acid and kynurenic acid in HIV-1 infection. In: Guidotti A, ed. *Neurotoxicity of Excitatory Amino Acids*. New York: Raven, 1990:217–221.

102. Heyes MP, Brew BJ, Saito K, et al. Inter-relationships between quinolinic acid, neuroactive kynurenines, neopterin and $\beta2$-microglobulin in cerebrospinal fluid and serum of HIV-1–infected patients. *J Neuroimmunol* 1992;40:71–80.

103. Heyes MP, Mefford IN, Quearry BJ, Dedhia M, Lackner A. Increased ratio of quinolinic acid to kynurenic acid in cerebrospinal fluid of D retrovirus-infected rhesus macaques: relationship to clinical and viral status. *Ann Neurol* 1990;27:666–675.

104. Heyes MP, Rubinow D, Lane C, Markey SP. Cerebrospinal fluid quinolinic acid concentrations are increased in acquired immune deficiency syndrome. *Ann Neurol* 1989;26:275–277.

105. Heyes MP, Saito K, Crowley S, et al. Quinolinic acid and kynurenine pathway metabolism in inflammatory and non-inflammatory neurological disease. *Brain* 1992;115:1249–1273.

106. Ho DD, Moudgil T, Alam M. Quantitation of human immunodeficiency virus type 1 in the blood of infected persons. *N Engl J Med* 1989;321:1621–1625.

107. Ho DD, Rota TR, Schooley RT, et al. Isolation of HTLV-III from cerebrospinal fluid and neural

tissues of patients with neurological syndromes related to the acquired imunodefiency syndrome. *N Engl J Med* 1985;313:1493–1497.

108. Ho DD, Sarngadharan MG, Resnick L, et al. Primary human T-lymphotrophic virus type III infection. *Ann Intern Med* 1985;103:880–883.

109. Hollander H, Levy JA. Neurological abnormalities and recovery of human immunodeficiency virus from cerebrospinal fluid. *Ann Intern Med* 1987;106:692–695.

110. Huber C, Batchelor J, Fuchs D. Immune response-associated production of neopterin release primarily under the control of interferon gamma. *J Exp Med* 1984;160:310–316.

111. Imberciadori G, Piersantelli N, Bo A, et al. Study of beta 2-microglobulin and neopterin in serum and cerebrospinal fluid of HIV-infected patients. *Acta Neurol (Napoli)* 1990;12:58–61.

112. Ivinson AJ, Taylor GR. PCR in genetic diagnosis. In: McPherson MJ, Quirke P, Taylor GR, eds. *PCR: A Practical Approach.* New York: Oxford University Press, 1991:15–27.

113. Jaton K, Sahli R, Bille J. Development of polymerase chain reaction assays for detection of *Listeria monocytogenes* in clinical cerebrospinal fluid samples. *J Clin Microbiol* 1992;30:1931–1936.

114. Johnson J, Zolla-Pazner S. Detection of HTLV-III antibody in cerebrospinal fluid from patients with AIDS and pre-AIDS with the use of a commercial test system. *Am J Clin Pathol* 1987;88: 351–353.

115. Johnson R. *Viral Infections of the Nervous System.* New York: Raven, 1982.

116. Johnson RT, McArthur JC, Narayan O. The neurobiology of human immunodeficiency virus infections. *FASEB J* 1988;2:2970–2981.

117. Kaiser R, Dörries R, Lüer W, et al. Analysis of oligoclonal antibody bands against individual HIV structural proteins in the CSF of patients infected with HIV. *J Neurol* 1989;236:157–160.

118. Katz RL, Alappattu C, Glass JP, Bruner JM. Cerebrospinal fluid manifestations of the neurological complications of human immunodeficiency virus infection. *Acta Cytol* 1989;33:233–244.

119. Kira J, Itoyama Y, Koyanagi Y. Presence of HTLV-I proviral DNA in central nervous system of patients with HTLV-I associated myelopathy. *Ann Neurol* 1992;31:39–45.

120. Kirchner H. Interferon gamma. *Prog Clin Biochem Med* 1984;1:169–203.

121. Kovacs JA, Kovacs AA, Polis M, et al. Cryptococcosis in the acquired immunodeficiency syndrome. *Ann Intern Med* 1985;103:533–538.

122. Koyanagi Y, Miles S, Mitsuyasu RT, Merrill JE, Vinters HV, Chen IS. Dual infection of the CNS by AIDS viruses with distinct cellular tropisms. *Science* 1987;236:819–822.

123. Laguna F, Arados M, Ortega A, Gonzalez-Lahoz J. Tuberculous meningitis with acellular cerbrospinal fluid in AIDS patients. *AIDS* 1992;6:1165–1167.

124. Lange JMA, de Wolf F, Krone WJA, Danner SA, Coutinho RA, Goudsmit J. Decline of antibody reactivity to outer viral core protein p17 is an earlier serological marker of disease progression in human immunodeficiency virus infection than anti-p24 decline. *AIDS* 1987;1:155–159.

125. Larsson M, Hagberg L, Norkrans G, Forsman A. Indole amine deficiency in blood and cerebrospinal fluid from patients with human immunodeficiency virus infection. *J Neuroscience Res* 1989;23: 441–446.

126. Lefvert AK, Link H. IgG production within the central nervous system: a critical review of proposed formulae. *Ann Neurol* 1985;17:13–20.

127. Levy JA, Bredesen DE. Central nervous system dysfunction in acquired immunodeficiency syndrome. *J AIDS* 1988;1:41–64.

128. Levy JA, Shimabukuro J, Hollander H, Mills J, Kaminsky L. Isolation of AIDS-associated retroviruses from cerebrospinal fluid and brains of patients with neurological symptoms. *Lancet* 1985;2: 586–588.

129. Levy RM, Bredesen DE, Rosenblum ML. Neurological manifestations of the acquired immunodeficiency syndrome (AIDS): experience at UCSF and review of the literature. *J Neurosurg* 1985;62: 475–495.

130. Lillo F, Cao Y, Concedi D, OE V. Improved detection of serum HIV p24 antigen after acid dissociation of immune complexes. *AIDS* 1993;7:1331–1336.

131. Liu PY-F, Shi Z-Y, Lau Y-J, Hu B-S. Rapid diagnosis of tuberculous meningitis by a simplified nested amplification protocol. *Neurology* 1994;44:1161–1164.

132. Lloyd A, Wakefield D, Robertson P, Dwyer JM. Antibodies to HIV are produced within the central nervous system of all subjects with all categories of HIV infection. *Aust N Z J Med* 1988;18: 854–860.

133. Lucey D, McGuire S, Clerici M, et al. Comparison of spinal fluid β2-microglobulin levels with CD4 + T cell count in 163 neurologically normal adults infected with the HIV-1. *J Infect Dis* 1991; 163:971–975.

134. Lüer W, Poser S, Weber T, Jürgens S, Eichenlaub D, Phole HD, Felgenhauer K. Chronic HIV encephalitis-I. Cerebrospinal fluid diagnosis. *Klin Wochenschr* 1988;66:21–25.

135. MacDonell KB, Chmiel JS, Poggensee L, Wu S. Predicting progression to AIDS: combined usefulness of CD4 lymphocyte counts and p24 antigenemia. *Am J Med* 1990;89:706–712.

136. Margolick JB, McArthur JC, Scott ER, et al. Flow cytometric quantitation of cell phenotypes in

cerebrospinal fluid and peripheral blood of homosexual men with and without antibodies to human immunodeficiency virus type I. *J Neuroimmunol* 1988;20:73–81.

137. Marshall DW, Brey RL, Butzin CA, Lucey DR, Abbadessa SM, Bosswell RN. CSF changes in a longitudinal study of 124 neurologically normal HIV-1 infected U.S. Air Force personel. *J AIDS* 1991;4:777–781.

138. Marshall DW, Brey RL, Cahill WT. Cerebrospinal fluid (CSF) findings in asymptomatic (AS) individuals infected by human immunodeficiency virus (HIV). *Neurology* 1988;38:167–168.

139. Marshall DW, Brey RL, Cahill WT, Houk RW, Zajac RA, Boswell RN. Spectrum of cerebrospinal fluid findings in various stages of HIV infection. *Arch Neurol* 1988;45:945–958.

140. Martin A, Heyes MP, Salazar AM, et al. Progressive slowing of reaction time and increasing cerebrospinal fluid concentrations of quinolinic acid in HIV-infected individuals. *J Neuropsychiatry Clin Neurosci* 1992;4:270–279.

141. Martin SB, Tracey KJ. *Tumour Necrosis Factor (TNF) in Neuroimmunology.* New York: Pergamon, 1992.

142. Martinez-Maza O, Crabb E, Mitsuyasu RT, Fahey JL, Giorgi JV. Infection with the human immunodeficiency virus (HIV) is associated with an in vitro increase in B lymphocyte activation and immaturity. *J Immunol* 1987;138:3720–3724.

143. Mastroianni CM, Paoletti F, Massetti AP, Falciano M, Vullo V. Elevated levels of tumor necrosis factor (TNF) in the cerebrospinal fluid from patients with HIV-1 associated neurological disease. *Acta Neurol* 1990;12:66–67.

144. Mastroianni CM, Paoletti F, Valenti C, Vullo V, Jirillo E, Delia S. Tumour necrosis factor (TNF-alpha) and neurological disorders in HIV infection. *J Neurol Neurosurg Psychiatry* 1992;55: 219–221.

145. Mathiesen T, Sonnerborg A, von Sydow M, Gaines H, Wahren B. IgG subclass reactivity against human immunodeficiency virus (HIV) and cytomegalovirus in cerebrospinal fluid and serum from HIV-infected patients. *J Med Virol* 1988;25:17–26.

146. McArthur JC. Neurological manifestations of AIDS. *Medicine* 1987;66:407–437.

147. McArthur JC, Cohen BA, Farzedegan H, et al. Cerebrospinal fluid abnormalities in homosexual men with and without neuropsychiatric findings. *Ann Neurol* 1988;23(suppl):34–37.

148. McArthur JC, Nance-Sproson TE, Griffin DE, et al. The diagnostic utility of elevation in cerebrospinal fluid β2-microglobulin in HIV-1 dementia. *Neurology* 1992;42:1707–1712.

149. McArthur JC, Sipos E, Cornblath DR, et al. Identification of mononuclear cells in CSF of patients with HIV infection. *Neurology* 1989;39:66–70.

150. Merrill J, Koyanagi Y, Chen I. Interleukin-1 and tumor necrosis factor alpha can be induced from mononuclear phagocytes by human immunodeficiency virus type 1 binding to the CD4 receptor. *J Virol* 1989;63:4404–4408.

151. Merrill J, Matsushima K. Production of and response to interleukin-1 by cloned human oligodendroglioma cell lines. *J Biol Regul Homeost Agents* 1988;2:77–86.

152. Michael NL, Vahey M, Burke DS, Redfield RR. Viral DNA and mRNA expression correlate with the stage of human immunodeficiency virus (HIV) type 1 infection in humans: evidence for viral replication in all stages of HIV disease. *J Virol* 1992;66:310–316.

153. Michaels J, Sharer LR, Epstein LG. Human immunodeficiency virus type 1 (HIV-1) infection of the nervous system: a review. *Immunodefic Rev* 1988;1:71–104.

154. Miles SA, Balden E, Magpantay L, et al. Rapid serological testing with immune-complex dissociated HIV P24 antigen for early detection of HIV infection in neonates. *N Engl J Med* 1993;328:297–302.

155. Mintz M, Rapaport R, Oleske JM, et al. Elevated serum levels of tumor necrosis factor are associated with progressive encephalopathy in children with acquired immunodeficiency syndrome. *Am J Dis Child* 1989;143:771–774.

156. Moeller AA, Pirke KM. Metabolites of serotonin and catecholamines in the cerebrospinal fluid of patients in advanced stages of HIV-1 infection. *J Neurol* 1990;237:124.

157. Monaghan DT, Cotman CW. Distribution of N-Methyl-D-aspartate–sensitive L-[3H] glutamate–binding sites in rat brain. *J Neurosci* 1985;5:2909–2919.

158. Morfeldt-Manson J, Julander I, von Steding KLV, Wasserman J, Nilsson B. Elevated serum beta-2-microglobulin. A prognostic marker for development of AIDS among patients with persistent generalized lymphadenopathy. *Infection* 1988;16:109–110.

159. Nathan C. Peroxide and pteridine: a hypothesis on the regulation of macrophage antimicrobial activity by interferon gamma. *Interferon* 1986;7:125–143.

160. Nathan C, Murray H, Wiebe M, Rubin B. Identification of interferon-gamma as the lymphokine that activates human macrophage oxidative metabolism and antimicrobial activity. *J Exp Med* 1983; 158:670–689.

161. Norfolk D, Child J, Roberts B, Forbes M, EH C. Serum beta-2-microglobulin in disorders of myeloid proliferation. *Acta Haematol* 1983;69:361–368.

162. Öhman S, Ernerudh J, Forsberg P, Henriksson A, von Schenck H, Vrethem M. Comparison of seven formulae and isoelectric focusing for determination of intrathecally produced IgG in neurological disease. *Ann Clin Biochem* 1992;29:405–410.

163. Oka S, Urayama K, Hirabayashi Y, et al. Quantitative analysis of human immunodeficiency virus type-1 DNA in asymptomatic carriers using the polymerase chain reaction. *Biochem Biophys Res Commun* 1990;167:1–8.
164. Ortona L, Tamburrini E, Antinori A, Ventura G. Neurological features in AIDS patients: studies on cerebrospinal fluid. *Ital J Neurol Sci* 1988;9:567–572.
165. Pang S, Koyangi Y, Miles S, Wiley C, Vinters HV, Chen ISY. High levels of unintegrated HIV-1 DNA in brain tissue of AIDS dementia patients. *Nature* 1990;343:85–89.
166. Pang S, Vinters H, Akashi T, O'Brien W, Chen I. HIV-1 Env sequence variation in brain tissue of patients with AIDS-related neurological disease. *J AIDS* 1991;4:1082–1092.
167. Perrella O, Carrieri P, Izzo E, et al. Cerebrospinal fluid beta-2-microglobulin in HIV-1 infection as a marker of neurological involvement. *Neurol Res* 1991;13:131–132.
168. Perrella O, Carrieri PB, Guarnaccia D, Soscia M. Cerebrospinal fluid cytokines in AIDS dementia complex. *J Neurol* 1992;239:387–388.
169. Peter JB, McKeown KL, Barka NE, Tourtellotte WW, Singer EJ, Syndulko K. Neopterin and β2-microglobulin and the assessment of intra–blood-brain-barrier synthesis of HIV-specific and total IgG. *J Clin Lab Anal* 1991;5:317–320.
170. Peter JB, Tourtellotte WW. Modest serum contamination of cerebrospinal fluid (CSF) invalidates the calculation of intra–blood-brain barrier (BBB) IgG synthesis and intra–BBB albumin formation but not unique CSF oligoclonal IgG bands. *Ann Neurol* 1986;20.
171. Petito C, Cash K. Blood–brain barrier abnormalities in the acquired immunodeficiency syndrome: immunohistochemical localization of serum proteins in postmortem brain. *Ann Neurol* 1992;32: 658–666.
172. Pfefferkorn E, Rebhun S, Eckel M. Characterization of an indoleamine-2,3 dioxygenase induction by gamma-interferon in cultured human fibroblasts. *J Interferon Res* 1986;6:267–279.
173. Portegies P, Enting RH, de Gans J, et al. Presentation and course of AIDS dementia complex: 10 years of follow-up in Amsterdam, The Netherlands. *AIDS* 1993;7:669–675.
174. Portegies P, Epstein LG, Hung ST, de Gans J, Goudsmit J. Human immunodeficiency virus type 1 antigen in cerebrospinal fluid. Correlation with clinical neurological status. *Arch Neurol* 1989; 46:261–264.
175. Porter S, Sande M. Toxoplasmosis of the central nervous system in the acquired immunodeficiency syndrome. *N Engl J Med* 1992;327:1643–1648.
176. Power C, Kong PA, Crawford TO, et al. Cerebral white matter changes in acquired immunodeficiency syndrome dementia: alterations of the blood-brain-barrier. *Ann Neurol* 1993;34:339–350.
177. Rapoport SI. Passage of proteins from blood to cerebrospinal fluid: model for transfer by pores or vesicles. In: Woods, JH, ed. *Neurobiology of Cerebrospinal Fluid*. New York: Plenum, 1983.
178. Reboul J, Schuller E, Pialoux G, Rey MA, Lebon P, Allinquant B. Immunoglobulins and complement components in 37 patients infected by HIV-1: comparison of general (systemic) and intrathecal immunity. *J Neurol Sci* 1989;89:243–252.
179. Redfield R, Wright DC, Tramont EC. The Walter Reed staging classification for HTLV-III/LAV infection. *N Engl J Med* 1986;314:131–132.
180. Reiber H, Felgenhauer K. Protein transfer at the blood cerebrospinal fluid barrier and the quantitation of the humoral immune response within the central nervous system. *Clin Chim Acta* 1987;163: 319–328.
181. Resnick L, Berger JR, Shapshak P, Tourtellotte WW. Early penetration of the blood-brain-barrier by HTLV-III/LAV. *Neurology* 1988;38:9–14.
182. Resnick L, DiMarzo-Veronese F, Schopbach J, et al. Intra–blood-brain-barrier synthesis of HTLV-III specific IgG in patients with AIDS or AIDS-related complex. *N Engl J Med* 1985;313:1498–1504.
183. Rhodes R. Evidence of serum-protein leakage across the blood–brain barrier in the acquired immunodeficiency syndrome. *J Neuropathol Exp Neurol* 1991;50:171–183.
184. Rolfs A, Schumaker HC. Early findings in the cerebrospinal fluid of patients with HIV-1 infection of the central nervous system. *N Engl J Med* 1990;323:418–419.
185. Sadat-Sowti B, Debre P. Cytokines and HIV infection. *Eur Cytokine Netw* 1992;3:515–521.
186. Scalzini A, Scura G, Stellini R, Cristini G. HIV1-Ag in cerebrospinal fluid during AIDS. *Acta Neurol* 1990;12:53–57.
187. Schechter MT, Neumann PW, Weaver MS, et al. Low HIV-1 proviral DNA burden detected by negative polymerase chain reaction in seropositive individuals correlates with slower disease progression. *AIDS* 1991;5:373–379.
188. Scheld W. Drug delivery to the central nervous system: general principles and relevance to therapy for infections of the central nervous system. *Rev Infect Dis* 1989;11(suppl):1669–1690.
189. Schmid P, Conrad A, Syndulko K, et al. Quantifying HIV-1 proviral DNA using the polymerase chain reaction on cerebrospinal fluid and blood of seropositive individuals with and without neurological abnormalities. *J AIDS* 1995;10(4):425–435.
190. Schuller E, Sagar HJ. Local synthesis of CSF immunoglubulins. *J Neurol Sci* 1981;51:361–370.
191. Schuller EAC, Benabdallah S, Sagar HJ, Reboul JAM, Tompe LC. IgG synthesis within the central nervous system. *Arch Neurol* 1987;44:600–604.

192. Schwarcz R, Kohler C. Differential vulnerability of central neurons of the rat to quinolinic acid. *Neurosci Lett* 1983;38:85.
193. Selmaj KW, Raine CS. Tumor necrosis factor mediates myelin and oligodendrocyte damage *in vitro. Ann Neurol* 1988;23:339–346.
194. Shankar P, Manjuanth N, Mohan K, et al. Rapid diagnosis of tuberculous meningitis by polymerase chain reaction. *Lancet* 1991;337:5–7.
195. Shaskan EG, Thompson RM, Price RW. Undetectable tumor necrosis factor-alpha in spinal fluid from HIV-1–infected patients [Letter]. *Ann Neurol* 1992;31:687–689.
196. Shaunak S, Albright RE, Klotman ME, Hnery SC, Bartlett JA, Hamilton JD. Amplification of HIV-1 provirus from cerebrospinal fluid and its correlation with neurological disease. *J Infect Dis* 1990; 161:1068–1072.
197. Shoji H, Hondra Y, Murai I, Sato Y, Oizumi K, Hondo R. Detection of varicella-zoster virus DNA by polymerase chain reaction in cerebrospinal fluid of patients with herpes zoster meningitis. *J Neurol* 1991;239:69–70.
198. Simmonds P, Balfe P, Peutherer JF, Ludlam CA, Bishop JO, Leigh Brown A. Human immunodeficiency virus–infected individuals contain provirus in small numbers of peripheral mononuclear cells and at low copy numbers. *J Virol* 1990;64:867–872.
199. Sinclair E, Scaravilli F. Detection of HIV proviral DNA in cortex and white matter of AIDS brains by non-isotopic polymerase chain reaction: correlation with diffuse poliodystrophy. *AIDS* 1992;6: 925–932.
200. Singer E, Wilkins J, Syndulko K. Altered cerebrospinal fluid levels of cortisol and biogenic amines in acquired immunodeficiency syndrome dementia complex versus asymptomatic seropositives: partial correction with zidovudine therapy. *Ann Neurol* 1990;28:280–281.
201. Singer EJ, Ruane P, Syndulko K, Fahy-Chandon B, Resnick L, Tourtellotte WW. Search for laboratory markers of CNS disease in HIV-seropositive individuals. *Neurology* 1989;39(suppl 1):420.
202. Singer EJ, Syndulko K, Fahy-Chandon B, et al. Cerebrospinal fluid p24 antigen levels and intrathecal immunoglobulin G synthesis are associated with cognitive disease severity in HIV-1. *AIDS* 1994; 8(2):197–204.
203. Singer EJ, Syndulko K, Fahy-Chandon B, et al. Intrathecal IgG synthesis and albumin leakage are increased in subjects with HIV-1 neurological disease. *J AIDS* 1994;7:265–271.
204. Skotzek B, Sander TH, Zimmermann J. Oligoclonals bands in serum and cerebrospinal fluid of patients with HIV infection. *J Neuroimmunol* 1988;20:151–152.
205. Snider WD, Simpson DM, Nielson S, Gold JWM, Metroka C, Posner JB. Neurological complications of acquired immune deficiency syndrome: analysis of 50 patients. *Ann Neurol* 1983;14:403–418.
206. Sönnerborg A, Ehrnst A, Strannegard O. Relationship between the occurrence of virus in plasma and cerebrospinal fluid of HIV-1 infected individuals. *J Med Virol* 1989;27:258–263.
207. Sönnerborg AB, Ehrnst AC, Bergdahl SKM, Pehrson PO, Skoldenberg BR, Strannegärd OO. HIV isolation from cerebrospinal fluid in relation to immunological and neurological symptoms. *AIDS* 1988;2:89–93.
208. Sönnerborg AB, Johansson B, Strannegard O. Detection of HIV-1 DNA and infectious virus in cerebrospinal fluid. *AIDS Res Hum Retrovir* 1991;7:369–373.
209. Sönnerborg AB, von Stedingk LV, Hansson LO, Strannegärd OO. Elevated neopterin and beta 2-microglobulin levels in blood and cerebrospinal fluid occur early in HIV-1 infection. *AIDS* 1989; 3:277–283.
210. Sönnerborg AB, von Sydow MA, Forsgren M, Strannegärd OO. Association between intrathecal anti–HIV-1 immunoglobulin G synthesis and occurrence of HIV-1 in cerebrospinal fluid. *AIDS* 1989;3:701–705.
211. Spector SA, Hsia K, Pratt D, et al. Virological markers of human immunodeficiency virus type 1 in cerebrospinal fluid. The HIV Neurobehavioral Research Center Group. *J Infect Dis* 1993;168: 68–74.
212. Staugaitis SM, Shapshak P, Tourtellotte WW, Lee MM, Reiber HO. Isoelectric focusing of unconcentrated cerebrospinal fluid: application to ultrasensitive analysis of oligoclonal immunoglobulin-G. *Electrophoresis* 1985;6:287–291.
213. Steuler H, Munzinger S, Wildemann B, Stroch-Hagenlocher B. Quantitation of HIV-1 proviral DNA in cells from cerebrospinal fluid. *J AIDS* 1992;5:405–408.
214. Steuler H, Storch-Haglenlocher B, Wildemann B. Distinct populations of human immunodeficiency virus type 1 in blood and cerebrospinal fluid. *AIDS Res Hum Retrovir* 1992;8:53.
215. Sykes P, Neoh S, Brisco M. Quantitation of targets for PCR by use of limiting dilution. *Biotechniques* 1992;13:444–449.
216. Syndulko K, Tourtellotte E, Conrad A, Izquierdo G. Trans–blood-brain-barrier albumin leakage and comparisons of intrathecal IgG synthesis calculations in multiple sclerosis patients. *J Neuroimmunol* 1993;46:185–192.
217. Tartaglione TA, Collier AC, Coombs RW, et al. Acquired immunodeficiency syndrome. Cerebrospinal fluid findings in patients before and during long-term oral zidovudine therapy. *Arch Neurol* 1991;48:695–699.

218. Taylor G. Polymerase chain reaction: basic principles and automation. In: McPherson M, Quirke P, Taylor G, eds. *PCR: A Practical Approach.* New York: Oxford University Press, 1991:1–14.
219. Tibbling G, Link H, Öhman S. Principles of albumin and IgG analyses in neurological disorders. *Scand J Clin Lab Invest* 1977;37:385–390.
220. Tomberlin M, Holtom P, Owens J, Larsen R. Evaluation of neurosyphilis in human immunodeficiency virus–infected individuals. *Clin Infect Dis* 1994;18:288–294.
221. Tornatore C, Chandra R, Berger J, Major E. HIV-1 infection of subcortical astrocytes in the pediatric central nervous system. *Neurology* 1994;44:481–487.
222. Torre D, Zeroli C, Ferraro G, et al. Cerebrospinal fluid levels of IL-6 in patients with acute infections of the central nervous system. *Scand J Infect Dis* 1992;24:787–791.
223. Tourtellotte WW. Cerebrospinal fluid in multiple sclerosis. In: Vinken P, Bruyn GW, eds. *Handbook of Clinical Neurology.* Amsterdam: North Holland, 1970:324–382.
224. Tourtellotte WW. Multiple sclerosis cerebrospinal fluid. In: Hallpike JF, Tourtellotte WW, Raine CS, eds. *Multiple Sclerosis. Pathology, Diagnosis and Management.* 2nd ed. London: Chapman & Hall, 1993.
225. Tourtellotte WW, Henderson WG, Tucker RP, Gilland O, Walker JE, Kokman E. A randomized, double-blind clinical trial comparing the 22 versus 26 gauge needle in the production of the post-lumbar puncture syndrome in normal individuals. *Headache* 1972;12:73–78.
226. Tourtellotte WW, Izquierdo G, Syndulko K, Baumhefner GW, Ellison GW, Myers LW. Intra–blood-brain-barrier IgG synthesis in multiple sclerosis: comparison of formulas after treatment. *Ann Neurol* 1989;26:178.
227. Tourtellotte WW, Potvin AR, Potvin JH, Ma BI, Baumhefner RW, Syndulko K. *Multiple Sclerosis De Novo Central Nervous System IgG Synthesis: Measurement, Antibody Profile, Significance, Eradication, and Problems.* New York: Springer-Verlag, 1980.
228. Tourtellotte WW, Shapshak P, Osborne MA, Rubinshtein G, Lee M, Staugaitis SM. New formula to calculate the rate of albumin blood-brain-barrier leakage. *Ann Neurol* 1989;26:176.
229. Tyor WR, Glass JD, Griffin JW, et al. Cytokine expression in the brain during the acquired immunodeficiency syndrome. *Ann Neurol* 1992;31:349–360.
230. Ujhelyi E, Fuchs D, Krall G, et al. Age dependency of the progression of HIV disease in haemophiliacs: predictive value of T cell subset and neopterin measurements. *Immunol Lett* 1990;26:67–74.
231. van Snick J. Interleukin-6: an overview. *Annu Rev Immunol* 1990;8:253–278.
232. Van Wielink G, McArthur JC, Moench T, et al. Intrathecal synthesis of anti HIV IgG correlation with increasing duration of HIV-1 infection. *Neurology* 1990;40:816–819.
233. Vazeux R. AIDS encephalopathy and tropism of HIV for brain monocytes/macrophages and microglial cells. *Pathobiology* 1991;59:214–218.
234. Vitkovic L, da Cunha A, Tyor W. Cytokine expression and pathogenesis in AIDS brain. In: Price R, Perry S, eds. *HIV, AIDS and the Brain.* New York: Raven, 1994.
235. Weber T, Butner W, Felgenhauer K. Evidence for different immune responses to HIV in CSF and serum? *Klin Wochenschr* 1987;65:259–263.
236. Werner E, Werner-Felmayer G, Fuchs D, Reibengger G, Wachter H. Parallel induction of tetra-hydrobiopterin biosynthesis and indoleamine 2,3-dioxygenase activity in human cells and cell line by interferon gamma. *Biochem J* 1989;262:861–866.
237. Werner ER, Bitterlich G, Fuchs D, et al. Human macrophages degrade tryptophan upon induction by interferon-gamma. *Life Sci* 1987;41:273–280.
238. Werner ER, Fuchs D, Hausen A, et al. Tryptophan degradation in patients infected by human immunodeficiency virus. *Biol Chem Hoppe Seyler* 1988;369:337–340.
239. Wiley CA, Achim CL, Schrier RD, Heyes MP, McCutchan JA, Grant I. Relationship of cerebrospinal fluid immune activation associated factors to HIV encephalitis. *AIDS* 1992;6:1299–1307.
240. Wiley CA, Schrier RD, Nelson JA, Lampert PW, Oldstone MBA. Cellular localization of human immunodeficiency virus infection within the brains of acquired immune deficiency syndrome patients. *Proc Natl Acad Sci U S A* 1986;83:7089–7093.
241. Yoshioka M, Shapshak P, Srivastava A, et al. Expression of HIV-1 and interleukin-6 in lumbosacral dorsal root ganglia of patients with AIDS. *Neurology* 1994;44:1120–1130.

AIDS and the Nervous System, Second Edition,
edited by J. R. Berger and R. M. Levy.
Lippincott-Raven Publishers, Philadelphia © 1997.

12

Clinical Neurophysiological Testing in Human Immunodeficiency Virus Infection

Colin D. Hall, John A. Messenheimer, and Bradley V. Vaughn

*Department of Neurology, University of North Carolina at Chapel Hill,
University of North Carolina Hospitals, Chapel Hill, North Carolina 27599*

In the decade since the first descriptions of the neurological effects of human immunodeficiency virus (HIV) infection, the whole gamut of standard clinical neurophysiological tests has been applied to groups of HIV-infected subjects. Studies have involved the central nervous system (CNS) and peripheral nervous system, as well as the the autonomic nervous system (ANS). Information from these studies is at times critical in the clinical diagnosis and treatment of individuals. However, as with most other diseases, clinical neurophysiological studies are generally nonspecific, and their major role has been as research tools in attempting to define the parameters of this new and devastating scourge of the human nervous system. Electrophysiological studies have proven to be particularly sensitive tools in the investigation of the degree of neurological dysfunction and the rate of its progression at various stages of systemic infection. Much of this work has concentrated on questions discussed elsewhere in this book: how frequent and how widespread are the nervous system effects of HIV; how early can signs of neurological dysfunction be seen in HIV-infected subjects, and in particular, are there subtle nervous system changes in the systematically asymptomatic stages; how rapidly does neurological dysfunction progress once it can be detected; is HIV-associated dementia a condition of rapid onset in the late stages of infection or is it preceded by protracted and initially subtle decline in neurological function; and are there any predictors for dementia that may be used to initiate early effective treatment as this becomes available. These questions have not yet been answered adequately, but the emerging picture owes a good deal to the evidence gathered from the studies to be addressed here.

This chapter discusses the clinical utility and reviews the research role of a variety of clinical neurophysiological tools, including routine and quantitative electroencephalography (EEG), a battery of evoked potential (EP) studies, studies of ANS function, and evaluation of sleep. Nerve conduction and electromyography are discussed in Chapter 9.

ELECTROENCEPHALOGRAPHY

Routine EEG

Changes in EEG may occur with many of the large variety of secondary complications of the CNS that occur in HIV infection. These include opportunistic infection, tumor, stroke, and metabolic and toxic complications of systemic disease. The changes lack specificity and match those found in similar diseases in the patient not infected with HIV. As such, their clinical value is limited to situations in which they would be of diagnostic and therapeutic use for these other conditions. Generalized and partial seizures have been reported in up to 11% of infected patients; in half of these there is no clear etiology other than HIV infection itself (72). In this setting, the EEG plays its customary role in contributing to the evaluation of seizure disorders.

A number of studies have addressed cross-sectional and longitudinal EEG changes in cohorts of HIV-positive subjects. In general there is a higher than expected incidence of diffuse rhythmical slowing in both asymptomatic and symptomatic patients, changes that are usually associated with diffuse gray, rather than white, matter involvement. These abnormalities are nonspecific etiologically, and their presence cannot be assumed to result from direct effects of HIV infection; they may result from one or more of the many secondary nervous system processes associated with the disease. Enzensberger first reported slowing associated with dementia in acquired immunodeficiency syndrome (AIDS) and suggested that the EEG may be a sensitive tool for the onset of encephalopathy (18). Other studies also have found association between the development of encephalopathy and loss of amplitude of the EEG, often with the appearance of additional slowing. Gabuza et al. (21) reported routine EEG findings in a group of patients with AIDS and AIDS-related complex (ARC). The most frequent abnormality was intermittent or continuous rhythmic theta or delta slowing, which was generalized, bifrontal or bitemporal in distribution. Overall, 67% of patients with AIDS and 36% of those with ARC had EEG abnormalities. Harden et al. retrospectively reviewed the EEGs from 13 patients with AIDS and four who were HIV-positive without AIDS and compared them with 17 age-matched controls with a variety of nonspecific neurological complaints. One HIV-positive patient had background slowing; all other abnormalities were found in the AIDS group. The EEGs were generally of unusually low amplitude, slow, and featureless. Loss of posterior rhythms was common. Some had increases in arrhythmic slowing, primarily in the delta range. Jabarri found a similar correlation in a longitudinal study of HIV-positive military personnel (31). Schnurbus et al., reviewing 370 records from 167 patients, found a progressive increase in background slowing with advancing disease (64). In our own longitudinal cohort studies, >40% of subjects with AIDS had intermittent or continuous, generalized or focal, theta or delta range slowing (41). Only 10% of asymptomatic subjects had abnormal EEGs. In those subjects who became demented, no routine EEG changes were seen in the evaluation 6 months before the onset of dementia.

Thus, there appears to be general agreement that in the later stages of infection there are EEG abnormalities, the severity of which generally match other manifestations of illness, particularly changes in neuropsychological performance. It also appears that progression to HIV encephalopathy is not predictable on the basis of EEG changes.

There have been more conflicting studies on possible changes in routine EEG during the systemically and neurologically asymptomatic stages of HIV infection.

Moeller et al. reported that almost 60% of unselected infected patients had slowing on EEG (44). When subdivided, 83% of those showing signs of neurological dysfunction, 54% with a history of neurological symptoms but no signs, and 36% of those without either were abnormal. There was no clear correlation with Walter Reed disease staging. Koralnik et al. reported in 1990 that a significant percentage of asymptomatic HIV-positive patients showed EEG abnormalities not seen in matched controls (35). However, several of the EEG changes the group classified as abnormalities were not generally accepted by other workers in the field as being of electrophysiological or clinical significance (50). Elovaara analyzed the EEG of 67 HIV-positive patients at various disease stages and found significant, predominantly anterior slowing (17). This was much more evident with advanced disease, but was already present in early disease. The Multicenter AIDS Cohort Study (MACS) group found no statistical difference between infected and asymptomatic uninfected subjects (49). There was increased slowing in the neuropsychologically impaired patients, but this was true in both HIV-positive subjects and HIV-negative controls. It was felt that neuropsychological impairment should be considered a confounding factor in evaluating EEG abnormality. Jabarri et al. found that in infected military personnel only 3% of asymptomatic subjects had abnormalities on initial EEG evaluation, and the development of abnormalities over time occurred in conjunction with perceptible declines in neuropsychological function (4). Arendt et al. compared 100 HIV-positive subjects in all stages of disease with age-matched controls. No statistically relevant differences in EEG were found between the groups (2). Similarly, Ragazzoni et al. found no difference in EEG between neurologically asymptomatic HIV-positive and HIV-negative subjects (61). In our own studies, only 11 of 177 records from asymptomatic subjects have shown abnormalities, and we have not found routine EEG to be of any predictive value for future neurological decline (26,41,68). Based on these more recent studies, a consensus is now emerging that routine EEG in asymptomatic HIV-positive patients does not differ from that in matched uninfected patients. Nor does it appear to provide a predictive marker for future clinical neurological disease.

Quantitative EEG

Quantitative EEG (QEEG) refers to the methodology where selected EEG epochs are subjected to computerized analysis in order to more precisely quantify the data. The major advantage of this approach is in providing greater sensitivity in detecting changes over time in the same subjects and cross-sectional changes between different patient groups. This method also may be sensitive to changes in the topography of EEG abnormalities. QEEG cannot stand by itself as a diagnostic tool (3) and must be interpreted in the context of a simultaneously obtained routine EEG. However, a number of studies have demonstrated the increased sensitivity of QEEG examinations when compared with routine visual analysis of EEG in a number of clinical conditions (33). In Alzheimer's disease, in which progressive degeneration is associated with dementia, quantitative studies have confirmed the earliest manifestations of involvement to be an increase in background theta activity, with alpha activity unaffected (8,60). Thus, QEEG has the potential to be much more sensitive than routine EEG in demonstrating early effects of HIV in the CNS. Unfortunately, QEEG methodology has not been standardized, and considerable variation in methodology is the rule. In many instances, investigators fail to provide sufficient details of their methods to permit reasonable assessment of their results. Although QEEG is potentially more objective than routine EEG, it is not completely free of bias. One of the major limitations is the fact that a number of EEG epochs of fixed length are averaged together to obtain an estimate of the frequency range of the data. The selection of which epochs are to be analyzed is performed manually and is subject to considerable bias unless techniques are in place to prevent this from happening (e.g., blinding). If epochs are selected correctly, artifacts or transient EEG abnormalities (spikes) are excluded from the average. However, intermittent abnormalities such as intermittent slowing may be lost in the averaging process. Several of the studies described here do not offer detailed methodology, and the results must therefore be interpreted with great caution.

To date, few studies of QEEG changes in HIV infection have been reported. QEEG studies are not always comparable with each other due to significant methodological differences, and in many of the available studies in HIV disease the investigators have not included sufficient methodological information to permit adequate assessment of the reported results. This is the case with the report of Parisi et al. (54). QEEG was performed on 101 HIV-positive patients with various stages of disease progression. Thirty seven had asymptomatic HIV infection (Asx), 19 had AIDS related complex (ARC), and 45 were Walter Reed stage IVA or above. There was an increase in EEG slowing with progression of disease. Koralnik et al. found increased anterior theta activity in the asymptomatic HIV-positive group when compared with controls (35).

Nuwer carried out a careful analysis of routine EEG and QEEG changes in a subset of HIV-positive asymptomatic subjects from the MACS study. There was no difference between this group and HIV-negative at-risk controls in either routine EEG or QEEG (49).

We have performed longitudinal QEEG evaluations on cohorts of adults and hemophilic children, averaging data from eight parasagittal electrodes (F3/F4 to O1/O2) referred to joined ears. Subjects have been followed for up to 3 years. In the adults, the AIDS and ARC subjects have higher absolute theta than did a control group or HIV-positive asymptomatic subjects. Repeated evaluations at 6-month intervals have shown a trend for reduction in alpha power over time, as well as statistically significant decreases in absolute delta, absolute theta, and relative delta. Asymptomatic adult subjects showed no reduction in alpha power over time. However, asymptomatic subjects who progressed to a symptomatic condition (ARC or AIDS) during the time of the study showed statistically significant increases in theta activity.

Quantitative EEG was evaluated for a pediatric hemophilic cohort in a manner similar to that of the adults and compared with a carefully matched HIV-negative hemophilic control group. The HIV-positive pediatric subjects have differed significantly from the controls due to a failure to increase their theta frequency over time, as well as a tendency to show more background delta frequency. These changes increase the possibility of subtle disease progression in this group but require further longitudinal observation.

Four subjects have developed AIDS encephalopathy during the course of this study. Each of these subjects has shown qualitatively similar changes in QEEG parameters (Fig. 1). Each has shown a marked decrease in total EEG power with a relative increase, or less of a decrease, in the theta band, such that the mean frequency decreased overall. This appears quite different from the changes observed in Alzheimer patients, who have increases in theta power with no change in alpha as the initial involvement.

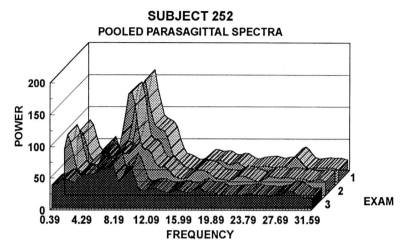

FIG. 1. EEG frequency spectra from a subject who developed AIDS dementia between his second and third examination. The spectra are an average of data obtained from eight parasaggital electrodes (F3/4–O1/2) referenced to joined ears. The patient was awake with eyes closed during the recording. Note that the spectra are very similar at examinations 1 and 2, before the development of dementia. At point 3, there is a notable decrease in EEG power and a shift toward lower frequencies. Examinations at 6-month intervals did not establish any QEEG parameters that were predictive of the development of dementia.

Given the known generators of EEG, it would be expected that the EEG would be sensitive to any process affecting dendritic morphology. The changes we are describing correlate well with the neuronal and dendritic loss that has been reported in HIV encephalopathy (38).

In summary, routine EEG has clinical applications in HIV disease that are similar to those in other diseases of the CNS. Lack of sensitivity has limited its use as a research tool in evaluating direct effects of HIV on the brain. QEEG has no clear role in the evaluation and care of HIV-positive subjects in a clinical setting. However, it has shown promise as a research tool in evaluating disease progression and perhaps in prediction of neurological dysfunction. There is QEEG support for progressive subclinical neurological dysfunction during the systemically asymptomatic stages of the disease.

EVOKED POTENTIAL STUDIES

As with EEG, EP studies may show abnormalities associated with many of the secondary neurological illnesses that accompany HIV infection. However, there is a dearth of information regarding the effects of these secondary diseases on EPs, mainly because specificity is low, making it unlikely that EPs will be of high clinical value.

On the other hand, EP studies have the potential to be helpful in the evaluation of the neurological effects of HIV itself. They are functional as opposed to anatomical tests. They are particularly sensitive to white matter abnormalities, as have been clearly implicated in HIV-related cognitive/motor disorders. They have been demonstrated in other diseases to be more sensitive to change than radiological evaluations or even clinical signs and symptoms (7,51). A further advantage of EP studies is that they are for the most part objective. We review the reported findings from a number of studies using some or all of a battery of EPs in HIV-infected cohorts. Because this is a rapidly evolving field, many of these reports have been presented in abstract form and lack careful peer review. It also should be emphasized that the changes reported in EPs are slight and nonspecific. Although they can tell us much about the progression of HIV-related nervous system disease and its effects on physiological systems, it is doubtful they will have significant value in the clinical management of the patients. However, from all sources there is growing evidence to indicate that EPs may be among the most sensitive tools available to the clinical researcher for evaluating the onset and progression of direct HIV-induced nervous system disease.

Somatosensory EP Responses

In 1988, Helweg-Larsen et al. studied 23 patients, all with AIDS. Sixteen had clinical signs of neurological dysfunction, almost all of which involved the lower extremities (27). Tibial nerve SEPs showed slowing of peripheral, thoracic, and cortical responses in all patients, suggesting a mixture of peripheral and CNS abnormalities. Later that year, they described an increase in the mean thoracic component (N24) of posterior tibial SEPs in 15 healthy, neurologically asymptomatic HIV-positive subjects when compared with controls (66). These patients all had normal peripheral nerve conduction velocities, and the investigators concluded that the findings were indicative of HIV-related changes in the region of the dorsal root ganglia. Two years later, 12 of these subjects were reexamined. Four had advanced in disease stage, eight were unchanged. In all but one subject there was an increase in the latency of the response to tibial stimulation at the T12 level, and there were increases in median wrist to cervical spine latency. However, central conduction times to the cortex remained normal. Although some of the change could be attributed to peripheral nerve slowing, the primary change was in the gluteal–T12 segment in the legs and the Erb's point—C7 segment in the legs. There was no relationship to disease stage, duration of established HIV infection, or CD4 T-lymphocyte counts (CD4 + counts). They concluded that these results indicated a mild and slowly progressive axonal neuropathy and a more severe progressive myelopathy or myeloradiculopathy (32).

Other groups also have found SEP changes. In their 73 neurologically asymptomatic patients, Jabarri et al. found seven with abnormalities on the first evaluation, and three more developed abnormalities in 2 years of follow-up (31). Six of the 10 had delayed ankle–cortex latencies on tibial stimulation, three had both tibial and median latency abnormalities, and one had median abnormalities alone. In three of the ten, the peripheral latencies were abnormal, two of these developed clinical peripheral neuropathy over the duration of the study. The others showed central deficits not associated with clinical disease of the brain or spinal cord. Koralnik et al. found mild differences in median nerve–cortical latencies in their group of 29 HIV-positive asymptomatic subjects when compared with HIV-negative controls (35). There was no significant change at 6–9 months follow-up. They did not study tibial potentials. Husstedt et al. reported that 37% of tibial and 15% of median nerve SEPs were abnormal in 355 patients studied (29). Both peripheral and central segments had abnormalities. Kamaijin et al. evaluated 60 asymptomatic and 11 symptomatic subjects and 23 controls and found slight but significant slowing of spinal conduction in both infected groups (34). Over 2 years, the lower extremities showed progression of both peripheral and central slowing, and the upper extremities showed progression of central slowing.

Other studies have not demonstrated any abnormalities of SEP. A group of 95 HIV-positive subjects in the United Kingdom was compared with 32 HIV-negative controls (39). None had neurological disease, and 15 were systemically symptomatic. Posterior tibial SEPs demonstrated no difference between controls and infected subjects in either peripheral or central conduction. A cross-sectional evaluation of 55 HIV-positive and 37 HIV-negative men in San Francisco showed no difference in median SEP evaluation (6). The infected subjects showed no difference when stratified according to immune status. None had progressed to a diagnosis of AIDS.

In our own study there was a 15% abnormality in posterior tibial SEP (PTSEP) on initial evaluation of subjects across the spectrum of severity of systemic disease. Of all modalities, the PTSEP had the highest rate of abnormality in these patients. Most of the conduction delay was in the lower lumbar region and may have been attributable to root or root entry zone lesions with much less evidence of central cord involvement. On follow-up for up to 2 years, a significant effect of time was not found for any of the PTSEP parameters. The median nerve sensory EPs showed an increase over time that was only marginally statistically significant and only when considering the total wrist–cortex segment.

More recently, Iragui et al. reported SEP differences between at-risk controls, asymptomatic HIV-positive, and ARC/AIDS groups (30). They found that only 8% of asymptomatic individuals but 43% of patients with ARC/AIDS had abnormal (>2.5 SD from control mean) PTSEPs. Peripheral conduction in the lower extremity, as indexed by the latency of the N22 lumbar potential, was increased only in the ARC/AIDS group. However, means of central conduction from lumbar cord to cortex were statistically significantly longer in both the asymptomatic and the ARC/AIDS groups than in the controls. The investigators indicated that these results support early involvement of central somatosensory pathways before any clinical neurophysiological evidence of peripheral involvement. Median nerve stimulation in the ARC/AIDS group demonstrated prolonged peripheral conduction and cortical (N20) latencies but normal central conduction times. This is consistent with our findings and those of others indicating much less involvement of median nerve sensory pathways.

In summary, SEPs, particularly PTSEPs, have the highest rates of abnormality of all EPs in HIV-positive subjects. The rate of abnormality ranges from 8% to 43% and is highest in symptomatic subjects, particularly those with clinical symptoms and signs of sensory dysfunction. The relationship of changes in the spinal segments to the development of clinical myelopathy has not been adequately studied, but it does appear that many subjects with abnormalities in this area do not develop overt myelopathy.

Visual EP Responses

In general, cross-sectional and longitudinal analyses of visual EP (VEP) in HIV-positive subjects have not demonstrated significant variations from the norm. This includes the studies by Koralnik et al. (35), Jabbari et al. (31), and Perelli et al. (56). Kamijin et al. (34) found abnormalities only in symptomatic subjects and found no deterioration in VEP over 1 and 2 years. Smith et al. (66) found that patients with

AIDS had statistically significantly longer latency than did both a control group and HIV-infected subjects who had not advanced to AIDS. Similarly, Iraqui et al. found statistically significant group differences in pattern reversal VEP (P100 latency) between their ARC/AIDS group and both controls and asymptomatic infected subjects (30).

VEPs in our own cohort also have been generally within normal limits and have been abnormal (3 SD from control values) in only 4% of subjects. Over time, however, the mean latency for the group has increased from 101.8 at the initial examination to 105.7 after 2 years follow-up, and highly significant ($p < 0.00005$) increases in the latency of the VEP have consistently been observed with repeated measures at 12, 18, and 24 months. When subcategories were evaluated, this progression was true for the systemically and neurologically asymptomatic as well as the symptomatic groups. There is a clear disease effect, and subjects who remain asymptomatic have significantly less mean increases (101.8–104.2 ms) than do those who develop ARC or AIDS (103.1–109.7 ms). It should be reinforced that despite these statistically significant changes, the absolute values overwhelmingly remain within the range of normal. These changes occur in the absence of any signs or symptoms related to the visual system. The findings are of little if any clinical value, but they do support the presence of continuous HIV-related physiological dysfunction involving the visual system, probably in myelinated fibers.

Brain Stem Auditory EP Responses

Of all EP modalities, brain stem auditory EP (BAEP) responses have shown the least significant change. Findings in different studies at various stages of disease have shown inconsistent results. In 15 neurologically asymptomatic infected patients who had not advanced to AIDS, Smith found that three had BAEPs in the abnormal range; the group as a whole had a delayed mean latency of peak V and the I–V interpeak latency when compared with controls, suggesting a defect of central conduction (66). Of 73 HIV-positive subjects, Jabarri et al. reported that only two had initial abnormalities, and three others developed central abnormalities within 6 months (31). Ragazzoni et al. found no difference between HIV-positive and control groups (61). Kamijin et al. found neither abnormalities in HIV-positive compared with controls nor changes over 2 years in the HIV-positive group (34). Perelli et al. found 22% abnormal BAEPs in their study, and abnormalities increased with increasing systemic disease (56). Boccellari et al. found increased wave III–V interpeak latency in 55 HIV-positive subjects when compared with controls (6). There was a relationship to immune function: the lower the CD4+ count, the greater the slowing. In addition, 85% with CD4+ counts less than and only 15% with CD4+ counts greater than $0.40 \times 10^9/L$ had abnormalities.

In our own studies, although the BAEP latencies have remained within the range of normal, I–III, III–IV, and I–V interpeak latencies have shown statistically significant increases over time (41). Significant increases in the amplitude ratio of I/V due to a decrease in the amplitude of wave V also have occurred over time. Both of these changes also correlate with disease staging. Thus, in our cohort, the BAEPs indicate a prolongation in conduction from the low pons to the midbrain over time, in both asymptomatic and symptomatic subjects. This strongly suggests that there is subclinical nervous system disease progression in all stages of the disease.

P3 Event-Related Potentials

Unlike the EPs described above, the P300, or P3 EP depends on conscious input from the subject. It is named after the latency of its major component, which is positive over the central and parietal scalp 300 ms after the subject detects a rare but expected stimulus (52). The classical method of eliciting the response is the auditory odd-ball paradigm in which the subject is asked to count infrequent and pseudorandom tones that are different in pitch from a more frequent tone. On recording at CZ, using an ear reference, the response to the frequent tone consists of a negative wave (N1) at 100 ms and a positive wave (P2) at 150 ms after delivery. The response to the infrequent tone consists of these peaks plus a second negativity (N2) at 200 ms and a large positive wave (P3) at 300 ms (all times approximate). Examples are given in Fig. 2. These N2 and P3 responses are dependent on age but not on the particular characteristic of the stimulus; for example, they also can be obtained by presenting the subject with a visual stimulus.

P3 has the potential to be particularly useful in addressing some of the questions related to the dementia that may accompany HIV infection. Although there is still debate as to its exact significance (24,57), most investigators have found abnormalities of the P3 latency in a majority of patients with a variety of dementing illnesses, including Alzheimer's and Huntington's diseases (28,58). Furthermore, there is evidence to indicate that abnormalities of P3 can distinguish cortical (Alzheimer's disease) from subcortical (Huntington's and Parkinson's diseases) dementias. The endogenous N2 and P3 components are delayed in the cortical forms (23,67), whereas in the subcortical forms both the exogenous (N1 and P2) and endogenous components are delayed (4,56,67). Thus, it is particularly relevant to ask whether this technique can identify subclinical cortical dysfunction and/or can predict late dementia.

There are a number of reports of event-related potentials (ERPs) in HIV, and most show that significant changes accompany the infection. Goodin et al. found prolongation of all ERP component latencies in a cross-sectional analysis of 41 asymptomatic and 14 symptomatic patients, nine of whom had dementia (24). Seventy-eight percent of the demented and 28% of the nondemented patients had a delay outside the normal range in the latency of at least one component of ERP. N1, N2, and P3 were particularly involved, and abnormalities were more severe in more advanced disease. By contrast, the EEG was normal in all asymptomatic patients, and abnormal (mild slowing) in only five of the demented patients. Ollo et al. evaluated a small group, nine asymptomatic HIV-positive subjects and nine with ARC/AIDS (53). None had clinical neurological disease. They were matched to a control group. Subjects were given both auditory and visual stimuli. Reduced amplitudes and increased latencies for P3 were observed for both visual and auditory stimuli in the ARC/AIDS group and for visual stimuli alone in the asymptomatic group. Delays in P2 latency with the auditory stimuli were found in the ARC/AIDS group. When compared with the controls, neither of the infected groups showed any difference in neuropsychological test performance.

Arendt et al. have reported on two ERP studies in HIV infection. The first was a cross-sectional evaluation of three groups: asymptomatic HIV-positive subjects, demented HIV-positive subjects, and controls (2). Seventy-nine percent of the demented and 28% of the asymptomatic subjects showed some abnormality of ERPs. Demented patients had a significant prolongation of N2 and P3 latencies when compared with the other groups. N2–P3 amplitudes were reduced in both infected groups,

SUBJECT 323

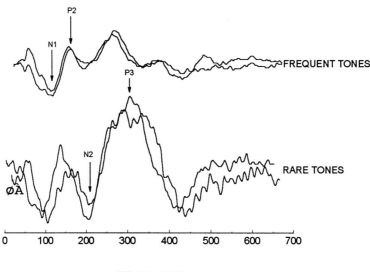

SUBJECT 305

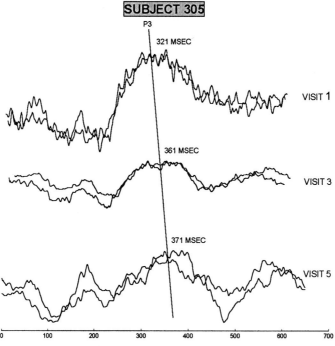

FIG. 2. Auditory oddball P3 responses from two HIV-positive patients. A normal response is shown **(A)**. Peaks labelled N1 and P2 are components of the reponses to frequent and rare tones. The N2 and P3 components are only seen with detection of the rare tones (PZ-A2, positivity at the PZ is upward). **B:** A series of responses from a patient seen five times at 6-month intervals. A progressive increase in P3 latency is evident in this patient, who did not show neuropsychological decline. (PZ-A2, positivity at the PZ is upward).

more markedly in the demented patients. Although subjects with dementia performed more poorly in neuropsychological testing, there was no correlation between this and the degree of abnormality of the ERPs.

The second study reported by Arendt was of 100 HIV-positive subjects across all parameters of systemic disease, but without evidence of CNS involvement or drug or alcohol abuse (1). They were contrasted to an age-matched control group in ERP responses, EEG, and psychometric testing. It is not clear how many of these subjects also had been involved in the prior study. There was a statistically significant reduction in N2–P3 amplitude in the patient group; 43% had abnormalities, deteriorating with advancing disease stage. ERP latencies were not significantly delayed in either of the infected groups. Ten of the patients had some abnormality of psychometric testing, and all these had prolongation of P3 latencies as well as either amplitude reduction or complete abolition of ERP peaks. Nine of the patients had slowing of the background EEG, and all of these also had markedly abnormal ERPs. Ragazzoni et al. found abnormalities, including longer P2, N2, and P3 latencies and reduced P3 amplitudes, in 28% of the HIV-positive subjects, more marked with more advanced disease (61).

Other researchers have found abnormalities in their cohorts to be less prevalent. In their 39 neurologically asymptomatic patients, Jabbari et al. found prolongation of P3 and N2 latency ERP abnormalities in five (31). One further subject developed abnormalities on follow-up of unspecified time. Goodwin et al., in a cohort of 206 Scottish HIV-positive drug users, found longer latency and reduced amplitude of P3 when compared with normal controls (25). When compared with HIV-seronegative drug users, however, only those in U.S. Centers for Disease Control and Prevention (CDC) stage IV showed a lower P3 amplitude. Fifty percent of the subjects had follow-up studies performed at 1 year. There was significant lengthening of P3 latency only in those with stage IV disease. More recently, Connolly et al. reported no difference in P3 latencies between symptomatic and asymptomatic HIV-positive subjects and an HIV-negative control group (12). They also found no decline in EPs in a subgroup of infected subjects over an average of 2 years.

We have evaluated auditory ERPs in our cohort of HIV-positive subjects. Thirty-seven were asymptomatic, and 41 were systemically symptomatic (ARC/AIDS). They have undergone follow-up evaluation at 6-month intervals. Seventy-eight have been examined at least twice, 54 three times, and 32 four times. Latencies were increasingly prolonged over time for the later (N2 and P3) components, but not for the earlier components (Fig. 2). Larger increases were seen for the symptomatic than for the asymptomatic group, but the difference was not statistically significant (40–42). We also have examined the relationship between changing P3 latency and performance on neuropsychological testing. Increasing P3 latency correlated with decreasing performance on tests measuring memory and speed of central processing.

Thus, evaluations of P3 EPs have elicited mixed results. Some, but not all investigators, have found changes in P3 latency over time and that more significant findings are present in symptomatic subjects. It is not clear whether they represent one or more processes that may be affecting gray and white matter independently. If further studies confirm these changes, they will add support to the premise that there are progressive neurophysiological changes over the course of time and disease stage.

In summary, a number of cross-sectional and ongoing longitudinal studies have evaluated the effects of EPs in HIV infection. Most have shown a significant increase in abnormal EPs of all types with advanced systemic disease, particularly with the presence of neurological disease. Findings in the asymptomatic stages of disease have been less consistent. Reasons for the discrepant results in different studies are not obvious. They cannot be easily explained by patient selection, confounding factors, or differences in test performance. However, these tests that show progressive decline support the contention that there is some progression of CNS function during earlier stages of HIV infection.

TESTING OF AUTONOMIC NERVOUS SYSTEM FUNCTION

The function of the ANS depends on the integrity of autonomic neurons and pathways in the brain, spinal cord, and peripheral nervous system. Because each of these structures may be damaged in the course of HIV infection, it is not surprising that there have been a number of reports of clinical autonomic dysfunction in HIV-infected patients (19). Symptoms that have been postulated as possibly due to autonomic dysfunction include syncope and hypotension (9), cardiac dysrhythmia (13), alterations of sweating (37), and bladder, bowel, and sexual dysfunction (5,11). Again, secondary infection, tumor, inflammatory and immune diseases, and vascular disease all may precipitate or accentuate autonomic involvement. A number of medications also may have autonomic effects.

Once again, ANS function testing may be used to elucidate or confirm the causes of such symptoms in individual patients. Generally, the role of ANS disease can be established by history and physical examination, and electrophysiological tests do not add a great deal to clinical care. As with the other studies described, more emphasis has been placed on using these tests as a research tool to define the degree of neurological involvement at various stages in the infection. Electrophysiological studies have the potential to be more sensitive to early ANS abnormalities and to subtle progression than does clinical examination alone.

Review of the literature on autonomic testing in HIV infection shows the same problems that exist with other testing. Much of the work is cross-sectional, and results are often only available in abstract form. In addition, there is no universally accepted standard as to what constitutes an abnormality. Different groups of tests have been used by different examiners, and different degrees of variation from the norm have been used to signify disease.

Studies reported have included postural and effort-related changes in blood pressure, postural changes in heart rate, cardiovascular responses to the Valsalva maneuver, heart rate period variability during deep breathing, sudomotor response, cold pressor responses, and tests of sweating. Investigators have generally performed a battery of such studies and arbitrarily designated that a certain number of abnormalities (usually one or two) in individual subtests indicates the presence of disease.

Cohen et al. performed ANS testing on five subjects with orthostatic hypotension (10). All were men, and one was an intravenous (IV) drug abuser. CDC disease staging was III in one and IVC in four. All had clinical neurological abnormalities, and four had cognitive deficits. All had evidence of generalized autonomic dysfunction. In a different study, Cohen evaluated 10 HIV-positive subjects without autonomic symptomatology and found that five showed both parasympathetic and sympathetic abnormalities on ANS testing (9). All five were in CDC group IV. Villa et al. compared autonomic function testing in 37 HIV-positive subjects with that in 18 HIV-negative controls (70). Both groups were intravenous heroin abusers. Nine of the subjects were in CDC group II, 23 were in group III, and five were in group IV. All subjects in CDC group IV had moderate or severe abnormalities, as did 44% in group II and 56% in group III. Seventeen subjects were followed over 10–13 months, and nine showed decline in ANS testing. Ruttimann et al. compared testing in 25 seropositive subjects with that in 10 controls (63). In the control group, only three intravenous drug users had abnormal studies. In the infected group, 72% with advanced disease and 29% with earlier disease had abnormalities. There was no difference between drug users and homosexuals in the infected group. In a cross-sectional study of 26 infected patients and 22 controls, Freeman et al. found a significant decline in infected subjects, as well as a progressive decline with advanced HIV disease (20). The most severe abnormalities were found in subjects with clinical neurological disease. In a cohort of 22 men, 19 with homosexual transmission and three intravenous drug users, Scott et al. found only one with definite abnormalities of ANS testing (65). Thirteen of the group were asymptomatic, seven showed only persistent generalized lymphadenopathy, and two had Kaposi's sarcoma.

In our own series, we performed ANS studies on 32 HIV-infected subjects (16) and compared them with nerve conduction studies. Twenty had abnormalities of ANS function. Of these, 55% had evidence of neuropathy on nerve conduction, as compared with 8% of those without ANS dysfunction. Seventy percent of those with abnormal studies had ARC/AIDS.

In summary, in a limited number of studies, there has been a high frequency of abnormalities of ANS function in patients in advanced stages of HIV disease, particularly when other neurological abnormalities are present. There also appears to be a relatively high prevalence of ANS abnormality in patients who are in the earlier stages of systemic disease, including those without symptomatic autonomic or neurological dysfunction.

EVALUATION OF SLEEP DISORDERS

HIV-positive patients have a high prevalence of sleep-related complaints, ranging from difficulty initiating and maintaining sleep to profound excessive daytime sleepiness. Darko found 71% of subjects with CDC stage IV disease to feel unrested upon awakening compared with 16% of normal controls (14). Prenzlauer et al. found 79% of a mixed group of 68 HIV-positive patients to have abnormalities on the Pittsburgh Sleep Quality Index (59). As might be expected in such a complex clinical illness, multiple etiologies have been proposed for these complaints, including depression, anxiety, sleep schedule disturbance, primary or secondary cerebral insults, systemic manifestations of infection, and effects of recreational drugs or medications. There are conflicting results on the possible role of zidovudine. Richman et al. found a higher rate of insomnia in subjects taking zidovudine than in those on placebo control (62), but Moeller et al., in a retrospective study, found no such difference (43).

The most important tool for the clinician in evaluating clinical sleep disturbance remains a detailed history and physical examination to search for clues of treatable sleep disorders. Historical clues may suggest that the sleep disruption comes from poor sleep hygiene, sleep schedule disturbance, or psychological stress. Polysomnography may be clinically helpful when the history and physical examination do not clearly delineate an underlying cause. Snoring, observed apneas, or symptoms of restless legs may suggest the need for an overnight sleep study to confirm treatable causes such as sleep apnea or periodic limb movements of sleep. The overnight polysomnogram should be tailored to maximize the potential in delineating the underlying cause of sleep disturbance.

Multiple sleep latency studies may be useful in evaluating patients with excessive daytime sleepiness, quantitating the ability of the patient to fall asleep during the day, and demonstrating daytime rapid eye movement (REM) sleep. Four to five naps are taken at 2-hour intervals, and each nap is examined for the time to sleep onset and the presence of REM sleep. A mean sleep latency is calculated for the total study. A mean sleep latency of >10 minutes is normal, <5 minutes indicates pathological sleepiness, and 5–10 minutes is a gray zone. Normal individuals do not enter REM sleep during the daytime naps. In most patients, this correlates with subjective sleepiness, but clearly there are some individuals for whom the objective findings do not match the subjective complaints.

Sleep is a systematically organized function of the CNS, and the evaluation of sleep is an important factor in demonstrating alteration in the function of the CNS. The clinical neurophysiological evaluation of sleep as a research tool has been used to evaluate clinical and subclinical involvement of the CNS at various stages of HIV infection. Using overnight polysomnographic evaluations, Kubicki et al. reported that five patients with AIDS, all with CNS changes on magnetic resonance imaging studies, had disturbed sleep, including prolonged sleep latency and REM latency, increased wakefulness and stage 1 sleep, decreased total sleep time, and decreased stage 2, 3, 4, and REM sleep (36). They also found an increased number of arousals, decreased number of spindles, and severely disturbed sleep architecture. Later, the same researchers reported that 15 subjects, with various cerebral manifestations, showed decreased power in the 11.5- to 13-Hz band in non–rapid eye movement (NREM) sleep. Coherence was used as a way to measure synchronous electrocerebral activity and demonstrated decreased interfrontal coherence in the 0- to 12-Hz band in NREM and REM sleep. The coherence factors were consistently found in all patients. The exact significance of this finding is unknown. These patients all had advanced disease with neurological manifestations and clearly could have multiple reasons for sleep disturbance.

In 1991, Wiegand et al. reported on 14 subjects with CDC stage III and IV who had no opportunistic CNS infections and had a higher incidence of impaired sleep, including longer sleep latency, reduced total sleep time, and greater amount of time spent awake and in stage 1 sleep than control subjects (71). They also found decreased stage 2 sleep and reduced number of sleep spindles. In patients with depressive symptoms, they found a negative correlation of these symptoms to REM latency. Decreased quality of sleep correlated with increased ventricular size and with cortical atrophy as measured by cortical sulcal width. They also found a correlation of sleep quality to plasma but not cerebrospinal fluid tryptophan levels. In a subsequent study of 26 subjects, 14 treated with zidovudine, the alterations in sleep parameters did not correlate with administration of zidovudine (45).

Polysomnography has also indicated sleep disturbance in asymptomatic HIV-infected subjects. First in eight, then in 14 asymptomatic individuals, Norman et al. demonstrated reduced sleep efficiency, increased sleep fragmentation, and increased awake and stage 1 sleep. They also found increased slow-wave sleep percentage for the whole night and abundant slow-wave sleep in the later half of the night (47,48). In a subsequent study, the same group confirmed the abnormal slow-wave sleep but were unable to demonstrate an increased percentage of slow-wave sleep (46).

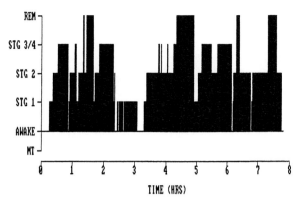

FIG. 3. Hypnogram from an asymptomatic HIV infected 42-year-old male who demonstrated an increased predominance of stage 3 and 4 sleep in the later portion of the sleep period, the longest REM period in the middle third of the sleep period, and several arousals throughout the night.

In our own study of 12 HIV-infected subjects who did not have a history of CNS lesions, affective disorders, or known drug abuse, we found an increased percentage of stage 1 sleep, slow-wave sleep, and REM sleep, decreased stage 2 sleep, and more frequent arousals (15). We also found greatly disturbed sleep architecture, with four of our subjects having increased slow-wave sleep in the latter half of the night and six of our subjects having an even distribution of REM throughout the night (Fig. 3). We found a correlation of the event-related P300 latency with the sleep efficiency, independent of age (69). Although immune function is closely tied to sleep (55), our study group showed no correlation between CD3, CD4, or CD8 T-lymphocyte cell counts and any of the changes in sleep parameters.

Multiple Sleep Latency Study

Only one group has addressed multiple sleep latencies in this patient population. Norman et al. included mean sleep latency in 10 asymptomatic HIV subjects using a four-nap protocol (65). They found that of the seven subjects who complained of excessive daytime sleepiness, only one individual had a short mean sleep latency (5 minutes). The remaining subjects had sleep latencies ranging from 9.25 to 15 minutes. No REM episodes were noted in the group.

SUMMARY

Both asymptomatic and symptomatic patients infected with HIV have objectively demonstrated disruption of sleep. Abnormal findings have included decreased total sleep time, reduced sleep efficiency, increased stage 1 sleep, reduced stage 2 sleep, and diminution in occurrence and frequency of sleep spindles. In addition, these individuals have disruption of the sleep cycle and architecture with increased slow-wave sleep in the latter half of the night and a more even distribution of REM sleep. Although this constellation of findings is unusual for other disorders disturbing sleep, the abnormalities are nonspecific. Further study in HIV-infected individuals is needed to clarify the possible mechanisms underlying the alterations in the immune and neurological systems resulting in a disturbance of sleep.

REFERENCES

1. Arendt G, Hefter H, Lablonowski H. Acoustically evoked event-related potentials in HIV-associated dementia. *Electroencephalogr Clin Neurophysiol* 1993;86:152–169.
2. Arendt G, Hefter H, Nelles HW, Hilperath F, Strohmeyer G. Age-dependent decline in cognitive information processing of HIV-positive individuals detected by event-related potential recordings. *J Neurol Sci* 1993;115:223–229.
3. Assessment: EEG brain mapping. *Neurology* 1989:39;1100–1101.
4. Ball SS, Marsch JT, Schubarth G, Brown WS, Strandburg R. Longitudinal P300 changes I Alzheimer's disease. *J Gerontol* 1989;44:M195–200.
5. Blanshard C, Ellis DS, Tovey G, Gazzard BG. Electron microscopy of rectal biopsies in HIV-positive individuals. *J Pathol* 1993;169:79–87.
6. Boccellari AA, Dilley JW, Yingling CD, et al. Relationship of CD4 counts to neurophysiological function in HIV-1 infected homosexual men. *Arch Neurol* 1993;50:517–521.
7. Chiappa KH. Pattern shift visual evoked potentials: interpretation. In: Chiappa KH, ed. *Evoked Potentials in Clinical Medicine.* 2nd ed. New York: Raven, 1990:126–127.
8. Coben LA, Chi D, Snyder AZ, Storandt M. Replication of a study of frequency analysis of the resting awake EEG in mild probable Alzeheimer's disease. *Electroencephalogr Clin Neurophys* 1990;75:148–154.
9. Cohen J, Laudenslager M. Autonomic nervous system involvement in patients with human immunodeficiency virus infection. *Neurology* 1989;39:1111–1112.
10. Cohen JA, Miller L, Polish L. Orthostatic hypotension in human immunodeficiency virus infection may be the result of generalized autonomic nervous system dysfunction. *J AIDS* 1991;4:31–33.
11. Coker RJ, Horner P, Bleasdale-Barr K, Harris JR, Mathias CJ. Increased gut parasympathetic activity and chronic diarrhoea in a patient with the acquired immunodeficiency syndrome. *Clin Auton Res* 1992;2:295–298.
12. Connolly S, Manji H, McAllister RH, et al. Long-latecy event-related potentials in asymptomatic human immunodeficiency virus type 1 infection. *Ann Neurol* 1994;35:189–196.
13. Craddock C, Pasvol G, Bull R, Protheroe A, Hopkin J. Cardiorespiratory arrest and autonomic neuropathyin AIDS. *Lancet* 1987;2:16–18.
14. Darko DF, McCutchan JA, Kripke DF, Gillin JC, Golshan S. Fatigue, sleep disturbance, disability and indices of progression of hiv infection. *Am J Psychiatry* 1992;149:514–520.
15. D'Cruz, Vaughn BV, Robertson K, Ehle A, Hall C. Analysis of sleep architecture in asymptomatic human immunodeficiency (HIV) infected patients. *Abstracts of the American Electroencephalographic Society.* 1993:112.
16. Donovan MK, Rogers OL, Robertson KR, Hall CD. Autonomic nervous system dysfunction in patients with human immunodeficiency virus (HIV) infection. Presented at the American Neurological Association Annual General Meeting, 1993.
17. Elovaara I, Saar P, Sirkka-Liisa V, Hokkanen L, Ilvanainen M, Lahdevirta J. EEG in early HIV-1 infection is characterized by anterior dysrhythmicity of low maximal amplitude. *Clin Electroencephalogr* 1991;22:131–140.
18. Enzensberger W, Fischer PA, Helm EB, Stille W. Value of electroencephalography in AIDS. *Lancet* 1985;1:1047–1048.
19. Freeman R, Cohen JA. Autonomic failure in AIDS. In: Philip Law, ed. *Autonomic Dysfunction.* 1991:677–683.
20. Freeman R, Roberts M, Friedman L, Broadbridge C. Autonomic function and human immunodeficiency virus infection. *Neurology* 1990;40:575–580.
21. Gabuza DH, Levy SR, Chiappa KH. Electroencephalography in AIDS and AIDS-related complex. *Clin Electroencephalogr* 1988;19:1–6.
22. Goodin DS. Clinical utility of long latency cognitive event-related potentials (P3): the pros. *Electroencephalogr Clin Neurophysiol* 1990;76:2–5.
23. Goodin DS, Aminoff MJ. Electrophysiological differences between subtypes of dementia. *Brain* 1991;1103–1113.
24. Goodin DS, Aminoff MJ, Chernoff DN, Hollander H. Long latency event-related potentials in patients infected with human immunodeficiency virus. *Ann Neurol* 1990;27:414–419.
25. Goodwin GM, Chiswick A, Egan V, St. Clair D, Brettle RP. The Edinburgh cohort of HIV-positive drug users: auditory event-related potentials show progressive slowing in patients with Centers for Disease Control stage IV disease. *AIDS* 1990;4:1243–1250.
26. Hall C, Robertson K, Messenheimer J, Wilkins J, Whaley R, Kwock L. Progression of nervous system

dysfunction in the systemically asymptomatic stages of human immunodeficiency virus infection. Presented at the IXth International Conference on AIDS, June 7–11, 1993, Berlin.

27. Helweg-Larsen S, Jakobsen J, Boesen F, et al. Myelopathy in AIDS: a clinical, neuroradiological and electrophysiological study of 23 Danish patients. *Acta Neurol Scand* 1998;77(1):64–73.

28. Homberg V, Hefter H, Granseyer G, Strauss W, Lange H, Hennerici M. Event related potentials in patients with Huntington's disease and the relatives at risk in relation to detailed psychometry. *Electroencephalogr Clin Neurophysiol* 1986;63:552–569.

29. Husstedt IW, Grotemeyer KH, Busch H, Kidek W. Somatosensory evoked potentials in HIV-infected patients. Abstracts of the IXth International Conference on AIDS, 1993, Berlin, PO-B16–1686.

30. Iragui VJ, Kalmijn J, Thal LJ, Grant I, HNRC Group. Neurological dysfunction in asymptomatic HIV-1 infected men: evidence from evoked potentials. *Electroencephalogr Clin Neurophys* 1994;92:1–10.

31. Jabbari B, Coats M, Salazar A, Martin A, Scherokman B, Laws W. Longitudinal study of EEG and evoked potentials in neurologically asymptomatic HIV infectes subjects. *Electroencephalogr Clin Neurophysiol* 1993;86:145–151.

32. Jakobsen J, Smith T, Gaub J, Helweg-Larsen S, Trojaborg W. Progressive neurological dysfunction during latent HIV infection. *Br Med J* 1989;299:225–228.

33. John ER, Pricheps LS, Easton P. Neurometrics; computer-assisted differential diagnosis of brain dysfunctions. *Science* 1988;239:162–169.

34. Kamijin J, Iragui-Madoz V, Thal L, Wallace M, Grant I, HNRC Group. Evoked potentials detect central nervous deficits in all HIV + subjects and peripheral deficits in symptomatic HIV + subjects. Abstracts IXth International Conference on AIDS, 1993, Berlin PO-B16–1733.

35. Koralnik IJ, Beaumanoir A, Hausler R, et al. A controlled study of early neurological abnormalities in men with asymptomatic human immunodeficiency virus infection. *N Engl J Med* 1990;323:864–870.

36. Kubicki ST, Henkes H, Terstegge K, Ruf B. AIDS related sleep disturbances—a preliminary report. In: *HIV and the Nervous System.* In, Kubicki, Henkes, Bienzle, Pohle, eds. New York: Gustav Fischer, 1988.

37. Lin-Greenberger A, Taneja-Uppal N. Dysautonomia and infection with human immunodeficinecy virus. *Ann Intern Med* 1987;106:167.

38. Masliah E, Achim CL, Ge N, DeTeresa R, Terry RD, Wiley CA. Spectrum of human immunodeficiency virus–associated neocortical damage. *Ann Neurol* 1992;32:321–329.

39. McAllister RH, Herns MV, Harrison MJG, et al. Neurological and neuropsychological performance in HIV seropositive men without symptoms. *J Neurol Neurosurg Psychiatry* 1992;55:143–148.

40. Messenheimer JA, Robertson KR, Kalkowski JC, Hall CD. Event related potentials (P3) in AIDS. *Am J EEG Technol* 1992;32:147–160.

41. Messenheimer JA, Robertson KR, Kalkowski JC, Hall CD. Longitudinal EEG, QEEG and evoked potential changes in HIV sero-positive patients with and without AIDS. American Presented at the Electroencephalographic Society Annual General Meeting, September 18–20, 1992, San Francisco, CA.

42. Messenheimer JA, Robertson KR, Wilkins JW, Kalkowski JC, Hall CD. Event related potentials in human immunodeficiency virus infection. *Arch Neurol* 1992;49:396–400.

43. Moeller AA, Oechsner M, Backmund HC, Popescu M, Emminger C, Holsboer F. Self-reported sleep quality in HIV infection: correlation to the stage of infection and zidovudine therapy. *J AIDS* 1991;4:1000–1003.

44. Moeller AA, Simon O, Jaeger H. AIDS and EEG with special aspect of hemophiliacs. In: Kubicki, Henkes, Bienzle, Pohle, eds. *HIV and the Nervous System.* New York: Gustav Fischer, 1988:81.

45. Moeller AA, Wiegand M, Oechsner M, Krieg JC, Holsboer F, Emminger C. Effects of zidovudine on EEG sleep in HIV-infected men. *J AIDS* 1992;5:636–637.

46. Norman SE, Chediak AD, Freeman C, et al. Sleep disturbances in men with asymptomatic human immunodeficiency (HIV) infection. *Sleep* 1992;15:150–155.

47. Norman SE, Chediak AD, Kiel M, Cohn MA. Sleep disturbances in HIV-infected homosexual men. *AIDS* 1990;4:775–781.

48. Norman SE, Resnick L, Cohn M, Duara R, Herbst J, Berger JR. Sleep disturbances in HIV-seropositive patients. *JAMA* 1988;260:922.

49. Nuwer MR, Miller EN, Visscher BR, et al. Asymptomatic HIV infection does not cause EEG abnormalities: results form the multicenter AIDS cohort study (MACS). *Neurology* 1992;42:1214–1219.

50. Nuwer MR, Miller EN, Visscher BR, Satz P. Early neurological abnormalities in HIV infection. *N Engl J Med* 1991;324:492–493.

51. Nuwer MR, Packwood JW, Myers LW, Ellison GW. Evoked potentials predict the clinical changes in a multiple sclerosis drug study. *Neurology* 1988;37:1754–1761.

52. Oken BS. Endogenous event related potentials. In: Chiappa KH, ed. *Evoked Potentials in Clinical Medicine.* 2nd ed. New York: Raven, 1990:563–592.

53. Ollo C, Johnson R, Grafman J. Signs of cognitive change in HIV disease: an event-related brain potential study. *Neurology* 1991;41:209–215.

54. Parisi A, Di Perri G, Strosselli M, Nappi G, Minoli L, Rondanelli EG. Usefulness of computerized

electroencephalography in diagnosing, staging and monitoring AIDS dementia complex. *AIDS* 1989; 3:209–213.

55. Payne LC, Krueger JM. Interactions of cytokines with the hypothalamic pituitary axis. *J Immunother* 1992;12:171–173.

56. Perelli F, Soldati G, Zambardi P, et al. Electrophysiological study (VEP, BAEP) in HIV-1 seropisitive patients with and without AIDS. *Acta Neurol Belg* 1993;93:78–87.

57. Pfefferbaum A, Ford JM, Kraemer HC. Clinical utility of long latency cognitive event-related potentials (P3): the cons. *Electroencephalogr Clin Neurophysiol* 1990;76:6–12.

58. Polich J, Ladish C, Bloom FE. P300 assessment of early Alzheimer's disease. *Electroencephalogr Clin Neurophysiol* 1990;77:179–189.

59. Prenzlauer SL, Bogdonoff L, Tiamson MLA, Bialer PA, Wilets I. Sleep and HIV illness. Abstracts IXth International Conference on AIDS, 1993, Berlin, PO-B16–1752.

60. Rae-Grant A, Blume W, Lau C, Hachinski UC, Fisman M, Merskey H. The electroencephalogram in Alzheimer-type dementia. *Arch Neurol* 1987;44:50–54.

61. Ragazzoni A, Grippo A, Ghidini P, et al. Electrophysiological study of neurologically asymptomatic HIV1 seropositive patients. *Acta Neurol Scand* 1993;87:47–51.

62. Richman DD, Fischl MA, Grieco MH, AZT Collaborative Working Group. The toxicity of azidothymidine (AZT) in the treatment of patients with AIDS and AIDS-related complex. *N Engl J Med* 1987;317:192–197.

63. Ruttimann S, Hilti P, Spinas G, Dubach U. High frequency of human immunodeficiency virus–associated autonomic neuropathy and more severe involvement in advanced stages of human immunodeficiency virus disease. *Arch Intern Med* 1991;151:2441–2443.

64. Schnurbus R, Hartmann M, Henkes H, et al. EEG findings (background activity and response to hyperventilation) in early stages of the HIV-infection. In: Kubicki, Henkes, Bienzle, Pohle, eds. *HIV and the Nervous System*. New York: Gustav Fischer, 1988:93–96.

65. Scott G, Piaggesi A, Ewing D. Sequential autonomic function testing in HIV infection. *AIDS* 1990; 4:1279–1282.

66. Smith T, Jakobsen J, Gaub J, Helweg-Larsen S, Trojaborg W. Clinical and electrophysiological studies of human immunodeficiency seropositive men without AIDS. *Ann Neurol* 1988;23:295–297.

67. Syndulko K, Hansch EC, Cohen SN, et al. Long-latency event related potentials in normal aging and dementia. In: Courjon J, Mauguiere F, Revol M, eds. *Clinical Applications of Evoked Potentials in Neurology*. New York: Raven, 1982:279–285.

68. Tennison M, Messenheimer J, Whaley R, et al. Neurological status of HIV-positive hemophiliac children. Presented at the meeting of Neuroscience of HIV infection, Basic and Clinical Frontiers, July 14–17, 1992, Amsterdam, The Netherlands.

69. Vaughn BV, Messenheimer JA, D'Cruz OF, Robertson KR, Kalkowski JC, Hall CD. Comparison of P3 and sleep parameters in asymptomatic HIV infected males, American Electroencephalographic Society 1993:130.

70. Villa A, Foresti V, Confalonieri F. Autonomic nervous system dysfunction associated with HIV infection in intravenous heroin users. *AIDS* 1992;6:85–89.

71. Wiegand M, Moller AA, Schreiber W, Kreig J-C, Holsboer F. Alterations of nocturnal sleep in patients with HIV infection. *Acta Neurol Scand* 1991;83:141–142.

72. Wong MC, Suite ND, Labar DR. Seizures in human immunodeficiency virus infection. *Arch Neurol* 1990;47:640–642.

AIDS and the Nervous System, Second Edition,
edited by J. R. Berger and R. M. Levy.
Lippincott-Raven Publishers, Philadelphia © 1997.

13

Neuroimaging of Acquired Immunodeficiency Syndrome

Michelle L. Hansman Whiteman, M. Judith Donovan Post, and
Evelyn M.L. Sklar

*Department of Radiology, Neuroradiology Section, University of Miami School of
Medicine, Jackson Memorial Hospital, Miami, Florida 33136*

Neuroradiology plays an integral role in the investigation of the patient with acquired immunodeficiency syndrome (AIDS) with central nervous system (CNS) disease. Clinical findings are often nonspecific; thus, neuroimaging is an instrumental tool in the diagnosis and management of these patients. Neurological disease may be the harbinger of systemic infection because 10–20% of patients with AIDS will present with neurological disturbance as the initial manifestation of AIDS (24,143). Various reports have estimated that 31–63% of patients with AIDS will develop neurological dysfunction as a complication of their disease (24,33,40,143,146,255). Autopsy series have found CNS involvement in 73–87% of cases (118,143,175).

Neurological disturbance in these patients often indicates significant intracranial pathology, and the most frequent signs and symptoms include headache, encephalopathy, seizures, ataxia, and focal motor or sensory deficit.

The most commonly used imaging modalities for documentation of CNS pathology are computed tomography (CT) and magnetic resonance imaging (MRI). Conventional angiography is rarely performed; it is used primarily for AIDS-related cerebrovascular disease and is particularly useful in the evaluation of vasculitis. MR angiography (MRA), a noninvasive technique for vascular imaging, may be used as an alternative to conventional angiography or in conjunction with conventional angiography in certain cases. Myelography is also rarely used but is currently used for patients who are poor candidates for MRI due to the presence of metal, pacemakers, or patient motion despite sedation or in the event the MRI is unavailable. Nuclear medicine imaging can provide critical information in defining mass lesions. Thallium-201 brain single-photon emission computed tomography (SPECT) can be used to differentiate inflammatory from neoplastic lesions and is thus extremely useful in differentiating toxoplasmic encephalitis from CNS lymphoma, which are the primary considerations in this population. MR spectroscopy, although still in its infancy, may be an indicator of subtle biochemical abnormalities in the brains of human immunodeficiency virus (HIV)-seropositive individuals.

What type of pathology is seen in HIV-infected patients, and what is the best way to image this pathology? DeLaPaz and Enzmann (69) reviewed a number of CT series encompassing a total of 443 cases. All studies were obtained on patients with

AIDS with neurological dysfunction. Atrophy was demonstrated in 33%, focal lesions in 38%, and normal results were evident in 29% (69). Pathological correlates of these focal lesions included toxoplasmosis (in 50–70% of focal lesions, depending on the series), primary CNS lymphoma (10–25% of focal lesions), and progressive multifocal leukoencephalopathy (PML) (in ~10–22%). Other reported focal lesions evident on CT of patients with AIDS have included *Candida albicans* (123,147) cryptococcoma (305), metastatic Kaposi's sarcoma (KS) (123,147), tuberculous (TB) abscess (204), aspergillosis, herpes simplex virus type 2 (HSV-2), encephalitis (69), as well as nocardia (278).

Double-dose delayed (DDD) CT is preferable to single-dose contrast CT for detection of parenchymal lesions. Single-dose and DDD CT were compared in patients with AIDS with neurological symptoms and documented CNS pathology (204). The DDD (78 g iodinated contrast via bolus/drip infusion with a 1-hour delay in scanning) technique was found to greatly increase the sensitivity of CT (204). The DDD studies detected an increased number of lesions and demonstrated greater enhancement and size of many lesions as compared with those on single-dose scans. DDD CT scans appear to be most useful in detecting focal parenchymal lesions and are less successful in demonstration of meningeal disease or white matter disease.

MRI performed on patients with AIDS with symptoms of neurological dysfunction (n = 125) demonstrated focal lesions in 54%, atrophy in 14%, bilateral diffuse white matter disease in 10%, and a normal scan in 22% (69). Definitive diagnosis was obtained in a number of these focal lesions, showing that 53% of focal lesions were due to toxoplasmosis and 16% of focal lesions represented primary CNS lymphoma (69).

How do MRI and CT compare? MRI and CT examinations on 98 patients with AIDS and symptoms of CNS pathology were evaluated and compared (69). MRI demonstrated greater sensitivity than did CT, particularly for diffuse white matter disease (69,207). In 22% of these patients, the MRI was abnormal, whereas the CT failed to demonstrate any abnormality. In another 22% of cases, the MRI demonstrated an increased number of focal lesions as compared with the corresponding CT.

The superiority of MRI over CT is due in part to its greater contrast resolution, and this greater sensitivity permits earlier diagnosis and treatment (102,143,207,243). A prospective study of CT and MRI (207) compared the imaging findings in 14 patients with AIDS and neurological symptoms. Plain and contrast high-resolution CT was compared with noncontrast MRI. In three of 17 cases, abnormalities were evident on MRI, whereas the CT was negative (207). However, there were no instances in which the CT was positive and the MRI was negative. MRI is particularly useful in demonstration of white matter disease, and postgadolinium images with multiplanar imaging are helpful in detection of meningeal pathology. Both pre- and postgadolinium images (including T2-weighted images [T2WIs]) are necessary in the evaluation of neurologically symptomatic patients with AIDS in order to avoid missing significant lesions (32). In this chapter, T2WIs refer to a TR of 1,500–3,000 ms and a TE of 80–120 ms. T1-weighted images (T1WIs) refer to a TR of 300–700 ms and a TE of 10–30 ms. Proton density images (PDIs) refer to a TR of 1,500–3,000 ms and a TE of 10–30 ms.

In a clinical study of 132 patients with AIDS, 20% had neurological symptoms as the initial presentation of AIDS. Sixty-three percent of the 132 patients ultimately developed neurological complications (24). Although *Pneumocystis carinii* pneumonia was found to be the most frequent presenting manifestation of AIDS, neurological disease was the second most common presenting disorder (24). In this clinical series, toxoplasmosis was by far the most common cause of neurological abnormality during the period under study. The most frequent neurological disorders found in this study (in descending order) included toxoplasmic encephalitis, cryptococcal meningitis, subacute encephalitis, peripheral neuropathy, cytomegalovirus (CMV) retinitis, metabolic encephalopathy, PML, myopathy, CNS lymphoma, and TB meningitis. In patients with neurological disease as the initial presentation of AIDS, toxoplasmosis was also the most frequent etiology. In contrast, neuropathological findings in autopsy series have demonstrated the most common disorders to be (in descending order) vacuolar myelopathy, subacute encephalitis, CMV encephalitis, nonspecific encephalitis, toxoplasmic encephalitis, primary CNS lymphoma, cryptococcal meningitis, PML, varicella-zoster encephalitis, and herpes simplex ventriculitis (188,189).

The ensuing pages address the most commonly encountered pathological entities present on imaging of the CNS in patients with AIDS, with a descriptive analysis of the radiographic appearance of these disorders using various neuroimaging techniques.

INFECTION

Viruses

HIV

The neurological manifestations of HIV infection in the absence of superimposed infection or neoplasm include encephalopathy, myelopathy, peripheral neuropathy, and myopathy (8,58,143,173,188,246). The presence of HIV-1, an RNA virus of the retrovirus group, within the CNS has been documented in 73% of adults and children with AIDS (102). In the brain, replicating HIV is most frequently associated with macrophages and multinucleated giant cells (188). These cells appear to be the chief targets of infection by HIV and the cause of the progressive encephalopathy seen in AIDS (83,85,129,240). Polymorphic microglia are also frequently infected. Astrocytes and oligodendrocytes are infrequently infected by HIV, and neurons are rarely infected (83,85).

The most common neurological complication of AIDS is subacute encephalitis (33,118,143,173,175,255). This is present in 28% of adult AIDS autopsies (189). Clinically, this subacute encephalitis presents with progressive dementia and motor and/or behaviorial dysfunction (173). Early difficulties with concentration and memory are followed by apparent apathy and social withdrawal and may be mistaken for symptoms of depression (101). Headache is also a common complaint. Seizures occur in ~10% (144). This subacute encephalitis has been attributed in some cases to CMV (175,243), although HIV itself appears to be the responsible agent in the majority of cases (173,240,243). The pathological correlate of HIV encephalopathy appears to be myelin pallor in association with HIV-infected multinucleated giant cells (199), microglial nodules, gliosis, and vacuolar degeneration (102). These multinucleated giant cells contain retrovirus particles on electron microscopy, and their presence strongly correlates with AIDS dementia complex (ADC) (173). Electron microscopy shows sparse infiltrates of lipid-laden macrophages, gemistocytic astrocytes, and lymphocytes (189). Diffuse atrophy is usually present. The multinucleated giant cells may be scattered within the cortex, basal ganglia, and white matter (58,188).

Lesions are present initially within the white matter, and with disease progression there is extension to the basal ganglia and cortex. In some patients the white matter lesions predominate, whereas in others the gray matter is more severely affected (265). Lesions also may be found in the brainstem, cerebellum, and spinal cord (172).

Although foci of demyelination are present, this is a secondary and comparatively late finding (30). The white matter contains occasional microglial cells, focal vacuolation, perivascular infiltrate, and frequent small, ill-defined foci of demyelination interspersed in a general pattern of myelin pallor (211). There is little edema and a paucity of inflammatory cells (30). The majority of intracranial lesions directly due to HIV are usually not apparent on gross examination except for atrophy (208). Milder cases show reactive astrocytosis within the white matter, with myelin pallor in the absence of multinucleated giant cells, inflammation, or atrophy (159).

HIV may also directly result in acute encephalitis (42), acute meningitis, or chronic meningitis (24,102). The viral meningitis usually presents with headache, fever, and meningeal signs. It usually remits spontaneously but can recur (265). Results of CT and MRI are usually negative (143,146).

CT may be negative or demonstrate atrophy in patients with subacute encephalitis. White matter abnormalities are infrequently identified on CT in patients with HIV encephalopathy (37,143,147,173,255) (Fig. 1). In some cases in which HIV has been cultured from brain tissue, the MRI has shown diffuse white matter disease, but the CT has been negative (85). In general, the clinical diagnosis of HIV encephalitis

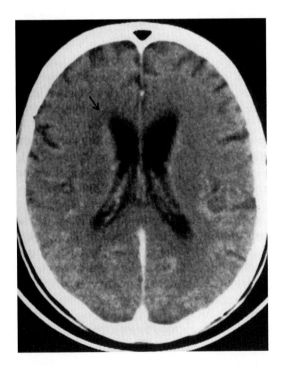

FIG. 1. HIV encephalitis (autopsy proven). Postcontrast axial CT scan demonstrates cortical atrophy and mild ventricular dilatation. Minimal white matter hypodensity is present (arrow).

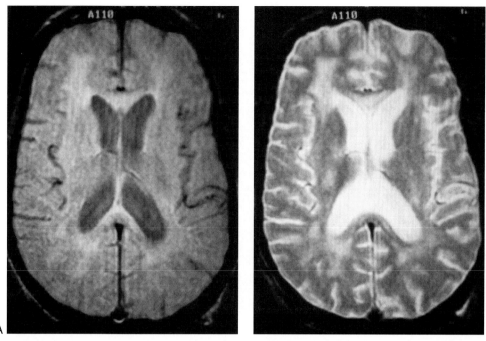

FIG. 2. HIV demyelination (autopsy proven). Proton density **(A)** and T2-weighted **(B)** axial MRIs demonstrate patchy areas of increased signal predominantly in the periventricular white matter but also with some involvement of the subcortical white matter. There is no mass effect. Also note central and cortical atrophy.

significantly antedates radiographic evidence of the disease (179,197,208). Detection of meningeal disease requires contrast administration (199).

Undoubtedly, the effects of cerebral HIV infection are more evident on MRI than on CT (159,173). Cortical atrophy is the most common MRI abnormality and is usually the only early finding (52,208). Both cortical and central atrophy progress on serial MRI examinations (52,208). Hyperintense lesions without mass effect are seen on T2WIs in the periventricular white matter and centrum semiovale, which correspond to foci of demyelination and vacuolation (30) (Fig. 2). Lesions vary from scattered, isolated, unilateral foci to large, confluent bilateral involvement (30) (Fig. 3). The extent of disease roughly parallels the clinical progression of the neurological disorder (208).

A multicenter AIDS cohort study has shown sulcal prominence and scattered foci of increased signal within the white matter on T2WIs in 63% of asymptomatic HIV-seropositive homosexual men compared with 48% of seronegative homosexual men (160). In another study, the MRI was abnormal in ~50% of patients with AIDS-related complex and 69% of patients with AIDS (91). These abnormalities included sulcal and ventricular enlargement, as well as bilateral patchy areas of increased signal without mass effect in the white matter on T2WIs (Fig. 4). These patchy areas become more diffuse, homogenous, and confluent with clinical progression from subtle cognitive changes to gross dementia (91) (Fig. 5). Small lesions (<1 cm) are less common (179). Using quantitative neuroimaging with MRI, Aylward et al. demonstrated that reductions in basal ganglia volume correlated best with the pres-

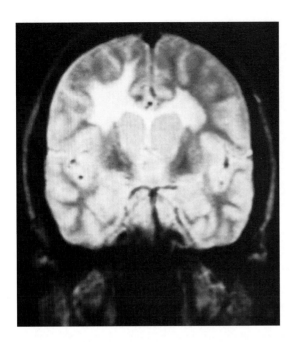

FIG. 3. HIV encephalitis. Coronal T2-weighted MRI shows confluent, high-intensity signal abnormality in the periventricular and subcortical white matter, without mass effect. There is involvement across the corpus callosum.

ence of HIV dementia (6). Although MRI may demonstrate atrophy and signal changes in the white matter, it cannot detect the microglial nodules and multinucleated giant cells seen on histological sections (197). Other researchers have found abnormal MRI results in ~13% of asymptomatic HIV-seropositive patients and 46% of symptomatic HIV-seropositive patients (205). MRI findings only appeared to correlate well in those who were symptomatic. Increasing cerebral atrophy and white

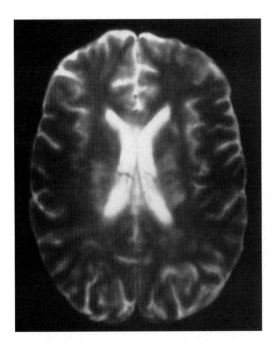

FIG. 4. HIV encephalitis. Axial T2-weighted MRI of an HIV-infected patient with clinical evidence of HIV encephalitis. Note symmetric, periventricular signal abnormality of the white matter. (From Bowen BC, Post MJD. Intracranial infection. In: Atlas S, ed. *Magnetic Resonance Imaging of the Brain and Spine.* New York: Raven, 1991:506; with permission.)

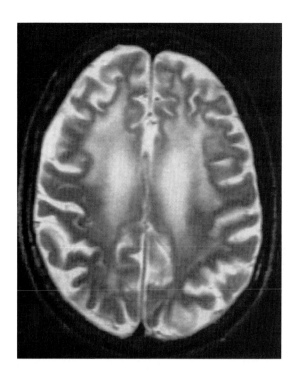

FIG. 5. HIV encephalitis. Axial T2-weighted MRI shows symmetric increased signal within the periventricular white matter with extension to subcortical regions as well. Clinically, this patient had evidence of HIV-related encephalopathy.

matter disease paralleled the development of clinically evident neurological disease (205).

Initial and repeat examinations performed at 2–4 years on asymptomatic HIV-seropositive patients have shown 80% of these studies to be normal and to remain normal (198). Twenty percent had minor abnormalities that were static and stable. Similar follow-up on patients with mild neurological symptoms showed that 50% of MRI scans were mildly abnormal but remained stable (198). Thus, a far greater number of symptomatic patients will have abnormal scans than will those who are asymptomatic. The MRI findings of minor abnormalities in asymptomatic HIV-seropositive patients may not be clinically significant because they apparently remain stable. Zidovudine therapy has shown partial reduction of HIV-related white matter changes on MRI with associated improvement in cognitive function (179).

Functional neuroimaging, either positron emission tomography (PET) or SPECT may offer earlier diagnosis than MRI or CT in patients with HIV encephalitis. These modalities have the potential to detect abnormalities before structural damage occurs. Iodine-123 MP-SPECT imaging of patients with ADC has shown multiple focal cortical perfusion abnormalities and has demonstrated these abnormalities prior to alterations evident by CT or MRI (193,301). The abnormalities on ^{123}I MP-SPECT developed in association with symptoms of dementia in these patients (193). Other ^{123}I MP studies have suggested a progression of ADC on ^{123}I MP-SPECT from subcortical asymmetry to cortical defects to more global cerebral perfusion deficits (131).

Technetium-99m HMPAO studies have shown regional abnormalities of cerebral blood flow in patients with ADC, and several of these had normal imaging studies (268). Other HIV-infected patients without ADC also had cerebral blood flow abnormalities with normal CT/MRI findings. In early HIV-related dementia there may be increased ^{99m}Tc HMPAO activity in the basal ganglia and thalamus (156). In later stages, these same regions may show decreased activity.

PET–18-F fluorodeoxyglucose studies have been conducted on asymptomatic HIV-seropositive patients, and results are similar to those of controls. These studies measured mean brain glucose metabolic rates (187). Similar findings have been seen in patients with ADC. However, regional metabolic patterns have been abnormal on PET scanning of patients with ADC. In one study, ADC was characterized by early subcortical hypermetabolism progressing to decreased glucose use in subcortical and cortical gray matter (226). Although the results of these studies are promising, continued research is necessary to determine the clinical utility of these procedures.

Proton MRI spectroscopy also has been used to detect cerebral abnormalities in HIV-infected patients. One study (113) found N-acetyl aspartate/creatine (NAA/Cr) significantly reduced in the patient group compared with the control group, and this ratio was lower in symptomatic compared with asymptomatic patients. The mean choline (Cho)/Cr ratio was significantly elevated in the patient population compared with the control group. Ten control spectra were found to be normal to "blinded" readers, whereas 12 of 15 patient spectra were determined to be abnormal. MRI of these same individuals showed no significant differences in the white matter of the patients versus those of the controls (113). Thus, proton spectroscopy holds a promise of early diagnosis of biochemical alterations in HIV-infected patients. Additional research is necessary to determine the reliability of these findings as well as their clinical utility.

Chong et al. obtained cerebral proton spectroscopy on 103 HIV-seropositive patients and 23 control subjects (50). Significant reductions in NAA/Cho and NAA/CR ratios were seen in the immunosuppressed patients with neurological abnormalities (50). NAA is a putative neuronal marker; thus, the reduced ratios support the theory that neuronal loss (and/or dysfunction) underlies ADC. These reduced ratios correlated with the presence of diffuse abnormalities on MRI, but not with focal lesions (50). Cho/Cr also was elevated in patients with low CD4 + counts and abnormal MRI studies. In this study, among 25 patients with normal MRIs who underwent clinical neurological evaluation, NAA/Cr was significantly lower (16% lower) in patients with neurological signs compared with patients without neurological abnormalities. Thus, spectroscopy indicated biochemical alterations that were not apparent on MRI of patients with neurological disease. Of the 103 HIV-infected patients, 11 had normal MRIs but abnormal spectra and 22 had normal spectra and abnormal images. Thus, the information provided by these two techniques appears to be complementary.

Pediatric HIV

Seventy percent of pediatric AIDS is secondary to congenital infection via maternal transmission (60). By the age of $4\frac{1}{2}$ years, $>90\%$ of children with congenital HIV infection develop neurological symptoms with a static or progressive encephalopathy (60). Other pediatric manifestations include microcephaly, cognitive defects, spasticity, seizures, and ataxia. Pediatric HIV infection may result in a progressive encephalopathy with loss of motor milestones and intellectual abilities, the development of weakness, and pyramidal tract signs (19,78). This progressive encephalopathy is estimated to occur in 30–50% of HIV-seropositive children (77). The majority of subacute encephalitis seen in the pediatric AIDS population is most likely due directly to HIV infection (20,241,243). Histopathological examination shows large multinucleated cells infected with HIV present in the brains of these children, along with inflammatory cell infiltrates and extensive calcific vasopathy, primarily involving small vessels in the basal ganglia, but also present in the pons and cerebral white matter (20,188,241). It is postulated that during the acute phase of HIV infection, there is damage to the vessel walls of small and medium-sized arteries with secondary calcium deposition in the walls and adjacent brain (20,241). Diminished brain volume is probably due to myelin loss or reduced myelination because neuronal loss is uncommon (265).

CT of these children most commonly shows atrophy and ventricular enlargement (20,60,77,78). Hypodensity of the white matter is seen infrequently. Basal ganglia calcification is often present and is usually bilateral (Fig. 6). Basal ganglia enhancement also has been reported (20,77,78,201). Calcification also may be present in the periventricular white matter of the frontal lobes (Fig. 7) (77). Treatment with zidovudine has resulted in improvement of atrophic changes on serial CT scanning (60). Patchy areas of white matter disease may be seen on MRI, and progression of this white matter disease on serial MRI studies correlates well with the progression of dementia.

Although CMV, toxoplasmosis, and PML all have been reported in the pediatric population (19,78,201,289), opportunistic infections are not seen as frequently as

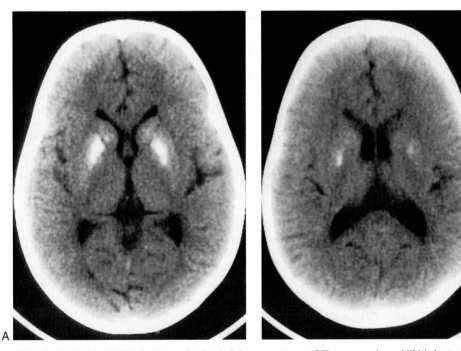

A   B

FIG. 6. Pediatric HIV infection. **A, B:** Axial noncontrast CT scans of an HIV-infected child demonstrate symmetric calcification of the basal ganglia related to underlying calcific vasopathy. There is also central and cortical atrophy. (From Whiteman MLH et al. AIDS-related white matter diseases. *Neuroimag Clin North Am* 1993;3:331–359; with permission.)

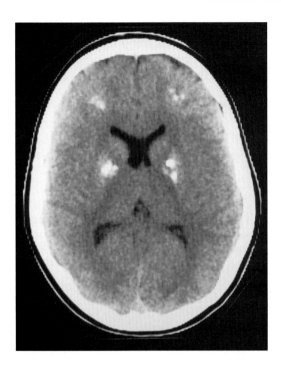

FIG. 7. Pediatric HIV infection. Non-contrast CT scan of a child with congenital HIV infection. Note symmetric calcification of the basal ganglia and frontal lobes. (From Whiteman MLH et al. AIDS-related white matter diseases. *Neuroimag Clin North Am* 1993;3: 331–359; with permission.)

they are in adults (19,78,201,241). Approximately 15% of CT and MRI of pediatric patients with AIDS demonstrate a focal abnormality secondary to opportunistic infection or CNS lymphoma (77,188).

CMV

CMV is a frequent pathogen in the AIDS population, not only in the CNS but throughout the body, involving a multitude of sites. CMV more commonly presents outside the CNS, involving the respiratory tract, liver, gastrointestinal tract, genitourinary tract, or hematopoietic system (199). This virus exists in a latent form in the vast majority of the population. Nearly 90% of adults have antibodies to CMV (138). Reactivation usually results in a subclinical or mild infection mimicking mononucleosis (31,296). In a minority of immunocompromised patients, however, reactivation can result in disseminated infection and/or severe necrotizing meningoencephalitis (33,202,255) and ependymitis (202).

CMV may involve the central and/or peripheral nervous system (10,282,292,293). Neurological manifestations of CMV include acute or chronic meningoencephalitis, cranial neuropathy, vasculitis, retinitis, myelitis, brachial plexus neuropathy and peripheral neuropathy (33,70,73,130,169,224,255).

Approximately 15–30% of adult patients with AIDS show CMV on neuropathological examination (11,172,189). Eighteen percent of patients with AIDS who undergo CT examination have pathological evidence of intracranial CMV (204). CMV may coexist with other lesions, including toxoplasmosis and cryptococcosis, and may be clinically silent when coexistent with other CNS infections (202).

The pathological hallmark of CMV is the "owl's eye," an enlarged cell with a distended nucleus containing eosinophilic viral inclusions and surrounded by a halo, resulting in the characteristic appearance (202). The owl's eye appearance may be seen in ependymal cells, subependymal astrocytes, oligodendroglia, endothelial cells, and neurons. CMV commonly involves the ependyma but, rarely, can result in extensive destruction of gray and white matter (199). Other typical histopathological findings include well-circumscribed microglial nodules and, rarely, focal parenchymal or ventricular necrosis (189). CMV intranuclear inclusions also may be found in the spinal cord, spinal nerves, and retina (202).

CMV meningoencephalitis may be seen in patients with HIV infection, as well as in otherwise healthy adults (290). It may be subclinical in immunocompetent and immunosuppressed patients (11,172,189,235). Less often, symptoms develop over days to months and include fever, altered mental status, confusion, memory loss, and progressive dementia (202). It is most commonly seen in transplant patients (234) and in patients with AIDS. In some cases of encephalitis there is diffuse brain involvement, not limited to the subependymal regions (138,146). Cerebrospinal fluid (CSF) findings and complement fixation blood titers are nonspecific, and the clinical diagnosis may thus be difficult (33).

CT is often insensitive in imaging of CMV encephalitis (202). Atrophy is the most frequent finding (33,146,255). Infrequently, hypodensity of the white matter may be apparent (213,255). Ring-enhancing lesions also have been described (146). One study of autopsy-proven CMV cases demonstrated that only 30% had CT abnormalities attributable to CMV (202). CT grossly underestimates the degree of involvement (199). In addition to diffuse white matter hypodensity and atrophy, periventricular and subependymal enhancement may be present (199) and is best visualized with DDD technique (213) (Fig. 8). Immunodeficient HIV-seropositive children with con-

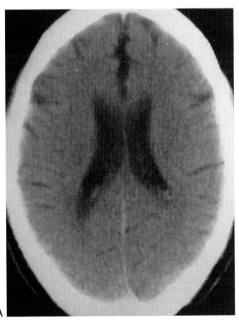 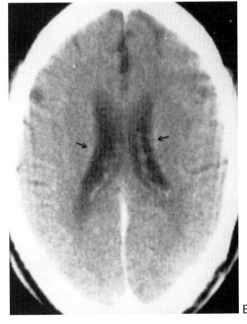

FIG. 8. CMV ventriculitis (pathologically proven). **A:** Axial noncontrast CT scan demonstrates mild cortical atrophy and ventricular enlargement. **B:** Postcontrast study shows faint subependymal enhancement *(arrows)*.

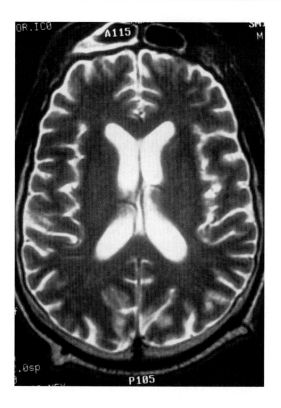

FIG. 9. CMV meningoencephalitis (pathologically proven). T2-weighted (2,400/80) axial MRI demonstrates cortical atrophy and ventricular enlargement in this patient with AIDS with evidence of CMV infection of the CNS at autopsy.

genital CMV infection may have reactivation of CMV infection, resulting in periventricular and white matter enhancement with edema seen on CT imaging (201).

MRI has greater sensitivity than CT in detection of CNS CMV (202). In addition to atrophy (Fig. 9), MRI may demonstrate increased signal on T2WIs in the periventricular white matter (213), which may be thick and is sometimes nodular (265,266). Infrequently, subependymal enhancement is seen and, if present, is a valuable diagnostic clue (Fig. 10) (202). Fat-suppressed MRI with gadolinium may show a thickened and enhancing choroid/retina in patients with CMV retinitis (273), a hemorrhagic retinitis frequently seen in the AIDS population.

HSV-1

HSV-1 is the causative agent in 95% of herpetic encephalitis and is the most common cause of fatal sporadic encephalitis (56,57,284). HSV-1 is found in the subependymal regions of 2% of AIDS autopsy cases in which a ventriculitis is present (189).

In adults, this infection usually arises in those with preexisting antibodies and thus represents viral reactivation. In children, HSV-1 acquisition is usually postnatal, and in neonates HSV-2 is much more frequent than HSV-1, accounting for 80–90% of neonatal herpesvirus infections and almost all of the congenital herpesvirus infections (242). Clinical symptoms in adults include a nonspecific alteration in mental status, a decreasing level of consciousness associated with focal neurological deficit, and fever (274). The CSF is nonspecific, and isolation of HSV from the CSF is rare

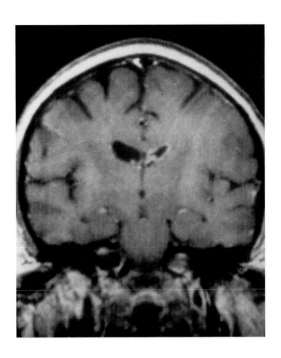

FIG. 10. CMV meningoencephalitis. Subependymal enhancement of the left lateral ventricle is evident on this coronal T1-weighted (600/20) MRI scan. Clinical and laboratory evidence confirmed CMV infection.

(287). CSF antibodies to HSV occur later in the disease (287). Electroencephalography (EEG) demonstrates activity localized to the temporal lobes (274). Definitive diagnosis can be made on the basis of brain biopsy (168). Polymerase chain reaction (PCR), a DNA amplification technique, may prove useful as a means of prompt diagnosis (227).

In patients without AIDS, HSV-1 infection can result in a necrotizing encephalitis of the temporal lobes and orbital surfaces of the frontal lobes (125). Involvement may extend to the insular cortex, cerebral convexity, and posterior occipital cortex (125). Disease is usually bilateral, with sparing of the basal ganglia (237). The cingulate gyrus may be involved later in the course of the disease (119). Location along the medial aspect of the temporal lobes and frontal lobes suggests that intracranial spread occurs along small meningeal branches of cranial nerve V arising in the trigeminal ganglion (274). Rhombencephalitis (pontine infection) is not unusual in HSV-1 and is possibly related to retrograde viral transmission along the cisternal portion of cranial nerve V to the brain stem (257).

CT of patients without AIDS but who are infected with HSV-1 demonstrates hypodense lesions in the temporal lobes with or without frontal lobe disease. Enhancement and hemorrhage are infrequent (99). Patchy parenchymal/gyral enhancement is occasionally seen on CT and/or MRI (119) (Fig. 11). Abnormal signal on T2WIs is usually evident before the development of this enhancement (119). Correlation of CT, MRI, EEG, and CSF results indicates the greater sensitivity of MRI as compared with CT (86). MRI demonstrates the early edematous changes of herpes encephalitis, with increased signal seen in the temporal and frontal lobes on T2WIs (10,174) (Fig. 12). MRI is thus considered the study of choice in imaging of HSV encephalitis (274). Focal hemorrhage is consistently present at autopsy, yet is often not detected or is less apparent on CT (30) (Fig. 13). MRI is more sensitive to this subacute hemorrhage (263). MRI also can be used to monitor response to treatment with acyclovir (141).

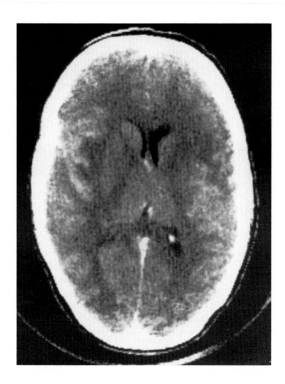

FIG. 11. Early herpes encephalitis occurring in a virology laboratory technician. There is mass effect on the right lateral ventricle due to temporal lobe involvement. Patchy enhancement along the right sylvian fissure is noted. This patient was not immunocompromised.

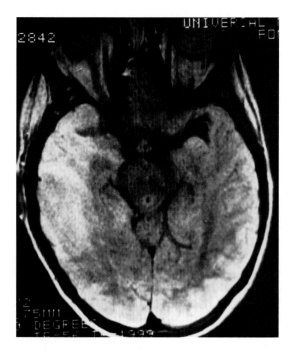

FIG. 12. Herpes encephalitis. Axial T2WI (1,999/56) of same patient seen in Fig. 11. There is a focal region of increased signal present in the right temporal lobe.

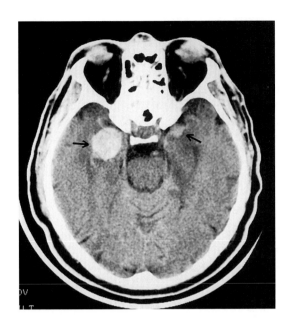

FIG. 13. Herpes encephalitis. Noncontrast CT in this patient with clinical symptoms of viral encephalitis demonstrates bilateral hemorrhagic involvement of the temporal lobes **(arrows)**.

Infection with HSV-1 and HSV-2 has been reported in patients with AIDS (119,199) but is an infrequent complication of AIDS, occurring in 2% of AIDS autopsy cases (189). In patients with AIDS, HSV often results in diffuse rather than temporofrontal inflammation (119). Both mild and severe forms of encephalitis due to HSV-1 and HSV-2 have been seen (143) and may coexist with other infections (143,147,189). Typical pathological findings of necrotizing encephalitis may be absent in the patient with AIDS, even when HSV-1 or HSV-2 is cultured from the brain tissue (199). CT scanning in patients with AIDS who are infected with HSV most often is normal or shows atrophy only (199). HSV-1 is a rare cause of myelitis in AIDS and may be associated with a dermatomal rash (287). MRI can demonstrate an intramedullary signal abnormality that correlates well with the neurological symptoms and the involved dermatome (74).

VZV

VZV is the cause of two distinct clinical syndromes, varicella (chicken pox) and herpes zoster infection (shingles) (274). Both result in similar histopathological findings in the skin (287). CNS infection may be seen in both entities and may result in hemorrhagic necrosis with intranuclear inclusions (287). Varicella-zoster encephalitis is seen in ~2% of adult AIDS autopsies after thorough neuropathological examination (189).

Zoster infection may result in encephalitis, neuritis, myelitis, and/or herpes ophthalmicus (274). These rarely complicate the clinical course of healthy adults with shingles, but there is increased risk of CNS involvement in immunocompromised patients (274). Although cranial and peripheral nerve palsies are the most common neurological disorders associated with zoster in patients without AIDS (87), diffuse encephalitis is the most frequent CNS complication seen in those immunosuppressed patients with CNS zoster infection (214). Latent virus residing in the ganglia of cranial nerves (especially cranial nerves V and VII) can reactivate and with retrograde extension traverse the brain stem, resulting in encephalitis. Fever, meningismus, and altered mental status in a patient with shingles should suggest the diagnosis (274). CSF shows a mild lymphocytic pleocytosis, a slightly elevated protein level, and normal glucose level. MRI may demonstrate increased signal in the brain stem and supratentorial gray matter (274), despite a negative CT result (64,82) (Fig. 14).

Although CNS complications are seen in 5% of patients with infectious mononucleosis (EBV) there does not appear to be an increased frequency of this disorder in HIV-seropositive individuals (274).

PML

PML is a progressive demyelinating disorder arising from CNS infection with a papovavirus. The causative agent is a human polyomavirus, the JC virus, which belongs to the papova family of CNS viruses (*pa*pilloma, *po*lyoma, *va*cuolating virus) (220).

PML was first described by Astrom et al. in 1958 (34). In 1965, using electron microscopy, ZuRhein and Chou (308) and, independently, Silverman and Rubenstein (245) found innumerable viruslike particles within inclusion bodies of oligodendrocytic nuclei. In 1971, Padgett et al. (182) isolated a virus from the postmortem brain of a patient with PML by using this tissue as a source of inoculum in cell cultures derived from human fetal brain. The initials of the donor patient were JC, and thus the virus was termed the JC virus.

Seroepidemiological studies indicate that the JC virus infects 80% of the human population before adulthood without producing overt illness (92). Antibodies to the JC virus are nearly ubiquitous among the adult population worldwide (283,289). The virus typically remains latent unless there is reactivation due to immunodeficiency (283).

Before the era of AIDS, PML was seen in association with other immunodeficient disorders, including renal transplantation, autoimmune disease, TB, sarcoidosis, Whipples' disease, nontropical sprue, and lymphoproliferative disorders (34). Patients receiving chemotherapy are also at increased risk for PML.

In 1982, Miller et al. reported on a homosexual man with a T cell immunodeficiency with biopsy-proven PML (165). In 1984, Bernick and Gregorios described PML in a patient with recognized AIDS (25). PML appears to have a stronger association with AIDS than with any other immunosuppressive disorder (260), and 55–85% of recent PML cases are attributable to AIDS (23,134). PML is evident in 5.3% of patients with AIDS at autopsy (289).

The target of the JC virus in PML is the oligodendrocyte, which forms and maintains the myelin sheath (207). Infection of the oligodendrocyte causes cytolytic destruction and thus results in myelin loss (154). The axon is usually spared. Electron microscopy can identify intranuclear inclusions consisting of JC virus particles (158,306,307). Enlarged abnormal astrocytes are also a feature of PML. These astrocytes are multinucleated with numerous large processes (92). Microscopic foci of scattered demyelination enlarge over time and coalesce (154). Gross examination of the brain shows a gray or brownish discoloration of the white matter as a result of myelin loss (289).

The clinical presentation of PML includes memory loss, personality change, cogni-

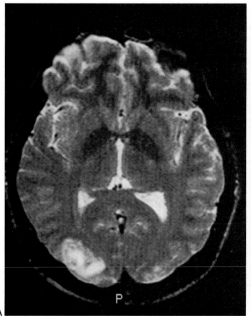
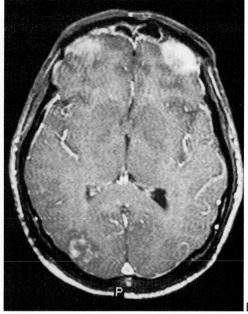
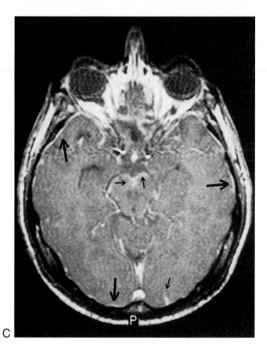

FIG. 14. Herpes zoster encephalitis in an HIV-seropositive patient (autopsy proven). **A:** Axial T2-weighted (2,200/80) MRI demonstrates hyperintense signal abnormality of both occipital lobes, right greater than left. **B:** T1-weighted (600/30) axial MRI obtained after gadolinium administration (0.1 mmol/kg) shows patchy enhancement in the right occipital lobe. **C:** At the level of the midbrain, enhancement of the prepontine and interpeduncular cisterns is apparent *(small arrows)*, as is enhancement in the left occipital lobe *(small arrow)*. Diffuse meningeal enhancement is also present *(large arrows)*. This patient did not have shingles in the months preceding his encephalitis. CSF cultures were negative. The right occipital lobe lesion was examined via biopsy, and the specimen showed only necrotic and inflammatory tissue. The patient's condition deteriorated rapidly. Postmortem examination showed evidence of herpes zoster encephalitis. Multiple focal areas of parenchymal necrosis were identified, including the right occipital lobe.

tive and speech disturbances, visual deficit, altered mental status, and motor and/or sensory abnormalities, with progressive neurological decline (29,34). Less frequent signs and symptoms include vertigo, seizures, headache, and aphasia (23,34). The progression of disease is relentless, although the time course is somewhat variable, with death often occurring within 9 months of symptom onset (34). The most common symptoms of PML are hemiparesis, visual impairment, and altered mentation, not only at presentation but during disease progression as well (23,60). Patients with lesions of the posterior fossa may exhibit ataxia, dysarthria, and dysmetria (117,186). Homonymous hemianopsia is the most frequent visual deficit. Spinal cord involvement is uncommon (16,138).

Neurological dysfunction is often an indicator of underlying immunodeficiency in patients who are otherwise asymptomatic (24). PML is thus the initial manifestation of AIDS in up to 47% of patients who present with PML (289).

On CT, PML appears as a focal area of hypodensity within the white matter, without mass effect and usually without enhancement (Fig. 15). Most frequently, both periventricular and subcortical lesions are present, although involvement also may be isolated to either the subcortical or periventricular location (289). Serial scans demonstrate extension of disease. Patchy enhancement is seen occasionally (289) (Fig. 16). CT may be negative in some cases, especially in early lesions (204).

MRI demonstrates greater sensitivity than CT in the imaging of PML in defining both the extent and number of lesions (207,289). MRI is thus the procedure of choice for imaging of PML (207). On T2WIs, lesions demonstrate increased signal intensity in the periventricular and/or subcortical white matter. Lesions may be small in size initially but often progress to larger areas of involvement (Fig. 17). A multifocal distribution is seen, and although PML may be unilateral, it is more frequently bilateral (289). There is no associated mass effect and lesions rarely enhance. When

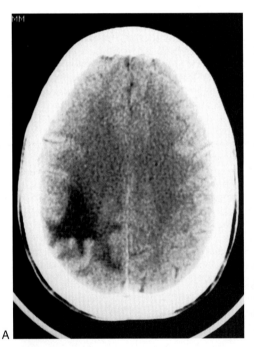 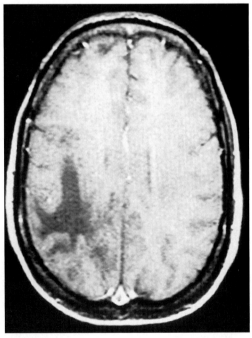

A   B

FIG. 15. PML (pathologically proven). **A:** Noncontrast axial CT demonstrates focal hypodensity in the right parietal region, conforming to the distribution of white matter. **B:** Postgadolinium (600/20) MRI of same patient shows similar hypointense signal involving the centrum semiovale and subcortical white matter of the parietal lobe. There is no mass effect or significant enhancement.

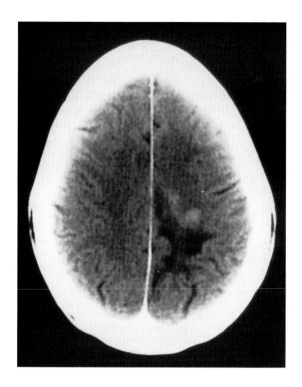

FIG. 16. PML (pathologically proven). Postcontrast CT scan demonstrates faint, nodular enhancement at the periphery of the lesion. (From Whiteman MLH et al. Progressive multifocal leukoencephalopathy in 47 HIV seropositive patients. *Radiology* 1993;187:233–240; with permission.)

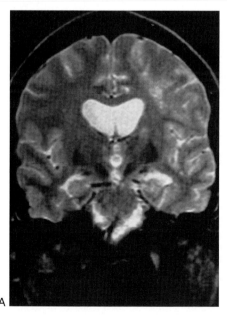

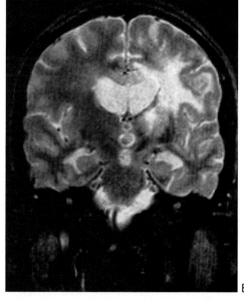

A   B

FIG. 17. PML (pathologically proven). **A:** Coronal T2-weighted (2,400/80) MRI shows faint signal abnormality in the left frontal subcortical white matter. **B:** Same patient, 3 months later. There is far greater involvement at this time, with both periventricular and subcortical disease, with extension as well to the left basal ganglia. There is early involvement of the corpus callosum. This radiographic progression paralleled the patient's clinical deterioration.

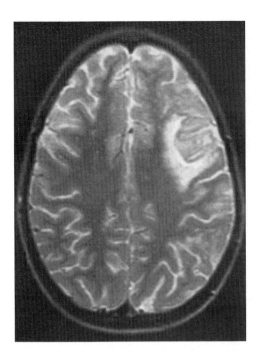

FIG. 18. PML (pathologically proven). Scalloped appearance of the subcortical white matter due to the involvement by PML. There is no mass effect.

enhancement is seen, it is faint and peripheral (289). The subcortical PML lesions have a quite characteristic appearance. The involvement follows the gray–white interface resulting in a "scalloped" (30) (Fig. 18) appearance as the demyelination affects the subcortical subcortical U-fibers (289). On T1WI the lesions are most often hypointense to parenchyma (Fig. 19), although early lesions may be isointense.

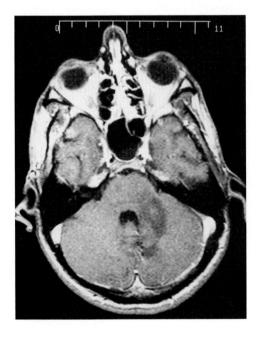

FIG. 19. PML (pathologically proven). T1-weighted (600/30) postgadolinium axial MRI demonstrates hypointense lesion involving the left middle cerebellar peduncle, extending into the cerebellar white matter. Note absence of mass effect on the fourth ventricle as well as the lack of enchancement.

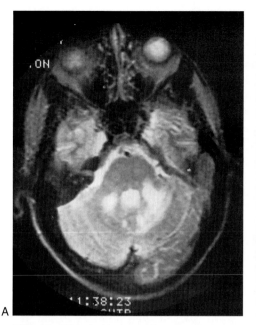
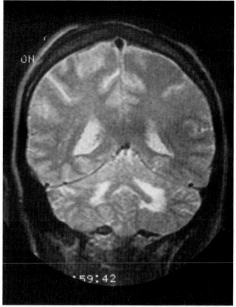

FIG. 20. PML (pathologically proven). T2-weighted axial MRI (2,400/80) **(A)** and T2-weighted coronal (2400/80) MRI **(B)** show bilateral posterior fossa involvement, left greater than right. There is involvement of the middle cerebellar peduncles bilaterally, with extension to the cerebellar white matter. PML also involves the pons on the left. There is no mass effect on the fourth ventricle.

Any lobe may become involved, but the frontal and parietooccipital locations are most common (289).

PML lesions also may be present in the deep gray structures (155,266,289). This is chiefly due to involvement of very small myelinated fibers that course through the basal ganglia and adjacent structures (289). Involvement of the posterior fossa is common and is present in approximately one third of PML cases (289) (Fig. 20). Usually there are additional supratentorial lesions, although PML isolated to the infratentorial structures does occur in ~10% of cases (265).

Radiographically, PML may be difficult to distinguish from HIV-related demyelination. The latter is more often diffuse, symmetric, and periventricular in location, whereas PML is more often multifocal, asymmetric, and with greater predilection for the subcortical white matter. The lesions of PML may be hypointense on T1WIs, whereas those of HIV-related demyelination are isointense. Clinical correlation is essential because HIV encephalitis most often presents with global disturbance and dementia, whereas PML in contrast presents with focal neurological deficits (290). Dementia infrequently dominates the clinical picture.

Bacteria

Syphilis

Syphilis is a chronic infection with three well-characterized stages. Descriptions of syphilis in the medical literature date back many centuries. The causative agent is *Treponema pallidum*, a spirochete. Between 1986 and 1989, the incidence of syphilis increased sharply in both men and women, largely as a consequence of AIDS (275). Without treatment, 5–10% of patients develop clinical evidence of neurosyphilis. One study of patients with AIDS with neurosyphilis found that 44% of all patients diagnosed with neurosyphilis over a 42-month period were also HIV infected (121). Several studies have documented an increased incidence of positive syphilis serology in HIV-infected patients compared with HIV-seronegative patients (122). An increased occurrence of syphilis in HIV-infected patients also has been reported by other investigators (248). In patients with AIDS, the course of neurosyphilis appears to be accelerated (122) and the disease may be more aggressive (121). A comparative study of patients with neurosyphilis, which included both HIV-seropositive and -seronegative patients found the HIV-seropositive group to be younger and to have a greater tendency to have features of secondary syphilis, such as rash, fever, adenopathy, headache, and meningitis (122). Syphilitic meningitis was more commonly seen in the HIV-infected group and CSF abnormalities were more striking in this group, with a higher number of white cells, a higher mean CSF protein level, and a lower mean glucose level in the HIV-positive group (122).

Neurosyphilis is most often asymptomatic. CNS involvement may occur at almost any stage of systemic infection (275). Neurosyphilis can occur weeks to decades after initial infection, and occurs in one third of patients who progress to the late stages of syphilis (275). Symptomatic patients with AIDS most often present with hemiparesis and visual disturbance (121), as well as fever, skin rash, headache, and weight loss (122).

There are two major clinical categories of symptomatic neurosyphilis: meningovascular and parenchymatous. Mixed features are common in the nonimmunosuppressed host. The parenchymatous manifestations include general paresis and tabes dorsalis. The usual interval from time of infection to symptom onset in nonimmunosuppressed individuals is 5–10 years for meningovascular syphilis, 20 years for general paresis, and 25–30 years for tabes dorsalis, although this time course appears to be accelerated in HIV-infected patients (122). Syphilitic eye disease also may be present and is more commonly seen in patients with AIDS with neurosyphilis as compared with HIV-seronegative patients with neurosyphilis (122).

In patients with AIDS, acute syphilitic meningitis and meningovascular neurosyphilis are the most commonly encountered forms (121). Meningeal neurosyphilis may present as an acute meningitis and may result in hydrocephalus, cranial neuritis, and/or formation of gummas (275). Vascular neurosyphilis is usually characterized by headache and focal neurological deficit related to a vascular event, with abnormal CSF findings. Meningovascular syphilis results in widespread thickening of the meninges, meningeal lymphocytic infiltrates, and perivascular lymphocytic infiltrates surrounding small blood vessels (185). Cranial nerve involvement most commonly occurs in cranial nerves II and VIII.

Two types of vascular involvement are seen in neurosyphilis: Heubner's endarteritis and Nissl-Alzheimer endarteritis. The arteritis seen in neurosyphilis is more commonly of the Heubner type, affecting large and medium-sized arteries with resultant irregular luminal narrowing and ectasia (30). Less frequently, the Nissl-Alzheimer type of arteritis is evident, primarily involving small vessels in which a luminal narrowing occurs as a consequence of intense proliferation of endothelial and adventitial cells (30). Thus, both types of arteritis may result in vascular occlusion.

Syphilitic gummas are circumscribed masses of granulation tissue surrounded by mononuclear epitheloid and fibroblastic cells with occasional giant cells and perivasculitis. Gummas are created by an intense localized leptomeningeal inflammatory reaction early in the meningeal phase of neurosyphilis (120). Gummas originate from the meningeal connective tissue and blood vessels with spread into the adjacent parenchyma (30). The gummas are usually seen overlying the cerebral convexitis, adherent to both dura and brain parenchyma. The lesions vary from 1 mm to 4 cm in size (185) and may be multiple but are most often solitary. There may be central caseous necrosis within the lesion, but spirochetes are rarely present (185). Any organ may be involved, with the most common sites being the skin, skeletal system,

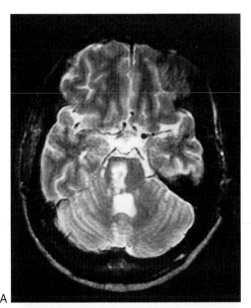

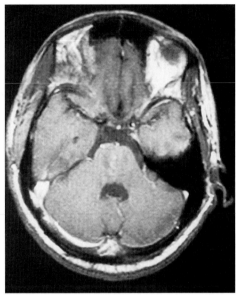

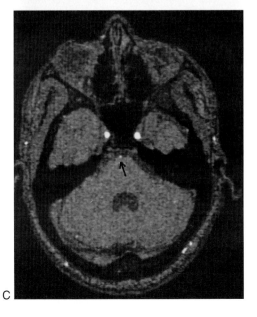

FIG. 21. Syphilis. **A:** T2-weighted (2,550/80) axial MRI demonstrates focal signal abnormality in the right pons. **B:** Postgadolinium T1-weighted (600/30) axial MRI shows a region of hypointense signal in the right pons with faint enhancement in the midline, at the edge of the lesion. This enhancement is presumably on the basis of subacute infarction. **C:** 3D time of flight MR angiogram (45/10, 20°) demonstrates marked reduction in the caliber of the basilar artery *(arrow)* due to meningovascular syphilis. (From Whiteman MLH et al. AIDS-related white matter diseases. *Neuroimag Clin North Am* 1993;3:331–359; with permission).

mouth and upper respiratory tract, larynx, liver, and stomach. CNS gummas are seen infrequently.

Just as the histopathological appearance of syphilitic involvement is varied, so are the radiographic manifestations. On CT, one third of studies are negative and one third show only cerebral atrophy (89,110). Small infarcts or foci of ischemia secondary to the vasculitis seen in meningovascular syphilis may be apparent on both CT and MRI. On MRI, multiple focal hyperintensities are seen on T2WIs involving both gray and white matter in cortical and subcortical locations (30). Multiple arterial distributions are affected involving both supratentorial and infratentorial structures (30) with predilection for the basal ganglia. MRI is superior to CT in demonstration of these ischemic regions (105,107). CT may show a solitary focus, whereas MRI can show multiple infarcts in the same patient, suggesting the possibility of a vasculitis (105). Postgadolinium images may show enhancement in areas of subacute infarction (89,105) (Fig. 21), and meningeal enhancement also may be present, again seen to better advantage on MRI than on CT (30).

On CT, gummas may appear as a mass lesion, with nodular or ring enhancement, at the brain surface (Fig. 22). Adjacent meningeal enhancement may be evident. In patients with AIDS, both meningeal enhancement and parenchymal enhancement are more often seen on CT, as compared with patients without AIDS who have neurosyphilis (122). The MRI appearance is similar (Fig. 23). Lesions also may appear as intraparenchymal nonenhancing masses (89,120).

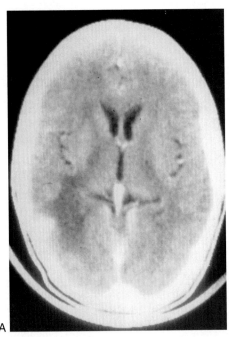 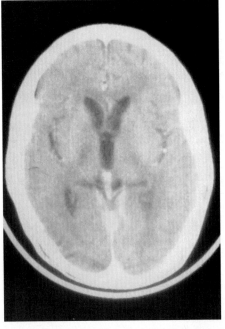

A   B

FIG. 22. Syphilis. **A:** Postcontrast axial CT scan demonstrates a peripheral enhancing lesion in the right temperooccipital region with surrounding edema. Clinical examination, CSF, and serum studies were consistent with neurosyphilis in this HIV-seropositive patient, and toxoplasmosis antibody titers were negative. **B:** After treatment with aqueous penicillin G complete resolution of the lesion is noted with residual ventricular dilitation. (From Berger JR, et al. *Syphilitic gumma with HIV infection. Neurology* 1992;42:1282–1287; with permission.)

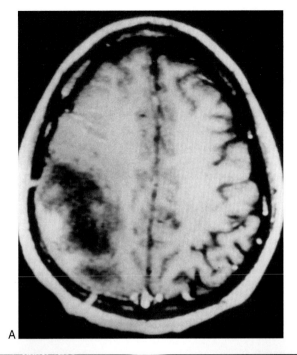

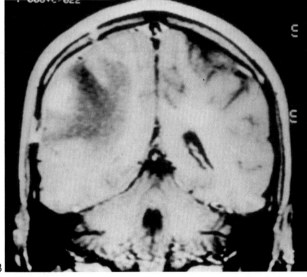

FIG. 23. Syphilis (pathologically proven). **A:** Axial post–gadolinium DTPA MRI scan shows peripheral parenchymal and meningeal enhancement surrounded by extensive edema and mass effect. **B:** Coronal image of the same patient shows an enhancing right parietal lesion with meningeal enhancement, edema, and mass effect. Treatment with i.v. aqueous penicillin resulted in marked clinical and radiographic improvement. (From Berger JR, et al. Syphilitic gumma with HIV infection. *Neurology* 1992;42:1282–1287; with permission.)

Mycobacteria

In the United States there has been an increase in the number of TB cases since 1986 (45,221,222) as well as an increase in extrapulmonary manifestations (162), which may be attributed to the AIDS epidemic. Extrapulmonary TB (including CNS TB) is currently included in the U.S. Centers for Disease Control and Prevention criteria for a diagnosis of AIDS in an HIV-seropositive patient (231). Of patients with AIDS who have TB, 70% have extrapulmonary manifestations (231). The incidence of *Mycobacterium tuberculosis* and *Mycobacterium avium-intracellulare* occurring in the AIDS population varies considerably with the type of population studied and the locale. Some investigators estimate that the mycobacterioses (TB and MAI) occur in 10–18% of all patients with AIDS (192). Nontuberculous mycobacteria occur one fifth as commonly as does TB in patients with AIDS (178). Five to 9% of patients with AIDS have TB (all sites included) (45,151,276). Conversely, information derived from clinic-based studies in Miami and San Francisco suggests that 28–31% of patients with TB are HIV seropositive (191,270). The relative risk of TB is >100 times higher in patients with AIDS as compared with the general population (276). Among HIV-infected intravenous drug users, there is a 20% incidence of TB (261). Intracranial TB occurs in 1% of all patients with AIDS (2). CNS TB occurs in 2–5% of all patients with TB (21,61) and in 10% of those with AIDS-related TB (21,26).

In the past, adult TB has been primarily a postprimary infection, whereas in children the majority of cases have been due to the primary infection (259). Reactivation of latent TB is the major mechanism for TB among HIV-seropositive individuals (238), although 10–30% of current TB cases in adults are due to primary infection (124,166,297). Latent TB often becomes clinically evident early on in HIV-related immunodeficiency; thus, TB usually precedes other AIDS-defining opportunistic infections in HIV-seropositive patients (184,192). Thus, TB usually develops in HIV-seropositive patients before full-blown AIDS is apparent (46,221). This suggests that less immunosuppression is needed to manifest TB than other HIV-related disorders. Unlike TB, which is often diagnosed early in the course of HIV infection (before a clinical diagnosis of AIDS), MAI is usually diagnosed well after the development of AIDS (231).

CNS TB may take a variety of forms, including TB meningitis, abscess focal cerebritis, and tuberculoma, and a subacute encephalitis may be present with MAI (26,143,204). The most common radiographic findings associated with CNS TB in patients with AIDS include enhancement of the basal cisterns, granulomas, abscess, calcifications, meningeal enhancement, hydrocephalus (usually of the communicating type), and basal ganglia infarcts, either bland or hemorrhagic. Other sites of infarction may be seen as well.

In 25–83% of patients with CNS TB, there is coexistent pulmonary disease (7,71). Eight-six percent of patients with TB and without AIDS have isolated pulmonary disease, whereas only 60% of patients with AIDS and TB have disease restricted to pulmonary involvement (221). Of all patients with TB, those with AIDS as well are more likely to have a disseminated form of the disease (221).

Leptomeningitis is the most frequent form of CNS TB encountered in HIV-infected patients (281) although cryptococcus is a more frequent pathogen in HIV-related meningitis. Fever, headache, and altered mental status are the most frequent presenting symptoms (21,281). Meningeal signs may be absent in one third of patients with AIDS-related TB meningitis.

Two different mechanisms are proposed for the pathogenesis of TB meningitis (244,266,304). The first mechanism suggests rupture of subependymal or subpial granulomas into the CSF. The second proposed pathogenesis involves penetration of the walls of meningeal vessels by hematogenous spread, usually from a pulmonary or gastrointestinal source.

This basal meningitis results in a thick gelatinous exudate involving the basal cisterns (65). Arteries that course through this exudate can become directly involved by the inflammatory infiltrate or indirectly by reactive endarteritis obliterans. Both processes may occur. Spasm results, and intimal alterations often lead to thrombosis and infarction (30). Arteritis is present in ~28–41% of cases with basilar meningitis (139). Infarctions are even more common in children (236). The MCA and small perforating branches to the basal ganglia are affected most often (244). Both MRI and CT can demonstrate these areas of infarction, although there is earlier detection with MRI.

Both CT and MRI also can document communicating hydrocephalus, a common sequela of TB meningitis (48). In a study of 35 patients with AIDS with proven intracranial TB, hydrocephalus was the most common imaging finding, present in 51% of the cases (281). Meningeal enhancement was present in 45%, parenchymal disease in 37%, vascular complication in 23%, and a normal result in 23% (281). Cisternal enhancement is often striking and may be seen well on both CT and MRI (Fig. 24). Meningeal enhancement is far better demonstrated on postgadolinium MRI than on CT (30).

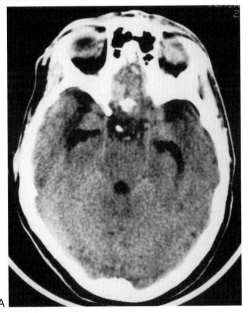
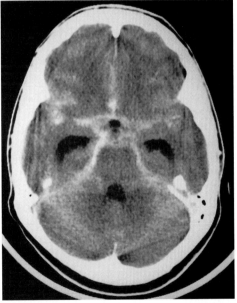

A B

FIG. 24. TB meningitis (culture proven). **A:** Noncontrast axial CT scan demonstrates enlargement of the temporal horns and slight dilitation of the fourth ventricle, suggesting a communicating hydrocephalus. **B:** Postcontrast CT scan shows diffuse cisternal enhancement as well as enhancement within the right sylvian fissure. Findings are compatible with a diffuse meningitis resulting in communicating hydrocephalus. Cultures grew MTB.

In a study of 232 cases of TB meningitis in the general population, acid-fast bacilli were found in the CNS in only 45% of cases (271). CSF typically shows a pleocytosis with a low glucose and slightly elevated protein, although this may be inconsistent in patients with AIDS. Elevated ADA (adenosine deaminase) levels (>9 U/L CSF) in the CSF may be helpful in establishing an early diagnosis because cultures take time and may delay urgent therapy, resulting in irreversible damage (4,164,218). The amplification of *Mycobacteria tuberculosis* DNA by polymerase chain reaction is also helpful in establishing an early diagnosis of TB meningitis.

Overall mortality for TB meningitis was >25% in the pre-AIDS era and even higher in children, with pediatric mortality rates reported between 17% and 71.9% (7,271). The mortality rate among HIV-seropositive patients treated for TB meningitis is ~21% (21). Those who survive are frequently left with significant deficits. The long-term morbidity rate among patients with TB meningitis (patients without AIDS) is 66% (271). These sequelae include mental retardation, paralysis, rigidity, cranial nerve palsy, seizures, and speech or visual deficits (271). These complications result from hydrocephalus, infarction, and/or TB involvement of the brain parenchyma and cranial nerves (271). Long-term morbidity in patients with AIDS is difficult to assess because patients may succumb to other opportunistic infections or malignancies. In one study of 24 patients who were treated for CNS TB and survived, four had persistent neurological sequelae (21).

In one study, parenchymal involvement was noted in 37% of patients with AIDS with CNS TB (281). TB granulomas (tuberculomas) are one form of parenchymal intracranial TB. Granulomas may be secondary to hematogenous spread of systemic disease or may evolve from extension of CSF infection into the adjacent parenchyma via cortical veins or small penetrating arteries (185). Pathologically, the granuloma is composed of a central zone of solid caseation necrosis, surrounded by a capsule of collagenous tissue, epithelioid cells, multinucleated giant cells, and mononuclear inflammatory cells (30). Few tubercle bacilli are seen on smears (277,291) but may be demonstrated in the necrotic center and throughout the capsule (62). Outside the capsule there is parenchymal edema and astrocytic proliferation (62). Tuberculomas may be found in the cerebrum, cerebellum, subarachnoid space, or subdural or epidural space (30). Parenchymal disease most often involves the corticomedullary junction and periventricular regions, as expected for hematogenous dissemination. The majority of tuberculomas are supratentorial (71,281). Parenchymal disease can occur with or without coexistent meningitis and may cause a focal cerebritis (264).

On CT, tuberculomas are seen in only a minority of patients with TB meningitis (244). Of those patients with parenchymal tuberculoma, 10–34% have multiple lesions (7,116). Contrast CT demonstrates a ring-enhancing lesion correlating to the pathological process of central necrosis and peripheral organization (95). One third of patients may demonstrate the "target sign," which appears as a central calcification or punctate enhancement surrounded by a region of hypodensity with surrounding rim enhancement (279). This sign is not pathognomic for TB but may be suggestive.

On noncontrast MRI, granulomas appear isointense to gray matter on T1WIs and may have a slightly hyperintense rim (possibly secondary to the presence of paramagnetic species, which shorten the T1 relaxation time) (95). On T2WIs, tuberculomas exhibit variable signals. They are often iso- or hypointense to brain parenchyma, and it is postulated that this relative hypointensity is related to T2 shortening by paramagnetic free radicals produced by macrophages that are heterogenously distributed throughout the caseous granuloma (266). Alternatively, the diminished signal on T2WIs may be attributed to the mature tuberculoma, being of greater density than the brain (95). Granulomas also may be hyperintense to brain on T2WIs, and this is likely due to a greater degree of central liquefactive necrosis in these lesions (30). There is usually associated mass effect and edema, and the edema surrounding tuberculomas is more prominent in the early stages of formation (95).

Postgadolinium images of TB granulomas demonstrate intense nodular and ring-like enhancement (30). Although communicating hydrocephalus may result from TB meningitis, an obstructive hydrocephalus may result from a focal parenchymal lesion and associated mass effect (281). Obstructive hydrocephalus also may be caused by entrapment of a ventricle by granulomatous ependymitis (185,244,304).

Healed tuberculomas may calcify in up to 23% of cases, and these are usually more evident on CT than on MRI (116). Atrophy is frequently a long-term sequela of TB CNS infection. Full resolution of cerebral tuberculoma requires months to years of medical therapy. The length of time required is related more to the size of the original lesion than to any other single factor (116).

TB abscess is a rare complication (244). In contrast to the solid caseation seen in the granuloma (with few tubercle bacilli present), the abscess is formed by semiliquid pus that is teeming with tubercle bacilli (277,291). The wall of a TB abscess lacks the giant cell epithelioid granulomatous reaction of a TB granuloma (298). It is postulated that the abscess may be due to liquefactive breakdown of a more typical caseated tuberculoma (298) (Fig. 25). TB abscesses are larger than tuberculomas and have a more accelerated clinical course (299). The appearance is similar to that of a bacterial abscess (266), although there is frequently less surrounding edema as compared with a pyogenic abscess (223). On CT the TB abscess is hypodense with edema and mass effect. Postcontrast images demonstrate ring enhancement that is usually thin and uniform, but less often may be somewhat irregular and thick. The appearance is related to the central zone of liquefactive necrosis with pus and surrounding inflammation. This central area is thus of increased signal on T2WIs (266). Lesions also may be multiloculated (26,204).

A comparison of CT scans of HIV-seropositive and -seronegative patients with TB meningitis showed hydrocephalus in 42% of the HIV-seropositive cases and in 44% of the HIV-seronegative cases (21). Nonenhancing lesions (presumably infarcts) were seen in 27% of the HIV-seropositive group but only in 6% of the HIV-seronegative group. Meningeal enhancement was also more prominent in the HIV-seropositive group, present in 23% of cases, and was seen in only 6% of the HIV-seronegative group. Enhancing parenchmyal lesions were noted in 15% of the HIV-seropositive scans, whereas no focal parenchymal lesions were seen in the HIV-seronegative group. Thus, infarction, meningeal enhancement, and parenchymal disease appear to be more common in patients with TB meningitis who are also HIV infected. This is supported by the results of another comparative study, which found mass lesions on imaging studies in 60% of the HIV-infected patients with TB meningitis but in only 14% of the non-HIV patients with TB meningitis (72).

Approximately 16% of both HIV-seronegative and HIV-seropositive patients demonstrate resistance to at least one of the drugs (isoniazid, rifampin, streptomycin, ethambutol) commonly used to treat TB (239). This resistance indicates transmission of resistant organisms from patients with TB who have received inadequate or inappropriate treatment (44).

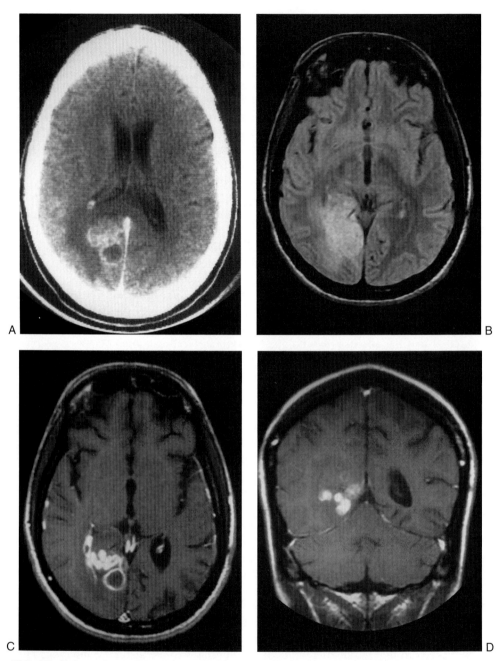

FIG. 25. Tuberculomas/TB abscess (biopsy proven). **A:** Postcontrast axial CT scan demonstrates focal, multiloculated enhancement in the right occipital lobe with a mild degree of surrounding edema. There is mass effect on the right lateral ventricle and anterior displacement of the occipital horn. **B:** Proton density (2,400/20) image of the same patient shows hyperintense signal in the right occipital lobe and compression of the atrium of the right lateral ventricle. **C:** Post–gadolinium DTPA MRI (600/20) shows both nodular and ring enhancing lesions. Biopsy showed a TB abscess. **D:** Coronal postgadolinium images (600/20) again shows a mixed pattern of both nodular and ring enhancing lesions.

Nocardia

The primary immunological defect in patients with AIDS is that of cell-mediated immunity rather than humoral immunity. This may account for the paucity of pyogenic CNS infection in these patients. Infection with *Escherichia coli*, *Salmonella* organisms, and *Nocardia* organisms have been reported (3,143,204,265). *E. coli* CNS infection may result in meningitis or meningoencephalitis, but is rare (143,204). Communicating hydrocephalus may be a sequela (199).

Nocardia species is an unusual infection that has been seen more frequently in recent years, likely related to the increasing number of patients with AIDS. *Nocardia* represents 0.3–1.8% of all infections seen in patients with AIDS (109,278). *Nocardia* also is seen in other patients with immunosuppressive disorders, including autoimmune disease, sarcoidosis, silicosis, chronic obstructive pulmonary disease, cancer, chronic granulomatous disease, and ulcerative colitis, and is also seen in transplant patients, patients on steroids, and patients undergoing chemotherapy treatment (3,14). *Nocardia asteroides* is an aerobic gram-positive filamentous rod that is variably acid fast and exhibits true branching and beading of the filaments, which may break up to form bacillary or coccobacillary forms (14). *Nocardia* is a true bacteria, not a fungus. *Nocardia* was first recognized as a pathogen (in cattle) by Nocard in 1888 (176). In 1890, the first nocardial infection in a human was reported (76).

The saprophytic nocardiaciae are common soil organisms. Infection most often results from inhalation into the lungs but may be due to direct innoculation related to trauma. Three types are known to be human opportunistic pathogens: *N. asteroides*, *N. brasiliensis*, and *N. caviae*. *N. asteroides* is the most common and is associated with lung, skin and brain abscesses. *N. brasiliensis* primarily involves the skin and lymphocutaneous sites, whereas *N. caviae* is rare (14). Most cases associated with HIV infection have involved *N. asteroides* (136,278). Approximately 75% of nocardial infections cases occur in individuals who are immunocompromised (14).

There is a strong association between nocardiosis in HIV-infected patients and intravenous drug use (114,278). Fever may be present, and a history of respiratory tract infection is common with nocardial infection. The pulmonary manifestations are protean. Respiratory colonization by *Nocardia* organisms occurs in 44–51% of immunocompromised patients (247). Eight-one percent of all nocardial infections are pulmonary (183). Cerebral nocardia abscess is associated with an 80% mortality rate (210). Survival depends on appropriate antimicrobial treatment, the degree of immunocompetence (81), and prompt surgical intervention when necessary.

In North America, the CNS is the second most common site of *N. asteroides*, accounting for 15–30% of cases (17,96). Five percent of *Nocardia* cases present with the CNS disease, without evidence of systemic infection (17). CNS disease is most often due to hematogenous spread from a primary site, usually the lungs (35). In one study of HIV-infected patients with nocardial infection (n = 19), 42% presented with nocardial infection as the initial opportunistic infection (114). Symptoms of CNS nocardial infection are nonspecific and include fever, headache, confusion, and seizures. CD4+ counts are usually low (114), and nocardiosis usually occurs among patients with advanced HIV disease (278). A review of nocardial meningitis in patients without AIDS, a rare disorder, found altered mental status, fever >101°F, stiff neck, and headache as the most common signs and symptoms (35). The disease is more frequent in men (35). Of patients with meningitis, 43% have brain abscesses. Typical CSF findings include a low glucose level, elevated protein, and a neutrophilic

CSF pleocytosis (35). Meningitis may be due to a ruptured abscess with ventricular spread of infection or may be due to direct hematogenous seeding (35).

The most common manifestation of CNS nocardia in both HIV-seropositive and seronegative patients is abscess, which is often multiple, involving the cerebrum, cerebellum, and deep gray structures (17,36,136). Spinal abscess and meningitis also have been described (253), as has mycotic aneurysm (96). Organisms are seldom isolated from the CSF in patients with cerebral nocardial abscess (253). This is due to a dilutional effect and may be overcome by hyperconcentration of the CSF. A neutrophilic CSF pleocytosis is often present (136).

CT imaging may demonstrate a ring-enhancing lesion, which can be multiple or multiloculated (136). There is surrounding edema and mass effect. Subependymal abscess formation also may be seen. Similar findings are seen on MRI (Fig. 26). The central cavity and surrounding edema are of increased signal intensity on T2WIs and are hypointense on T1WIs.

Culture of *Nocardia* requires 2–4 weeks of incubation, often resulting in a delayed diagnosis especially if clinical suspicion is not high. The diagnosis of nocardial infection is frequently delayed or missed due to the nonspecific nature of the clinical presentation. The low incidence of nocardial infection in patients with AIDS may be due in part to a lack of recognition (278). Because nocardial infection is not an AIDS-defining condition, it is likely underreported (278). A timely diagnosis of nocardial infection is only feasible if clinicians are aware of this disorder and maintain a high level of suspicion. The diagnosis should be suspected in any patient with an intracranial lesion and a cavitary lung infiltrate (136). Additionally, if an HIV-infected patient has been treated with antitoxoplasmosis medication and CNS lesions persist despite adequate therapy, nocardial infection may be considered.

Treatment of CNS nocardial infection is problematic due to variations in sensitivity as a result of inoculum size, strain type, and assay technique. Cerebral penetration is also difficult to predict (14), as is penetration of the abscess cavity (3). Trimethoprim-sulphamethoxazole (TMP-SMX) is currently the treatment of choice (136), with good CSF penetration. A variety of other drugs have been used against *Nocardia* and may be quite effective: ampicillin, erythromycin, minocycline, and amikacin. Minimum duration of therapy with TMP-SMX is probably 6 months in the general population, with a longer course needed for patients with AIDS (136). TMP-SMX is used as prophylaxis against *P. carinii* pneumonia in patients with advanced HIV disease. This use may protect against nocardial infection and may account, in part, for the low incidence of nocardiosis among patients with AIDS (109).

Mortality from nocardial infection among patients with AIDS is seen in two thirds of those affected. The cause of this high mortality rate is multifactorial. Delay in culture results in delayed diagnosis and treatment, allowing widespread dissemination (278). If treatment is discontinued, relapse may occur rapidly and the disease may become resistant to medical therapy (278). Poor prognosis is also related to severe host immune dysfunction (278). Thus, prolonged and perhaps lifelong treatment may be needed in patients with AIDS.

Bacillary Angiomatosis

Bacillary angiomatosis recently has been recognized as a multisystem infectious disease occurring primarily in HIV-infected patients. The etiological agent is a gram-

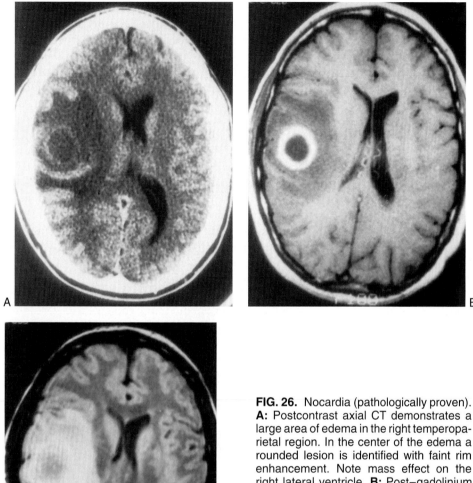

FIG. 26. Nocardia (pathologically proven). **A:** Postcontrast axial CT demonstrates a large area of edema in the right temperoparietal region. In the center of the edema a rounded lesion is identified with faint rim enhancement. Note mass effect on the right lateral ventricle. **B:** Post–gadolinium DTPA T1-weighted (600/20) axial MRI scan demonstrates the lesion with a thick, smooth rim of enhancement. Note central area of hypointensity, suggestive of pus within the abscess cavity. Surrounding edema is hypointense. **C:** Proton density (2,400/20) axial MRI demonstrates high-intensity edema surrounding the lesion, which is of lower signal intensity. A hypointense rim may also be discerned.

negative bacillus known as *Rochalimaea,* similar to the agent of cat scratch fever (*Afipia felis*) (128). Either of two *Rochalimaea* species—*R. quintana* or *R. henselae*—can be isolated from lesions or blood (128). This disease most commonly presents with cutaneous lesions: angiomatous, tender papules that may resemble KS on occasion (137). Subcutaneous nodules and cellulitic plaques also may be seen (15). Systemic symptoms include fever, chills, night sweats, and weight loss (15). Osteolytic lesions may be found at a number of sites, are often symptomatic, and may present before the skin lesions, predating cutaneous manifestations by several months (15). In addition to bony involvement, the liver, spleen, lymph nodes, conjunctiva, and respiratory tract may be involved (15). Local complications such as airway obstruction may occur, or overwhelming infection may result from multiple organ involvement (55).

Pathological examination of cutaneous and visceral lesions demonstrates a proliferation of capillaries in an edematous stroma, with many polymorphonuclear leukocytes (15). There are clear pathological distinctions between this lesion and KS (55). Culture of the causative organism *Rochalimaea* is quite difficult, but is possible (128).

The bone lesions are often painful and are symptomatic in approximately one third of patients with cutaneous lesions (15). Lytic lesions may result in cortical destruction and permeation of medullary bone with aggressive periosteal reaction (15). Bone scan shows increased uptake at affected sites. The lesions are also well seen on CT (Fig. 27).

Because AIDS-related KS does not involve bone, the finding of a cutaneous lesion in association with a painful bone lesion should suggest the diagnosis of bacillary angiomatosis (15). Bone scan shows not only symptomatic foci but also asymptomatic areas of involvement (15) and can be used to suggest the diagnosis of bacillary angiomatosis in a patient with a cutaneous lesion (15).

Treatment is administered with erythromycin, and in some instances other antibiotics are used. Adequate therapy results in symptomatic improvement, with resolution of cutaneous and osseous lesions.

Fungal Disease

Cryptococcosis

Fungal disease may affect the immunocompromised as well as the immunocompetent. Those fungi generally affecting only the immunosuppressed are *Aspergillus, Candida,* and *Mucor.* Other fungal diseases that may occur in both the immunocompromised host and in the normal host include cryptococcosis (41), coccidiomycosis, histoplasmosis, and blastomycosis (152). *Cryptococcus, Aspergillus, Candida,* and *Mucor* are ubiquitous fungi, whereas the remainder are endemic to particular geographic locations (127). CNS infection by the systemic mycoses results in granulomatous reaction with a variable degree of suppuration (185). Intracranial vessels, leptomeninges, and/or the parenchyma may be involved, resulting in a CT and/or MRI appearance that is indistinguishable from that of TB (266).

The mycotic lesions seen in the CNS vary in appearance with the fungal forms (185). Fungi growing in infected tissue as yeast cells (cryptococcosis, histoplasmosis) spread hematogenously to the microvasculature of the meninges, penetrate the vessel walls, and result in acute or chronic leptomeningitis (185). Less often, parenchymal disease such as granulomas or abscesses are seen.

Fungi grown as hyphae only (*Aspergillus, Mucor*) or pseudohyphae (*Candida*) involve the parenchyma to a greater degree than the meninges because the larger forms have limited access to the meningeal circulation (185).

Hyphae form mycelial colonies capable of vascular invasion and obstruction of large, medium, and small arteries, resulting in infarction and cerebritis (185). Pseudohyphae are adherent yeast cells and their progeny, and they are smaller than true hyphae. *Candida* infection therefore results in scattered granulomatous microab-

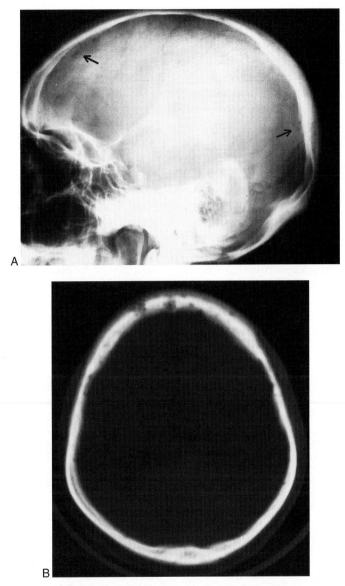

FIG. 27. Bacillary angiomatosis (pathologically proven). **A:** Lateral plain radiograph of the skull demonstrates multiple ill-defined lytic lesions *(arrows)*. **B:** Bone window of an axial CT scan on the same patient demonstrates multiple lytic lesions of the cranium. This patient had widespread bony disease at the time of diagnosis.

scesses secondary to small vessel (arteriole) occlusion and tissue breakdown (304). CNS *Candida* gains access to the meninges by penetration of the meningeal microvasculature by individual or small groups of yeast cells (30).

Cryptococcus neoformans is the most frequent fungus to involve the CNS in patients with AIDS (69). It is clinically evident in 6–7% of patients with AIDS (63), and in 45% of the patients with AIDS who have cryptococcosis it is the first manifestation of their immunodeficiency (63). Inhalation is the usual mode of infection. Cryptococcal infection of the meninges results in a basilar granulomatous meningitis (69). Cryptococcal meningitis is usually a subacute meningitis, with headache the most common and sometimes the sole symptom (143). In one study of 35 patients with CNS cryptococcal infection (including 28 patients with AIDS), 66% complained of headache, altered mental status was noted in 29%, and fever was present in 26% (195). Clinical presentation also may include neck stiffness (195), seizures, and signs and symptoms of increased intracranial pressure (33). Diagnosis is made via India ink preparation, detection of cryptococcal antigen in the CSF, or fungal CSF culture.

Imaging findings in cryptococcal meningitis are often unremarkable. CT is frequently negative (204,255), and positive findings are most often nonspecific atrophy and communicating hydrocephalus (146,204,286). Meningeal enhancement may occur but is usually absent (123,204) (Fig. 28). MRI also may be negative in cryptococcal meningitis (207). Gadolinium-enhanced studies may show meningeal enhancement, which is inapparent on noncontrast images (219).

The route of spread of infection to the parenchyma may be either via hematogenous dissemination or direct spread of meningeal infection to the cortex (30). Parenchymal disease in cryptococcal infection may take a variety of forms, and the literature is somewhat confusing on this topic. Four patterns may be encountered: (a) parenchymal mass lesions, also known as cryptococcomas; (b) dilated Virchow-Robin spaces; (c) parenchymal/leptomeningeal nodules; and (d) a mixed pattern. The symptoms and pathological findings in patients with AIDS with cryptococcal disease are often

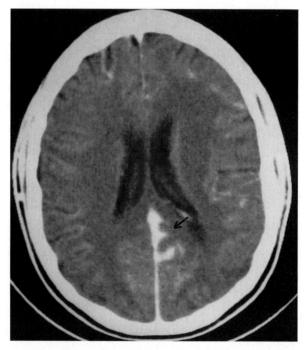

FIG. 28. Cryptococcal meningitis. Postcontrast axial CT scan demonstrates meningeal enhancement *(arrows)* in this patient with AIDS who also had recurrent cryptococcal meningitis. Cryptococcal antigen was detected in the CSF. Ventricular dilatation was new compared with the results of prior studies.

muted, perhaps due to the inability to mount a significant cell-mediated immune response (265). This also may account for the paucity of radiographic findings in many cases (265).

Dilated Virchow-Robin spaces are perivascular spaces that may become filled with fungus. As the vessels extend from the basal cisterns to the brain substance, fungal invasion results in enlargement of the perivascular spaces, which is most evident in the basal ganglia. In such cases, the infectious agent is outside the parenchyma and therefore does not incite a significant inflammatory response. The parenchymal/leptomeningeal nodules represent small cortical granulomas (265).

Cryptococcomas represent a collection of organisms, inflammatory cells, and gelatinous mucoid material (157). The relative amount of each constituent may vary and may result in an imaging appearance that has been termed "gelatinous pseudocyst." However, the constituents may vary in relative concentration, and the lesion can thus appear as an isodense or isointense mass lesion on imaging studies. Pathological study of both the gelatinous pseudocysts and the more solid-appearing lesions show pseudocystic spaces filled with mucoid material (157). There is little inflammatory response (195). Intraventricular cystic cryptococcomas also have been described (195).

The imaging findings in cryptoccal disease may differ according to the patient population. In a study of patients without AIDS (n = 20), 50% had normal CT scans, 25% had hydrocephalus, 15% had focal nodules, 15% demonstrated gyral enhancement, and 5% demonstrated patchy contrast uptake (267). In contrast, a study of immunocompromised patients (n = 29, with 28 of 29 HIV infected) found that 31% had normal CT scans, 45% showed atrophy, 10% had nonenhancing mass lesions, and 7% had enhancing lesions (272). Another study of 35 patients (28 with AIDS) showed atrophy in 34%, a normal study in 43%, mass lesions in 11%, and hydrocephalus in only 9% (195). Thus, it appears that hydrocephalus is less common in the immunocompromised patient, and abnormal enhancement is also less frequent. The absence of hydrocephalus may be attributed to the lack of inflammatory leptomeningeal reaction and the paucity of resulting adhesions within the basal cisterns, which often result in hydrocephalus in the nonimmunocompromised host.

Infrequently, CT may demonstrate hypodense lesions with solid or ring enhancement, particularly in the basal ganglia (305). Parenchymal disease in cryptococcosis is less widely distributed and incites less edema than toxoplasmic encephalitis (9). Peripheral, small enhancing nodules may be seen consistent with cortical granulomas. These may contain punctate calcifications. More often, focal hypodensities without enhancement can be seen in the basal ganglia, representing dilated perivascular spaces inhabited by collections of *Cryptococcus* organisms (Fig. 29). Cystic masses with septations representing gelatinous pseudocysts also can be seen in the basal ganglia, which do not demonstrate significant enhancement but may produce mild mass effect (Fig. 30).

MRI may demonstrate tiny clustered foci of signal abnormality that are isointense to CSF, compatible with dilated Virchow-Robin spaces (Fig. 31). These are located in the basal ganglia bilaterally, are relatively symmetric, and also may be seen in the midbrain (272). These do not enhance with gadolinium. Multiple miliary enhancing parenchymal and leptomeningeal nodules may be seen (272), suggestive of granulomas.

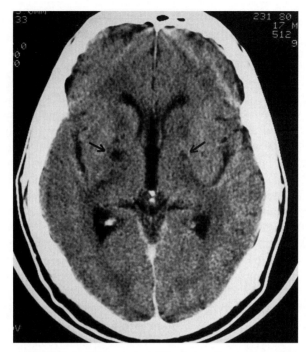

FIG. 29. Cryptococcal disease. Postcontrast CT of a patient with a history of cryptococcal meningitis. Rounded hypodensities *(arrows)* seen in the basal ganglia represent dilated Virchow-Robin spaces, filled with organisms.

Coccidioidomycosis

Coccidioides immitis infection results from hematogenous spread of endospores from a pulmonary source (30). CNS infection may manifest as a basilar, granulomatous meningitis or as microabscesses. The meningeal inflammation may be associated with caseous granulomas (185). A vasculitis also may result, with infarction, although complete vascular occlusion is rare (126). Coccidioidomycosis can be rapidly progressive and fatal. Diagnosis is based on CSF complement fixation titers.

CT most often demonstrates mild atrophy, without any enhancing lesion. Rarely, CT and MRI may demonstrate enhancement of the meningeal surfaces at the convexities and basal cisterns or communicating hydrocephalus (223). Entrapment of any portion of the ventricular system may occur secondary to ependymitis, resulting in obstructive hydrocephalus (223). Less commonly seen are enhancing granulomas in the white matter or deep gray matter.

Mucormycosis

Mucormycosis is a phycomycosis of the genus *Mucor*. CNS involvement is seen most often in diabetic patients and in those who are immunocompromised and has been reported in association with AIDS (54,59). Mucormycosis is usually of the rhinocerebral (craniofacial) type, with spread along the perivascular and perineural channels. Extension through the cribriform plate may result in frontal lobe infection,

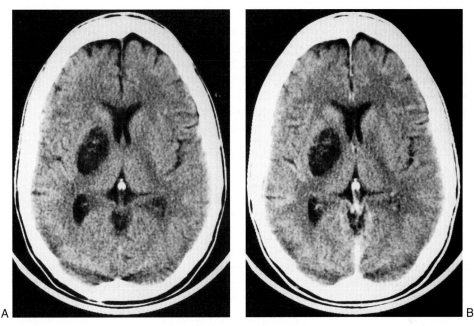

FIG. 30. Cryptococcal gelatinous pseudocysts. **A:** Noncontrast axial CT demonstrates gelatinous pseudocysts in the right basal ganglia of a patient with AIDS. **B:** There is no enhancement of the lesion after contrast administration. The appearance of this lesion and the lack of enhancement is related to the inability of the host to mount a significant inflammatory response.

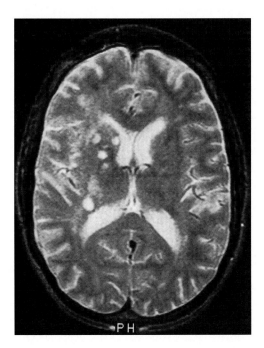

FIG. 31. Cryptococcal disease. T2-weighted (2,400/80) axial MRI shows multiple rounded foci of increased signal intensity in the right caudate, thalamus, and basal ganglia. These represent dilated Virchow-Robin spaces, containing the cryptococcal fungi.

and involvement at the orbital apex may result in extension to the cavernous sinus (30). The paranasal sinuses also may demonstrate mucosal thickening. Bone destruction occurs late (84). CNS *Mucor* infection may result in infarction or abscess, usually at the base of the brain and cerebellum, after invasion of the infratemporal fossa or orbit (84) (Fig. 32). Infarction or abscess may occur at a site remote from the primary focus due to vascular dissemination (30). Relative hypointensity of the lesion on T2-weighted MRIs is a helpful diagnostic clue (54).

Aspergillosis

CNS aspergillosis has been reported to occur rarely in patients with AIDS (33,143). CNS disease may result from direct extension of nasal and paranasal infection or may result from hematogenous spread. CNS aspergillosis (usually via *Aspergillus fumigatus*) is more often due to hematogenous spread from a pulmonary focus (185). *Aspergillus* hyphae invade cerebral vessels resulting in occlusion and hemorrhagic infarction (30). Septic infarcts may be associated with focal cerebritis and abscess formation (30) (Fig. 33). These infarcts are usually in the anterior circulation, anterior cerebral artery, or middle cerebral artery distribution (30).

Involvement of the circle of Willis may lead to direct extension to the cavernous sinus with angiitis, thrombosis, and infarction (30). Extension to the subarachnoid space may result in meningitis and meningoencephalitis (203,304).

Candidiasis

Candida is a common pathogen in patients with AIDS outside the CNS, but is uncommon in the CNS (123,143). Rarely, *Candida* infection may be seen within the CNS and may take a variety of forms, including meningitis (69), meningoencephalitis (143), abscess (143), microabscess (143), and granulomatoma (69).

On CT, the microabscesses appear iso- or hypointense on noncontrast scans and show multiple punctate-enhancing nodules on contrast studies (69). Granulomas may appear as hyperdense nodules on CT (69) with surrounding edema and nodular or ring (123) enhancement. CT often underestimates the extent of pathology in patients with widespread fungal disease (75).

A "target" appearance may be seen on MRI (69). Lesions may demonstrate a central, well-demarcated, hypointense signal with surrounding hyperintensity (edema) on T2WIs (266). MRI also may demonstrate evidence of meningitis, granulomas, abscess, vasculitis, and infarction but is unable to differentiate between the types of fungal disease.

Parasites

Toxoplasmic Encephalitis

Opportunistic infection of the CNS is a common complication of AIDS, seen in ~50% of adult AIDS autopsy series (140,170,189). A number of patients have two or more infections (189). Toxoplasmic encephalitis is caused by the obligate intracellular protozoan *Toxoplasma gondii*, with a worldwide distribution (30). Seropositivity

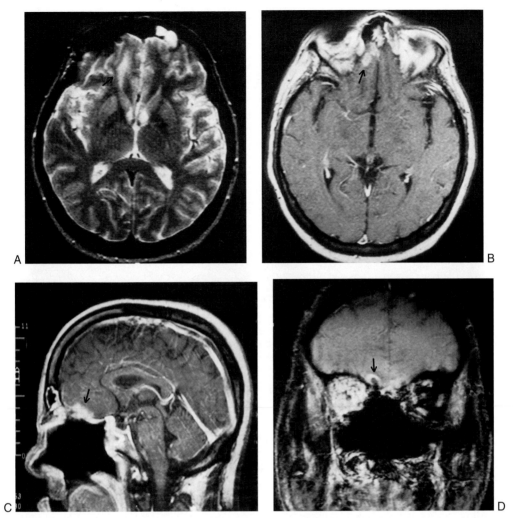

FIG. 32. Mucormycosis. **A:** T2-weighted axial MRI (2,650/80) demonstrates edema in the right frontal lobe *(arrow).* Inflammatory changes in the left frontal sinus is evident as high signal intensity. **B:** Axial post–gadolinium DTPA MRI (600/30) shows focal enhancement in the right frontal lobe (arrow). **C:** This patient (same patient as in **A** and **B**) had recently undergone extensive facial and paranasal sinus resection for mucormucosis with right orbital exenteration. This sagittal image (600/30) demonstrates the enhancement of the gyrus rectus *(arrow),* indicating extension of infection into the adjacent brain parenchyma. **D:** This is a coronal T1-weighted (750/15) postcontrast study performed with fat suppression. Note the left orbital fat has been supressed and appears dark. On the right, an orbital extenteration has been performed. Marked enhancement of the right orbit is due to a combination of postsurgical and inflammatory changes. Note focal intracranial enhancement *(arrow).* After intensive antibiotic therapy, the patient showed significant clinical improvement.

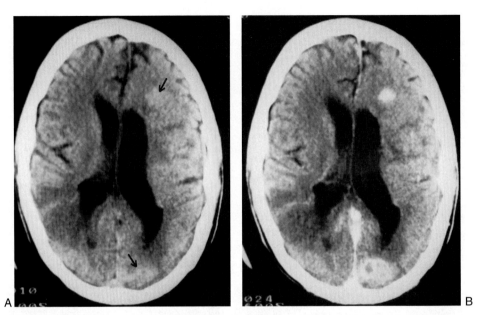

FIG. 33. Aspergillosis. **A:** Noncontrast CT demonstrates ventricular dilatation as well as vague areas of hyperdensity in the left frontal lobe and in the left occipital pole *(arrows)*. The hyperdensity likely indicates pettechial hemorrhage. There is also a wedge-shaped hypodensity in the right parietooccipital region, which suggests an area of ischemic infarction. **B:** Postcontrast CT shows focal enhancement in the left frontal and left occipital lobes. The patient expired several days later and the autopsy showed multiple intracranial abscesses due to aspergillus as well as areas of hemorrhage and infarction.

for adults in the United States ranges from 20% to 70% (143,185). In the immunocompetent patient, infection may be subclinical or may result in a benign course with self-limiting adenopathy, with or without fever (41,133,185,216,280). Before the era of AIDS, fulminant necrotizing encephalitis as a result of *Toxoplasma* species infection occurred only in those patients with significant immunodeficiency such as collagen vascular disease, underlying malignancy, organ transplantation, and patients maintained on steroids or undergoing chemotherapy or radiation treatment (41,133,216,280). The major mode of transmission of *Toxoplasma* organisms is via raw meat (75,147). Transmission is also possible via bodily secretions, raw milk, transfusions, organ transplantation, contaminated needles, cat feces, and *in utero* exposure (147).

In patients with HIV infection, toxoplasmic encephalitis results in a progressive and often fatal encephalitis if untreated (33,143,200). The clinical course includes altered mental status, confusion, lethargy, headache, fever, seizure, and focal neurological deficit (33,143,200). Toxoplasmosis is the most commonly reported opportunistic brain infection in patients with AIDS, presenting with altered mental status, fever, seizure, and/or focal neurological deficit (69,123,143,199,200,286). It is present in 10% of adult AIDS autopsies (189). Because seropositivity for toxoplasmosis is so widespread, a positive titer is nondiagnostic, only indicating past or recent exposure. However, a negative titer in a patient with an intracranial mass lesion should arouse suspicion of other possible etiologies. However, up to 22% of patients with AIDS with toxoplasmic encephalitis may not have detectable anti–*Toxoplasma* IgG antibodies (196). CSF findings in toxoplasmosis are nonspecific.

Pathologically, toxoplasmic encephalitis infection contains three distinct zones without a capsule (200). The central portion is a solid and coagulated avascular necrotic center with few organisms. The intermediate zone contains an intense inflammatory reaction with patchy areas of necrosis. This zone is engorged with blood vessels. Endothelial cell swelling and proliferation with cuffing of venules by lymphocytes, plasma cells, and macrophages are evident. In this zone are numerous free extracellular and intracellular tachyzoites. Encysted forms are rare, and there are fewer areas of necrosis in this zone (200). The peripheral zone contains more encysted forms (bradyzoites) and fewer free tachyzoites. Vascular lesions are few, and necrosis is rare in this zone. Leptomeningitis is present only directly adjacent to an area of encephalitis. Vascular involvement may lead to small vessel thrombosis and necrosis (200). There is no arteritis of the larger vessels (200).

Pathological diagnosis is made on hematoxylin and eosin (HE) stains or Giemsa stains. In more diagnostically difficult cases, electron microscopy of formalin-fixed material or standard immunoperoxidase procedures may be used (200).

Early imaging of patients with acute neurological deterioration is imperative because the results often dictate clinical management, and appropriate therapy can be instituted promptly. The characteristic appearance of toxoplasmic encephalitis on noncontrast CT is that of multiple areas of iso- or hypodensity with a predilection for the basal ganglia (in 75–88%) and the corticomedullary junction (147,200). Lesions also may involve the posterior fossa (204). The lesions may vary in size from <1 cm to >3 cm (200). Hemorrhage has been reported (75,147), although it is uncommon. There is surrounding edema and mass effect, of variable degree (204).

Postcontrast CT demonstrates ring, solid, or nodular enhancement (Fig. 34). Ring enhancement is most common, with central hypodensity. The rings are usually thin and smooth but may be thick and irregular (200), especially in the larger lesions. The DDD technique has been found to be extremely effective in detection of lesions of toxoplasmic encephalitis (143,200,204,207) (Fig. 35). The DDD technique permits maximal enhancement, and the central portion of the ring lesions may fill in on delayed scans (204).

The radiographic appearance correlates well with the pathological findings, with the central hypodensity representing the region of avascular coagulation necrosis. The enhancing ring corresponds to the region of intense inflammation, and the peripheral zone may appear radiographically as edema (200). Pathological radiological correlation has shown that the pathological extent of these lesions is often greater than the area of contrast enhancement evident on CT (200).

Toxoplasmic encephalitis is effectively treated with pyramethamine and sulfadiazide with dramatic clinical improvement (33,143,146,204). Serial scans obtained after the patient is on therapy demonstrate a decrease in the number and size of the lesions, with a reduction in edema and mass effect (Fig. 36). These changes usually occur within 2–4 weeks after initiation of treatment (123,146,204) but may take up to 6 months to fully resolve (143,147) Treated lesions have a variable appearance on CT. The areas of prior involvement may appear normal, may demonstrate encephalomalacia and focal atrophy, or may calcify (204). The larger complex lesions with mass effect tend to resolve more slowly than other lesions and often result in encephalomalacia. Despite radiographic resolution, in the presence of a persistent cellular immunodeficiency, toxoplasmic encephalitis frequently recurs if treatment is discontinued; therefore, lifelong maintenance therapy is required (143,204).

Spin-echo MRI without and with gadolinium is more sensitive to both new and

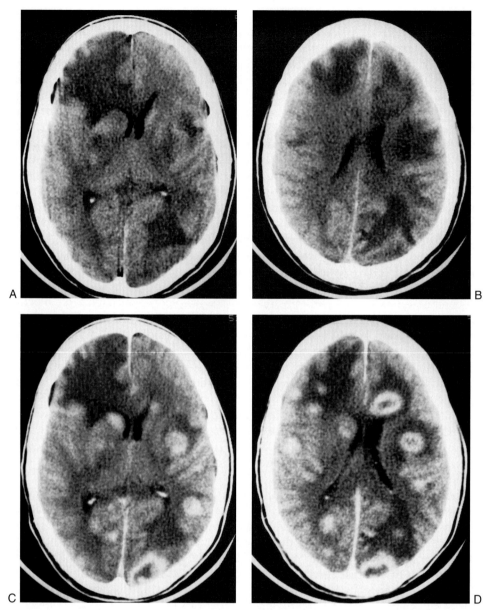

FIG. 34. Toxoplasmic encephalitis. **A, B:** Noncontrast CT images of an HIV-seropositive patient with toxoplasmic encephalitis. Lesions are isodense to hypodense, with extensive mass effect and edema. Lesions are difficult to separate from surrounding edema without the use of contrast. Toxoplasmic encephalitis. **C, D:** Postcontrast (DDD technique) images demonstrate multiple enhancing lesions. Some toxoplasmic lesions show nodular enhancement, whereas others demonstrate ring enhancement. (From Whiteman MLH et al. AIDS-related white matter diseases. *Neuroimag Clin North Am* 1993;3:331–359; with permission.)

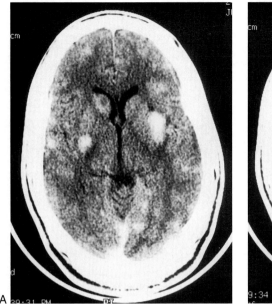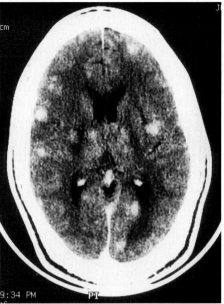

FIG. 35. Toxoplasmic encephalitis. Postcontrast (DDD) CT images demonstrate multiple areas of nodular enhancement. Less edema is present than is seen in Fig. 1. A ring-enhancing lesion is noted in the head of the right caudate nucleus. Lesions are primarily located at the gray–white junction and in the basal ganglia. (From Whiteman MLH et al. Progressive multifocal leukoencephalopathy in 47 HIV seropositive patients. *Radiology* 1993;187:233–240; with permission.)

old lesions of toxoplasmic encephalitis than is postcontrast CT (143,147,207). On T2WIs, active lesions are of variable intensity. The lesions may be hyperintense to parenchyma and thus indistinguishable from high-intensity surrounding edema (Fig. 37) or may be isointense or hypointense to brain parenchyma centrally surrounded by high signal edema (207,265). This latter appearance has been referred to as a target sign (207) and is nonspecific.

On T1WIs the lesions appear as focal areas of iso- or hypointensity. Postgadolinium (0.1 mm/kg) MRIs show ring or nodular enhancement in active lesions, clearly distinguishable from surrounding hypointense (low signal) edema (Fig. 38). The enhancement pattern seen is similar to that on CT (204). Hemorrhage in toxoplasmic lesions is uncommon.

MRI has a greater sensitivity compared with CT, especially for small lesions at the corticomedullary junction. Lesions are commonly encountered in the basal ganglia and are often multiple. As a result of greater sensitivity, MRI is able to detect a greater number of toxoplasmic lesions as compared with CT. Additionally, the MRI may be positive, whereas the CT is completely negative (143,147). On contrast MRI examination, only 14% of patients with toxoplasmosis demonstrate a solitary lesion (196). Thus, the lack of multiplicity on a high-quality MRI scan should prompt a suspicion of other possible pathology.

Treated lesions may become mineralized (calcified) and may thus show small foci of decreased signal on T1WIs and T2WIs. However, detection may be easier on CT (5). Some treated lesions may show bright signal on T1WIs and T2WIs, possibly

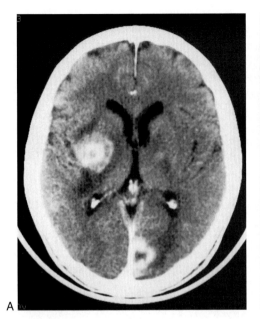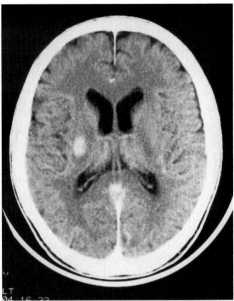

A   B

FIG. 36. Resolving toxoplasmic encephalitis. **A:** Enhancing lesions are identified in the right basal ganglia and left occipital lobe. **B:** After 2 weeks of treatment with pyramethamine and sulfadiazine, the occipital lesion is almost completely resolved and the basal ganglia lesion is diminished in size with a reduction in edema and mass effect. Lesions should be followed to complete resolution, if clinically feasible.

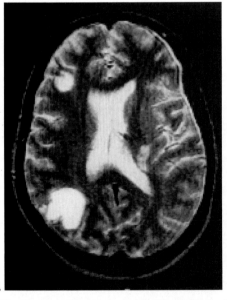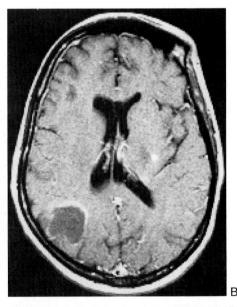

A   B

FIG. 37. Toxoplasmic encephalitis (pathologically proven). **A:** T2-weighted (2,550/80) MRI demonstrates multiple foci of increased signal intensity, inseparable from surrounding edema. **B:** Postgadolinium T1WI (600/20) shows both nodular and ring-enhancing lesions involving the corticomedullary junction and basal ganglia.

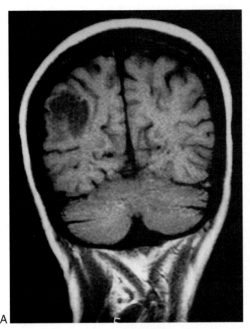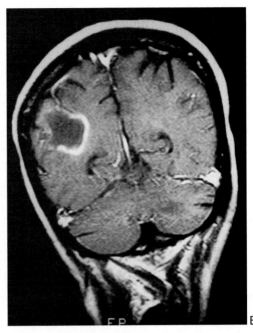

A   B

FIG. 38. Toxoplasmic encephalitis (pathologically proven). **A:** Noncontrast T1-weighted coronal MRI demonstrates focal hypointensity in the right parietal region with mild mass effect. **B:** Postgadolinium T1WI demonstrates rim enhancement of the lesion. The rim is slightly irregular and appears to be incomplete.

due to mineralization with paramagnetic species (i.e., manganese, iron, copper, etc.) (5). Mineralized lesions may therefore have foci of increased or decreased signal on MRI. High-intensity areas also may represent variation in the deposition of calcium hydroxyapatite or subacute hemorrhage (13).

In the past, early biopsy of these enhancing lesions was advocated in order to establish the diagnosis and promptly institute appropriate therapy (143,146,200). For the past several years, these cases have been handled conservatively. Because toxoplasmic encephalitis is common in these patients, individuals who present with typical clinical and radiographic findings are placed on appropriate medical therapy and follow-up scans are obtained in 10 days to 2 weeks. Consistent improvement on serial scans is presumptive evidence of toxoplasmic encephalitis. However, an important caveat is that all lesions must be followed to resolution because multiple pathologies may be present in any individual patient (Fig. 39). Lack of considerable improvement should prompt biopsy because a focal enhancing mass lesion may represent primary CNS lymphoma or possibly another type of infection. A second caveat is that it is impossible to accurately assess lesion activity if the patient is on steroids.

Primary CNS lymphoma may be quite difficult to distinguish from toxoplasmic encephalitis on CT and MRI. Although toxoplasmic lesions are often multiple but may be solitary, primary CNS lymphoma is often a solitary lesion but may be multifocal as well (Fig. 40). Treatment of these disorders is radically different; thus, it becomes important for the radiologist and the clinician to distinguish between these two entities. Thallium-201 brain SPECT imaging has become invaluable in making

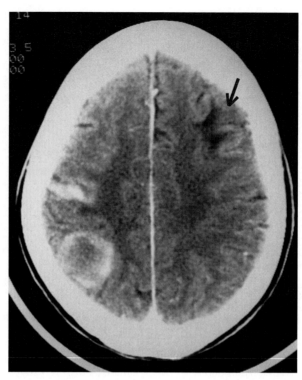

FIG. 39. Coexistent lesions of PML and toxoplasmic encephalitis (pathologically proven). This HIV-seropositive patient had multiple lesions on CT and MRI, some demonstrating enhancement and some without appreciable enhancement. Thallium-201 brain SPECT was negative, suggesting an inflammatory process. Improvement on antitoxoplasmosis therapy was sluggish, and biopsy was therefore obtained. Both toxoplasmic encephalitis (enhancing lesions) and PML *(arrow)* were present on biopsy.

this distinction. Metabolically active tissue, such as tumor, demonstrates increased uptake relative to surrounding parenchyma (228), whereas infectious lesions do not (Fig. 41). Although ^{201}Tl brain SPECT will be positive for many tumor types, in this population a positive study is most likely to indicate a primary CNS lymphoma (228) (Fig. 42). This study can be obtained quickly after clinical presentation and may preclude the need for 10–14 days of therapy and reevaluation. Patients with AIDS who now present with typical clinical and radiographic findings suggestive of toxoplasmosis or lymphoma are sent for nuclear imaging with ^{201}Tl brain SPECT. Positive scans are suspicious for primary CNS lymphoma and biopsy is encouraged. Negative ^{201}Tl scans are presumed to be due to infectious etiologies, and patients are placed on anti–*Toxoplasma* medical therapy with follow-up scans obtained in 10–14 days. However, it should be noted that the sensitivity of the thallium scan is limited by resolution, and tumors <6–8 mm in size may not be detected (228). Also, lymphomatous lesions in a subependymal location may not be detected.

Cysticercosis

Cysticercosis is the most common parasitic infection of the human CNS worldwide (66). It occurs in both immunocompetent and immunosupressed persons from en-

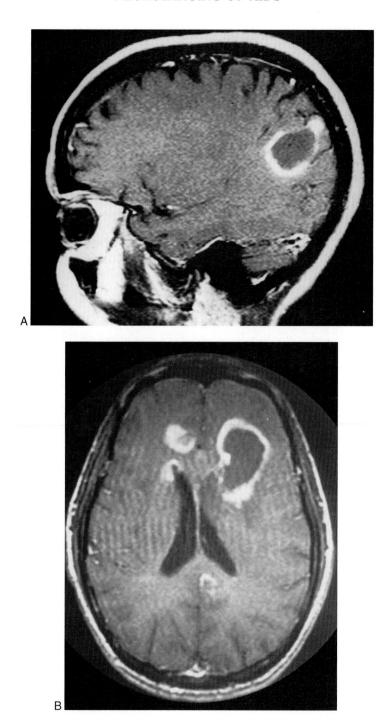

FIG. 40. Toxoplasmic encephalitis versus CNS lymphoma. **A:** Irregular ring-enhancing lesion in a patient with pathologically proven toxoplasmic encephalitis. Additional lesions were present on other sections. **B:** Note striking similarity to this patient, with pathologically proven primary CNS lymphoma, which is multicentric. This patient had negative toxoplasmic titers.

demic areas. Although it is not an opportunistic infection and is not indicative of HIV status, cysticercosis is described here because it is seen in both seronegative and seropositive patients from endemic regions and therefore must be recognized by the neuroradiologist and considered as part of a differential diagnosis.

Neurocysticercosis is endemic in Mexico, Central and South America, India, and China. Cases are also reported from Eastern Europe, Portugal, Africa, and Asia (66). Immigration has resulted in an increased prevalence of this disease in the United States (66).

The causative agent is the pork tapeworm, *Taenia solium.* The life cycle of this tapeworm will be reviewed here briefly to generate better understanding of the pathogenesis of this disease. Humans can be the definitive hosts in this cycle (infected with a tapeworm) or can be the intermediate host (infected with cysticercus, the larval form) (66).

When humans ingest inadequately cooked pork that contains viable larvae of *T. solium* (cysticerci) they become the definitive hosts for the tapeworm (66). Humans are the only definitive host for this cestode (66). After ingestion, the cysticercus develops in the small intestine into a tapeworm, 1-8 m in length. This presence of the tapeworm itself usually does not induce symptoms in the host, but the tapeworm releases eggs that pass into the stool (66). If these ova contaminate food or water that is eaten by the pig, the life cycle continues in the pig as the intermediate host (66).

In a similar fashion, humans may become the intermediate hosts after ingestion of contaminated food or water. Gastric juices within the stomach dissolve the thick outer shell of the ova to release the oncosphere (66). These oncospheres, the primary larvae, penetrate the stomach and intestinal mucosa and enter the blood stream. The oncospheres may then lodge in any tissue but show a predilection for the brain (66). Less common sites include the retina, heart, skeletal muscle, and subcutaneous tissue (66). In the brain, the oncospheres may burrow into brain parenchyma, meninges, ependyma, and choroid plexus. Spinal cord involvement is seen but is distinctly unusual (161). There are four types of neurocysticercosis: parenchymal, subarachnoid, intraventricular, and mixed (39). The parenchymal type is probably the most common (223).

Initial infection of the brain by the larva is usually asymptomatic and results in a small edematous lesion (149). The secondary larvae or cysticerci then develop into cysts, and 2–3 months after original host ingestion of ova, mature parenchymal cysts have developed (66) (Fig. 43). This is often asymptomatic but can result in seizures. The cysts each have a protoscolex, and the cysts measure 3–18 mm in diameter (79).

When alive, the cyst provokes a minimal surrounding inflammatory reaction and remain viable for 2–6 years after infestation (66). As the cyst dies, antigens and metabolic products leak from the wall into the surrounding brain, inciting an intense inflammatory reaction in adjacent tissues (Fig. 44). Edema develops and the lesion may become symptomatic with seizures or focal neurological signs. The clear cyst fluid becomes turbid and gelatinous (79). The cyst then collapses, degenerates, and often calcifies (66).

If oncospheres lodge in the meninges or choroid plexus, the infection may involve the ventricular system and/or subarachnoid space (66). Within the subarachnoid space, the cysts may become multiloculated, resembling a cluster of grapes. This is known as the racemose form, which measures 5 mm to 9 cm in size (66). The

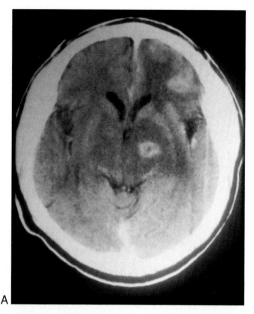

A

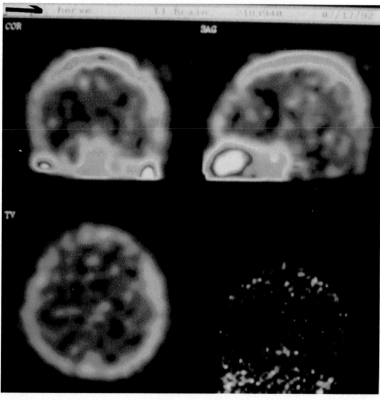

B

FIG. 41. Thallium-201 brain SPECT imaging of toxoplasmic encephalitis. **A:** Postcontrast CT demonstrates ring-enhancing lesions in the left frontal lobe and in the left thalamus with associated mass effect and edema. **B:** Thallium-201 brain SPECT (coronal, sagittal, axial, and planar images). No focal uptake is identified. Subsequent CT scans showed resolution of lesions on antitoxoplasmosis therapy. (From Whiteman MLH, Bowen BC, Post MJD, Bell MD. Intracranial infection. In: Atlas SW, ed. *Magnetic Resonance Imaging of the Brain and Spine, 2nd edition.* Philadelphia: Lippincott-Raven, 1996:707–772.)

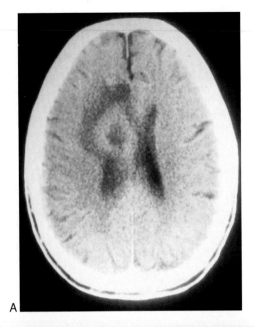

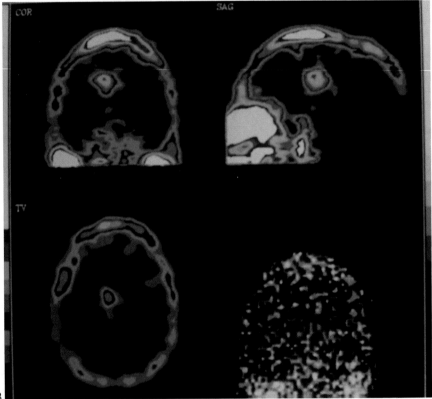

FIG. 42. Thallium-201 brain SPECT imaging of CNS lymphoma. **A:** Noncontrast CT scan demonstrates a hyperdense lesion with a necrotic center in the pericallosal region with surrounding edema and mass effect. **B:** Brain SPECT images with thallium-201 (coronal, sagittal, axial, and planar images) demonstrate a focal region of increased uptake corresponding to the same location as the lesion seen on CT. This is a biopsy-proven lymphoma. (From Whiteman MLH, Bowen BC, Post MJD, Bell MD. Intracranial infection. In: Atlas SW, ed. *Magnetic Resonance Imaging of the Brain and Spine, 2nd edition.* Philadelphia: Lippincott-Raven, 1996:707–772.)

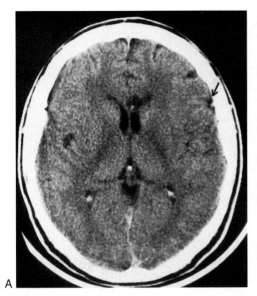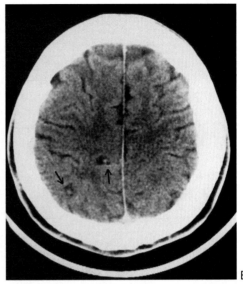

A   B

FIG. 43. Cysticercosis. **A:** Noncontrast CT scan demonstrates a cystic lesion in the corpus callosum with a high-density peripheral nodule, representing the scolex. A peripheral cyst is also noted *(arrow)*. **B:** Additional lesions are seen *(arrows)* in the same patient. This patient, who had recently left Mexico was asymptomatic, and was scanned because of a history of head trauma. Note absence of mass effect. There is no edema.

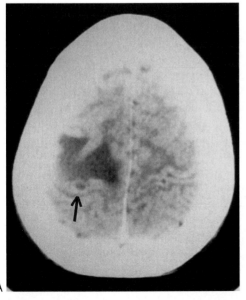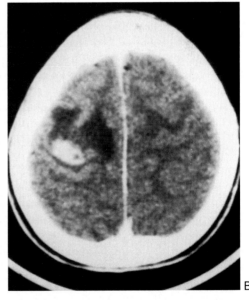

A   B

FIG. 44. Cysticercosis. **A:** Noncontrast CT of a 10-year-old child from Honduras demonstrates edema in the right parietal lobe. A thick-walled ring lesion is also noted *(arrow)*. This patient presented with seizures. **B:** Postcontrast CT demonstrates intense, focal enhancement. This is compatible with a degenerating cysticercus.

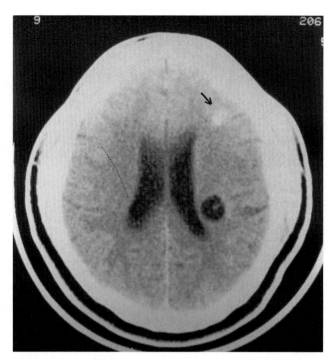

FIG. 45. Cysticercosis. Noncontrast CT demonstrates a viable cyst with scolex as well as a calcified lesion *(arrow)*, indicating various stages of evolution in neurocysticercosis.

protoscolex is absent from the racemose form (161). Chronic meningitis and/or ventriculitis can occur over years, possibly as a consequence of leakage of cysticercus antigens into the CSF (66). The racemose cyst can thus form a mass and result in hydrocephalus (148). The racemose cyst does not usually calcify after degeneration. Intraventricular cysts may be solitary or of the racemose form.

In endemic regions, there may be recurrent ingestion of ova; thus, the intracranial cysts can be found in different stages of evolution (Fig. 45). The entire process for resolution of a single lesion in the untreated patient is ~2–10 years (66).

CSF is abnormal in ~50% of cases (66). A lymphocytic pleocytosis may be present (232). Opening pressure of >200 m H_2O is present in ~40% of cases.

Imaging findings are usually characteristic. Initial infection results in small edematous lesions that are hypodense on CT and hyperintense on T2-weighted MRIs and do not enhance (132). Nodules may then appear which enhance mildly (132). These nodules represent protoscoleces within cysticerci but without cyst fluid. When mature cysts form, they are readily demonstrated by CT and MRI and measure 5–20 mm in diameter (150). This is the vesicular stage. Cysts may be near the gray–white junction but also can be found in the basal ganglia, cerebellum, and brain stem (Fig. 46). The cyst wall is thin and smooth. There is little if any edema. The protoscolex is often identified as a focal nodule within the cyst and can be seen better on MRI than on CT, although it may be seen on both studies. The mural nodule is best seen on proton density MRI (150,262,269). The cyst wall only occasionally enhances at this stage. The cysts are isointense to CSF on all MRI sequences and of fluid density on CT. MRI often demonstrates a greater number of viable lesions than does CT.

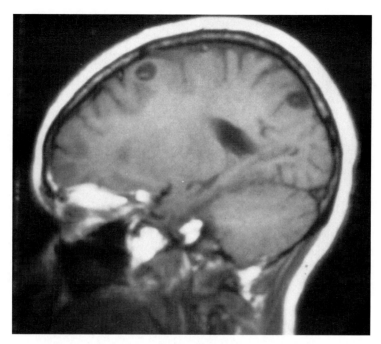

FIG. 46. Cysticercosis. Sagittal T1-weighted MRI (600/30) demonstrates cysts at the corticomedullary junction. Note absence of mass effect and edema.

As the larva dies, the host inflammatory response results in formation of a fibrous capsule that often demonstrates ring enhancement on CT and MRI. Degenerating cysts may be hyperintense on both T1- and T2-weighted MRIs due to the debris and proteinaceous material accumulated within the cyst (258). This is the colloidal vesicular stage. Degenerating cysts incite surrounding edema, which is evident on MRI as increased signal on T2WIs and on CT as surrounding hypodensity (Fig. 47). In the granular nodular stage, the cyst retracts and forms a granulomatous lesion that may show nodular or ring enhancement (49).

In the final nodular calcified stage the lesion becomes mineralized. The granulomatous nodules are replaced by gliosis and eventually calcification (49). Calcified lesions are easier to identify on CT but may show focal hypointense signal on MRI.

Intraventricular and subarachnoid cysts are difficult to identify on CT because they are isodense to CSF and do not enhance. These lesions are better seen on MRI, especially because the fourth ventricle is the most common site of intraventricular cysticercosis (38,40,150,212,262) (Fig. 48). Hydrocephalus is often demonstrated. Within the subarachnoid space, the cerebellopontine angle and suprasellar cisterns are the most common locations (30). Infestation of the subarachnoid space can result in communicating hydrocephalus due to chronic meningitis, and MRI may show enhancement of basal cisterns (30). Radiographs of the extremities may show calcification within skeletal muscle, suggestive of cysticercosis (160).

Diagnosis of neurocysticercosis can be made on the basis of clinical, radiographic, and serological indicators. Treatment is administered with praziquantel or albendazole. Intraventricular cysts may not respond as well as parenchymal cysts. Lesions that result in ventricular obstruction may be treated by surgical removal.

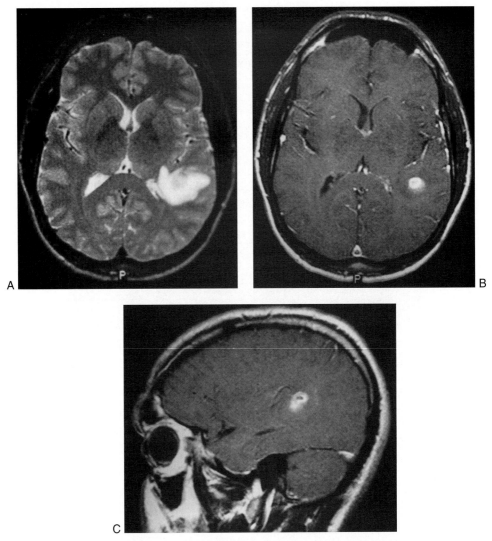

FIG. 47. Degenerating cysticerci. **A:** Axial T2-weighted MRI (2,650/80) demonstrates a degenerating cyst, which is slightly hyperintense to gray matter. High-intensity surrounding edema is evident, with compression of the atrium of the left lateral ventricle. **B:** Axial postgadolinium T1WI (600/20) demonstrates enhancement of a thick ring with isointense signal present centrally. **C:** Sagittal image (600/20) also demonstrates the ring enhancing lesion with surrounding inflammatory reaction consistent with a degenerating cyst.

NEOPLASMS

Lymphoma

Primary CNS lymphoma (PCNSL) is the most frequent CNS neoplasm seen in HIV-infected patients. It is seen in 6.4% of patients with AIDS who present with CNS disease and in 6% of all AIDS autopsies (189). The first reported association between AIDS and CNS lymphoma was in 1983 by Snider et al. (290). PCNSL in an HIV-seropositive individual is considered an AIDS-defining condition (229).

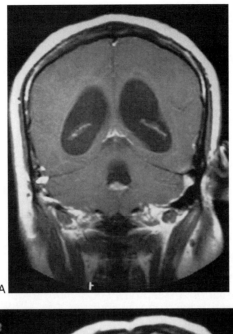

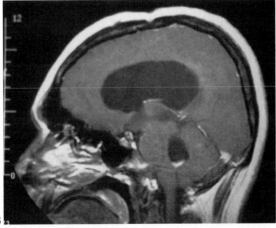

FIG. 48. Intraventricular cysticercosis. **A, B:** Coronal and sagittal T1-weighted MRIs (600/20) with gadolinium demonstrate enhancement at the outlet of the fourth ventricle, resulting in obstructive hydrocephalus. No other intracranial lesions were present. At surgery, a cysticercus cyst was removed from the distal portion of the fourth ventricle.

PCNSL is usually of B cell origin (256). In AIDS-related CNS lymphoma, the most common types are diffuse immunoblastic lymphoma (215), diffuse large cell lymphoma (215), and small-cell noncleaved lymphoma (177,225,256). In contrast, diffuse mixed-cell and diffuse large-cell lymphomas are the most common types of PCNSL in patients without AIDS (180). AIDS-related CNS lymphoma tends to demonstrate necrosis more often than does non–AIDS-related CNS lymphoma (215). Although hemorrhage is not often evident radiographically, these lesions are commonly hemorrhagic and necrotic at pathology (111).

Lesions are usually centrally located, involving the basal ganglia, thalamus, corpus callosum, cerebellar vermis, and periventricular regions. Subependymal spread may be evident (30). However, AIDS-related CNS lymphomas are more frequently peripheral in location as compared with non–AIDS-related lymphomas. Up to 25% of CNS lymphomas occur infratentorially (180). These lymphomas begin as a perivascular infiltrate with centrifugal spread and eventual parenchymal invasion (180). The histological hallmark of this entity is multiplication of the basement membranes of vessels with lymphomatous involvement. This is well demonstrated by silver reticulum stains (98,180).

PCNSL has a number of manifestations, including solitary or multiple masses or nodules, diffuse meningeal or periventricular lesions, vitreous involvement, and/or focal intradural masses (103). Spinal cord involvement with PCNSL is rare (97,98,103). In clinical studies, intracranial masses are multicentric in at least 25–50% (97,215), but autopsy data suggest that multicentric disease is present in 72% of cases (215).

AIDS-related PCNSL most often presents with a focal neurological deficit. Additional symptoms include confusion, lethargy, memory loss, and B symptoms (unexplained fever, night sweats, weight loss) (215,225). Seizures may occur in up to one third of cases (225). Other symptoms include headache, nausea, and vomiting. Comparative studies of AIDS-related and non–AIDS-related CNS lymphoma have shown that constitutional or B symptoms occur more frequently in AIDS (33% vs. 8%). Also, there is a greater male predominance and a younger age at presentation (34 vs. 59 years old) in AIDS-related lymphomas (215).

CSF protein is usually elevated, and pleocytosis may be present (97,98,215). Decreased glucose is seen less often. The frequency with which CSF cytology is abnormal varies from 4% to 43.5% (180,215) in non-AIDS lymphoma and has been reported to be 20–25% in AIDS-related PCNSL (215).

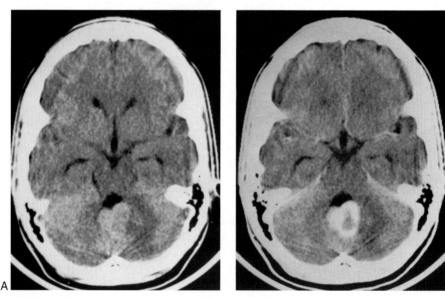

FIG. 49. AIDS-related primary CNS lymphoma. **A:** Noncontrast CT demonstrates a hyperdense mass in the cerebellar vermis with compression of the posterior aspect of the fourth ventricle. **B:** Postcontrast image shows intense inhomogenous enhancement of the lesion. Biopsy showed lymphoma.

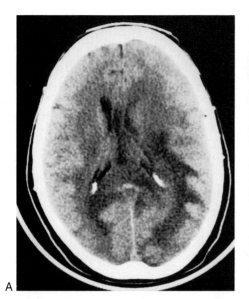 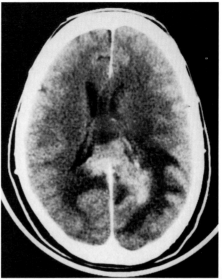

A   B

FIG. 50. Lymphoma. **A:** The splenium of the corpus callosum appears hypodense, and the ventricles appear splayed apart. Vasogenic edema is seen posteriorly and bilaterally. **B:** Post-contrast study shows intense enhancement of this biopsy-proven CNS lymphoma. The corpus callosum is a common site of lymphomatous involvement, in both patients with AIDS and patients without AIDS. (From Whiteman MLH et al. AIDS-related white matter diseases. *Neuroimag Clin North Am* 1993;3:331–359; with permission.)

Non-AIDS lymphomas appear as hyperdense masses on noncontrast CT examination, related to the cellularity of these lesions, with little associated edema (30,43,108,115). In AIDS-related CNS lymphoma, lesions may appear hyperdense or hypodense on noncontrast CT (Figs. 49 and 50) (80,88,146,181). Hypodensity often may be related to the greater degree of necrosis present in AIDS-related lymphomas. Hypodense lesions often have hyperdense rims where there is less necrosis (290). Hemorrhage in these lesions is uncommonly seen on CT. Calcification is rare (303). There is usually mass effect of a variable degree, and edema is also present, but to a variable degree. The pattern of edema cannot be used to reliably distinguish between toxoplasmosis and lymphoma.

Postcontrast images demonstrate dense enhancement. This is homogenous in non-AIDS lymphoma but may be homogenous, heterogenous, or ring enhancing in AIDS-related lymphoma. This again may relate to the greater frequency of necrosis in the latter. Up to 50% of AIDS-related CNS lymphoma may show ring enhancement (215), often making distinction from toxoplasmic encephalitis difficult. Periventricular enhancement suggests subependymal spread of tumor (Fig. 51) and is often a valuable clue in the radiographic diagnosis of CNS lymphoma. A solitary lesion does not necessarily favor lymphoma over toxoplasmosis. Forty-seven percent of AIDS-related PCNSL is multicentric by CT, and almost all cases are multicentric at autopsy (256). Conversely, 59% of the toxoplasmosis cases showed only a single lesion on CT imaging (147). Another study found that 14% of patients with toxoplasmic encephalitis had solitary lesions on MRI (196).

Traditionally, patients with AIDS with enhancing lesions on CT were placed on antitoxoplasmosis therapy, and follow-up scans were obtained in 10–14 days. Contin-

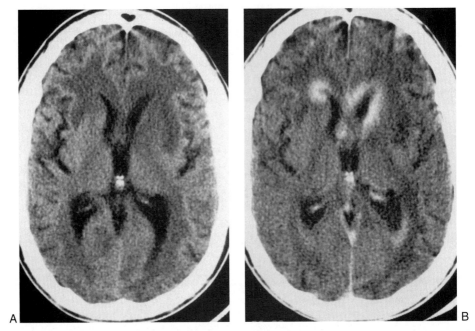

A   B

FIG. 51. Lymphoma. **A:** Noncontrast CT demonstrates atrophy as well as vague hypodensity in the frontal lobes bilaterally and in the left periatrial region. **B:** Postcontrast image shows periventricular enhancement consistent with subependymal spread of lymphoma.

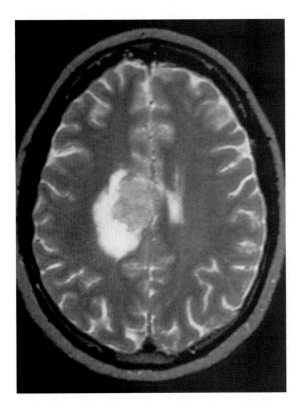

FIG. 52. Lymphoma. T2-weighted (2,550/80) axial MRI shows a lesion of the body of the corpus callosum that is isointense to gray matter. Surrounding hyperintensity represents edema.

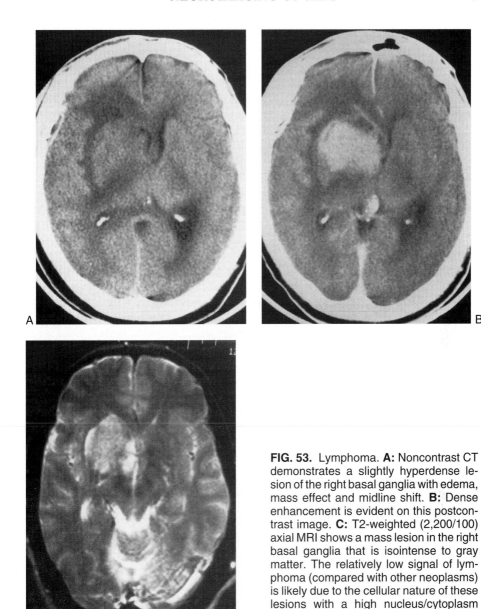

FIG. 53. Lymphoma. **A:** Noncontrast CT demonstrates a slightly hyperdense lesion of the right basal ganglia with edema, mass effect and midline shift. **B:** Dense enhancement is evident on this postcontrast image. **C:** T2-weighted (2,200/100) axial MRI shows a mass lesion in the right basal ganglia that is isointense to gray matter. The relatively low signal of lymphoma (compared with other neoplasms) is likely due to the cellular nature of these lesions with a high nucleus/cytoplasm ratio. Hyperintensity at the periphery of the lesion is edema.

ued improvement and ultimate resolution of these lesions on therapy indicated a presumptive diagnosis of toxoplasmosis. Lesions that did not improve were then examined via biopsy.

More recently, the use of ^{201}Tl brain SPECT has reduced the delay in biopsy for many of these patients. Patients with AIDS who have enhancing lesions of at least 6–8 mm promptly undergo ^{201}Tl brain SPECT imaging, which permits differentiation of tumor (most likely lymphoma) from infection (most commonly toxoplasmic encephalitis) (228). Neoplasms demonstrate increased uptake of thallium, due to metabolic activity, whereas infections do not (Fig. 42). However, lesions of <6–8 mm may not be resolved (subependymal lesions also may fail to demonstrate thallium uptake). A positive ^{201}Tl brain SPECT study strongly suggests lymphoma (or another neoplasm) in a patient with AIDS, and biopsy is then obtained for confirmation. A negative result suggests infection, most likely toxoplasmic encephalitis, and medical treatment is begun immediately. In our experience, the thallium study thus eliminates the delay in biopsy for patients with suspected CNS lymphoma. Patients with enhancing CNS lesions and negative thallium studies should be followed by CT to complete resolution because (a) multiple pathologies are often coexistent and (b) small lymphomatous lesions may not be apparent on the thallium study.

Treatment of CNS lymphoma with steroids may reduce enhancement and mask the underlying pathology. Additionally, if patients with abnormal CT scans are placed on both steroids and antitoxoplasmosis therapy, it becomes unclear whether improvement is due to infection responding to appropriate treatment or to lymphoma with rapid response to steroids. It is therefore imperative for accurate interpretation of these studies to know what treatment the patient has received.

Although many neoplastic lesions appear bright on T2-weighted MRI, the dense cellularity of lymphoma renders these lesions isointense or hypointense to parenchyma on all MRI sequences (Fig. 52) (303). These signal characteristics may strongly suggest the diagnosis in the appropriate clinical setting (Fig. 53). Administration of gadolinium-DTPA results in solid or ringlike enhancement (Fig. 54). Ring enhancement is more frequently associated with necrotic lesions. As on CT, lesions are most often centrally located and often multicentric, although lesions in patients with AIDS may be peripherally located. The pattern of edema is again variable, although there is usually some mass effect.

Cerebral angiography is no longer performed in the diagnosis of lymphoma, having been supplanted by CT and MRI. In the past, angiographic findings were nonspecific and included mass effect, vascular irregularity and faint tumor blush.

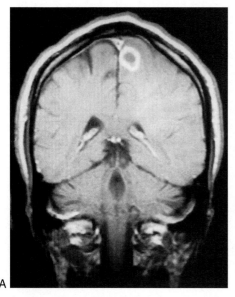 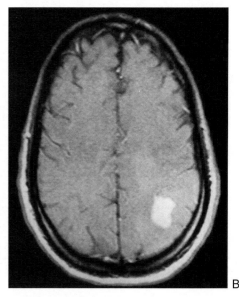

A   B

FIG. 54. Lymphoma. **A:** Postcontrst coronal T1-weighted (900/30) MRI study shows a ring-enhancing lesion in a parasagittal location. **B:** Axial MRI of the same patient (900/30) shows another lesion that demonstrates a solid pattern of enhancement.

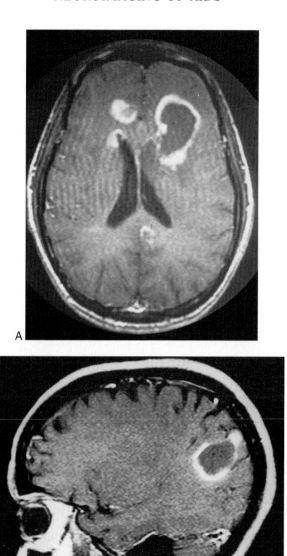

FIG. 55. Lymphoma versus toxoplasmic encephalitis. **A:** Post–gadolinium DTPA T1-weighted axial MRI (600/30) of a CNS lymphoma demonstrates both solid and ring-enhancing lesions, as well as subependymal enhancement. The ring enhancement may be due to central necrosis of the lesion (same image as Fig. 7B). **B:** Note similarity to this patient with biopsy-proven toxoplasmosis. Thallium-201 brain SPECT can be used to differentiate the patient in **A** from the patient in **B**. The patient in **B** did have a thallium study consistent with toxoplasmosis; however, the patient had a sluggish response to medical therapy and biopsy therefore was obtained, which showed toxoplasmic encephalitis.

Differential diagnosis includes toxoplasmic encephalitis (Fig. 55) as well as other infectious etiologies. Primary brain tumors also may be considered. Thallium-201 brain SPECT often can differentiate infection from neoplasm (for lesions of >6–8 mm), and the signal characteristics on MRI frequently differentiate lymphoma from other tumors.

Overall, the median length of survival for patients with AIDS-related primary CNS lymphoma is 2–3 months (215). Supportive care alone results in survival of <1 month (88). Radiation is the primary treatment for these patients (230,233). Chemotherapy may be used as an adjuvant to radiation (103). However, treatment of patients with AIDS with immunosuppressive drugs is limited by the underlying immunodeficiency (215). The multicentric nature of intracranial lymphoma suggests that a surgical approach would be impractical. Neurosurgical involvement is primarily directed toward biopsy. Rarely, AIDS-related CNS lymphomas may disseminate outside the CNS to bone marrow or lymph nodes (88,215).

In addition to primary CNS lymphoma, systemic non-Hodgkins lymphoma (NHL) a common complication of AIDS, may infrequently involve the CNS secondarily, usually via meningeal spread. Symptoms may therefore include cranial nerve neuropathy and radiculopathy, as well as headache and mental status changes (265). Frank parenchymal metastases are far less common. Secondary CNS involvement is reported in ~20% of AIDS-related systemic lymphomas (118,265) (Fig. 56). CT and MRI are usually negative, although MRI has considerable advantage over CT in demonstration of leptomeningeal disease (303). Spinal cord compression by epidural lymphomatous masses also has been reported in patients with AIDS (143,255) (Fig. 57).

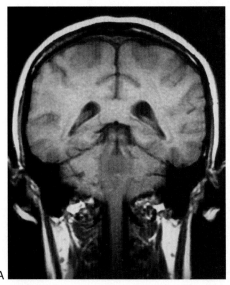 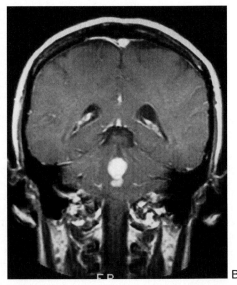

FIG. 56. Systemic lymphoma with spread to the fourth ventricle. **A:** Coronal T1-weighted (600/20) MRI shows a soft-tissue mass in the fourth ventricle. This patient had a history of systemic (non-CNS) NHL. **B:** Post–gadolinium-DTPA study shows intense enhancement of the mass within the fourth ventricle. The lesion may be due to spread of the systemic NHL to the meninges and CSF with deposition of tumor in the ventricle.

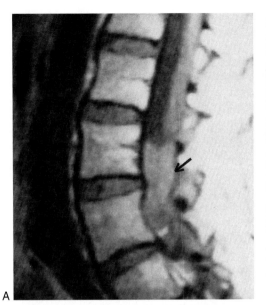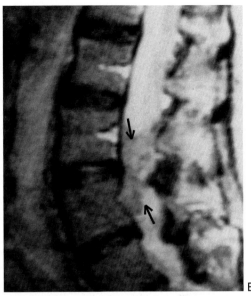

A   B

FIG. 57. Epidural lymphoma. **A:** T1-weighted (600/20) sagittal MRI shows an epidural soft-tissue mass in the lumbar region *(arrow)* with compression of the thecal sac. **B:** T2-weighted (2,400/80) sagittal image demonstrates the soft-tissue mass, which is of intermediate signal intensity *(arrows)*.

Glioma

Glioma is another primary brain neoplasm that may be seen in these patients, although the vast majority are due to PCNSL. Although gliomas have been reported to occur in HIV-positive patients (47,171), it is unclear at present whether there is an overall increased incidence of this neoplasm in HIV-infected patients as compared with the general population.

Radiographically, glioma may be indistinguishable from PCNSL or a solitary lesion of toxoplasmosis. On CT these lesions are usually hypodense, with surrounding edema and mass effect. Postcontrast images demonstrate solid or ring enhancement. The ring is usually thick and irregular. Necrotic areas are more common in the higher grade (III–IV) gliomas. Calcification and hemorrhage are infrequent.

On MRI, these lesions are usually hypointense on T1WIs and hyperintense on T2WIs. The pattern of enhancement is similar to that seen on CT. The periphery of these tumors may be ill defined, and malignant cells may be found outside the area of enhancement, within the surrounding edema.

Gliomas may be located anywhere within the cerebrum and cerebellum, but unlike lymphoma, do not often follow the ventricular outline. A location that is common to both glioma and PCNSL is the corpus callosum, which results in the so-called butterfly lesion. In such cases, MRI may be able to distinguish between glioma and PCNSL on the basis of signal characteristics. A lymphoma of the corpus callosum usually demonstrates intermediate signal on T2WIs, whereas a glioma is hyperintense. However, necrotic lymphomas also can appear hyperintense; thus, glioma and PCNSL may be radiographically indistinguishable in some cases, necessitating biopsy. Most gliomas also demonstrate uptake on ^{201}Tl scans, except for very low grade or small (<2 cm) lesions.

Kaposi's Sarcoma

KS may metastasize to the brain, although this is rare (123,143,204). It has been reported in both the cerebrum and cerebellum (123,143,207). Lesions tend to be hemorrhagic (123,143,204). CT imaging may show a solitary, hypodense, parenchymal mass with uniform nodular enhancement that is indistinguishable from lymphoma or toxoplasmosis (123,147,204). MRI also demonstrates a parenchymal mass with a nonspecific appearance.

HEAD AND NECK IMAGING IN HIV-INFECTED PATIENTS

Imaging of the head and neck has become an important aspect of neuroradiology in recent years. Certain radiographic findings in the head and neck regions are often apparent in HIV-infected individuals. Cervical adenopathy may be present and may be indicative of lymphoma, mycobacterial infection, metastatic disease, or diffuse reactive adenopathy.

Hyperplastic intraparotid lymph nodes and cysts (lymphoepithelial cysts) have been described in patients with AIDS (254). These may be unilateral or bilateral. On CT the nodes are homogenous in density without necrosis (254). The cysts are somewhat lower in density and may be single or multiple. On MRI both the cysts and intraparotid nodes are hypointense on T1W1 and hyperintense on T2W1 (Fig. 58). The cysts may vary in size from 5 mm to 4 cm in diameter. These parotid cysts are often present in association with suprahyoid adenopathy.

Sinusitis is present in at least 10–20% of patients with AIDS (106). Sinonasal infection in these patients is usually polymicrobial. Kaposi's sarcoma (KS) has been reported to occur in the nasal and oral cavities (106). Involvement of the oropharynx is reported in up to 20% of patients with cutaneous KS (1,93).

Lymphoma may be seen within the pharynx, especially in the nasopharynx, in association with Waldeyer's ring. This results in bulky submucosal masses and may be radiographically indistinguishable from the lymphoid proliferation of the nasopharynx, which is seen frequently in HIV-seropositive patients (106) (Fig. 59).

Both *M. tuberculosis* and atypical mycobacterium may cause lymphadenitis (scrofula) in HIV-seropositive patients. Three species of atypical mycobacterium can result in cervical adenopathy: *M. kansasii*, *M. avium-intracellulare*, and *M. scrofulaceum* (254). Clinical presentations may differ, depending on the causative agent. Atypical *Mycobacterium* infection occurs primarily in children. Common sites of entry in children are the oropharynx and conjunctiva and thus account for the majority of nodes occurring in tonsilar tissue and submandibular, parotid, preauricular, and upper cervical nodes (254). Few constitutional symptoms are present, and nodes are usually unilaterally involved. These organisms do not respond to antituberculous treatment; therefore, surgery is the therapy of choice, with removal of involved nodes and overlying skin (254). In contrast, cervical adenopathy due to *M. tuberculosis* is a local manifestation of a systemic infection (254). Many patients have a history of previous TB. This disorder occurs primarily in young people 20–30 years of age but can occur at any age. Few constitutional symptoms are present. The nodes are

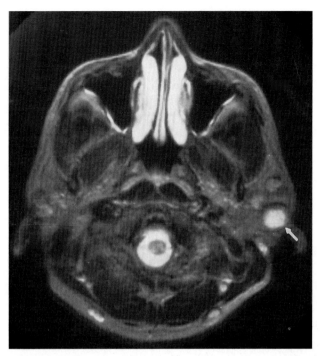

FIG. 58. T2-weighted (2,400/80) axial MRI demonstrates several well-circumscribed masses in the left parotid gland. The largest of these *(arrow)* is of increased signal intensity and is compatible with either a lymphoepithelial cyst or an intraparotid lymph node.

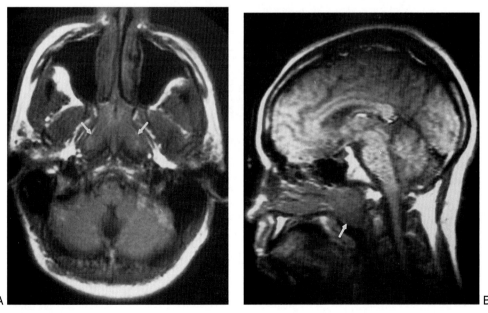

A   B

FIG. 59. Lymphoid hyperplasia of the nasopharynx. Note bulky, homogenous soft tissue present in the nasopharynx on axial **(A)** and sagittal **(B)** T1-weighted (600/20) MRIs *(arrows)* of this HIV-seropositive patient.

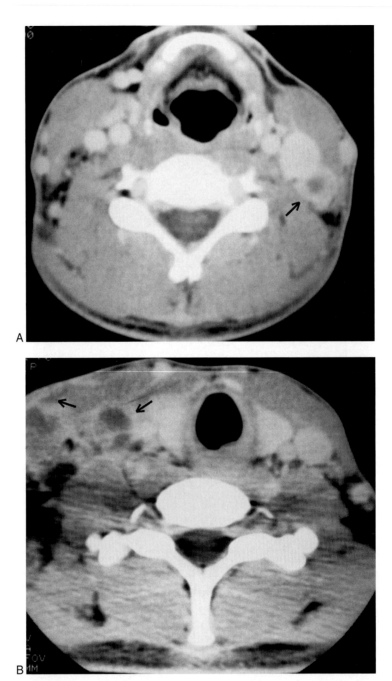

FIG. 60. TB adenitis. **A:** Postcontrast axial CT scan of the neck at the level of the hyoid bone shows a lymph node in the left jugular chain *(arrow)* with rim enhancement and central hypodensity. **B:** Lower in the neck, at the level of the thyroid gland, multiple rim-enhancing lymph nodes are evident on the right and inflammatory changes are seen in the subcutaneous tissues *(arrows)*.

firm and nontender (254). Symptoms of a neck mass may be present from days to years (254). Posterior triangle nodes are often involved bilaterally (Fig. 60). Nodes that are located lower in the cervical region are more likely to be associated with concomitant pulmonary disease (295).

If TB adenitis is clinically suspected, an excisional biopsy is preferred over an incisional biopsy because the latter is more often associated with fistula formation and poor wound healing (254). Caseating granulomas are considered diagnostic because acid-fast bacilli are not always identified and may not be cultured from the specimen (254).

On CT these nodes may be homogenous in density or have central necrosis and may calcify. Peripheral enhancement of the nodes may be present, and the rim can be thick and irregular. The nodes may coalesce to form a single necrotic mass—the "cold abscess" (254)—with obliteration of adjacent fascial planes. Often, however, dermal thickening and induration are absent (254). Triple-drug antituberculous therapy is the usual treatment for *M. tuberculosis* (254).

CEREBROVASCULAR DISEASE

HIV-infected patients are at increased risk for cerebral infarction. A large study of patients with AIDS (n = 1,286) found 1.6% to have cerebrovascular complications (142). The annual incidence of infarction in the general population 35–45 years of age is 0.025% (94). Neuropathological series show a frequency of infarction in patients with AIDS of 8–34% (22,145). There is a broad spectrum of etiologies, but in many cases the pathogenesis of this is unclear. Cerebral granulomatous angitis due to HIV can result in vascular occlusive disease (300). In this disorder, granulomatous inflammation in the walls of large and medium-sized vessels can result in thrombosis and infarction (63). Both intracerebral and leptomeningeal arteries may be involved (63). As noted previously, VZV infection (255) as well as syphilis may produce cerebral infarction. Nonbacterial thrombotic endocarditis also may be responsible in a number of cases (199).

CT and MRI may show the sequelae of cerebrovascular disease, including parenchymal hemorrhage, infarction, subarachnoid hemorrhage, and communicating hydrocephalus. Hypodensity is seen on CT, involving both gray and white matter, conforming to a vascular distribution. Variable enhancement of infarcted territories is seen on CT after 5–7 days and diminishes after several weeks (63). MRI often demonstrates infarction before detection by CT, with increased signal seen on proton density and T2WIs. Enhancement of arterial structures on MRI may indicate sluggish flow (63) and may be an early sign of infarction.

In the past, conventional cerebral angiography has been used to evaluate suspected vasculitis and/or mycotic aneurysms in HIV-infected patients. Currently, conventional angiography is used infrequently in the diagnostic evaluation of these patients (Fig. 61). MRA is a useful, noninvasive technique that can be used to demonstrate vascular stenosis and/or occlusion (Fig. 21C). MRA can be obtained in conjunction with conventional spin-echo MRIs. Studies can be performed with or without the use of gadolinium. The intracranial vasculature as well as the cervical vessels can be evaluated. MRA can determine vascular patency (arterial or venous), can demonstrate vascular stenosis and thrombosis, and can detect the presence of aneurysms >3–4 mm. In some cases, both conventional angiography and MRA may be obtained

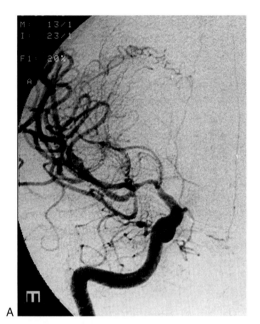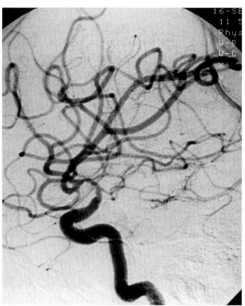

A   B

FIG. 61. Meningovascular syphilis. AP **(A)** and lateral views **(B)** of a right internal carotid angiogram show beading of the supraclinoid carotid and the M1 segment of the middle cerebral artery. Note that the anterior cerebral artery is not opacified, due to either occlusion or severe spasm related to syphilitic vasculitis.

and correlated and patients can be followed with MRA, avoiding repeated invasive procedures.

DISEASES OF THE SPINE AND SPINAL CORD

HIV-related infections also may involve the spine and spinal cord. Twenty-nine percent of adult AIDS autopsies demonstrate vacuolar myelopathy of the spinal cord. Symptoms of vacuolar myelopathy include weakness, incontinence, ataxia, and spastic paraparesis (199). Pathological examination shows vacuolization of spinal cord white matter in association with lipid-laden macrophages, swelling of the myelin sheaths, and axonal degeneration (189,190). There is myelin loss and spongy degeneration. Inflammation is absent (189). The mid- and lower thoracic spine is most often affected (190). Results of MRI are most often negative but may show increased signal on T2WIs in some cases (12). VZV, *T. gondii*, and TB also have been reported to involve the spinal cord in patients with AIDS (51,163,194), although these cases are rare. Findings on MRI are nonspecific, with increased signal on T2WIs. Toxoplasmic and TB lesions of the cord may demonstrate enhancement, but the appearance may be indistinguishable from other intramedullary mass lesions.

CMV polyradiculomyelitis is an uncommon disorder consisting of radicular pain, rapidly progressive paraparesis, and urinary retention (288) and occurs in ~2% of all patients with AIDS who also have neurological disease (67). The syndrome also has been described as CMV-related Guillain-Barré syndrome, subacute polyneuropathy, polyradiculopathy, polyradiculoneuropathy, myelitis with radiculopathy, and acute myeloradiculitis (18,27,112,153,249). There is rapid development of flaccid paraparesis, beginning distally and ascending (288). Deep tendon reflexes are significantly reduced or absent. There is early urinary retention and sensory alterations in lumbar and sacral dermatomes ("saddle anesthesia") (288). Sensory impairment is less prominent than motor deficits. Upper extremities are minimally affected, whereas the lower extremities are paretic (288). Leg and/or back pain are frequent presenting complaints. There is no spasticity (288).

Diagnosis is chiefly a clinical one, although the CSF characteristically demonstrates a polymorphonuclear pleocytosis (68). Cultures are often negative, despite definitive CMV infection (292). More recently, PCR, a DNA amplification technique, has become available and may provide a fairly rapid diagnosis (within 24 hours). This has shown great utility in recent studies (53,90,294) and should be performed on patients suspected of having CMV polyradiculitis to establish the diagnosis so that prompt therapy may be instituted. The results of PCR are often positive when viral cultures are negative (53,90,294). MRI demonstrates diffuse enhancement of the cauda equina and surface of the conus (288). Nerve roots may show clumping. Cord signal is normal on T2WIs and on noncontrast T1WIs, and thus the diagnosis is easily missed without the use of gadolinium (Fig. 62). Patients are usually treated with ganciclovir, although foscarnet is used if symptoms are resistant to ganciclovir. Recovery is variable, depending on the degree of involvement and the duration of symptoms.

Descriptions of TB spondylitis date back to 3000 B.C. and can be found in the writings of Hippocrates (450 BC) (100,252,302). The first complete account of the disease was in 1779 by Pott (209). L1 is the site most frequently involved in spinal TB (104), with a predilection for the thoracolumbar junction. Sacral and cervical spinal TB is infrequent. More than one vertebral level is usually involved, with infection predominantly in the anterior portion of the vertebral body (285). Spinal TB results from hematogenous spread of infection, more likely via the paravertebral venous plexus of Batson than via arterial dissemination (104).

Most often, TB spondylitis begins in the anterior aspect of the vertebral body, adjacent to the subchrondral bone (217). The disk space may then become involved via a number of routes. Extension may occur along the anterior or posterior longitudinal ligaments or by a direct extension through the endplate. The process is much more indolent compared with pyogenic infection, and the posterior elements are rarely involved (217). Eventually, long segments of the spine may be involved. Collapse of a vertebral body, particularly in the anterior segment, may result in TB kyphosis or gibbus deformity (217).

Spinal TB infection frequently extends into adjacent ligaments and soft tissues, most often occurring anterolaterally. However, extension into the spinal canal also may occur, resulting in an epidural mass with compression of the thecal sac (217). Subligamentous extension may result in infection of bone or disk at sites remote from the initial focus, with intervening "skip" areas that are not involved (217). This can mimic metastatic disease. In the lumbar region, paraspinal infection may extend to the psoas muscle, resulting in a psoas abscess that can then extend into the groin and thigh (217).

TB psoas abscesses often contain calcification (217), whereas nontuberculous psoas abscesses rarely calcify. Psoas abscess complicates TB spondylitis in ~5% of cases (217). Symptoms of TB spinal infection may be present for many months. Clinical data suggesting TB over pyogenic infection include insidious onset of symp-

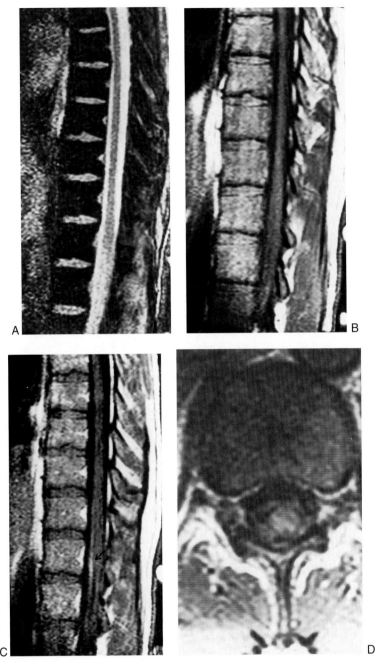

FIG. 62. CMV polyradiculomyelitis. **A:** Gradient echo (700/18, 25°) sagittal image through the conus demonstrates no evidence of signal abnormality within the cord. **B:** Sagittal T1-weighted (600/20) MRI also demonstrates no focal abnormality. **C:** Post–gadolinium MRI demonstrates nerve root enhancement of the cauda equina *(arrow)*. **D:** Noncontrast axial MRI (600/20) through the conus tip again shows no definite abnormality.

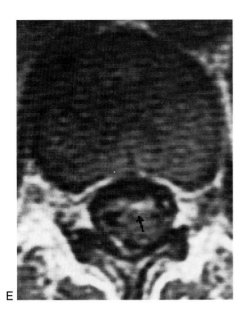

E

FIG. 62. *Continued.* **E:** Axial post–gadolinium MRI (600/20) shows marked enhancement of the cauda equina *(arrow).*

toms, characteristic pattern on chest radiograph, and late onset of paraplegia after several months of back pain (28). TB also may have a better prognosis than pyogenic spinal infection (250).

Radiographic features suggestive of TB include osseous destruction with delayed involvement of the disk space, calcified paravertebral mass, and infection primarily occurring in the anterior aspect of the vertebral body. MRI can detect infection earlier than other modalities. Modic et al. (167) found enhanced MRI to have a sensitivity of 96%, a specificity of 92%, and an accuracy of 94% in vertebral osteomyelitis. Evidence of osteomyelitis appears on MRI at approximately the same time as on bone and gallium scans (167). T1WIs show hypointense signal of the involved vertebral bodies. T2WIs show increased signal intensity at sites of involvement. If the disk space is involved, it will also demonstrate increased signal on T2WIs and may be narrowed. Extension into paraspinal soft tissues also will be obvious and can be seen well on both CT and MRI. On MRI the infected soft tissues demonstrate increased signal on T2WIs (Fig. 63). CT is useful in demonstration of paraspinal calcification and can show evidence of gas within a psoas abscess. CT is also useful in delineation of bony detail.

MRI with gadolinium demonstrates enhancement of infected bone and disk space and is of particular value in cases in which the diagnosis is uncertain. MRI also can be used to follow response to medical therapy. Psoas abscesses show inhomogenous or ring enhancement.

Symptoms of epidural abscess include back pain, radicular pain, stiffness, cramping, and paresthesias. Weakness and paralysis appear later and may be irreversible (135) if appropriate treatment is not instituted promptly. These abscesses may progress rapidly over a few hours or days, but some may show a more chronic progression, over weeks to months (135). Prompt diagnosis is essential to preservation of neurological function. MRI is the study of choice for imaging these patients because MRI can distinguish epidural abscess from tumor, disk, and hematoma (251).

On T1WIs, epidural abscess is iso- or hypointense to spinal cord and of increased

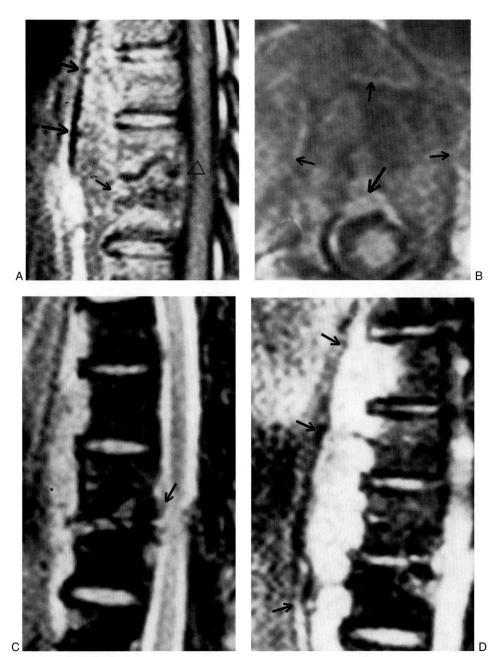

FIG. 63. TB spondylitis with epidural extension. **A:** Sagittal T1-weighted MRI (600/20) shows end-plate irregularity and loss of the disk space at T9–10 *(small arrow)*. A large prevertebral mass extends anteriorly over multiple lower thoracic vertebral bodies *(large arrows)* beneath the anterior longitudinal ligament (linear black structure). There is mild extension of the inflammatory process posteriorly into the epidural space *(arrowhead)*. **B:** Axial T1-weighted (600/20) MRI without contrast demonstrates the prevertebral and paravertebral *(small arrows)* extension of the TB infection. Involvement of the ventral epidural space is also evident, with slight compression of the thecal sac *(large arrow)*. **C:** Gradient echo (600/18, 25°) sagittal image in the midline again demonstrates end-plate irregularity with disk space narrowing at T9–10. Increased signal intensity is seen in the prevertebral soft tissues. Epidural extension into the spinal canal is also demonstrated *(arrow)*. **D:** Sagittal gradient echo (600/18, 25°) image to the right of midline demonstrates very bright signal in the prevertebral soft tissues, extending over many vertebral bodies *(arrows)*.

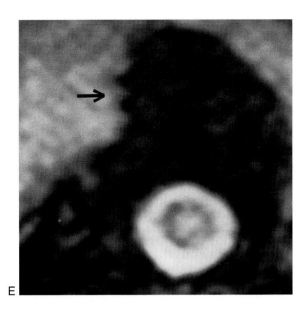

E

FIG. 63. *Continued.* **E:** Axial gradient echo image (100/18, 25°) depicts the prevertebral and paravertebral TB infection of the soft tissues, as well as bony destruction *(arrow).*

signal intensity on T2WIs (206). Contrast enhancement shows homogenous or ring enhancement. The abscess may be contiguous, with a disk space or vertebral infection or may occur as a result of hematogenous spread, without spinal involvement. The causative organism in both HIV-infected patients and HIV-seronegative patients is most commonly *Staphylococcus aureus* (250). Other bacteria, TB, as well as fungi can all result in epidural abscess formation (250).

Treatment of the epidural abscess depends on its size, the presence or absence of neurological deficit, and the degree of patient debilitation. A small abscess may be treated conservatively with antibiotics in the appropriate clinical setting. However, aspiration may be indicated in these patients to determine the causative organism. Larger, symptomatic abscesses require surgical debridement as well as antibiotics.

REFERENCES

1. Abeymayor E, Calcterra T. Kaposi's sarcoma and community acquired immunodeficiency syndrome: an update with emphasis on its head and neck manifestations. *Arch Otolaryngol* 1983;109:536–542.
2. Abos J, Graus F, Miro JM, Mallolas J, et al. Intracranial tuberculomas patients with AIDS. *AIDS* 1991;5:461–462.
3. Adair JC, Beck AC, Apfelbaum RI, Baringer JR. Nocardial cerebral abscess in the acquired immunodeficiency syndrome. *Arch Neurol* 1987;44:548–550.
4. Alvarez S, McCabe WR. Extrapulmonary tuberculosis revisited: a review of experience at Boston City and other hospitals. *Medicine* 1984;63:25–55.
5. Atlas SW, Grossman RI, Hackney DB, et al. Calcified intracranial lesions: detection with gradient echo acquisition rapid MR imaging. *AJNR* 1988;9:253–259.
6. Aylward EH, Henderer JD, McArthur JC, et al. Reduced basal ganglia volume in HIV-I associated dementia: results from quantitative neuroimaging. *Neurology* 1993;43:2099–2104.
7. Bagga A, Kalra V, Ghai OP. Intracranial tuberculoma. *Clin Pediatr* 1988;27:487–490.
8. Bailey R, Baltch A, Venkatish R, et al. Sensory motor neuropathy associated with AIDS. *Neurology* 1988;38:886–891.
9. Balakrishnnen J, Becker PS, Kumar AJ, et al. Acquired immunodeficiency syndrome: correlation of radiological and pathological findings in the brain. *Radiographics* 1990;10:201– 216.
10. Bale JF, Anderson RD, Grose C. Magnetic resonance imaging of the brain in childhood herpes virus infections. *Pediatr Infect Dis J* 1987;6:644–647.

11. Bale JF Jr. Human cytomegalovirus infection and disorders of the nervous system of patients with the acquired immune deficiency syndrome. *Arch Neurol* 1984;41:310–320.
12. Barakos JA, Mark AS, Dillon WP, Norman D. MR imaging of acute transverse myelitis and AIDS myelopathy. *J Comput Assist Tomogr* 1990;14:45–50.
13. Barkovich AJ, Atlas SW. Magnetic resonance of intracranial hemorrhage. *Radiol Clin North Am* 1988;26:801–820.
14. Barnicoat MJ, Wierzbicki AS, Norman PM. Cerebral nocardiosis in immunosuppressed patients: five cases. *Q J Med* 1989;268:689–698.
15. Baron AL, Steinbach LS, LeBoit PE, et al. Osteolytic lesions and bacillary angiomatosis in HIV infection: radiological differentiation from AIDS-related Kaposi sarcoma. *Radiology* 1990;177: 77–81.
16. Bauer W, Chamberlain W, Horenstein S. Spinal demyelination in progressive multifocal leukoencephalopathy. *Neurology* 1987;19:287.
17. Beaman B, Burnside J, Edwards B, Causey W. Nocardial infection in the United States. 1972–1974. *J Infect Dis* 1976;134:286–289.
18. Behar R, Wiley C, McCutchan JA. Cytomegalovirus polyradiculoneuropathy in acquired immune deficiency syndrome. *Neurology* 1987;37:557–561.
19. Belman AL, Novick B, Ultmann MH, et al. Neurological complications in children with acquired immune deficiency syndrome. *Ann Neurol* 1984;16:414.
20. Belman AL, Ultmann MH, Horoupian D, Novick B, et al. Neurological complications of infants and children with acquired immune deficiency syndrome. *Ann Neurol* 1985;18:560– 566.
21. Berenguer J, Moreno S, Laguna F, Vicente T, et al. Tuberculous meningitis in patients infected with the human immunodeficiency virus. *N Engl J Med* 1992;326:668–672.
22. Berger JR, Harris JO, Gregorios J, Norenberg M. Cerebrovascular disease in AIDS: a case control study. *AIDS* 1990;4:239–244.
23. Berger JR, Kaszowitz B, Post MJD, Dickinson G. Progressive multifocal leukoencephalopathy associated with human immunodeficiency virus infection. A review of the literature with a report of sixteen cases. *Ann Intern Med* 1987;78–87.
24. Berger JR, Moskowitz L, Fischl M, Kelley RE. Neurological disease as the presenting manifestation of acquired immunodeficiency syndrome. *South Med J* 1987;80:683–686.
25. Bernick C, Gregorios JB. Progressive multifocal leukoencephalopathy in a patient with acquired immune deficiency syndrome. *Arch Neurol* 1984;41:780–783.
26. Bishburg E, Sunderam G, Reichman LB, Kapila R. Central nervous system tuberculosis with the acquired immunodeficiency syndrome and its related complex. *Ann Intern Med* 1986;105:210–213.
27. Bishopric CG, Bruner J, Butler J. Guillain-Barre syndrome with cytomegalovirus infection of peripheral nerves. *Arch Pathol Lab Med* 1985;109:1106–1108.
28. Blacklock JWS. Injury as aetiological factor in tuberculosis. *Proc R Soc Med* 1957;50:61.
29. Blum LW, Chambers RA, Schwartzman RJ, Streletz LJ. Progressive multifocal leukoencephalopathy in acquired immune deficiency syndrome. *Arch Neurol* 1985;42:137–139.
30. Bowen BC, Post MJD. Intracranial infection. In: Atlas SW, ed. *Magnetic Resonance Imaging of the Brain and Spine*. New York: Raven. 1991:501–538.
31. Boyd JF. Adult cytomegalic inclusion disease. *Scott Med J* 1980;25:266–269.
32. Brant-Zawadzki M, Berry I, Osaki L, et al. Gd-DTPA in clinical MR of the brain. I. Intraaxial lesions. *AJNR* 1986;7:781–788.
33. Britton CB, Miller JR. Neurological complications of acquired immunodeficiency syndrome (AIDS). *Neurol Clin* 1984;2:315–339.
34. Brooks BR, Walker DL. Progressive multifocal leukoencephalopathy. *Neurol Clin* 1984;2:299–313.
35. Bross JE, Gordon G. Nocardial meningitis: case reports and review. *Rev Infect Dis* 1991;13:160–165.
36. Bryne E, Brophy BP, Perret LV. Nocardia cerebral abscess: new concepts in diagnosis, management and prognosis. *J Neurol Neurosurg Psychiatry* 1979;42:1038–1045.
37. Bursztyn EM, Lee BCP, Bauman J. CT of acquired immunodeficiency syndrome. *AJNR* 1984;5: 711–714.
38. Byrd SE, Locke GE, Biggers S, Percy AK. The computed tomographic appearance of cerebral cysticercosis in adults and children. *Radiology* 1982;144:819–823.
39. Carbajal JR, Palacios E, Azar-kia B, et al. Radiology of cysticercosis of the central nervous system including computed tomography. *Radiology* 1977;125:127–131.
40. Cardenas JC. Cyticercosis of the nervous system: pathological and radiological findings. *J Neurosurg* 1962;19:635–640.
41. Carey RM, Kimball AC, Armstrong D, Lieberman PH. Toxoplasmosis. Clinical experiences in a cancer hospital. *Am J Med* 1973;54:30–38.
42. Carne CA, Tedder RS, Smith A, et al. Acute encephalopathy coincident with seroconversion for anti–HTLV-III. *Lancet* 1985;2:1206–1208.
43. Cellerier P, Chiras J, Gray F, et al. Computed tomography in primary lymphoma of the brain. *Neuroradiology* 1984;26:485–492.

44. Centers for Disease Control. Primary resistance to antituberculous drugs—United States. *MMWR* 1983;32:521–523.
45. Centers for Disease Control. Tuberculosis and acquired immunodeficiency syndrome—New York City. *MMWR* 1987;36:785–795.
46. Chaisson RE, Slutkin G. Tuberculosis and human immunodeficiency virus infection. *J Infec Dis* 1989;159:96–100.
47. Chamberlain MC. Gliomas in patients with acquired immune deficiency syndrome. *Cancer* 1994; 74:1912–1914.
48. Chang K-H, Han M-H, Roh JK, et al. Gd-DTPA enhanced MR imaging in intracranial tuberculosis. *Neuroradiology* 1990;32:19–25.
49. Chang K-H, Lee JH, Han MH, Han MC. The role of contrast-enhanced MR imaging in the diagnosis of neurocysticercosis. *AJNR* 1991;128:509–512.
50. Chong WK, Sweeney B, Wilkinson I, et al. Proton spectroscopy of the brain in HIV infection: correlation with clinical, immunological, and MR imaging findings. *Radiology* 1993;188:119–124.
51. Chretien F, Gray F, Lescs MC, et al. Acute varicella-zoster virus ventriculitis and meningo-myelo-radiculitis in acquired immunodeficiency syndrome. *Acta Neuropathol (Berl)* 1993;86:659–665.
52. Chrysikopoulous HS, Press GA, Grafe MR, et al. Encephalitis caused by human immunodeficiency virus: CT and MR imaging manifestations with clinical and pathological correlation. *Radiology* 1990;175:185–191.
53. Cinque P, Vago L, Brytting M, et al. Cytomegalovirus infection of the central nervous system in patients with AIDS: diagnosis by DNA amplification from cerebrospinal fluid. *J Infect Dis* 1992; 166:1408–1411.
54. Clinicopathological conference. *N Engl J Med* 1990;323:1823–1833.
55. Cockerell CJ, Webster GF, Whitlow MA, et al. Epithelial angiomatosis: a distinct vascular disorder in patients with the acquired immunodeficiency syndrome or AIDS-related complex. *Lancet* 1987; 2:265–266.
56. Corey L, Spear PG. Infection with herpes simplex viruses. Part I. *N Engl J Med* 1986;314:686–691.
57. Corey L, Spear PG. Infection with herpes simplex viruses: Part 2. *N Engl J Med* 1986;314:749–757.
58. Cornblath D, McArthur J. Predominantly sensory neuropathy in patients with AIDS and AIDS-related complex. *Neurology* 1988;38:794–796.
59. Cuadrado LM, Guerrero A, et al. Cerebral mucormycosis in two cases of acquired immunodeficiency syndrome. *Arch Neurol* 1988;45:109–111.
60. Curless RG. Congenital AIDS: review of neurological problems. *Child Nerv Syst* 1987;5:9–11.
61. Curless RG, Mitchell CD. Central nervous system tuberculosis in children. *Pediatr Neurol* 1991; 7:270–274.
62. Dastur DK. Neurotuberculosis. In: Minckler J, ed. *Pathology of the Nervous System.* Vol. 3. New York: McGraw-Hill, 1972:2412–2422.
63. Davenport C, Dillon WP, Sze G. Neuroradiology of the immunosuppressed state. *Radiol Clin North Am* 1992;30:611–637.
64. Davidson HD, Steiner RE. Magnetic resonance imaging of infections of the central nervous system. *AJNR* 1985;6:499–504.
65. Davis JM, Davis KR, Kleinman GN, et al. Computed tomography of herpes simplex encephalitis with clinico-pathological correlation. *Radiology* 1978;129:409–416.
66. Davis LE, Kornfeld M. Neurocysticercosis: neurological, pathogenic, diagnostic and therapeutic aspects. *Eur Neurol* 1991;31:229–240.
67. de Gans J, Portegies P. Neurological complications of infection with human immunodeficiency virus type I: a review of literature and 241 cases. *Clin Neurol Neurosurg* 1989;91:197–217.
68. de Gans J, Tiessens G, Portegies P, Tutnarima JA, Troost D. Predominance of polymorphonuclear leukocytes in cerebrospinal fluid of AIDS patients with cytomegalovirus polyradiculomyelitis. *J AIDS* 1990;3:1155–1158.
69. DeLaPaz RL, Enzmann D. Neuroradiology of acquired immunodeficiency syndrome. In: Rosenblum ML, et al, eds. *AIDS and the Nervous System.* New York: Raven, 1988:121–153.
70. Dorfman LJ. Cytomegalovirus encephalitis in adults. *Neurology* 1973;23:136–144.
71. Draouat S, Abdenabi B, Ghanem M, Bourjat P. Computed tomography of cerebral tuberculoma. *J Comput Assist Tomogr* 1987;11:594–597.
72. Dube MP, Holtom PD, Larsen RA. Tuberculous meningitis in patients with and without human immunodeficiency virus infection. *Am J Med* 1992;93:520–524.
73. Duchowny M, Caplan L, Siber G. Cytomegalovirus infection of the adult nervous system. *Ann Neurol* 1979;5:458–461.
74. Endoh J, Ogasawara N, Yamamoto M. Encephalo-myelo-radiculitis with high HSV-1 antibody index of CSF. *Rinsho Shinkeigaku* 1990;30:1133–1136.
75. Enzmann DR, Brant-Zawadzki M, Britt RH. CT of central nervous system infections in immuno-compromised patients. *AJR* 1980;135:263–267.
76. Eppinger H. Ueber eine neue pathogene Cladothrix und eine durca sie nervorgerufene Pseudotuberculosis (Cladothrichica). *Beitr Pathol Anat Allgem Pathol* 1890;9:287–328.

77. Epstein LG, Sharer LR, Goudsmit J. Neurological and neuropathological features of human immuno-deficiency virus infection in children. *Ann Neurol* 1988;23(suppl 6):19–23.
78. Epstein LG, Sharer LR, Joshi VV. Progressive encephalopathy in children with acquired immune deficiency syndrome. *Ann Neurol* 1985;17:488–496.
79. Escobar A. The pathology of neurocysticercosis. In: Palacios E, Rodriguez-Carbajal J, Taveras JM, eds. *Cysticercosis of the Central Nervous System.* Springfield, IL: Charles C Thomas, 1983:27–59.
80. Formenti SC, Gill PS, Lean E, et al. Primary central nervous system lymphoma in AIDS. Results of radiation therapy. *Cancer* 1989;63:1101–1107.
81. Frazier AR, Rosenow EC, Roberts GD. Nocardiosis. A review of 25 cases occurring during 24 months. *Mayo Clin Proc* 1975;50:657–663.
82. Furman JM, Brownstone PK, Balch RW. Atypical brainstem encephalitis: magnetic resonance imaging and oculographic features. *Neuroradiology* 1985;35:438–440.
83. Gabuzda DH, Ho DD, dela Monte SM, et al. Immunohistochemical identification of HTLV-III antigen in brains of patients with AIDS. *Ann Neurol* 1986;20:289–295.
84. Gamba JL, Woodruff WW, Djang WT, Yeates AE. Craniofacial mucormycosis: assessment with CT. *Radiology* 1986;160:207–212.
85. Gartner S, Markovits P, Markovits DM, et al. Virus isolation from and identification of HTLV-III/LAV-producing cells in brain tissue from a patient with AIDS. *JAMA* 1986;256:2365–2371.
86. Gasecki AP, Steg RE. Correlation of early MRI with CT scan, EEG and CSF: analyses in a case of biopsy proven herpes simplex encephalitis. *Eur Neurol* 1991;31:372–375.
87. Gershon A, Steinberg S, Greenberg S, et al. Varicella-zoster associated encephalitis: detection of specific antibody in cerebrospinal fluid. *J Clin Microbiol* 1980;12:764–767.
88. Gill PS, Levine AM, Meyer PR, et al. Primary central nervous system lymphoma in homosexual men. Clinical, immunological and pathological features. *Am J Med* 1985;78:742– 748.
89. Godt P, Stoeppler L, Wischer U, Schroeder HH. The value of computed tomography in cerebral syphilis. *Neuroradiology* 1979;18:197–200.
90. Gozlan J, Salord J-M, Roullet E, et al. Rapid detection of cytomegalovirus DNA in cerebrospinal fluid of AIDS patients with neurologic disorders. *J Infect Dis* 1992;166:1416–1421.
91. Grant I, Atkinson JH, Hesselink JR, et al. Evidence for early central nervous system involvement in the acquired immunodeficiency syndrome (AIDS) and the human immunodeficiency virus (HIV) infections. *Ann Intern Med* 1987;107:828–836.
92. Greenfield JG. *Greenfield's Neuroapathology.* 4th ed. New York: Wiley, 1984:261–288.
93. Grepp DR, Chandler W, Hyams V. Primary Kaposi's sarcoma of the head and neck. *Ann Intern Med* 1984;100:107–114.
94. Grindal AB, Cohen RJ, Saul RF, et al. Cerebral infarction in young adults. *Stroke* 1978;9:39–42.
95. Gupta RK, Jena A, Sharma DK, et al. MR imaging of intracranial tuberculomas. *J Comput Assist Tomogr* 1988;12:280–285.
96. Hadley MN, Spetzler RF, Martin NA, Johnson PC. Middle cerebral artery aneurysm due to nocardia asteroides: case report of aneurysm excision and extracranial–intracranial bypass. *Neurosurgery* 1988;22:923–928.
97. Helle TL, Britt RH, Colby TV. Primary lymphoma of the central nervous system. Clinicopathological study of experience at Stanford. *J Neurosurg* 1984;60:94–103.
98. Henry JM, Heffner RR Jr, Dillard SH, et al. Primary malignant lymphomas of the central nervous system. *Cancer* 1974;34:1293–1302.
99. Hindmarsh T, Lindquist M, Olding-Stenkvist E, et al. Accuracy of computed tomography in the diagnosis of herpes simplex encephalitis. *Acta Radiol* 1986;369:192–196.
100. Hippocrates. *The genuine works of Hippocrates.* [Translated by F Adams]. London: Sydenham Society, 1849.
101. Ho DD, Bredesen DE, Vinters HV, et al. The acquired immunodeficiency syndrome (AIDS) dementia complex. *Ann Intern Med* 1989;111:400.
102. Ho DD, Rota TR, Schooler RT. Isolation of HLTV-III from cerebrospinal fluid and neuronal tissue of patients with neurological sydromes related to the acquired immunodeficiency syndrome. *N Engl J Med* 1985;313:1493–1497.
103. Hochberg FH, Miller DC. Primary central nervous system lymphoma. *J Neurosurg* 1988;68:835–853.
104. Hodgson AR. Infectious disease of the spine. In: Rothman RH, Simeone FA, eds. *The Spine.* Philadelphia: WB Saunders, 1975:567.
105. Holland BA, Perrett LV, Mills CM. Meningovascular syphilis: CT and MR findings. *Radiology* 1986;158:439–442.
106. Holliday RA. Manifestations of AIDS in the oromaxillofacial region. The role of imaging. *Radiol Clin North Am* 1993;31:45–60.
107. Holmes KK. Syphilis. In: Isselbacher KJ, Adams RD, Braunwald E, Petersdorf RG, Wilson JD, eds. *Harrison's Principles of Internal Medicine.* 9th ed. New York: McGraw-Hill, 1980:716–726.

108. Holtus S, Nyman U, Cronquist S. Computed tomography of malignant lymphoma of the brain. *Neuroradiology* 1984;26:33–38.

109. Holtz HA, Lavery DP, Kapila R. Actinomycetales infection in the acquired immunodeficiency syndrome. *Acta Neuropathol* 1985;66:203–205.

110. Ihmeidan IH, Post MJD, Katz D, et al. Radiographic findings in HIV+ patients with neurosyphilis. *AJNR* 1989;10:896.

111. Ioachim HL, Dorsett B, Cronin W, et al. Acquired immunodeficiency syndrome-associated lymphomas: clinical, pathological, immunological and viral characteristics of 111 cases. *Hum Pathol* 1991;22:659–673.

112. Jacobson MA, Mills J, Reish J, et al. Failure of antiviral therapy for acquired immunodeficiency syndrome-related cytomegalovirus myelitis. *Arch Neurol* 1988;45:1090–1092.

113. Jarvik JG, Lenkinski RE, Grossman RI, et al. Proton MR spectroscopy of HIV-infected patients: characterization of abnormalities with imaging and clinical correlation. *Radiology* 1993;186: 739–744.

114. Javaly K, Horowitz HW, Wormser GP. Nocardiosis in patients with human immunodeficiency virus infection. Report of 2 cases and review of the literature. *Medicine* 1992;71:128–138.

115. Jiddane M, Nicole F, Diaz P, et al. Intracranial malignant lymphoma. Report of 30 cases and review of the literature. *J Neurosurg* 1986;65:592–599.

116. Jinkins JR. Computed tomography of intracranial tuberculosis. *Neuroradiology* 1991;33:126–135.

117. Jones HR, Hedley-Whyte T, Friedberg SR, et al. Primary cerebellopontine progressive multifocal leukoencephalopathy diagnosed premortem by cerebellar biopsy. *Ann Neurol* 1982;11:199–202.

118. Jordan BD, Navia BA, Petito C, et al. Neurological syndromes complicating AIDS. *Front Radiat Ther Oncol* 1985;19:82–87.

119. Jordan J, Enzmann DR. Encephalitis. In: Hesselink JR, ed. *Neuroimaging Clin North Am* 1991;1: 17–38.

120. Kaplan JG, Sterman AB, Horoupian D, et al. Luetic meningitis with gumma: clinical, radiographic, and neuropathological features. *Neurology* 1981;31:464–467.

121. Katz DA, Berger JR. Neurosyphilis in acquired immunodeficiency syndrome. *Arch Neurol* 1989; 46:895–898.

122. Katz DA, Berger JR, Duncan RC. Neurosyphilis. A comparative study of the effects of infection with human immunodeficiency virus. *Arch Neurol* 1993;50:243–249.

123. Kelly WM, Brant-Zawadzki M. Acquired immunodeficiency syndrome: neuroradiological findings.- *Radiology* 1983;149:485–491.

124. Khan MA, Kovnat DM, Bachus B, Whitcomb ME, et al. Clinical and roentgenographic spectrum of pulmonary tuberculosis in the adult. *Am J Med* 1977;62:31–38.

125. Kissane JM. *Anderson's Pathology*. Vol. 2, 9th ed. St. Louis: CV Mosby, 1990:2160–2161.

126. Kobayaski RM, Coel M, Niwayama G, et al. Cerebral vasculitis in coccidoidal meningitis. *Ann Neurol* 1977;1:281–284.

127. Kobayshi GS. Fungi. In: Davis BD, Dulbecco R, Eisen HN, Ginsbert HS, eds. *Microbiology*. New York: Harper & Row, 1980:817–850.

128. Koehler JE, Quinn FD, Berger TG, et al. Isolation of rochalimaea species from cutaneous and osseous lesions of bacillary angiomatosis. *N Engl J Med* 1992;327:1625–1631.

129. Koenig S, Gendelman HE, Orenstein JM, et al. Detection of AIDS virus in macrophages in brain tissue from AIDS patients with encephalopathy. *Science* 1986;233:1089–1093.

130. Koppen AH, Lansing LS, Renk SK, Smith RS. Central nervous system vasculitis in cytomegalovirus infection. *J Neurol Sci* 1981;51:395–410.

131. Kramer EL, Sanger JJ. Central nervous system complications of the acquired immunodeficiency syndrome on I-123 iodoamphetamine brain SPECT. *Adv Funct Neuroimaging* 1989;1:15–19.

132. Kramer LD, Locke GE, Byrd SE, et al. Cerebral cysticercosis: documentation of natural history with CT. *Radiology* 1989;171:459–462.

133. Krick JA, Remington JS. Current concepts in parasitology. Toxoplasmosis in the adult—an overview. *N Engl J Med* 1978;298:550–553.

134. Krupp LB, Lipton RB, Swerdlow ML, et al. Progressive multifocal leukoencephalopathy; clinical and radiographic features. *Ann Neurol* 1985;17:344–349.

135. Lasker BR, Harter DH. Cervical epidural abscess. *Neurology* 1987;37:1747.

136. LeBlang SD, Whiteman MLH, Post MJD, et al. CNS nocardia in AIDS patients: CT and MRI with pathologic correlation. *J Comput Assist Tomgr* 1995;19:15–22.

137. LeBoit PE, Berger T, Egbert BM, et al. Bacillary angiomatosis: the histopathology and differential diagnosis of a pseudoneoplastic infection in patients with HIV infection. *Am J Surg Pathol* 1989; 13:909–920.

138. Leestma JE. Viral infections of the nervous system. In: Davis RL, Robertson DM, eds. *Textbook of Neuropathology*. Baltimore: Williams & Wilkins, 1985:704–787.

139. Leiguarda R, Berthier M, Starkstein S, et al. Ischemic infarction in 25 children with tuberculous meningitis. *Stroke* 1988;19:200–204.

140. Lemann W, Cho E-S, Nielsen SL, et al. Neuropathological findings in 104 cases of acquired im-

munedeficiency syndrome (AIDS): an autopsy study [Abstract]. *J Neuropathol Exp Neurol* 1985; 44:349.

141. Lester JW, Carter MP, Reynolds TL. Herpes encephalitis: MR monitoring of response to acyclovir therapy. *J Comput Assist Tomogr* 1988;12:941–943.

142. Levy RM, Bredesen DE. Central nervous system dysfunction in the acquired immunodeficiency syndrome. *J AIDS* 1988;1:41.

143. Levy RM, Bredesen DE, Rosenblum ML. Neurological manifestations of the acquired immunodeficiency syndrome (AIDS): experience at UCSF and review of the literature. *J Neurosurg* 1985;62: 475–495.

144. Levy RM, Bredesen DE, Rosenblum ML, et al. Central nervous system disorders in AIDS. In: Levy JA, ed. *AIDS Pathogenesis and Treatment.* New York: BC Dekker, 1988:371.

145. Levy RM, Janssen RS, Bush TJ, et al. Neuroepidemiology of acquired immunodeficiency syndrome. In: Rosenblum ML, ed. *AIDS and the Nervous System.* New York, Raven, 1988:13–28.

146. Levy RM, Pons VG, Rosenblum ML. Central nervous system mass lesions in the acquired immunodeficiency syndrome (AIDS). *J Neurosurg* 1984;61:9–16.

147. Levy RM, Rosenbloom S, Perrett LV. Neuroradiological findings in the acquired immunodeficiency syndrome (AIDS): a review of 200 cases. *AJNR* 1986;7:833–839.

148. Lobato RD, Lamas E, Portillo JM, et al. Hydrocephalus in cerebral cysticercosis. *J Neurosurg* 1981; 55:786–793.

149. Lopes-Hernandez A. Clinical manifestations and sequential computed tomographic scans of cerebral cysticercosis in childhood. *Brain Dev* 1983;5:269–277.

150. Lotz J, Hewlett R, Alheit B, Bowen R. Neurocysticercosis: correlative pathomorphology and MR imaging. *Neuroradiology* 1988;30:35–41.

151. Louie E, Rice LB, Holzman RS. Tuberculosis in non-Haitian patients with acquired immunodeficiency syndrome. *Chest* 1986;90:542–545.

152. Lyons RW, Andriole VT. Fungal infections of the CNS. *Neurol Clin* 1986;159–170.

153. Mahieux F, Gray F, Fenelon G, et al. Acute myeloradiculitis due to cytomegalovirus as the initial manifestation of AIDS. *J Neurol Neurosurg Psychiatry* 1987;52:270–274.

154. Major EO, Amemiya K, Tornatore CS, et al. Pathogenesis and molecular biology of progressive multifocal leukoencephalopathy, the JC virus–induced demyelinating disease of the human brain. *Clin Micro Rev* 1992;5:49–73.

155. Mark AS, Atlas SW. Progressive multifocal leukoencephalopathy in patients with AIDS: appearance on MR images. *Radiology* 1989;173:517–520.

156. Masdeu SC, Yudd A, Van Heertum RL, Grundman M, et al. Single-photon emission computed tomography in human immunodeficiency virus encephalopathy: a preliminary report. *J Nucl Med* 1991;1471–1475.

157. Mathews VP, Alo PL, Glass JD, Kumar AJ, McArthur JC. AIDS-related CNS cryptococcosis: Radiological–pathological correlation. *AJNR* 1992;13:1477–1486.

158. Mazlo M, Tariska I. Morphological demonstration of the first phase of polyomavirus replication in oligodendroglia cells of human brain in progressive multifocal leuko-encephalopathy (PML). *Neuropathology* 1980;49:133–143.

159. McArthur JC, Becker PS, Parisi JE, et al. Neuropathological changes in early HIV-1 dementia. *Ann Neurol* 1989;26:681–684.

160. McArthur JC, Cohen BA, Selnes OA, et al. Low prevalence of neurological and neuropsychological abnormalities in otherwise healthy HIV-1 infected individuals: results from the multicenter AIDS Cohort Study. *Ann Neurol* 1989;26:601–611.

161. McCormick GF. Cysticercosis: review of 230 patients. *Bull Clin Neurosci* 1985;50:76–101.

162. Mehta JB, Dutt A, Harvill L, et al. Epidemiology of extrapulmonary tuberculosis. A comparative analysis with pre-AIDS era. *Chest* 1991;99:1134–1138.

163. Melhem ER, Wang H. Intramedullary spinal cord tuberculoma in a patient with AIDS. *Am J Neuroradiol* 1992;13:986–988.

164. Meyers BR. Tuberculous meningitis. *Med Clin North Am* 1982;66:755–762.

165. Miller JR, Barett RE, Britton CB, et al. Progressive multifocal leukoencephalopathy in a male homosexual with Tcell immunodeficiency. *N Engl J Med* 1982;307:1436–1438.

166. Miller WT, MacGregor RR. Tuberculosis: frequency of unusual radiographic findings. *AJR* 1978; 130:867–875.

167. Modic MT, Feiglin DH, PIraino DW, et al. Vertebral osteomyelitis: assessment using MR. *Radiology* 1985;151:157.

168. Morawetz RB, Whitley RJ, Murphy DM. Experience with brain biopsy for suspected herpes encephalitis: review of forty consecutive cases. *Neurosurgery* 1983;12:654–657.

169. Moskowitz LB, Gregorios JB, Hensley GT, Berger JR. Cytomegalovirus induced demyelination associated with acquired immune deficiency syndrome. *Arch Pathol Lab Med* 1984;108:873–877.

170. Moskowitz LB, Hensley GT, Chan JC, et al. The neuropathology of acquired immune deficiency syndrome. *Arch Pathol Lab Med* 1984;108:867.

171. Moulignier A, Mikol J, Pialoux G, et al. Cerebral glial tumors and human immuno-deficiency virus–1 infection. More than a coincidental association. *Cancer* 1994;686–692.

172. Navia BA, Cho E-S, Petito CK, Price RW. The AIDS dementia complex: II. Neuropathology. *Ann Neurol* 1986;19:525–535.

173. Navia BA, Jordan BD, Price RW. The AIDS dementia complex 1. Clinical features. *Ann Neurol* 1986;19:517–524.

174. Neils EW, Lukin R, Tomsick TA, Tew JM. Magnetic resonance imaging and computerized tomography scanning of herpes simplex encephalitis; report of two cases. *J Neurosurg* 1987;67:592–594.

175. Nielsen SL, Petito CK, Urmacher CD, Posner JB. Subacute encephalitis in acquired immune deficiency syndrome: a postmortem study. *Am J Clin Pathol* 1984;82:678–682.

176. Nocard ME. Note sur la maladie des boeufs de la Guadeloupe connue sous le nom de farcin. *Ann Inst Pasteur* 1888;2:293–302.

177. Non-Hodgkins lymphoma pathological classification project: National Cancer Institute sponsored study of classifications of non-Hodgkins lymphomas. Summary and description of a working formula for clinical usage. *Cancer* 1982;49:2112–2135.

178. O'Brien RJ. The epidemiology of nontuberculous mycobacterial disease. *Clin Chest Med* 1989;10:407–418.

179. Olsen WL, Longo FM, Mills CM, Norman D. White matter disease in AIDS: findings at MR imaging. *Radiology* 1988;169:445–448.

180. O'Neil BP, Illig JJ. Primary central nervous system lymphoma. *Mayo Clin Proc* 1989;64:1005–1020.

181. Orron DE, Kuhn MJ, Malholtra V, et al. Primary cerebral lymphoma in acquired immunodeficiency (AIDS)—CT manifestations. *Comput Med Imag Graphics* 1989;13:207–214.

182. Padget BL, Walker DL, ZuRhein GM, et al. Cultivation of papova-like virus from human brain with progressive multifocal leukoencephalopathy. *Lancet* 1971;1257–1260.

183. Palmer DL, Harvey RL, Wheeler JK. Diagnostic and therapeutic considerations in *Nocardia asteroides* infection. *Medicine* 1974;53:391–401.

184. Pape JW, Liautaud B, Thomas F, et al. Characteristics of the acquired immunodeficiency syndrome (AIDS) in Haiti. *N Engl J Med* 1983;309:945–950.

185. Parker JC Jr, Dyer MC. Neurological infection due to bacteria, fungi and parasites. In: Doris RL, Robertson DM, eds. *Textbook of Neuropathology*. Baltimore: Williams & Wilkins, 1985:632–703.

186. Parr J, Horoupian DS, Winkelman C. Cerebellar form of progressive multifocal leukoencephalopathy (PML). *Can J Neurol Sci* 1979;6:123–128.

187. Pascal S, Resnick L, Yoshii F, et al. FDG/PET scan metabolic asymmetry in asymptomatic HIV seropositive subjects: correlation with disease onset. *J Nucl Med* 1990;31:826.

188. Petito CK. Review of central nervous system pathology in human immunodeficiency virus infection. *Ann Neurol* 1988;23(suppl) 54–57.

189. Petito CK, Cho E-S, Lemann W, Navia BA, Price RW. Neuropathology of acquired immunodeficiency syndrome (AIDS): an autopsy review. *J Neuropathol Exp Neurol* 1986;45:635–646.

190. Petito CK, Navia BA, Cho E-S, et al. Vacuolar myelopathy pathologically resembling subacute combined degeneration in patients with the acquired immunodeficiency syndrome. *N Engl J Med* 1985;312:874–879.

191. Pitchenik AE, Burr J, Suarez M, Fertel D, et al. Human Tcell lymphotropic virus–III (HTLV-III) seropositivity and related disease among 71 consecutive patients in whom tuberculosis was diagnosed: a prospective study. *Am Rev Respir Dis* 1987;135:875–879.

192. Pitchenik AE, Cole C, Russell BW, Fischl MA, et al. Tuberculosis, atypical mycobacteriosis, and the acquired immunodeficiency syndrome among Haitian and non-Haitian patients in South Florida. *Ann Intern Med* 1984;101:641–645.

193. Pohl P, Vogl G, Fill H, Rossler H, Zangerle R, Gerstenbrand F. Single photon emission computed tomography in AIDS dementia complex. *J Nucl Med* 1988;29:1382–1386.

194. Poon TP, Tchertkoff V, Pares GF, et al. Spinal cord toxoplasma lesion in AIDS. MR findings. *J Comput Assist Tomogr* 1992;16:817–819.

195. Popovich MJ, Arthur RH, Helmer E. CT of intracranial cryptococcosis. *AJNR* 1990;11:139–142.

196. Porter SB, Sande MA. Toxoplasmosis of the central nervous system in the acquired immunedeficiency syndrome. *N Engl J Med* 1993;2:1643–1648.

197. Post MJD. Neuroimaging in various stages of human immunodeficiency virus infection. *Curr Opin Radiol* 1990;2:73–79.

198. Post MJD, Berger JR, Duncan R, Quencer RM, Pall L, Winfield D. Asymptomatic and neurologically symptomatic HIV-seropositive subjects: results of long–term MR imaging and clinical follow-up. *Radiology* 1993;188:727–733.

199. Post MJD, Berger JR, Hensley GT. The radiology of central nervous system disease in the acquired immunodeficiency syndrome. In: Taveras JM, Ferrucci JT, eds. *Radiology: diagnosis–imaging–intervention*. Vol. 3. Philadelphia: JB Lippincott, 1988:1–26.

200. Post MJD, Chan JC, Hensley GT, Hoffman TA, et al. Toxoplasma encephalitis in Haitian adults with acquired immunodeficiency syndrome: a clinical–pathological–CT correlation. *AJR* 1983;140:861–868.

201. Post MJD, Curless RG, Gregorios JB, et al. Reactivation of congenital cytomegalic inclusion disease in an infant with HTLV-III associated immunodeficiency: a CT–pathological correlation. *J Comput Assist Tomogr* 1986;10:533–536.
202. Post MJD, Hensley GT, Moskowitz LB, Fischl M. Cytomegalic inclusion virus encephalitis in patients with AIDS: CT, clinical and pathological correlation. *AJR* 1986;146:1229–1234.
203. Post MJD, Hoffman TA. Cerebral inflammatory disease. In: Rosenberg RN, ed. *The Clinical Neurosciences*. Heinz ER, ed. *Neuroradiology*. Vol. 4. New York: Churchill-Livingstone, 1984:525–594.
204. Post MJD, Kursunoglu SJ, Hensley GT, et al. Cranial CT in acquired immunodeficiency syndrome: spectrum of diseases and optimal contrast enhancement technique. *AJNR* 1985;6:743–754.
205. Post MJD, Levin BE, Berger JR, et al. Sequential cranial MR findings of asymptomatic and neurologically symptomatic HIV positive subjects. *AJNR* 1992;13:359–370.
206. Post MJD, Quencer RM, Montalvo BM, et al. Spinal infection: evaluation with MR imaging and intraoperative US. *Radiology* 1988;169:765.
207. Post MJD, Sheldon JJ, Hensley GT, et al. Central nervous system disease in acquired immunodeficiency syndrome: prospective correlation using CT, MR imaging and pathological studies. *Radiology* 1986;158:141–148.
208. Post MJD, Tate LG, Quencer RM, et al. CT, MR and pathology in HIV encephalitis and meningitis. *AJNR* 1988;9:469–476.
209. Pott P. *Remarks on that kind of palsy of the lower limbs which is frequently found to accompany a curvature of the spine*. London: J Johnson, 1779.
210. Presant CA, Wiernik PH, Serpick AA. Factors affecting survival in nocardiosis. *Am Rev Respir Dis* 1973;108:1444–1448.
211. Price RW, Navia BA, Cho E-S. AIDS encephalopathy. *Neurol Clin* 1986;4:285–301.
212. Rabiela-Cerrantes MT, Rivas-Hernandez A, Rodriques-Ebarra J, et al. Anatomopathological aspects of human brain cysticercosis: In: Flisser A, Williams K, Larralde C, et al., eds. *Cysticercosis: Present State of Knowledge and Perspective*. New York: Academic, 1982:179–200.
213. Ramsey RG, Geremia GK. CNS complications of AIDS: CT and MR findings. *AJR* 1988;151: 449–454.
214. Reichman RC. Neurological complications of varicella-zoster infection. In: Dolin R, ed. Herpes-zoster varicella infections. *Am Intern Med* 1978;89:375–388.
215. Remick SC, Diamond C, Migliozzi JA, et al. Primary central nervous system lymphoma in patients with and without the acquired immune deficiency syndrome. A retrospective analysis and review of the literature. *Medicine* 1990;69:345–360.
216. Remington JS. Toxoplasmosis in the adult. *Bull NY Acad Med* 1978;50:211–227.
217. Resnick D, Niwayama G. Osteomyelitis, septic arthritis, and soft tissue infection: the organisms. In: Resnick D, Niwayama G, eds. *Diagnosis of Bone and Joint Disorders*, Vol. 4. 2nd ed. Philadelphia: WB Saunders, 1988.
218. Ribera E, Martinez-Vasquez JM, Ocana I, et al. Activity of Adenosine deaminase in cerebrospinal fluid for the diagnosis and follow–up of tuberculous meningitis in adults. *J Infect Dis* 1987;155: 603–607.
219. Riccio TJ, Hesselink JR. Gd-DTPA enhanced MR of multiple cryptococcal brain abscesses. *AJNR* 1989;10:565–566.
220. Richardson EP Jr. Progressive multifocal leukoencephalopathy 30 years later. *N Engl J Med* 1988; 318:315–317.
221. Rieder HL, Cauthen GM, Bloch AB, et al. Tuberculosis and acquired immunodeficiency syndrome—Florida. *Arch Intern Med* 1989;149:1268–1273.
222. Reider HL, Cauthen GM, Kelly GD, et al. Tuberculosis in the United States. *JAMA* 1989;262: 385–389.
223. Rodriguez-Carbajal J, Palacios E, Naidich TA. Infections and parasitic disorders—supratentorial. In: Taveras JM, Ferucci JT, eds. *Radiology: Diagnosis–Imaging–Intervention*. Vol. 3. Philadelphia: JB Lippincott, 1986:1–22.
224. Rosen PP. Cytomegalovirus infection in cancer patients. *Pathol Ann* 1978;13:175–208.
225. Rosenblum ML, Levy RM, Bredesen DE, et al. Primary central nervous system lymphomas in patients with AIDS. *Ann Neurol* 1988;23(suppl):13–16.
226. Rottenberg DA, Moeller JR, Strother SC, et al. The metabolic pathology of the AIDS dementia complex. *Ann Neurol* 1987;22:700–706.
227. Rowley AH, Whitley RJ, Lakemar FD, Wolinsky SM. Rapid detection of herpes-simplex virus DNA in cerebrospinal fluid of patients with herpes simplex encephalitis. *Lancet* 1990;335:440–441.
228. Ruiz A, Ganz WI, Post MJD, et al. Use of Thallium-201 brain SPECT to differentiate cerebral lymphoma from toxoplasma encephalitis in AIDS patients. *Am J Neuroradiol* 1994;15:1885–1894.
229. Safai B, Diaz B, Schwartz J. Malignant neoplasms associated with human immunodeficiency virus infection. *CA Cancer J Clin* 1992;42:74–96.
230. Sagerman RH, Cassady JR, Chang CH. Radiation therapy for intracranial lymphoma. *Radiology* 1967;88:552–554.

231. Sathe SS, Reichman. Mycobacterial disease in patients infected with the human immunodeficiency virus. *Clin Chest Med* 1989;10:445–463.
232. Scharf D. Neurocysticercosis. *Arch Neurol* 1988;45:777–780.
233. Schaumburg HH, Plank CR, Adams RD. The reticulum cell sarcoma–microglioma group of brain tumors. A consideration of their clinical features and therapy. *Brain* 1972;95:199–212.
234. Schneck SA. Neuropathological features of human organ transplantation: I. Possible cytomegalovirus infection. *J Neuropathol Exp Neurol* 1965;24:415–429.
235. Schober R, Herman MM. Neuropathology of cardiac transplantation. Survey of 31 cases. *Lancet* 1973;1:962–967.
236. Schoeman J, Hewlett R, Donald P. MR of childhood tuberculous meningitis. *Neuroradiology* 1988; 30:473–477.
237. Schroth G, Gawehn J, Thron A, Vallbracht A, Voigt K. Early diagnosis of herpes simplex encephalitis by MRI. *Neurology* 1987;37:179–183.
238. Selwyn PA, Hartel D, Lewis VA, et al. A prospective study of the risk of tuberculosis among intravenous drug users with human immunodeficiency virus infection. *N Engl J Med* 1989;320: 545–550.
239. Shafer RW, Chirgwin KD, Glatt AE, et al. HIV prevalence, immunosuppression and drug resistance in patients with tuberculosis in an area endemic for AIDS. *AIDS* 1991;5:399–405.
240. Sharer LR, Cho E-S, Epstein LG. Multinucleated giant cells and HTLV-III in AIDS encephalopathy. *Hum Pathol* 1985;16:760.
241. Sharer LR, Epstein LG, Joshi VV, Rankin LF. Neuropathological observations in children with AIDS and with HTLV-III infection of brain. *J Neuropathol Exp Neurol* 1985;44:350.
242. Shaw DWW, Cohen WA. Viral infection of the CNS in children: imaging features. *AJR* 993;160: 125–133.
243. Shaw GM, Harper ME, Hahn BH, et al. HTLV-III infection in brains of children and adults with AIDS encephalopathy. *Science* 1985;227:177–181.
244. Sheller JR, Des Prez RM. CNS tuberculosis. *Neurol Clin* 1986;4:143–158.
245. Silverman L, Rubinstein LJ. Electron microscopic observation on a case of progressive multifocal leukoencephalopathy. *Acta Neuropathol (Berl)* 1965;5:215–224.
246. Simpson DM, Bender AN. Human immunodeficiency virus–associated myopathy: analysis of 11 patients. *Ann Neurol* 1988;24:78–84.
247. Simpson OL, Stinson EB, Egger MJ, Remington JS. Nocardial infection in the immunocompromised host: a detailed study in a defined population. *Rev Infect Dis* 1981;3:492–507.
248. Sindrup JH, Weismann K, Wantzin GL. Syphilis in HTLV-III infected male homosexuals. *AIDS Res* 1986;2:285–288.
249. Singh BM, Levine S, Yarrish RL, et al. Spinal cord syndromes in the acquired immune deficiency syndrome. *Acta Neurol Scand* 1986;73:590–598.
250. Sklar EML, Post MJD, Lebwohl NH. Imaging of infection of the lumbosacral spine. *Neuroimag Clin North Am* 1993;3:577–590.
251. Smith AS, Blaser SI. Infections and inflammatory processes of the spine. *Radiol Clin North Am* 1991;29:809.
252. Smith EG, Davison WR. *Egyptian Mummies.* London: G Allen & Unwin, 1924:157.
253. Smith PW, Steinkraus GE, Henricks BW, Madsen EC. CNS nocardiosis: response to sulfamethoxazole–trimethoprim. *Arch Neurol* 1980;37:729–730.
254. Smoker WRK, Harnsberger HR, Reede DL, et al. The neck. In: Som PM, Bergeron RT, eds. *Head and Neck Imaging.* 2nd ed. St. Louis: CV Mosby, 1991:572–576.
255. Snider WD, Simpson DM, Nielsen S, et al. Neurological complications of acquired immune deficiency syndrome: analysis of 50 patients. *Ann Neurol* 1983;14:403–418.
256. So YT, Choucair A, Davis RL, et al. Neoplasms of the central nervous system in acquired immunodeficiency syndrome. In: Rosenblum ML, Levy RM, Bredesen DE, eds. *AIDS and the Nervous System.* New York: Raven, 1988.
257. Soo MS, Tien RD, Gray L, Andrews PI, Friedman H. Mesenrhombencephalitis: MR findings in nine patients. *AJR* 1993;160:1089–1093.
258. Spickler EM, Lufkin RB, Teresi L, Lanman T, Levesque M, Benston JR. High-signal intraventricular cysticercosis on T1 weighted MR imaging. *AJNR* 1989;10(suppl):64.
259. Starke JR. Modern approach to the diagnosis and treatment of tuberculosis in children. *Pediatr Clin North Am* 1988;35:441–464.
260. Stoner G, Ryschkewitsch CF, Walker DL, Webster HD. JC papovavirus large tumor (T)-antigen expression in brain tissue of acquired immune deficiency syndrome (AIDS) and non-AIDS patients with progressive multifocal leukoencephalopathy. *Proc Natl Acad Sci U S A* 1986;23:2271–2275.
261. Sunderam G, McDonald RJ, Maniatis T, Oleske J, et al. Tuberculosis as a manifestation of the acquired immunodeficiency syndrome (AIDS). *JAMA* 1986;256:362–366.
262. Suss RA, Maravilla KR, Thompson J. MR imaging of intracranial cysticercosis: comparison with CT and anatomopathological features. *AJNR* 1986;7:235–242.

263. Switzer P, Gomori JM, Eliashiv S. Gd-DTPA enhanced MRI of herpes simplex encephalitis: a case report. *Clin Imag* 1991;15:121–124.
264. Sze G. Infection and inflammatory diseases. In: Stark DD, Bradley WG Jr, eds. *Magnetic Resonance Imaging*. St. Louis: CV Mosby, 1988:316–343.
265. Sze G, Brant-Zawadzki MN, Norman D, Newton HT. The neuroradiology of AIDS. *Semin Roentgenol* 1987;22:42–53.
266. Sze G, Zimmerman RD. The magnetic resonance imaging of infections and inflammatory diseases. *Radiol Clin North Am* 1988;26:839–859.
267. Tan CT, Kuan BB. Cryptococcus meningitis, clinical CT scan considerations. *Neuroradiology* 1987; 29:43–46.
268. Tatsch K, Schielke E, Einhaupl KM, et al. Tc-99m HMPAO SPECT in early stages of HIV infection. *J Nucl Med* 1990;31:827.
269. Teitelbaum GP, Otto RW, Lin M, et al. MR imaging of neurocysticercosis. *AJR* 1989;153:857–866.
270. Theuer CP, Hopewell PC, Elias D, et al. Human immune deficiency virus infection in tuberculosis patients. *J Infect Dis* 1990;162:8–12.
271. Thomas MD, Chopra JS, Walia BNS. Tuberculous meningitis (TBM). *J Assoc Phys Ind* 1977;25: 633–639.
272. Tien RD, Chu PK, Hesselink Jr, et al. Intracranial cryptococcosis in immunocompromised patients: CT and MR findings in 29 cases. *AJNR* 1991;12:283–289.
273. Tien RD, Chu PK, Hesselink JR, Szumowski J. Intra- and para-orbital lesions: value of fat suppression MR imaging with paramagnetic contrast enhancement. *AJNR* 1991;12:245–247.
274. Tien RD, Feldberg GJ, Osumi AK. Herpesvirus infections of the CNS: MR findings. *AJR* 1993; 161:167–176.
275. Tien RD, Gean-Marton AD, Mark AS. Neurosyphilis in HIV carriers: MR findings in six patients. *AJR* 1992;158:1325–1328.
276. Tuberculosis and AIDS—Connecticut. *MMWR* 1987;36:133–135.
277. Tyson G, Newman P, StrachenWE. Tuberculous brain abscess. *Surg Neurol* 1978;10:323–325.
278. Uttamchandani RB, Daikos GL, Reyes RR, et al. Nocardiosis in 30 patients with advanced human immunodeficiency virus infection. Clinical features and outcome. *Clin Infect Dis* 1994;18:348–353.
279. van Dyk A. CT of intracranial tuberculosis with specific reference to the ''target sign.'' *Neuroradiology* 1988;30:329–336.
280. Vietzke WM, Gelderman AH, Grimley PM, Valsamis MP. Toxoplasmosis complicating malignancy. Experience at the National Cancer Institute. *Cancer* 1968;21:816–827.
281. Villoria MF, de la Torre J, Munoz L, et al. Intracranial tuberculosis in AIDS: CT and MRI findings. *Neuroradiology* 1992;34:11–14.
282. Vinters HV, Kwok MK, Ho HW, et al. Cytomegalovirus in the nervous system of patients with the acquired immune deficiency syndrome. *Brain* 1989;112:245–268.
283. Walker DL. Progressive multifocal leukoencephalopathy. In Vinken PJ, Bruyn GW, Klawans HL, eds. *Handbook of Clinical Neurology*. Vol. 47. Demyelinating Diseases. Amsterdam: Elsevier Science, 1985:503–524.
284. Weiner LP, Fleming JO. Viral infections of the nervous system. *J Neurosurg* 1984;61:207–224.
285. Westermark N, Forssman G. The roentgen diagnosis of tuberculous spondylitis. *Acta Radiol* 1938; 19:207.
286. Whelan MA, Kricheff II, Handler M, et al. Acquired immunodeficiency syndrome: cerebral computed tomographic manifestations. *Radiology* 1983;149:477–484.
287. Whitley RJ, Schlitt M. Encephalitis caused by herpesviruses, including B virus. In: Scheld WM, Whitley RJ, Durack DT, eds. *Infection of the Central Nervous System*. New York: Raven, 1991: 41–86.
288. Whiteman MLH, Dandapani BK, Shebert RP, Post MJD. MRI of AIDS-related polyradiculomyelitis. *J Comput Assist Tomogr* 1994;18:7–11.
289. Whiteman MLH, Post MJD, Berger JR, Tate LG, et al. Progressive multifocal leukoencephalopathy in 47 HIV-seropositive patients: neuroimaging with clinical and pathological correlation. *Radiology* 1993;187:233–240.
290. Whiteman MLH, Post MJD, Bowen BC, Bell MD. AIDS-related white matter diseases. *Neuroimag Clin North Am* 1993;3:331–359.
291. Whitener DR. Tuberculous brain abscess: report of a case and review of the literature. *Arch Neurol* 1978;35:148–155.
292. Wiley CA, Nelson JA. Role of human immunodeficiency virus and cytomegalovirus in AIDS encephalitis. *Am J Pathol* 1988;133:73–81.
293. Wiley CA, Schrier RD, Denaro FJ, et al. Localization of cytomegalovirus proteins and genome during fulminant central nervous system infection in an AIDS patient. *J Neuropathol Exp Neurol* 1986;45:127–139.
294. Wolf DG, Spector SA. Diagnosis of human cytomegalovirus central nervous system disease in AIDS patients by DNA amplification from cerebrospinal fluid. *J Infect Dis* 1992;166:1412–1415.

295. Wong ML, Jefek BW. Cervical mycobacterial disease. *Trans Am Acad Ophthalmol Otolaryngol* 1974;78:75.
296. Wong T-W, Warner NE. Cytomegalic inclusion disease in adults. Report of 14 cases with review of literature. *Arch Pathol Lab Med* 1962;74:403–422.
297. Woodring JH, Vandiviere HM, Fried AM, et al. Update: the radiographic features of pulmonary tuberculosis. *AJR* 1986;146:497–506.
298. Wouters EFM, Hupperts RMM, Vreeling FW, et al. Successful treatment of tuberculous brain abscess. *J Neurol* 1985;23:118–119.
299. Yang PJ, Reger KM, Seeger JF, et al. Brain abscess: an atypical CT appearance of CNS tuberculosis. *AJNR* 1987;8:919–920.
300. Yankner BA, Skolnik PR, Shoukimas GM, et al. Cerebral granulomatous angiitis associated with isolation of human T-lymphotropic virus type III from the central nervous system. *Ann Neurol* 1986; 20:362–364.
301. Yudd AP, Van Heertum RL, O'Connell RA, et al. I-123 SPECT brain scanning in patients with HIV positive encephalopathy. *J Nucl Med* 1987;30:811.
302. Zimmerman MR. Pulmonary and osseous tuberculosis in an Egyptian mummy. *Bull NY Acad Med* 1979;55:604.
303. Zimmerman RA. Central nervous system lymphoma. *Radiol Clin North Am* 1990;28:697– 721.
304. Zimmerman RA, Bilaniuk LT, Sze G. Intracranial infection. In: Brant-Zawadzki M, Norman D, eds. *Magnetic Resonance Imaging of the Central Nervous System*. New York: Raven, 1987:235–257.
305. Zuger A, Louis E, Holzman RS, et al. Cryptococcal disease in patients with the acquired immunodeficiency syndrome. Diagnostic features and outcome of treatment. *Ann Intern Med* 1986;104:234–240.
306. ZuRhein GM. Polyoma-like virions in a human demyelinating disease. *Acta Neuropathol* 1967;8: 57–68.
307. ZuRhein GM. Association of papovavirus with a human demyelinating disease (progressive multifocal leukoencephalopathy) *Prog Med Virol* 1969;11:185–247.
308. ZuRhein GM, Chou E-S. Particles resembling papovaviruses in human cerebral demyelinating disease. *Science* 1965;148:1477–1479.

AIDS and the Nervous System, Second Edition,
edited by J. R. Berger and R. M. Levy.
Lippincott-Raven Publishers, Philadelphia © 1997.

14

Neuroophthalmology of Acquired Immunodeficiency Syndrome

Janet L. Davis

Department of Ophthalmology, University of Miami School of Medicine, Bascom Palmer Eye Institute, Ann Bates Leach Hospital, Miami, Florida 33136

The high rate of opportunistic infections, degenerative disorders, and neoplasms in the central nervous systems (CNS) of patients with human immunodeficiency virus (HIV) disease produces a similarly high rate of neuroophthalmic signs and symptoms. If the eye is considered as part of the nervous system, an estimated 40–90% of patients with acquired immunodeficiency syndrome (AIDS) will have clinically apparent ocular or neuroophthalmic manifestations (32,33,51,52,64,65,87,90,98). Disorders affecting primarily the ocular tissue also may affect the CNS. The common cytomegalovirus (CMV) infection of the retina, which affects 20–50% of HIV-infected patients (32,52,58,59,61,84,87,90,98,103) may be associated in some cases with encephalitis (90) or peripheral neuropathy (5). Several other infections, such as toxoplasmosis, cryptococcosis, and syphilis, also infect both the nervous system and the eye.

The ocular disorders associated with HIV infection are usually grouped in four major categories: retinal vascular disease, opportunistic ocular infections, neoplasms, and neuroophthalmic abnormalities without direct pathological alteration of ocular tissue (59).

RETINAL VASCULAR DISEASE

Autopsy series have demonstrated changes in the retinal microvasculature in all persons dying with HIV disease (84,90). Ultrastructurally, the changes resemble diabetic retinopathy, with swelling of endothelial cells, thickening of the basal lamina, degeneration and loss of pericytes, and narrowing of capillary lumina. Retinal microaneurysms (90), small intraretinal hemorrhages (84), and nerve fiber layer infarcts (cotton-wool spots) may be seen. The prevalence of microangiopathy increases with greater immune deficiency (13,16,17) so that 16% of patients with CD4+ lymphocyte counts (CD4+ counts) of >50 cells/mm^3 and 45% of those with CD4+ counts of <50 are involved (68). Disturbance of the blood–retina barrier has been detected by fluorophotometry before the appearance of any clinical lesions (15).

The cause of the microvascular abnormalities is unclear. Infection with CMV as a precursor to cotton-wool patches has been excluded (91). Cotton-wool spots have been analyzed for the presence of immunoglobulin (Ig)G, IgA, IgM, and C3b without

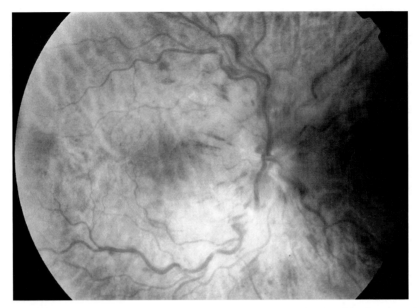

FIG. 1. Central retinal vein occlusion that occurred in an otherwise healthy 32-year-old man with HIV infection. The retinal veins are distended, and intraretinal hemorrhages are present in all four quadrants of the fundus. HIV testing should probably be included in the list of testing for systemic disease with retinal vascular occlusive disease occurring in the young.

any evidence that they are the result of humoral immunity or immune complex deposition (91). HIV virus has been localized to human retinal endothelial cells (93), leading to speculation that intravascular HIV infection might lead to retinal ischemia. HIV infection also has been proposed as the cause of severe retinal dysfunction in three patients with vitritis but without focal lesions (12). In addition to decreased electroretinographic amplitudes, arteriolar narrowing was noted in one of the cases.

Investigation for hemorrheological abnormalities in 22 patients with HIV infection showed an association with higher fibrinogen levels in the patients who had cotton-wool patches, but no conclusive differences in hematocrit, viscosity, immune complexes, or immunoglobulins were determined (26). The natural history of cotton-wool spots includes periodic appearance in crops of lesions (32) and rapid fading over a median of 6–7 weeks (72). The capillary disease is patchy rather than diffuse as in diabetic retinopathy. These features suggest that another factor, possibly infectious, may play a role in the appearance of cotton-wool patches.

More severe retinal vascular alterations occur in some patients who may develop central or branch retinal vein occlusions or arteriolar occlusions (57) (Fig. 1). Anterior ischemic optic neuropathy has been reported (11).

OPPORTUNISTIC INFECTIONS

CMV Retinitis

CMV is the most important opportunistic infection of the eye in HIV infection both in frequency and as a source of visual morbidity. Numerous comprehensive reviews and clinical trial data have been published (38,45,58,112).

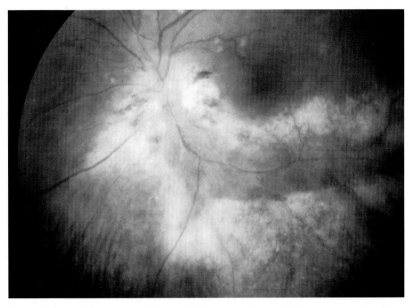

FIG. 2. Granular, superficial, necrotizing retinitis involving the inferotemporal arcade and optic nerve. Such an appearance is typical for CMV retinitis in the posterior pole and suggests that long sections of retinal vascular endothelium may become infected with virus, which then spreads into contiguous retina in the typical brush-fire pattern. Small, round patches of CMV retinitis that are not associated with major vessels may indicate infection of smaller caliber vessels.

Spread into the eye is presumed to be along blood vessels (Fig. 2). Damage to the endothelium by intravascular HIV or human herpesvirus 6 infection may predispose to retinal infection with CMV during periods of CMV viremia (95). At autopsy, intraocular infection was always accompanied by extraocular CMV infection, and evidence of extraocular disease occurred about two times more commonly than CMV retinitis in one study before effective antiviral treatment for CMV (90). However, infection of the brain by CMV is probably less common than CMV retinitis. In an autopsy series of HIV-infected patients, eight of 31 had CMV retinitis, but only three of the eight had evidence of cerebral cytomegalic inclusion bodies and subacute encephalitis (46). A comparison of findings at autopsy in the eyes and brains of 18 HIV-infected patients showed a similar pattern of infection, with histopathological evidence of CMV infection in the eyes of eight patients of whom two also had both CMV encephalitis and visceral involvement (21). One each had CMV retinitis with either encephalitis or visceral involvement, but not both, and two patients had CMV encephalitis without retinitis.

The clinical significance of these findings is less clear. Clinically manifested disease due to cerebral or visceral involvement with CMV is less common than CMV retinitis, due either to a predilection for the eye or to the prominent awareness of impairment in vision. A prospective study to determine characteristics associated with the emergence of CMV disease in 1,009 patients followed for a median of 600 days showed that 93 patients developed CMV retinitis compared with 20 cases of gastrointestinal disease and one case of biopsy-proven encephalitis (35). Patients with homosexual risk factors were more likely to develop CMV disease, as were those already diagnosed with AIDS and those with CD4+ counts of <100 cells/ mm^3. It is unknown whether untreated (or uncontrolled) CMV retinitis predisposes to spread of infection to other organs including the brain. CMV encephalitis may occur despite treatment with antiviral medicines for CMV retinitis (104). Similarly, the importance of treating CMV systemically when only the eye has clinically significant disease is unclear. Development of effective local (intraocular) therapy for the control of CMV retinitis would permit clinical trials to determine the relative risks and benefits of systemic treatment of CMV in patients with symptomatic eye disease but no other signs of disease (1,74,102). Local therapy with the intravitreal ganciclovir device may prove to be more efficacious than intravenous treatment because higher intravitreal drug levels are achieved (74).

Standard treatment for CMV retinitis currently involves intravenously administered ganciclovir or foscarnet on a daily basis for life. Based on protocols developed for clinical trials, retinitis progression is defined as movement of the retinitis border by 750 μm along at least a 750-μm span (112). Retinitis progression or new lesions are a trigger for reinduction with higher drug levels for 2 weeks, usually followed by a higher daily maintenance level, although the labelling for ganciclovir does not acknowledge higher doses than 5 mg/kg/day as safe, and the toxicity of foscarnet generally prohibits its use at >120 mg/kg/day. The drugs appear to be equivalent in their efficacy in controlling retinitis, which in both cases is quite poor, with median time to retinitis progression of ~60 days for both (113). A survival advantage may exist for patients who take foscarnet rather than ganciclovir (112), possibly because of its weak anti-HIV effect.

Despite inexorable, slow progression (53), central visual acuity is preserved in most patients, although peripheral field loss may occur (113). Patients with lower CD4+ counts at initiation of treatment have a greater risk of visual loss (113). Severe visual loss may occur when the optic nerve is involved. Among 10 cases of cytomegalic papillitis, those associated with limited retinitis contiguous with the papilla tended to do well visually, whereas those with isolated, primary cytomegalic papillitis did poorly despite treatment with intravenous ganciclovir (39). Treatment of cytomegalic papillitis with retrobulbar corticosteroids and intravitreal ganciclovir in addition to standard intravenous antiviral therapy may improve visual outcome (117).

Noncytomegalic Necrotizing Herpetic Retinitis

Varicella zoster virus and herpes simplex virus may cause a rapidly progressive necrotizing retinitis that differs from CMV retinitis in that it appears to affect the deeper layers of the retina initially and quickly spreads to form a confluent, full-thickness necrosis with a high rate of bilaterality, retinal detachment, and vision loss (24,25,31). It develops in at least 10% of patients with herpes zoster ophthalmicus who are infected with HIV (106). Herpes zoster ophthalmicus in a person <50 years of age should increase the suspicion of HIV infection and also merits surveillance for the development of potentially blinding posterior segment disease (62,106). Acyclovir appears to be poorly effective for the control of necrotizing herpetic retinitis (25). Alternative antiviral regimens with combinations of foscarnet, ganciclovir, and intravitreal injections of ganciclovir may provide better control of the retinitis. It is known from animal models of herpes simplex retinitis that the virus probably spreads from one eye to the other via the visual pathways, including the optic nerves and Edinger-Westphal nucleus (118). Histological evidence of spread of varicella zoster via synaptic connections throughout the visual pathways to the occipital lobes was also documented in one HIV-infected patient who died with bilateral necrotizing herpetic retinitis and varicella encephalitis (100). In contrast to CMV retinitis, necrotizing herpetic retinitis seems likely to spread to the CNS (Fig. 3). Prolonged treatment with effective antiviral agents may be indicated even if vision is destroyed by the retinitis. Optimal therapy for herpetic encephalitis or meningitis in HIV infection is not clear. By analogy to the treatment failures seen in retinitis (25), acyclovir may not be adequate, particularly if given orally.

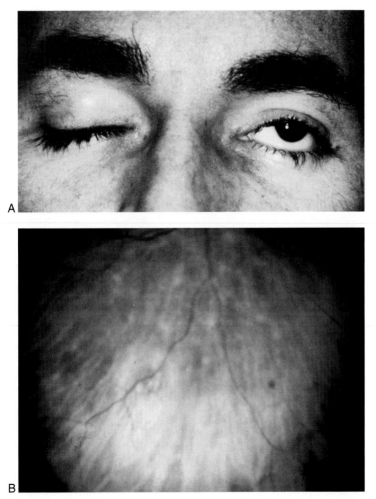

FIG. 3. A: This 35-year-old man with HIV infection presented with sudden total loss of vision in the left eye, decreased hearing on the left, and a prior Bell's palsy interpreted as a Ramsey-Hunt syndrome from varicella zoster infection. Photo was taken on attempted lid closure. **B:** Examination showed bilateral, confluent, necrotizing retinitis. The ground-glass appearance, rapid progression, and lack of scarring is atypical for CMV retinitis. Vision loss in the left eye was attributed to retrobulbar neuritis. Intensive antiviral therapy with intravenous ganciclovir and foscarnet and intravitreal ganciclovir was initiated, but vision did not improve in the left eye. Vision was ultimately lost in the right eye from a hemorrhagic retinal detachment.

Toxoplasmic Chorioretinitis

Toxoplasmosis is a relatively uncommon cause of necrotizing retinitis in AIDS and is definitely less common than intracranial infection with toxoplasmosis. In a series of 445 HIV-infected Brazilians, there was a 25% prevalence of CMV retinitis, 22% had cerebral toxoplasmosis, and only 8.5% had evidence of toxoplasmic chorioretinitis (80). In Australia, 39 cases of cerebral toxoplasmosis yielded only two cases of ocular toxoplasmosis (110). In a series of autopsies in France, where toxoplasmosis is also common, 11 of 25 subjects had cerebral toxoplasmosis but no eye infections were found (21). The presence of ocular toxoplasmosis suggests a high risk of cerebral toxoplasmosis. In one series, 29% of ocular toxoplasmosis cases (13 of 45 patients) were concurrently diagnosed with cerebral toxoplasmosis (17). Neuroimaging studies are probably indicated in patients with AIDS who present with ocular toxoplasmosis.

Clinical aspects of ocular toxoplasmosis in AIDS may differ from the disease in immunocompetent patients. Bilateral or multifocal infection appears to be more common, and anterior segment and vitreous inflammatory reactions may be less intense (10,17,50). Active areas of retinochoroiditis may appear in areas of the fundus where there is no preexisting chorioretinal scar (50) (Fig. 4). Fulminant infections with widespread areas of retinal necrosis have been reported (10,34,41,44,88). This form of infection is most likely to be confused with CMV retinitis or other necrotizing herpetic retinitis. Uncontrolled infection may lead to orbital cellulitis, panophthalmitis, and papillitis (41,78). Unlike other types of necrotizing retinitis, severe toxoplasmic infection may produce ocular pain. Isolated toxoplasmic papillitis has been

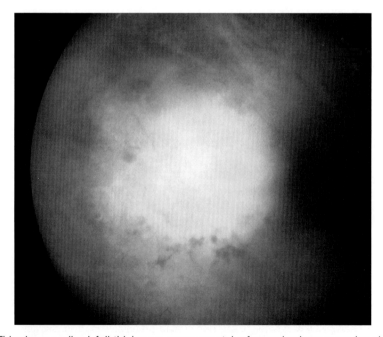

FIG. 4. This circumscribed, full-thickness, opaque patch of very slowly progressive chorioretinitis with overlying vitreous inflammatory reaction is typical of toxoplasmic chorioretinitis. Diagnosis was delayed because of knowledge of the patient's HIV status with suspicion of viral retinitis and because no typical preexisting chorioretinal scar was present.

reported as the presenting manifestation of HIV infection (27). Iridocyclitis presumed due to toxoplasmic cysts in the iris may occur in the absence of toxoplasmic retino-choroiditis (96).

Treatment with conventional antitoxoplasmosis agents such as pyrimethamine combined with sulfadiazine or clindamycin is generally effective in healing the reti-nochoroiditis (17,34,49). Relapse may occur despite continued low-dose maintenance therapy in 20% (17). Trimethoprim-sulfamethoxazole, tetracyclines, or atovaquone (82) are alternatives for patients who are intolerant or do not respond to standard regimens or may be useful to maintain remission.

Syphilis

Although syphilitic uveitis is relatively rare among patients with AIDS (0.6% in one series [80]), it is a common manifestation of secondary or tertiary treponemal disease. Serological evidence of past disease may be considerably more common; in one series in which 61 patients were tested, 26 had positive rapid plasma reagin titers (73). Six of 11 patients in a recent series of neurosyphilis presented with ocular manifestations, most typically uveitis, although one patient presented with a retinitis (37). Half of the patients who presented with eye findings also had mucocutaneous manifestations such as rash or alopecia, although rash was less common in another large series (4). CNS involvement has been common in patients who present with syphilitic uveitis, retinitis, or optic neuritis (4,77). Syphilitic uveitis should be consid-ered an indication for HIV testing: among the 17 of 25 patients with syphilitic uveitis who agreed to HIV testing, 12 were found to be HIV positive (71%) (4). This is higher than the rate of HIV positivity (23%) found in a case-control study of patients presenting with syphilis and may account for the tendency for more HIV-positive patients to present with secondary syphilis (56). Although seronegative cases have been reported (42,47,77,89), serological testing appears to be highly reliable as a means of identifying syphilitic uveitis (4).

Severity of syphilitic uveitis is increased in HIV-infected patients (4). Of 12 pa-tients with syphilitic uveitis, 11 were bilateral, four had optic neuropathies, four had disk edema, three had neuroretinitis, and two had branch retinal vein occlusions (4). Syphilitic perineuritis or swelling of the optic disk may occur with or without marked visual disturbance and resolve slowly after treatment is initiated (14,116). Poor vision or visual field defects persist in some cases (66,89). Optic disk edema with visual loss may also rarely occur secondary to solid gumma (syphiloma) in the anterior optic nerve sheath (109). Retrobulbar optic neuritis with sudden loss of vision, includ-ing bilateral blindness, has been reported (120,121).

HIV infection probably makes syphilis more difficult to treat and leads to failure of standard treatment regimens (81). Penicillin G benzathine treatment has failed in several cases to prevent progression to ocular or neurological disease (6,37,54,77).

Recurrence of panuveitis 1 year after treatment with 10 days of intravenous penicil-lin (24 million U/day) has been reported (4). Meningeal involvement with pleocytosis and cranial nerve palsies may occur with uveitis and meningovascular disease mani-festing as strokelike events. Gumma may form early in the disease despite the relative impairment in cell-mediated immunity (54,109).

Cryptococcosis

Infection with *Cryptococcus neoformans* occurs in ~7% of patients with AIDS (16,59), causes a substantial portion of neurological disease (70) and is often the presenting opportunistic infection (16,63). One series in San Francisco reported 16 of 128 (12.5%) neurologically symptomatic patients to have cryptococcal disease, second only to toxoplasmosis (70). Cryptococcal disease is probably even more common in Africa. The largest series of ophthalmic manifestations of cryptococcosis is from Kigali, Rwanda (63). Sixty-one of 80 (76%) HIV-infected patients with cryptococcal disease had abnormal eye examinations. Papilledema was the most common finding (25 patients, 31%), followed by decreased visual acuity, and abducens nerve palsy, seven patients (9%) each. This rate of neuroophthalmic findings was similar to that in a smaller study in the United States (59). Optic atrophy, optic neuropathy, and cortical blindness caused severe visual loss in six patients, in four of whom the loss was bilateral (63). Lesser degrees of optic nerve involvement also were found with marked disk edema with hemorrhages and nerve fiber layer infarcts in four patients (5%), moderate disk edema in six (7.5%), and blurred disk margins in 15 (19%). One patient had a chorioretinal granuloma thought to be a cryptococcoma.

The rates of papilledema and abducens palsy are similar to those in a series reported before AIDS (86), but the rate of severe visual loss was less than one half as much. Kestelyn et al. surmised that the relative lack of inflammatory response in HIV infection protected the nerve or that treatment was more prompt in HIV disease (63). Evidence suggests that severe visual loss in cryptococcal meningitis and encephalitis correlates with invasion of the visual pathways with cryptococci rather than with papilledema (67). Adhesive arachnoiditis from proliferation of cryptococci within the optic nerve sheath may cause papilledema with moderate to severe vision loss and abnormal visual fields (71); less severe degrees of involvement may respond to decompression of the optic nerve sheath (36). The cause of vision loss in individual cases may be difficult to determine clinically or with neuroimaging studies (71).

Chorioretinitis from hematogenous spread to intraocular tissue is much less common than optic nerve manifestations or cranial nerve palsies in both HIV-infected and non–HIV-infected patients (59,63,86). When it occurs, it is usually accompanied by signs of CNS involvement such as disk edema or cranial nerve palsies (13,99,119).

Tuberculosis

Chorioretinal lesions are uncommon. Miliary choroidal involvement has been reported in the last week of life of a patient with disseminated *Mycobacterium tuberculosis* infection (9). More typical multifocal choroiditis due to *M. tuberculosis* also has been reported (92). Skin tests for hypersensitivity to tubercular antigens may be negative (18). Although choroidal nodules due to infection with the atypical mycobacteria have been reported (90), recognition of clinically important disease due to these organisms is rare.

Other Infections

Papovavirus and *Mucor* are examples of opportunistic infections that may affect the visual system through involvement of the CNS without direct ocular involvement

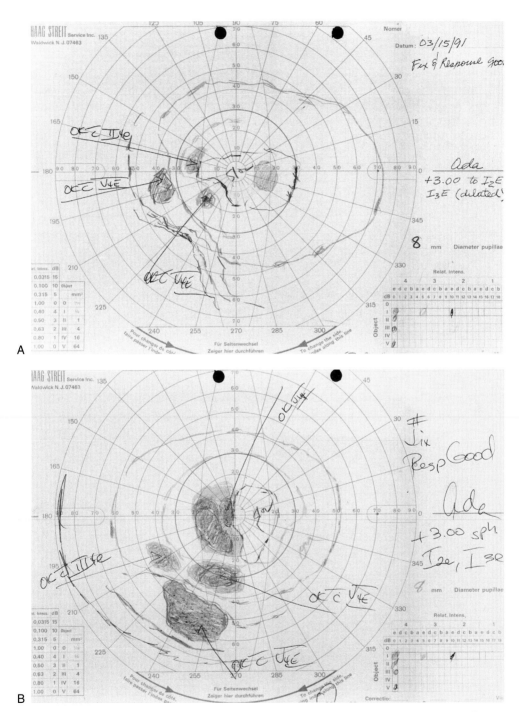

FIG. 5. A: This 40-year-old HIV-infected patient complained of poor vision and spots in front of his eyes. Vision was 20/20 and 20/25. The visual field of the right eye showed multiple scotomata. A CT scan of the brain was normal, but an MRI of the brain was consistent with PML. **B:** Visual field of the left eye showing multiple scotomata.

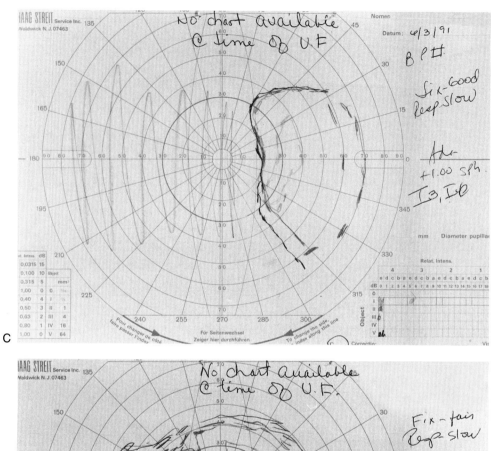

C

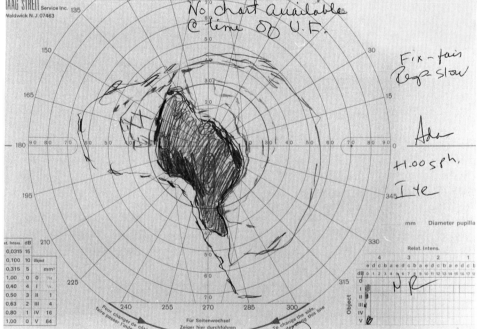

D

FIG. 5. *Continued.* **C:** Three months later there was progressive loss of visual field with mark-edly decreased acuity (see also **B**).

(7,19). Progressive multifocal leukoencephalopathy, papovavirus CNS infection commonly presents with visual confusion, simultagnosia, and Balint's syndrome (inability to gaze or scan in the peripheral visual field, failure of hand–eye coordination, and visual disorientation) (3) (Fig. 5).

NEOPLASMS

Lymphoma

Orbital or CNS lymphoma may produce cranial nerve palsies (60,87), papilledema, or multifocal intracranial, parenchymal mass lesions (87) (Fig. 6). The clinical manifestations and computed tomographic (CT) and magnetic resonance imaging (MRI) studies of CNS lymphoma and inflammatory lesions such as cerebral toxoplasmosis can be indistinguishable. Serological studies may be negative in >20% of cases of toxoplasmic encephalitis (94). Thallium-enhanced single-photon emission CT shows intense focal uptake in histologically confirmed CNS lymphoma, whereas toxoplasmic encephalitis, proven by response to antitoxoplasmosis treatment, shows no thallium uptake (101).

Intraocular non-Hodgkin's lymphoma has been described in only a small number of HIV-infected patients (48,76,105,111). Histologically, CNS lymphoma in HIV infection resembles that in nonimmunocompromised patients (69). Aspects of some case reports that differ from the involvement in non–HIV-infected patients (20,107)

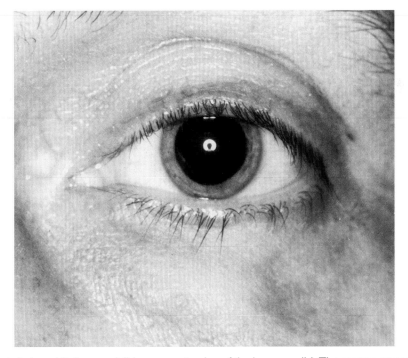

FIG. 6. Inferior orbital mass visible as a protrusion of the lower eyelid. The mass was confirmed by biopsy to be lymphoma. The patient did not complain of diplopia because the other eye was nonseeing from advanced CMV retinitis. Visual acuity in this eye was normal.

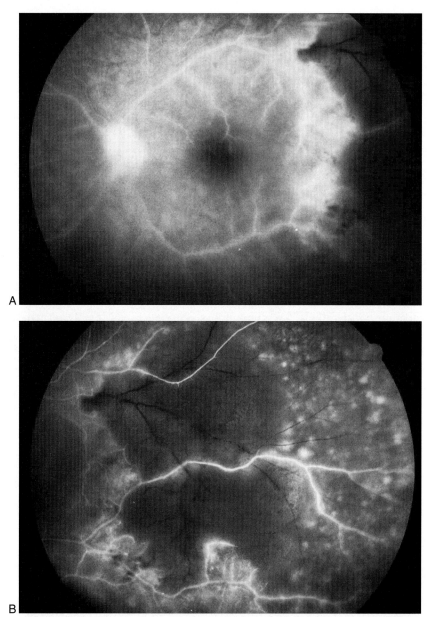

FIG. 7. A: This intraocular lymphoma was originally thought to be a viral retinitis. The late stages of a fluorescein angiogram are shown. The leaking vessels are sheathed with inflammatory material. **B:** Fluorescein angiography directly over the yellow–white lesion shows vascular occlusions over the lesion and late staining of the walls of the remaining patent vessels. The characteristic solid retinal pigment epithelial detachments are visible as mottled areas in the region of greatest nonperfusion. More peripherally, punctate staining is seen in the retinal pigment epithelium due to irregular infiltration by malignant lymphocytes. A large intracranial lymphomatous mass was diagnosed by neuroimaging studies and brain biopsy; the patient died ~6 weeks later. (From Duker J, Davis JL. Non-Hodgkin lymphoma of the posterior segment complicating human immunodeficiency virus (HIV) infection. *Ophthalmology* 1991;98(suppl): 112; with permission.)

are orbital extension with displacement of the globe (76) and very rapid growth (105). Bilateral ocular and concomitant brain involvement has been reported (111). Immunophenotyping showed large B cell lymphoma in one case (48); in general, most lymphomas in AIDS are B cell in origin (69,79).

Discriminating between opportunistic infection of the retina and lymphoma can be difficult because some lesions may have an appearance consistent with necrotizing retinitis (Fig. 7) (23). Concomitant retinal involvement with lymphoma and CMV has been reported (111). Treatment with radiation produces an initial response in brain lymphoma (30), but experience with radiation treatment for intraocular involvement in patients with AIDS is limited.

NEUROOPHTHALMIC MANIFESTATIONS

Table 1 displays the neuroophthalmic manifestations associated with common opportunistic infections in AIDS. Optic neuritis is commonly accompanied by retinitis or chorioretinitis but may be isolated. Other reported neuroophthalmological manifestations arise from CNS disorders without direct ocular involvement.

A small number of observational studies have been performed that show clinically significant neuroophthalmological findings to occur in ~7–8% of those with HIV infection. The largest series of 200 patients found cranial nerve palsy or motility

TABLE 1. *Neuroophthalmic manifestations of opportunistic infections in HIV disease*

Infection	Manifestation	References
CMV	Optic neuritis	39,40,73,83
	Retrobulbar neuritis	33
	Internuclear ophthalmoplegia	55
	Cranial nerve palsy	5,75
	Slowed saccades	75
Herpes simplex encephalitis	Parinaud's syndrome	65
Varicella-zoster	Optic neuritis	100,119
	Cortical blindness	100
	Cranial nerve palsy	87
Toxoplasmosis	Optic neuritis	50
	Papilledema	50,73,87
	Cranial nerve palsy	2,28,32,50,70,73
	Horner's syndrome	43
	Gaze palsy	43,73
	Visual field defect	73
Syphilis	Optic neuritis	14,66,89
	Perineuritis	119
	Retrobulbar neuritis	120,121
	Cranial nerve palsy	43
	Internuclear ophthalmoplegia	43
Cryptococcosis	Papilledema	73,87
	Perineuritis	71
	Photophobia	22
	Cranial nerve palsies	32,87
	Ocular dipping	97
	Cortical blindness	73
	Visual field defect	73
Tuberculosis	Cortical blindness	8
Papovavirus (PML)	Visual loss (field defects)	7,108
	Blindness	7
Mucormycosis	Gaze palsy	19

disturbance in 4%, optic neuropathy in 2.5%, and papilledema in 1.5% (59). The deficits were most commonly due to cryptococcosis. Ten of 127 patients (7.9%) had neuroophthalmic findings (73) and three of 40 (7.5%) had cranial nerve palsies (87) due to toxoplasmosis, cryptococcosis, or lymphoma in other, smaller series. Neurological manifestations appeared to be more common in advanced stages of AIDS because none of 50 patients with AIDS-related complex had any neuroophthalmic findings (73).

Neuroophthalmological disorders also may occur in the absence of any definite CNS infection or neoplasm. Some of these disorders may be degenerative or related in some unknown way to infection with the human immunodeficiency virus itself. Axonal loss averaged 40% in optic nerves from patients dying with AIDS who did not have opportunistic infections of the retina (114). Mean axonal diameters were not different from the mean diameters of axons from normal nerves, which was interpreted as evidence that no single class of axons was disproportionately affected. Sectoral nerve loss also was absent. The changes were therefore most similar to the loss of axons seen with normal aging. Decreased saccadic velocities (85) and motor slowing in visual scanning (29) have been reported. Impairment in saccadic eye movements detected by clinical examination has been suggested as one of a tetrad of neurological signs that foreshadow the development of AIDS dementia complex (115).

SUMMARY

Infectious diseases account for most of the visual system morbidity in HIV infection. Some infections preferentially affect the intraocular structures (e.g., CMV) whereas others more commonly cause intracranial disease (e.g., cryptococcus and toxoplasmosis). The intraocular features of disease are generally distinctive enough that diagnosis of the cause of a retinitis or chorioretinitis can be made on the basis of physical examination of the eye by an experienced ophthalmoscopist. CNS disease, in contrast, may cause similar neuroophthalmic manifestations for diseases as disparate as lymphoma and toxoplasmic encephalitis. Neuroimaging studies and invasive biopsy may be necessary to reach a satisfactory diagnosis. Retinal vasculopathy and neurodegenerative diseases do not have known infectious causes, although it has been proposed that they are the result of tissue infection with HIV itself.

Fundus examination should be conducted by an experienced ophthalmologist because the examination possible with a direct ophthalmoscope misses ~80% of the retinal surface area. Neuroophthalmic examination is useful to guide the subsequent diagnostic work-up in patients with visual complaints without fundus findings.

ACKNOWLEDGMENT

Dr. Norman Schatz provided valuable assistance in reviewing the manuscript.

REFERENCES

1. Anand R, Nightingale SD, Fish RH, Smith TJ, Ashton P. Control of cytomegalovirus retinitis using sustained release of intraocular ganciclovir. *Arch Ophthalmol* 1993;111:223–227.

2. Antworth MV, Beck RW. Third nerve palsy as a presenting sign of acquired immune deficiency syndrome. *J Clin Neuroophthalmol* 1987;7:125.
3. Ayuso-Peralta L, Jiménez-Jiménez FJ, Tejeiro J, et al. Progressive multifocal leukoencephalopathy in HIV infection presenting as Balint's syndrome. *Neurology* 1994;44:1339–1340.
4. Becerra LI, Ksiazek SM, Savino PJ, et al. Syphilitic uveitis in human immunodeficiency virus-infected and noninfected patients. *Ophthalmology* 1989;96:1727–1730.
5. Behar R, Wiley C, McCutchan JA. Cytomegalovirus polyradiculoneuropathy in acquired immune deficiency syndrome. *Neurology* 1987;37:557–561.
6. Berger JR. Neurosyphilis in human immundeficiency virus type 1–seropositive individuals. A prospective study. *Arch Neurol* 1991;48:700–702.
7. Berger JR, Kaszovitz B, Post MJD, Dickinson G. Progressive multifocal leukoencephalopathy associated with human immunodeficiency virus infection. *Ann Int Med* 1987;107:78–87.
8. Bishburg E, Sunderam G, Reichman LB, Kapila R. Central nervous system tuberculosis with the acquired immunodeficiency syndrome and its related complex. *Ann Int Med* 1986;105:210–213.
9. Blodi BA, Johnson MW, McLeish WM, Gass JD. Presumed choroidal tuberculosis in a human immunodeficiency virus infected host. *Am J Ophthalmol* 1989;108:605–607.
10. Bottoni F, Gonnella P, Autelitano A, Orzalesi N. Diffuse necrotizing retinochoroiditis in a child with AIDS and toxoplasmic encephalitis. *Graefes Arch Clin Exp Ophthalmol* 1990;228:36–39.
11. Brack MJ, Cleland PG, Owen RI, Allen ED. Anterior ischaemic optic neuropathy in the acquired immune deficiency syndrome. *Br Med J [Clin Res]* 1987;295:696–697.
12. Brodie SE, Friedman AH. Retinal dysfunction as an initial ophthalmic sign in AIDS. *Br J Ophthalmol* 1990;74:49–51.
13. Carney MD, Combs JL, Waschler W. Cryptococcal choroiditis. *Retina* 1990;10:27–32.
14. Carter JB, Hamill RJ, Matoba AY. Bilateral syphilitic optic neuritis in a patient with a positive test for HIV. *Arch Ophthalmol* 1987;105:1485–1486.
15. Cellini M, Baldi A. Vitreous fluorophotometric recordings in HIV infection. *Int Ophthalmol* 1991; 15:37–40.
16. Chuck SL, Sande MA. Infections with *Cryptococcus neoformans* in the acquired immunodeficiency syndrome. *N Engl J Med* 1989;321:794–799.
17. Cochereau-Massin I, LeHoang P, Lautier-Frau M, et al. Ocular toxoplasmosis in human immunodeficiency virus–infected patients. *Am J Ophthalmol* 1992;114:130–135.
18. Croxatto JO, Mestre C, Puente S, Gonzalez G. Nonreactive tuberculosis in a patient with acquired immune deficiency syndrome. *Am J Ophthalmol* 1986;10.
19. Cuadrado LM, Guerrero A, Garcia Asenjo JAL, Martin F, Palau E, Garcia Urra D. Cerebral mucomycosis in two cases of acquired immunodeficiency syndrome. *Arch Neurol* 1988;45:109–111.
20. DeAngelis LM, Yahalom J, Heinemann MH, Cirrincione C, Thaler HT, Krol G. Primary CNS lymphoma: combined treatment with chemotherapy and radiotherapy. *Neurology* 1990;40:80–86.
21. DeGirolami U, Hénin D, Girard B, Katlama C, LeHoang P, Hauw JJ. Étude pathologique de 1 oeil et du systéme nerveux central dans 25 case de SIDA. *Rev Neurol (Paris)* 1989;145:819–828.
22. Dismukes WE. Cryptococcal meningitis in patients with AIDS. *J Infect Dis* 1988;157:624–628.
23. Duker J, Davis JL. Non-Hodgkin lymphoma of the posterior segment complicating human immunodeficiency virus (HIV) infection. *Ophthalmology* 1991;98(suppl):112.
24. Duker JS, Nielsen JC, Eagle RCJ, Bosley TM, Granadier R, Benson WE. Rapidly progressive acute retinal necrosis secondary to herpes simplex virus, type 1. *Ophthalmology* 1990;97:1638–1643.
25. Engstrom RE, Holland GN, Margolis TP, et al. The progressive outer retinal necrosis syndrome. A variant of necrotizing herpetic retinopathy in patients with AIDS. *Ophthalmology* 1994;101: 1488–1502.
26. Engstrom REJ, Holland GN, Hardy WD, Meiselman HJ. Hemorrheological abnormalities in patients with human immunodeficiency virus infection and ophthalmic microvasculopathy. *Am J Ophthalmol* 1990;109:153–161.
27. Falcone PM, Notis C, Merhige K. Toxoplasmic papillitis as the initial manifestation of acquired immunodeficiency syndrome. *Ann Ophthalmol* 1993;25:56–57.
28. Farkash AE, Maccabee PJ, Sher JH, Landesman SH, Hotson G. CNS toxoplasmosis in acquired immune deficiency syndrome: a clinical–pathological–radiological review of 12 cases. *J Neurol Neurosurg Psych* 1986;49:744–748.
29. Fitzgibbon ML, Cella DF, Humfleet G, Griffin E, Sheridan K. Motor slowing in asymptomatic HIV infection. *Percept Mot Skills* 1989;68:1331–1338.
30. Formenti SC, Gill PS, Lean E, et al. Primary central nervous system lymphoma in AIDS. Results of radiation therapy. *Cancer* 1989;15:1101–1107.
31. Forster DJ, Dugel PU, Frangieh GT, Liggett PE, Rao NA. Rapidly progressive outer retinal necrosis in the acquired immunodeficiency syndrome. *Am J Ophthalmol* 1990;110:341–348.
32. Freeman WR, Lerner CW, Mines JA, et al. A prospective study of the ophthalmological findings in the acquired immune deficiency syndrome. *Am J Ophthalmol* 1984;97:133–142.
33. Friedman AH. The retinal lesions of the acquired immune deficiency syndrome. *Trans Am Ophthalmol Soc* 1984;82:447–491.

34. Gagliuso DJ, Teich SA, Friedman AH, Orellana J. Ocular toxoplasmosis in AIDS patients. *Trans Am Ophthalmol Soc* 1990;88:63–86.
35. Gallant JE, Moore RD, Richman DD, Keruly J, Chaisson RE. Incidence and natural history of cytomegalovirus disease in patients with advanced human immunodeficiency virus disease treated with zidovudine. The Zidovudine Epidemiology Study Group. *J Infect Dis* 1992;166:1223–1227.
36. Garrity JA, Herman DC, Imes R, Fries P, Hughes CF, Campbell RJ. Optic nerve sheath decompression for visual loss in patients with acquired immunodeficiency syndrome and cryptococcal meningitis with papilledema. *Am J Ophthalmol* 1993;116:472–478.
37. Gordon SM, Eaton ME, George R, et al. The response of symptomatic neurosyphilis to high-dose intravenous penicillin G in patients with human immunodeficiency virus infection. *N Engl J Med* 1994;331:1469–1473.
38. Gross JG, Bozzette SA, Mathews WC, et al. Longitudinal study of cytomegalovirus retinitis in acquired immune deficiency syndrome. *Ophthalmology* 1990;97:681–686.
39. Gross JG, Sadun AA, Wiley CA, Freeman WR. Severe visual loss related to isolated peripapillary retinal and optic nerve head cytomegalovirus infection. *Am J Ophthalmol* 1989;108:691–698.
40. Grossniklaus HE, Frank KE, Tomsak RL. Cytomegalovirus retinitis and optic neuritis in acquired immune deficiency syndrome. *Ophthalmology* 1987;94:1601–1604.
41. Grossniklaus HE, Specht CS, Allaire G, Leavitt JA. Toxoplasma gondii retinochoroiditis and optic neuritis in acquired immune deficiency syndrome. Report of a case. *Ophthalmology* 1990;97:1342–1346.
42. Halperin LS. Neuroretinitis due to seronegative syphilis associated with human immunodeficiency virus. *J Clin Neuroophthalmol* 1992;12:171–172.
43. Hamed LM, Schatz NJ, Galetta SL. Brainstem ocular motility defects and AIDS. *Am J Ophthalmol* 1988;106:437–442.
44. Heinemann MH, Gold JM, Maisel J. Bilateral toxoplasma retinochoroiditis in a patient with acquired immune deficiency syndrome. *Retina* 1986;6:224–227.
45. Henderly DE, Jampol LM. Diagnosis and treatment of cytomegalovirus retinitis. *J AIDS* 1991;4:S6–10.
46. Hénin D, Duyckaerts C, Chaunu MP, et al. Étude neuropathologique de 31 cas de syndrome d'immuno-dépression acquise. *Rev Neurol (Paris)* 1987;10:631–642.
47. Hicks CB, Benson PM, Lupton GP, Tramont EC. Seronegative secondary syphilis in a patient infected with the human immunodeficiency virus (HIV) with Kaposi sarcoma. *Ann Int Med* 1987;107:492–495.
48. Hofman P, Le Tourneau A, Negre F, Michiels JF, Diebold J. Primary uveal B immunoblastic lymphoma in a patient with AIDS. *Br J Ophthalmol* 1992;76:700–702.
49. Holland GN. Ocular toxoplasmosis in the immunocompromised host. *Int Ophthalmol* 1989;13:399–402.
50. Holland GN, Engstrom RJ, Glasgow BJ, et al. Ocular toxoplasmosis in patients with the acquired immunodeficiency syndrome. *Am J Ophthalmol* 1988;106:653–667.
51. Holland GN, Gottlieb MS, Yee RD, Schanker HM, Pettet TH. Ocular disorders associated with a new severe acquired cellular immunodeficiency syndrome. *Am J Ophthalmol* 1982;93:393–402.
52. Holland GN, Pepose JS, Pettit TH, Gottlieb MS, Yee RD, Foos RY. Acquired immune deficiency syndrome. Ocular manifestations. *Ophthalmology* 1983;90:859–873.
53. Holland GN, Shuler JD. Progression rates of cytomegalovirus retinopathy in ganciclovir-treated and untreated patients. *Arch Ophthalmol* 1992;110:1435–1442.
54. Horowitz HW, Valsamis MP, Wicher V, et al. Brief report: cerebral syphilitic gumma confirmed by the polymerase chain reaction in a man with human immunodeficiency virus infection. *N Engl J Med* 1994;331:1488–1491.
55. Humphry RC, Weber JN, Marsh RJ. Ophthalmic findings in a group of ambulatory patients infected by human immunodeficiency vius (HIV): a prospective study. *Br J Ophthalmol* 1987;71:565–569.
56. Hutchinson CM, Hook EW, Shepherd Mr, Verley J, Rompalo AM. Altered clinical presentation of early syphilis in patients with human immunodeficiency virus infection. *Ann Intern Med* 1994;121:94–100.
57. Ismail Y, Nemechek PM, Arsura EL. A rare cause of visual loss in AIDS patients: central retinal vein occlusion. *Br J Ophthalmol* 1993;77:600–601.
58. Jabs DA, Enger C, Bartlett JG. Cytomegalovirus retinitis and acquired immunodeficiency syndrome. *Arch Ophthalmol* 1989;107:75–80.
59. Jabs DA, Green WR, Fox R, Polk BF, Bartlett JG. Ocular manifestations of acquired immune deficiency syndrome. *Ophthalmology* 1989;96:1092–1099.
60. Jack MK, Smith T, Collier AC. Oculomotor cranial nerve palsey associated with acquired immunodeficiency syndrome. *Ann Ophthalmol* 1984;16:460–462.
61. Jacobson MA, O Donnell JJ, Porteous D, Brodie HR, Feigal D, Mills J. Retinal and gastrointestinal disease due to cytomegalovirus in patients with the acquired immune deficiency syndrome: prevalence, natural history, and response to ganciclovir therapy. *Q J Med* 1988;67:473–486.

62. Kestelyn P, Stevens AM, Bakkers E, Rouvroy D, VandePerre P. Severe herpes zoster ophthalmicus in young African adults: a marker for HTLV-III seropositivity. *Br J Ophthalmol* 1987;71:806–809.

63. Kestelyn P, Taelman H, Bogaerts J, et al. Ophthalmic manifestations of infections with cryptococcus neoformans in patients with the acquired immunodeficiency syndrome. *Am J Ophthalmol* 1993;116: 721–727.

64. Kestelyn P, VandePerre P, Dominique R, et al. A prospective study of the ophthalmological findings in the acquired immune deficiency syndrome in Africa. *Am J Ophthalmol* 1985;100:230–238.

65. Khadem M, Kalish SB, Goldsmith J, et al. Ophthalmological findings in acquired immune deficiency syndrome (AIDS). *Arch Ophthalmol* 1984;102:201–206.

66. Kleiner RC, Najarian L, Levenson J, Kaplan HJ. AIDS complicated by syphilis can mimic uveitis and Crohn's disease. Case report. *Arch Ophthalmol* 1987;105:1486–1487.

67. Kupfer C, McCrane E. A possible cause of decreased vision in cryptococcal meningitis. *Invest Ophthalmol* 1974;13:801–804.

68. Kuppermann BD, Petty JG, Richman DD, et al. Correlation between CD4 + counts and prevalence of cytomegalovirus retinitis and human immunodeficiency virus–related noninfectious retinal vasculopathy in patients with acquired immunodeficiency syndrome. *Am J Ophthalmol* 1993;115: 575–582.

69. Levine AM, Gill PS. AIDS-related malignant lymphoma: clinical presentation and treatment approaches. *Oncology* 1987;4:41–46.

70. Levy RM, Bredesen DE, Rosenblum ML. Neurological manifestations of the acquired immunodeficiency syndrome (AIDS): experience at UCSF and review of the literature. *J Neurosurg* 1985;62: 475–495.

71. Lipson BK, Freeman WR, Beniz J, et al. Optic neuropathy associated with cryptococcal arachnoiditis in AIDS patients. *Am J Ophthalmol* 1989;107:523–527.

72. Mansour AH, Rodenko G, Dutt R. Half-life of cotton-wool spots in the acquired immunodeficiency syndrome. *Int J STD AIDS* 1990;1:132–133.

73. Mansour AM. Neuro-ophthalmic findings in acquired immunodeficiency syndrome. *J Clin Neuro Ophthalmol* 1990;10:167–174.

74. Martin DF, Parks DJ, Mellow SD, et al. Treatment of cytomegalovirus retinitis with an intraocular sustained-release ganciclovir implant. *Arch Ophthalmol* 1994;112:1531–1539.

75. Masdeu JC, Small CB, Weiss L, Elkin CM, Llena J, Mesa-Tejada R. Multifocal cytomegalovirus encephalitis in AIDS. *Ann Neurol* 1988;23:97–99.

76. Matzkin DC, Slamovits TL, Rosenbaum PS. Simultaneous intraocular and orbital non-Hodgkin lymphoma in the acquired immune deficiency syndrome. *Ophthalmology* 1994;101:850–855.

77. McLeish WM, Pulido JS, Holland S, Culbertson WW, Winward K. The ocular manifestations of syphilis in the human immunodeficiency virus type 1–infected host. *Ophthalmology* 1990;97: 196–203.

78. Moorthy RS, Smith RE, Rao NA. Progressive ocular toxoplasmosis in patients with acquired immunodeficiency syndrome. *Am J Ophthalmol* 1993;115:742–747.

79. Morgello S, Petito CK, Mouradian JA. Central nervous system lymphoma in the acquired immunodeficiency syndrome. *Clin Neuropathol* 1990;9:205–215.

80. Muccioli C, Lottenberg C, Lima J, Santos P, Kim M, Belfort R. Ophthalmological aspects of 445 HIV infected patients Sao Paulo, Brazil. *International Conference on AIDS* 1993;9:413.

81. Musher DM, Hamill RJ, Baughn RE. Effect of human immunodeficiency virus (HIV) infection on the course of syphilis and on the response to treatment. *Ann Intern Med* 1990;113:872–881.

82. Mutsch A, Klauss V, Muller-Lissner S, Rommel F. Ocular and cerebral toxoplasmosis in an AIDS-patient treatment with atovoquone (BW566C80). *International Conference on AIDS* 1993;9:386.

83. Neuwirth J, Gutman I, Hofeldt AJ, et al. Cytomegalovirus retinitis in a young homosexual male with acquired immunodeficiency. *Ophthalmology* 1982;89:805–808.

84. Newsome DA, Green WR, Miller ED, et al. Microvascular aspects of acquired immune deficiency syndrome retinopathy. *Am J Ophthalmol* 1984;98:590–601.

85. Nguyen N, Rimmer S, Katz B. Slowed saccades in the acquired immunodeficiency syndrome. *Am J Ophthalmol* 1989;107:356–360.

86. Okun E, Butler WT. Ophthalmological complications of cryptococcal meningitis. *Arch Ophthalmol* 1964;71:52–57.

87. Palestine AG, Rodrigues MM, Macher AM, et al. Ophthalmic involvement in acquired immunodeficiency syundrome. *Ophthalmology* 1984;91:1092–1099.

88. Parke DW, Font RL. Diffuse toxoplasmic retinochoroiditis in a patient with AIDS. *Arch Ophthalmol* 1986;104:571–575.

89. Passo MS, Rosenbaum JT. Ocular syphilis in patients with human immunodeficiency virus infection. *Am J Ophthalmol* 1988;106:1–6.

90. Pepose JS, Holland GN, Nestor MS, Cochran AJ, Foos RY. Acquired immune deficiency syndrome. Pathogenic mechanisms of ocular disease. *Ophthalmology* 1985;92:472–484.

91. Pepose JS, Nestor MS, Holland GN, Cochran AJ, Foos RY. An analysis of retinal cotton-wool spots

and cytomegalovirus retinitis in the acquired immunodeficiency syndrome [letter]. *Am J Ophthalmol* 1983;95:118–120.

92. Perez Blazquez E, Montero Rodriguez M, Mendez Ramos MJ. Tuberculous choroiditis and acquired immunodeficiency syndrome. *Ann Ophthalmol* 1994;26:50–54.

93. Pomerantz RJ, Kuritzkes DR, de la Monte SM, et al. Infection of the retina by human immunodeficiency virus type I. *N Engl J Med* 1987;317:1643–1647.

94. Porter SB, Sande MA. Toxoplasmosis of the central nervous system in the acquired immunodeficiency syndrome. *N Engl J Med* 1993;23:1643–1648.

95. Qavi HB, Green MT, SeGall GK, Font RL. Demonstration of HIV-1 and HHV-6 in AIDS-associated retinitis. *Curr Eye Res* 1989;8:379–413.

96. Rehder JR, Burnier MBJ, Pavesio CE, et al. Acute unilateral toxoplasmic iridocyclitis in an AIDS patient. *Am J Ophthalmol* 1988;106:740–741.

97. Rehman F, Mehler MF. Reverse ocular dipping. *Neurology* 1988;38:506.

98. Rosenberg PR, Uliss AE, Friedland GH, Harris CA, Small CB, Klein RS. Acquired immunodeficiency syndrome: ophthalmic manifestations in ambulatory patients. *Ophthalmology* 1983;90: 874–878.

99. Rosenblatt MA, Cunningham C, Teich S, Friedman AH. Choroidal lesions in patients with AIDS. *Br J Ophthalmol* 1990;74:610–614.

100. Rostad SW, Olson K, McDougall J, Shaw CM, Alvord EC. Transsynaptic spread of varicella zoster virus through the visual system: A mechanism of viral dissemination in the central nervous system. *Hum Pathol* 1989;20:174–179.

101. Ruiz A, Ganz WI, Post MJD, et al. Use of thallium-201 brain SPECT to differentiate cerebral lymphoma from toxoplasma encephalitis in AIDS patients. *Am J Neuroradiol* 1994;15:1885–1894.

102. Sanborn GE, Anand R, Torti RE, et al. Sustained-release ganciclovir therapy for treatment of cytomegalovirus retinitis. Use of an intravitreal device. *Arch Ophthalmol* 1992;110:188–195.

103. Schuman JS, Orellana J, Friedman AH, Teich SA. Acquired immunodeficiency syndrome (AIDS). *Surv Ophthalmol* 1987;31:384–410.

104. Schwarz TF, Loeschke K, Hanus I, Jäger G, Feiden W, Stefani FH. CMV encephalitis during ganciclovir therapy of CMV retinitis. *Infection* 1990;18:289–290.

105. Seerp Baarsma G, Roland Smit LM. Presumed intraocular lymphoma in a 60-year-old man with AIDS. *Eur J Ophthalmol* 1992;2:203–204.

106. Sellitti TP, Huang AJ, Schiffman J, Davis JL. Association of herpes zoster ophthalmicus with acquired immunodeficiency syndrome and acute retinal necrosis. *Am J Ophthalmol* 1993;116: 297–301.

107. Siegel MJ, Dalton J, Friedman AH, Strauchen J, Watson C. Ten-year experience with primary ocular reticulum cell sarcoma (large cell non-Hodgkin's lymphoma). *Br J Ophthalmol* 1989;73:342–346.

108. Slavin ML, Mallin JE, Jacob HS. Isolated homonymous hemianopsia in the acquired immunodeficiency syndrome. *Am J Ophthalmol* 1989;108:198–200.

109. Smith JL, Byrne SF, Cambron CR. Syphiloma/gumma of the optic nerve and human immunodeficiency virus seropositivity. *J Clin Neuro Ophthalmol* 1990;10:175–184.

110. Speirs G, Mirch AS, Lucas CR, Druce JD, Hayes K. CNS toxoplasmosis in AIDS: a clinical, pathological, serological and radiological review of 39 cases. *International Conference on AIDS* 1991;7:186.

111. Stanton CA, Sloan Bd, Slusher MM, Greven CM. Acquired immunodeficiency syndrome–related primary intraocular lymphoma. *Arch Ophthalmol* 1992;110:1614–1617.

112. Studies of the Ocular Complications of AIDS Research Group. Mortality in patients with the acquired immunodeficiency syndrome treated with either foscarnet or ganciclovir for cytomegalovirus retinitis. *N Engl J Med* 1992;326:213–220.

113. Studies of the Ocular Complications of AIDS Research Group. Foscarnet–ganciclovir cytomegalovirus retinitis trial. 4. Visual outcomes. *Ophthalmology* 1994;101:1250–1261.

114. Tenhula WN, Xu S, Madigan MC, Heller K, Freeman WR, Sadun AA. Morphometric comparisons of optic nerve axon loss in acquired immunodeficiency syndrome. *Am J Ophthalmol* 1992;113: 14–20.

115. Teschke RS. A tetrad of neurological signs sensitive to early human immunodeficiency virus brain disease [Letter]. *Arch Neurol* 1987;44:693.

116. Toshniwal P. Optic perineuritis with secondary syphilis. *J Clin Neuroophthalmol* 1987;7:6–10.

117. Ussery Fd, Gibson SR, Conklin RH, Piot DF, Stool EW, Conklin AJ. Intravitreal ganciclovir in the treatment of AIDS-associated cytomegalovirus retinitis. *Ophthalmology* 1988;95:640–648.

118. Vann VR, Atherton SS. Neural spread of herpes simplex virus after anterior chamber inoculation. *Invest Ophthalmol Vis Sci* 1991;32:2462–2472.

119. Winward KE, Hamed LM, Glaser JS. The spectrum of optic nerve disease in human immunodeficiency virus infection. *Am J Ophthalmol* 1989;107:373–380.

120. Zaidman GW. Neurosyphilis and retrobulbar neuritis in a patient with AIDS. *Ann Ophthalmol* 1986; 18:260–261.

121. Zambrano W, Perez GM, Smith JL. Acute syphilitic blindness in AIDS. *J Clin Neuro Ophthalmol* 1987;7:1–5.

AIDS and the Nervous System, Second Edition,
edited by J. R. Berger and R. M. Levy.
Lippincott-Raven Publishers, Philadelphia © 1997.

15

Neuropsychological Changes in Human Immunodeficiency Virus Infection

[°†§]Frederick A. Schmitt, [°†]Mary M.C. Wetherby, and [‡]Yaakov Stern

[°†]*Departments of Neurology,* [§]*Psychiatry, and Psychology,* [†]*Sanders-Brown Center on Aging, University of Kentucky Medical Center, Lexington, Kentucky 40536–4337; and* [‡]*Departments of Neurology and Psychiatry, College of Physicians and Surgeons, Columbia University, Presbyterian Hospital, Sergievsky Center, New York, New York 10032*

When acquired immunodeficiency syndrome (AIDS) was first identified, clinical and basic research centered on the host of opportunistic infections associated with this disease. Given the progressive and fatal suppression of the immune system caused by human immunodeficiency virus (HIV) infection of T-4 helper cells, pathological and radiological investigations focused on the identification of opportunistic infections of the central nervous system (CNS). Although many patients acquired *Pneumocystis carinii* pneumonia, Kaposi's sarcoma, and other opportunistic infections, several patients infected with HIV described mental slowing and other generalized cognitive deficits as their primary presenting symptoms.

Early reports of changes in mentation focused on both seropositive individuals who were asymptomatic for other opportunistic infections as well as those with more obvious symptoms of HIV disease. This work resulted in the recognition that neurological changes, particularly cognitive dysfunction, could be a defining feature of AIDS. The U.S. Centers for Disease Control and Prevention (CDC) (7) criteria consider the presence of dementia sufficient for the diagnosis of AIDS in persons who are HIV positive. HIV is found in the CNS, including within the cerebrospinal fluid (CSF) and the brain. A good deal of data have suggested that the impact of HIV on the CNS may be the result of neurotoxic factors linked either directly to the virus or to infected macrophages (15) (see Chapter 4 for reviews).

Since the initial recognition of cognitive changes in persons who are HIV seropositive, neuropsychological research reports have documented changes in HIV-positive asymptomatic persons as well as in persons with more obvious symptoms of HIV infection. Navia and Price (39) have reported that up to 25% of patients with early HIV disease may present with neurological symptoms. Neurological symptoms also may appear before neuroradiological detection of HIV-related CNS processes (and often before other AIDS-related illnesses) in up to 10% of HIV infected individuals (28). Cognitive changes become more prevalent as HIV infection becomes more severe. For example, Saykin et al. (48) reported no statistically significant correlations between neuropsychological test data and magnetic resonance imaging (MRI) volumetric indices. However, their study population did show neuropsychological impairments (48). One might therefore hypothesize that changes in neurocognitive function may provide an early indicator of CNS involvement of HIV.

Neurobehavorial manifestations of HIV include both cognitive and affective changes. Given the recent and fairly comprehensive compendium of the neuropsychiatric aspects of HIV disease (16), this review provides a brief summary of the cognitive effects and possible confounding variables that can lead to problems in interpreting cognitive changes in persons with HIV. Furthermore, this review will attempt to provide a brief chronological history of the early data that demonstrated changes in cognition in persons with HIV infection. More recent information regarding subtle changes in mentation is included, followed by a brief discussion of evolving areas of research. Although a comprehensive review of methodological issues and assessment procedures is beyond the scope of this review, Table 1 provides examples of several common measures used to track cognitive changes in HIV infection. For greater detail regarding these clinical and related research instruments, the reader is directed to texts by Lezak (29), Hannay (18), and Heilman and Valenstein (19). Pediatric HIV assessment approaches also recently have been reviewed by Brouwers et al. (5), and a review by Fennell (10) describes a newly developed and comprehensive National Institute of Mental Health–sponsored neurodevelopmental assessment battery that is currently being used in a study by the AIDS Clinical Trials Group (ACTG, protocol 188). Discussions of methodological issues associated with the evaluation of neuopsychological changes in adults and children with HIV infection can be found in articles by Bornstein (2), Van Gorp et al. (64), and Fletcher et al. (13).

Early Studies

One of the early reports involving neuropsychologic tests and HIV was presented by Grant et al. (15), who obtained MRI data as well as cognitive data from four small groups of homosexual men. These men were divided into categories of asymptomatic but seropositive, AIDS-related complex (ARC), and AIDS. The three groups were then compared with a small group of HIV-negative homosexual men with demographic characteristics similar to those of the persons who were seropositive. Neuropsychological performance data were based on blind clinical ratings and suggested that almost half of the HIV-positive asymptomatic patients exhibited neuropsychological abnormalities. Furthermore, the trend of impairment across the four groups showed a fairly low prevalence of impairment for the seronegative group (9%). The seropositive but asymptomatic patients showed a rate of impairment of approximately 44%. The more symptomatic patients showed a prevalence of impairment of >50% for ARC and 87% impairment for persons diagnosed with AIDS. Although these data suggested that neurocognitive deficits may occur in HIV-seropositive but asymptomatic individuals, the criteria for impairment were based on the existence of at least one test that was "definitely impaired" or two cognitive tests that were "probably impaired." This type of clinical rating might be considered a liberal definition of cognitive deficit (53). In addition, the investigators reported only a statistical trend for increased percentage of defective performance across groups, as opposed to significant differences between particular groups.

The suggestion of early neurocognitive abnormalities was seen as controversial and has served as a driving force for much of the subsequent neuropsychological

TABLE 1. *Examples of commonly used adult and pediatric procedures*

Test instrument	Domain/Use	Test battery	Patient activity
General			
Symbol Digit Modalities Test	Psychomotor speed, attention, concentration	MACS	Copy appropriate numbers according to a given symbol code in 90 s (trial 1); trial 2, orally repeat numbers to code
Digit Symbol (WAIS-R)	Same as above	ACTG/AAN	Copy symbols according to a given number code in 90 s
Trail Making Test (parts A & B)	Visual perceptual, attention, ability to switch mental sets	ACTG/MACS/AAN	Numbers and letters are connected in sequences (timed to completion, errors tallied)
Memory			
California Verbal Learning Test	Verbal memory/learning	AAN	Learning and recall of categorized words with immediate and delayed recall
Digital Span (WAIS-R or WMS-R)	Attention and immediate memory	MACS	Subject must remember increasingly lengthy sequences of numbers (both forward and backward recall)
Logical Memory (WMS)	Verbal memory/learning	AAN	Recall of a story tested immediately and after 30-min delay
Rey Auditory–Verbal Learning Test	Learning and memory for word lists	ACTG/AAN/MACS	Five learning/recall trials plus recall after a word interference list and 20-min delayed recall and recognition testing
Visual Reproduction (WMS)	Visual memory	AAN	Geometric designs presented with recall tested by redrawing design immediately and after 30-min delay
Language			
Vocabulary subtest (WAIS-R)	Premorbid IQ, language	ACTG/AAN	Give definitions of words
Animal Naming (fluency)	Language	AAN	Subject names as many animals as possible within a 1-min period
Boston Naming Test	Language	AAN	Subject names presented pictures
Controlled Oral Word Association Test	Language	MACS/AAN	Name as many words as possible beginning with a given letter in 1 min
Motor			
Timed gait	Motor functioning	ACTG	Walk a 10-yard distance as quickly as possible, both ways, while being timed
Grooved pegboard	Motor speed and manual dexterity	ACTG/MACS/AAN	Place pegs in board while being timed
Finger tapping	Motor functioning	ACTG/AAN	Multiple 10-s trials to tap with index finger (dominant and nondominant) as many times as possible

(continued)

TABLE 1. (*continued*)

Test instrument	Domain/Use	Test battery	Patient activity
Other functions			
Paced Auditory Serial Addition Test	Processing speed	AAN	Subject must add last 2 numbers in subsets of numbers rapidly presented at different intervals
Wisconsin Card Sorting Test	Abstraction, reasoning, problem solving	AAN	Rules must be deduced by correctly matching cards to four key cards with only "yes" or "no" clues from examiner
Halstead Category Test	Abstraction, reasoning, problem solving	AAN	Rules must be deduced in order to correctly respond to stimuli with only "correct" or "incorrect" feedback
Continuous Performance Test	Attention, concentration and vigilance	AAN	Key must be pushed on computer/apparatus when a specified target appears
Block Design (WAIS-R)	Visuospatial/ constructional praxis	AAN	Designs reproduced with colored/patterned blocks while timed
General			
Bayley Scales of Infant Development (Mental Scale)	Cognitive ability	Infant (to 42 mo on 2nd edition)	Specific behaviors (e.g., point to the doggie on the picture card) are scored
Stanford-Binet Intelligence Scale	Cognitive abilities (global)	School age	Vocabulary, bead memory, quantitative, memory for sentences, pattern analysis, comprehension
Wechsler Intelligence Scale for Children (WISC III)	Cognitive abilities (global)	11 mo to 16 yr 11 mo	Subtests consist of *Verbal* (Vocabulary, Comprehension, Arithmetic, Similarities, Information); *Performance* (Coding, Picture Arrangement, Block Design, Object Assembly, Picture Completion)
McCarthy Scales of Children's Abilities	Cognitive abilities (global) overall development	30 mo to 8 yr 6 mo	*Verbal Scale* (Pictorial Memory, Word Knowledge, Verbal Memory, Verbal Fluency, Opposite Analogue); *Perceptual-Performance Scale* (Block Building, Puzzle Solving, Tapping Sequence, Right-left Orientation, Draw-a-Design, Draw-a-Child, Conceptual Grouping); *Quantitative Scale* (Number Questions, Numerical Memory, Counting, and Sorting)
Achievement			
Woodcock-Johnson Tests of Achievement–Revised	Academic achievement	School age	*Letter-Word Identification:* Child reads presented letters & words. *Word Attack:* Child reads aloud letter combinations that are linguistically logical in English but that do not form actual words or are low-frequency words. *Passage Comprehension:* Child reads passage to him/herself and identifies a missing key word or picture.

Test	Construct	Age	Description
Memory			
Wide Range Assessment of Memory and Learning	Immediate recall and story memory	School age	*Verbal Learning:* Four learning/recall trials. *Story Memory:* Child repeats story previously read to him or her. Two stories.
Language			
Gardner Expressive One-Word Picture Vocabulary	Expressive single word vocabulary	School age	Using auditory and visual perceptions, the child is required to verbally identify a series of pictures
Gardner Receptive One-Word Picture Vocabulary	Receptive single word vocabulary	School age	The child identifies pictures that match words spoken by the examiner
Peabody Picture Vocabulary Test	Receptive single word vocabulary	School age	Child identifies a picture that matches a word spoken by the examiner
Motor			
Bayley Pegboard	Motor	Infant	Pegs are placed in board during allotted time
Purdue Pegboard	Gross and fine motor	School age	Pegs are placed in board during 30 s trials for right, left, and both hands
Beery Development Test of Visual-Motor Integration	Constructional visuospatial abilities	School age	Geometric forms of increasing complexity are copied with paper and pencil
Bayley Motor Scale	Motor	Infant	Specific behaviors requiring motor functioning are rated by the examiner
McCarthy Motor Scale	Gross and fine motor coordination	30 mo to 8 yr 6 mo	Leg coordination, arm coordination, initiative action, draw-a-design, draw-a-child

ACTG, AIDS Clinical Trial Group's adult battery; MACS, Multicenter AIDS Cohort Study's test battery; AAN, American Academy of Neurology AIDS Working Group's test examples/suggestions for cognitive assessment.

research in this area. Approximately 2 years after the Grant et al. (15) report, Goethe et al. (14) presented data from a larger U.S. Air Force study. This study had some weaknesses given the use of control group samples of convenience. When the performance of 83 HIV-seropositive men was compared with that of 18 HIV-seronegative controls with a history of head injury, no differences in test performance emerged between these two groups. Another study that failed to find significant differences on neuropsychological performance between seropositive and seronegative individuals (24) also suggested that neurocognitive changes in early HIV disease were fairly uncommon.

This view was further strengthened from several reports generated by the Multicenter AIDS Cohort Study (MACS), in which McArthur et al. (35) compared nearly 200 seronegative controls to >200 seropositive asymptomatic patients. They found that there were no significant differences on any of the neuropsychological tests between asymptomatic seropositive and seronegative individuals when the effects of depression, education, and age were controlled in the analyses. Furthermore, only 5.5% of the seropositive but asymptomatic subjects were "outliers" on a brief neuropsychological screening battery. These data therefore suggested that the rate of impairment in early HIV disease was ~6%. On the other hand, a study by Wilkie et al. (63) found support for early cognitive impairment in HIV-positive men. This study found that 43% of HIV-positive but asymptomatic individuals scored one standard deviation below the mean on four or more tests of cognitive speed and memory. In contrast, only 8% of the seronegative individuals showed performance that was impaired.

The primary differences between these early studies appear to involve several methodical issues. These include the criteria that were used to establish impairment, choice of tests, control groups, and subject factors such as overall health, HIV risk factors, history of drug use, and affective symptoms. The importance of these confounding factors in neuropsychological research has been discussed in several articles and reviews (2,59,65). These methodological issues appear to have contributed to the different estimates of the incidence and prevalence of mental impairment in individuals with HIV infection. Clearly, sensitivity of the tests used to document cognitive dysfunction, the demographic characteristics of infected individuals, as well as their current health status influence the detection of cognitive changes as a result of HIV infection. These methodological differences would also impact on the detection of potential changes in brain functioning as a result of the natural history of HIV disease progression or treatment with antiretroviral therapies.

However, the early studies of cognitive dysfunction with early HIV infection have served to focus attention on two primary factors that appear to contribute to impairment in HIV disease. First, clear differences in the type and extensiveness of tests used to evaluate persons with HIV result in different estimates of the incidence, prevalence, and severity of cognitive dysfunction. A second factor that has also emerged from this research is that of disease severity (Table 2). The proportion of HIV-positive persons who show cognitive impairment appears to increase with severity of HIV disease as it progresses from a seropositive but asymptomatic stage to AIDS. These data also support the fact that a small proportion of asymptomatic but seropositive persons show subtle changes in mentation as measured by tests of speeded performance as well as memory and other complex neuropsychological tests independent of affective symptoms (17,22,62). Furthermore, longitudinal data in asymptomatic seropositive patients suggests relative stability in performance at least for periods ranging from 6 to 18 months (51,56). More recent longitudinal data from Stern et al. (55) shows that HIV-positive subjects perform more poorly on memory tests than HIV-negative controls. However, over a 4.5-year interval, practice effects were seen for both groups on semi-annual assessments. Nevertheless, practice effects were either attenuated or not seen for those persons with lower CD4 + counts. More advanced HIV disease was associated with poorer executive and memory functioning, and findings on neurological examination were associated with memory impairment and the lack of learning or practice effects on cognitive testing.

A number of studies have focused on risk factors for HIV infection in an attempt to control for potential confounding variables that might contribute to test-based estimates of impairment in HIV-seropositive individuals. Many of these studies have compared HIV-negative subjects with HIV-positive individuals while attempting to match groups on drug use history, medical history, affective status, and demographic variables. For example, Stern et al. (57) evaluated >200 gay men using both neuro-psychological and neurological methods. When HIV-positive patients were compared with HIV-negative persons, clear differences emerged. Frontal lobe (executive) functioning was assessed, as were verbal memory tasks. These included tests of episodic memory (word list learning) and verbal fluency (language and semantic memory). Intriguingly, this study showed that the presence of neurological signs and symptoms correlated with the neuropsychological test measures only in persons who were HIV seropositive. Additionally, impairment in test performance for HIV-seropositive persons was associated with the frequency of self-reports or complaints of cognitive dysfunction.

These data as well as data from other studies support the assertion that mild neurocognitive symptoms can be detected in some persons who are HIV seropositive. Mild neurocognitive symptoms have therefore been incorporated into the American Academy of Neurology AIDS Task Force's (66) nomenclature for neurological aspects of HIV-1 infection (HIV-1–associated minor cognitive/motor disorder). These early neurological and neuropsychological symptoms have been documented as being associated with HIV disease. However, the existence of this early stage of neurocognitive dysfunction has not been thoroughly investigated as a potential predictor of the later development of dementia symptoms commonly referred to as AIDS dementia complex (ADC), HIV-1–associated dementia complex, or HIV encephalopathy (1).

Risk Factors for Impaired Cognition

Before turning to a discussion of the symptoms associated with dementia and HIV infection, it is important to evaluate a salient cofactor that may partially explain the rate of neuropsychological impairment in HIV infection. One important factor has emerged from the MACS data (47). This MACS evaluation focused on education as a possible predictive factor in HIV-associated neurocognitive impairments. The findings from this cohort suggest that the rates of neuropsychological impairment are fairly low and rather similar when education levels are considered. Essentially, serostatus does not contribute differentially to the rate of impairment in highly educated persons (more than high school education). However, education levels of high school and below result in an approximate doubling in the frequency of cognitive impairment in seropositive persons when they are compared with seronegative individuals with similar risk factors.

TABLE 2. Neuropsychological assessment in HIV infection

Study	Sample	Test battery (or cognitive domain)	Findings/conclusions
Early studies			
Rubinow et al. (45)	13 AIDS, 9 HIV+, 4 HIV+, and 5 HIV− with hepatitis, 6 healthy controls	Wechsler Adult Intelligence Scale, Category Test, Trailmaking Part B, cancellation tasks	Focal and global cognitive impairment plus motivational changes in patients with AIDS relative to seropositive patients and controls
Goethe et al. (14)	11 adults: Walter Reed stages 1–5 vs. mild head injury control subjects	Controlled Oral Word Association (COWA), Paced Serial Addition Test (PASAT), Selective Reminding Test, Continuous Visual Memory Test, finger tapping, Trails B	Cognitive dysfunction does not precede immunological decline
McArthur et al. (35)	270 HIV+ men: CDC stages II and III	Verbal skills, problem solving, verbal and visual memory recognition and delayed recall, visuo-constructional abilities, psychomotor speed, attention, concentration	Prevalence of dementia and other HIV-1–related neurological disorders very low among healthy HIV+ homosexual men
Disease status			
Wilkins et al. (65)	40 adults: CDC stages II, III, IVa	Test measuring verbal and figural recent memory; language; visuospatial and constructional ability; concentration and speed of processing; initiation, inhibition and mental flexibility; fine motor functions	Early stages of HIV disease are not associated with a high frequency of cognitive impairment if confounding (premorbid) variables are taken into consideration
Selnes et al. (51)	238 HIV+ men: CDC stages II and III	Digit Span, Symbol Digit Modalities, Rey Auditory Verbal Learning Test, Verbal Fluency, Grooved Pegboard, Brief Symptom Inventory	Gradual cognitive decline does not occur during the early, asymptomatic stages of HIV infection
Miller et al. (37)	811 HIV+ men: CDC stages II, III, IV	Tests of attention, memory, psychomotor speed	Frequency of neuropsychological abnormalities in asymptomatic HIV-1–infected homosexual men low and not statistically different from that of seronegative controls
Wilkie et al. (63)	59 gay men: 46 with lymphadenopathy with CD4 counts below 700 versus 13 seronegative controls	Language, memory, visuospatial processes, information processing speed, reasoning, attention, reaction time (Sternberg paradigm), mental status	Cognitive inefficiency occurs in a subsample of individuals during early HIV infection
Bornstein et al. (3)	29 asymptomatic HIV+ men (initial CD4 mean = 575) and 18 HIV+ men with ARC and AIDS (initial CD4 mean = 443)	Selective Reminding Test, Trail Making Test, Grooved Pegboard, reaction time measures	Faster rates of decline in percent CD4 lymphocytes predicts poorer performance on measures of memory and reaction time. Rate of CD4 loss may be a risk factor for the development of HIV-related neurobehavioral deficits
Miller et al. (36)	993 gay/bisexual men: CDC stages II, III, IV	Attention, reaction time, memory, psychomotor speed	Frequency of cognitive abnormalities in asymptomatic HIV infected men is low and not statistically different from HIV− controls

Study	Subjects	Tests	Findings
Stern et al. (57)	208 men: 84 HIV−, 49 HIV+ asymptomatic, 29 HIV+ mildly symptomatic, 46 HIV+ with significant symptoms (not sufficient for AIDS)	Mental status, attention, general intelligence and visuospatial reasoning, abstract reasoning, memory, language, verbal fluency, executive function, visuospatial function, motor speed, praxis	Subjective and objective neuropsychological and neurologic findings suggest a definable syndrome associated with HIV infection in asymptomatic individuals
Marder et al. (30)	Adult male and female IV drug users; 99 HIV− and 122 HIV+	Tests of general intelligence, memory, language, executive functions, visuospatial abilities, attention, motor speed	Subtle neurologic and neuropsychological abnormalities may precede clinical evidence of AIDS in intravenous drug users and may be more evident in those with head injury
Law et al. (27)	26 asymptomatic seropositive adults and 23 HIV− controls	Working memory, reaction time, Beck Depression Inventory, Spielberger State-Trait Anxiety Scale	Seropositive persons with significantly slowed reaction times did not show working memory deficits
Subjective ratings van Gorp et al. (58)	479 adult men: CDC stages II and III	Tests measuring attention, motor speed, psychomotor speed, verbal memory, verbal fluency, depression and Cognitive Failures Questionnaire	Presence of depressed mood, independent of serostatus or actual neuropsychological impairment, associated with increased cognitive complaints
Wilkins et al. (64)	131 subjects: CDC stages II, III, and IV	Tests measuring visual-motor integration and alternation between stimulus sets, confrontational naming, memory, motor functioning, depression and anxiety, psychiatric diagnoses, and subjective complaints	Cognitive complaints are associated with psychiatric symptoms but not cognitive performance. Motor complaints are associated with decreased motor performance but not psychiatric symptoms
Depressed mood van Gorp et al. (58)	298 men: CDC stages II and III	Tests measuring motor and cognitive processing, spatial processing, verbal cognitive and language functioning, verbal memory, depression and anxiety	Three subgroups were identified: unimpaired depressed with psychomotor slowing and memory dysfunction, and generally impaired subjects with normal mood
Hinkin et al. (22)	54 men: CDC stages II, III, and IV	Measured intelligence, attention and concentration, language visuospatial functions, verbal and nonverbal memory, executive functions, motor/psychomotor speed, mood	Presence of clinically significant levels of depression in a non-elderly HIV-1–seropositive sample does not necessarily lead to significant neuropsychological dysfunction
Grant et al. (17)	139 men: CDC stages II, III, and IV	PASAT, auditory and visual memory, Category Test, Trails B, estimate of verbal intelligence	There are no systematic relationships between depression and neuropsychological impairment
Marsh and McCall (33)	30 men: CDC stages II and III	Tests measuring intellectual functioning, language, attention, memory, learning, visuospatial constructional ability	Subtle neuropsychological impairment is present early in the course of infection. Variability in HIV+ subjects' performance confirms the need for development of specific criteria for defining neuropsychological impairment in HIV+ individuals.

It has been suggested that these data support the concept of cognitive reserve (46) as a factor that contributes to the vulnerability of the CNS to the early effects of HIV as well as other neurological and dementing disorders (26). Therefore, if the concept of cognitive or cerebral reserve actually reflects observable differences in brain structure and function, persons with lower reserve (education as a surrogate marker) might be at a greater risk of impairment in HIV disease if other potentially confounding variables are controlled. This would suggest that measures of cognitive reserve, as partially indexed by education and occupation, could account for a larger proportion of the variance in predicting which individuals could develop cognitive dysfunction and dementia for a wide range of neurological diseases (54).

Recent evidence suggests that the caudate nucleus and basal ganglia are primary areas of HIV pathogenesis (32,44,60) (Table 3). This line of investigation has used tests that are sensitive to basal ganglia dysfunction (as demonstrated in persons with Huntington's and Parkinson's disease). These neuropsychological procedures evaluate motor skill learning through the use of a pursuit-rotor task (32). Performance on the pursuit-rotor task is compared with markers of immune system status as well as CSF changes based on the neurotoxin quinolinic acid (20,21).

In this research, Martin et al. (32) evaluated 29 seropositive and 15 seronegative controls. By carefully matching controls and seropositive subjects on age, education, and overall intellectual functioning, these investigators were able to evaluate their subjects' ability to learn the pursuit-rotor task. The data showed that seropositive individuals could be divided into two groups: those who could adequately learn the task and those who had difficulties learning. Interestingly, those seropositive individuals who were classified as "good learners" of the pursuit-rotor task showed performance that was essentially identical to that of seronegative controls. Seropositive subjects who were classified as "poor learners" on the pursuit-rotor learning task demonstrated additional impairments on simple and choice reaction time measures.

Although these tasks of learning and reaction time are clearly sensitive to early effects of HIV infection on the brain, the most interesting finding from this study is the association between CSF levels of quinolinic acid, learning, and reaction time (31,32). Fairly robust and positive correlations were found between CSF quinolinic acid and slowing of reaction time. On the other hand, immunological status as indexed by CD4+ counts and CD4:CD8 ratios were not associated with the performance of the seropositive subjects. These data provide a robust test of the occurrence of cognitive changes in asymptomatic but seropositive individuals. More importantly, these findings link changes in brain functioning to a marker of an endogenous neurotoxic activity as a potential indicator of HIV effects on the CNS. However, it remains to be seen whether persons with elevated CSF quinolinic acid levels and accompanying neurocognitive symptoms demonstrate a progression in cognitive dysfunction as a result of quinolinic acid or other HIV-associated neurotoxic effects.

HIV and Dementia

The most dramatic impact of HIV on the CNS is often seen in the form of dementing symptoms. Initially reported as HIV-encephalopathy, this constellation of symptoms was renamed the AIDS dementia complex by Price et al. (43) and HIV–associated cognitive/motor complex (66). Initial reports suggested that these dementia symptoms were secondary to opportunistic infections, CNS tumors, and other medical

TABLE 3. *Neuropsychological measures and CNS markers of HIV activity*

Study	Sample	Test battery (or cognitive domain)	Outcome
MRI			
Grant et al. (15)	55 men: HIV−, HIV+ asymptomatic, ARC, and AIDS	Intelligence, attention, abstraction, cognitive flexibility, parallel processing, PASAT, logical memory, visual memory, associate learning	CNS involvement of HIV may begin early in the course of AIDS and cause mild cognitive deficits in otherwise asymptomatic persons. Agreement rate between MRI and neuropsychologic tests substantially better than chance.
Saykin et al. (48)	33 HIV+ men meeting CDC criteria for persistent generalized lymphadenopathy	Tests assessing memory, language, psychomotor speed, intellectual abilities, perceptual and motor processes, personality, affective state	Neuropsychological findings not correlated with duration of lymphadenopathy syndrome, absolute T-helper values, or MRI volumetric measures. Findings indicate that psychometric testing may provide the first sign of CNS involvement in HIV infection.
PET			
van Gorp et al. (60)	31 men with AIDS (CDC IVa)	Wechsler Adult Intelligence Scale-Revised, Trails A and B, Rey-Osterrieth Complex Figure, COWA, Rey Auditory Verbal Learning Test, Boston Naming, Grooved Pegboard	Basal ganglia, thalamus, and temporal lobe regions selectively affected in AIDS. Significant correlations found between cerebral metabolic activity and specific neuropsychologic measures.
Quinolinic acid			
Martin et al. (31)	52 adults from Walter Reed stages 1 through 5	Visual reaction time, attention, coding speed, motor dexterity, visuospatial/construction, language, memory/learning, problem solving.	Cerebrospinal fluid concentrations of quinolinic acid elevated in HIV-infected individuals and correlated with reaction time.
Martin et al. (32)	44 adults from Walter Reed stages 1 through 5	Pursuit-rotor tasks, reaction time tasks, Vocabulary, Block Design, Beck Depression Inventory, Speilberger Anxiety Scale	A subgroup of HIV-infected subjects exhibits slowing and impaired acquisition of a motor skill. Impaired motor speed and learning are related to increased concentrations of quinolinic acid in cerebrospinal fluid, but not CD4 counts or CD4:CD8 ratio.

conditions associated with advancing HIV disease. Additional studies showed that this dementia syndrome was also associated with cortical atrophy. Neuroimaging and neuropathological studies further demonstrated that this dementia was closely associated with atrophy in the basal ganglia and caudate nucleus (9,40). Neuronal loss has been described in persons with cognitive dysfunction and HIV infection. Data have suggested that over two thirds of patients (before death) can present with dementing symptoms. Furthermore, roughly one fourth to one third of patients could present with symptoms of dementia as an early sign of HIV infection (39). Although the neuropathological (38) as well as neuroimaging (9,44,60) data show involvement of cortical and subcortical regions, the general cognitive pattern associated with HIV-associated cognitive and motor complex tends to resemble a subcortical dementia (8). This pattern of deficits is based on the data that document memory dysfunction and slowed motor performance as the primary cognitive manifestations of HIV infection.

Clinical Staging Criteria and Cognition

The study of neurocognitive symptoms associated with HIV infection has resulted in the creation of a number of staging schemes as mentioned above, including Price and Brew's (43) conceptualization of ADC. A discussion of the clinical criteria for dementia associated with HIV infection is beyond the scope of this chapter (1). What is important to the study of HIV is the apparent increased incidence of dementia across different age groups (e.g., persons in their 20s and 30s to persons >75 years of age). Janssen et al. (23) reported on data collected by the CDC that suggest that age is an important risk factor in the development of HIV-associated cognitive and motor symptoms.

Another, more direct test of age as a risk factor for cognitive impairment in HIV infection was undertaken by the MACS investigators (61). They presented two studies that evaluated >2,000 subjects from the MACS cohort who were either HIV seropositive or seronegative. Using this large sample, performance on a number of neuropsychological and reaction time measures was analyzed. Analyses showed a significant main effect for age on reaction time and timed tests of cognitive function but no interaction between age and serostatus. This suggests that age and serostatus appear to be separate contributors to cognitive impairment. Advanced age in seropositive individuals does not appear to increase the risk of impairment. The second study evaluated a different group of >75 seropositive men who ranged in age from 29 to 55 and 47 matched seronegative control subjects. Analyses of the data from this second study replicated the findings from the larger cohort suggesting no increased risk of dysfunction with advancing age in seropositive persons.

Neuropsychological Findings with Treatment

A final issue to be briefly discussed is that of the treatment of cognitive symptoms in HIV infection (Table 4). Two treatments with beneficial effects on cognition have appeared in the literature. These involve treatment with antiretroviral agents that cross the blood–brain barrier and result in improvement in cognitive functioning (42,49,52) and methylphenidate with resulting brain metabolism changes (11). Given that there are several recent reviews concerning treatment of HIV and the effects on

TABLE 4. *Neuropsychologic evidence of treatment efficacy*

Study	Population	Test battery (or cognitive domain)	Outcomes
Zidovudine (ZDV)			
Schmitt et al. (49)	281 adults with advanced ARC or AIDS	Tests measuring attention, memory, visual-motor skills, mood and affect	HIV-associated cognitive abnormalities may be partially ameliorated after the administration of ZDV
Pizzo et al. (42)	21 children ages 14 mo to 12 yr, CDC stage P2	Tests measuring general abilities, adaptive behavior, language, attention and motor speed, memory and learning, visual and perceptual abilities, problem solving	ZDV therapy results in increased IQ scores. Changes in cognitive function may be among earliest signs of AIDS encephalopathy.
Yarchoan et al. (67)	7 adults with ARC and AIDS	Test measuring attention, memory, coordination	ZDV theory results in improvement in tests of attention, fine motor coordination, and memory
Brouwers et al. (4)	13 children ages 14 mo to 12 yr, CDC stage P2	Tests measuring general level of cognitive functioning, adaptive behavior	Neuropsychological functioning significantly improved with continuous infusion of ZDV
Sidtis et al. (52)	40 adults with a clinical diagnosis of mild to severe AIDS dementia complex (ADC)	Verbal Fluency, Timed Gait, Trailmaking Parts A and B, Digit Symbol, Finger Tapping	Extended previous findings that ZDV exerts therapeutic effect on ADC, with substantial improvement in neuropsychological test performance in some patients
Dideoxycytidine (ddC)			
Pizzo et al. (41)	15 children ages 6 mo to 13 yr, CDC stage P2	General intelligence, language, attention and motor speed, memory and learning, problem solving, visual perceptual abilities, social behavior	Alternating regimen of ddC and ZDV may prove beneficial for patients with definite or possible hematologic intolerance to ZDV
Dideoxyinosine (ddl)			
Butler et al. (6)	43 children ages 3 mo to 18 yr, CDC stage P2	Tests measuring general ability, adaptive behavior, language, attention and motor speed, memory and learning, visual and perceptual abilities, problem solving	Significant correlation between plasma levels of ddl and improvement in IQ score. Promising antiretroviral activity in HIV-infected children from ddl treatment.
Methylphenidate			
Fernandez et al. (11)	19 adult men with ARC	Mini-Mental State Exam, Trail Making Tests, verbal memory	Cognitive, affective, and behavioral impairments respond to psychostimulant therapy; both qualitative and quantitative improvement seen

neurocognitive functioning (5,12,50), the interested reader is directed to these chapters for a more detailed discussion. What is important, however, is the fact that the mild and distressing cognitive and motor symptoms that are seen in persons with HIV infection do respond to pharmacological treatment. Positive effects of treatment have been replicated in adults as well as children. The magnitude of the effect appears to be associated with the degree of penetration of the antiretroviral agent across the blood–brain barrier. Success of these treatments suggests that persons who have neurological and neurocognitive symptoms as a result of their HIV infection could be treated and monitored for improvement through the use of neuropsychological methods.

Several articles have emerged in the literature documenting attempts to develop brief assessment batteries to document either the progression of the AIDS cognitive and motor complex or the response to therapeutic interventions. One important approach, developed by Sidtis and Price (52), has been incorporated in the ACTG studies of neurological dysfunction. Another approach is the screening battery that is used by the MACS group. More recently, a brief battery that focuses on executive functioning, attention, and episodic memory has been proposed as a brief screening instrument that could be useful for the diagnosis of the dementia syndrome associated with AIDS (34).

Conclusions

Neuropsychological impairment has been clearly recognized for over a decade as a consequence of HIV infection. Deficits in neurocognitive functioning have been described at different stages of infection. The incidence and severity of dysfunction increases as HIV infection progresses. Primary questions concerning the natural history in the progression of neurocognitive deficits in HIV infection have been a focus of the MACS investigations. These data suggest, at least in the short term, that the prevalence and progression of cognitive dysfunction in seropositive but asymptomatic individuals is fairly rare and limited. On the other hand, data from other studies suggest that once a person has developed the full range of dementia symptoms associated with HIV infection, there is rapid progression of symptoms leading to mortality.

Methodological issues surrounding the evaluation of the neurocognitive symptoms associated with HIV infection are important. The search for additional risk factors and confounding factors that might over- or underrepresent the occurrence of cognitive symptoms in seropositive persons remains an important area of study. Furthermore, documenting the nature and extent of these neurocognitive deficits is clearly important in patient care, particularly when it concerns decisions regarding occupational status, financial matters, and daily living skills.

Questions remain, however, as to the association between neurocognitive symptoms and biological markers of HIV activity in the brain. Although work such as that by Martin et al. (32) is enlightening, there are a number of other potential neurotoxic processes associated with HIV infection that need to be evaluated in light of their potential contribution to the mental changes in HIV disease. It is possible that the use of new and fairly specialized measures of attention and reaction time may shed additional light into the incidence and prevalence of impairment in seropositive but asymptomatic individuals. Furthermore, these measures might be used in a prospective fashion to evaluate the risk of developing a dementia as a result of HIV infection. In conjunction with other neuropsychological measures, tests of attention and reaction time also might be used to evaluate the impact of various contributing factors to the development of a dementia syndrome in AIDS. These factors could include such areas as premorbid neurological status, reserve capacity, and recreational and intravenous drug use (30), as well as occurrence of other systemic diseases associated with immune system depression.

A final area of research that should prove fruitful in the future is similar to work that is currently being published in the field of Alzheimer's disease and related dementias. Here, neuropathological changes in the brain could be evaluated in light of neurological and neuropsychological measures. For example, measures of cognitive function that are being obtained throughout life from HIV-positive persons could be evaluated for associations between clinical and neuropathological findings. In the meantime, insights into brain and behavior as impacted by HIV continues to be evaluated with advanced imaging technology (25). This research produces quantifiable data of regional changes in the brain, particularly those areas such as the basal ganglia, which appear to be dramatically impacted by HIV. As additional information regarding neurotoxic processes in HIV disease becomes available, persons with HIV could be evaluated for associations between their neuropsychiatric symptoms and neurotoxic activity in the brain. In all, the past decade has seen an increase in knowledge about the neurobehavioral effects of HIV. The next decade should see a continued increase in our understanding of the effects of HIV on brain functioning and potential treatments for this disease and its neurocognitive symptoms.

REFERENCES

1. Becker JT, Martin A, Lopez OL. The dementias and AIDS. In: Grant I, Martin A, eds. *Neuropsychology of HIV infection*. New York: Oxford University Press, 1994:133–145.
2. Bornstein RA. Methodological and conceptual issues in the study of cognitive change in HIV infection. In: Grant I, Martin A, eds. *Neuropsychology of HIV infection*. New York: Oxford University Press, 1994:146–160.
3. Bornstein RA, Nasrallah HA, Para MF, Fas RJ, Whitacre CC, Rice RR. Rate of CD4 decline and neuropsychological performance in HIV infection. *Arch Neurol* 1991;48:704–707.
4. Brouwers P, Moss J, Wolters P, Eddy J, Balis F, Poplack DG, Pizzo PA. Effect of continuous-infusion zidovudine therapy on neuropsychological functioning in children with symptomatic human immunodeficiency virus infection. *J Pediatr* 1990;117:980–985.
5. Brouwers P, Moss H, Wolters P, Schmitt F. Developmental deficits and behavioral change in pediatric AIDS. In: Grant I, Martin A, eds. *Neuropsychology of HIV Infection*. New York: Oxford University Press, 1994:310–338.
6. Butler KM, Husson RM, Balis FM, et al. Dideoxyinosine in children with symptomatic human immunodeficiency virus infection. *N Engl J Med* 1991;324:137–144.
7. Centers for Disease Control. Revision of the CDC surveillance case definition for acquired immunodeficiency syndrome. *MMWR* 1987;34:3–15.
8. Cummings JL, Benson DF. Subcortical dementia. Review of an emerging concept. *Arch Neurol* 1984; 41:874–879.
9. Dal Pan GJ, McArthur JH, Aylward E, et al. Patterns of cerebral atrophy in HIV-1–infected individuals: results of a quantitative MRI analysis. *Neurology* 1992;42:2125–2130.
10. Fennell EB. Assessing neurobehavioral changes in HIV + infants and children. A methodological approach. *Ann NY Acad Sci* 1993;693:141–150.
11. Fernandez F, Adams F, Levy JK, Holmes VF, Neidhart M, Mansell PWA. Cognitive impairment due to AIDS-related complex and its response to psychostimulants. *Psychosomatics* 1988;29:38–46.
12. Fernandez F, Levy JK, Ruiz P. The use of methylphenidate in HIV patients: a clinical perspective. In: Grant I, Martin A, eds. *Neuropsychology of HIV Infection*. New York: Oxford University Press, 1994:295–309.
13. Fletcher JM, Francis DJ, Pequengnat W, et al. Neurobehavioral outcomes in diseases of childhood: individual change models for pediatric human immune viruses. *Am Psychol* 1991;46:1267–1277.

14. Goethe KE, Mitchell JE, Marshall DW, et al. Neuropsychological and neurological function of human immunodeficiency virus seropositive asymptomatic individuals. *Arch Neurol* 1989;46:129–133.
15. Grant I, Atkinson JH, Hesselink JR, et al. Evidence for early central nervous system involvement in the acquired immunodeficiency virus (HIV) infections. *Ann Intern Med* 1987;107:828–836.
16. Grant I, Martin A, eds. *Neuropsychology of HIV infection.* New York: Oxford University Press, 1994.
17. Grant I, Olshen RA, Atkinson JH, et al. Depressed mood does not explain neuropsychological deficits in HIV-infected persons. *Neuropsychology* 1993;7:53–61.
18. Hannay HJ. *Experimental Techniques in Human Neuropsychology.* New York: Oxford University Press, 1986.
19. Heilman KM, Valenstein E, eds. *Clinical Neuropsychology.* 2nd ed. New York: Oxford University Press, 1985.
20. Heyes MP, Brew BJ, Martin A, et al. Quinolinic acid in cerebrospinal fluid and serum in HIV infection: relationship to clinical and neurological status. *Ann Neurol* 1991;29:202–209.
21. Heyes MP, Jordan EK, Lee K, et al. Relationship of neurological status in macaques infected with the simian immunodeficiency virus to cerebrospinal fluid quinolinic acid and kynurenic acid. *Brain Res* 1992;570:237–250.
22. Hinkin CH, van Gorp WG, Satz P, Weisman JD, Thommes J, Buckingham S. Depressed mood and its relationship to neuropsychological test performance in HIV-1 seropositive individuals. *J Clin Exp Neuropsychol* 1992;14:289–297.
23. Janssen RS, Nwanyanwu OC, Selik RM, Stehr-Green JK. Epidemiology of human immunodeficiency virus encephalopathy in the United States. *Neurology* 1992;42:1472–1476.
24. Janssen RS, Saykin AJ, Cannon L, et al. Neurological and neuropsychological manifestations of HIV-1 infection: associations with AIDS-related complex but no asymptomatic HIV-1 infection. *Ann Neurol* 1989;26:592–600.
25. Jernigan TL, Archibald SL, Berhow MT, et al. MRI morphometric analysis of cerebral volume loss in HIV infection. *Arch Neurol* 1993;50:250–255.
26. Katzman R, Terry R, DeTeresa R, et al. Clinical, pathological, and neurochemical changes in dementia: a subgroup with preserved mental status and numerous neocortical plaques. *Ann Neurol* 1988; 23:138–144.
27. Law WA, Martin A, Mapou RL, et al. Working memory in individuals with HIV infection. *J Clin Exp Neuropsychol* 1994;16:173–182.
28. Levy RM, Bredesen DE, Rosenblum ML. Neurological manifestations of the acquired immunodeficiency syndrome (AIDS): experience at UCSF and review of the literature. *J Neurosurg* 1985;62: 475–495.
29. Lezak MD. *Neuropsychological Assessment.* 2nd ed. New York: Oxford University Press, 1983.
30. Marder K, Stern Y, Malouf R, et al. Neurological and neuropsychological manifestations of human immunodeficienct virus infection in intravenous drug users without AIDS: relationship to head injury. *Arch Neurol* 1992;49:1169–1175.
31. Martin A, Heyes MP, Salazar AM, et al. Progressive slowing of reaction time and increasing cerebrospinal fluid concentrations of quinolinic acid in HIV-infected individuals. *J Neuropsychiatry Clin Neurosci* 1992;4:270–279.
32. Martin A, Heyes MP, Salazar AM, Law WA, Williams J. Impaired motor-skill learning, slowed reaction time, and elevated cerebrospinal fluid quinolinic acid in a subgroup of HIV-infected individuals. *Neuropsychology* 1993;7:149–157.
33. Marsh NV, McCall DW. Early neuropsychological change in HIV infection. *Neuropsychology* 1994; 8:44–48.
34. Maruff P, Currie J, Malone V, McArthur-Jackson C, Mulhall B, Benson E. Neuropsychological characterization of the AIDS dementia complex and rationalization of a test battery. *Arch Neurol* 1994;51:689–695.
35. McArthur JC, Cohen BA, Selnes OA, et al. Low prevalence of neurological and neuropsychological abnormalities in otherwise healthy HIV-1–infected individuals: results from the multicenter AIDS cohort study. *Ann Neurol* 1989;26:601–611.
36. Miller EN, Satz P, Visscher B. Computerized and conventional neuropsychological assessment of HIV-1–infected homosexual men. *Neurology* 1991;41:1608–1616.
37. Miller EN, Selnes OA, McArthur JC, et al. Neuropsychological performance in HIV-1–infected homosexual men: the multicenter AIDS cohort study (MACS). *Neurology* 1990;40:197–203.
38. Navia BA, Cho ES, Petito CK, Price RW. The AIDS dementia complex. II. Neuropathology. *Ann Neurol* 1986;19:525–535.
39. Navia BA, Price RW. The acquired immunodeficiency syndrome dementia complex as the presenting or sole manifestation of human immunodeficiency virus infection. *Arch Neurol* 1987;44:65–69.
40. Petito CK. What causes brain atrophy in human immunodeficiency virus infection. *Ann Neurol* 1993; 34:128–129.
41. Pizzo PA, Butler K, Balis F, et al. Dideoxycytidine alone and in an alternating schedule with zidovudine in children with symptomatic human immunodeficiency virus infection. *J Pediatr* 1990;117: 799–808.

42. Pizzo PA, Eddy J, Falloon J, et al. Effect of continuous intravenous infusion of zidovudine (AZT) in children with symptomatic HIV infection. *N Engl J Med* 1988;319:889–896.
43. Price RW, Brew BJ. The AIDS dementia complex. *J Infect Dis* 1988;158:1079–1083.
44. Rottenberg DA, Moeller JR, Strother SC, et al. The metabolic pathology of the AIDS dementia complex. *Ann Neurol* 1987;22:700–706.
45. Rubinow DR, Berrettini CH, Brouwers P, Lane HC. Neuropsychiatric consequences of AIDS. *Ann Neurol* 1988;23(suppl):24–26.
46. Satz P. Brain reserve capacity on symptom onset after brain injury: a formulation and review of evidence for threshold theory. *Neuropsychology* 1993;7:273–295.
47. Satz P, Morgenstern H, Miller E. Low education as a possible risk factor for cognitive abnormalities in HIV-1: findings from the multicenter AIDS cohort study. *J AIDS* 1993;6:503–511.
48. Saykin AJ, Janssen RS, Sprehn GC, Kaplan JE, Spira TJ, Weller P. Neuropsychological dysfunction in HIV-infection: characterization in a symphadenopathy cohort. *Int J Clin Neuropsychol* 1988;10: 1988.
49. Schmitt FA, Bigley JW, McKinnis R, et al. Neuropsychological outcome of zidovudine (AZT) treatment of patients with AIDS and AIDS-related complex. *N Engl J Med* 1988;319:1573–1578.
50. Schmitt FA, Dixon LR, Brouwers P. Neuropsychological response to antiretroviral therapy in HIV infection. In: Grant I, Martin A, eds. *Neuropsychology of HIV Infection.* New York: Oxford University Press, 1994:276–294.
51. Selnes OA, Miller E, McArthur J, et al. HIV-1 infection: no evidence of cognitive decline during the asymptomatic stages. *Neurology* 1990;40:204–208.
52. Sidtis JJ, Gatsonis C, Price RW, et al. Zidovudine treatment of the AIDS dementia complex: results of a placebo-controlled trial. *Ann Neurol* 1993;33:343–349.
53. Stern Y. The impact of human immunodeficiency virus on cognitive function. *Ann NY Acad Sci* 1991;640:219–223.
54. Stern Y, Gurland B, Tatemichi TK, Tang MX, Wilder D, Mayeux R. Influence of education and occupation on the incidence of Alzheimer's disease. *JAMA* 1994;271:1004–1010.
55. Stern Y, Liu X, Marder K, Todak G, Sano M, Ehrhardt A, Gorman J. Neuropsychological changes in a prospectively followed cohort of gay and bisexual men with and without HIV. *Neurology* 1995; 43:467–472.
56. Stern Y, Marder K, Bell K, et al. Stability of neuropsychological changes in HIV-positive gay men. Presented at the conference on neurological and neuropsychological complications of HIV infection: update 1990. Monterey, CA, 1990.
57. Stern Y, Marder K, Bell K, et al. Multidisciplinary baseline assessment of homosexual men with and without human immunodeficiency virus infection. *Arch Gen Psychiatry* 1991;48:131–138.
58. van Gorp WG, Hinkin C, Satz P, Miller EN, Weisman J, Holston S, Drebing C, Marcotte TD, Dixon W. Subtypes of HIV-related neuropsychological functioning: a cluster analysis approach. *Neuropsychology* 1993;7:62–72.
59. van Gorp WG, Lamb D, Schmitt FA. Methodological issues in neuropsychological research with HIV-spectrum disease. *Arch Clin Neuropsychol* 1993;8:17–33.
60. van Gorp WG, Mandelkern MA, Gee M, et al. Cerebral metabolic dysfunction in AIDS: findings in a sample with and without dementia. *J Neuropsychiatry* 1992;4:280–287.
61. van Gorp WG, Miller EN, Marcotte TD, et al. The relationship between age and cognitive impairment in HIV-1 infection: findings from the multicenter AIDS cohort study and clinical cohort. *Neurology* 1994;44:929–935.
62. van Gorp WG, Satz P, Hinkin C, et al. Metacognition in HIV-1 seropositive asymptomatic individuals: self-ratings versus objective neuropsychological performance. *J Clin Exp Neuropsychol* 1991;13: 812–819.
63. Wilkie FL, Eisdorfer C, Morgan R, Loewenstein DA, Szapocznik J. Cognition in early human immunodeficiency virus infection. *Arch Neurol* 1990;47:433–440.
64. Wilkins JW, Robertson KR, Snyder CR, Robertson WK, van der Horst C, Hall CD. Implications of self-reported cognitive and motor dysfunction in HIV-positive patients. *Am J Psychiatry* 1991;148: 641–643.
65. Wilkins JW, Robertson KR, van der Horst C, Robertson WT, Fryer JG, Hall CD. The importance of confounding factors in the evaluation of neuropsychological changes in patients infected with himan immunodeficiency virus. *J AIDS* 1990;3:938–942.
66. Working Group of the American Academy of Neurology AIDS Task Force. Nomenclature and research case definitions for neurological manifestations of human immunodeficiency virus-type 1 (HIV-1) infection. *Neurology* 1991;41:778–785.
67. Yarchoan R, Thomas RV, Grafman J, et al. Long-term administration of 3′-azido-2′,3′-dideoxythymidine to patients with AIDS-related neurological disease. *Ann Neurol* 1988;23(suppl):82–87.

AIDS and the Nervous System, Second Edition, edited by J. R. Berger and R. M. Levy. Lippincott-Raven Publishers, Philadelphia © 1997.

16

Neuropsychiatry of Human Immunodeficiency Virus Infection

J. Hampton Atkinson and Igor Grant

Department of Psychiatry, University of California San Diego, Veterans Affairs Medical Center, La Jolla, California 92093

A fundamental tenet of modern neuropsychiatry is that emotional life and behaviors are shaped by a dynamic rendezvous of neurobiology, "personal" factors, and the broader social context. This interplay is exquisitely evident in the neuropsychiatry of human immunodeficiency virus (HIV) infection, and it is crucial to diagnosis and treatment selection that this interplay become part of the practitioner's model of HIV disease.

Accordingly one can use three interrelated models of understanding the origin of neuropsychiatric states observed in the course of infection and illness from HIV. The biologic model posits that HIV involvement of the CNS (particularly its subcortical effects) may lead not only to neurocognitive impairment but may precipitate anxiety or depression syndromes or psychotic phenomenon. Alternatively, individuals may react to early HIV-associated neurocognitive decline with anxiety or depression symptoms, much as is seen in the natural history of Parkinsonism (19). The transition model proposes that adverse psychologic phenomena (e.g., the worried-well, adjustment disorders, mood disorders, anxiety disorders) might be precipitated at key nodal points in the HIV experience: these key transitions include discovery of seroconversion; commencement of antiretroviral treatment; detection of physical symptoms; progression in HIV illness stage; or HIV-related bereavement. In this case psychiatric symptoms or syndromes may be reflecting a breakdown in coping capacities. A third conceptualization may be termed the background model. It emphasizes that a primary psychiatric disorder that preceded HIV infection also may emerge during the course of an individual's HIV illness, for reasons not necessarily associated with HIV biology or transitions. Furthermore, it takes note of evidence gathered from diverse medical illness populations that stressful life events unrelated to the medical condition itself may elicit emotional distress more strongly than do illness-related events. It is this model that demands the most careful history taking. Each of these models in turn may be conceptualized as evolving from three related contexts relevant to HIV.

NEUROBIOLOGICAL CONTEXT OF HIV

The neurobiological context can be composed of either primary or secondary neurocognitive complications of HIV infection.

The primary neurobiological complications are those that can be attributed directly to HIV infection of the central nervous system (CNS) or to immunopathological events (e.g., autoimmune phenomena) precipitated by HIV infection.

Secondary neurobiological complications include infections and neoplasms facilitated by the immunodeficiency state; cerebrovascular complications; and toxic states produced either by HIV-associated medical illnesses (e.g., hypoxemia due to pneumocystic pneumonia) or toxic effects of various therapeutic agents (e.g., myopathy due to zidovudine).

PSYCHOLOGICAL CONTEXT OF HIV

In North America and Europe, the two major groups that have been at highest risk for infection with HIV—homosexual men and intravenous drug–using (IDU) men and women—may be at elevated risk for selected psychiatric disorders that precede seroconversion (3,53). In failing to take a careful history, one can make the error of ascribing to HIV infection and its consequences psychological disorders that may have little direct relation to infection as such, and whose natural history and response to treatment may therefore follow the familiar lines of primary psychiatric disorders.

In Western industrialized societies, men with hemophilia are the third traditional risk group. Although there is no evidence of pre-HIV psychological vulnerability in hemophiliacs as a group, vulnerability to emotional distress (anxiety and depressive symptoms) appears to be associated with the personal or family history of psychiatric disorder, perception of low social support, use of passive and avoidant coping approaches, and the experience of stressful life events apart from HIV itself, along with demographic characteristics of youth, low education, and unemployment (22).

SOCIAL CONTEXT OF HIV

Social stigmatization and fear of HIV and acquired immunodeficiency syndrome (AIDS) is widespread. Despite some increased tolerance, the practical consequences of infection still include loss of employment, denial of medical benefits or life insurance, and roadblocks to career aspirations. Clinicians treating HIV-infected persons must be careful not to underestimate these social phenomena and their impact on individual patients.

Beyond society's response to HIV, it is important to consider the quality of the individual's immediate social network because social support moderates the effect of illness and of adverse life events on mood and function. Thus, regardless of the U.S. Centers for Disease Control and Prevention (CDC) stage, HIV-seropositive individuals with satisfying and stable social networks, especially those who cope actively with these adverse life events, will be significantly less distressed than individuals with unsatisfying or inconsistent support (22).

The reward for applying these models is a sound understanding of the likely diagnosis and subsequent course of neuropsychiatric disorder presenting in HIV-infected individuals. Given our model and its context—the diagnosis and treatment of major neurocognitive and psychiatric disorders—the neuropsychiatry of HIV can now be reviewed. Wherever applicable, this review is presented using the nomenclature of the newly introduced fourth edition of the *Diagnostic and Statistical Manual of Mental Disorders* (DSM-IV) (1) because this nosology will be the coin of the realm for the foreseeable future. In cases in which rigorous diagnostic standards are already widely used (e.g., the American Academy of Neurology criteria for HIV-associated cognitive disorders), these criteria will be used and the overlap with DSM-IV described.

HIV-ASSOCIATED NEUROCOGNITIVE DISORDERS

From a neuropsychiatric perspective, the most important of the primary neurobiological complications are the HIV-associated neurocognitive disorders. The cardinal feature of these disorders is impairment in cognitive functioning. Associated features include motor slowing or incoordination and, sometimes, affective disturbances.

In DSM-IV, disorders formerly called ''organic mental disorders'' have been grouped into three sections: (a) dementia, delirium, amnestic, and other cognitive disorders; (b) mental disorders whose etiopathogenesis is due to a general medical condition (anxiety, mood, psychotic, and catatonic disorders due to a medical condition), including personality changes due to a general medical condition; and (c) substance-induced disorders (anxiety, mood, psychotic, and cognitive disorders). Whereas each phenomena has distinct cardinal features, their one common criterion is that to be termed a disorder the condition must be severe enough to cause disruption in everyday life activity.

Classification and Diagnostic Criteria for Neurocognitive Disorders

Epidemiology and Diagnosis

From a historical perspective, there has been considerable confusion about the occurrence and features of the neurocognitive disorders, primarily because precise diagnostic criteria were not laid out until recently. For example, one of the earliest terms was ''HIV encephalopathy,'' a designation derived from early pathological studies, which noted presence of encephalitic features in the brains of many patients dying with AIDS (9,45,87). Another term was ''AIDS dementia complex'' (ADC), which suggested a constellation of cognitive, motor, and affective–behavioral complications (69). The difficulty with the ADC designation was that many clinicians and investigators tended to use it somewhat indiscriminately, not bearing in mind, for instance, that the term ''dementia'' connotes severe disability. Undesirable consequences of this inexact usage were failure to recognize milder cognitive disorders or reluctance on the part of clinicians to diagnose patients for fear of stigmatizing them with the ADC label.

''Neurocognitive disorder'' refers to a disturbance in function resulting from presence of a neurocognitive impairment. A neurocognitive (neuropsychological) impairment exists when there is deficient performance in some area of cognitive functioning, which can include attention/speed of information processing, verbal/language skills, abstracting (executive abilities), complex perceptual/motor abilities, psychomotor skills, sensory/perceptual ability, and memory functions (including learning and recall of information). To classify performance on a cognitive task as being impaired, it is necessary to establish a criterion (or cutpoint) beyond which performance is considered to be abnormal.

According to the World Health Organization (WHO), a disability exists when certain impairments interfere with a person's functioning. Thus, the term "disorder" (as in neurocognitive disorder) should be reserved for those individuals who have neurocognitive impairments that are significant enough to produce disability, i.e., to interfere to some extent at least with day-to-day functioning. Unfortunately, there is still insufficient systematic study on the implications of reliably determined neuropsychological impairment on day-to-day functioning.

Accepting for a moment the definition that a person has a neurocognitive disorder if he or she has neuropsychological impairment sufficient to interfere to some degree with everyday functioning, how should these disorders be classified? There are two basic strategies, one based on considerations of severity of impairment and its duration and the other on presumed etiology.

Based on severity/time course considerations, three forms of neurocognitive disorder can be found in HIV-infected persons. These are mild neurocognitive disorder (MND), HIV-associated dementia (HAD), and delirium associated with HIV disease. The criteria used by the San Diego HIV Neurobehavioral Research Center (HNRC) for each of these disorders are presented in Tables 1–3. Tables 1 and 2 also provide a summary of criteria proposed by the Working Group of the American Academy of Neurology AIDS Task Force (95) for dementia (HIV-1–associated dementia complex) and mild neurocognitive disorder (HIV-1–associated minor cognitive/motor disorders).

The use of criteria presented in Tables 1–3 to ascertain the presence of MND, dementia, or delirium in HIV-1–infected persons greatly facilitates both basic descriptive/epidemiological work as well as theoretical research into the neurocognitive complications of HIV disease. In the past, failure to make these distinctions has led to wildly differing estimates of "dementia" in HIV-infected persons. For example, a WHO report indicated that 8–66% of persons with AIDS might develop ADC. Price and Brew (75) suggested that prevalence in patients with AIDS might be on the order of 33%, whereas data from the CDC suggested a rate of 6.5% of all cases of AIDS reported to the CDC between September 1, 1987 and December 31, 1988 (48).

The recent practice of using structured diagnostic criteria, either based on DSM-IV, the International Classification of Diseases (ICD), or the AAN Working Group Criteria (all of which have essential features in common), has led to much more comparable estimates for dementia among recent reports. For example, one small series indicated an annual dementia incidence among symptomatic HIV-infected patients of 14% using DSM-III criteria; another (64), reporting on data from the Multi-Center AIDS Cohort Study (MACS), noted an annual incidence of 7.1% using DSM-III–like criteria; and a WHO series (57), reporting on data from Munich, Sao Paolo, Kinshasa, and Nairobi, found a prevalence among symptomatic HIV-infected persons ranging from 4.4% to 6.5% (DSM-III-R criteria) or 5.4–6.9% (ICD-10 criteria). Clearly, the use of well-defined criteria for dementia appears to have led to more reliable (and convergent) estimates for the prevalence of dementia both in the United States and internationally.

Unfortunately, the concept of mild neurocognitive disorder (minor cognitive motor disorder) has been articulated only recently. Therefore, comparable data on its prevalence are not available at this time. Similarly, although the concept of delirium was articulated in more or less its present form in 1980, it appears not to have been regularly used in work with patients with AIDS. Hopefully, this practice will change

TABLE 1. *HIV-1 associated cognitive disorders*

As defined by Grant and Atkinson	As proposed by AAN Working Group
HIV-1 associated neurocognitive disorders	HIV-1 associated cognitive/motor complex
A. HIV-1 associated dementia (HAD)	A. Probable[a] HIV-1 associated dementia complex
1. Marked acquired impairment in cognitive functioning, involving at least two ability domains (e.g., memory, attention); typically the impairment is in multiple domains, especially in learning of new information, slowed information processing, and defective attention/concentration. The cognitive impairment can be ascertained by history, mental status examination, or neuropsychological testing.	1. Acquired abnormality in at least two of the following cognitive abilities (present for at least 1 month): attention/concentration; sped of information processing; abstraction/reasoning; visuospatial skills; memory/learning; speech/language. Cognitive dysfunction causes impairment in work or activities of daily living.
2. The cognitive impairment produces marked interference with day to day functioning (work, home life, social activities).	2. At least one of the following: a. acquired abnormality in motor functioning b. decline in motivation or emotional control or change in social behavior
3. The marked cognitive impairment has been present for at least 1 month.	3. Absence of clouding of consciousness during a period long enough to establish presence of #1.
4. The pattern of cognitive impairment does not meet criteria for delirium (e.g., clouding of consciousness is not a prominent feature); or, if delirium is present, criteria for dementia need to have been met on a prior examination when delirium was not present.	4. Absence of another cause of the above cognitive, motor, or behavioral symptoms or signs (e.g., active CNS opportunistic infection or malignancy, psychiatric disorders, substance abuse).
5. There is no evidence of another, pre-existing etiology that could explain the dementia, e.g., other CNS infection, CNS neoplasm, cerebrovascular disease, pre-existing neurological disease, or severe substance abuse compatible with CNS disorder.	

[a] The designation probable is used when criteria are met, there is no other likely cause, and data are complete. The designation possible is used if another potential etiology is present whose contribution is unclear, or where a dual diagnosis is possible, or when the evaluation is not complete.

(From Grant I, Martin A. Neuropsychology of HIV infection. New York: Oxford University Press, 1994;362.)

TABLE 2. *HIV-1 associated cognitive disorders*

As defined by Grant and Atkinson	As proposed by AAN Working Group

HIV-1 associated neurocognitive disorders
B. HIV-1 associated mild neurocognitive disorder (MND)
1. Acquired impairment in cognitive functioning, involving at least two ability domains, documented by performance of at least 0.5 standard deviations below age-education-appropriate norms on standardized neuropsychological tests. The neuropsychological assessment must survey at least the following abilities: verbal/language; attention/speeded processing; abstraction; memory (learning, recall); complex perceptual-motor performance; motor skills.
 	
2. The cognitive impairment produces at least mild interference in daily functioning (at least one of the following):
  a. Self-report of reduced mental acuity, inefficiency in work, homemaking, or social functioning.
  b. Observation by knowledgeable others that the individual has undergone at least mild decline in mental acuity with resultant inefficiency in work, homemaking, or social functioning.
 	
3. The cognitive impairment has been present at least one month.
 	
4. Does not meet criteria for delirium or dementia.
 	
5. There is no evidence of another pre-existing cause for the MND.[b]
	HIV-1 associated cognitive/motor complex
	B. Probable[a] HIV-1 associated minor cognitive/motor disorder
	1. Acquired cognitive/motor/behavior abnormalities (must have both a and b):
	  a. At least two of the following symptoms present for at least one month verified by a reliable history:
	    i. impaired attention or concentration
	    ii. mental slowing
	    iii. impaired memory
	    iv. slowed movements
	    v. incoordination
	  b. Acquired cognitive/motor abnormality verified by clinical neurologic examination or neuropsycho-logical testing.
	2. Cognitive/motor/behavioral abnormality causes mild impairment of work or activities of daily living (objectively verifiable or by report of key informant).
	3. Does not meet criteria for HIV-1 associated dementia complex or HIV-1-associated myclopathy.
	4. Absence of another cause of the above cognitive/motor/behavioral abnormality (e.g., active CNS opportunistic infection or malignancy, psychiatric disorders, substance abuse).

[a] The designation *probable* is used when criteria are met, there is no other likely cause, and data are complete. The designation *possible* is used if another potential etiology is present whose contribution is unclear, or where a dual diagnosis is possible, or when the evaluation is not complete.

[b] If the individual with suspected MND also satisfies criteria for a *major depressive episode* or *substancedependence*, the diagnosis of MND should be deferred to a subsequent examination conducted at a time when the major depression has remitted or at least 1 month has elapsed following termination of dependent-substance use.

(From Grant I, Martin A. Neuropsychology of HIV infection. New York: Oxford University Press, 1994;362–363.)

TABLE 3. *Delirium associated with HIV-1 disease*

1. Clouding of consiousness (examples: reduced alertness, disturbed awareness, disorientation).

2. Marked acquired impairment in cognitive functioning, involving at least two ability domains. Typically the impairment is in multiple domains, with defective attention/ concentration and difficulty in learning and retaining information prominent. The cognitive impairment can be ascertained by history, mental status examination, or neuropsychological testing.

3. The marked impairment develops rapidly (i.e., over hours to days).

4. If dementia or mild neurocognitive disorder was previously diagnosed, there must be significant rapid cognitive worsening to support the additional diagnosis of delirium.

5. There is evidence from the history, physical exam, or laboratory findings of a neurological or medical condition to account for the delirium.

in the near future so that the epidemiology of this serious neurocognitive complication also can be defined.

Most observers agree that symptomatic HIV-1 infection is accompanied by an increased rate of neuropsychological impairment (34). Exactly how much of an increased risk patients with AIDS experience is not yet agreed upon. Some studies have indicated that at least a third of persons with symptomatic HIV infection have at least mild neuropsychological impairment (31,40,55,78,90). Other studies, although documenting neuropsychological impairment in AIDS, have estimated somewhat lower rates, i.e., on the order of 20% (6,67). A few studies have failed to detect any differences in rate of impairment between patients with AIDS and controls (79). A recent review study of patients with AIDS found that the rate of neurocognitive impairment ranged from 12% to 87% (median 53%) (39).

With respect to the asymptomatic phase of HIV disease, neuropsychological results have been mixed. Initially, there were reports of an increased prevalence of impairment among asymptomatic persons (31). This was followed by a number of reports, including some from very large studies, indicating no differences in neuropsychological status between asymptomatic HIV-seropositive persons and controls (17,62,63,67,79). More recently, newer studies have again detected performance differences between asymptomatic individuals and controls (6,36,40,57,59,60,89). For those recent studies reporting an elevated rate of impairment among asymptomatic persons, the rates have been estimated to range from a low of 9.1% in the WHO Neuropsychiatric AIDS Study (57) to 30.5% in the San Diego HNRC Cohort. A review of 29 studies with data on rates of neuropsychological impairment in asymptomatic carriers and controls showed a median rate of 12% impaired among samples of HIV-seronegative controls (range 0–42%) and 35% for asymptomatic HIV-seropositive individuals (range, 0–50%) (93).

Course

The progression of neurocognitive complications is poorly understood. Some investigators have found no evidence for cognitive decline in asymptomatic patients followed for ~2 years (85). On the other hand, studies following a group of patients with AIDS-related complex and AIDS for about a year concluded that the seropositive subjects declined significantly on neuropsychological tests compared with seronegative controls (24).

In the HNRC series we have completed at least 2 years of follow-up in ~150 participants (33). The annual rate of neuropsychological decline among seropositive individuals is on the order of 20%. Several studies suggest that the risk of decline is not strongly associated with stage of disease (24,33). Thus, neither initial CDC classification nor whether they progressed from one CDC stage to the other was associated with likelihood of neurocognitive decline.

There is even less information on the likelihood of neuropsychological change as a function of estimated date of seroconversion. In the HNRC series, our preliminary estimate is that the annual hazard of neurocognitive impairment in the first 3 years after seroconversion is on the order of 10% (33).

There has been considerable interest in ascertaining neurological and psychiatric variables that may increase or attenuate risk of developing neurocognitive disorders in the context of HIV-1 infection. In addition, it is important to realize that psychiatric disorder also may complicate the course of neurocognitive conditions. It is theoretically possible that advancing age and lower intelligence might decrease "cerebral reserve" (81) in HIV-infected persons, allowing subtle impairments to be detected more easily; but at present, the few systematic studies have not detected convincing interactions between age or education and serostatus so long as age-adjusted norms are applied to the neuropsychological data (32,91,92).

From a strictly neuropsychiatric perspective, most interest has focused on pre-HIV alcohol or other substance abuse and on an interaction with depression (because severe mood disorders by themselves are known to impair cognitive function) (16).

Drug Abuse

Because both alcoholism (28) and nonalcohol substance use disorders (30,77) are associated with neuropsychological impairment, it may be speculated that heavy concurrent or previous substance use might facilitate the emergence of HIV-associated neurocognitive disorder.

At this point there is no convincing evidence to suggest that this is the case. For example, one review (93) compared findings from seven neuropsychological studies of HIV-seropositive IDUs and 35 studies involving sexual transmission. They concluded that the rates of impairment were comparable from both sets of studies. Indeed, this overview concluded that the likelihood of detecting impairment in seropositive asymptomatic individuals depended largely on comprehensiveness of the neuropsychological assessment and not on issues such as risk factor, sample size, and data analytic methodology (93).

In the HNRC sample, reports of cumulative lifetime and current year use of alcohol (expressed in mg/day) or other psychoactive agents (e.g., barbiturates or benzodiazapines in diazepam [Valium®] mg/day equivalents) were compared for neuropsychologically "impaired" and "unimpaired" men. The cumulative estimates of experience with various classes of drugs did not differ between neuropsychologically impaired and unimpaired persons (39).

Mood Disorder

For some time there was considerable speculation that depressed mood might contribute to or in some way explain neuropsychological impairment in HIV-seropositive persons, especially those who were asymptomatic. However, several studies have now failed to detect a clinically significant association between mood disturbance and neuropsychological impairment in seropositive individuals (34,35). Therefore, although lifetime prevalence mood disorder is certainly increased both in seropositive individuals and those coming from risk groups for HIV infection (3), the presence of mood disturbance does not appear to contribute meaningfully to the neurocognitive deficits detected by testing these populations (41).

Alternatively complaints of problems with memory are prevalent in individuals with depressed mood (and in those with major depression). In some series (35), complaints of problems with memory in HIV-seropositive persons are just as likely to reflect underlying depressive mood as they are to signify neurocognitive disorder. This indicates that psychiatric evaluation is essential in HIV populations with subjective complaints of difficulties with remembering or other cognitive problems.

Psychiatric and Neurocognitive Comorbidity

One study suggests that individuals with neurocognitive impairment are significantly more likely to demonstrate a current, coexisting major depression than are unimpaired men (14% vs. 5%) (39). Thus, although depressed mood does not explain neurocognitive impairment in HIV, the individual with neurocognitive deficits is likely to be vulnerable to a major depressive syndrome. Rates of current major depression in persons with syndromic diagnoses of minor cognitive/motor disorder or HAD are not available. The importance of psychiatric and neurological comorbidity is that affected persons are doubly at risk for untoward social outcomes and may represent especially difficult treatment cases.

Treatment

The enthusiasm that surrounded preliminary work of a neuroprotective effect by zidovudine (74) has been tempered by more recent findings pointing toward protective efficacy of zidovudine only for dosages exceeding 1,000 mg daily (64), and then perhaps only for a limited time (25).

DELIRIOUS STATES

Epidemiology

The prevalence and incidence of delirium in HIV illness is unknown, although it is generally one of the most frequent diagnoses made by neurology and psychiatric consultation services when evaluating hospitalized HIV-infected patients (23). It is likely that deliria are as underdiagnosed and undertreated in HIV populations as it is in the ''usual'' medical or surgical patient.

Etiology

The combination of systemic illness, underlying neurocognitive impairment, and multiple medications with CNS effects is the recipe for delirium in patients with the usual major neurological diseases. The same is true for persons with symptomatic HIV disease. Therapeutic agents are likely to be associated with delirium. Often implicated are medications with anticholinergic properties, such as amitriptyline (Elavil®) and chlorpromazine (Thorazine®), along with antiemetic agents (scopolamine [Donnatal®] and prochlorperazine [Compazine®]), as well as the antihistamines and benzodiazepines. Similarly, delirium has occasionally been reported as a complication of zidovudine and ganciclovir (Cytovene®). Opportunistic or other infections (reviewed above), metabolic factors (hypoxemia, hypercarbia, electrolyte imbalances, hypoglycemia), hepatic and renal dysfunction, surgical intervention, and psychoactive substance use, and withdrawal states can all contribute to the likelihood of delirium.

Pneumocystis corinii pneumonia can be complicated by hypoxemia, which can lead to clouding of consciousness. Other causes of delirium in late-stage AIDS include severe nutritional deficiencies (e.g., vitamin B12) and electrolyte imbalance (e.g., hyponatremia).

Diagnosis

As treatments and technologies for advanced HIV disease have improved, critically ill patients at high risk for delirium are now encountered in ambulatory settings. A high index of suspicion for subtle presentation of delirium is warranted in all symptomatic HIV-infected patients, especially given the consequences of failing to recognize this neurological emergency. The DSM-IV diagnostic criteria focus on two cardinal symptoms: (a) reduced clarity of awareness of the environment and reduced ability to focus, shift, or sustain attention; and (b) a change in cognition (e.g., memory deficit, disorientation, language disturbance or perceptual disturbances like misinterpretations, illusions, hallucinations) not better explained by dementia. The disturbance must develop over a short period and fluctuate. Findings that in DSM-III and III-R were core criteria (e.g., disturbance in sleep–wake cycle, psychomotor agitation or retardation) are now relegated to auxiliary status, termed ''associated features.''

Course

The course and prognosis of deliria in the HIV-infected patient appears to mimic that found in other medical illnesses. There is a prodromal phase that may be brief or of several days' duration, an acute phase during which the diagnosis is made, and then either prompt resolution or a more persisting subacute phase that may last for several days or weeks or occasionally longer. Excess morbidity from delirium beyond its neuromedical etiology may result from suicide, falls while fleeing delusional dangers, or assault based on paranoid perception of caretakers. If delirium is associated with an underlying HIV dementia, then the prognosis may be especially grave (86).

Treatment

Symptoms of delirium in HIV illness can be effectively managed with low doses of either low-potency neuroleptics such as chlorpromazine 10–25 mg once to three times daily or with high-potency agents such as haloperidol (Haldol®) 0.25–5 mg once to three times daily. There may well be an increased incidence of extrapyramidal symptoms associated with high-potency agents in advanced HIV illness, and patients with underlying HIV-associated dementia appear to be at highest risk for extrapyramidal side effects. For patients who do not respond to low-dose oral therapy, excellent results have been reported with intravenous haloperidol given in individual boluses ranging from 2 to 10 mg every hour or, in extreme instances, up to 150 mg haloperidol daily. Some clinicians also have had good results with a combination of intravenous haloperidol and lorazepam (Ativan®), with an average daily intravenous dose of <50 mg of haloperidol and 10 mg lorazapam. In general, no serious adverse effects have been noted with these more aggressive intravenous regimens, although nearly one half of the patients treated may have extrapyramidal symptoms (28).

Benzodiazapines alone (e.g., lorazepam) do not appear to be effective in delirious states and may accentuate confusion (7).

PSYCHIATRIC DISORDERS AND HIV

The diversity of psychiatric conditions associated with HIV illness can conveniently be categorized into adjustment disorders, anxiety and mood disorders, psychosis, and substance use disorders.

Adjustment Disorders

Epidemiology

Epidemiological studies generally have not included examination for prevalence of adjustment disorder in the general population. In the context of HIV, the rates of adjustment disorders with depressed, anxious, or mixed features differ according to the population studied and appear to vary across key transition points. As might be expected, rates are highest in the days and weeks after an individual tests seropositive and may be elevated especially in workplace settings where testing is mandatory (e.g., military populations). Here rates of an adjustment disorder approach 15–20% (12,70). By contrast, among individuals who have been voluntarily tested and have known their serostatus on average for at least 1 year, rates of adjustment disorder are only 5%, even though these persons may be dealing with other HIV disease progression or treatment concerns (94).

Etiology

In terms of our proposed models of psychiatric phenomena in HIV, adjustment disorders neatly fit the ''background'' and ''transition'' models. By definition, a stressor is the etiological agent of an adjustment disorder; the magnitude of stressor(s) is not specified in the DSM-IV diagnostic criteria. The stressor may be acute (as in testing HIV positive) or chronic (as in the stress of adapting to chronic illness). What is generally being referred to is a major adverse life event. These may include social factors (which may be non-HIV related), such as termination of a romantic relationship, loss of employment, or business duress; or the stressor may be a signal ''transition'' medical event, such as testing seropositive or being informed of a precipitous decline of CD4+ lymphocytes counts. The emotional anguish of bereavement is generally not regarded as an adjustment disorder unless the emotional response is unusually severe, long-lived (>2 months), and associated with marked impairment of function.

Diagnosis

The core feature of an adjustment disorder is the development of clinically significant emotional (e.g., anxiety, depression, or mixed features) or behavior symptoms (e.g., fighting, binge alcohol or drug use, quitting a job) in response to an identifiable stressor within 3 months of the onset of the stressor. By definition, the adjustment disorder must resolve within 6 months after off-set of the stressor or its consequences.

(The diagnosis may still be made if the symptoms last longer than 6 months in response to a chronic stressor, as in a chronic disabling medical condition.)

Course

Most often adjustment disorders in HIV appear to last only a few weeks or months. For example, adjustment disorders with mixed anxious and depressive features in response to serotesting positive for HIV appear to resolve within 3 months (71,72).

Treatment

Nonpharmacological therapy should be attempted first, before pharmacotherapy is used. Indicated is a crisis management approach (88), which includes (a) addressing either avoidance and denial or its counterpart of unrealistic hopelessness ("This means I'm going to be dead soon" or "There is probably no treatment so I might as well not even be diagnosed"); (b) understanding and stating the anger that often follows adversity; and (c) providing information and problem-solving suggestions. Arranging assistance from HIV self-help groups also may be extremely therapeutic. If the predominant mood is depressed, but a major depressive disorder is not present, the usual approach is to withhold antidepressant pharmacotherapy (because response is delayed and improvement rates low for adjustment disorder).

If anxiety is predominant and it interferes with daily function for 5–7 days, pharmacotherapy may be added. Psychopharmacological treatment of anxiety is usually conceptualized as being brief, lasting no more than 2–6 weeks, and is presented with the view that most episodes of anxiety will remit within that time. For physically asymptomatic seropositive individuals, the usual choice may be an intermediate or long-acting benzodiazapine (e.g., diazepam [Valium] 20–40 mg a day or lorazepam 0.5 mg every 8 hours). For individuals with physically more symptomatic disease, agents with short to intermediate half-lives that have no active metabolites, such as lorazepam 0.5 mg every 8 hours or oxazepam (Serax®) 10 mg every 6 hours, are preferable.

For longer acting agents, the dosing strategy is to select a dose that promotes restful sleep and is associated with relief of anxiety without oversedation in daytime. For example, if diazepam were used, one would give 5 mg at bedtime and then seek a dose that provides sleep without daytime sedation. The night-time dose would be doubled each night until the goal is achieved, up to a maximum of 40 mg (43). To an extent, the same strategy may be used for lorazepam, starting with 0.5 mg. Here the night-time dose may be repeated up to every 8 hours.

In general, evidence of a therapeutic effect should be expected within 1 week of starting treatment. Treatment failure despite adequate dosages suggests that a major depressive disorder or substance use disorder (e.g., alcohol abuse) is the true underlying disorder, and reconsideration of the diagnosis or treatment is warranted.

For individuals with recent histories of alcohol or nonalcohol substance use disorders, the use of benzodiazepines may be desirable. Busprione hydrochloride (Buspar®) or hydroxyzine (Vistaril®) are reasonable alternatives. The delayed onset of therapeutic effect makes buspirone less suitable for cases of acute severe anxiety.

Similarly, panic disorder in physically asymptomatic or more symptomatic phases responds to standard therapy, which includes education, cognitive therapy, and pharmacological intervention (e.g., desipramine). In physically symptomatic persons, doses of benzodiazopines or cyclic antidepressants start at as little as one third of those used for the physically healthy individual and should be increased cautiously.

Anxiety Disorders

Epidemiology

The rates of the major anxiety disorders in HIV—panic disorder, obsessive–compulsive disorder, and generalized anxiety disorder—appear to have lifetime and current prevalences within the range expected from community epidemiological studies (e.g., 1–2%) (50,80) and to be similar in prevalence across all disease stages.

Etiology

The neurobiology of major anxiety disorder is under intense investigation, and the role of serotonergic and noradrenergic mechanisms have been recently reviewed (38,83). Interestingly, there is little evidence indicating that HIV infection of the brain produces a disorder with features reminiscent of the major anxiety disorders. Occasionally HIV may be the focus of the stated content of the anxiety (e.g., obsessions about being HIV infected despite repeated negative tests).

Diagnosis

The diagnosis and clinical features of the major anxiety disorders usually are straightforward, and because these disorders are infrequent and are usually the object of specialized psychiatric treatment, their specific diagnosis will not be reviewed here; instead reference is made to standard psychiatric texts (49). The main point often overlooked is that the panic, obsession, or other anxiety symptom may be associated with an underlying major depression that requires treatment if any progress is to be made. A second point is that episodes of anxiety that do not meet DSM-IV criteria for a disorder may be prevalent (66). One study noted that up to 20% of HIV-infected individuals (and at-risk controls) had episodes of anxiety lasting at least 1 month on 1 year follow-up (4).

Course and Treatment

The course is generally favorable and similar to that expected in non-HIV samples. The specifics of treatment are reviewed in standard texts (49). For bouts of anxiety that do not reach criteria for a disorder, the treatment approaches described for adjustment disorders are applicable.

Mood Disorders

Mood disorders in HIV can be classified as primary or secondary. ''Primary'' means that onset preceded the medical illness and is physiologically unrelated to the medical illness or that the condition preceded onset of psychoactive substance use disorders (alcohol, CNS depressants, stimulants) or use of medications. Primary mood disorder may have a strong biological basis (e.g., bipolar disorder, some major depression disorders) or may be precipitated by actual or symbolic loss or adversity. Major depression and bipolar disorder are the signal primary disorders in DSM-IV. Secondary mood disorders chronologically appear after onset of a medical or substance use disorder and are physiologically linked to that disorder. The relevant diagnostic nomenclature in the DSM-IV is "mood disorder due to a general medical condition" and "substance-induced mood disorder." Here the cardinal symptom is a prominent and persistent abnormality in mood that is judged to be the direct physiological cause of the medical (e.g., HIV) illness or a psychoactive substance. The subtypes are (a) with depressive features (if full criteria for major depression are not met); (b) with major depressionlike episode (if full criteria for major depression are evident); (c) with manic features (if mood is euphoric); and (d) with mixed features (if symptoms of depression and mania are present but neither predominates). This diagnostic scheme permits classification of mood states that are attributed directly to HIV-related physiological changes. Their prevalence, course, and treatment characteristics of these conditions are only now being outlined.

Major Depression

Epidemiology

Large-scale community surveys indicate a lifetime prevalence of major depressive disorder among men at 3–13% and for women at 5–21% (50,80). When men at highest risk for HIV are considered (homosexual or IDU men), the lifetime prevalence is estimated to range between 25% and 35%. Some studies suggest that in the majority of cases the first episode of major depression preceded the date of seroconversion (3,94). Similarly, women at highest risk for HIV (IDUs or partners of IDUs) have lifetime rates approaching 40% (53). The point prevalence of major depression in the general population is ~3% for men and 5% for women (80). In high-risk groups for HIV, the rates have generally been in the range of 4–8% for seropositive homosexual/ bisexual or IDU men. Interestingly, these rates of major depression are similar across asymptomatic HIV-seropositive, moderately symptomatic, and individuals with AIDS, at least in ambulatory populations (3,71,72,94). Hospitalized individuals with advanced HIV disease appear to have higher rates, but these are consistent with a high prevalence of major depression generally in the hospitalized medically ill person (73).

In summary, individuals at risk for HIV infection appear to have elevated rates of major depression that preceded infection; after infection, their risk of major depression is at least in line with rates in populations of other chronic medical and neurological illness (e.g., stroke, multiple sclerosis, Alzheimer's disease, Huntington's disease, Parkinson's disease) (19). Patients with primary bipolar disorder (manic–depressive disorders) are believed to be at increased risk for HIV infection due to sexual sprees, poor judgment, and the disinhibiting effects of concurrent alcohol or drug use (e.g., 3,94).

Etiology

The neurobiology of primary mood disorders is reviewed elsewhere (49). In terms of the biological model, it is unlikely that HIV itself increases the likelihood of major depression because rates after HIV infection are in the range found in other chronic medical diseases and are equivalent across asymptomatic, mildly symptomatic, and advanced CDC stages (3). HIV infection can be associated with anergic/apathetic fatigue states, presumably mediated by release of somnogenic lymphokines, but this is not to be confused with major depression. Decline of immunocompetence as reflected by lower CD4+ count does not seem to be associated with depressive mood disorder per se (56). When the relative etiological weights of the transition model (e.g., initiating antiretroviral therapy, noting the onset of constitutional symptoms, diagnosis of frank AIDS) and the background model are considered (such as adverse life events independent of HIV infection or preexisting mood disorder), the evidence suggests that most major depression in HIV stems from recurrence of a pre-HIV mood disorder (2).

Diagnosis

The DSM-IV diagnosis of major depression requires that five (or more) of nine symptoms are present nearly every day for the same 2-week period. At least one of these symptoms must be (a) depressed mood or (b) loss of interest or pleasure in usually pleasurable activity. Furthermore, the symptom complex must cause meaningful distress or impairment in daily activities, including social or occupational obligations. Finally, these symptoms must be attributable to psychological factors: they cannot be the products of medications, drug or alcohol use, or medical illness.

The nine criterion symptoms are (a) subjective report of depressed mood, or observation by other (tearfulness); (b) diminished interest or pleasure in almost all activities; (c) unintended weight loss or gain (>5% of body weight in a month) or diminished appetite; (d) insomnia or hypersomnia; (e) observable psychomotor retardation or agitation; (f) fatigue or loss of energy; (g) feelings of absolute worthlessness or excessive guilt (not simply self-reproach or guilt about being ill); (h) diminished ability to think, concentrate, or be decisive; and (i) recurrent thought of death (not just fear of dying), or suidical ideation or plans.

The diagnosis of major depressive disorder is straightforward in most HIV illness, especially because the person in the lengthy asymptomatic stage has few medical symptoms and generally well-preserved cognitive capacities. In the instance of symptomatic HIV disease, far too much has been made of the difficulty of making a diagnosis of depression in medical illness or of the potential for overdiagnosis by confounding somatic symptoms of physical illness and depression. If one seeks the cardinal symptoms (depressed mood or low interest) and applies proper severity criteria (e.g., almost all activities are less interesting; true worthlessness is present, not merely lowered self-esteem), several studies indicate that confounding by somatic symptoms does not affect diagnostic validity (15).

Thus, in the presence of somatic or neurocognitive symptoms (e.g., fatigue or forgetfulness), the diagnosis of major depression should not be made unless there is prominent and pervasive sadness, diminished interest or pleasure, feeling of worthlessness or guilt, indecisiveness, and morbid preoccupation with death. In particular, diminished activity based on fatigue must be discriminated from withdrawal from lack of interest or pleasure. The interviewer must be careful to distinguish a true sense of worthlessness from one of disappointment at not being able to perform at full capacity; likewise, persisting guilty rumination must be distinguished from episodic guilt associated with drug use or from having a sexually transmitted disease and from regret over lost opportunity. In terms of evaluating thoughts of death, which might be expected to occur in individuals with HIV illness, one must assess the level of morbid preoccupation and a change of focus from usual thoughts or attitudes or fears about death. Because many HIV-positive individuals have considered suicide at some point in the illness, the interviewer must note whether suicidal ideation is held out as a plan to potentially use at some future date (as a way of maintaining control or of euthanasia) or if it represents a self-destructiveness based on a morbid sense of failure, worthlessness, or past transgressions indicative of depression.

Obviously cognitive complaints of mental slowing and lack of concentration can be a part of a depressive picture or can be evidence of mild neurocognitive disorder or dementia. Studies indicate that ambulatory seropositive individuals (including those with frank AIDS) with depression scores in the moderate range do not differ from nondepressed seropositive individuals on detailed neuropsychological assessment of attention, language, visual spatial function, memory, or speeded information processing, although they may be somewhat slower in motor functioning (91). Conversely, individuals with mild neurocognitive disorder documented by neuropsychological testing have higher rates of current mood disorder that their nonimpaired counterparts (39). Therefore, the full evaluation of cognitive complaints requires both detailed psychiatric assessment and neuropsychological testing.

Course

Preliminary studies indicate that the cumulative 2-year incidence of major depressive disorder is ~25% and is equivalent across asymptomatic, mildly symptomatic, and individuals with frank AIDS (2). Again, the majority of these incident cases are recurrent disorder rather than new onset, as might be expected given the high lifetime base rates in certain high-risk groups (e.g., homosexual/bisexual men, IDUs) (2). The course of individual episodes is variable and is similar to that found in major depression in psychiatric populations; most individuals have infrequent episodes spaced widely apart, whereas a few have a frequent episodes (two or more annually). In an important minority of cases, a more chronic course ensues (2). Whether major depression is more severe or intractable in the neurocognitively impaired person is unknown.

Treatment

Therapy of a major depressive episode in the physically asymptomatic individual with HIV disease is straightforward. Clinical experience and randomized trials (76) indicate that the usual therapeutic doses with standard antidepressant agents are generally safe and effective in physically asymptomatic or moderately symptomatic individuals, although there are few data on maintenance treatment and longer term follow-up. The most important treatment consideration is the avoidance of agents with high anticholinergic properties (e.g., amitriptyline). Some clinicians prefer tricyclic agents with low anticholinergic properties profiles (e.g., desipramine [Nor-pramin®]) because of their familiarity with these agents; others choose the newer selective serotonin reuptake inhibitors (SSRI) drugs, such as fluoxetic (Prozac®), paroxetine (Paxil®), or sertraline (Zoloft®) because of their even more favorable side effect profiles.

Whichever agent is chosen, the clinician must be certain to apply the same caution to the physically symptomatic HIV-infected patient as would be used when treating the usual geriatric neurological patient or the individual with a major neurological illness (e.g., Parkinson's disease, multiple sclerosis). In physically symptomatic individuals, starting dosages are usually about one third to one half those given to the customary physically well patient (e.g., desipramine 25 mg daily, fluoxitine 10 mg daily, or paroxetine 10 mg daily). The most prevalent side effects of desipramine are the same as in non-HIV samples (e.g., agitation or sedation, dry mouth, constipation, urinary retention), although they are likely be of greater magnitude, and it is noted that up to 25% of outpatients with frank AIDS experience severe side effects (42). Some of the SSRI antidepressants may have specific disadvantages in the physically ill. For example, fluoxitine may be associated with agitation, insomnia, and weight loss. Lower dosages or slower rates of increase usually solve this problem, or compa-rable agents with more sedating properties may be used (e.g., sertraline). Another drawback is that some SSRI agents have drug interactions with other medications (e.g., fluoxetine increases serum concentrations of other antidepressants, and benzo-diazepines interfere with cytochrome P450 hepatic oxidative metabolism).

Physically asymptomatic individuals probably show the best rates of response. There may be somewhat reduced efficacy in patients with frank AIDS, suggesting that overall health factors influence response to therapy (96). This reduced efficacy in later stage illness is consistent with reports of a response rate of ~40% in hospital-ized, non-HIV medically ill patients with major depression. The possibility of more limited efficacy in later stage disease also has been related to loss of social support and the psychological burden of advancing physical illness. Is the person with neuro-cognitive impairment (with or without physical symptoms) also "treatment resis-tant"? This is unknown, although experience with geriatric populations suggests that major depression in the context of cognitive deficit is especially difficult to treat (16).

Physically ill patients with major depression who are unable to tolerate or do not respond to cyclic antidepressant regimens may respond to psychostimulants such as methylphenidate (Ritalin®), dextroamphetamine (Dexedrine®), or pemoline (Cyl-ert®). The usual starting dose is 5–10 mg daily in a divided dose in the morning and early afternoon with increases daily or every other day up to 20–30 mg/day. Some authorities prefer methylphenidate because dextroamphetamine may produce severe tremor or a persisting movement disorder in later stage patients (44).

Electroconvulsive therapy (ECT) is effective in patients whose depression requires urgent treatment, in those who have not responded to pharmacological therapies, or in those with major depression with psychotic features (82). With judicious use, good outcomes may be expected even in individuals with neurocognitive impairment, much in the same way that elderly patients with dementia and major depression respond positively. Neurological examination and brain imaging are necessary to rule out opportunistic brain disease and increased intracranial pressure before com-mencing ECT.

Mania

Manic episodes with or without hallucinations, delusions, or a disorder of thought process occur rarely; although mania can complicate any stage of HIV infection, it is most often a late-stage event.

Epidemiology

Manic episodes appear to be rare, and informal estimates put the point prevalence at 0.01–1.5% (84).

Etiology

Our biological and background approaches provide useful explanatory models of mania. Most manic episodes are attributable to therapeutic dosages of medications, or substances of abuse, or occasionally to HIV-related neurological conditions such as stroke, meningitis, and tumor. Steroids, zidovudine, and ganciclovir are the most frequently reported iatrogenic causes (13). In these instances the manic phenomenon is probably best conceptualized as a prodrome or presentation of a delirium or withdrawal; intoxication states from alcohol, benzodiazepines, barbituates, or stimulants (e.g. cocaine, methamphetamines) also produce manic symptoms. In terms of the background model, men and women with bipolar disorder are at a heightened risk of HIV infection and must always be screened for HIV. There are reports of manic syndromes in individuals without substance-induced mania who also had no previous personal or family history of mood disorder. In these cases the etiology is presumed to be HIV or associated viral coinfections, along with intersecting adverse life circumstances—an intersection of biological vulnerabilities and background stress.

Diagnosis

DSM-IV provides two diagnostic categories encompassing most cases of HIV mania. Criteria for a full manic episode requires a 1-week period of an abnormally elevated, expansive, or irritable mood (or of any duration if hospitalization is required because of the mood abnormality). At least three of the following symptoms (four if the mood is irritable but not elevated) must be concurrent: (a) highly inflated self-esteem or grandiosity; (b) diminished need for sleep (e.g., feels rested after only 2 or 3 hours sleep); (c) increased talkativeness; (d) subjective sense of racing thoughts or rapid shifting from thought to thought (flight of ideas); (e) distractibility; (f) increased activity (either aimless agitation or in goal-directed work, school, social, or sexual activity); and (g) excessive involvement in pleasurable activity at high risk for adverse consequences (e.g., buying sprees, sexual sprees).

Typical case reports involve individuals previously described as stable who over a period of days or weeks undergo a change in personality (e.g., become pompous, belittling, and sexually inappropriate), and then progress into a full manic picture. In this instance the diagnosis is manic episode due to HIV. Most often fewer associated symptoms are present, and if so, the diagnosis is mood disorder due to HIV, with manic features. The DSM IV category "mood disorder due to HIV, with manic features'' requires only the presence of an abnormal mood that meaningfully effects function. In most HIV cases the mood is elevated rather than irritable, and there is associated grandiosity. Diminished need for sleep, loquaciousness, teeming thoughts, and unrealistic personal or financial schemes may be present. Case reports assert that mental status examinations do not disclose neurocognitive deficit, but detailed neuropsychological examinations have not been reported; therefore, mild neurocognitive disorder as a predisposing factor cannot be excluded. The neuromedical evaluation is generally unremarkable apart from findings expected for HIV disease (14).

Treatment

Acute manic states may be managed with neuroleptics in low doses, such as chlorpromazine 25–150 mg/day or haloperidol 0.5–5 mg daily. Clonazepam (Klonipin®), up to 10 mg/day, also has been found to be effective for acute mania and may be especially useful in patients who cannot tolerate neuroleptics or lithium (13). If the manic picture is the presentation of a delirium from the patient's general medical condition, however, benzodiazepines should be avoided because they simply heighten confusion and disorientation and obscure the diagnosis. Maintenance therapy with standard mood-stabilizing agents (e.g., lithium [Eskalith®], valproate [Divalproex®], carbamazepine [Tegretol®]) may be indicated for patients with recurrent episodes, family history of bipolar disorder, or, of course, personal history of bipolar illness. Lithium carbonate has been used to treat patients who develop a manic episode induced by zidovudine, and the resulting control of symptoms should allow the patient to continue antiretroviral therapy.

Psychotic Disorders

Epidemiology

Prevalence estimates vary widely depending on study methodology. If one considers the prevalence of HIV infection for patients with schizophrenia being admitted to psychiatric hospitals in urban epicenters of the AIDS epidemic, perhaps 10% of schizophrenic persons are infected (18). When the psychotic disorder is due to HIV, large-scale surveys find a prevalence of <0.5%, whereas chart review methods find frequencies ranging from 3% to 15% in persons from whom obvious causes (e.g., delirium) have been excluded (37,86). Thus, psychotic symptoms may be uncommon, but not rare, in HIV-infected populations without an underlying primary psychosis.

Etiology

In terms of our model, the detection of psychotic symptoms or disorders should most often trigger a search for background factors (e.g., primary schizophrenia, psychostimulant abuse, or major depression with psychotic features) or biological factors (e.g., deliria; neurological vascular disease, opportunistic infection, or neoplasm; and iatrogenic causes). Alternatively, psychosis has been attributed to direct effects of HIV on the brain or from coinfection with other CNS viruses such as cytomegalovirus or herpes simplex virus (37). The predilection of HIV for subcortical or temporal regions may be etiologically related to psychotic symptoms.

The etiological role of stressful HIV transitions as precipitating psychosis seems to be minor, although signal medical events may provoke psychotic episodes in vulnerable persons.

Diagnosis

The core concept of psychotic syndromes defined in DSM-IV is the presence of delusions, hallucinations, disorganized speech, thought, or behavior. These phenomena can occur in HIV illness despite intact consciousness and memory (i.e., in the absence of delirium and dementia). Delusions (falsely held beliefs that cannot be influenced by reason or contradictory evidence) may either be nonbizarre (involving circumstances that occur in everyday existence, such as being pursued or nominated for high elected office) or bizarre (involving fantastic situations outside of real experience, such as being controlled by aliens, being able to control others by mental telepathy). Disorganized speech is that in which statements are not logically connected and whose content makes no sense; loose associations and incoherence are examples of disorganized speech (and presumably thought). Disorganized behavior is random, disconnected, or odd (26).

When delusions or hallucinations develop only in the course of HIV-associated dementia, the diagnosis is HAD with delusions (or hallucinations). If psychotic symptoms result from exposure to medication or drug of abuse (e.g., amphetamine), the DSM-IV designates the picture as a "substance-induced psychotic disorder." For psychosis attributable to physiology of a physical illness, the DSM-IV classification "psychotic disorder due to general medical condition (e.g., HIV)" would apply. Such psychotic states, sometimes known as noniatrogenic new onset psychosis in the HIV literature, are usually later stage complications of HIV infection, require immediate medical and neurological evaluation, and often require neuroleptic management.

The clinical presentation in "psychotic disorder due to HIV infection" is extremely variable. The most prevalent symptom seems to be delusions (occurring in almost 90% of cases in some series) with persecutory, grandiose, or somatic components. Persecutory themes can be quite elaborate, with patients proclaiming messianic themes or believing that they have been accorded superhuman powers by God. Somatic delusions may include being shot through with electricity or lasers. Delusions of thoughts being inserted into ones mind by outside forces, thought broadcasting (one's thought being audible to others), and of physical acts controlled by aliens are also described. Most patients experience auditory hallucinations, with perhaps half of these also experiencing visual hallucinations. A majority of series also report disorders of thought process, including looseness of associations or frankly disorganized thinking (37,86).

Disturbances of mood commonly coexist, with anxiety being the most prevalent symptom, followed by depressed mood, euphoria, or irritability, and mixed depressed and euphoric states. Lability, flatness, and inappropriate laughter or anger are also described (37).

Disorganized and even bizarre behavior may be evident. Individuals may turn to eating dirt to "conquer their fear of germs" (86). One of our patients painted himself and his entire apartment, including furniture and appliances, with green paint in order to "celebrate life."

Bedside examination shows impairment in memory or other cognitive functions in up to one third of patients with psychosis (86); more comprehensive and formal neuropsychological assessment would likely detect neurocognitive difficulties in a larger proportion of cases, but many psychotic individuals are unable to submit to such examinations.

Other neurological findings are infrequent and nonspecific, usually consisting of ataxia, mild increases in motor tone, hyperreflexia, and tremor, but bizarre grimaces and posturing can be present. Cerebrospinal fluid is generally unremarkable, except for the mild pleocytosis common to HIV infection. Diffuse cortical slowing has been reported in about half of those patients who submitted to electroencephalography. Computed tomography and magnetic resonance imaging scans can show nonspecific cerebral atrophy in about half of the cases. Rarely, focal abnormalities are evident, suggesting tumor, opportunistic infection, or vascular etiology.

Course

The course and prognosis are highly variable and depend partly on whether specific complicating conditions coexist. For example, coexisting HIV dementia (HAD with delusions or hallucinations) indicates a poor prognosis. Here the course may be one of rapid deterioration with death often within 6 months or less (5). On the other hand, when neurocognitive abnormalities are not detected or are mild, individuals have been followed for up to 2 years in a stable, treated course (86). Overall, there is some evidence that death occurs earlier in those experiencing psychosis compared with nonpsychotic patients who have similarly advanced HIV disease (86).

Treatment

Treatment of new-onset psychotic symptoms attributable to HIV is applied using neuroleptics. In the short term, prognosis with regard to symptom control is reasonably favorable, with most patients responding to low-dose regimens of neuroleptics. The major therapeutic concern is choosing an agent with the lowest incidence of side effects because in randomized comparative studies high-potency (e.g., haloperidol [Haldol®]) and low potency agents (thioridazine [Mellaril®]) were equally effective in ameliorating symptoms (86).

The usual therapeutic dose is one tenth to one third that used for psychoses in psychiatric settings (e.g., schizophrenia), with the mean daily dose being ~150 mg in chlorpromazine equivalents (e.g., 1–10 mg daily of haloperidol or fluphenazine [Prolixin®]). Positive symptoms of psychosis (delusions, hallucinations) are much more likely to respond than are the so-called negative symptoms (withdrawal, apathy) (86). Because negative symptoms may be particularly disabling, risperidone [Risperidal®] may be a desirable agent, given their putative efficacy for negative symptoms. The time course of response is similar to that observed in schizophrenia, with the majority of improvement occurring within the first 6 weeks of therapy. It is unclear why such low-dose regimens are adequate but may be related to pharmacokinetic changes associated with chronic disease, or to HIV-associated damage to subcortical limbic or basal ganglia structures. This latter explanation also has been thought to be the source of sensitivity of patients with HIV-associated psychosis to medication-induced extrapyramidal side effects (46). Interestingly, movement disorder attributable to subcortical damage can appear in HIV-infected persons not taking neuroleptics and include myoclonus, paroxysmal dystonia, parkinsonian features, essential tremors, hemiballism, and hemichorea.

If high-potency neuroleptics are used, extrapyramidal side effects will be universal—and bothersome enough to require treatment. Even with low-potency agents, ~60% of patients will develop extrapyramidal signs (86). In general, extrapyramidal side effects can be managed with low doses of benztropine mesylate (Cogentin®), 1–3 mg daily, but amantadine (Symmetrel®) 50–100 mg twice daily can be used instead to avoid the "deliriogenic" anticholinergic effects of benztropine mesylate. Other authorities advocate molindone (Moban®) 10–15 mg daily as the primary neuroleptic because of its lower likelihood of producing extrapyramidal syndromes (27).

Substance Use Disorders

Substance use disorders are important to detect for at least three reasons. First, abuse or dependence can heighten likelihood of transmitting HIV by sharing of infected "works" by IDUs. And even among non-IDUs, drug or alcohol abuse seems to be associated with having sex with multiple anonymous partners and reduced use of condoms. Second, intoxication or withdrawal syndromes can complicate the neuropsychiatric presentation of the HIV-infected patient. And third, substance use disorders often complicate mood or psychotic disorders and make this extremely difficult or impossible.

Epidemiology

In the general population, the lifetime prevalence of alcohol dependence ranges from 20% (for men) to 8% (for women); nonalcohol drug dependence prevalences are 9% for men and 6% for women (50). The lifetime rates of alcohol use disorders in the major risk groups—homosexual/bisexual men and IDU men and women—range from 20% to >40%. Although some studies show higher current rates of substance use disorders among seropositive gay and bisexual individuals compared with those expected from community samples, others show roughly comparable or only slightly higher rates (e.g., 5%) (3,72,94).

Etiology

The etiology of substance abuse in those at risk for HIV infection is no better understood than it is for substance abuse generally. It has been speculated that at least among homosexual/bisexual individuals the developmental stresses of establishing an alternate sexual identity and of negotiating this within the context of family expectations and stigmatization by society may contribute to substance use as a way of mastering distress. The low rates of active substance use disorders in AIDS may reflect alcohol intolerance due to debilitating illness. Preliminary data also suggest that the stress of HIV infection does not necessarily lead to an increased risk of developing an alcohol or nonalcohol substance use disorder.

Diagnosis

The major substance use disorders in DSM-IV are abuse and dependence. Criteria for abuse focus on behavioral problems from use rather than quantity or frequency of use. One or more of the following must be present: (a) failure to fulfill a major role obligation (e.g., poor work performance or absences; neglect of children or household; school expulsion); (b) recurrent use in situations involving physical hazard (e.g., driving an automobile); (c) substance-related legal problems (e.g., arrest); and (d) continued use despite social problems resulting from use (e.g., arguments with spouse about intoxication).

Dependence requires at least three of the following: (a) tolerance; (b) withdrawal syndrome; (c) intake of substance in larger amounts for longer periods than was intended; (d) desire to cut down or control use; (e) a great deal of time is taken up obtaining the substance, using it or recovering from its effects; (f) reduction in usual social, occupational, or recreational activities; and (g) continued use despite presence of persistent or recurrent physical or psychological problem due to the substance.

Diagnosis depends on a high index of suspicion based either on obvious current findings (e.g., unexplained deterioration in work or relationships; intermittent hypertension [due to stimulant use]; elevated GGT [from alcohol]), or a past history of abuse or dependence. Sometimes direct inquiry about criterion symptoms can lead to frank revelation of difficulty; more often the patient grossly underestimates the impact of abuse or dependence on everyday life. This has led some astute clinicians to note that the first rule of taking an alcohol or drug history is "Never believe the history." More valid data may come from family informants or significant others and from urine toxicology or other laboratory findings.

Course

Preliminary studies of HIV-seropositive homosexual/bisexual participants (with follow-ups of 2 years' duration) suggest the incident alcohol and nonalcohol substance use disorders represent relapses of disorders whose original onset preceded likely date of seroconversion. Furthermore, seropositive and seronegative homosexual/bisexual men were equally likely to experience an episode of the disorder within the follow-up period. Incident rates are generally <5% annually and are equivalent across asymptomatic and symptomatic groups, although those with frank AIDS have even lower rates. It may be that, at least within homosexual/bisexual communities, the emphasis on health promotion and education about the adverse health consequences of alcohol and other drugs of abuse has had a positive effect.

Treatment

Although diverse psychological, behavioral, and pharmacological approaches to treating substance use disorders are available, the mainstay of treatment is still self-help groups (e.g., Alcoholics Anonymous). This should be combined with a vigorous assessment for likely comorbid psychiatric disorders (e.g., major depression), which if undetected can thwart rehabilitation.

OTHER NEUROPSYCHIATRIC TOPICS

Suicide

Individuals with advanced HIV disease may have a 30-fold risk of committing suicide compared with seronegative individuals matched for age and social position (51,61). These rates exceed even the heightened risk for suicide in other neurological diseases, such as Huntington's disease. Psychiatric disorder is strongly implicated in suicide, attempted suicide and suicidal ideation in HIV populations, and psychiatric histories are evident in almost 50% of suicide cases (61).

Suicide attempt and suicidal ideation are correlated most often with histories of major depressive disorder or substance use disorders and in the majority of cases these suicidal behaviors commenced before likely date of seroconversion (4,65). Women may be at elevated risk for suicidal ideation (10,11). Thus, although debate over the distinction between suicide and the right to choose death or to refuse unwanted treatment are important issues, it is imperative that individuals expressing suicidal behaviors or ideas should be examined for a major psychiatric disorder and be offered appropriate treatment.

Fatigue–Anergia States

Fatigue–anergia–apathy syndromes also can complicate advanced disease in its middle and later stages. These syndromes are not necessarily accompanied by depressive symptomatology or marked neurocognitive impairment. Although release of various lymphokines (e.g., tumor necrosis factor; various interleukins) may be primarily responsible, some investigators have suggested that there could be a psychodynamic component of this syndrome—a conservation-withdrawal response in the face of loss of control. Beyond assuring that nutrition and medical management are optimal, simple measures such as encouragement and support, allowing a patient to participate in treatment decisions, and providing activities outside the hospital room can be helpful, with a response usually occurring within 1 week. Psychostimulants in dosages used from patients with neurocognitive disorder (e.g., methylphenidate, 10–20 mg daily) have achieved gratifying results in other groups of patients, but there are no controlled studies available.

Neuroleptic Malignant Syndrome

It is thought that patients with AIDS generally, and those with HIV-associated dementia in particular, may be at increased risk for the most serious side effect of antipsychotic drugs, the neuroleptic malignant syndrome. This condition may present with subtle signs, and the diagnosis should be entertained in any patient on neuroleptics who develops rigidity, akinesia, mutism, lethargy, fever, autonomic instability, and increased creatine kinase (CK) activity. Neuroleptic malignant syndrome may be particularly associated with high-potency agents. Treatment is directed at discontinuing the neuroleptic and at supportive care (8).

Sleep Disorders

Decreased sleep quality, difficulty falling asleep, nighttime fragmented sleep, and early morning awakenings seem to increase as immune function and CD4 + lymphocytes diminish and may affect a substantial proportion of individuals with AIDS. The reports of increased sleep difficulty in men with later stage disease seem to be independent of zidovudine therapy or of psychological distress (20,68). Some have proposed that alterations in sleep architecture, such as increases in slow-wave sleep, may be an early marker of CNS involvement in HIV-infected persons. The therapeutic approach generally has been limited to symptomatic treatment using nonbenzodiazepine agents used as hypnotics, such as trazodone (Desyrel®).

Pain Syndromes

Pain is just as underrecognized and under-treated in HIV disease as it is in other life-threatening illnesses, such as cancer. The etiology and pathogenesis of pain in HIV-related disorders is only beginning to be understood (52,54). Psychiatric disorders may complicate persisting pain, and because no one specialty addresses pain syndromes, patient care is often fragmented between anesthesiologists, neurologists, internists, and psychiatrists.

Neuropathic pain related to HIV usually presents as a persisting, painful sensorimotor neuropathy with dysesthesia, stocking-glove sensory loss, diminished distal reflexes, and distal weakness. Similarly, postherpetic neuralgia (herpes zoster radiculitis) may involve pain of the face or trunk. Treatment of neuropathic pain syndromes is usually applied using low-dose tricyclic antidepressants, such as desipramine or nortriptyline, 10–25 mg/day. The typical steady-state dose is 50 mg, although some patients have required higher amounts (75–100 mg daily). A response often ensues within 1–2 weeks, but 4–6 weeks of treatment may be necessary before response occurs or another tricyclic agent is chosen. In general, tricyclic antidepressants are more effective than opiate analgesics for chronic neuropathic pain. Mexiletine, a congener of lidocaine and an agent used for treatment of ventricular arrhythmias, also may be effective for neuropathic pain (21). The maximum dose is 600 mg daily. A multicenter trial is currently assessing the efficacy compared with amitriptyline. Anticonvulsants such as diphenylhydantoin (Dilantin®) or carbamazepine also may be effective at usual therapeutic concentrations required for seizure management. Postherpetic neuralgia also may respond to clonazepam 1–5 mg daily.

Chronic headache may appear as a residual symptom from aseptic meningitis in seroconversion illness or as an effect of zidovudine (which may persist after drug discontinuation). It is known that imipramine (Tofranil®), desipramine, amitriptyline, and nortriptyline can be effective in treating migraine and mixed migraine-tension headache syndromes in the non-HIV population, and there is speculation that persisting headache after aseptic meningitis also may respond to low-dose regimens of these agents (e.g., nortriptyline or desipramine 10—25 mg daily with increase up to 75 mg). Among the rheumatological disorders are arthralgias, myalgias, and arthritides involving large joints of the leg. HIV-related arthralgias may respond to nonsteroidal antiinflammatory agents, although acetaminophen (Tylenol®) should be avoided because it may diminish metabolism of zidovudine. HIV also may be associated with a polymyositis, which involves pain, weakness, and elevated CPK, along with changes on electromyography indicating a myopathic process. Chronic zidovudine administration may produce a myositis that persists when the medication is discontinued. Psychopharmacological interventions are not of demonstrated efficacy in these states.

Multidisciplinary pain treatment approaches, which use coordinated efforts of experts in various disciplines, may be as useful in chronic HIV-related pain as they are in chronic, non–HIV-related pain syndromes. These approaches use education about the nature of persisting pain, activity scheduling, self-monitoring and relaxation training, and cognitive therapies to reduce disability related to pain.

CONCLUSION

Until 1981, acquired immune deficiency represented a rare disorder of concern mostly to medical subspecialists. As we approach the end of the twentieth century, we anticipate that there may be 40 million to 100 million men, women, and children worldwide infected with HIV-1. Given the current experience, at least 10 million of these will develop AIDS (58).

Neurobiological and psychobiological complications of AIDS and HIV infection promise to become one of the most prevalent sources of neuropsychiatric morbidity by the year 2000. These facts, coupled with our understanding that the proximate cause of HIV infection resides almost always in human behavior—some of it ordinary, some linked to psychopathology, but all of it potentially modifiable—poses unprecedented challenges and opportunities to scientists and clinicians working at the interfaces of biomedicine, public health, and neuropsychiatry.

ACKNOWLEDGMENT

This work was supported by Grant P50 MH45294 from the National Institute of Mental Health and by the Department of Veterans Affairs.

REFERENCES

1. American Psychiatric Association Committee on Nomenclature and Statistics. *Diagnostic and Statistical Manual of Mental Disorders.* 4th ed. Washington, DC: American Psychiatric Association Press, 1994.
2. Atkinson JH, Grant I. Natural history of neuropsychiatric manifestations of HIV disease. *Psychiatr Clin North Am* 1994;17:17–33.
3. Atkinson JH, Grant I, Kennedy CJ, Richman DD, Spector SA, McCutchan JA. Prevalence of psychiatric disorders among men infected with human immunodeficiency virus. *Arch Gen Psychiatry* 1988; 45:859.
4. Atkinson JH, Grant I, Patterson T, Gutierrez R, Brown S, McCutchan J. Longitudinal follow-up of psychiatric disorders in HIV. *Psychosom Med* 1991;53:232–233.

5. Boccellari AA, Dilley JW. Management and residential placement problems of patients with HIV-related cognitive impairment. *Hosp Commun Psychiatry* 1992;43:32–37.
6. Bornstein RA, Nasrallah HA, Para MF, Whitacre CC, Rosenberger P, Fass RJ. Neuropsychological performance in symptomatic and asymptomatic HIV infection. *AIDS* 1993;7:519–524.
7. Breitbart W. Psycho-oncology: depression, anxiety, delirium. *Semin Oncol* 1994;21:754–769.
8. Breitbart W, Marotta RF, Call P. AIDS and neuroleptic malignant syndrome. *Lancet* 1988;2: 1488–1499.
9. Britton CB, Marquardt MD, Koppel B, Garvey G, Miller JR. Neurological complications of the gay immunosuppressed syndrome: clinical and pathological features [Abstract]. *Ann Neurol* 1982;12:80.
10. Brown GR, Rundell JR. Suicidal tendencies in women with human immunodeficiency virus infection. *Am J Psychiatry* 1989;146:556.
11. Brown GR, Rundell JR. Prospective study of psychiatric morbidity in HIV-seropositive women without AIDS. *Gen Hosp Psychiatry* 1990;12:30.
12. Brown GR, Rundell JR, McManis SE, Kendall SN, Zachary R, Temoshok L. Prevalence of psychiatric disorders in early stages of HIV infection. *Psychosom Med* 1992;54:588–601.
13. Budman CL, Vandersall TA. Clonazepam treatment of acute mania in an AIDS patient. *J Clin Psychiatry* 1990;51:212.
14. Buhrich N, Cooper DA, Freed E. HIV infection associated with symptoms indistinguishable from functional psychosis. *Br J Psychiatry* 1988;152:649.
15. Chochinov HM, Wilson KG, Enns M, Lander S. Prevalence of depression in the terminally ill: effect of diagnostic criteria and symptom threshold judgements. *Am J Psychiatry* 1994;151:537–540.
16. Coffey CE, Cummings JL, eds. *Textbook of Geriatric Neuropsychiatry.* Washington, DC: American Psychiatric Press, 1994.
17. Collier AC, Marra C, Coombs RW, et al. Central nervous system manifestations of human immunodeficiency virus infection without AIDS. *J AIDS* 1992;5:229–241.
18. Cournos F, Empfield M, Horwath E, et al. HIV seroprevalence among patients admitted to two psychiatric hospitals. *Am J Psychiatry* 1991;148:1225.
19. Cummings JL, Trimble MR. *Concise Guide to Neuropsychiatry and Behavioral Neurology.* Washington, DC: American Psychiatric Association Press, 1995.
20. Darko DF, McCutchan JA, Kripke DF, Gillin JC, Golshan S. Fatigue, sleep disturbance, disability, and indices of progression of HIV infection. *Am J Psychiatry* 1992;149:514.
21. Dejgard A, Kastrup J, Petersen P. Mexiletine for treatment of chronic painful diabetic neuropathy. *Lancet* 1988;2:9–11.
22. Dew MA, Ragni MW, Nimorwicz P. Infection with human immunodeficiency virus and vulnerability to psychiatric distress: a study of men with hemophilia. *Arch Gen Psychiatry* 1990;47:737.
23. Dilley JW, Ochitill HN, Perl M, Volberding P. Findings in psychiatric consultations with patients with acquired immunodeficiency syndrome and related disorders. *Am J Psychiatry* 1985;142:82.
24. Dunbar N, Perdices M, Grunseit A, Cooper DA. Changes in neuropsychological performance of AIDS-related complex patients who progress to AIDS. *AIDS* 1992;6:691–700.
25. Dupont RM, Jernigan T, Lehr P, Lamoureux G, Halpern S, Grant I. Cerebrovascular response in HIV infection. *Annual meeting of the American Psychiatric Association.* Philadelphia, May 21–26, 1994.
26. Fauman MA. *Study Guide to DSM-IV.* Washington, DC: American Psychiatric Press, 1994.
27. Fernandez F, Levy JK, eds. *Psychiatric Diagnosis and Treatment Issues in the Patient with HIV Infection.* Washington, DC: American Psychiatric Press, 1990.
28. Grant, I. Alcohol and the brain-neuropsychological correlates. *J Consult Clin Psychol* 1987;55: 310–324.
29. Grant I. The neuropsychiatry of human immunodeficiency virus. *Semin Neurol* 1990;10:267.
30. Grant I, Adams KM, Carlin AS, Rennick P, Judd LL, Schooff K. The collaborative neuropsychological study of polydrug users. *Arch Gen Psychiatry* 1978;35:1063–1074.
31. Grant I, Atkinson JH, Hesselink JR, et al. Evidence for early central nervous system involvement in the acquired immunodeficiency syndrome (AIDS) and other human immunodeficiency virus (HIV) infections. Studies with neuropsychological testing and magnetic resonance imaging. *Ann Intern Med* 1987;107:828.
32. Grant I, Caun K, Kingsley DPE, Winer J, Trimble MR, Pinching AJ. Neuropsychological and NMR abnormalities in HIV infection. The St. Mary's-Queen Square study. *Neuropsych Behav Neurol* 1992; 5:185.
33. Grant I, Heaton RK, Deutsch R, McCutchan JA, Atkinson JH, Chandler J. Risk of neuropsychological impairment steadily rises from date of seroconversion: HNRC experience. Poster presentation at International Conference on AIDS, Yokohama, August 8–9, 1994, p. 193 (poster PB0200).
34. Grant I, Martin A. *Neuropsychology of HIV Infection.* New York: Oxford University Press, 1994.
35. Grant I, Olshen RA, Atkinson JH, et al. Depressed mood does not explain neuropsychological deficits in HIV-infected persons. *Neuropsychology* 1993;7:53–61.

36. Handelsman L, Aronson M, Maurer G, et al. Neuropsychological and neurological manifestations of HIV-1 dementia in drug users. *J Neuropsychiatry Clin Neurosci* 1992;4:21–28.
37. Harris J, Jeste DV, Gleghorn A, Sewell DD. New-onset psychosis in HIV-infected patients. *J Clin Psychiatry* 1991;52:369.
38. Hauger RL, Lupien S, Plotsky PM. Hypothalamic-pituitary-adrenocortical dysregulation in affective disorders: focus on stress neuroendocrinology, corticotropin-releasing factor receptors, and pituitary corticotrope function. In: Michels R, Cavenar JO, Cooper AM, Guze SB, Judd LL, Solnit AJ, eds. *Psychiatry.* Revised ed. Philadelphia: JB Lippincott, 1994:1–43.
39. Heaton RK, Velin RA, Atkinson JH, et al. Neuropsychological impairment in an HIV-positive male cohort. In: Stein M, Baum A, eds. *Perspectives on Behavioral Medicine.* East Sussex, England: Lawrence Erlbaum, 1995⊥. 79–93.
40. Heaton RK, Velin RA, McCutchan JA, et al. Neuropsychological impairment in human immunodeficiency virus-infection: implications for employment. *Psychosom Med* 1994;56:8–17.
41. Hinkin CH, van Gorp WG, Satz P, Weisman JD, Thommes J, Buckingham S. Depressed mood and its relationship to neuropsychological test performance in HIV-1 seropositive individuals. *J Clin Exp Neuropsychol* 1992;14:289.
42. Hintz S, Kuck J, Peterkin J, Volk DM, Zisook S. Depression in the context of human immunodeficiency virus infection: implications for treatment. *J Clin Psychiatry* 1990;51:497.
43. Hollister LE. Principles of therapeutic applications of benzodiazepines. In: Smith DE, Wesson DR, eds. *The Benzodiazepines. Current Standards for Medical Practice.* Lancaster, England: MTP Press, 1985:87–94.
44. Holmes V, Fernandez F, Levy JK. Psychostimulant response in AIDS-related complex (ARC) patients. *J Clin Psychiatry* 1989;50:5.
45. Horowitz SL, Benson DF, Gottlieb MS, Davos I, Bentson JR. Neurological complications of gay-related immunodeficiency disorder [Abstract]. *Ann Neurol* 1982;12:80.
46. Hriso E, Kuhn T, Masdeu JC, Grundman M. Extrapyramidal symptoms due to dopamine-blocking agents in patients with AIDS encephalopathy. *Am J Psychiatry* 1991;148:1558.
47. Janssen RS, Saykin AJ, Cannon L, et al. Neurological and neuropsychological manifestations of HIV-1 infection: association with AIDS-related complex but not asymptomatic HIV-1 infection. *Ann Neurol* 1989;26:592–600.
48. Janssen RS, Stehr-Green J, Starcher T. Epidemiology of HIV encephalopathy in the United States. Abstracts of the Vth International Conference on AIDS, 1989:50.
49. Kaplan HI, Saddock BJ, eds. *Comprehensive Textbook of Psychiatry.* 6th ed. Vol. 2. Psychiatric aspects of acquired immunodeficiency syndrome. Baltimore, MD: Williams & Wilkins, 1995.
50. Kessler RC, McGonagle KA, Zhao S, et al. Lifetime and 12-month prevalence of DSM III-R psychiatric disorders in the United States: results from the National Comorbidity Survey. *Arch Gen Psychiatry* 1994;51:8–19.
51. Kizer K, Green W, Perkins M. AIDS and suicide in California. *JAMA* 1988;259:1333–1337.
52. Lewis MS, Warfield CA. Management of pain in AIDS. *Hosp Pract* October 30, 1990.
53. Lipsitz JD, Williams JBW, Rabkin JG, et al. Psychopathology in male and female intravenous drug users with and without HIV infection. *Am J Psychiatry* 1994;151:1662–1668.
54. Lebovits AH, Lefkowitz M, McCarthy D, Simon R, et al. The prevalence and management of pain in patients with AIDS: a review of 134 cases. *Clin J Pain* 1989;5:245.
55. Lunn S, Skydsbjerg M, Schulsinger H, Parnas J, Pedersen C, Mathiesen L. A preliminary report on the neuropsychological sequelae of human immunodeficiency virus. *Arch Gen Psychiatry* 1991;48:139–142.
56. Lyketsos CG, Hoover DR, Guccione M, et al. Depressive symptoms as predictors of medical outcomes in HIV infection. *JAMA* 1994;270:2563–2567.
57. Maj M, Satz P, Janssen R, et al. WHO neuropsychiatric AIDS study, cross-sectional phase II: neuropsychological and neurological findings. *Arch Gen Psychiatry* 1994;51:51–61.
58. Mann J, Tarantola D, Netter TW. *AIDS in the World.* Cambridge, MA: Harvard University Press, 1992.
59. Martin A, Heyes MP, Salazar AM, Law WA, Williams J. Impaired motor-skill learning, slowed reaction time, and elevated cerebrospinal fluid quinolinic acid in a subgroup of HIV-infected individuals. *Neuropsychology* 1993;7:149–157.
60. Martin EM, Robertson LC, Edelstein HE, et al. Performance of patients with early HIV-1 infection on the Stroop task. *J Clin Exp Neuropsychol* 1992;14:857–868.
61. Marzuk PM, Tierney H, Tardiff K, et al. Increased risk of suicide in persons with AIDS. *JAMA* 1988;259:1333.
62. McAllister RH, Herns MV, Harrison MJG, et al. Neurological and neuropsychological performance in HIV seropositive men without symptoms. *J Neurol Neurosurg Psychiatry* 1992;55:143–148.
63. McArthur JC, Cohen BA, Selnes OA, et al. Low prevalence of neurological and neuropsychological abnormalities in otherwise healthy HIV-1–infected individuals: results from the Multicenter AIDS Cohort Study. *Ann Neurol* 1989;26:601–611.

64. McArthur JC, Hoover DR, Bacellar H, et al. Dementia in AIDS patients: incidence and risk factors. *Neurology* 1993;43:2245–2252.
65. McKegney FP, O'Dowd MA. Suicidality and HIV status. *Am J Psychiatry* 1992;149:396.
66. Miller D, Acton TG, Hedge B. The worried well: their identification and management. *J R Coll Physicians Lond* 1988;22:158.
67. Miller EN, Selnes OA, McArthur JC, et al. Neuropsychological performance in HIV-1–infected homosexual men: the Multicenter AIDS Cohort Study (MACS). *Neurology* 1990;40:197–203.
68. Moeller AA, Oechsner M, Backmund HC, Popescu M, Emminger C, Holsboer F. Self-reported sleep quality in HIV infection: correlation to the stage of infection and zidovudine therapy. *J AIDS* 1991; 4:1000.
69. Navia BA, Jordan BD, Price RW. The AIDS dementia complex: 1. Clinical features. *Ann Neurol* 1986;19:517–524.
70. Pace J, Brown GR, Rundell JR, Paolucci S, Drexler K, McManis S. Prevalence of psychiatric disorders in a mandatory screening program for infection with human immunodeficiency virus: a pilot study. *Milit Med* 1990;155:76.
71. Perry S, Jacobsberg L, Fishman B. Suicidal ideation and HIV testing. *JAMA* 1990;263:579.
72. Perry S, Jacobsberg LR, Fishman B, Frances A, Bobo J, Jacobsberg BK. Psychiatric diagnosis before serological testing for the human immunodeficiency virus. *Am J Psychiatry* 1990;147:89.
73. Perry SW, Tross S. Psychiatric problems of AIDS inpatients at the New York Hospital: preliminary report. *Public Health Rep* 1984;99:200.
74. Portegies P, de Gans J, Lange JM, et al. Declining incidence of AIDS dementia complex after introduction of zidovudine treatment [erratum in *Br Med J* 1989;299:1141]. *Br Med J* 1989;299: 819–821.
75. Price RW, Brew BJ. The AIDS dementia complex. J Infect Dis 1988;158:1079–1083.
76. Rabkin JG, Harrison WM. Effect of imipramine on depression and immune status in a sample of men with HIV infection. *Am J Psychiatry* 1990;147:495.
77. Reed RJ, Grant I. The long-term neurobehavioral consequences of substance abuse: conceptual and methodological challenges for future research. *NIDA Res Monogr* 1990;101:10–56.
78. Reinvang I, Froland SS, Skripeland V. Prevalence of neuropsychological deficit in HIV infection. Incipient signs of AIDS dementia complex in patients with AIDS. *Acta Neurol Scand* 1991;83: 289–293.
79. Riccio M, Pugh K, Jadresic D, et al. Neuropsychiatric aspects of HIV-1 infection in gay men: controlled investigation of psychiatric, neuropsychological and neurological status. *Psychosom Res* 1993; 37:819–830.
80. Robins LN, Regier DA, eds. *Psychiatric Disorders in America.* New York: The Free Press, 1991.
81. Satz P, Morgenstern H, Miller EN, et al. Low education as a possible risk factor for cognitive abnormalities in HIV-1: findings from the Multicenter AIDS Cohort Study (MACS). *J AIDS* 1993; 6:503–511.
82. Schaerf FW, Miller RR, Lipsey JR, McPherson RW. ECT for major depression in four patients infected with human immunodeficiency virus. *Am J Psychiatry* 1989;146:782.
83. Schatzberg AF, Nemeroff CB, eds. *Textbook of Psychopharmacology.* Washington DC: American Psychiatric Press, 1995.
84. Schmidt U, Miller D. Two cases of hypomania in AIDS. *Br J Psychiatry* 1988;152:839.
85. Selnes OA, Miller E, McArthur JC, et al. HIV-1 infection: no evidence of cognitive decline during the asymptomatic stages. *Neurology* 1990;40:204–208.
86. Sewell DD, Jeste DV, Atkinson JH, et al. HIV-associated psychosis: a prospective, controlled study of 20 cases. *Am J Psychiatry* 1994;151:237–242.
87. Snider IM, Simpson DM, Nielsen S, Gold JW, Metroka CE, Posner JB. Neurological complications of acquired immune deficiency syndrome: analysis of 50 patients. *Ann Neurol* 1983;14:403–418.
88. Stein EH, Murdaugh J, Macleod JA. Brief psychotherapy of psychiatric reactions to physical illness. *Am J Psychiatry* 1969;125:76–83.
89. Stern Y, Marder K, Bell K, et al. Multidisciplinary baseline assessment of homosexual men with and without human immunodeficiency virus infection: neurological and neuropsychological findings. *Arch Gen Psychiatry* 1991;48:131.
90. Tross S, Price RW, Navia B, Thaler HT, Gold J, Sidtis JJ. Neuropsychological characterization of the AIDS dementia complex: a preliminary report. *AIDS* 1988;2:81–88.
91. van Gorp WG, Mandelkern M, Gee M, et al. Cerebral metabolic dysfunction in AIDS: findings in a sample with and without dementia. *J Neuropsychiatry Clin Neurosci* 1992;4:280–287.
92. Velin RA, Grant I, Heaton RK, McCutchan JA, Chandler J. Effects of advancing age on neurocognitive functioning in HIV-infection. Symposium presentation at the 45th Annual Scientific Meeting of the Gerontological Society of America, Washington, DC, November 22, 1992.
93. White DA, Heaton RK, Monsch AU, HNRC Group. Neuropsychological studies of asymptomatic human immunodeficiency virus-type 1 infected individuals. *J Int Neuropsychol Soc* 1995; 1:304–315.

94. Williams JB, Rabkin JG, Remien RH, Gorman JM, Ehrhardt AA. Multidisciplinary baseline assessment of homosexual men with and without human immunodeficiency virus infection. *Arch Gen Psychiatry* 1991;48:124.
95. Working Group of the American Academy of Neurology AIDS Task Force. Nomenclature and research case definitions for neurological manifestations of human immunodeficiency virus-type I (HIV-1) infection. *Neurology* 1991;41:778.
96. Zisook S, DeVaul RA, Click MA. Measuring symptoms of grief and bereavement. *Am J Psychiatry* 1982;34:1550–1593.

AIDS and the Nervous System, Second Edition,
edited by J. R. Berger and R. M. Levy.
Lippincott-Raven Publishers, Philadelphia © 1997.

17

The Neuropathology of Human Immunodeficiency Virus Infection of the Spinal Cord

Carol K. Petito

*Department of Pathology, University of Miami School of Medicine,
Miami, Florida 33136*

Clinical manifestations of spinal cord disease usually occur during the later stages of acquired immunodeficiency syndrome (AIDS) (7), although, rarely, an acute transverse myelopathy may develop at the time of human immunodeficiency virus (HIV) seroconversion (9). Because spinal cord signs and symptoms may be overshadowed by systemic illnesses or other nervous system diseases, their true incidence is not precisely known. McArthur noted a 7% incidence of clinical myelopathies in a total of 186 HIV-infected patients (24), whereas none of 50 patients with AIDS reported by Snider et al. had clinical myelopathies (42). We previously estimated that the incidence of myelopathies in patients with AIDS may reach 20% because 60% of patients with vacuolar myelopathy (VM), a disorder with autopsy incidence of 30%, have myelopathic signs and symptoms (29) (see Chapter 8).

Although clinical myelopathies are not common, the incidence of spinal cord diseases at postmortem examination is high (16,17,19,22,31,33). Large autopsy series that specifically have examined their distribution and frequency in adults show abnormalities in approximately half of the cases (19,33). In contrast, only 11% of consecutively autopsied patients with neither HIV infection nor AIDS have pathological abnormalities of this structure (21).

Spinal cord diseases in HIV-seropositive patients can be grouped into several major categories: those due to direct HIV infection (HIV myelitis); those due to opportunistic infections or lymphomas; those associated with HIV infection but whose etiology is unknown or not firmly established; and, lastly, those related to vascular or metabolic disorders. Table 1 reviews their distribution in five postmortem studies in which disease incidence was specifically examined (16,17,19,22,33). VM is by far the most common, although, as reviewed by Henin et al. (19), its reported incidence varies from 1% to 50%. Next in frequency are opportunistic infections, which occur in 8–15% of patients. Cytomegalovirus (CMV) and fungal myelitides predominate, although varicella zoster virus (VZV), herpes simplex virus, toxoplasmosis, bacteria (including *Mycobacterium tuberculosis*), syphilis, and progressive multifocal leukoencephalopathy may involve the spinal cord. Myelitis due to direct HIV infection, slightly less common than opportunistic infections or lymphomas, occurs in 5–8% of all spinal cords. The incidence of HIV and opportunistic infections,

TABLE 1. *Incidence of spinal cord diseases in adult patients with AIDS*

	Grafe and Wiley (16)	Kure (22)	Henin (19)	Petito (27)	Gray (17)
Total No. of patients	26	120	138	178	13
HIV myelitis[a]	8%[a] (15%*†)	6%[a] (21%†)	8%*†	5%*	8%
Vacuolar myelopathy	31%	14%	17%	29%	54%
Opportunistic infections	8%		8%	15%	8%
CMV	8%		3%	5%	8%
HSV				2%	
VZV				1%	
Fungal			4%	4%	
Bacterial				2%	
Toxoplasmosis			1%	1%	
Nonspecific myelitis	38%		7%	10%	
Lymphoma			4%	2%	8%
Other[b]		5%	2%	1%	8%
Chronic meninigitis			9%		
Normal	NS	NS	59%	52%	NS

NS, not stated.
[a] Diagnosed on basis of multinucleated cells* for HIV immunoreactivity†.
[b] Including infarcts, progressive multifocal leukoencephalopathy, and gracile tract degeneration.

as well as lymphoma, in the spinal cord is lower than in the brain, and, in general, spinal cord infections and tumors are rare in the absence of brain involvement (33).

Two studies specifically have examined the distribution of spinal cord disorders in pediatric patients with AIDS (11,40). In contrast to adults, children with AIDS rarely develop opportunistic infection or VM. Their incidence of HIV myelitis varies. It was absent in one of the studies (11) but encountered in almost half of the spinal cords from the other (40). A delay in the normal myelination of the corticospinal tracts, a unique feature of the pediatric group, was highlighted by Dickson et al. (11).

HIV MYELITIS

The inflammatory lesions of HIV may produce a myelitis, especially in cases in which brain involvement is severe and widespread (30). In our experience, the discrete microglial nodules with their accompanying multinucleated cells usually are found in the gray matter (Fig. 1). However, when these inflammatory lesions are

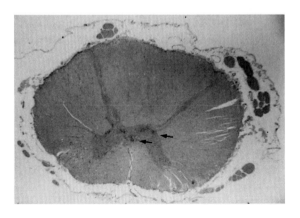

FIG. 1. HIV myelitis. Focal hyperdensities, two of which are indicated by arrows, represent microglial nodules containing immunoreactive monocytes and macrophages. They are more numerous in gray matter than in white matter. HIV immunohistochemistry with hematoxylin counterstain. (Original magnification ×10.)

located in white matter, focal vacuolation may be severe (Fig. 2). This vacuolation usually can be distinguished from VM by its focality and its association with HIV-immunoreactive microglial nodules. HIV myelitis occasionally may be confined to the spinal cord, in the absence of brain lesions (14,33). Its etiological relationship to VM is not clear; however, the typical lesions of HIV myelitis are infrequent in patients with VM. By itself, HIV myelitis is unlikely to be symptomatic unless the lesions are widely disseminated, as occurred in one reported case (14). Preliminary data reported by Brew suggests that HIV myelitis, but not VM, responds to zidovudine therapy (5).

VASCULAR MYELOPATHY

A spongy degeneration in the spinal cord white matter was initially described in one patient in the original study of the neurological complications of AIDS (42). Its resemblance to subacute combined degeneration of vitamin B12 deficiency was noted in that time and in a later report (15). When we subsequently reported the clinical and pathological features of this disorder in 20 patients with AIDS (32), we used the descriptive term vacuolar myelopathy in recognition of the histological appearance because its pathogenesis was not yet understood and there was no apparent relationship with either HIV myelitis or opportunistic infections.

VM is the most frequent cause of the spinal cord symptoms of spastic paraparesis and ataxia, the course of which usually is slowly progressive. In our initial study, 60% of the 20 reported patients were symptomatic, and most had moderate or severe VM at autopsy. Electrophysiological studies on patients with AIDS show delayed nerve conduction within the spinal cord that is most pronounced when associated with ataxia and paraparesis (18,41).

White discoloration and slight swelling are detected in the fasciculus gracilis and lateral columns in cases of severe VM, whereas the gross examination is unremarkable with less severe disease. Microscopically, white matter vacuolation, arising from intramyelin swellings, is present in the lateral and posterior columns and tends to be most severe in the lower half of the thoracic spinal cord (Fig. 3). The lesions are due to intramyelin swelling. Axonal atrophy or degeneration may be secondary to compression by the swollen myelin (32) or may be related to primary macrophage-directed phagocytosis of otherwise intact axon cylinders (2). When severe, or perhaps in cases of long duration, Wallerian degeneration is present in the rostral posterior columns or caudal corticospinal tracts. There is little evidence of a demyelinating component to VM, which contrasts with the pathology of HTLV-I–associated myelopathy (HAM). This other human retroviral-associated myelopathy displays multifocal regions of inflammation and demyelination (1,28), mediated perhaps by cytotoxic T-lymphocytes (25). Although rare cases of HAM have been reported in HIV-infected patients (37), patients with AIDS with VM are not coinfected with HTLV-I (6).

Macrophage infiltration and reactive astrocytosis are variable and correlate with the severity and duration of the disorder (Fig. 4). However, microglial cell proliferation can be intense, especially when immunohistochemistry is used to facilitate detection of these cells (22). Tyor et al. have demonstrated that cytokines and cytokine messenger RNAs are increased in the spinal cords of HIV-infected patients, with or without VM, and hypothesize that this may contribute to or even initiate the spinal

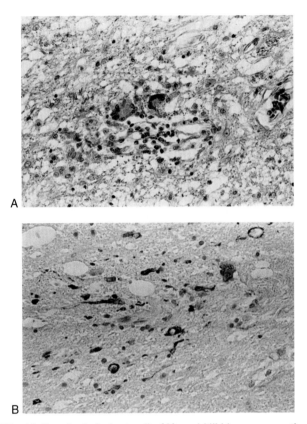

FIG. 2. HIV myelitis. Multinucleated giant cells **(A)** and HIV-immunoreactive monocytes and giant cells **(B)** are characteristic of this infection. (Original magnification ×200.)

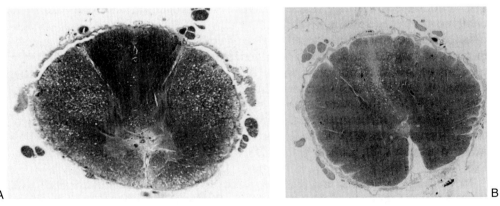

FIG. 3. VM. **A:** Concentration of vacuoles in lateral columns. **B:** Necrosis of *F. gracilis* with moderate vacuolation in remainder of the posterior columns and only minor vacuolation in lateral columns. Luxol-fast blue. (HE, original magnification ×10.)

cord damage (43). Programmed cell death, or apoptosis, is a possible mechanism of myelin damage because it is present in the CNS of patients with AIDS (31) and because it is the process whereby cytokines induce oligodendrocyte damage *in vitro* (39).

The nonuniform distribution of the vacuolation among cases may indicate different etiologies. Severe vacuolation in the *F. gracilis*, with or without actual tissue necrosis (Fig. 3B), suggests that the initial sites of injury are peripheral nerves, posterior nerve roots, or dorsal root ganglia (DRG) at lumbosacral levels. Wallerian degeneration in the *F. gracilis* and secondary spinal cord edema in adjacent lateral columns would then explain the apparent changes of VM. In contrast, vacuolation concentrated in the lateral columns (Fig. 3A) may reflect a primary insult originating in more rostral aspects of the CNS.

The relationship between VM and local HIV infection has been debated since we initially reported a total or relative absence of the inflammation characteristic of HIV. Some investigators have localized HIV-infected macrophages to regions of VM by immunohistochemistry, *in situ* hybridization, and electron microscopy (12,23,35,40,45). Others have been unable to make such correlations using the same or similar techniques (16,19,22,33,36,38,42a). In a study of 70 patients with AIDS who also had VM, we found no correlation between VM and the presence of either HIV antigen or genomic material in the spinal cord (33). However, there is a very strong association between HIV encephalitis and VM, especially when the VM is severe (19,31,33). This association could indicate that VM is secondary to HIV encephalitis in the brain. More likely, the association could be fortuitous and reflect the fact that both disorders occur during the later stages of the AIDS illness.

At least 25% of patients with AIDS have vitamin B12 deficiency (3), which may have etiological significance in some cases of VM. Certainly, the histopathology of the two disorders can be strikingly similar. Clinical–pathological studies show that at least some patients with VM have evidence of B12 deficiency (3,30) and preliminary data from one clinical report has associated vitamin B12 deficiency with myelopathy in patients with AIDS (4).

GRACILE TRACT DEGENERATION

In 1988, Rance et al. described four patients with AIDS and sensory neuropathies whose spinal cords showed atrophy of the posterior columns (34). The pathology includes loss of both myelin and axons in the gracile tract of the upper thoracic or cervical cord, as depicted in Fig. 5. These investigators hypothesize that the degeneration was secondary to lesions in the DRG. A subsequent quantitative study by Scaravilli et al. (38) confirmed the relationship between neuronal loss in DRGs in patients with AIDS and pallor of the gracile tracts of the spinal cord.

If the diagnosis of GTD is confined to those cases with *F. gracilis* atrophy, this disorder can be readily distinguished from VM. However, the pathological distinction between GTD and VM is blurred when the medial *F. gracilis* is necrotic and is associated with vacuolation of the more lateral portion of the posterior columns together with mild vacuolation of the lateral columns (Fig. 3B). At present we group such cases under the heading of VM with *F. gracilis* necrosis. However, it is possible, or indeed probable, that such cases represent an early form of GTD.

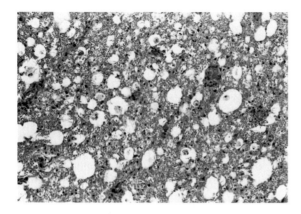

FIG. 4. VM. Lipid-laden macrophages are usually located within the vacuoles. (HE, original magnification ×200.)

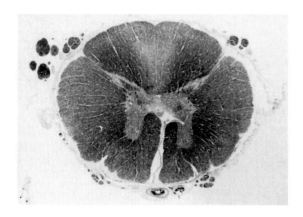

FIG. 5. Gracile tract degeneration. Atrophy of posterior columns with myelin (and axonal) loss usually occurs in the more medial portions of the *F. gracilis.* Luxol-fast blue. (HE, original magnification ×10.)

OPPORTUNISTIC INFECTIONS

The overall autopsy incidence of opportunistic infections of the spinal cord averages ~10%. CMV and fungi are the most common, but others, including herpes simplex, VZV, *M. tuberculosis*, syphilis, toxoplasmosis, progressive multifocal leukoencephalopathy and measles virus, have been described. The spinal cord is rarely the sole site of CNS involvement (33). As in the brain, multiple infections of spinal cord may occur. This is especially true of CMV that can be associated not only herpes simplex virus but also with VZV (personal observation).

The pathological changes in the spinal cord in these infections are similar to those observed in the brain and described elsewhere in this chapter. However, the specific anatomy of the spinal cord, as well as the route of entry and spread of particular organisms, are responsible for certain characteristics of lesion localization in the spinal cord. For example, CMV enters the CNS by hematogenous dissemination but, in the presence of CMV ventriculitis, cerebrospinal fluid is likely (26). Thus, a subpial localization in the spinal cord and lower medulla is common (Figs. 6 and 7). VZV myelitis, on the other hand, typically involves the posterior horn(s) because this infection arises from reactivation of a latent infection of the DRG. Its characteristic spread along axonal pathways is responsible for the frequent concentration of

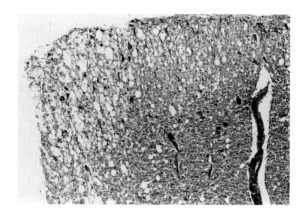

FIG. 6. CMV myelitis. Concentration of lesions in subpial area. (HE, original magnification ×100.)

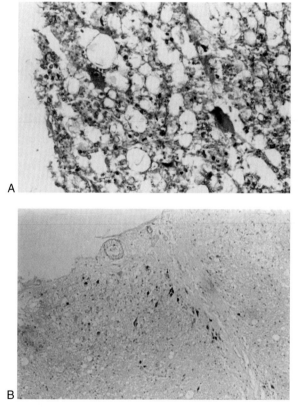

FIG. 7. CMV myelitis. **A:** Enlarged cells with eosinophilic intranuclear inclusions. (Original magnification ×400.) **B:** CMV-immunoreactive cells. (Original magnification ×100.)

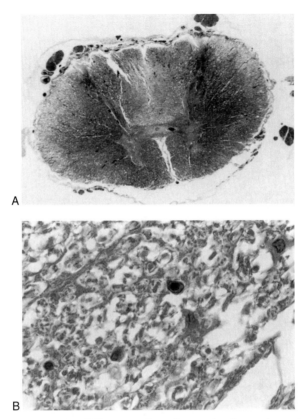

FIG. 8. Varicella zoster myelitis. Diffuse myelin pallor predominates in posterior columns **(A)**. Cowdry type A intranuclear inclusions of VZV displace the chromation to the nuclear membrane **(B)**. **A:** Luxol-fast blue, (HE, original magnification ×10.) **B:** (HE, original magnification ×1,000.)

lesions in the posterior columns (Fig. 8A). A variety of pathological changes can accompany VZV myelitis, including focal or diffuse necrosis (10). In addition, hemorrhages, demyelination, and vasculitis have been described in the spinal cord as well as in the brain. Cowdry type A intranuclear inclusions of VZV (Fig. 8B) may be few and difficult to discern on routine hematoxylin and eosin stains.

NEOPLASMS

Primary or secondary lymphomas of the spinal cord are not common. Their postmortem incidence ranges from 2% to 4%, whereas they are encountered in 10% or 15% of brains. However, in those patients with AIDS who also have brain lymphoma, the spinal cord is involved in ~25% of cases (27). Systemic lymphomas also may involve the spinal cord and usually do so by meningeal infiltration rather than by parenchymal infiltration and mass effect (19). Epidural spread of systemic lymphoma, with secondary cord or root compression, also may occur in selected cases. Because the frequency of AIDS lymphomas is increasing (20), we may see more spinal cord involvement in the future.

MISCELLANEOUS

Single case reports or small series of cases have described a variety of spinal cord disorders in HIV infection that are in addition to or modifications of those described above. Acute myelopathies have been associated with seroconversion (9) and multifocal HIV myelitis (14). Ischemic myelopathy attributable to disseminated intravascular coagulopathy may occur (13) and theoretically also could be related to anticardiolipin antibodies that may develop in patients with AIDS (8). Focal regions of axonal swellings, similar or identical to those described in the brain and brain stem (44), also may be seen in the spinal cord. The absence of any detectable infectious etiology and the similarity of these lesions to small infarcts suggests an ischemic etiology, possibly related to a hypercoagulable state.

ACKNOWLEDGMENT

The secretarial help of Ms. Lee Ann Moffett is gratefully acknowledged. This article was supported in part by the National Institutes of Health (NINDS RO1-NS27416).

REFERENCES

1. Akizuki S, Setoguchi M, Nakazato O, et al. An autopsy case of human T-lymphotrophic virus type I-associated myelopathy. *Hum Pathol* 1988;19:988–990.
2. Artigas J, Grosse G, Niedobitek F. Vacuolar myelopathy in AIDS. A morphological analysis. *Path Res Pract* 1990;186:228–237.
3. Beach RS, Morgan R, Wilkie F, et al. Plasma vitamin B_{12} level as a potential cofactor in studies of human immunodeficiency virus type-I–related cognitive changes. *Arch Neurol* 1992;49:501–506.
4. Berger JR, Pall LM, Strickman-Stein N, Duncan RC, Winfield D. The relationship of B_{12} deficiency to HIV-1 associated myelopathy. 4th International Neuroscience Meeting of HIV infection, Amsterdam, 1992.
5. Brew BJ. HIV-1 related neurological disease. *J AIDS* 1993;6:510–515.
6. Brew BJ, Hardy W, Zuckerman E, et al. AIDS-related vacuolar myelopathy is not associated with co-infection by human T-lymphotropic virus type one. *Ann Neurol* 1989;26:679–681.
7. Brew BJ, Sidtis J, Petito CK, Price RW. The neurological complications of AIDS and human immunodeficiency virus infection. In: Plum F, ed. *Advances in Contemporary Neurology*. Philadelphia: FA Davis, 1989:1–49.
8. Brey RL, Arroyo R, Boswell RN. Cerebrospinal fluid anti-cardiolipin antibodies in patients with HIV-1 infection. *J AIDS* 1991;4:435–441.
9. Denning DW, Anderson J, Rudge P, Smith H. Acute myelopathy associated with primary infection with human immunodeficiency virus. *Br Med J* 1987;294:143–144.
10. Devinsky O, Cho E-S, Petito CK, Price RW. Herpes zoster myelitis. *Brain* 1991;114:1181–1196.
11. Dickson DW, Belman AL, Kim TS, Horoupian DS, Rubinstein A. Spinal cord pathology in pediatric acquired immunodeficiency syndrome. *Neurology* 1989;32:227–235.
12. Eilbott DJ, Peress N, Burger H, et al. Human immunodeficiency virus type I in spinal cords of acquired immunodeficiency syndrome patients with myelopathy: expression and replication in macrophages. *Proc Natl Acad Sci U S A* 1989;85:3337–3341.
13. Fenelon G, Gray F, Scaravilli F, et al. Ischemic myelopathy secondary to disseminated intravascular coagulation in AIDS. *J Neurol* 1991;238:51–54.
14. Geny C, Gherardi R, Boudes P, et al. Multifocal multinucleated giant cell myelitis in an AIDS patient. *Neuropathol Appl Neurobiol* 1991;17:157–162.
15. Goldstick L, Mandybur TI, Bode R. Spinal cord degeneration in AIDS. *Neurology* 1985;35:103–105.
16. Grafe MR, Wiley CA. Spinal cord and peripheral nerve pathology in AIDS: the roles of cytomegalovirus and human immunodeficiency virus. *Ann Neurol* 1988;25:561–566.
17. Gray F, Geny C, Lionnet F, et al. Etude neuropathologique de 135 cas adults de syndrome d'immuno-déficience acquise (SIDA). *Ann Pathol* 1991;11:236–247.
18. Helweg-Larsen S, Jakobsen J, Boesen F, et al. Myelopathy in AIDS. A clinical and electrophysiological study of 23 Danish patients. *Acta Neurologica Scand* 1988;77:64–73.

19. Hénin D, Smith TW, DeGirolami U, Sughayer M, Hauw J-J. Neuropathology of the spinal cord in the acquired immunodeficiency syndrome. *Hum Pathol* 1992;23:1106–1114.
20. Ioachim HL, Dorsett B, Cronin W, Maya M, Wahl S. Acquired immunodeficiency syndrome–associated lymphoma. *Hum Pathol* 1991;22:659–673.
21. Kamin SS, Petito CK. Vacuolar myelopathy in immunocompromised nonAIDS patients. *J Neuropathol Exp Neurol* 1988;47:385.
22. Kure K, Llena JF, Lyman WD, et al. Human immunodeficiency virus-1 infection of the nervous system. *Hum Pathol* 1991;22:700–710.
23. Maier H, Budka H, Lassmann H, Pohl P. Vacuolar myelopathy with multinucleated giant cells in the acquired immune deficiency syndrome (AIDS). Light and electron microscopic distribution of human immunodeficiency virus (HIV) antigens. *Acta Neuropathol* 1989;78:497–503.
24. McArthur JC. Neurological manifestations of AIDS. *Medicine* 1987;66:407–437.
25. Moore GRW, Traugott U, Scheinberg LC, Raine CS. Tropical spastic paraparesis: a model of virus-induced, cytotoxic T-cell–mediated demyelination? *Ann Neurol* 1989;26:523–530.
26. Morgello S, Cho E-S, Nielsen S, Devinsky O, Petito CK. Cytomegalovirus encephalitis in patients with acquired immunodeficiency syndrome: an autopsy study of 30 cases and a review of the literature. *Hum Pathol* 1987;18:289–297.
27. Morgello S, Petito CK, Mouradian JA. Central nervous system lymphoma in the acquired immunodeficiency syndrome. *Clin Neuropathol* 1990;9:205–215.
28. Ohama E, Horikawa Y, Shimizu T, et al. Demyelination and remyelination in spinal cord lesions of human lymphotropic virus type I–associated myelopathy. *Acta Neuropathol* 1990;81:78–83.
29. Petito CK. Myelopathies. In: Scaravilli F, ed. *The Neuropathology of HIV Infection*. New York: Springer-Verlag, 1993:187–199.
30. Petito CK, Cho E-S, Lemann W, Navia BA, Price RW. Neuropathology of acquired immunodeficiency syndrome (AIDS): an autopsy review. *J Neuropathol Exp Neurol* 1986;45:635–646.
31. Petito CK, Roberts B. Evidence of apoptotic cell death in HIV encephalitis. *Am J Pathol* 1995;146:1121–1130.
32. Petito CK, Navia BA, Cho E-S, et al. Vacuolar myelopathy pathologically resembling subacute combined degeneration in patients with the acquired immunodeficiency syndrome. *N Engl J Med* 1985;312:874–879.
33. Petito CK, Vecchio D, Chen Y-T. HIV antigens and DNA in AIDS spinal cords correlate with macrophage infiltration but not with vacuolar myelopathy. *J Neuropathol Exp Neurol* (in press).
34. Rance NE, McArthur JC, Cornblath DR, Landstrom DL, Griffin JW, Price DC. Gracile tract degeneration in patients with sensory neuropathy and AIDS. *Neurology* 1988;38:265–271.
35. Rhodes RH, Ward JM, Cowan RP, Moore PT. Immunohistochemical localization of human immunodeficiency viral antigens in formalin-fixed cords with AIDS myelopathy. *Clin Neuropathol* 1989;8:22–27.
36. Rosenblum M, Scheck AC, Cronin K, et al. Disassociation of AIDS-related vacuolar myelopathy and productive HIV infection of the spinal cord. *Neurology* 1989;39:892–896.
37. Rosenblum MK, Brew BJ, Hahn B, et al. Human T-lymphotropic virus type I–associated myelopathy in patients with the acquired immunodeficiency syndrome. *Hum Pathol* 1991;23:513–519.
38. Scaravilli F, Sinclair E, Arango JC, Manji H, Lucas S, Harrison MJG. The pathology of the posterior root ganglia in AIDS and its relationship to the pallor of the gracile tract. *Acta Neuropathol* 1991;84:163–170.
39. Selme K, Raine CS, Farooq M, Norton WT, Brosnan CF. Cytokine cytotoxicity against oligodendrocytes. Apoptosis induced by lymphotoxin. *J Immunol* 1991;147:1522–1529.
40. Sharer LR, Dowling PC, Michaels J, et al. Spinal cord disease in children with HIV-1 infection: a combined molecular biological and neuropathological study. *Neuropathol Appl Neurobiol* 1990;16:317–331.
41. Smith T, Jakobsen J, Trojaborg W. Myelopathy and HIV infection. *AIDS* 1990;4:589–591.
42. Snider WD, Simpson DM, Nielsen S, Gold JWM, Metroka CE, Posner JB. Neurological complications of the acquired immunodeficiency syndrome: analysis of 50 patients. *Ann Neurol* 1989;14:403–418.
42a. Tan SV, Guiloff RJ, Scaravilli, F. AIDS-associated vascular myelopathy. A morphometric study. *Brain* 1995;118:1247–1261.
43. Tyor WR, Glass JD, Baumrind, N et al. Cytokine expression of macrophages in HIV-1–associated vacuolar myelopathy. *Neurology* 1993;43:1002–1009.
44. Vinters HV, Anders KH, Barach P. Focal pontine leukoencephalopathy in immunosuppressed patients. *Arch Pathol Lab Med* 1987;111:192–196.
45. Weiser B, Peress N, LaNeve D, Eibott DJ, Seidman R, Burger H. Human immunodeficiency virus expression in the central nervous system correlates directly with extent of disease. *Proc Natl Acad Sci U S A* 1990;87:3997–4001.

AIDS and the Nervous System, Second Edition,
edited by J. R. Berger and R. M. Levy.
Lippincott-Raven Publishers, Philadelphia © 1997.

18

Neuropathology of Human Immunodeficiency Virus-1 Infection of the Brain

*Leroy R. Sharer, †Yoshihiro Saito, and †Benjamin M. Blumberg

*Department of Pathology and Laboratory Medicine, New Jersey Medical School,
Newark, New Jersey 07103; and †Department of Neurology, University of
Rochester Medical Center, Rochester, New York 14642

Since the time of the first descriptions of neurological abnormalities associated with acquired immunodeficiency syndrome (AIDS) (70), investigators have attempted to comprehend the neuropathological changes that are associated with this condition. Early reports attributed the cognitive-motor impairments that were seen in many people with AIDS to opportunistic infections, such as cytomegalovirus (CMV) (76,103). The discovery of human immunodeficiency virus type 1 (HIV-1) (2,41) and the recognition of infection of the central nervous system (CNS) by this virus (101) greatly facilitated our understanding of this problem. This chapter summarizes current knowledge about brain infection by HIV-1, covering a broad spectrum of HIV-1–related neuropathology.

GROSS NEUROPATHOLOGICAL FEATURES

Atrophy of the brain is a prominent feature of both HIV-1–associated cognitive–motor impairment in adults and progressive encephalopathy in children on neuroimaging studies (32,40). At postmortem examination in adult subjects, however, atrophy is often less apparent. The average brain weights in adults with AIDS dementia complex has been reported to be within the normal range (74); nevertheless, there is often mild to moderate enlargement of the ventricles, more noticeable in the lateral and third ventricles than in the aqueduct and fourth ventricle (Fig. 1). Enlargement of the sulci, as is commonly seen in degenerative disorders such as Alzheimer's disease, is generally less apparent (43). It has been speculated that both the lack of sulcal enlargement and the relatively normal brain weights in adults might be related to terminal clinical events that produce brain swelling in many patients (74). Examples of HIV-1 encephalitis have been described that have shown severe atrophy of the cerebral cortex (17,44,49,96), in some cases with abundant viral particles on electron microscopy (17,44,68), but these cases are rare.

In children with AIDS, brain weights are generally reduced for the age of the child (61), correlating well with head circumferences that are smaller than normal in affected younger children (32). In addition, the brains of young children with

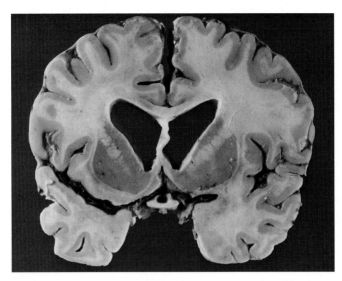

FIG. 1. Coronal section of rostral cerebral hemispheres in a 42-year-old man with severe HIV-1 encephalitis, with enlargement of the lateral ventricles. The sulci are not enlarged.

HIV-1 infection may appear immature, with less myelination and less gyral and sulcal development than expected for age (31).

White matter changes are common in the brains of people with HIV-1 infection, both on neuroimaging studies (40,78,83) and on microscopical examination of the brain (92). However, on gross inspection the white matter is usually normal, with no evidence of reduced myelination. Rarely there may be small foci of white matter necrosis that can coalesce to become grossly visible, with cystic degeneration (94).

MICROSCOPICAL NEUROPATHOLOGY

A variety of microscopical features has been described in association with HIV-1 infection. These are delineated separately, under separate subheadings.

Inflammatory Cell Infiltrates

One of the most common histopathological features in the brain of a subject with AIDS is the presence of loose collections of microglial and inflammatory cells (Fig. 2), which are often located around blood vessels and which may contain reactive astrocytes. The presence of HIV-1 often can be demonstrated within these cell collections by the use of various techniques, such as immunocytochemistry for HIV-1 antigens and *in situ* hybridization for HIV-1–specific nucleic acid sequences (92). The infected cells in these lesions can be shown to be either monocytes, macrophages, or microglial cells. These cellular lesions bear some resemblance to microglial, or glial–microglial, nodules that are a hallmark of virus infection of the CNS, although they tend to be more loose than the classically tight microglial nodule, and they are often located in the vicinity of blood vessels. Rarely, the glial–microglial inflammatory lesions may have disruption of the neuropil and incipient small necrotic foci

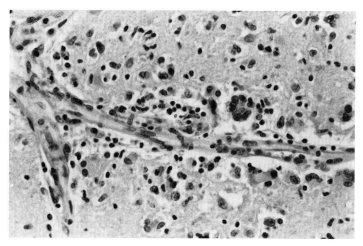

FIG. 2. Loose collection of cells, termed inflammatory cell infiltrate, about a blood vessel in the cerebral cortex, same patient as in Fig. 1. Many mononuclear cells are present, with a multinucleated cell just above the vessel, on the right side of the image. (HE ×262.5.)

within them (Fig. 3). Inflammatory cells within the lesions consist chiefly of lymphocytes, with occasional plasma cells. Multinucleated giant cells, another hallmark of HIV-1 infection, also may be present in these cell collections. The inflammatory collections most often are found in the white matter of the cerebral hemispheres, the basal ganglia, the diencephalon, and the brain stem, although they may be seen in any part of the CNS, from the cerebral cortex to the gray and white matter of the spinal cord (92). Recently Achim et al. (1) stressed the viral burden of HIV-1 in brain, on the basis of semiquantitative immunocytochemistry for p24 core protein

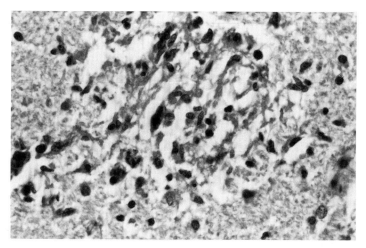

FIG. 3. Inflammatory cell collection with disruption of the neuropil and incipient necrosis and cerebellar white matter in a 36-year-old man with HIV-1 encephalitis. The tissue within the infiltrate is loosened, compared with the more normal appearance of the adjacent, uninvolved neuropil. (HE ×420.)

of the virus, with the highest amount of virus in the basal ganglia, in agreement with the topographical distribution of these cellular lesions.

Inflammatory cell infiltrates must be distinguished from glial–microglial nodules produced by opportunistic viruses, particularly CMV. If characteristic features, such as intranuclear inclusions (with CMV or other viruses), cytomegaly (with CMV), or multinucleated cells (with HIV-1), are lacking, and if specific viral antigens or nucleic acid sequences cannot be demonstrated, as is frequently the case in autopsy tissue, it may be impossible to determine the exact cause of such lesions. In patients with AIDS, occasional glial–microglial nodules may even be seen with nonviral opportunistic infections, including *Toxoplasma gondii* (48,98) and *Cryptococcus neoformans* (98), although the offending organism usually can be recognized on microscopical examination of the lesions in these instances.

Multinucleated Giant Cells

The most characteristic feature of HIV-1 encephalitis is the multinucleated (syncytial) giant cell (95), which is a major site of productive infection of virus within the CNS (70). Multinucleated cells, which are derived from cells of monocytic origin and retain monocytic cell markers, range in size and appearance from large, giant cells with copious cytoplasm, resembling Langhans or foreign-body type giant cells (Fig. 4), to those with scanty cytoplasm and clusters of nuclei (nuclear cluster cells) (96) (Fig. 5). The giant cells have pale, faintly granular cytoplasm, and they also may have dense, eosinophilic centers (47). Within the giant cells, the nuclei can be either scattered throughout the cytoplasm or clustered at one edge of the cell. In some instances the nuclei are attached to each other by small tails of basophilic nucleoplasm, so-called nuclear bridges (71). Although the latter appearance might suggest development of these cells by amitotic division, it is much more likely that the multinucleated cells arise through a process of fusion of infected cells, probably of microglia and monocytes/macrophages (24,69). Retroviruses, including HIV-1

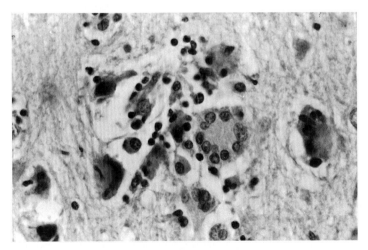

FIG. 4. Multinucleated giant cells in the cerebral cortex of the same patient as in Fig. 1. There are also scattered lymphocytes and other mononuclear cells in the field. (HE ×420.)

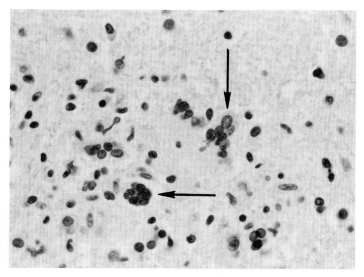

FIG. 5. Two nuclear cluster cells *(arrows)* in the cerebellar white matter in the same patient as in Fig. 1. Cells of this sort can be shown to have scanty cytoplasm that stains positively by lectin histochemistry using the *Ricinus communis* agglutinin-1 (RCA−1), indicating that they are derived from monocytes/macrophages (99). (HE ×470.)

(82), are well known as fusion agents. Syncytial formation is an *in vitro* growth characteristic of certain strains of HIV-1, called syncytium-inducing (SI) variants (106) in lymphocytes; and SI variants have been shown to correlate with a more rapid course of immune deficiency (22,57).

Multinucleated giant cells are often located adjacent to blood vessels, although in some instances their relationship to vessels is not apparent. Their topographical distribution is similar to that of the HIV-1–related inflammatory cell infiltrates, with a location most commonly in cerebral white matter, basal ganglia, and brain stem. Multinucleated cells are occasionally seen in non-CNS tissues in people with HIV-1 infection, but this is much less frequent than their occurrence in the CNS, even in the same individual. The presence of multinucleated giant cells in brain on routine histological examination is considered to be sufficient for a diagnosis of HIV-1 encephalitis, if other means to demonstrate the presence of virus, such as immunocytochemistry or *in situ* hybridization, are not available or are unsuccessful (11). It should be obvious that the finding of multinucleated giant cells, while allowing a diagnosis of HIV-1 encephalitis, does not exclude the possibility that other infectious agents also may be present (50).

Multinucleated giant cells similar to those that occur in the CNS in people infected with HIV-1 also can be seen in the CNS in rhesus macaques infected with simian immunodeficiency virus (SIV), a non-human primate immunodeficiency virus that is related to HIV-1 (93). Multinucleated cells also are seen in the brains of humans with encephalitis due to HIV-2 (56), another primate immunodeficiency virus that is more closely related to SIV than to HIV-1 (53).

Multinucleated giant cells are a diagnostic feature of granulomatous disease of the CNS; and when they are present, the pathologist must exclude other possibilities, including sarcoidosis, the *Mycobacterium tuberculosis* variety of hominis infection, *Coccidioides immitis,* and *Histoplasma capsulatum,* among other conditions. True granulomas have epithelioid cells and other features that are not typical for HIV-1 encephalitis; hence, the differential diagnosis is usually not difficult. Other viruses are rarely associated with multinucleated giant cells in the CNS. Measles virus (MV) may produce giant cells in the brain (33), but human CMV does not, compared with CMV in guinea pigs (6).

White Matter Pathology

Most cases of HIV-1 infection in both adults and children exhibit microscopical pallor of the white matter of the cerebral hemispheres. It is generally accepted that this white matter pallor is the histopathological correlate of the increased signal intensities in the white matter that are detected by magnetic resonance imaging scans (78,80). White matter pallor must be distinguished from the different condition of myelin loss, or true demyelination, which is a less common feature of HIV-1 infection. The white matter pallor is defined by pale staining of the white matter by the use of routine techniques, including hematoxylin and eosin staining and myelin stains. However, staining of myelin components, such as myelin basic protein, is normal (83). The pallor is usually accompanied by an astrocytic gliosis, which can be readily demonstrated in affected brains by the use of immunocytochemistry for glial fibrillary acidic protein (GFAP) (Fig. 6). Some investigators have preferred to use the term HIV leukoencephalopathy to describe this disorder (9), although strictly speaking this term encompasses myelin loss and the presence of macrophages (11), in addition to pallor and astrocytosis. It should be added that some cases of HIV-1 infection also exhibit astrocytosis in the cerebral cortex (16,111), a phenomenon considered to be part of the entity of diffuse poliodystrophy (9,10).

Current evidence suggests that oligodendrocytes are not infected by HIV-1, al-

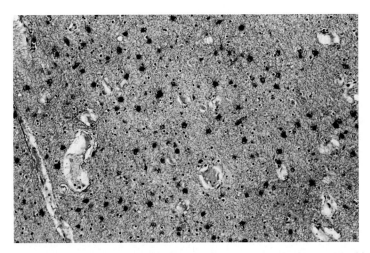

FIG. 6. Reactive astrocytosis in cerebral white matter of a 13-month-old girl with AIDS. The hypertrophic astrocytes are uniformly distributed throughout the field. On routine stains, there was also generalized pallor of the white matter in this case. (Immunocytochemistry for GFAP, diaminobenzidine chromogen, hematoxylin counterstain ×105.)

though these cells have been demonstrated to have increased proliferating cell nuclear antigen in the brains of subjects with HIV-1 infection (72). Several investigators have noted the presence of serum proteins in the abnormal, pale white matter, leading to the conclusion that there is a chronic alteration of the blood–brain barrier (BBB) in these cases (80,83). It is currently uncertain whether this apparent breakdown of the BBB is related to infection of endothelial cells by HIV-1.

Neuropathological Features of Pediatric AIDS

Certain neuropathological findings are more prominent in the brains of children with HIV-1 infection than in adults, of which the most common are vascular or juxtavascular calcifications. These calcifications are more correctly termed mineralizations because substances other than calcium salts, such as iron-containing compounds, usually can be demonstrated within them. In children with AIDS, they are especially numerous in the basal ganglia, particularly the putamen and globus pallidus, as well as the frontal white matter. Such mineralizations constituted the single most common histopathological feature in a series of 37 children with HIV-1 infection that we described, occurring in 34 (92%) of the cases (94). When dense, these mineralizations can be seen on computerized tomographic (CT) scans (23), although they are more frequently detected on microscopical examination at autopsy.

Microscopically, the mineralizations are often small and basophilic, occurring either adjacent to or within the walls of small blood vessels (Fig. 7). In some instances the smaller mineralizations are eosinophilic, suggesting that they are proteinaceous exudates that are becoming mineralized. Less commonly the walls of larger vessels, either small to medium-sized arteries, are involved. In extreme examples in the basal ganglia, there can be large, extracellular, basophilic nodules of mineral material.

The pathogenesis of the formation of these mineralizations is unknown. Only in rare instances is there evidence of inflammation of the walls of the vessels about which the mineralizations form (96). However, imaging studies of a child who devel-

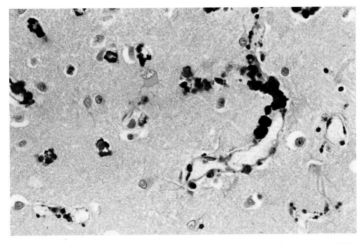

FIG. 7. Basophilic, juxtavascular mineralizations in the putamen of a 5-year-old boy with AIDS. The nodules are extracellular, and they involve capillaries as well as small vessels. Reactive astrocytes are also apparent in the field. (HE ×262.5.)

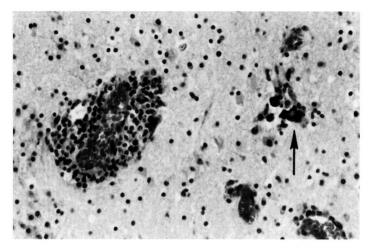

FIG. 8. Inflammation of the wall of a small vein, left side of the image, in the cerebral white matter of a 25-month-old boy with severe HIV-1 encephalitis (Case 4 of Sharer et al. [96]). The inflammatory cells have filled and distended the perivascular space. Extracellular, basophilic mineralization is present on the right side *(arrow)*, and reactive astrocytes are also present. (HE ×262.5.)

oped mineralizations associated with basal ganglia symptoms suggested that their occurrence was related to a transient alteration in the BBB (28). DeCarli et al. (23) have suggested that calcifications on CT scans are seen only with perinatally acquired HIV-1 infection and not after parenteral infection. However, analysis of our own cases, of which only a small number were infected through blood transfusions, indicates that mineralizations can occur in both clinical settings (LR Sharer, unpublished observation).

Other vascular changes, not associated with mineralizations, also have been described in the brains of children with HIV-1 infection more often than in the brains of adults (94,96). These include inflammation of the walls of intraparenchymal vessels and intimal thickening in larger leptomeningeal arteries. The former change (Fig. 8) tends to resemble a vasculitis, and in some cases there are multinucleated giant cells within the inflammation in the vessel walls. Vascular inflammation tends to occur in less than one third of the cases that come to postmortem examination (94). Intimal thickening of large to medium-sized leptomeningeal vessels, an infrequent finding in the brains of children with AIDS (15,79), can be associated with infarcts in the brain. This intimal change also has been described in a few adults with AIDS (15).

INFECTION OF CELLS WITHIN THE BRAIN BY HIV-1

There is abundant neuropathological evidence for HIV-1 infection of CNS cells of monocyte lineage, including on the basis of immunocytochemistry, *in situ* hybridization, and electron microscopy (92). This infection, whether of microglial cells, macrophages, or multinucleated giant cells, is often productive (92), with the formation of immature and mature, as well as morphologically defective, particles (68)

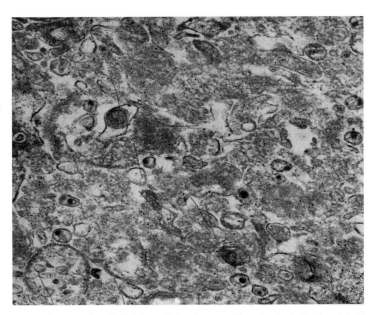

FIG. 9. Electron micrograph of HIV-1 particles in a multinucleated giant cell in the brain of a 6-year-old boy with severe HIV-1 encephalitis (same patient as reported by Meyenhofer et al. [68]). The particles vary greatly in appearance, with some of them having the classic bullet-shaped arrangement of the core, whereas in others the core is beneath the envelope, suggesting that they are defective. (magnification ×42,660.)

(Fig. 9). It is of interest that, on the basis of molecular studies, defective HIV-1 progeny may preponderate in the CNS (63) and may be significant in pathogenesis (112).

Infection of other cell types in the CNS is more controversial. There were several early reports of infection of astrocytes (30,60,84,86,104,115). However, they often could not be confirmed, using probes and antibodies that detected structural genes or gene products. Recently we and others (89,107) reported the identification of HIV-1 infection of astrocytes in white matter of brain tissue from children with AIDS. This result was obtained by targeting the HIV-1 regulatory gene *nef*, using both nucleic acid probes specifically containing this sequence, and antisera for the *nef* protein, an especially good target for immunocytochemistry because it is both overexpressed and membrane anchored (89). We have termed this phenomenon restricted HIV-1 infection because we believe that it is analogous to *in vitro* active infection of glial cells in which the normal temporal regulation of HIV-1 transcripts is blocked by binding of the HIV-1 regulatory protein *rev* to a glial cellular protein (18), thus blocking expression of structural gene products. These characteristics of restricted infection have been demonstrated in neuroectodermally derived cells *in vitro*, in both glioblastoma cells (7) and fetal astrocytes (108). At present there is little evidence for the occurrence of restricted HIV-1 infection of astrocytes in adults (85) and no evidence to suggest that the astrocytosis that often accompanies the white matter pallor is related to direct, restricted infection, although this problem has not been studied exhaustively. In contrast to the situation with astrocytes, reports of infection of oligodendrocytes have been sporadic and generally unconfirmed.

Whether neurons are infected *in vivo* has, if anything, been even more controversial. Scattered reports through the years have indicated neuronal infection (104,110), but most investigators have not been able to confirm these findings using similar techniques. Recently Nuovo et al., using the new and powerful technique of DNA amplification by polymerase chain reaction (PCR), followed by *in situ* hybridization, so-called *in situ* PCR, have demonstrated HIV-1 infection of pyramidal neurons within the cerebral cortex (77). These findings have yet to be confirmed, and our own preliminary studies, using a modification of this technique, have not supported them as yet (100). Infection of differentiated neurons is theoretically possible because recent data indicate that HIV-1 DNA can integrate into the chromatin of postmitotic cells (12,62). It is important to note that, if neurons are infected, the data of Nuovo et al. imply that this infection is latent and does not give rise to any gene products capable of triggering neuronal death, for example by apoptosis (42).

As mentioned previously, infection of brain capillary endothelial cells also has been controversial. *In vitro* and animal data suggest that such infection should occur (64,73), but in practice it has been difficult to separate endothelial cell infection from infection of tightly applied pericytic cells, which are of monocyte origin and hence are likely to be able to support HIV-1 infection at some point in the course of the disease. Double labeling studies using monocyte and endothelial cell markers, which are fraught with technical and interpretative difficulties, have not clarified this point.

INTERACTION OF OTHER VIRUSES WITH HIV-1

The immunosuppression attendant on HIV-1 infection may stimulate activation of other viruses that adventitiously inhabit the CNS (51), leading to either coinfection or interaction with HIV-1 and contributing to encephalopathy and neuropathology. We briefly consider three such viruses that we have studied in our laboratories: human CMV, measles virus (MV), and human herpesvirus 6 (HHV6). These viruses interact in different ways with HIV-1, leading to characteristically different neuropathological pictures that provide additional insights into the pathogenesis of AIDS and the significance of restricted HIV-1 infection in astrocytes (5,89).

Reactivation of CMV, a herpesvirus that is often latent in brains of normal individuals, is a common complication of late-stage AIDS in adults, causing severe retinal infection in up to 25% of patients, as well as encephalitis (38,76). In the brain, CMV has a wide cell tropism, infecting neurons, astrocytes, and endothelial cells, among other cells; coinfection of individual cells with HIV-1 has been observed (75). Our colleagues have recently adapted our *in vivo* xenograft model system (19) for the study of CMV infection of neuroectodermal cells derived from the retina, using human fetal retinal tissue grafted into the anterior chamber of the eyes of immune-deficient mice (25). Infection of this tissue with CMV produced focal cytopathology with spreading disruption of retinal cell rosettes, typical "owl's eye" inclusion bodies in heavily involved regions, and many infectious progeny virus, as measured by electron microscopy and by reisolation of virus from cultured graft tissue (25).

The IE2 protein of CMV transactivates the HIV-1 promoter (21), and the HIV-1 *tat* protein stimulates CMV replication (54). Thus, accelerated outgrowth of both viruses is favored during AIDS. In this milieu, neither virus dominates the neuropathological picture (114); this situation may be reflected in the difficulty of diagnosing CMV encephalitis clinically, when HIV-1 encephalopathy coexists with it (39,55). CMV coinfection of up to 26% of mononuclear cells productively infected with

HIV-1 has been demonstrated in AIDS brain tissues with double-labeling techniques (75). The recent identification of restricted HIV-1 infection of astrocytes (89,107) suggests that more HIV-1 may have been present in these tissues than originally thought and raises the additional possibility of coinfection in astrocytes.

We have recently studied the contribution of HHV6, the agent of roseola, to neuropathology in AIDS. Because HHV6 infection is universally acquired by 2 years of age, this virus may be a cofactor in pediatric AIDS, and it persists in the adult CNS (14). HHV6 shares tropism for the CD4 receptor with HIV-1, and it is also neurotropic. In children, febrile episodes may often be related to subacute HHV6 encephalitis (52). In brain tissues from four of five pediatric patients with AIDS, HHV6 was less prevalent in brain than was HIV-1, although HHV6 was far more prevalent in AIDS brains than in controls (88). In these cases, HHV6 DNA was detected by *in situ* hybridization, mostly in white matter and often in perivascular regions that also had HIV-1 infection, as determined both by HIV-1 p24 immunocyto-chemistry and by the presence of multinucleated giant cells.

Persistent HHV6 infection may become disseminated during late-stage AIDS in adults (59). We detected HHV6 DNA in monocytes, oligodendrocytes, and neurons, but not in astrocytes in pediatric AIDS brain tissue (88); coinfection by both HIV-1 and HHV6 was identified in monocytic cells in only two cases of the five HIV-1–positive cases. Therefore, restricted HIV-1 infection of astrocytes probably has no connection with HHV6. In our pediatric cases, HHV6 antigens were not detectable by immunocytochemistry, using monoclonal antibodies for early and late proteins. We have concluded from these observations that HHV6 infection of cells in the brain of children with HIV-1 infection is normally latent; HHV6 replication in peripheral monocytes appears to be activated by HIV-1, but this replication is suppressed in the inflammatory milieu of the HIV-1–infected brain. *In vitro* studies on activation of HIV-1 by HHV6 have yielded contradictory results (13,27). Our neuropathological studies suggest that HHV6 is most likely to act as a cofactor for HIV-1 in the early stages of its replication and during early phases of HIV-1 infection.

We have also studied the neuropathology in CNS tissues from four pediatric patients with AIDS who died from opportunistic CNS MV infection (97). MV, the causative agent of subacute sclerosing panencephalitis (3), is well known to infect oligodendrocytes and neurons, as well as astrocytes and monocytes/microglia (33,67). Neuropathological examination of our cases showed necrosis, severe neuronal loss, and inflammation, with characteristic eosinophilic intranuclear inclusion bodies in involved areas. Immunocytochemistry for MV nucleocapsid protein showed intense signal in inclusion bodies and in the cytoplasm of many oligodendrocytes, neurons, astrocytes, and monocytes. HIV-1–infected cells were not associated with regions containing MV infection; indeed, there was little, if any, local interaction between HIV-1 and MV. Restricted HIV-1 infection of astrocytes appears to be merely coinci-dental to MV infection. This finding was not unexpected because the replication cycle of paramyxoviruses is relatively self-contained, although MV may have some specific interaction with host cell proteins (4).

NEURONAL LOSS IN HIV-1 INFECTION

Several groups of investigators, using varied techniques, have demonstrated loss of neurons in the cerebral cortex in adult patients with HIV-1 infection (37,58,113).

By contrast, asymptomatic subjects, with presumably early systemic HIV-1 infection, have not shown evidence of cortical neuronal loss by use of the same techniques (34). In all of these studies there was no attempt to correlate neuronal loss with either clinical dementia or cognitive–motor impairment. One group has been unable to confirm these findings, noting similar cortical neuronal populations in demented patients with AIDS and age-matched, non–HIV-1–infected controls (91).

Despite the one negative study, the weight of the published evidence strongly favors that there is loss of neurons in the cerebral cortex in patients with AIDS. The neuronal loss seems to be more severe in some portions of the cortex than in others, particularly in the frontal cortex, although the parietal and occipital cortices are involved as well (35). In addition, Masliah et al. have described decreased synaptic density by immunocytochemistry for synaptophysin, decreased dendritic branching on Golgi staining, and dendritic degenerative changes (vacuolation, etc.) on electron

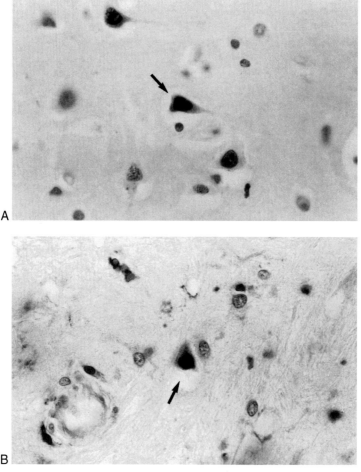

FIG. 10. Neurons with apoptotic, dark-staining nuclei *(arrows)*, cerebral cortex **(A)**, and globus pallidus **(B)** in a 5-year-old boy with HIV-1 encephalitis. Nuclear detail is lost in both of these neurons, whereas it is retained in other nuclei. (Apoptag terminal end-labeling technique, nickel-enhanced diaminobenzidine chromogen, no counterstain ×420.)

microscopy (65,113). It has been suggested that these changes are related to the pathogenesis of dementia or cognitive–motor impairment, but as yet they have not all been correlated with clinical impairment. Indeed, a recent postmortem study, while confirming neuronal loss in HIV-1–infected patients versus noninfected controls, has failed to demonstrate a correlation of neuronal loss with dementia in patients who were clinically evaluated for neurological impairment antemortem (36).

Assessment of neuronal loss is extremely difficult in children, in whom the brain is growing, making age matching of controls an even more critical factor in such an evaluation than it is in adults. Preliminary data have been presented from one center to suggest that, instead of neuronal loss (or decrease in neuronal density), there is an increase in the density of all cells, including neurons, in the cerebral cortex in children with AIDS, when compared with control, HIV-1–negative children, possibly related to a decrease in the intercellular matrix in the brain (8).

The mechanism of cortical neuronal cell loss in people with HIV-1 infection is not understood. Recent evidence from several investigators studying the brains of adults and children with HIV-1 infection suggests a role for apoptosis or programmed cell death in producing neuronal loss. It has been noted that neuronal cells *in vitro* are extremely sensitive to low concentrations of the cytokine tumor necrosis factor-alpha (TNF-α), with neuronal death occurring as apoptosis (105). It has been proposed that cytokines, including TNF-α, elaborated by either infected macrophages, stimulated (or infected) astrocytes, or both, play a role in the pathogenesis of AIDS dementia (29). Our own studies on CNS tissues from children with AIDS have noted an association between the presence of HIV-1 encephalitis and apoptosis of neurons, using the terminal transferase end-labeling technique for DNA (42) (Fig. 10). Others have reported similar findings using comparable techniques (81). A role for direct infection of neurons in producing nerve cell loss is not excluded by these studies, but as mentioned it is currently uncertain whether infection of cortical neurons with HIV-1 occurs.

THE RELATIONSHIP OF NEUROPATHOLOGICAL FINDINGS TO ENCEPHALOPATHY

Several investigators have noted a discrepancy between clinical dementia and the neuropathological features of HIV-1 encephalitis (45,74,87). Glass et al. found that routine histopathology fails to detect HIV-1–related changes in 50% of demented adults at autopsy (45). In their series, only 25% of patients with prospectively documented dementia had multinucleated giant cells in the brain, although none of the nondemented patients had multinucleated giant cells. They found some correlation for diffuse white matter pallor and dementia, with 50% of the demented patients in their series having either multinucleated giant cells, white matter pallor, or both. In our own pediatric material, the great majority of cases have had an excellent correlation with changes of active HIV-1 encephalitis and clinical progressive encephalopathy. However, even we have seen exceptions to this rule, with rare cases of nonstatic, progressive encephalopathy without HIV-1 changes in the brain. Those few patients with encephalopathy that have not shown either inflammatory cell collections, multinucleated giant cells, or both, have nevertheless had other changes, particularly mineralizations in basal ganglia and white matter pallor and gliosis (LR Sharer, unpublished observation).

Whether there is latent or restricted HIV-1 infection, for example in astrocytes, in cases of dementia without multinucleated giant cell encephalitis has not been established. However, the pathological findings have raised the issue of direct versus indirect effects, with the former meaning direct effects of infection by HIV-1 itself, and the latter effects either of viral products, such as the envelope glycoprotein (gp)120, or of activated macrophages and astrocytes, mediated through cytokines or other agents. The various pathogenetic theories are discussed in Chapter 4 of this book.

EFFECTS OF ANTIRETROVIRAL THERAPY ON HIV-1 ENCEPHALITIS

Several recent publications have attempted to determine whether the use of antiretroviral therapy, with agents such as zidovudine (ZDV; or azidothymidine [AZT]), dideoxycytidine (ddC), and dideoxyinosine (ddI), has any effect on the incidence of neuropathological changes observed at postmortem examination. It has been noted for some time that there may be a reduction in the severity of cognitive-motor dysfunction (116), including on objective testing (90,102), after the institution of drugs directed against retroviruses. In some cases these effects may be dramatic, with rapid improvement of neuroimaging findings (66). It is currently uncertain how these effects occur. Clinical–neuropathological studies have several limitations in this area, including accurate assessment of the dose of antiretroviral therapy taken, cessation of therapy at varying times before death, and inadequate clinical neurological information in many cases.

Despite these problems, several studies from Europe and the U.S. have indicated that there is a reduction in the frequency of either multinucleated giant cell encephalitis (46), diffuse white matter pallor (leukoencephalopathy), or both (45,109) in treated patients, compared with untreated, age-matched, control, HIV-1–positive patients. However, not all studies have agreed on this point, with some investigators finding no difference in the incidence of the HIV-1–related neuropathological changes in the treated cases (20) (and CK Petito, personal communication). The reasons for the discrepancy in findings are not immediately apparent.

Our own studies of a small number (n = 12) of children who were treated versus untreated, control, HIV-1–infected children (n = 38) indicates a diminished incidence of multinucleated giant cells in the brain (25% vs. 60.5%), as well as of inflammatory cell infiltrates (41% vs. 74%) in treated versus untreated children. However, there was a similar incidence of white matter pathology (83% vs. 76%) and mineralizations (92% vs. 92%) in the two groups. Only three of the 12 children who were treated had multinucleated cells in the brain. It is of interest that two of these three children had initially been treated with ZDV but were then switched to ddC, because of disease progression in one child and intolerance to the medication in the other. Our untreated cases are predominantly historical and not contemporaneous controls because only a small number of children coming to postmortem at our institution since 1988 remained untreated with antiretroviral drugs. It is possible that one reason for the difference in findings in Petito's adult series and our pediatric series is the relatively higher doses of antiretroviral therapy that are used to treat children with HIV-1 infection than are used to treat adults (M Mintz, personal communication). If antiencephalitic effects of antiretroviral therapy are dose-related, it might be prudent to use higher doses of antiretroviral agents, particularly ZDV, in those adults who can tolerate them and in those who have not developed resistant viral strains (26).

ACKNOWLEDGMENT

Dr. Leon G. Epstein provided helpful comments about the manuscript. Markus Meyenhofer supplied the electron micrograph. This work was supported in part by P01 NS 31492 and R01 NS5-25141. B.M.B. was the recipient of a University of Rochester SCRC Grant, and Y.S. is a Pediatric AIDS Foundation Scholar.

REFERENCES

1. Achim CL, Wang R, Miners DK, Wiley CA. Brain viral burden in HIV infection. *J Neuropathol Exp Neurol* 1994;53:284–294.
2. Barré-Sinoussi F, Chermann JC, Rey F, et al. Isolation of a T-lymphotropic retrovirus from a patient at risk for acquired immune deficiency syndrome (AIDS). *Science* 1983;220:868–871.
3. Billeter MA, Cattaneo R, Spielhofer P, et al. Generation and properties of measles virus mutations typically associated with subacute sclerosing panencephalitis. *Ann NY Acad Sci* 1994;724:367–377.
4. Blumberg BM, Chan J, Udem S. Function of paramyxovirus 3′ and 5′ end sequences (in theory and practice). In: Kingsbury DW, ed. *The Paramyxoviruses*. New York: Plenum, 1991:235–247.
5. Blumberg BM, Gelbard HA, Epstein LG. HIV-1 infection of the developing nervous system: central role of astrocytes in pathogenesis. *Virus Res* 1994;32:253–267.
6. Booss J, Kim JH. Cytomegalovirus encephalitis: neuropathological comparison of the guinea pig model with the opportunistic infection in AIDS. *Yale J Biol Med* 1989;62:187–195.
7. Brack-Werner R, Kleinschmidt A, Ludvigsen A, et al. Infection of human brain cells by HIV-1: restricted virus production in chronically infected human glial cell lines. *AIDS* 1992;6:273–285.
8. Brudkowska J, Kozlowski PB, Kozielski R, Tarnawski M, Wisniewski HM. Neuronal density of the frontal cortex in HIV infected children with microencephaly [Abstract]. *Brain Pathol* 1994;4:482.
9. Budka H. Neuropathology of human immunodeficiency virus infection. *Brain Pathol* 1991;1:163–175.
10. Budka H, Costanzi G, Cristina S, et al. Brain pathology induced by infection with the human immunodeficiency virus (HIV): a histopathological, immunocytochemical, and electron microscopical study of 100 autopsy cases. *Acta Neuropathol* 1987;75:185–198.
11. Budka H, Wiley CA, Kleihues P, et al. HIV associated disease of the nervous system: review of nomenclature and proposal for neuropathology based terminology. *Brain Pathol* 1991;1:143–152.
12. Bukrinsky MI, Haggerty S, Dempsey MP, et al. A nuclear targeting signal within HIV-1 matrix protein governs infection of non-dividing cells. *Nature* 1993;365:666–669.
13. Carrigan DR, Knox KK, Tapper MA. Suppression of human immunodeficiency virus type 1 replication by human herpesvirus six. *J Infect Dis* 1990;162:844–851.
14. Caserta MT, Hall CB, Schnabel K, et al. Neuroinvasion and persistence of human herpesvirus 6 in children. *J Infect Dis* 1994;170:1586–1589.
15. Cho E-S, Sharer LR, Peress NS, Little B. Intimal proliferation of leptomeningeal arteries and brain infarcts in subjects with AIDS [Abstract]. *J Neuropathol Exp Neurol* 1987;46:385.
16. Ciardi A, Sinclair E, Scaravilli F, Harcourt-Webster NJ, Lucas S. The involvement of the cerebral cortex in human immunodeficiency virus encephalopathy: a morphological and immunohistochemical study. *Acta Neuropathol* 1990;81:51–59.
17. Clague CPT, Ostrowski MA, Deck JHN, Harnish DG, Colley EA, Stead RH. Severe diffuse necrotizing cortical encephalopathy in acquired immune deficiency syndrome (AIDS): an immunocytochemical and ultrastructural study [Abstract]. *J Neuropathol Exp Neurol* 1988;47:346.
18. Constantoulakis P, Campbell M, Felber BK, Nasioulas G, Afonina E, Pavlakis GN. Inhibition of Rev-mediated HIV-1 expression by an RNA binding protein encoded by the interferon-inducible 9-27 gene. *Science* 1993;259:1314–1318.
19. Cvetkovich TA, Lazar E, Blumberg BM, et al. Human immunodeficiency virus type 1 (HIV-1) infection of neural xenografts. *Proc Natl Acad Sci U S A* 1992;89:5162–5166.
20. Davies J, Everall I, Bell J, et al. Does azidothymidine alter HIV associated neuropathology [Abstract]? *Clin Neuropathol* 1993;12(suppl 1):9–10.
21. Davis MG, Kenney SC, Kamine J, Pagano JS, Huang E-S. Immediate-early gene region of HCMV trans-activates the promoter of HIV. *Proc Natl Acad Sci U S A* 1987;84:8642–8646.

22. De Wolf F, Hogervorst E, Goudsmit J, et al. Syncytium-inducing and non–syncytium-inducing capacity of human immunodeficiency virus type 1 subtypes other than B: phenotypic and genotypic characteristics. *AIDS Res Hum Retrovir* 1994;10:1387–1400.

23. DeCarli C, Civitello LA, Brouwers P, Pizzo PA. The prevalence of computed tomographic abnormalities of the cerebrum in 100 consecutive children symptomatic with the human immune deficiency virus. *Ann Neurol* 1993;34:198–205.

24. Dickson DW. Multinucleated giant cells in acquired immunodeficiency syndrome encephalopathy: origin from endogenous microglia? *Arch Pathol Lab Med* 1986;110:967–968.

25. DiLoreto D, Epstein LG, Lazar ES, Britt WJ, del Cerro M. Cytomegalovirus infection of human retinal tissue: an *in vivo* model. *Lab Invest* 1994;71:141–148.

26. Di Stefano M, Norkrans G, Chiodi F, Hagberg L, Nielsen C, Svennerholm B. Zidovudine-resistant variants of HIV-1 in brain. *Lancet* 1993;342:865

27. Ensoli B, Lusso P, Schachter F, et al. Human herpes virus-6 increases HIV-1 expression in co-infected T cells via nuclear factors binding to the HIV-1 enhancer. *EMBO J* 1989;8:3019–3027.

28. Epstein LG, Berman CZ, Sharer LR, Khademi M, Desposito F. Unilateral calcification and contrast enhancement of the basal ganglia in a child with AIDS encephalopathy. *Am J Neuroradiol* 1987; 8:163–165.

29. Epstein LG, Gendelman HE. Human immunodeficiency virus type 1 infection of the nervous system: pathogenetic mechanisms. *Ann Neurol* 1993;33:429–436.

30. Epstein LG, Sharer LR, Cho E-S, Meyenhofer M, Navia B, Price RW. HTLV-III/LAV-like retrovirus particles in the brains of patients with AIDS encephalopathy. *AIDS Res* 1985;1:447–454.

31. Epstein LG, Sharer LR, Goudsmit J. Neurological and neuropathological features of human immunodeficiency virus infection in children. *Ann Neurol* 1988;23(suppl):19–23.

32. Epstein LG, Sharer LR, Oleske JM, et al. Neurological manifestations of human immunodeficiency virus infection in children. *Pediatrics* 1986;78:678–687.

33. Esiri MM, Oppenheimer DR, Brownell B, Haire M. Distribution of measles antigen and immunoglobulin-containing cells in the CNS in subacute sclerosing panencephalitis (SSPE) and atypical measles encephalitis. *J Neurol Sci* 1982;53:29–43.

34. Everall I, Gray F, Barnes H, Durigon M, Luthert P, Lantos P. Neuronal loss in symptom-free HIV infection [Letter]. *Lancet* 1992;340:1413

35. Everall I, Luthert P, Lantos P. A review of neuronal damage in human immunodeficiency virus infection: its assessment, possible mechanism and relationship to dementia. *J Neuropathol Exp Neurol* 1993;52:561–566.

36. Everall IP, Glass JD, McArthur J, Spargo E, Lantos P. Neuronal density in the superior frontal and temporal gyri does not correlate with the degree of human immunodeficiency virus-associated dementia. *Acta Neuropathol* 1994;88:538–544.

37. Everall IP, Luthert PJ, Lantos PL. Neuronal loss in the frontal cortex in HIV infection. *Lancet* 1991; 337:1119–1121.

38. Faber DW, Wiley CA, Lynn GB, Gross JG, Freeman WR. Role of HIV and CMV in the pathogenesis of retinitis and retinal vasculopathy in AIDS patients. *Invest Ophthalmol Vis Sci* 1992;33:2345–2353.

39. Fiala M, Singer FJ, Graves MC, et al. AIDS dementia complex complicated by cytomegalovirus encephalopathy. *J Neurol* 1993;240:223–231.

40. Flowers CH, Mafee MF, Crowell R, et al. Encephalopathy in AIDS patients: evaluation with MR imaging. *AJNR* 1990;11:1235–1245.

41. Gallo RC, Salahuddin SZ, Popovic M, et al. Frequent detection and isolation of cytopathic retroviruses (HTLV-III) from patients with AIDS and at risk for AIDS. *Science* 1984;224:500–502.

42. Gelbard HA, James HJ, Sharer LR, et al. Apoptotic neurons in brains from paediatric patients with HIV-1 encephalitis and progressive encephalopathy. *Neuropathol Appl Neurobiol* 1995;21(3): 208–217.

43. Gelman BB, Guinto FC. Morphometry, histopathology, and tomography of cerebral atrophy in the acquired immunodeficiency syndrome. *Ann Neurol* 1992;32:31–40.

44. Giangaspero F, Scanabissi E, Baldacci MC, Betts CM. Massive neuronal destruction in human immunodeficiency virus (HIV) encephalitis: a clinico-pathological study of a pediatric case. *Acta Neuropathol* 1989;78:662–665.

45. Glass JD, Wesselingh SL, Selnes OA, McArthur JC. Clinical-neuropathological correlation in HIV-associated dementia. *Neurology* 1993;43:2230–2237.

46. Gray F, Bélec L, Keohane C, et al. Zidovudine therapy and HIV encephalitis: a 10-year neuropathological survey. *AIDS* 1994;8:489–493.

47. Gray F, Gherardi R, Scaravilli F. The neuropathology of the acquired immune deficiency syndrome (AIDS): a review. *Brain* 1988;111:245–266.

48. Gray F, Gherardi R, Wingate E, et al. Diffuse "encephalitic" cerebral toxoplasmosis in AIDS: report of four cases. *J Neurol* 1989;236:273–277.

49. Gray F, Haug H, Chimelli L, et al. Prominent cortical atrophy with neuronal loss as correlate of human immunodeficiency virus encephalopathy. *Acta Neuropathol* 1991;82:229–233.

50. Gray F, Sharer LR. Combined pathologies. In: Gray F, ed. *Atlas of the Neuropathology of HIV Infection.* Oxford, England: Oxford University Press, 1993:162–172.

51. Haase AT, Stowring L, Ventura P, et al. Detection by hybridization of viral infections of the human central nervous system. *Ann NY Acad Sci* 1984;436:103–108.

52. Hall CB, Long CE, Schnabel KC, et al. Human herpesvirus-6 infection in children: a prospective study of complications of reactivation. *N Engl J Med* 1994;331:432–438.

53. Hirsch VM, Olmsted RA, Murphey-Corb M, Purcell RH, Johnson PR. An African primate lentivirus (SIVsm) closely related to HIV-2. *Nature* 1989;339:389–392.

54. Ho W-Z, Ayyavoo V, Srinivasan A, Stinski MF, Plotkin SA, Gonozol E. Human immunodeficiency virus type 1 *tat* gene enhances human cytomegalovirus gene expression and viral replication. *AIDS Res Hum Retrovir* 1991;7:689–695.

55. Holland NR, Power C, Mathews VP, Glass JD, Forman M, McArthur JC. Cytomegalovirus encephalitis in acquired immunodeficiency syndrome (AIDS). *Neurology* 1994;44:507–514.

56. Hormingo A, Bravo-Marques JM, Souza-Ramalho P, Pimental J, Teixeira C, Martins R. Uveomeningoencephalitis in a human immunodeficiency virus type 2-seropositive patient. *Ann Neurol* 1988; 23:308–310.

57. Japour AJ, Fiscus SA, Arduino J-M, Mayers DL, Reichelderfer PS, Kuritzkes DR. Standardized microtiter assay for determination of syncytium-inducing phenotypes of clinical human immunodeficiency virus type 1 isolates. *J Clin Microbiol* 1994;32:2291–2294.

58. Ketzler S, Weis S, Haug H, Budka H. Loss of neurons in the frontal cortex in AIDS brains. *Acta Neuropathol* 1990;80:92–94.

59. Knox KK, Carrigan DR. Disseminated active HHV-6 infections in patients with AIDS. *Lancet* 1994; 343:577–578.

60. Koenig S, Gendelman HE, Orenstein JM, et al. Detection of AIDS virus in macrophages in brain tissue from AIDS patients with encephalopathy. *Science* 1986;233:1089–1093.

61. Kozlowski PB, Sher JH, Dickson DW, et al. Central nervous system in pediatric HIV infection: experience from a multicenter study. In: Kozlowski PB, Snider DA, Vietze PM, Wisniewski HM, eds. *Brain in Pediatric AIDS.* Basel, Switzerland: Karger, 1990:132–146.

62. Lewis P, Emerman M. Passage through mitosis is required for oncoretroviruses but not for the human immunodeficiency virus. *J Virol* 1994;68:510–516.

63. Li Y, Kappes JC, Conway JA, Price RW, Shaw GM, Hahn BH. Molecular characterization of human immunodeficiency virus type 1 cloned directly from uncultured human brain tissue: identification of replication-competent and -defective viral genomes. *J Virol* 1991;65:3973–3985.

64. Mankowski JL, Spelman JP, Ressetar HG, et al. Neurovirulent simian immunodeficiency virus replicates productively in endothelial cells of the central nervous system *in vivo* and *in vitro. J Virol* 1994;68:8202–8208.

65. Masliah E, Achim CL, Ge N, DeTeresa R, Terry R, Wiley CA. Spectrum of human immunodeficiency virus–associated neocortical damage. *Ann Neurol* 1992;32:321–329.

66. Matthes J, Walker LA, Watson JG, Bird AG. AIDS encephalopathy with response to treatment. *Arch Dis Child* 1988;63:545–547.

67. McQuaid S, Kirk J, Zhou A-L, Allen IM. Measles virus infection of cells in perivascular infiltrates in the brain in subacute sclerosing panencephalitis: confirmation by non-radioactive *in situ* hybridization, immunocytochemistry and electron microscopy. *Acta Neuropathol* 1993;85:154–158.

68. Meyenhofer MF, Epstein LG, Cho ES, Sharer LR. Ultrastructural morphology and intracellular production of human immunodeficiency virus (HIV) in brain. *J Neuropathol Exp Neurol* 1987;46: 474–484.

69. Michaels J, Price RW, Rosenblum MK. Microglia in the giant cell encephalitis of acquired immune deficiency syndrome: proliferation, infection and fusion. *Acta Neuropathol* 1988;76:373–379.

70. Michaels J, Sharer LR, Epstein LG. Human immunodeficiency virus type 1 (HIV-1) infection of the nervous system: a review. *Immunodeficiency Rev* 1988;1:71–104.

71. Mizusawa H, Hirano A, Llena J. Nuclear bridges within multinucleated giant cells in subacute encephalitis of acquired immunodeficiency syndrome (AIDS). *Acta Neuropathol* 1988;76:166–169.

72. Morris CS, Esiri MM, Sprinkle TJ, Gregson N. Oligodendrocyte reactions and cell proliferation markers in human demyelinating diseases. *Neuropathol Appl Neurobiol* 1994;20:272–281.

73. Moses AV, Bloom FE, Pauza CD, Nelson JA. Human immunodeficiency virus infection of human brain capillary endothelial cells occurs via a CD4/galactosylceramide-independent mechanism. *Proc Natl Acad Sci U S A* 1993;90:10474–10478.

74. Navia BA, Cho E-S, Petito CK, Price RW. The AIDS dementia complex: II. Neuropathology. *Ann Neurol* 1986;19:525–535.

75. Nelson JA, Reynolds-Kohler C, Oldstone MBA, Wiley CA. HIV and HCMV coinfect brain cells in patients with AIDS. *Virology* 1988;165:286–290.

76. Nielsen SL, Petito CK, Urmacher CD, Posner JB. Subacute encephalitis in acquired deficiency syndrome: a postmortem study. *Am J Clin Pathol* 1984;82:678–682.

77. Nuovo GJ, Gallery F, MacConnell P, Braun A. *In situ* detection of polymerase chain reaction–ampli-

fied HIV-1 nucleic acids and tumor necrosis factor-α RNA in the central nervous system. *Am J Pathol* 1994;144:659–666.

78. Olsen WL, Longo FM, Mills CM, Norman D. White matter disease in AIDS: findings at MR imaging. *Radiology* 1988;169:445–448.

79. Park YD, Belman AL, Kim TS, et al. Stroke in pediatric acquired immunodeficiency syndrome. *Ann Neurol* 1990;28:303–311.

80. Petito CK, Cash KS. Blood–brain barrier abnormalities in the acquired immunodeficiency syndrome: immunohistochemical localization of serum proteins in postmortem brain. *Ann Neurol* 1992;32: 658–666.

81. Petito CK, Falangola MF, Roberts B. Programmed cell death in brains of patients with AIDS [Abstract]. *Brain Pathol* 1994;4:485.

82. Popovic M, Sarngadharan MG, Read E, Gallo RC. Detection, isolation, and continuous production of cytopathic retroviruses (HTLV-III) from patients with AIDS and pre-AIDS. *Science* 1984;224: 497–500.

83. Power C, Kong P-A, Crawford TO, et al. Cerebral white matter changes in acquired immunodeficiency syndrome dementia: alterations of the blood–brain barrier. *Ann Neurol* 1993;34:339–350.

84. Pumarola-Sune T, Navia BA, Cordon-Cardo C, Cho E-S, Price RW. HIV antigen in the brains of patients with the AIDS dementia complex. *Ann Neurol* 1987;21:490–496.

85. Ranki A, Ovod V, Haltia M, Nyberg M, Aavik E, Krohn K. High expression of *nef* protein in HIV-infected brain astrocytes associated with rapidly progressing CNS disease [Abstract]. VII International Conference on AIDS 1991; Abstract TuA10.

86. Rhodes RH, Ward JM, Cowan RP, Moore PT. Immunohistochemical localization of human immunodeficiency virus antigens in formalin-fixed spinal cords with AIDS myelopathy. *Clin Neuropathol* 1988;8:22–27.

87. Rosenblum MK. Infection of the central nervous system by the human immunodeficiency virus type 1: morphology and relation to syndromes of progressive encephalopathy and myelopathy in patients with AIDS. *Pathol Annu* 1990;1:117–169.

88. Saito Y, Sharer LR, Dewhurst S, Blumberg BM, Hall CB, Epstein LG. Cellular localization of human herpesvirus-6 in the brains of children with AIDS encephalopathy. *J Neurovirol* 1995;1: 30–39.

89. Saito Y, Sharer LR, Epstein LG, et al. Overexpression of *nef* as a marker for restricted HIV-1 infection of astrocytes in postmortem pediatric central nervous tissues. *Neurology* 1994;44:474–481.

90. Schmitt FA, Bigley JW, McKinnis R, Logue PE, Evans RW, Drucker JL. Neuropsychological outcome of zidovudine (AZT) treatment of patients with AIDS and AIDS-related complex. *N Engl J Med* 1988;319:889–896.

91. Seilhean D, Duyckaerts C, Vazeux R, et al. HIV-1–associated cognitive/motor complex: absence of neuronal loss in the cerebral neocortex. *Neurology* 1993;43:1492–1499.

92. Sharer LR. Pathology of HIV-1 infection of the central nervous system [Review]. *J Neuropathol Exp Neurol* 1992;51:3–11.

93. Sharer LR. Neuropathology and pathogenesis of SIV infection of the central nervous system. In: Price RW, Perry SW, eds. *HIV, AIDS and the Brain*. New York: Raven, 1994:133–145.

94. Sharer LR, Cho E-S. Pathology of the central nervous system in children with HIV-1 infection. In: Moran C, ed. *AFIP Fascicle, Synopsis of AIDS Pathology in Children*. Washington, DC: AFIP (in press).

95. Sharer LR, Cho ES, Epstein LG. Multinucleated giant cells and HTLV-III in AIDS encephalopathy. *Hum Pathol* 1985;16:760.

96. Sharer LR, Epstein LG, Cho ES, et al. Pathological features of AIDS encephalopathy in children: evidence for LAV/HTLV-III infection of brain. *Hum Pathol* 1986;17:271–284.

97. Sharer LR, Fischer B, Blumberg BM, et al. Opportunistic measles virus infection of the CNS in children with AIDS [Abstract]. *Brain Pathol* 1994;4:480.

98. Sharer LR, Kapila R. Neuropathological observations in acquired immunodeficiency syndrome (AIDS). *Acta Neuropathol* 1985;66:188–198.

99. Sharer LR, Mintz M. Neuropathology of AIDS in children. In: Scaravilli F, ed. *The Neuropathology of HIV Infection*. Berlin: Springer Verlag, 1993:201–214.

100. Sharer LR, Saito Y, Epstein LG, Blumberg BM. Detection of HIV-1 DNA in pediatric AIDS brain tissue by two-step ISPCR. *Adv Neuroimmunol* 1994;4:283–285.

101. Shaw GM, Harper ME, Hahn BH, et al. HTLV-III infection in brains of children and adults with AIDS encephalopathy. *Science* 1985;227:177–182.

102. Sidtis JJ, Gatsonis C, Price RW, et al. Zidovudine treatment of the AIDS dementia complex: results of a placebo controlled trial. *Ann Neurol* 1993;33:343–349.

103. Snider WD, Simpson DM, Nielsen S, Gold JW, Metroka CE, Posner JB. Neurological complications of acquired immune deficiency syndrome: analysis of 50 patients. *Ann Neurol* 1983;14:403–418.

104. Stoler MH, Eskin TA, Benn S, Angerer RC, Angerer LM. Human T-cell lymphotropic virus type III infection of the central nervous system: a preliminary in situ analysis. *JAMA* 1986;256:2360–2364.

105. Talley AK, Dewhurst S, Perry S, et al. Tumor necrosis factor alpha induces apoptosis in human

neuronal cells: protection by the antioxidant N-acetylcysteine and the genes *bcl-2* and *crmA*. *Mol Cell Biol* 1995;15(5):2359–2366.

106. Tersmette M, de Goede REY, Al BJM, et al. Differential syncytium-inducing capacity of human immunodeficiency virus isolates: frequent detection of syncytium-inducing isolates in patients with acquired immunodeficiency syndrome (AIDS) and AIDS-related complex. *J Virol* 1988;62: 2026–2032.

107. Tornatore C, Chandra R, Berger JR, Major EO. HIV-1 infection of subcortical astrocytes in the pediatric central nervous system. *Neurology* 1994;44:481–487.

108. Tornatore C, Meyers K, Atwood W, Conant K, Major E. Temporal patterns of human immunodeficiency virus type 1 transcripts in human fetal astrocytes. *J Virol* 1994;68:93–102.

109. Vago L, Castagna A, Lazzarin A, Trabattoni G, Cinque P, Costanzi G. Reduced frequency of HIV-induced brain lesions in AIDS patients treated with zidovudine. *J AIDS* 1993;6:42–45.

110. Walker DG, Itagaki S, Berry K, McGeer PL. Examination of brains of AIDS cases for human immunodeficiency virus and human cytomegalovirus nucleic acids. *J Neurol Neurosurg Psychiatry* 1989;52:583–590.

111. Weis S, Haug H, Budka H. Astroglial changes in the cerebral cortex of AIDS brains: a morphometric and immunohistochemical investigation. *Neuropathol Appl Neurobiol* 1993;19:329–335.

112. Weiss RA. Defective viruses to blame [Editorial]? *Nature* 1989;338:458.

113. Wiley CA, Masliah E, Morey M, et al. Neocortical damage during HIV infection. *Ann Neurol* 1991; 29:651–657.

114. Wiley CA, Nelson JA. Role of human immunodeficiency virus and cytomegalovirus in AIDS encephalitis. *Am J Pathol* 1988;133:73–81.

115. Wiley CA, Schrier RD, Nelson JA, Lampert PW, Oldstone MBA. Cellular localization of human immunodeficiency virus infection within the brains of acquired immune deficiency syndrome patients. *Proc Natl Acad Sci U S A* 1986;83:7089–7093.

116. Yarchoan R, Brouwers P, Spitzer AR, et al. Response of human immunodeficiency virus associated neurological disease to 3′-azido-3′-deoxythymidine. *Lancet* 1987;1:132–135.

AIDS and the Nervous System, Second Edition,
edited by J. R. Berger and R. M. Levy.
Lippincott-Raven Publishers, Philadelphia © 1997.

19

Neuropathology of Human Immunodeficiency Virus Related Opportunistic Infections and Neoplasms

Johann A. Hainfellner and Herbert Budka

Institute of Neurology, University of Vienna, A-1097 Wien, Austria

The frequency of neuropathological changes of all types in the brains of HIV-1–infected patients as found at autopsy has been reported to range between 55% and 95%. Among these, opportunistic infections are the most frequent complications with a frequency between 25% and 65% (3,29,40,60,84,117,118,121,134,166,178,229). The frequency of the different forms of opportunistic infections according to the results of several large autopsy series (3,40,60,84,117,118,121,134,166,178), including our own data from an autopsy series of 165 patients, is summarized in Table 1.

The wide range between different autopsy series is due to the considerable variation of the local frequency of the specific infection, whereas the spectrum of infections is roughly similar. The frequency of each opportunistic infection depends on many factors, including age, sex, risk group, geographic factors, socioeconomic conditions, previous and/or present treatment, sample size, bias in sampling, and different diagnostic criteria (84,229). Often multiple coexisting processes develop in the same patient, but there are no combinations observed more frequently than others. Women do not differ from men with regard to types and incidence of opportunistic central nervous system (CNS) infections (117). Compared with adults, children have fewer opportunistic infections (34,56,117). In infants with congenital AIDS, opportunistic infections are exceptional.

Stereotactic brain biopsy is a highly accurate and safe diagnostic tool to ascertain the nature of cerebral lesions in patients with AIDS, especially of opportunistic infections or neoplasms (2,7,39,66,108,152,164,244). Brain biopsy is usually undertaken when a mass lesion shows a poor clinical and/or radiological response to anti-*Toxoplasma* therapy.

Since 1989, 55 stereotactic biopsies in 54 patients with AIDS have been performed in our center. In 47 of 55 biopsies (85%), an etiological diagnosis could be established. The diagnoses are 18 (33%) progressive multifocal leukoencephalopathy (PML), 15 (27%) toxoplasmic encephalitis, 11 (20%) non-Hodgkin's lymphoma of the CNS (CNS-NHL), one (2%) tuberculosis, one (2%) *Aspergillus* infection, and one (2%) combined HIV encephalitis and HIV leukoencephalopathy. Eight (14%) showed necroses or inflammation of undefined character. Despite this clear-cut diagnostic value, the inability to treat neither PML nor CNS-NHL has been considered

TABLE 1. *Comparison of the occurrence of CNS opportunistic infections*

	Present series (1983–1994)	Drlicek et al. (1993)	Matthiessen et al. (1992)	Chimelli et al. (1992)	Kure et al. (1991)
Total n	165	184	174	252	221
Opportunistic infections					
Protozoal					
Toxoplasmosis	17	23.4	37.3	34.1	13.1
Trypanosomiasis	—	—	—	0.4	—
Fungal					
Cryptococcus	7	2.7	5.8	13.5	9
Candida	1.2	4.3	0.6	—	0.9
Aspergillus	—	1.6	—	0.4	0.9
Histoplasmosis	—	—	—	0.4	0.9
Bacterial					
Tuberculosis	1.2	—	0.6	0.8	1.4
Mycoabacterium avium-intracellulare	—	—	—	—	—
Treponemal infection	—	—	—	—	—
Bacterial infections	—	2.7	—	2	0.5
Viral					
CMV	16	17.4	14.3	7.9	12.7
PML/JCV	11	5.4	2.8	0.8	5.4
HSV	0.6	0.5	—	—	0.9
VZV	—	—	—	—	0.9
Measles virus	0.6	—	—	—	—
Nodular encephalitis	28[a]	1.6[b]	?	6.7[b]	—
Neoplasma					
Primary lymphoma	8	6	17.9	4	5.4
Secondary lymphoma	—	1.1	1.7	0.4	1.4
Kaposi's sarcoma	—	—	0.6	—	—
Lymphomatoid granulomatosis	—	—	—	—	—
Glioma	—	—	1.7	—	—

[a] In 13 cases the etiologic agent was either CMV, *Toxoplasma*, or HSV; in 15 cases no agent was detectable.
[b] No etiologic agent detectable.
[c] Including apparently cases of HIV encephalitis.

to argue against the regular use of brain biopsy patients with late-stage AIDS (61). However, even in patients with CNS-NHL, radiotherapy prolongs survival and improves quality of life. Therefore, it has been proposed that brain biopsy should be reserved for CNS mass lesions in patients with a good quality of life (7).

The present overview summarizes the vast amount of data about opportunistic infections and neoplasms of the CNS in HIV-1 infection. As to the more recently described HIV-2, information on associated nervous system pathology is scarce (128). In our experience, the spectrum of HIV-2–related neuropathology is indistinguishable from that of HIV-1 (125).

OPPORTUNISTIC INFECTIONS

Viral Infections

Viral infections are frequent complications of AIDS. The nervous system is mainly affected by two groups of viruses: the herpesviruses (primarily cytomegalovirus [CMV] and, less frequently, varicella zoster virus [VZV] and herpes simplex virus *and neoplasms in different autopsy series (%)*

Gray et al. (1991)	Lang et al. (1989)	Rhodes (1987)	Petito et al. (1986)	Anders et al. (1986)	Levy et al. (1985)	All series
135	135	100	153	89	128	1736
40.7	25.9	5	10.5	6.7	14.1	22.2
—	—	—	—	—	—	0.06
4.5	3.7	5	2.6	12.4	12.5	7.3
—	—	2	1.3	—	1.6	1.1
0.7	0.7	—	—	—	—	0.5
—	—	—	0.7	1.1	—	0.3
—	—	—	—	—	—	0.5
1.5	—	—	—	—	0.8	0.2
—	0.7	1	—	4.5	0.8	0.4
0.7	1.5	17	—	—	—	1.8
16.3	10.4	12	26.1	15.7	?	14.5
0.7	6.7	—	2	6.7	1.6	3.9
—	0.7	1	2	—	6.3	0.9
1.5	—	—	2	—	0.8	0.5
—	—	—	—	—	—	0.06
?	13.3[b]	47[c]	17	63[c]	—	8.9
11.1	3	8	5.9	3.4	7	6.3
0.7	3.7	5	2	1.1	1.6	1.2
—	—	—	—	—	1.6	0.06
—	—	—	—	1.1	—	0.06
—	—	—	—	—	—	0.2

[HSV]), and papovavirus. The herpesviruses cause variable neuropathological manifestations, whereas the JC papovavirus produces a single well-defined disease: PML.

CMV

CMV particles consist of a core containing double-stranded DNA, an icosahedral capsid, and a surrounding envelope. CMV infections are common, but CMV disease rarely occurs in immunologically uncompromised adults, in whom it may present as meningoencephalitis (45). It is more common in fetuses and neonates after *in utero* exposure. It then may produce congenital malformations and progressive neurological disease after birth (15).

The most severe and pathologically varied manifestations of CMV infection of the nervous system are found in patients with AIDS. CMV disease of the CNS usually develops in association with disseminated systemic CMV infection (117,220). CMV disease in AIDS may be due to reactivation of latent virus or infection with exogenous virus, which may be transmitted by contact with individuals who are shedding virus (115). Rarely, CMV infection of the CNS occurs in infants with congenital AIDS (20). Historically, CMV was the first pathogen to be linked to the microglial nodules, which are commonly observed in brains from patients with AIDS (155).

CMV probably enters the brain from the blood and then disseminates via the

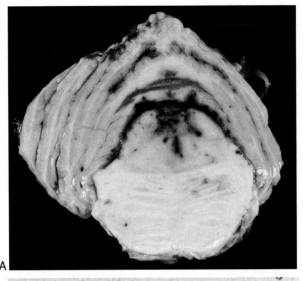

A

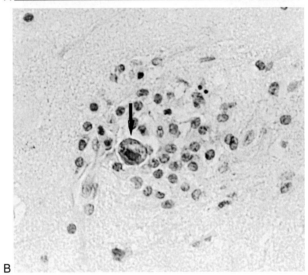

B

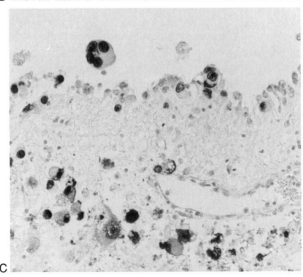

C

cerebrospinal fluid (CSF) before invasion into the brain parenchyma (143). CMV is able to replicate in several cell types of the nervous system, including astrocytes, ependymal cells, choroid plexus epithelium, vascular endothelium, and neurons. In the peripheral nervous system, Schwann cells may be infected (18). Cell infection does not always result in cytomegaly. Antigen-negative and structurally normal neurons and glial cells were shown to contain human CMV DNA fragments, indicating restricted intracellular replication of CMV (240). Except for meningomyeloradiculitis causing a cauda equina syndrome, clinical presentation of CMV infection of the CNS is uncharacteristic. In some cases, CMV infection of the CNS was diagnosed by immunocytochemical demonstration of infected cells in CSF (204). Amplification of CMV DNA by polymerase chain reaction (PCR) in the CSF has proven to be a rapid and reliable diagnostic method to detect CMV infection of the CNS (43,79).

Macroscopically, CMV-infected brains show either no changes, focal parenchymal necrosis, or hemorrhagic necrosis lining the ventricles and cerebral surfaces (Fig. 1A). Histologically, the most common finding is microglial nodules scattered diffusely in gray more than white matter, with (Fig. 1B) or often without detectable CMV inclusion-bearing cells in many nodules. The description and discussion of nodular encephalitis are given in more detail on pages 490 and 491. Focal parenchymal necrosis and necrotizing ventriculoencephalitis are characterized by a variable degree of inflammation accompanied by cytomegaly with intranuclear and intracytoplasmic CMV inclusions in glial, ependymal, and endothelial cells and neurons (Fig. 1C). Frequently, the necrotizing lesions are associated with CMV nodular encephalitis in the same brain. Rarely, inclusion-bearing cells occur in an otherwise normal parenchyma. CMV inclusions can be readily identified by their characteristic size and shape in conventional light microscopy and by immunocytochemistry and *in situ* hybridization (193). The latter techniques show that normal appearing cells at the edges of the lesions may contain virus. Focal parenchymal necrosis, ventriculoencephalitis, and isolated inclusion-bearing cells seem to be specific features of CMV brain disease in AIDS. Ventriculoencephalitis may give rise to necrotizing radiculomyelitis by seeding via the CSF (18,143).

A few cases present with polyradiculomyelitis or spinal ganglionitis. The clinical correlate is rapidly ascending polyradiculoneuropathy similar to Guillain-Barré syndrome (139,222) but with a granulocytic CSF pleocytosis.

Both productive CMV and HIV infections may develop within the same brain (238). However, CMV is usually restricted to necrotizing lesions or microglial nodules, whereas HIV products are mostly confined to lesions of HIV encephalitis (28,30,190). Exceptionally, coinfection of multinucleated giant cells by HIV and CMV has been demonstrated using immunocytochemical double-labeling techniques (18,19). In our hands, double-labeling applied to several coinfected brains did not show cellular colocalization.

FIG. 1. CMV infection. **A:** Gross specimen of pons and cerebellum in generalized ventriculitis. Hemorrhagic necrosis surrounds the fourth ventricle and extends to the surfaces of the tegmentum pontis and cerebellar folia. **B:** CMV nodular encephalitis. The microglial nodule surrounds one cytomegalic cell *(arrow)* with an intranuclear inclusion (hematoxylin and eosin, original magnification ×400). **C:** CMV ventriculoencephalitis. There is patchy loss of ependymal lining and necrosis. An anti-CMV antibody strongly labels the intranuclear inclusions of cytomegalic cells that include ependymal cells. (Original magnification ×200.)

HSV

HSV-1 is the most frequent causative agent in man's sporadic acute encephalitis in temperate parts of the world, with an untreated mortality rate of 51–76% (64). The natural prevalence of HSV-1 infection increases gradually, beginning in childhood, reaching 70–80% in later adult years (46). HSV remains in a latent state in the trigeminal, superior cervical, and vagal ganglia (52,227). The virus is transported intraaxonally to neurons of second and third order (6). In AIDS, HSV encephalitis is surprisingly rare. In our autopsy series we identified only one case with nodular encephalitis and HSV DNA within the nodules (190). HSV encephalitis does not seem to occur much more frequently in AIDS than in immunocompetent individuals; its clinical and pathological features seem to be identical to those well known in immunocompetent patients.

HSV-2 caused culture-proven encephalitis in two homosexual men with persistent lymphadenopathy (57) and thoracic myelitis in one patient with AIDS (25).

A rapid, noninvasive method for the routine laboratory diagnosis of CNS infection due to HSV is PCR of CSF (12).

VZV

VZV infects nearly 100% of the population in temperate parts of the world (231,232). During a chickenpox outbreak, VZV apparently spreads into sensory ganglia via contiguous exteroceptive nerves. Herpes zoster is assumed to be due to reactivation of a latent infection of the sensory ganglia (70). There may be frequent involvement of the CNS in herpes zoster presenting as encephalitis and encephalomyelitis (167,191), perivenous encephalomalacia (137), leukoencephalopathy with and without brain stem involvement (137,185), nodular brain stem encephalitis (191), and vasculopathy (62). Although there is a strong association between immunosuppression and herpes zoster, only a few patients with AIDS with neurological complications associated with VZV have been reported. Presentations of VZV disease in AIDS have included multifocal leukoencephalitis with and without a noninflammatory vasculopathy (86,142); encephalomyelitis, mainly involving the gray matter, possibly secondary to transsynaptic spread to the brain or spinal cord from VZV ophthalmicus (183), trigeminal (181), dermatomal (136), or myotomal (191) infection; ependymitis/ventriculitis mimicking CMV infection with (41) and without (72) secondary meningomyeloradiculitis; and fulminant ascending myeloradiculopathy (221). Eosinophilic intranuclear inclusions of Cowdry type A are found in oligodendrocytes, astrocytes, occasional neurons, ependymal cells, endothelial cells, and Schwann cells. VZV infection is verified by immunocytochemical and/or *in situ* hybridization techniques (191). The occurrence of a cutaneous herpes zoster eruption before, or concomitant with, the onset of neurological signs is a useful, although unreliable, diagnostic clue (86). PCR of CSF for detection of VZV DNA has been proposed as a useful tool for the early diagnosis of VZV-associated neurological disease (172).

Epstein-Barr Virus

No specific disorder of the nervous system has convincingly been linked to Epstein-Barr virus (EBV). However, there is strong evidence that EBV is implicated in the pathogenesis of CNS lymphoma, both in the presence and absence of AIDS (16,37,51,89,131,141,163).

PML

Papovaviruses cause PML, with an autopsy incidence in patients with AIDS of 2–11%. These DNA viruses include three different subtypes: BK virus, JC virus, and SV40 virus. PML has been linked to the latter two viruses, although almost all or all are caused by JC virus, whereas any role of SV40 virus has remained controversial (192).

Antibodies against JC virus are found in 70% of normal adults (158). It is still unclear how the primary infection takes place, where the virus resides in seropositive, asymptomatic persons, and how it reaches the CNS (14). However, JC virus was found in extraneural sites, including the kidney, spleen, and bone marrow (58,98). During the primary infection, JC virus may reach the CNS via the blood and from infected vascular endothelial cells, or during immunosuppression, latent JC virus dormant in the kidney and bone marrow may be reactivated and invade the brain (14). Within the CNS, oligodendrocytes are fully permissive to infection, whereas astrocytes show a restricted infection (32,87,135,196). The cell type specificity is regulated by the enhancer element (127) and transcription factors (98). *In vitro* studies suggest that CMV might serve as a helper virus for JC virus replication in otherwise nonpermissive cells (92).

PML is exclusively a disease of the human CNS and was first described in 1958 in patients with chronic lymphocytic leukemia and Hodgkin's disease (13). The ultrastructural studies of Zu Rhein and Chou (245) first demonstrated papovavirus within oligodendroglial nuclei, and JC virus was isolated from infected brain tissue in 1971 (159).

PML is found in a broad spectrum of different forms of immunosuppression, including AIDS; in the pre-AIDS era it occurred in 11.1% of persons without obvious compromising conditions (32). In HIV-seropositive patients, PML has been noted in the absence of other clinical manifestations of immunodeficiency (102). JC virus has been detected in brains of patients with AIDS without clinically evident PML (173). Although rare, PML is among the neurological complications of HIV-1–infected children (22). Neurological symptoms are unspecific, including focal signs and/or dementia (224). Patients usually have a relentless downhill course. CT scans show low-density nonenhancing white matter lesions, and magnetic resonance imaging (MRI) demonstrates high-intensity signals on T2-weighted spin-echo images.

Macroscopically, the white matter features multiple, bilateral, irregular, and ill-defined patches of discoloration and granular destruction (Fig. 2A). Lesions range in size from a few millimeters to extensive involvement of cerebral and cerebellar hemispheres. Parietooccipital regions are most frequently involved. Whole-brain histological sections stained for myelin demonstrate the characteristic multifocal lesions of moth-eaten appearance (Fig. 2B).

Histologically, there are confluent foci of demyelination, with many lipid-laden macrophages and reactive gliosis with bizarre, giant astrocytic nuclei in the center. Mainly at the edge of the lesion, greatly enlarged oligodendroglial nuclei are pathognomonic ("PML cells" [32]); their chromatin is replaced by glassy amphophilic viral inclusion material. Abundant JC virus products are demonstrable by immunocy-

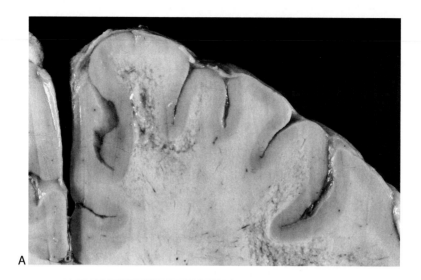

A

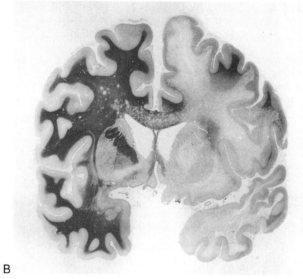

B

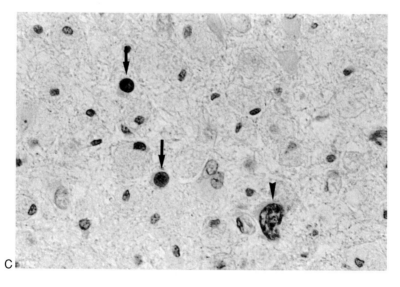

C

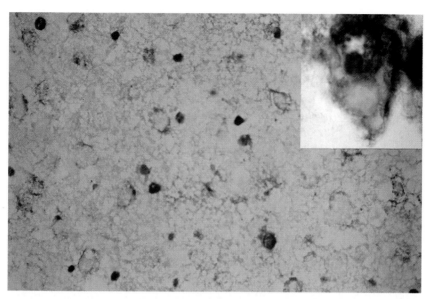

FIG. 3. PML. Local HIV coinfection of PML lesions. In a PML lesion with numerous glial nuclei labeled with an antipapovavirus antiserum (32) (blue label), numerous infiltrating macrophages are labeled at the cell surface with a monoclonal antibody against HIV p17 antigen (28) (brown label). (Original magnification ×250.) **Inset:** Colocalization of HIV and JC virus products in a single cell. A macrophage in a PML lesion is labeled at the cell surface with an antibody against HIV p24 antigen (28) (brown) and shows additional nuclear staining with antipapovavirus serum (blue). (Original magnification ×900.)

tochemistry (32) and *in situ* DNA hybridization (192) in these cells (Fig. 2C). There is a varying degree of inflammation that may also be absent. The cortex is usually spared, although lesions can extend to the cortex white matter junction. Rarely, the white matter of the spinal cord may be affected.

PML lesions in AIDS are usually similar to those occurring with other basic diseases (116,192,224). However, changes in AIDS may be atypically extensive, necrotic, unilateral, or asymmetrical and may involve regions classically spared such as the temporal lobes, basal ganglia, brain stem, or cerebellum (Fig. 2B). Inflammation is often mild or absent, and viral inclusions may be remarkably abundant (1). Macrophages infiltrating the demyelinating PML lesions may be infected by HIV-1 (192,217,237). In our autopsy series, four patients with PML had unusually extensive and necrotic lesions infiltrated with abundant macrophages that expressed HIV antigens (Fig. 3). Combined anti-SV40 and anti-HIV immunocytochemistry did not show cellular colocalization of JC virus and HIV in those cases. However, another case from our biopsy series displayed a PML lesion infiltrated by HIV infected

←───────────────────────────────────────

FIG. 2. PML. **A:** Gross brain specimen. The white matter shows multiple confluent and poorly circumscribed patches of granular destruction. **B:** Whole mount coronal section of the cerebral hemispheres. Extensive predominantly unilateral demyelination including the basal ganglia, temporal lobe, and commissura anterior. The corpus callosum and contralateral white matter are demyelinated in a moth-eaten distribution. **C:** Immunocytochemistry using an anti-papovavirus serum (32) labels oligodendroglial nuclei *(arrows)* and an astroglial nucleus *(arrowhead)* (original magnification ×400).

macrophages, and immunocytochemical double labeling showed colocalization of JC virus and HIV in a single macrophage (Fig. 3 inset). The increase in damage to tissue in AIDS brains may be due to transactivation of one virus by the other (71,192). On the one hand, JC virus DNA may transactivate the HIV long terminal repeat sequence; on the other hand, the HIV-1 regulatory protein *tat* may enhance the JC virus lytic cycle in glial cells by stimulating JC virus gene expression (212).

The diagnosis may be done morphologically on brain tissue examined via biopsy; immunocytochemistry and/or *in situ* hybridization techniques or electron microscopy confirm the histological diagnosis. Ultrastructurally, the virus particles are round or elongated and sometimes arranged in crystalline arrays. Virus particles and antigen are usually located in nuclei. A new promising method for identification of JC virus in neurological disease is PCR of CSF (140,228).

Measles Virus

Encephalitis is a rare complication of measles infection manifesting as (a) acute encephalitis, (b) subacute sclerosing panencephalitis, and (c) subacute measles encephalitis in the immunosuppressed (156). Patients of the latter group usually have a history of contact with measles or an actual attack from which they recover fully. Several months later, encephalitic signs, seizures, myoclonus, stupor, and coma develop. Histologically, diagnostic features are eosinophilic intranuclear inclusion bodies in neurons and oligodendrocytes (50) and the presence of measles virus antigen (30).

Despite the ubiquity of measles infection, its complications in AIDS are exceptional. We observed productive measles virus encephalitis in a 15-year-old male hemophilic patient with AIDS who suddenly developed encephalitic signs without any CSF abnormalities. Brain autopsy showed significant diffuse gliosis and perivascular inflammatory infiltrates in gray and white matter with maximum in the mesencephalon and diencephalon. Numerous cells had intranuclear and intracytoplasmic eosinophilic inclusions, which were strongly immunoreactive with an antimeasles virus antiserum. Electron microscopy showed nuclear inclusion bodies with the typical appearance of smooth paramyxovirus nucleocapsids with tubular structure and mean diameter of 150 nm (31). Previous reports have described measles virus in myelitis (197) and encephalitis (149) in AIDS, although in the latter report productive infection was not demonstrated.

Unspecified Nodular Encephalitis

In many brains of HIV-1–infected patients, the only histological finding is the presence of gliomesenchymal nodules (GMNs). These nodules, composed of lymphocytes, microglia, and macrophages, with adjacent reactive astrocytes, are scattered more in the gray matter than in the white matter (162). GMNs are not detectable radiologically (80). Nodular encephalitis in AIDS has already been described as ''AIDS subacute encephalitis'' and has been frequently confused with HIV encephalitis, from which it is distinguished by the different distribution of foci (the cortex being preferentially involved), by the different composition (more densely packed

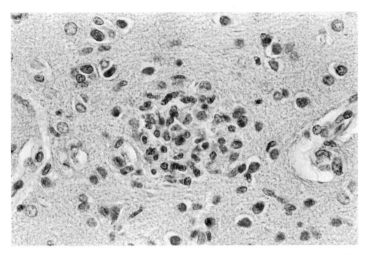

FIG. 4. Microglial nodule in the cerebral cortex in unspecified nodular encephalitis. The nodule shows a compact arrangement of mostly rounded cells. (Hematoxylin and eosin, original magnification ×440.)

rounded cells in GMNs [Fig. 4] vs. the usually looser arrangement of elongated microglia in HIV encephalitis [29]), and by the lack of multinucleated giant cells (33) and HIV antigens (28). The most frequent cause of nodular encephalitis is CMV (109), although cytomegalic cells are only sporadically found within the nodules (118). In some of our cases, numerous small blocks did not show the infectious agent, whereas large sections demonstrated cytomegalic cells or other agents. In some cases, *Toxoplasma* organisms or HSV were shown as the underlying cause of nodular encephalitis by immunocytochemistry and/or *in situ* hybridization (29,190).

Fungal Infections

Fungal infections of the CNS associated with HIV infection are similar to those seen in individuals not immunocompromised by AIDS (96) and include cryptococcosis, aspergillosis, mucormycosis, and candidiasis (122,130). In addition, endemic fungi (e.g., histoplasmosis in the southeastern and coccidiomycosis in the southwestern United States) may involve the CNS. Signs and symptoms associated with fungal infections are often subtle. Evaluation of serum and CSF antibodies and culture assays or morphological identification are mandatory for the diagnosis of fungal infections.

Cryptococcus neoformans

Cryptococcus neoformans is the most common fungus to infect the brain and the leptomeninges in AIDS. The incidence ranges between 3% and 13.5% in autopsy series. Fifty percent to 85% of the patients have documented evidence of systemic cryptococcal infection (117,246). *Cryptococcus* is a common soil contaminant, being excreted in bird feces. Primary infection is usually localized to the lung and subsequent septicemia occurs almost exclusively in immunocompromised states. Cryptococcal spread to the brain manifests mostly as a leptomeningitis and less commonly as meningoencephalitis. Signs and symptoms of CNS cryptococcal infection evolve over days or weeks, are nonspecific, and include malaise, fever, headache, nausea, vomiting, and mental status changes (207,246). Focal abnormalities are infrequent. Neuroradiological investigations are only contributory when cryptococcomas are present. On computed tomography (CT) and MRI, the latter are confined to the cerebral hemispheres and appear as mass lesions lacking specific features. The diagnosis relies on demonstration of cryptococcal antigen in the CSF. Moreover, the organisms may be directly visualized in cytological CSF preparations (Fig. 5A). Recurring relapses of cryptococcal meningitis after antifungal therapy are common (130,246). There is strong evidence that recurrence of cryptococcal meningitis results from the original infecting strain (203). CSF olfactory pathways may contain sequestered reservoirs of cryptococci and may be a possible source of meningeal relapse (126).

Macroscopically, the brain appears normal or shows gelatinous clouded to opacified meninges. The basal meninges are most typically affected, and obstruction of CSF outflow at the foramina of Luschka and Magendie can give rise to hydrocephalus. On sectioning, perivascular spaces sometimes show cystic enlargement. Many brains have one or multiple cryptococcomas containing soft gray mucoid material with a diameter of up to a centimeter (220). In rare instances cryptococcomas may present as massive space-occupying lesions (117). Cryptococcomas have no fibrous capsule. Granuloma formation and necrosis are infrequent. Histologically, the subarachnoid and expanded Virchow-Robin spaces show diffuse accumulations of fungal organisms (Fig. 5B). Inflammation is usually minimal or absent. The fungi are spherical to oval, vary in diameter from 2 to 15 μm, and have a thick, clear halo around each organism due to the presence of an abundant mucopolysaccharide capsule. The capsules can be readily demonstrated with the mucicarmine and periodic acid-Schiff (PAS) stains. *Cryptococcus* is a budding yeast, and the organisms are usually extracellular; however, in one patient we saw a prominent histiocytic infiltrate with phagocytosis of fungi, as has also been observed by others (3). Even macrophages producing HIV antigen were seen to phagocytose cryptococci (28). There may be minimal inflammatory response in the neighborhood of the capsules, but often no inflammation is present.

Candida albicans

Candida albicans is an oval budding yeast without a capsule and with production of pseudohyphae. It is ubiquitous, being found on many plants and as normal flora of the alimentary tract and mucocutaneous membranes of humans, and may cause mild to severe infections of the skin, nails, and mucous membranes in individuals with normal immune defenses and serious deep-seated infections in debilitated hosts (226). It is an infrequent CNS pathogen in patients with an intact neutrophilic response. Therefore, infection of CNS is relatively rare, even in AIDS (1–4% in autopsy series). It may occur as a terminal event and is usually associated with systemic infection. Gross anatomical examination of the brain shows either nonspecific changes or small to large abscesses or hemorrhagic necroses scattered in gray and white matter. Histologically, a central necrosis is invaded by pseudohyphae and small oval to spherical blastospores, and surrounded by a variably developed mixture of

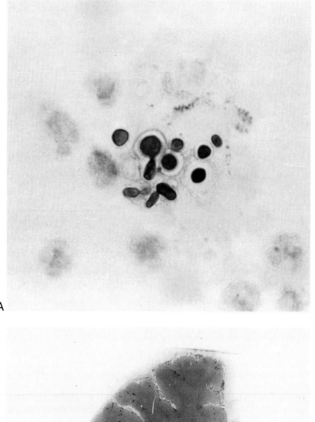

A

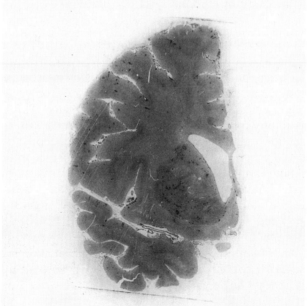

B

FIG. 5. A: Cryptococci including a budding spore in a CSF cytospin preparation. (Grocott's silver methenamine stain, original magnification ×440.) **B:** Cryptococcosis. On this whole mount coronal section of a cerebral hemisphere, abundant darkly stained deposits of fungal organisms are evident, most prominently in the basal ganglia. These fungal accumulations are localized in meninges and perivasal spaces within the brain (Alcian blue stain).

mononuclear and polymorphonuclear inflammatory cells. *Candida* infection also may present as meningitis.

Aspergillus

Aspergillosis is among the most common fungal infections requiring hospitalization (68). *Aspergillus* species may (a) colonize without extension in preformed cavities and debilitated tissues within the respiratory tract; (b) superficially infect the skin, paranasal sinuses, burn eschars, nail, and other sites; (c) cause invasive, inflammatory, granulomatous, necrotizing infection of the lungs; or (d) manifest as systemic and fatal disseminated disease (179). In a published report on AIDS, *Aspergillus* species occasionally caused brain infection (242). Clinically, typical symptoms were fever and headache. Terminally, focal signs were present. CSF examination was nondiagnostic. Neuroradiology showed multiple hypodense nonenhancing lesions. Grossly, the brains showed abscesses or areas of hemorrhagic necrosis. Microscopically, there were tissue necrosis, a neutrophilic inflammatory infiltrate, and septate hyphae branching dichotomously at acute angles with prominent blood vessel invasion. The infection may also present as meningitis and meningoencephalitis (220). One atypical case presented with basal meningitis with pontine infarction secondary to invasive *Aspergillus* sinusitis (35). In one case of our biopsy series, *Aspergillus* was detected as the cause of multiple focal cerebral lesions.

Mucormycosis

Mucormycosis is an opportunistic infection caused by nonseptate fungi belonging to the class Zygomycetes and the order Mucorales (55). Zygomycetes are widespread in soil, fruits, and decomposing plants and animal matter. The ubiquitous nature provides an opportunity for invasion of the body through the skin and mucous membranes. CNS infection is usually secondary, due to hematogenous spread after primary infection of the nasopharynx, the skin, and the gastrointestinal tract (150). Zygomycetes are uncommon pathogens in AIDS (49,122). The few cases reported were found exclusively among intravenous drug abusers. The infection is usually fulminant and rapidly fatal, despite antifungal therapy. Grossly, CNS lesions are confined to the deep cerebral gray and white matter and often are multiple. The pattern of lesion is similar to that seen with *Aspergillus*, with marked angioinvasion by fungal hyphae, thrombosis of infected vessels, and infarction of the surrounding brain tissue. Silver-methenamine stains the Zygomycetes, showing broad, nonseptate hyphae of irregular width branching at right angles (49).

Coccidioidomycosis

The dimorphic fungus *Coccidioides immitis* is a common soil contaminant in the southwestern United States and Central and South America (160). Coccidial infection is usually subclinical or produces subacute respiratory symptoms (233). Solitary or multiple discrete lesions beyond the thorax are infrequent (54). In the setting of immunological deficiency, fungemia with widespread dissemination may occur (26). Single cases and small series of *Coccidioides* infection in AIDS have been reported

(26,121,122). The disease is either due to reactivation of a latent infection or may result from an extreme vulnerability to the acquisition of the primary infection. CNS infection is uncommon and manifests as meningitis or multiple abscesses. The diagnosis can be made in the presence of high serum antibody levels, positive culture of CSF, blood, bronchial washings, or biopsy tissue, or histologically. Response to antifungal therapy is poor (26).

Histoplasmosis

The dimorphic fungus Histoplasma capsulatum is endemic in the central United States, mid-Atlantic states, and central Florida and is found also in other areas throughout the world (226). It occurs in soil with high nitrogen concentrations, especially related to droppings of starlings, chickens, and bats (77,130) and causes a variety of self-limiting diseases in normal hosts, but commonly disseminates in those who are immunosuppressed (234). Several small series document an increased incidence of disseminated histoplasmosis in patients with AIDS in endemic areas (24,106,214,235). Disseminated histoplasmosis is most accurately diagnosed by bone marrow or blood cultures. Serum antibody titers to *Histoplasma* are usually elevated. CSF culture is often negative. Response to antifungal therapy is poor. CNS involvement by *Histoplasma* presents as meningitis, granulomatous encephalitis with solitary or multiple lesions, and progressive disseminated histoplasmosis with multiple small microglial nodules and poorly formed granulomas scattered throughout the brain (220).

Cladosporiosis

A single case of cladosporiosis has been observed in a male intravenous drug–abusing patient with AIDS. CT showed multiple contrast-enhancing lesions. Autopsy showed focal suppurative and granulomatous lesions, one in the deep cerebral gray matter and one in the brain stem, with pathognomonic pigmented budding yeasts and hyphae (47).

Parasitoses

Toxoplasmosis is by far the most common form of parasitic brain infestation in patients with AIDS, and only a few scattered reports describe other brain parasites.

Toxoplasma gondii

Toxoplasma gondii is a protozoan parasite that is a rare cause of disease in the general population (114). In patients with AIDS, infection of the brain by *Toxoplasma gondii* is one of the most common causes of neurological dysfunction and morbidity and is the most common process producing focal brain lesions (121,129).

Toxoplasma gondii is distributed worldwide and is an obligate intracellular parasite. Humans acquire the initial infection via ingestion of encysted bradyzoites in poorly cooked or undercooked meat (177). After invasion of the gut, the organisms are disseminated to all organs, including the brain. The parasites actively invade a wide range of host cells (200) and reside there engulfed in a cell membrane–derived so-called parasitophorous vacuole. More than 90% of primary infections are subclinical, but toxoplasmic cysts persist in tissue. Experimental data indicate that protective immunity is mainly mediated by CD8 + cytotoxic T cells producing interferon-gamma and interleukin-2 (111). An immunosuppressed state may lead to parasitic activation.

CNS involvement in AIDS has been reported in 4–41% of AIDS autopsy cases. Most patients have no evidence of systemic toxoplasmosis, which suggests reactivation of a latent local infection (117,205). The mechanism of the cerebral localization in immunosuppressed patients with reactivated toxoplasmosis is not clear. Its presence in the CNS may be enhanced by a relative lack of host defense in the brain, which experimentally has been shown to be mediated by cytokine-activated microglial cells (38), as compared with systemic organs (211,223). Furthermore, experimental data show an effect of the strain of *Toxoplasma gondii* on the development of toxoplasmic encephalitis (210). However, geographical location and risk factor subgroup seem to be the most important determinants of prevalence of this infection in patients with AIDS (220,229). Indeed, there are striking differences in the incidence of toxoplasmic encephalitis between Europe (17–40.7%), North America (5–14,1%), and Latin America (34.1%). Haitian patients are at greatest risk for developing toxoplasmosis (122). In children with AIDS, only a few cases of CNS toxoplasmosis have been reported (56). The clinical symptoms are typically subacute, evolve over 7–14 days, and may be both focal and diffuse. Some patients develop dementia and coma, which clinically can mimic the AIDS dementia complex (153). The presence of immunoglobulin M antibody and high anti-*Toxoplasma* titers in the serum generally indicate active infection. In the absence of serum antibody to *Toxoplasma,* it is unlikely but not excluded that a cerebral mass lesion represents toxoplasmosis. Organisms are rarely detected in centrifuged CSF. A fourfold or greater increase of antibody titer in repeat CSF taps is highly suggestive of active CNS infection (129). A study of 37 patients with cerebral toxoplasmosis showed a 62% frequency of CSF *Toxoplasma* antibodies (171). The frequent involvement of the choroid plexus may be responsible in part for the high frequency of CSF anti-*Toxoplasma* antibodies (65).

Neuroradiology shows usually multiple mass lesions, which are sometimes irregular or hypodense but most commonly rounded and ring-enhancing and associated with a hypodense area of edema. These findings are not pathognomonic, and similar changes may be associated with CNS lymphomas, tuberculosis, or fungal infections. MRI is much more sensitive than CT at detecting smaller lesions (123).

CNS toxoplasmosis is fatal unless treated. Clinical and neuroradiological improvement is usually demonstrable within a few days after initiating therapy. Because relapses are common, often life-long therapy is indicated (129).

Macroscopically, lesions appear as more or less sharply demarcated zones of necrosis that are sometimes hemorrhagic (Fig. 6). They are usually multiple and most common in the deep gray matter and at the peripheral cortical gray–white matter junction. The infratentorial structures are less frequently affected, and the spinal cord is least frequently affected. Some cases show lesions in the choroid plexus, which also may be the sole site of CNS infection (65,83). Involvement of the leptomeninges is rare and exclusively found in association with a contiguous parenchymal lesion. The lesions range in size between a few millimeters and a few centimeters.

Histologically, the CNS may show either latent or active infection. Latent infection

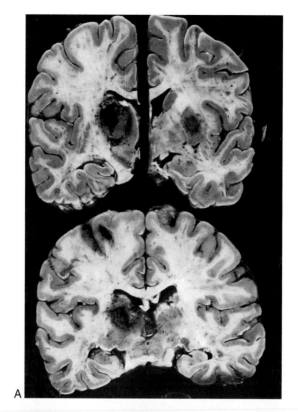

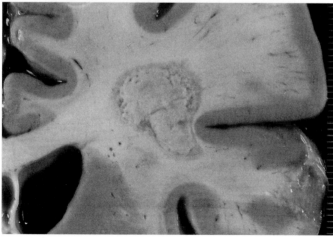

FIG. 6. Toxoplasmosis. **A:** Early lesion. Coronal sections of the cerebral hemispheres show poorly circumscribed hemorrhagic and necrotic lesions predominantly in basal ganglia. **B:** Chronic lesion. A gross specimen shows a well-demarcated necrotic lesion of the white matter without mass effect.

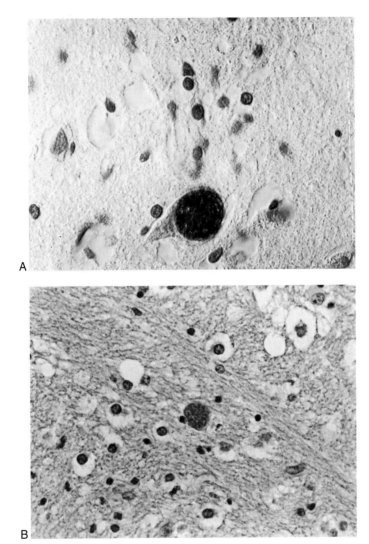

FIG. 7. Toxoplasmosis. **A:** Latent state. Encysted bradyzoites are localized in the cytoplasm of a neuron. (Anti-*Toxoplasma* immunocytochemistry, Nomarski contrast, original magnification ×1,000.) **B:** Latent state. Encysted organisms in the cerebral parenchyma without necrosis and inflammation. (Hematoxylin and eosin, original magnification ×400.)

is characterized by intact cysts (bradyzoites) lying intracellularly (Fig. 7A) or free in tissue (Fig. 7B) without necrosis and inflammation. The clinically significant active infection shows three phases: (a) poorly circumscribed necrosis with variable petechial hemorrhages surrounded by acute and chronic inflammation, macrophage infiltration, vascular proliferation, tachyzoites, and encysted bradyzoites (acute infection, less than a few weeks' duration) (Figs. 6A and 7D); (b) organizing necroses with organisms in a minority of cases (several weeks to months); and (c) chronic necroses, well demarcated, with rare cysts at the periphery of the necrosis (after many months) (Fig. 6B). Some patients have both acute and chronic lesions that are, in our experience, frequently accompanied by toxoplasmic nodular encephalitis. In

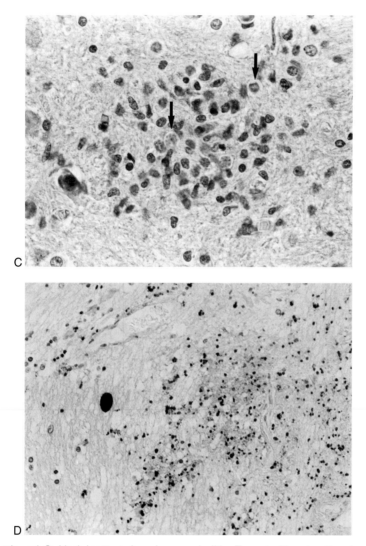

FIG. 7. *Continued.* **C:** Nodular toxoplasmic encephalitis. Encysted bradyzoites *(arrows)* within a microglial nodule. (Hematoxylin and eosin, original magnification ×440.) **D:** At the border of a recent necrotizing cerebral lesion, anti-*Toxoplasma* immunocytochemistry strongly labels free tachyzoites and encysted bradyzoites. (Original magnification ×400.)

more recent years, we have mainly observed chronic lesions. This corresponds with the observations of others and is ascribed to improved clinical management of patients (205). Blood vessels in the vicinity of acute lesions also can be invaded by organisms and show marked intimal proliferation or frank vasculitis with fibrinoid necrosis and thrombosis (99). In patients with acute cerebral lesions, tachyzoites are frequently found in the choroid plexus (65).

In addition to necroses or abscesses, CNS toxoplasmosis may present as nodular encephalitis (Fig. 7C). Toxoplasmic nodular encephalitis appears unique to AIDS and may be responsible for a treatable diffuse encephalopathy in these patients (85).

Unusual forms of cerebral toxoplasmosis include widespread microinfarcts due to parasitic emboli (83); ventriculitis and subependymal infection (117); necrotizing meningoencephaloventriculomyelitis, apparently after dissemination of the microorganism from a primary cerebral periventricular lesion through the CSF (11); necrotizing myelopathy (93,138,151); overwhelming fatal toxoplasmosis with toxoplasma cysts scattered throughout the brain and with multiple cerebral hemorrhages (236); and anergic disseminated fatal toxoplasmosis (10).

The pathogenesis of *Toxoplasma*-induced necroses is unclear. Cytotoxic products of *T. gondii* have not yet been isolated (225).

Immunohistochemical techniques are useful for the tissue diagnosis of toxoplasmosis, especially in the absence of encysted forms (Fig. 7D). One report proposed electron microscopy as a rapid and precise method of diagnosing CNS toxoplasmosis (213). The standard diagnostic method is the time-consuming mouse inoculation with biopsy tissue and subsequent smears after days of inoculation (220).

Amplification of genomic nucleic acid by PCR is a promising new diagnostic tool for diagnosis of toxoplasmosis (219).

Amebiasis

Free-living amebae of the genera *Naegleria* and *Acanthamoeba* are uncommon human pathogens (132). In the setting of an immunosuppressed host, various species of the genus *Acanthamoeba* may take the lungs, the skin, or the genitourinary tract as the route of entry and may secondarily, presumably hematogenously, cause a subacute to chronic granulomatous encephalitis (8,133). In AIDS, *Acanthamoeba* species caused acute meningoencephalitis in a few cases (69,76,239) and leptomyxoid ameba in one case (8). Commonly, focal signs and mental status abnormalities occur; meningism and headache are not prominent features. The CSF protein level is increased, the glucose is normal, and cytology is normal or shows polymorphonuclear leukocytosis (239). CT without contrast shows hypodense lesions (8) and with contrast shows enhancing lesions (69). Grossly, the brain exhibits hemorrhagic softenings. Histology shows necrotizing thromboocclusive angiitis, mainly in large veins. Amebic trophozoites and cysts infiltrate vessel walls and necrotic brain tissue between the vessels and are found at the edges of the lesions (8,69,76,239). The amebae may sometimes be difficult to distinguish from histiocytes. PAS or methenamine silver stains are helpful in visualizing the organisms, although definitive identification may ultimately depend on culture and/or immunocytochemical studies (8,69).

Trypanosomiasis

American trypanosomiasis, or Chagas' disease, is endemic in Latin America, caused by the flagellated, obligate intracellular protozoan *Trypanosoma cruzi,* and transmitted by hematophagous triatomid insects, or reduviid bugs (115). In the acute stage, the parasites seed to the skeletal and cardiac muscle. The involvement of the CNS is common, occurring mainly in children (202). However, fatal meningoencephalitis is rare. A subsequent indeterminate stage may last many years, and a few patients develop the chronic stage with cardiomyopathy and megaesophagus or megacolon. Reactivation of the indeterminate or chronic stages of Chagas' disease is uncommon and limited to immunosuppressed hosts (119). In association with AIDS, there are only three reported cases of acute exacerbation of chronic Chagas' disease with involvement of the CNS (53,74,180). Two cases presented with a cerebral mass lesion (53,74). In Gluckstein's patient (74), cranial CT scan demonstrated an irregular contrast-enhancing mass lesion with edema. In both patients, histology showed chronic inflammation and numerous intracellular amastigotes. In Gluckstein's patient (74), the diagnosis was confirmed by positive culture from a brain biopsy specimen. The third patient presented with diffuse meningoencephalitis (180). Histology showed microglial nodules scattered throughout the brain and brain stem. A few nodules contained amastigotes. The cerebellum showed large necrotic hemorrhagic areas with innumerable amastigotes lying free or located within macrophages or glial cells. Vascular necrosis was sometimes present, but no thromboses were observed. Amastigotes were confirmed immunohistochemically.

Prototothecosis

In a single patient with AIDS, achloric algae (*Prototheca*) caused meningoencephalitis (198).

Bacterial Infections

Bacterial infection of the CNS is relatively rare in AIDS. This seems to be due to the unimpaired neutrophilic response in AIDS. Mycobacterial infections are by far the most common bacterial pathogens encountered in the CNS of patients with HIV infection (36).

Mycobacterium avium-intracellulare

Mycobacterium avium-intracellulare (MAI) is a common environmental contaminant. Before the AIDS epidemic, disseminated infection with MAI rarely occurred, and primarily in immunocompromised patients (97). In contrast, disseminated MAI infection is common in patients with AIDS. Clinical symptoms are usually nonspecific. Some patients exhibit chronic diarrhea, abdominal pain, and chronic malabsorption, and histology shows clusters of mycobacteria within macrophages of the lamina propria of the small intestine, suggesting that the bowel might be the portal of entry for MAI in some patients (91). The diagnosis of infection is usually made by blood cultures. The brain is one of the organs least frequently seeded in mycobacteremia (3,91). CNS affection may manifest as chronic meningitis, brain abscesses, and, rarely, as diffuse encephalitis or cranial or peripheral neuropathy. The tissue reaction is characterized by mononuclear inflammatory cells and numerous large rounded histiocytes having abundant pale granular to slightly foamy cytoplasm. The macrophages are arranged in poorly formed aggregates. The cytoplasm of the macrophages is filled with bacilli, which are not readily stained with the Ziehl-Neelsen method, but with PAS stain (161). Because MAI is resistant to commonly used antimycobacterial chemotherapy, infection is associated with a poor prognosis (91).

Mycobacterium tuberculosis

Infection with the acid-fast *Mycobacterium tuberculosis* (MTB) has been shown to be significant among intravenous drug abusers (208) and Haitians (168) with

AIDS. As a direct consequence of the AIDS epidemic, an increase of MTB infection has been noted in the United States and Africa (67,220). In Europe, one report from the United Kingdom documents such an increase (67). Although MTB infection of the CNS is generally rare in developed countries, one study shows that intravenous drug abusers with AIDS are at high risk for CNS involvement with tuberculosis (23). The clinical presentation is meningitis, acute abscess formation, or chronic indolent mass lesion. Radiology shows either ring-enhancing or hypodense lesions. Because tuberculosis is potentially curable, it must be considered in the differential diagnosis of CNS space-occupying lesions in intravenous drug abusers with AIDS (23). The diagnosis can be made by biopsy with the demonstration of acid-fast bacilli.

Neurosyphilis

Neurosyphilis occurs in <10% of untreated patients with syphilis (44). In HIV infection, there is no evidence of an increased risk of progression of syphilis to neurosyphilis, but a retrospective study demonstrates differences in the clinical features of neurosyphilis in the presence and in the absence of HIV infection (110). The differences include younger age at presentation, more frequent occurrence of secondary syphilis, and differences in CSF measurements, including a higher mean white blood cell count, a higher mean protein level, a lower mean glucose level, and a more frequent occurrence of syphilitic meningitis in HIV-positive patients. The clinical presentations of neurosyphilis in HIV infection include optic neuritis, acute meningitis, meningoencephalitis, or myelopathy, but neurosyphilis also may be asymptomatic (105). Radiology may show strokelike lesions or a convexity mass (165,215); angiography may demonstrate areas of narrowing of cerebral arteries (148), and collateral perforating branches at the base of the brain may be hypertrophied in a ''puff of smoke'' appearance, typical of Moyamoya disease (144). Only a few cases of neurosyphilis in HIV infection have been studied pathologically: cerebral gummas were observed in two patients (83); one patient had meningovascular syphilis (165); and another patient had meningovascular syphilis and necrotizing encephalitis with massive treponemal invasion of the brain (144). Tabes dorsalis or general paresis have not been reported.

Miscellaneous Infections

In one hemophilic patient with AIDS, disseminated BK type polyomavirus infection caused subacute meningoencephalitis (216).

Listeria monocytogenes is frequently seen as a cause of neonatal meningitis and of meningitis in patients without AIDS who have impaired T cell immunity (9). A population-based surveillance has proven that patients with HIV infection are at increased risk of bacteremia and meningitis due to *L. monocytogenes* (107). Because *L. monocytogenes* is a food borne pathogen (189,195), HIV-infected individuals consuming raw milk products, soft cheeses, and poorly cooked meat products are at increased risk of listeriosis (107).

Nocardia asteroides usually causes a primary focus of infection in the lung and disseminates hematogenously in the immunosuppressed state. The CNS is involved with multiple abscesses. In AIDS, occasional cases of CNS abscesses due to *N. asteroides* have been reported (95,100,199).

Meningitis and microabscesses caused by *Escherichia coli* have been reported (147,230).

Infections with Gram-positive cocci in AIDS are rare. A single case of *Streptococcus pneumoniae* meningitis (90) was described in a homosexual man, and a single case of *Streptococcus milleri* meningitis secondary to endocarditis and septicemia was reported in an intravenous drug–abusing patient (241). In a polymicrobial brain abscess, one of the identified organisms was *Staphylococcus epidermidis* (169).

Whipple's disease was identified in the brain of one patient with AIDS. MRI showed two areas of increased density in the cerebral white matter, and brain biopsy showed PAS-positive rods with a negative MAI culture (103).

In one pediatric case of AIDS, *Pseudomonas* caused necrotizing meningoencephalitis (117).

AIDS-RELATED NEOPLASIA OF THE CNS

Ninety-five percent of the neoplasms in AIDS are either malignant NHL or Kaposi's sarcoma (KS) (120,186). These tumors are found in up to 40% of patients with AIDS in clinical series. Within the CNS, NHL is by far the most common tumor; a few cases of KS in the CNS have been reported (Table 1).

Malignant NHL

The incidence of primary CNS-NHL in patients with AIDS is between 3% and 10% in autopsy series. All risk factor subpopulations except for hemophiliacs are susceptible to CNS-NHL. AIDS is now becoming one of the major risk factors for CNS-NHL (21). The median age of presentation of CNS-NHL in AIDS is 35 years (176), whereas the median age in immunocompetent patients is 61 years (82). In pediatric AIDS, lymphoma is one of the most common intracerebral pathologies (34,56,117). Clinical signs and symptoms are unspecific and are usually secondary to increased intracranial pressure or are focal deficits related to supratentorial mass lesions (73,120,182,201). CNS-NHL generally occurs at a late stage of disease; however, it is the initial presenting manifestation of AIDS in 0.6% of the patients (182). Other CNS-NHLs are clinically unsuspected and an incidental autopsy finding in patients dying of opportunistic infections (3). The meninges are only rarely involved. Contrarily, secondary seeding from systemic lymphomas mainly involves the leptomeninges, extending along the Virchow-Robin spaces, the cranial and spinal nerve sheaths, and the CSF pathways. Neuroradiology of CNS-NHL shows nonspecific mass lesions with variable contrast enhancement. This appearance may be indistinguishable from that of toxoplasmosis or other opportunistic infections (75). The diagnosis can be made from stereotactic brain biopsy (7). Rarely, the tumor communicates directly with the CSF, and exfoliated cells may allow an occasional cytological diagnosis of lymphoma to be made on a CSF specimen (201). Recently it has been shown that PCR on CSF for EBV DNA is highly sensitive and specific for AIDS-associated CNS-NHL, and may be useful as a diagnostic tumor marker (42). In general, CNS-NHL is responsive to radiotherapy with resultant remission; however, some patients are not responsive to brain irradiation (17,75). Overall, the prognosis of CNS-NHL in AIDS is poor (82).

At brain cutting, CNS-NHL appear as unifocal or multifocal, often poorly deline-

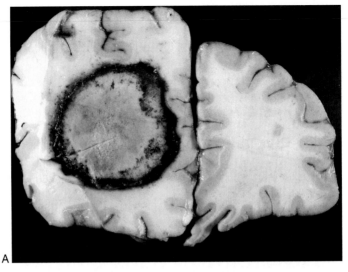

A

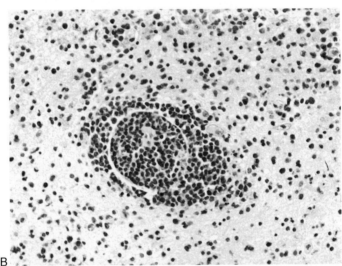

B

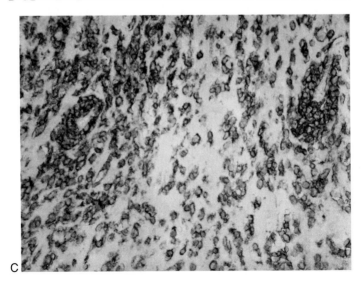

C

504

ated, soft, fleshy to granular mass lesions that may be localized anywhere in the brain. However, the lesions have a relative predilection for the deep cerebral gray matter, corpus callosum, periventricular white matter, and cerebellar vermis. The CNS-NHL may also be localized in the spinal cord and in the cauda equina (101,112). In some cases the cut surface presents a variegated picture with foci of yellow–white necrosis and hemorrhage. Necrosis may be extensive and may involve almost the whole tumor (Fig. 8A).

Histologically, the tumor is characterized by perivascular sheets of malignant cells that are separated by concentric circles of basal membrane constitutives such as reticulin and fibronectin (113); the adjacent brain tissue is infiltrated in a pseudoinflammatory pattern (Fig. 8B). The tumor may extend into the ventricles and/or subarachnoid space; the bone also may be invaded. Central parts of the tumor are frequently necrotic. There is a greater degree of difficulty in subclassifying CNS-NHL when compared with non-CNS sites (201); the updated Kiel classification is not applicable to many CNS-NHLs. This is due to the pleomorphic mixture of both neoplastic and reactive lymphoid cells present in many cases and/or a mixed tumor cell population observed in occasional cases. The neoplastic lymphoid cells may range from small, noncleaved cells with multiple nucleoli to the large cells of immunoblastic lymphoma (81,89,146,175,243). Most CNS-NHLs are high grade. Immunohistochemically, an appropriate staining pattern for B cell antigens such as CD20 (Fig. 8C) and positive staining for cytoplamic or cell surface immunoglobulins in the majority of CNS-NHLs confirms their B cell origin (81,201). Primary cerebral T cell lymphoma in AIDS has been sporadically reported (104,145,174). We observed one case of T cell CNS-NHL in our stereotactic brain biopsy series of patients with AIDS.

The pathogenesis of AIDS-related CNS-NHL is unclear. Compared with the nonimmunosuppressed population, there are probably differences in the etiological events leading to the development of AIDS associated CNS-NHL.

Viral infections have frequently been implicated as etiological agents of NHL (94,120,186,201). In recent years, EBV has emerged as the most probable candidate (16,37,51,89,131,141,163). Immunocytochemistry against EBV products such as latent membrane protein (16,37,131), EBNA-2 and viral capsid antigen (16), dot blotting using a ^{32}P-labeled *Bam*HI W fragment of EBV (163), *in situ* hybridization with a ^{35}S-labeled *Bam*HI-W probe (89) and a probe complementary to the EBER1 transcript (37,131), and PCR for the EBNA-1 region and the first internal repeat segment of the EBV genome (51,141) were positive in a high percentage of cases. Immunoblast-rich lesions are more commonly associated with EBV than Burkitt-type tumors (89). CNS-NHL in AIDS are frequently associated with macrophages and multinucleate giant cells that contain HIV (48). However, PCR for the *gag* region of HIV failed to detect virus in any case of a series of 12 AIDS-associated CNS-NHLs (141).

FIG. 8. Malignant non-Hodgkin lymphoma of the CNS. **A:** Coronal section through the frontal lobes shows a rounded, relatively well-circumscribed necrotic lesion in the white matter. **B:** Histologically, the tumor cells accumulate perivascularly and infiltrate diffusely the adjacent CNS tisssue. (Hematoxylin and eosin, original magnification ×200.) **C:** Labeling of tumor cells with monoclonal anti-CD20 antibody against B cells. (Original magnification ×100.)

Hodgkin's Disease

Primary cerebral Hodgkin's disease (HD) is a controversial entity. No unequivocal case has been reported yet (184).

In systemic HD, CNS involvement may occur. In one series of patients with HD, 15–20% experienced neurological symptoms during the course of the disease, most commonly from CNS involvement (188).

One HIV-positive patient with a history of intravenous drug abuse and stage IVB HD had, after drug-induced clinical remission, intracerebral mixed cellularity HD (88).

Angiotropic Large Cell Lymphoma

Angiotropic large cell lymphoma, formerly known as angioendotheliomatosis, is a peculiar type of lymphoma with a striking tendency for the tumor cells to remain confined to the lumina of blood vessels. Many organs are involved, but the skin and the nervous system tend to be selectively affected (206). In some cases, the disease is restricted to the CNS (209). Plugging of blood vessel lumina by tumor cells results in infarction of brain and spinal cord. Immunohistochemically, tumor cells are positive for leukocyte common antigen (157).

A single case of neoplastic angiotropic large cell lymphoma of the CNS in AIDS was described in a 12-year-old hemophilic boy who died after a clinical course characterized by progressive psychoorganic syndrome and opportunistic infections. In addition to the lymphoma, the brain showed giant cell encephalitis and meningocerebral cryptococcosis (59).

Lymphomatoid Granulomatosis

Lymphomatoid granulomatosis (LG), first described in 1972 (124), primarily affects the lung. The nervous system is usually involved as part of multisystem disease. A minority of patients survive more than 2 years. LG is frequently observed in the setting of an immunocompromised host. Some cases have been described to involve the CNS exclusively or preferentially (170,194).

In AIDS, LG confined to the CNS is a rare finding (4,5). The neurological features are extremely variable, depending on the location of the lesions.

Grossly, there are multifocal lesions scattered throughout the brain with softening and necrosis. Histologically, the lesions show an angiocentric mixed inflammatory infiltrate composed of lymphocytes, plasma cells, histiocytes, and scattered atypical mononuclear cells. The infiltrate may extend into the surrounding brain parenchyma. Loose aggregates of histiocytes may occur, but granuloma formation is rare. Increased numbers of bizarre mononuclear cells and numerous mitoses are associated with a poor prognosis. The process leads to expansion of affected vessel walls, usually small and medium-sized arteries and veins, necrosis of the walls, and luminal thrombosis. Consequently, infarction of brain tissue may be present. LG evolves into, or is frequently associated with, NHL (220). Some patients with LG recover without therapy (124).

Immunohistochemistry shows that the majority of the cells in LG are T-lymphocytes, mostly T-suppressor cells, and macrophages (4). The pathogenesis of LG is unclear. LG is considered as a reactive process stimulated by an antigen such as EBV (218) or as a T cell lymphoma (154).

Kaposi's Sarcoma

KS, the most common neoplasm associated with AIDS, develops in up to 30% of patients with AIDS (230). KS cells are of putative endothelial cell lineage showing angiogenic activity in culture (187). It has been proposed that KS is not a true sarcoma, but rather a proliferation of endothelial cells (27) stimulated by the *tat* protein, which is secreted by HIV (63). KS preferentially occurs in homosexual men and frequently manifests in a multicentric fashion (230). Intracranial KS, however, is an extremely uncommon tumor. Only three cases of KS metastatic to the CNS have been reported in patients with AIDS (78,121).

Grossly, metastatic CNS-KS presents with multiple hemorrhagic nodules in the cerebral cortex. Histologically, the tumor is characterized by an atypical spindle cell proliferation, with erythrocytes in slit-shaped vascular spaces and hemosiderin pigment in cells. This pattern is identical to that seen in non-CNS sites.

ACKNOWLEDGEMENT

We thank Helga Flicker for excellent technical assistance. This work has been done within the EC Biomed-1 Concerted Action on the Neuropathology of HIV Infection.

REFERENCES

1. Aksamit AJ, Gendelman HE, Orenstein JM, Pezeshkpour GH. AIDS-associated progressive multifokal leukoencephalopathy (PML): comparison to non-AIDS PML with *in situ* hybridization and immunohistochemistry. *Neurology* 1990;40:1073–1078.
2. Alesch F, Armbruster C, Budka H. Diagnostic value of stereotactic biopsy of cerebral lesions in patients with AIDS. *Acta Neurochir* 1995;134:214–219.
3. Anders KH, Guerra WF, Tomiyasu V, Verity MA, Vinters HV. The neuropathology of AIDS: UCLA experience and review. *Am J Pathol* 1986;124:537–558.
4. Anders KH, Latta H, Chang BS, Tomiyasu U, Ouddusi AS, Vinters HV. Lymphomatoid granulomatosis and malignant lymphoma of the central nervous system in the acquired immunodeficiency syndrome [Abstract]. *Hum Pathol* 1989;20:326–334.
5. Anders KH, Latta H, Vinters HV. Lymphomatoid granulomatosis and lymphoma in the central nervous system of patients with AIDS. *J Neuropathol Exp Neurol* 1988;47:386.
6. Anderson JR, Field HJ. The distribution of herpes simplex type 1 antigen in mouse central nervous system after different routes of inoculation. *J Neurol Sci* 1983;60:181–195.
7. Antinori A, Ammassari A, Murri R, et al. Primary central nervous system lymphoma and brain biopsy in AIDS. *Lancet* 1993;341:1411–1412.
8. Anzil AP, Rao C, Wrzolek MA, Visvesvara GS, Sher JH, Kozlowski PB. Amebic meningoencephalitis in a patient with AIDS caused by a newly recognized opportunistic pathogen—leptomyxid ameba. *Arch Pathol Lab Med* 1991;115:21–25.
9. Armstrong D, Wong B. Central nervous system infections in immunocompromised hosts. *Ann Rev Med* 1982;33:293–308.
10. Artigas J, Grosse G, Niedobitek F. Anergic disseminated toxoplasmosis in an AIDS patient. Case Report. *Arch Pathol Lab Med* 1994;117:540–541.
11. Artigas J, Grosse G, Niedobitek F, Kassner M, Risch W, Heise W. Severe toxoplasmic ventriculomeningoencephalomyelitis in two AIDS patients following treatment of cerebral toxoplasmic granuloma. *Clin Neuropathol* 1994;13:120–126.
12. Aslanzadeh J, Osmon DR, Wilhelm MP, Espy MJ, Smith TF. A prospective study of the polymerase

chain reaction for detection of herpes simplex virus in cerebrospinal fluid submitted to the clinical virological laboratory. *Mol Cell Probes* 1992;6:367–373.

13. Åström KE, Mancall EL, Richardson EP Jr. Progressive multifocal leukoencephalopathy. A hitherto unrecognized complication of chronic lymphatic leukaemia and Hodgkin's disease. *Brain* 1958;81: 93–111.

14. Åström KE, Stoner GL. Early pathological changes in progressive multifocal leukoencephalopathy: a report of two asymptomatic cases occurring prior to the AIDS epidemic. *Acta Neuropathol* 1994; 88:93–105.

15. Bale JF Jr. Human cytomegalovirus infection and disorders of the nervous system. *Arch Neurol* 1984;41:310–320.

16. Bashir R, Luka J, Cheloha K, Chamberlain M, Hochberg F. Expression of Epstein-Barr virus proteins in primary CNS lymphoma in AIDS patients. *Neurology* 1993;43:2358–2362.

17. Baumgartner JE, Rachlin JR, Beckstead JH, et al. Primary central nervous system lymphomas: natural history and response to radiation therapy in 55 patients with acquired immunodeficiency syndrome. *J Neurosurg* 1990;73:206–211.

18. Belec L, Gray F, Mikol J, et al. Cytomegalovirus (CMV) encephalomyeloradiculitis and human immunodeficiency virus (HIV) encephalitis: presence of HIV and CMV co-infected multinucleated giant cells. *Acta Neuropathol* 1990;81:99–104.

19. Belec L, Mhiri C, Belghiti D, Geny C, Boudes P, Gray F. Cytomegalovirus (CMV) and human immunodeficiency virus (HIV) co-infection, of multinucleated giant cells in acquired immunodeficiency syndrome (AIDS) encephalopathy. *Arch Anat Cytol Pathol* 1990;38:189–197.

20. Belec L, Tayot J, Tron P, Mikol J, Scaravilli F, Gray F. Cytomegalovirus encephalopathy in an infant with congenital acquired immuno-deficiency syndrome. *Neuropediatrics* 1990;21:124–129.

21. Beral V, Peterman T, Berkelman R, Jaffe H. AIDS associated non-Hodgkin lymphoma. *Lancet* 1991;337:805–809.

22. Berger JR, Scott G, Albrecht J, Belman AL, Tornatore C, Major ED. Progressive multifocal leukoencephalopathy in HIV-1–infected children. *AIDS* 1992;6:837–841.

23. Bishburg E, Sunderam G, Reichman LB, Kapila R. Central nervous system tuberculosis with the acquired immunodeficiency syndrome and its related complex. *Ann Intern Med* 1986;105:210–213.

24. Bonner JR, Alexander J, Dismukes WE, et al. Disseminated histoplasmosis in patients with the acquired immune deficiency syndrome. *Arch Intern Med* 1984;144:2178–2181.

25. Britton CB, Mesa-Tejada R, Fenoglio CM, Hays AP, Garvey GG, Miller JR. A new complication of AIDS: thoracic myelitis caused by herpes simplex virus. *Neurology* 1985;35:1071–1074.

26. Bronnimann DA, Adam RD, Galgiani JN, et al. Coccidioidomycosis in the acquired immunodeficiency syndrome. *Ann Intern Med* 1987;106:372–379.

27. Brooks JJ. Kaposi's sarcoma: hypothesis as reversible hyperplasia. *Lancet* 1986;2:1309–1311.

28. Budka H. Human immunodeficiency virus (HIV) envelope and core proteins in CNS tissues of patients with the acquired immune deficiency syndrome (AIDS). *Acta Neuropathol* 1990;79: 611–619.

29. Budka H, Costanzi G, Christina S, et al. Brain pathology induced by infection with the human immunodeficiency virus (HIV). A histological, immunocytochemical, and electron microscopical study of 100 autopsy cases. *Acta Neuropathol* 1987;75:185–198.

30. Budka H, Lassmann H, Popow-Kraupp T. Measles virus antigen in panencephalitis. *Acta Neuropathol* 1982;56:52–62.

31. Budka H, Urbantis S, Liberski P, Eichinger S, Popow-Kraupp T. Subacute measles virus encephalitis: a new and opportunistic infection in an AIDS patient. *Neurology* 1996; 46:586–587.

32. Budka H, Shah KV. Papovavirus antigens in paraffin sections of PML brains. *Clin Biol Res* 1983; 105:299–309.

33. Budka H, Wiley CA, Kleihues P, et al. HIV-associated disease of the nervous system: review of nomenclature and proposal for neuropathology-based terminology. *Brain Pathology* 1991;1: 143–152.

34. Burns DK. The neuropathology of pediatric acquired immunodeficiency syndrome. *J Child Neurol* 1992;7:332–346.

35. Carrazana EJ, Rossitch E Jr, Morris J. Isolated central nervous system aspergillosis in the acquired immunodeficiency syndrome. *Clin Neurol Neurosurg* 1991;93:227–230.

36. Centers for Disease Control. Diagnosis and management of mycobacterial infection and diseases in persons with human immunodeficiency virus infection. *Ann Intern Med* 1987;106:254–256.

37. Chang KL, Flaris N, Hickey WF, Johnson RM, Meyer JS, Weiss LM. Brain lymphomas of immunocompetent and immunocompromised patients: study of the association with Epstein-Barr virus. *Mod Pathol* 1993;6:427–432.

38. Chao CC, Gekker G, Hu S, Peterson PK. Human microglial cell defense against Toxoplasma gondii. The role of cytokines. *J Immunol* 1994;152:1246–1252.

39. Chappell ET, Guthrie BL, Orenstein J. The role of stereotactic biopsy in the management of HIV-related focal brain lesions. *Neurosurgery* 1992;30:825–829.

40. Chimelli L, Rosemberg S, Hahn MD, Lopes MB, Netto MB. Pathology of the central nervous system

in patients infected with the human immunodeficiency virus (HIV): a report of 252 autopsy cases from Brazil. *Neuropathol Appl Neurobiol* 1992;18:478–488.

41. Chrétien F, Gray F, Lescs MC, et al. Acute varicella-zoster virus ventriculitis and meningo-myelo-radiculitis in acquired immunodeficiency syndrome. *Acta Neuropathol* 1993;86:659–665.

42. Cinque P, Brytting M, Vago L, et al. Epstein-Barr virus DNA in cerebrospinal fluid from patients with AIDS-related primary lymphoma of the central nervous system. *Lancet* 1993;14:398–401.

43. Cinque P, Vago L, Brytting M, et al. Cytomegalovirus infection of the central nervous system in patients with AIDS: diagnosis by DNA amplification from cerebrospinal fluid. *J Infect Dis* 1992; 166:1408–1411.

44. Clark EG, Danbolt N. The Oslo study of the natural history of untreated syphilis: an epidemiological investigation based on a restudy of the Boeck-Bruusgaard material—a review and appraisal. *J Chronic Dis* 1955;2:311–344.

45. Cohen JI, Corey GR. Cytomegalovirus infection in the normal host. *Medicine* 1985;64:100–114.

46. Coleman RM, Pereira C, Bailey DP, Dondero D, Wickliffe C, Nahmias AJ. Determination of herpes simplex virus type-specific antibodies by enzyme-linked immunosorbent assay. *J Clin Microbiol* 1983;18:287–291.

47. Colon L, Lasala G, Kanzer MD, Parisi JE, DeVinatea ML, Macher AM. Cerebral cladosporiosis in AIDS [Abstract]. *J Neuropathol Exp Neurol* 1988;47:387.

48. Cornford M, Said J, Vinters H. Immunohistochemical localisation of human immunodeficiency virus (HIV) in central nervous system lymphoproliferative disorders of patients with AIDS. *Mod Pathol* 1991;4:232–238.

49. Cuadrado LM, Guerrero A, Asenjo JALG, Martin F, Palau E, Vira DG. Cerebral mucormycosis in two cases of acquired immunodeficiency syndrome. *Arch Neurol* 1988;45:109–111.

50. Dawson JR. Cellular inclusions in cerebral lesions of lethargic encephalitis. *Am J Pathol* 1933;9: 7–15.

51. DeAngelis LM, Wong E, Rosenblum M, Furneaux H. Epstein-Barr virus in acquired immune deficiency syndrome (AIDS) and non-AIDS primary central nervous system lymphoma. *Cancer* 1992; 70:1607–1611.

52. Deatly AM, Spivack JG, Lavi E, Fraser NW. RNA from an immediate early region of the type 1 herpes simplex virus genome is present in the trigeminal ganglia of latently infected mice. *Proc Natl Acad Sci U S A* 1987;84:3204–3208.

53. Del Castillo M, Mendoza G, Oviedo J, Bianco RPP, Anselmo AE, Silva M. AIDS and Chagas' disease with central nervous system tumor-like lesion. *Am J Med* 1990;88:693–694.

54. Deresinski SC, Stevens DA. Coccidioidomycosis in compromised hosts: experience at Stanford Univeristy Hospital. *Medicine* 1975;54:377–395.

55. Diamond RD, Bennet JE. Disseminated cryptoccosis in man: decreased lymphocyte transformation in response to *Cryptococcus neoformans. J Infect Dis* 1973;127:694–697.

56. Dickson DW, Llena JF, Nelson SJ, Weidenheim KM. Central nervous system pathology in pediatric AIDS. *Ann N Y Acad Sci* 1993;693:93–106.

57. Dix RD, Waitzman DM, Follansbee S, et al. Herpes simplex virus type 2 encephalitis in two homosexual men with persistent lymphadenopathy. *Ann Neurol* 1985;17:203–205.

58. Dörries K, ter Meulen V. Detection of papovavirus JC in kidney tissue. *J Med Virol* 1983;11: 307–311.

59. Dozic S, Suvakovic V, Cvetkovic D, Jevtovic D, Skender M. Neoplastic angioendotheliomatosis (NAE) of the CNS in a patient with AIDS subacute encephalitis, diffuse leukoencephalopathy and meningo-cerebral cryptococcosis. *Clin Neuropathol* 1990;9:284–289.

60. Drlicek M, Liszka U, Wondrusch E, Lintner F, Grisold W, Casati B. Pathology of the central nervous system in AIDS. A review of 184 autopsy cases. *Wien Klin Wochenschr* 1993;105:467–471.

61. Editorial. Brain biopsy for intracranial mass lesions in AIDS. *Lancet* 1992;340:1135.

62. Eidelberg D, Sotrel A, Horoupian DS, Neumann PE, Pumarola-Sune T, Price RW. Thrombotic cerebral vasculopathy associated with herpes zoster. *Ann Neurol* 1986;19:7–14.

63. Ensoli B, Barillari G, Salahuddin SZ, Gallo RC, Wong-Staal F. Tat protein of HIV-1 stimulates growth of cells derived from Kaposi's sarcoma lesions of AIDS patients. *Nature* 1990;345:84–86.

64. Esiri MM, Kennedy PGE. Viral diseases. In: Adams JH, Duchen LW, eds. *Greenfield's Neuropathology.* London: Edward Arnold, 1992:335–399.

65. Falangola MF, Petito CK. Choroid plexus infection in cerebral toxoplasmosis in AIDS patients. *Neurology* 1993;43:2053–2040.

66. Feiden W, Bise K, Steude U, Pfister HW, Moller AA. The stereotactic biopsy diagnosis of focal intracerebral lesions in AIDS patients. *Acta Neurol Scand* 1993;87:228–233.

67. Foley NM, Miller RF. Tuberculosis and AIDS: is the white plague up and coming? *J Infect* 1993; 26:39–43.

68. Fraser DW, Ward JI, Ajello L, Plikaytis BD. Aspergillosis and other systemic mycosis. *JAMA* 1979; 242:1631–1635.

69. Gardner HAR, Martinez AJ, Visvesvara GS, Sotrel A. Granulomatous amebic encephalitis in an AIDS patient. *Neurology* 1991;41:1993–1995.
70. Gelb LD. Varicella-zoster virus. In: Fields BN, Knipe DM, eds. *Virology*. New York: Raven, 1990: 2011–2054.
71. Gendelman HE, Phelps W, Feigenbaum L, et al. Trans-activation of the human immunodeficiency virus long terminal repeat sequence by DNA viruses. *Proc Natl Acad Sci U S A* 1986;83:9759–9763.
72. Gilden DH, Murray RS, Wllish M, Kleischmidt-DeMasters BK, Vafai A. Chronic progressive varicella-zoster virus encephalitis in an AIDS patient. *Neurology* 1988;38:1150–1153.
73. Gill PS, Levine AM, Meyer PR, et al. Primary central nervous system lymphoma in homosexual men. Clinical, immunological, and pathological findings. *Am J Med* 1985;78:742–748.
74. Gluckstein D, Cifferi F, Ruskin J. Chagas' disease: another cause of cerebral mass in the acquired immunodeficiency syndrome. *Am J Med* 1992;92:429–432.
75. Goldstein JD, Dickson DW, Moser FG, et al. Primary central nervous system lymphoma in acquired immune deficiency syndrome. A clinical and pathological study with results of treatment of radiation. *Cancer* 1991;1:2756–2765.
76. Gonzalez MM, Gould E, Dickinson G, et al. Acquired immunodeficiency syndrome associated with *Acanthamoeba* infection and other opportunistic organisms. *Arch Pathol Lab Med* 1986;110: 749–751.
77. Goodman NL, Larsh HW. Environmental factors and growth of *Histoplasma capsulatum* in soil. *Mycopathol Mycol Appl* 1967;33:145–156.
78. Gorin FA, Bale JF, Hacks-Miller M, Schwarts RA. Kaposi's sarcoma metastic to the CNS. *Arch Neurol* 1985;42:162–165.
79. Gozlan J, Salord JM, Roullet E, et al. Rapid detection of cytomegalovirus DNA in cerebrospinal fluid of AIDS patients with neurological disorders. *J Infect Dis* 1992;166:1416–1421.
80. Grafe MR, Press GA, Berthoty DP, Hesselink JR, Wiley CA. Abnormalities of the brain in AIDS patients: correlation of postmortem MR findings with neuropathology. *AJNR* 1990;11:905–911.
81. Grant JW, Isaacson PG. Primary central nervous system lymphoma. *Brain Pathol* 1992;2:97–109.
82. Grant JW, von Deimling A, Marcus RE, Weetman A, Gallagher PJ. Primary CNS lymphoma. A clinical and pathological study [Abstract]. *J Pathol* 1990;161:353.
83. Gray F. *Atlas of the Neuropathology of HIV Infection*. Oxford, England: Oxford University Press, 1993.
84. Gray F, Geny C, Lionnet F, et al. Neuropathologic study of 135 adult cases of acquired immunodeficiency syndrome (AIDS). *Ann Pathol* 1991;11:236–247.
85. Gray F, Gherardi R, Wingate E, et al. Diffuse "encephalitic" cerebral toxoplasmosis in AIDS. Report of four cases. *J Neurol* 1989;236:273–277.
86. Gray F, Mohr M, Rozenberg F, et al. Varicella zoster virus encephalitis in acquired immunodeficiency syndrome: report of four cases. *Neuropathol Appl Neurobiol* 1992;18:502–514.
87. Greenlee JE. Progressive multifocal leukoencephalopathy. *Curr Clin Top Infect Dis* 1989;10: 140–156.
88. Hair LS, Rogers JD, Chadburn A, Sisti MB, Knowles DM, Powers JM. Intracerebral Hodgkin's disease in a human immunodeficiency virus positive patient. *Cancer* 1991;67:2931–2934.
89. Hamilton-Dutoit SJ, Pallesen G, Franzmann MB, et al. AIDS-related lymphoma. Histopathology, immunophenotype, and association with Epstein-Barr virus as demonstrated by *in situ* nucleic acid hybridization. *Am J Pathol* 1991;138:149–163.
90. Havlir DV, Witt DM, Sande M. A 32-year-old man with the acquired immunodeficiency syndrome and pneumococcal meningitis. *West J Med* 1987;146:618–619.
91. Hawkins CC, Gold JWM, Whimbey E, et al. *Mycobacterium avium* complex infections in patients with the acquired immunodeficieny syndrome. *Ann Intern Med* 1986;105:184–188.
92. Heilbronn R, Albrecht I, Stephan S, Burkle A, zur-Hausen H. Human cytomegalovirus induces JC virus DNA replication in human fibroblasts. *Proc Natl Acad Sci U S A* 1993;90:11406–11410.
93. Herskovitz S, Siegel SE, Schneider AT, Nelson SJ, Goodrich JT, Lantos G. Spinal cord toxoplasmosis in AIDS. *Neurology* 1989;39:1552–1553.
94. Hochberg FH, Miller G, Schooley RT, Hirsch MS, Feorino P, Henle W. Central-nervous-system lymphoma related to Epstein-Barr virus. *N Engl J Med* 1983;309:745–748.
95. Holtz HA, Lavery DP, Kapila R. Actinomycetales infection in the acquired immunodeficiency syndrome. *Ann Intern Med* 1985;102:203–205.
96. Hooper DC, Pruitt AA, Rubin RH. Central nervous system infection in the chronically immunosuppressed. *Medicine* 1982;61:166–188.
97. Horsburgh CR Jr, Mason UG III, Farhi DC, Iseman MD. Disseminated infection with *Mycobacterium avium-intracellulare*: a report of 13 cases and a review of the literature. *Medicine* 1985;64:36–48.
98. Houff SA, Major EO, Katz DA, et al. Involvement of JC-virus infected mononuclear cells from the bone marrow and spleen in the pathogenesis of progressive multifocal leukoencephalopathy. *N Engl J Med* 1988;318:301–305.
99. Huang TE, Chou SM. Occlusive hypertrophic arteritis as the cause of discrete necrosis in CNS toxoplasmosis in the acquired immunodeficiency syndrome. *Hum Pathol* 1988;19:1210–1214.

100. Idemyor V, Cherubin CE. Pleurocerebral *Nocardia* in a patient with human immunodeficiency virus. *Ann Pharmacother* 1992;26:188–189.
101. Ioachim HL, Dorsett B, Cronin W, Maya M, Wahl S. Acquired immunodeficiency syndrome–associated lymphomas: clinical, pathological, immunological and viral characteristics of 111 cases. *Hum Pathol* 1991;22:659–673.
102. Jakobsen J, Diemer NH, Gaub J, Brun B, Helweg-Larsen S. Progressive multifocal leukoencephalopathy in a patient without other clinical manifestations of AIDS. *Acta Neurol Scand* 1987;75: 209–213.
103. Jankovic J. Whipple's disease of the central nervous system in AIDS. *N Engl J Med* 1986;315: 1029–1030.
104. Jellinger K, Paulus W. Primary central nervous system lymphomas—an update. *J Cancer Res Clin Oncol* 1992;119:7–27.
105. Johns DR, Tierney M, Felsenstein D. Alteration in the natural history of neurosyphilis by concurrent infection with the human immunodeficency virus. *N Engl J Med* 1987;316:1569–1572.
106. Johnson PC, Sarosi GA, Septimus EJ, Satterwhite TK. Progressive disseminated histoplasmosis in patients with the acquired immune deficiency syndrome: a report of 12 cases and a literature review. *Semin Respir Infect* 1986;1:1–8.
107. Jurado RL, Farley MM, Pereira E, et al. Increased risk of meningitis and bacteremia due to *Listeria monocytogenes* in patients with human immunodeficiency virus infection. *Clin Infect Dis* 1993;17: 224–227.
108. Kanavaros P, Mikol J, Nemeth J, et al. Stereotactic biopsy diagnosis of primary non-Hodgkin's lymphoma of the central nervous system. A histological and immunohistochemical study. *Pathol Res Pract* 1990;186:459–466.
109. Kato T, Hirano A, Llena JF, Dembitzer HM. Neuropathology of acquired immune deficiency syndrome (AIDS) in 53 autopsy cases with particular emphasis on microglial nodules and multinucleated giant cells. *Acta Neuropathol* 1987;73:287–294.
110. Katz DA, Berger JR, Duncan RC. Neurosyphilis. A comparative study of the effects of infection with human immunodeficiency virus. *Arch Neurol* 1993;50:243–249.
111. Khan IA, Ely KH, Kasper LH. A purified parasite antigen (p30) mediates CD8+ T cell immunity against fatal *Toxoplasma gondii* infection in mice. *J Immunol* 1991;147:3501–3506.
112. Klein P, Zientek G, VandenBerg SR, Lothman E. Primary CNS lymphoma: lymphomatous meningitis as a cauda equina lesion in an AIDS patient. *Can J Neurol Sci* 1990;17:329–331.
113. Kochi N, Budka H, Radaszkiewicz T. Development of stroma in malignant lymphomas of the brain compared with epidural lymphomas. *Acta Neuropathol* 1986;71:125–129.
114. Krick JA, Remington JS. Toxoplasmosis in the adult—an overview. *N Engl J Med* 1978;298: 550–553.
115. Krogstad DJ, Visvesvara GJ, Walls KW, Smith JW. Blood and tissue protozoa. In: Balows A, ed. *Manual of Clinical Microbiology*. Washington, DC: American Society for Microbiology, 1991: 727–750.
116. Kuchelmeister K, Gullotta F, Bergmann M, Angeli G, Masini T. Progressive multifocal leukoencephalopathy (PML) in the acquired immunodeficiency syndrome (AIDS). A neuropathological autopsy study of 21 cases. *Pathol Res Pract* 1993;189:163–173.
117. Kure K, Llena JF, Lyman WD, et al. Human immunodeficiency virus-1 infection of the nervous system: and autopsy study of 268 adult, pediatric, and fetal brains. *Hum Pathol* 1991;22:700–710.
118. Lang W, Miklossy J, Deruaz JP, et al. Neuropathology of the acquired immune deficiency syndrome (AIDS): a report of 135 consecutive autopsy cases from Switzerland. *Acta Neuropathol* 1989;77: 370–390.
119. Leiguarda R, Roncoroni A, Taratuto AL, et al. Acute CNS infection by *Trypanosoma cruzi* (Chagas' disease) in immunosuppressed patients. *Neurology* 1990;40:850–851.
120. Levine AM. Non-Hodgkin's lymphomas and other malignancies in the acquired immune deficiency syndrome. *Semin Oncol* 1987;14:34–39.
121. Levy RM, Bredesen DE, Rosenblum ML. Neurological manifestations of the acquired immunodeficiency syndrome (AIDS): experience at UCSF and review of the literature. *J Neurosurg* 1985;62: 475–495.
122. Levy RM, Bredesen DE, Rosenblum ML. Opportunistic central nervous system pathology in patients with AIDS. *Ann Neurol* 1988;23(suppl):7–12.
123. Levy RM, Mills CM, Posin JP, Moore SG, Rosenblum ML, Bredesen DE. The efficacy and clinical impact of brain imaging in neurologically symptomatic AIDS patients: a prospective CT/MRI study. *J AIDS* 1990;3:461–471.
124. Liebow AA, Carrington CRB, Friedman PJ. Lymphomatoid granulomatosis. *Hum Pathol* 1972;3: 457–538.
125. Lima C, Budka H, Champallimaud JL, Coelho R, Leitao O. The neuropathology of HIV-2 infection [Abstract]. *Clin Neuropathol* 1992;11:277.
126. Lima C, Vital JP. Olfactory pathways in three patients with cryptococcal meningitis and acquired immune deficiency syndrome. *J Neurol Sci* 1994;123:195–199.

127. Loeber G, Dörries K. DNA rearrangements in organ-specific variants of polyomavirus JC strain GS. *J Virol* 1988;62:1730–1735.
128. Lucas SB, Hounnou A, Peacock C, et al. The mortality and pathology of HIV infection in a West African city. *AIDS* 1993;7:1569–1579.
129. Luft BJ, Remington JS. Toxoplasmic encephalitis. *J Infect* 1988;157:1–6.
130. Lyons RW, Andriole VT. Fungal infections of the CNS. *Neurol Clin* 1986;4:159–170.
131. MacMahon EM, Glass JD, Hayward SD, et al. Epstein-Barr virus in AIDS-related primary central nervous system lymphoma. *Lancet* 1991;19:969–973.
132. Martinez AJ. Free-living amoebae: pathogenic aspects: a review. *Protozool Abstr* 1983;7:293–306.
133. Martinez AJ, Janitschke K. Acanthamoeba, an opportunistic microorganism: a review. *Infection* 1985;13:2–7.
134. Matthiessen L, Marche C, Labrousse F, Trophilme D, Fontaine C, Vedrenne C. Neuropathology of the brain in 174 patients who died of AIDS in a Paris hospital 1982–1988. *Ann Med Interne Paris* 1992;143:43–49.
135. Mázló M, Herndon RM. Progressive multifocal leukoencephalopathy: ultrastructural findings in two brain biopsies. *Neuropathol Appl Neurol* 1977;3:323–339.
136. McArthur JC. Neurological manifestations of AIDS. *Medicine* 1987;66:407–437.
137. McCormick WF, Rodnitzky RL, Schochet SS, McKee AP. Varicella-zoster encephalomyelitis: a morphological and virological study. *Arch Neurol* 1969;21:559–570.
138. Mehren M, Burns PJ, Mamani F, Levy CS, Laureno R. Toxoplasmic myelitis mimicking intramedullary spinal cord tumor. *Neurology* 1988;38:1648–1650.
139. Miller R, Storey J, Greco C, et al. Subacute radiculomyelopathy caused by cytomegalovirus in patients with AIDS [Abstract]. *Neurology* 1988;38:242.
140. Moret H, Guichard M, Matheron S, et al. Virological diagnosis of progressive multifocal leukoencephalopathy: detection of JC virus DNA in cerebrospinal fluid and brain tissue of AIDS patients. *J Clin Microbiol* 1993;31:3310–3313.
141. Morgello S. Epstein-Barr and human immunodeficiency viruses in acquired immunodeficiency syndrome–related primary central nervous system lymphoma. *Am J Pathol* 1992;141:441–450.
142. Morgello S, Block GA, Price RW, Petito CK. Varicella-zoster virus leukoencephalitis and cerebral vasculopathy. *Arch Pathol Lab Med* 1988;112:173–177.
143. Morgello S, Cho ES, Nielsen S, Devinsky O, Petito C. Cytomegalovirus encephalitis in patients with acquired immunodeficiency syndrome: an autopsy study of 30 cases and a review of the literature. *Hum Pathol* 1987;18:289–297.
144. Morgello S, Laufer H. Quaternary neurosyphilis in a Haitian man with human immunodeficiency virus infection. *Hum Pathol* 1989;20:808–811.
145. Morgello S, Maiese K, Petito C. T cell lymphoma in the CNS: clinical and pathological features. *Neurology* 1989;39:1190–1196.
146. Morgello S, Petito CK, Mouradian JA. Central nervous system lymphoma in the acquired immunodeficiency syndrome. *Clin Neuropathol* 1990;9:205–215.
147. Moskowitz LB, Hensley GT, Chan JC, Gregorios JB, Conley FK. The neuropathology of acquired immune deficiency syndrome. *Arch Pathol Lab Med* 1984;108:867–872.
148. Musher DM, Hamill RJ, Baughn RE. Effect of human immunodeficiency virus (HIV) infection on the course of syphilis and on the response to treatment. *Ann Intern Med* 1990;113:872–881.
149. Mustafa MM, Weitman SD, Winick NJ, Bellini WJ, Timmons CF, Siegel JD. Subacute measles encephalitis in the young immunocompromised host: report of two cases diagnosed by polymerase chain reaction and treated with ribavirin and review of the literature. *Clin Infect Dis* 1993;16:654–660.
150. Myer RD, Rosen P, Armstrong D. Phycomycosis complicating leukemia and lymphoma. *Ann Intern Med* 1972;77:871–879.
151. Nag S, Jackson AC. Myelopathy: an unusual presentation of toxoplasmosis. *Can J Neurol Sci* 1989;16:422–425.
152. Namiki TS, Nichols P, Young T, Martin SE, Chandrasoma P. Stereotaxic biopsy diagnosis of central nervous system lymphoma. *Am J Clin Pathol* 1988;90:40–45.
153. Navia BA, Petito CK, Gold JWM, Cho ES, Jordan BD, Price RW. Cerebral toxoplasmosis complicating the acquired immune deficiency syndrome: clinical and neuropathological findings in 27 patients. *Ann Neurol* 1986;19:224–238.
154. Nichols PW, Koss AM, Levine AM, Lukes RJ. Lymphomatoid granulomatosis: a T-cell disorder? *Am J Med* 1982;72:467–471.
155. Nielsen SL, Petito CK, Urmacher CD, Posner JB. Subacute encephalitis in acquired immune deficiency syndrome: a postmortem study. *Am J Clin Pathol* 1984;82:678–682.
156. Norrby E, Oxman MN. Measles Virus. In: Fields BN, Knipe DM, ed. *Fields Virology*. New York: Raven, 1990:1013–1014.
157. Ojeda VJ, Spagnolo DV. Neoplastic angioendotheliomatosis is, in fact, intravascular malignant lymphoma. *Acta Neuropathol* 1986;72:203.

158. Padgett BL, Walker DL. Prevalence of antibodies in human sera against JC virus an isolate from a case of progressive multifocal leukoencephalopathy. *J Infect Dis* 1973;127:467–470.

159. Padgett BL, Walker DL, Rhein GMZ, Echroade RJ. Cultivation of papova-like virus from human brain with progressive multifocal leucoencephalopathy. *Lancet* 1971;1:1257–1260.

160. Pappagianis D. Epidemiology of coccidioidomycosis. *Curr Top Med Mycol* 1988;2:199–238.

161. Pappolla MA, Mehta VT. PAS reaction stains phagocytosed atypical mycobacteria in paraffin sections. *Arch Pathol Lab Med* 1984;108:372–373.

162. Patsouris E, Kretzschmar HA, Stavrou D, Mehraein P. Cellular composition and distribution of gliomesenchymal nodules in the CNS of AIDS patients. *Clin Neuropathol* 1993;12:130–137.

163. Paulus W, Jellinger K, Hallas C, Ott G, Muller-Hermelink HK. Human herpesvirus-6 and Epstein-Barr virus genome in primary cerebral lymphomas. *Neurology* 1993;43:1591–1593.

164. Pell MF, Thomas DG, Whittle IR. Stereotactic biopsy of cerebral lesions in patients with AIDS. *Br J Neurosurg* 1991;5:585–589.

165. Peters M, Gottschalk D, Boit R, Pohle HD, Ruf B. Meningovascular neurosyphilis in human immunodeficiency virus infection as a differential diagnosis of focal CNS lesions: a clinicopathological study. *J Infect* 1993;27:57–62.

166. Petito CK, Cho ES, Lemann W, Navia BA, Price RW. Neuropathology of acquired immunodeficiency syndrome (AIDS): an autopsy review. *J Neuropathol Exp Neurol* 1986;45:635–646.

167. Pilz P, Budka H. Herpes Zoster. Neuropathologische Befunde und Gedanken zur Pathogenese. *Curr Top Neuropathol* 1982;7:119–127.

168. Pitchenik AE, Cole C, Russell BW, Fischl MA, Spira TJ, Snider DE Jr. Tuberculosis, atypical mycobacteriosis, and the acquired immunodeficiency syndrome among Haitian and non-Haitian patients in South Florida. *Ann Intern Med* 1984;101:641–645.

169. Pitlik SD, Fainstein V, Bolivar R, et al. Spectrum of central nervous system complications in homosexual men with acquired immune deficiency syndrome. *J Infect Dis* 1983;148:771–772.

170. Podlas HB, Gritzman MCD, Thomaides S, Roos H. CT of CNS lesions in lymphomatoid granulomatosis: case report. *AJNR* 1988;9:592–594.

171. Potasman I, Resnick L, Luft BJ, Remington JS. Intrathecal production of antibodies against *Toxoplasma gondii* in patients with toxoplasmic encephalitis and the acquired immunodeficiency syndrome (AIDS). *Ann Intern Med* 1988;108:49–51.

172. Puchhammer-Stöckl E, Popow-Kraupp T, Heinz FX, Mandl CW, Kunz C. Detection of varicella-zoster virus DNA by polymerase chain reaction in the cerebrospinal fluid of patients suffering from neurological complications associated with chicken pox or herpes zoster. *J Clin Microbiol* 1991;29:1513–1516.

173. Quinlivan EB, Norris M, Bouldin TW, et al. Subclinical central nervous system infection with JC virus in patients with AIDS. *J Infect Dis* 1992;166:80–85.

174. Rao C, Wrzolek M, Koslowski P. Primary T cell central nervous system lymphoma in AIDS [Abstract]. *J Neuropathol Exp Neurol* 1989;48:302.

175. Raphael M, Gentilhomme O, Tulliez M, Byron PA, Diebold J. Histopathological features of high-grade non-Hodgkin's lymphomas in acquired immunodeficiency syndrome. *Arch Pathol Lab Med* 1991;115:15–20.

176. Remick SC, Diamond C, Migliozzi JA, et al. Primary central nervous system lymphoma in patients with and without the acquired immune deficiency syndrome. *Medicine* 1990;69:345–360.

177. Remington JS, Jacobs L, Kaufman HE. Toxoplasmosis in the adult. *N Engl J Med* 1960;262:179–240.

178. Rhodes RH. Histopathology of the central nervous system in the acquired immunodeficiency syndrome. *Hum Pathol* 1987;18:636–643.

179. Rogers AL, Kennedy MJ. Opportunistic hyaline hyphomycetes. In: Balows A, ed. *Manual of clinical microbiology*. Washington, DC: American Society for Microbiology, 1991:659–673.

180. Rosemberg S, Chave CJ, Higuchi ML, Lopes MB, Castro LH, Machado LR. Fatal meningoencephalitis caused by reactivation of *Trypanosoma cruzi* infection in a patient with AIDS. *Neurology* 1992;42:640–642.

181. Rosenblum ML. Bulbar encephalitis complicating trigeminal zoster in the acquired immune deficiency syndrome. *Hum Pathol* 1989;20:292–295.

182. Rosenblum ML, Levy RM, Bredesen DE, So YT, Wara W, Ziegler JL. Primary central nervous system lymphomas in patients with AIDS. *Ann Neurol* 1988;23(suppl):13–16.

183. Rostad SW, Olson K, McDougall J, Shaw CM, Alvord EC Jr. Transsynaptic spread of varicella zoster virus through the visual system: a mechanism of viral dissemination in the nervous system. *Hum Pathol* 1989;20:174–179.

184. Russel DS, Rubinstein LJ. *Pathology of Tumours of the Nervous System*. London: Edward Arnold, 1989.

185. Ryder JW, Croen K, Kleinschmidt-Demasters BK, Ostrove JM, Straus SE, Cohn DL. Progressive encephalitis three months after resolution of cutaneous zoster in a patient with AIDS. *Ann Neurol* 1986;19:182–188.

186. Safai B, Lynfield R, Lowenthal DA, Koziner B. Cancers associated with HIV infection. *Anticancer Res* 1987;7:1055–1067.

187. Salahuddin SZ, Nakamura S, Biberfeld P, et al. Angiogenic properties of Kaposi's sarcoma–derived cells after long-term culture *in vitro*. *Science* 1988;242:430–433.
188. Scheithauer B. Cerebral metastasis in Hodgkin's disease. *Arch Pathol Lab Med* 1979;103:284–287.
189. Schlech WF III, Lavigne PM, Bortolussi RA, et al. Epidemic listeriosis—evidence for transmission by food. *N Engl J Med* 1983;308:203–206.
190. Schmidbauer M, Budka H, Ambros P. Herpes simplex virus (HSV) DNA in microglial nodular brainstem encephalitis. *J Neuropathol Exp Neurol* 1989;48:645–652.
191. Schmidbauer M, Budka H, Pilz P, Kurata T, Hondo R. Presence, distribution and spread of productive varicella zoster virus infection in nervous tissues. *Brain* 1992;115:383–398.
192. Schmidbauer M, Budka H, Shah KV. Progressive multifocal leukoencephalopathy (PML) in AIDS and in the pre-AIDS era. A neuropathological comparison using immunocytochemistry and *in situ* DNA hybridization for virus detection. *Acta Neuropathol* 1990;80:375–380.
193. Schmidbauer M, Budka H, Ulrich W, Ambros P. Cytomegalovirus (CMV) disease of the brain in AIDS and connatal infection: a comparative study by histology, immunocytochemistry and *in situ* hybridization. *Acta Neuropathol* 1989;79:286–293.
194. Schmidt BJ, Meagher-Villemure K, Carpio JD. Lymphomatoid granulomatosis with isolated involvement of the brain. *Ann Neurol* 1984;15:478–481.
195. Schuchat A, Deaver KA, Wenger JD, et al. Role of foods in sporadic listeriosis: 1. Case-control study of dietary risk factors. *JAMA* 1992;267:2041–2045.
196. Shah KV. Papovaviruses. In: Fields BN, ed. *Virology*. New York: Raven, 1985:371–391.
197. Sharer LR, Dowling PL, Michaels J, et al. Spinal cord disease in children with HIV-1 infection: a combined molecular biological and neuropathological study. *Neuropathol Appl Neurobiol* 1990;16:317–331.
198. Sharer LR, Kaminski Z, Cho ES, Ambros R. Case 1. Presented at the 28th Annual Diagnostic Slide Session, American Association of Neuropathologists. Seattle, Washington, 1987.
199. Sharer LR, Kapila R. Neuropathological observations in acquired immunodeficiency syndrome (AIDS). *Acta Neuropathol* 1985;66:188–198.
200. Sibley LD. Interactions between *Toxoplasma gondii* and its mammalian host cells. *Semin Cell Biol* 1993;4:335–344.
201. So YT, Beckstead JH, Davis RL. Primary central nervous system lymphoma in acquired immune deficiency syndrome: a clinical and pathological study. *Ann Neurol* 1986;20:566–572.
202. Spina-França A, Mattosinho-França LC. American trypansomiasis (Chagas' disease). In: Vinken PJ, Bruyn GW, eds. *Handbook of Clinical Neurology*. Amsterdam: Elsevier/North Holland, 1978:85–114.
203. Spitzer ED, Spitzer CG, Freundlich LF, Casadevall A. Persistence of initial infection in recurrent *Cryptococcus neoformans* meningitis. *Lancet* 1993;341:595–596.
204. Stark E, Haas J, Schedel I. Diagnosis of cytomegalovirus infections of the nervous system by immunocytochemical demonstration of infected cells in cerebrospinal fluid. *Eur J Med* 1993;2:223–224.
205. Strittmatter C, Lang W, Wiestler OD, Kleihues P. The changing pattern of human immunodeficiency virus–associated cerebral toxoplasmosis: a study of 46 postmortem cases. *Acta Neuropathol* 1992;83:475–481.
206. Strouth JC, Donohue S, Ross A, Aldred A. Neoplastic angioendotheliosis. *Neurology* 1965;15:644–648.
207. Sugar AM. Overview: cryptococcosis in the patient with AIDS. *Mycopathologia* 1991;114:153–157.
208. Sunderam G, McDonald RJ, Maniatis T, Oleske J, Kapila R, Reichman LB. Tuberculosis as a manifestation of acquired immunodeficiency syndrome. *JAMA* 1986;256:362–366.
209. Sunohara N, Mukoyama M, Satoyoshi E. Neoplastic angioendotheliosis of the central nervous system. *J Neurol* 1984;231:14–19.
210. Suzuki Y, Joh K. Effect of the strain of *Toxoplasma gondii* on the development of toxoplasmic encephalitis in mice treated with antibody to interferon-gamma. *Parasitol Res* 1994;80:125–130.
211. Suzuki Y, Orellana MA, Schreiber RD, Remington JS. Interferon-gamma: the major mediator of resistance against *Toxoplasma gondii*. *Science* 1988;240:516–518.
212. Tada H, Rappaport J, Lahgari M, Amini S, Wong-Staal F, Khalili K. Trans-activation of the JC virus late promoter by the *tat* protein of type 1 human immunodeficiency virus in glial cells. *Proc Natl Acad Sci U S A* 1990;87:3479–3483.
213. Tang TT, Harb JM, Dunne WM Jr, et al. Cerebral toxoplasmosis in an immunocompromised host. A precise and rapid diagnosis by electron microscopy. *Am J Clin Pathol* 1986;85:104–110.
214. Taylor MN, Baddour LM, Alexander JR. Disseminated histoplasmosis associated with the acquired immune deficiency syndrome. *Am J Med* 1984;77:579–580.
215. Tien RD, Gean-Marton AD, Mark AS. Neurosyphilis in HIV carriers: MR findings in six patients. *AJR* 1992;158:1325–1328.
216. Vallbracht A, Löhler J, Gossmann J, et al. Disseminated BK type polyomavirus infection in an AIDS patient associated with central nervous system disease. *Am J Pathol* 1993;143:29–39.

217. Vazeux R, Cumont M, Girard PM, et al. Severe encephalitis resulting from coinfections with HIV and JC virus. *Neurology* 1990;40:944–948.
218. Veltri RW, Raich PC, McClung JE, Shah SH, Sprinkle PM. Lymphomatoid granulomatosis and Epstein-Barr virus. *Cancer* 1982;50:1513–1517.
219. Verhofstede C, Reniers S, Colebunders R, van Wanzeele F, Plum J. Polymerase chain reaction in the diagnosis of *Toxoplasma* encephalitis. *AIDS* 1993;7:1539–1541.
220. Vinters HV, Anders KH. *Neuropathology of AIDS*. Boca Raton, FL: CRC Press, 1990.
221. Vinters HV, Guerra WF, Eppolito L, Keith PE III. Necrotizing vasculitis of the nervous system in a patient with AIDS-related complex. *Neuropathol Appl Neurobiol* 1988;14:417–424.
222. Vinters HV, Kwok MK, Ho HW, et al. Cytomegalovirus in the nervous system of patients with the acquired immune deficiency syndrome (AIDS). *Brain* 1989;112:245–268.
223. Vollmer TL, Waldor MK, Steinman L, Conley FK. Depletion of T-4+ lymphocytes with monoclonal antibody reactivates toxoplasmosis in the central nervous system: a model of superinfection in AIDS. *J Immunol* 1987;138:3737–3741.
224. von-Einsiedel RW, Fife TD, Aksamit AJ, et al. Progressive multifocal leukoencephalopathy in AIDS: a clinicopathological study and review of the literature. *J Neurol* 1993;240:391–406.
225. von-Lichtenberg F. Protozoal infection. In: von Lichtenberg F, ed. *Pathology of Infectious Diseases*. New York: Raven, 1991:243–295.
226. Walsh TJ, Mitchell TG. Dimorphic fungi causing systemic mycoses. In: Balows A, ed. *Manual of Clinical Microbiology*. Washington, DC: American Society for Microbiology, 1991:630–643.
227. Warren KG, Brown SM, Wroblewska Z, Gilden D, Koprowski H, Subak-Sharpe J. Isolation of latent herpes simplex virus from the superior cervical and vagus ganglions of human beings. *N Engl J Med* 1978;298:1068–1069.
228. Weber T, Turner RW, Frye S, et al. Specific diagnosis of progressive multifocal leukoencephalopathy by polymerase chain reaction. *J Infect Dis* 1993;169:1138–1141.
229. Weis S, Hippius H. *HIV-1 Infection of the Central Nervous System. Clinical, Pathological, and Molecular Aspects*. 1st ed. Seattle: Hogrefe & Huber, 1993.
230. Welch K, Finkbeiner W, Alpers CE. Autopsy findings in the acquired immune deficiency syndrome. *JAMA* 1984;252:1152–1159.
231. Weller TH. Varicella and herpes zoster: changing concepts of the natural history, control, and importance of a not-so-benign virus. Part 1. *N Engl J Med* 1983;309:1362–1368.
232. Weller TH. Varicella and herpes zoster: changing concepts of the natural history, control, and importance of a not-so-benign virus. Part 2. *N Engl J Med* 1983;309:1434–1440.
233. Werner SB, Pappagianis D, Heindl I, Mickel A. An epidemic of coccidioidomycosis among archeology students in northern California. *N Engl J Med* 1972;286:507–512.
234. Wheat LJ, Slama TG, Norton JA, et al. Risk factors for disseminated or fatal histoplasmosis. *Ann Intern Med* 1982;96:159–163.
235. Wheat LJ, Slama TG, Zeckel ML. Histoplasmosis in the acquired immune deficiency syndrome. *Am J Med* 1985;78:203–210.
236. Wijdicks EF, Borleffs JC, Hoepelman AI, Jansen GH. Fatal disseminated hemorrhagic toxoplasmic encephalitis as the initial manifestation of AIDS. *Ann Neurol* 1991;29:683–686.
237. Wiley CA, Grafe M, Kennedy C, Nelson JA. Human immunodeficiency virus (HIV) and JC virus in acquired immune deficiency syndrome (AIDS) patients with progressive multifocal leukoencephalopathy. *Acta Neuropathol* 1988;76:338–346.
238. Wiley CA, Nelson JA. Role of human immunodeficiency virus and cytomegalovirus in AIDS encephalitis. *Am J Pathol* 1988;133:73–81.
239. Wiley CA, Safrin RE, Davis CE, et al. Acanthamoeba meningoencephalitis in a patient with AIDS. *J Infect Dis* 1987;155:130–133.
240. Wiley CA, Schrier RD, Denaro FJ, Nelson JA, Lampert PW, Oldstone MBA. Localization of cytomegalovirus proteins and genome during fulminant central nervous system infection in an AIDS patient. *J Neuropathol Exp Neurol* 1986;45:127–139.
241. Witt DJ, Craven DE, McCabe WR. Bacterial infections in adult patients with the acquired immune deficiency syndrome (AIDS) and AIDS-related complex. *Am J Med* 1987;82:900–906.
242. Woods GL, Goldsmith JC. *Aspergillus* infection of the central nervous system in patients with acquired immunodeficiency syndrome. *Arch Neurol* 1990;47:181–184.
243. Ziegler JL, Beckstead J, Volderbing PA, et al. Non-Hodgkin lymphoma in 90 homosexual men: relation to generalized lymphadenopathy and the acquired immunodeficiency syndrome. *N Engl J Med* 1984;311:565–570.
244. Zimmer C, Marzhauser S, Patt S, et al. Stereotactic brain biopsy in AIDS. *J Neurol* 1992;239:394–400.
245. Zu Rhein GM, Chou SM. Particles resembling papova viruses in human cerebral demyelinating disease. *Science* 1965;148:1477–1479.
246. Zugger A, Louei E, Holzman RS, Simberkoff MS, Rahal JJ. Cryptococcal disease in patients with the acquired immunodeficiency syndrome. *Ann Intern Med* 1986;104:234–240

AIDS and the Nervous System, Second Edition,
edited by J. R. Berger and R. M. Levy.
Lippincott-Raven Publishers, Philadelphia © 1997.

20

Neurological Manifestations of Primary Human Immunodeficiency Virus-1 Infection

°*Bruce J. Brew and* †*Brett Tindall*

†*National Centre in HIV Epidemiology and Clinical Research,* °†*St. Vincent's Hospital, and Departments of* °*HIV Medicine and Neurology and* †*Centre for Immunology, University of New South Wales, Sydney, Australia 2010*

The neurological manifestations of primary human immunodeficiency virus 1 (HIV-1) infection are not rare and may challenge the diagnostic and management skills of the attending physician. This review will discuss first the features of the illness associated with seroconversion to HIV-1 and then the neurological manifestations that may complicate such an illness according to the anatomic level of the clinically dominant presentation. A discussion of possible pathogenetic mechanisms with the highlighting of one model that is considered most likely will follow. Lastly, there is a section on the practical approach to the management of such patients.

PRIMARY HIV INFECTION

Primary exposure to HIV-1 is associated with a clinical illness in approximately 70% of cases (Table 1). In a review of 139 published cases of primary HIV-1 infection (14) the most common physical symptoms and signs were fever (97%), adenopathy (77%), pharyngitis (73%), rash (70%), and myalgia or arthralgia (58%). Mucocutaneous ulceration may also be a frequent finding (23). The time from exposure to HIV-1 until the onset of the acute clinical illness is typically between 2 and 4 weeks (with a reported range from 6 days to 6 weeks). The clinical illness is acute in onset and generally lasts approximately 2 weeks (23,36).

In the majority of cases of primary HIV-1 infection, symptoms and signs rapidly resolve, and a period of asymptomatic infection that may last many months to years follows. It is not yet clear what factors influence the development of symptomatic primary HIV-1 infection (including neurological symptoms), but potential factors include the tropism, virulence, and inoculum of the infecting strain and the nature of the individual host immune response.

The clinical features of seroconversion to HIV-2 have not been well defined. Nonetheless, neurological complications have been rarely reported. One case of a neuropathy in association with primary HIV-2 infection has been described in a 50-

TABLE 1. *Characteristic features of primary HIV-1[a] infection*

Clinical findings	Laboratory findings
Fever	Lymphocytopenia (weeks 1–2)
Pharyngitis	Lymphocytosis (weeks 2–4)
Rash (usually truncal)	Thrombocytopenia (weeks 1–3)
Adenopathy	Positive serum/CSF[b] HIV-1 p24 antigen
Mucocutaneous ulceration	Positive or indeterminate serum/CSF HIV-1 antibody
Myalgia/arthralgia	Abnormal liver function tests

[a] Human immunodeficiency virus 1.
[b] Cerebrospinal fluid.

year-old French man, a resident of the Ivory Coast (41). No clinical details were provided. Only one other case of primary HIV-2 infection has been reported in the literature, and there was no evidence of neurological involvement in that case.

NEUROLOGICAL CLINICAL PRESENTATIONS

The neurological sequelae of primary HIV-1 infection are varied and affect almost all parts of the nervous system (Table 2). The clinical features always occur in the context of an acute febrile illness and not infrequently involve more than one part of the nervous system simultaneously.

Incidence

There are few data on the incidence of neurological manifestations of primary HIV-1 infection. In a review of 139 published cases of primary HIV-1 infection (14) encephalopathy and neuropathy were each reported in 8% of cases. Pedersen et al. 1989 (36) reported encephalitis in 4 (approximately 9%) of 46 subjects with primary HIV-1 infection. Headache has been reported in 30% to 45% of subjects (14,23,40) and in one series was associated with photophobia in 71% of cases (40).

The annual incidence of new HIV-1 infection in the United States is estimated to be 0.6 to 0.8 per thousand (approximately 40,000 new cases per annum) (13), and the frequency of symptomatic primary HIV-1 infection is generally estimated to be approximately 70% (i.e., 28,000 cases of symptomatic primary HIV-1 infection per annum) (23,50). Based on the above incidence data [16% (14)], it is therefore estimated that approximately 4,480 new cases of HIV-1 infection per annum in the United States alone would present with an appreciable neurological manifestation.

While this number stands in marked contrast to the relatively small number of

TABLE 2. *Neurologic syndromes of primary HIV-1 infection*

Clinical findings	Laboratory findings
Aseptic meningoencephalitis Myelopathy Cranial neuropathies (especially VII) Peripheral neuropathy	CSF mononuclear pleocytosis
Myalgia/rhabdomyloysis	Raised creatine kinase levels

cases reported in the literature, many cases of primary HIV-1 infection are not recognized due to the sometimes vague and transitory nature of symptoms and the lack of education among clinicians regarding this period of infection. Clark et al. (15) have pointed out that it is likely that many hundreds or thousands of patients present to primary care physicians annually but are not identified. Recognition of primary HIV-1 infection requires knowledge and a high index of suspicion on the part of the clinician, the ability to take a history that accurately identifies potential risk factors, and the time and facilities for review of such subjects.

Central Nervous System Syndromes

Central nervous system (CNS) manifestations of primary HIV-1 infection cover a wide spectrum from mild headache to severe meningoencephalitis.

Headaches are a frequent manifestation of primary HIV-1 infection. The occasional finding of retrobulbar pain, particularly on eye movement (32) and photophobia, suggests that in some patients the headache is more than one would expect from fever alone and may in fact be a mild form of meningoencephalitis.

The first reports of meningoencephalitis (12,29) in association with primary HIV-1 infection described subjects with a rapid onset of altered neurological status consisting of confusion progressing to obtundation and coma. These changes typically occurred within 2 weeks of onset of an acute febrile illness. Subsequent cases have demonstrated a wide spectrum of presentations. In some cases the manifestations have been mild with lethargy and disorientation (46), while others have been marked by dramatic neurological decompensation over a few days (5,27). Even in cases where subjects have progressed to a severely obtunded state (5), resolution typically occurs within 2 weeks of presentation.

Seizures may also complicate seroconversion, but importantly they occur in the context of the other clinical features of acute meningoencephalitis (12). This is in contradistinction to seizures occurring later in the course of HIV-1 infection where they may be the only neurological abnormality (57).

Investigations of patients with these manifestations are consistent with mild to moderate aseptic meningoencephalitis. Examination of cerebrospinal fluid (CSF) shows a mild to moderate mononuclear pleocytosis (5,28,29,44), which improves and sometimes resolves within 2 weeks. Protein levels may be increased (29) and may remain so for up to 6 weeks (44). The HIV-1 has been isolated from the CSF of some subjects with meningoencephalitis, sometimes within a day of presentation (28,29,44). Electroencephalographic (EEG) studies show generally diffuse changes that are consistent with the diagnosis of an aseptic meningoencephalitis (12,44). In those cases where computed tomography (CT) scan has been performed, it has not shown abnormalities.

Neuropsychological Impairment

There is a paucity of research to indicate whether neuropsychological impairment occurs at the time of primary HIV-1 infection. Certainly, acute personality and cognitive changes (10,12,46) have been documented in the context of presentation with aseptic meningoencephalitis, but it is not clear whether appreciable or permanent neuropsychological impairment may occur at this stage.

Carne et al. (12) reported one such patient who was forgetful at presentation and rapidly progressed into a state of incoherence and grand mal seizures. During the 3 weeks after discharge he remained "slightly forgetful," but psychometric assessment 6 months after admission did not show any residual impairment. We have previously reported a subject who presented initially with aggression and a moderately severe expressive dysphasia that resolved (10). Neuropsychological assessment 5 months after the illness revealed some minor impairment, which did not alter in the following 2 years. However, the absence of comparable testing data from the acute period prevents attribution of causation to HIV-1.

Myelopathy

One case of myelopathy has been reported (19) in which the subject presented with a stiff right leg, unsteady gait, and difficulty with micturition. Over the ensuing 2 weeks, severe lancinating pains in the back developed with a paraparesis, hyperreflexia of the arms, a pout reflex, and mild mental slowing. Full myelography and CT of the brain were normal and repeated CSF studies showed a mild mononuclear pleocytosis. The HIV-1 was isolated from CSF. The symptoms improved over 4 weeks; however, at the 2-month review obvious neurological signs persisted in legs and the gait remained unsteady.

Two further cases are suggestive of involvement of the lower segments of the spinal cord or the cauda equina. One patient presented with neurogenic urinary retention and sacral sensory loss which resolved over several weeks (58). A mononuclear CSF pleocytosis was present with normal protein concentration. Similarly, Gaines et al. (23) reported one case of urinary retention and asymmetric back pain which appeared on day 15 of illness and had resolved within 8 days. Primary HSV-2 infection was excluded, but the subject refused lumbar puncture, and it was not possible to further delineate the syndrome.

Neuropathies

Both cranial and peripheral neuropathies have been reported during primary HIV-1 infection. While some patients may develop a cranial neuropathy in the context of a generalized neuropathy, others have developed isolated cranial neuropathies. The most common reports have been of facial nerve palsy (1,35,39,56). Indeed, the first case of primary HIV-1 infection in the literature described a case of left facial palsy in a health care worker who was occupationally infected (1). In three of the reported cases the facial palsy has been associated with lower limb signs of a neuropathy, reflecting the potential for multiple sites of neurological involvement (35,39,56). Although some of the cases have documented clear evidence of axonal damage (e.g., 56), in others it is not clear whether these cases represent central involvement of the facial nerve nucleus, such as may occur in aseptic meningoencephalitis or cranial nerve inflammatory neuropathy per se (34).

As with CNS system syndromes, examination of CSF, when performed, showed only a mild to moderate mononuclear pleocytosis and a mild increase in protein levels.

Piette et al. reported two cases of facial palsy (39). The first case presented with facial diplegia, sensory and motor impairment of the legs with areflexia, and a short period of confusion with hallucinations. Sensory and motor impairment of the arms was noted. The EEG showed bilateral temporal slow waves. The CT scan was normal. There was a moderate mononuclear pleocytosis and slightly raised protein. Neurological symptoms and CSF indices resolved over 3 months, though causalgia and areflexia of legs persisted. The second case was an uncomplicated facial palsy that developed 8 weeks after initial presentation with a febrile illness and resolved within 4 weeks (39).

Wiselka et al. (56) reported a subject who developed facial nerve palsy and abdominal/flank pain approximately 2 weeks after onset of febrile illness and resolution within 3 weeks. Neurophysiological studies performed 2 days after the onset of the facial palsy revealed a partial lesion of left facial nerve with axonal damage.

Several cases of severe and rapidly progressive neuropathy resembling Guillain-Barré syndrome have been described (4,26,35,39,53). In general, the clinical features have been consistent with Guillain-Barré syndrome except that a CSF mononuclear pleocytosis may be found. In one subject quadriplegia and a facial diplegia evolved over a period of 3 weeks followed by hypoxia necessitating intubation (53). Cerebrospinal fluid examination was unremarkable except for a raised protein that peaked at 72.5 mg/dL. Neurophysiological studies showed slowing of nerve conduction studies with prolonged distal latencies. Treatment with steroids and plasmapheresis were ineffective. At the 6-month review the subject had improved but retained a moderate quadriparesis. Hagberg et al. (26) reported two cases in which ascending paresis developed 1 and 20 weeks following infection with HIV-1. The first case had symptoms limited to pain in both hands and paraparesis with resolution after 4 weeks. In the second case, paraesthesia of both hands and legs was followed by a progressive course with cranial nerve involvement necessitating assisted ventilation. Although the time from onset of the febrile illness to onset of the neurological signs in the second case was extended (20 weeks), at the time of neurological presentation the subject only showed low titers of serum HIV-1 antibody, which subsequently increased.

Two cases of acute bilateral brachial neuritis have been reported (10,11). In both, the neurological symptoms began approximately 2 weeks after onset of an acute febrile illness and resolved within several weeks. One of the reported patients was also confused at the time of the brachial neuritis, again illustrating the propensity for multifocal involvement.

Other sundry reports include prominent sensory neuropathy of the limbs with areflexia in 2 (17%) of 12 subjects with primary HIV-1 infection; no clinical details or data on long-term review were provided (48). One case of ataxic neuropathy (20) and one case of polyneuropathy (30) have been reported as being manifestations of primary HIV-1 infection, but in neither was a definite link with primary HIV-1 infection demonstrated.

Muscle Involvement

While involvement of the brain, spinal cord, and peripheral nerve has been reported numerous times, if one excludes the common finding of myalgia (14,23,36), primary muscle disease is unusual. Two cases of rhabdomyolysis affecting all limbs and with very high creatine kinase (CK) levels have been reported (18,33). The symptoms and the CK levels resolved within a few days and several weeks, respectively.

PATHOGENESIS

The pathogenesis of these neurological complications is unknown, but some insights may be had by a brief review of the systemic features of seroconversion to HIV-1. Primary HIV-1 infection is associated with high levels of infectious HIV-1 in plasma and peripheral blood mononuclear cells during the first few weeks followed by a rapid decline in viral load and a concomitant resolution of acute symptoms (14,17). The viral clearance is presumably related to the emergence of an effective host immune response that includes humoral, cellular, and cytokine responses.

With this general background, it is possible to speculate on likely pathogenetic mechanisms of neurological involvement. Before doing so, however, there are certain ''building blocks'' that may assist in approaching such an understanding. First, by and large the neurological sequelae occur several weeks after the primary illness. Second, in general, the brain is affected to some extent even in those without symptoms (49), and superimposed upon this is a more dominant abnormality in some other part of the nervous system. Third, CSF abnormalities are frequent and HIV-1 can be recovered from the CSF in a large number of patients. Fourth, autopsy studies on HIV-1-infected asymptomatic patients who have had accidental deaths have shown that no HIV-1 can be detected by polymerase chain reaction (PCR) in half of the patients, and in the remaining the levels of detectable virus are consistent with contamination from the systemic circulation (3). Last is the finding in limited pathological studies of nervous tissue from patients with a primary HIV-1 illness and neurological complications that productive infection is absent (16,24).

These findings point to a model of pathogenesis that is largely focused on indirect mechanisms of tissue damage driven but not directly caused by HIV-1 per se. It is proposed that the neurological sequelae of the primary HIV-1 infection illness are secondary to immune activation and that the brain itself is not infected at this time, contrary to previous considerations. It is further proposed that the CSF abnormalities reflect trafficking of infected cells through the nervous system [the Trojan Horse mechanism (38)]. In short, then, the nervous system is affected by HIV-1 but not infected.

The alternate hypothesis that the nervous system is infected at the beginning of the primary infection seems unlikely. The arguments against this are, first, that there is a delay in the expression of the neurological sequelae. If direct infection were the explanation, then one would expect that the neurological complications would occur in concert with the other manifestations. Second, the lack of productive infection from biopsies, albeit that the number of such samples is limited, argues against direct infection.

As to the cellular mechanisms of tissue damage, it is likely that the processes are similar to those that operate later in HIV-1 disease. Among these are gp120, which is known to be neurotoxic, and quinolinic acid, along with other as yet undefined neurotoxins. There have been no studies of quinolinic acid during primary HIV-1 infection. However, significant increases in serum and CSF quinolinic acid levels in the analogous rhesus monkey model of primary simian immunodeficiency virus (SIV) infection have been demonstrated. In these animals, primary SIV infection was associated with a significant increase in quinolinic acid levels, and animals who maintained high levels after the acute period appeared to have worse prognoses (31). The increased levels of quinolinic acid are presumably related to increased levels of virally elicited cytokines during primary infection such as occurs in primary HIV-1 infection (47,49,55).

The factors determining neurological involvement during primary HIV-1 infection also remain speculative. Nonetheless, it seems likely that strains of HIV-1 that are particularly neurotropic or monocytotropic have a high propensity to cause manifestations. Recent studies (43,59) have demonstrated that the isolates of HIV-1 obtained during primary HIV-1 infection are generally macrophage tropic and non–syncytium inducing (regardless of the phenotype of subjects who transmitted the virus). We have shown that HIV-1-infected macrophages can produce large quantities of quinolinic acid and that this production is dependent upon the degree of macrophage tropism of the HIV-1 isolate (8,9). It is therefore tempting to propose that neurological sequelae are more likely to occur with isolates that have greater degrees of macrophage tropism.

APPROACH TO MANAGEMENT

Primary HIV-1 infection should now be considered in the differential diagnosis of a wide range of acute neurological syndromes. In particular, it should be considered in any person with a known possible recent exposure to HIV-1 who presents with a febrile illness of acute onset followed by a neurological manifestation.

Primary HIV-1 infection is confirmed serologically by the appearance of serum antibodies that are directed against the specific internal and surface proteins that form HIV-1. Dependent upon the facilities available, a combination of rapid assays, standard enzyme-linked-immunosorbent assays (ELISAs), and Western blot (WB) can generally detect infection within the first 2 weeks following exposure. Antibodies within the CSF also appear during this period and may in some cases predate the development of serum antibodies (42). Assay for serum HIV-1 p24 antigen is also important when the differential diagnosis includes primary HIV-1 infection. The HIV-1 p24 antigen can be detected in both serum and CSF as early as 24 hours after onset of the acute clinical illness (21,25,54) and in some cases has been detected in the CSF prior to detection in serum. Although not part of the routine diagnostic armamentarium, virus isolation and PCR may in some cases prove useful or be for research purposes.

In addition to these definitive serological assays, other laboratory data may be helpful in alerting the clinician (Table 1). Primary HIV-1 infection may be associated with a transient but severe lymphopenia during the first week of illness followed by a lymphocytosis in the second to fourth weeks of illness (mainly constituted of CD8-lymphocytes) (22). Transient, mild to moderate thrombocytopenia is common in the first 2 weeks of illness (22). Elevated serum levels of hepatic transaminases are not uncommon during the acute illness but return to within normal limits rapidly (7).

In those cases where it is realized that the patient's illness is a consequence of primary HIV-1 infection, treatment is controversial. There is no clear evidence that the administration of zidovudine at this stage is useful (51,52). However, in practical terms it is often administered based on the rationale of diminishing viral replication that is the driving force behind the production of a viral-coded or host-mediated neurotoxin(s). The utility of immunomodulatory agents is unknown. While there is no clinical trial data on the efficacy of corticosteroids, anecdotal data exist to suggest that their use in primary HIV-1 infection leads to a more rapid progression to AIDS

(2,6,37,45). Therefore, use of corticosteroids cannot be recommended. No data exist as to the benefit of other immunomodulatory agents such as intravenous gammaglobulin.

CONCLUSION

There is an increasing need for the clinician to appreciate the neurological complications of primary HIV-1 infection. The clinical "signposts" of the typical seroconversion illness (Table 1) along with the characteristic multifocal nature of neurological involvement and the laboratory findings (Tables 1 and 2) should alert the physician. However, the importance of clinical recognition extends beyond individual patient management and affords a unique opportunity to understand the pathogenesis of the neurological complications of HIV-1 in general.

.

REFERENCES

1. Anonymous. Needlestick transmission of HTLV-III from a patient infected in Africa. *Lancet* 1984; ii:1376–1377.
2. Apperley JF, Rice SJ, Hewitt P, et al. HIV infection due to platelet transfusion after allogeneic bone marrow transplantation. *Eur J Haematol* 1987;39:185–189.
3. Bell JE, Busuttil A, Ironside JW, et al. Human immunodeficiency virus and the brain: investigation of virus load and neuropathological changes in pre-AIDS subjects. *J Infect Dis* 1993;168:818-824.
4. Beytout J, Llory JF, Clavelou P, Brunot A, Regnier A, Lafeuille H. Meningoradiculite a la phase de primoinfection a VIH. Interet de la plasmapherese. *La Presse Med* 1989;18:1031–1032.
5. Biggar RJ, Johnson BK, Musoke SS, et al. Severe illness associated with the appearance of antibody to human immunodeficiency virus in an African. *Br Med J* 1986;293:1210–1211.
6. Bismuth H, Samuel D, Gugeniem J, et al. Emergency liver transplantation for fulminant hepatitis. *Ann Intern Med* 1987;107:337–341.
7. Boag FC, Dean R, Hawkins DA, Lawrence AG, Gazzard BG. Abnormalities of liver function during HIV-1 seroconversion illness. *Int J STD AIDS* 1992;3:46–48.
8. Brew BJ, Corbeil J, Pemberton L, et al. Quinolinic acid production by macrophages infected with HIV-1 isolates from patients with and without AIDS dementia complex. *J Neurovirol* 1996;1(5/6): 369–374.
9. Brew BJ, Evans L, Byrne C, Pemberton L, Hurren L. The relationship between AIDS dementia complex and the presence of macrophage tropic and non syncytium inducing isolates of human immunodeficiency virus type 1 in the cerebrospinal fluid. *J Neurovirol* (in press).
10. Brew BJ, Perdices M, Darveniza P, et al. The neurological features of early and "latent" human immunodeficiency virus. *Austral N Z J Med* 1989;19:700–705.
11. Calabrese LH, Proffitt MR, Levin KH, et al. Acute infection with the human immunodeficiency virus (HIV-1) associated with acute brachial neuritis and exanthematous rash. *Ann Intern Med* 1987;107: 849–851.
12. Carne CA, Tedder RS, Smith A, et al. Acute encephalopathy coincident with seroconversion for anti-HTLV-III. *Lancet* 1985;ii:1206–1208
13. Centers for Disease Control. Estimates of HIV-1 prevalence and projected AIDS cases: summary of a workshop, October 31–November 1, 1989. *Morb Mortal Wkly* 1990;39:110–112,117–119.
14. Clark SJ, Saag MS, Decker WD, et al. High titers of cytopathic virus in plasma of patients with symptomatic primary HIV-1 infection. *N Engl J Med* 1991;324:954–960.
15. Clark SJ, Saag MS, Hahn BH, Shaw GM, Daar ES, Ho D. Primary HIV-1 infection (letter). *N Engl J Med* 1991;325:734–735.
16. Cornblath DR, McArthur JC, Kennedy PGE, Witte AS, Griffin JW. Inflammatory demyelinating peripheral neuropathies associated with human T-cell lymphotropic virus type III infection. *Ann Neurol* 1987;21:32–40.
17. Daar ES, Moudgil T, Meyer RD, Ho DD. Transient high levels of viremia in patients with primary human immunodeficiency virus type 1 infection. *N Engl J Med* 1991;324:961–964.
18. del Rio C, Soffer O, Widell JL, Judd RL, Slade BA. Acute human immunodeficiency virus infection temporally associated with rhabdomyolysis, acute renal failure, and nephrosis. *Rev Infect Dis* 1990; 12:82–285.

50. Tindall B, Cooper DA. Primary HIV infection. Primary human immunodeficiency virus infection: host responses and intervention strategies. *AIDS* 1991:5;1–14.
51. Tindall B, Carr A, Goldstein D, Cooper DA. Administration of zidovudine during primary HIV-1 infection may be associated with a less vigorous immune response. *AIDS* 1993;7:127–128.
52. Tindall B, Gaines H, Imrie A, et al. Zidovudine in the management of primary HIV infection. *AIDS* 1991;5:477–484.
53. Vendrell J, Heredia C, Pujol M, et al. Guillain-Barré syndrome associated with seroconversion for anti-LAV HTLV–III. *Neurology* 1987;37:544.
54. von Sydow M, Gaines H, Sonnerborg A, Forsgren M, Pehrson PO, Strannegard O. Antigen detection in primary HIV-1 infection. *Br Med J* 1988;296:238–240.
55. von Sydow M, Sonnerborg A, Gaines H, Strannegard T. Interferon-alpha and tumor necrosis factor-alpha in serum of patients in varying stages of HIV-1 infection. *AIDS Res Human Retroviruses* 1991; 7:375–380.
56. Wiselka MJ, Nicholson KG, Ward SC, Flower AJE. Acute infection with human immunodeficiency virus associated with facial nerve palsy and neuralgia. *J Infect* 1987;15:189–194.
57. Wong MC, Suite NA, Labar DR. Seizures in human immunodeficiency virus infection. *Arch Neurol* 1990;47:640–642.
58. Zeman A, Donaghy M. Acute infection with human immunodeficiency virus presenting with neurogenic urinary retention. *Genitourin Med* 1991;67:345–347.
59. Zhu T, Mo H, Wang N, et al. Genotypic and phenotypic characterization of HIV-1 in patients with primary infection. *Science* 1993;261:1179–1181.

19. Denning DW, Anderson J, Rudge P, et al. Acute myelopathy associated with primary i1 human immunodeficiency virus. *Br Med J* 1987;294:143–144.

20. Elder G, Dalakas M, Pezeshkpour G, Sever J. Ataxic neuropathy due to ganglioneuritis a acute human immunodeficiency virus infection. *Lancet* 1986;ii:1275–1276.

21. Gaines H, Albert J, von Sydow M, et al. HIV-1 antigenaemia and virus isolation from p primary HIV-1 infection. *Lancet* 1987;i:1317–1318.

22. Gaines H, von Sydow MAE, von Stedingk LV, et al. Immunological changes in pr infection. *AIDS* 1990;4:995–999.

23. Gaines H, von Sydow M, Pehrson PO, Lundbergh P. Clinical picture of primary HI' presenting as a glandular-fever-like illness. *Lancet* 1988;297:1363–1368.

24. Gherardi R, Lebargy F, Gaulard P, et al. Necrotising vasculitis and HIV-1 replication nerves. *N Engl J Med* 1989;321:685–686.

25. Goudsmit J, de Wolf F, Paul DA, et al. Expression of human immunodeficiency virus 1-Ag) in serum and cerebrospinal fluid during acute and chronic infection. *Lancet* 198

26. Hagberg L, Malmvall B-E, Svennerholm L, et al. Guillan-Barre syndrome as an early of HIV-1 central nervous system infection. *Scand J Infect Dis* 1986;18:591–592.

27. Hardy WD, Daar ES, Sokolov RT Jr, Ho DD. Acute neurological deterioration in a yo *Infect Dis* 1991;13:745–750.

28. Ho DD, Rota TR, Schooley RT, et al. Isolation of HTLV-III from cerebrospinal flu tisues of patients with neurological syndromes related to the acquired immunodeficien *N Engl J Med* 1985;313:1493–1497.

29. Ho DD, Sarngadharan MG, Resnick L, Dimarzo-Veronese F, Rota TR, Hirsch MS. P1 T-lymphotropic virus type III infection. *Ann Intern Med* 1985;103:880–883.

30. Hughes PJ, McLean KA, Lane RJM. Cranial polyneuropathy and brainstem disorder seroconversion in HIV-1 infection. *Int J STD AIDS* 1992;3:60–61.

31. Jordan EK, Heyes MP. Virus isolation and quinolinic acid in primary and chronic simiar ciency virus infection. *AIDS* 1993;7:1173–1179.

32. Lindskov R, Lindhardt BO, Weisman K, et al. Acute HTLV-III infection with rose *Lancet* 1986;i:447.

33. Mahe A, Bruet A, Chabin E, Fendler J-P. Acute rhabdomyolysis coincident with p infection. *Lancet* 1989;ii:454–455.

34. Parry GJ. Peripheral neuropathies associated with human immunodeficiency virus i *Neurol* 1988;23(Suppl):S49–S53.

35. Paton P, Poly H, Gonnaud P-M, et al. Acute meningoradiculitis concomitant with ser(human immunodeficiency virus type 1. *Res Virol* 1990;141:427–433.

36. Pedersen C, Lindhardt B, Jensen BL, et al. Clinical course of primary HIV-1 infection: for subsequent course of infection. *Br Med J* 1989;299:154–157.

37. Pedersen C, Nielsen JO, Dickmeiss E, Jordal R. Early progression to AIDS following infection. *AIDS* 1989;3:45–47.

38. Peluso R, Haase A, Stowring L, Edwards M, Ventura P. A trojan horse mechanism of visna virus in monocytes. *Virology* 1985;147:31–236.

39. Piette AM, Tusseau F, Vignon D, et al. Acute neuropathy coincident with seroconve LAV/HTLV-III. *Lancet* 1986;i:852.

40. Rabeneck L, Popovic M, Gartner S, et al. Acute HIV-1 infection presenting with pain1 and esophageal ulcers. *JAMA* 1990;263:2318–2322.

41. Ritter J, Chevallier P, Peyramond D, Sepetjan M. Serological markers during an a infection. *Vox Sanguine* 1990;59:244–245.

42. Rolfs A, Schumacher HC. Early findings in the cerebrospinal fluid of patients with H of the central nervous system. *N Engl J Med* 1990;323:418–419.

43. Roos MTL, Lange JMA, Goede REY, et al. Viral phenotype and immune response in p immunodeficiency virus type 1 infection. *J Infect Dis* 1992;165:427–432.

44. Ruutu P, Suni J, Oksanen K, Ruutu T. Primary infection with HIV-1 in a severely imm patient with acute leukemia. *Scand J Infect Dis* 1987;19:369–372.

45. Samuel D, Castaing D, Adam R, et al. Fatal acute HIV-1 infection with aplastic anaem by liver graft. *Lancet* 1988;i:1221–1222.

46. Scully RE, Mark EJ, McNeely WF, McNeely BU. Case Records of the Massachusetts (tal, Case 33—1989. *N Engl J Med* 1989;321:454–463.

47. Sinicco A, Biglino A, Sciandra M, et al. Cytokine network and acute primary HIV-1 i 1993;7:1167–1172.

48. Sinicco A, Palestro G, Caramello P, et al. Acute HIV-1 infection, clinical and biol(12 patients. *J Acquired Immune Deficiency Syndromes* 1990;3:260–265.

49. Sonnerborg AB, von Stedingk L-V, Hansson L-O, Strannegard OO. Elevated neopt(microglobulin levels in blood and cerebrospinal fluid occur early in HIV-1 infection 277–283.

19. Denning DW, Anderson J, Rudge P, et al. Acute myelopathy associated with primary infection with human immunodeficiency virus. *Br Med J* 1987;294:143–144.

20. Elder G, Dalakas M, Pezeshkpour G, Sever J. Ataxic neuropathy due to ganglioneuritis after probable acute human immunodeficiency virus infection. *Lancet* 1986;ii:1275–1276.

21. Gaines H, Albert J, von Sydow M, et al. HIV-1 antigenaemia and virus isolation from plasma during primary HIV-1 infection. *Lancet* 1987;i:1317–1318.

22. Gaines H, von Sydow MAE, von Stedingk LV, et al. Immunological changes in primary HIV-1 infection. *AIDS* 1990;4:995–999.

23. Gaines H, von Sydow M, Pehrson PO, Lundbergh P. Clinical picture of primary HIV-1 infection presenting as a glandular-fever-like illness. *Lancet* 1988;297:1363–1368.

24. Gherardi R, Lebargy F, Gaulard P, et al. Necrotising vasculitis and HIV-1 replication in peripheral nerves. *N Engl J Med* 1989;321:685–686.

25. Goudsmit J, de Wolf F, Paul DA, et al. Expression of human immunodeficiency virus antigen (HIV-1-Ag) in serum and cerebrospinal fluid during acute and chronic infection. *Lancet* 1986;ii:177–180.

26. Hagberg L, Malmvall B-E, Svennerholm L, et al. Guillan-Barre syndrome as an early manifestation of HIV-1 central nervous system infection. *Scand J Infect Dis* 1986;18:591–592.

27. Hardy WD, Daar ES, Sokolov RT Jr, Ho DD. Acute neurological deterioration in a young man. *Rev Infect Dis* 1991;13:745–750.

28. Ho DD, Rota TR, Schooley RT, et al. Isolation of HTLV-III from cerebrospinal fluid and neural tisues of patients with neurological syndromes related to the acquired immunodeficiency syndrome. *N Engl J Med* 1985;313:1493–1497.

29. Ho DD, Sarngadharan MG, Resnick L, Dimarzo-Veronese F, Rota TR, Hirsch MS. Primary human T-lymphotropic virus type III infection. *Ann Intern Med* 1985;103:880–883.

30. Hughes PJ, McLean KA, Lane RJM. Cranial polyneuropathy and brainstem disorder at the time of seroconversion in HIV-1 infection. *Int J STD AIDS* 1992;3:60–61.

31. Jordan EK, Heyes MP. Virus isolation and quinolinic acid in primary and chronic simian immunodeficiency virus infection. *AIDS* 1993;7:1173–1179.

32. Lindskov R, Lindhardt BO, Weisman K, et al. Acute HTLV-III infection with roseola-like rash. *Lancet* 1986;i:447.

33. Mahe A, Bruet A, Chabin E, Fendler J-P. Acute rhabdomyolysis coincident with primary HIV-1 infection. *Lancet* 1989;ii:454–455.

34. Parry GJ. Peripheral neuropathies associated with human immunodeficiency virus infection. *Ann Neurol* 1988;23(Suppl):S49–S53.

35. Paton P, Poly H, Gonnaud P-M, et al. Acute meningoradiculitis concomitant with seroconversion to human immunodeficiency virus type 1. *Res Virol* 1990;141:427–433.

36. Pedersen C, Lindhardt B, Jensen BL, et al. Clinical course of primary HIV-1 infection: consequences for subsequent course of infection. *Br Med J* 1989;299:154–157.

37. Pedersen C, Nielsen JO, Dickmeiss E, Jordal R. Early progression to AIDS following primary HIV infection. *AIDS* 1989;3:45–47.

38. Peluso R, Haase A, Stowring L, Edwards M, Ventura P. A trojan horse mechanism for the spread of visna virus in monocytes. *Virology* 1985;147:31–236.

39. Piette AM, Tusseau F, Vignon D, et al. Acute neuropathy coincident with seroconversion for anti-LAV/HTLV-III. *Lancet* 1986;i:852.

40. Rabeneck L, Popovic M, Gartner S, et al. Acute HIV-1 infection presenting with painful swallowing and esophageal ulcers. *JAMA* 1990;263:2318–2322.

41. Ritter J, Chevallier P, Peyramond D, Sepetjan M. Serological markers during an acute HIV-1-2 infection. *Vox Sanguine* 1990;59:244–245.

42. Rolfs A, Schumacher HC. Early findings in the cerebrospinal fluid of patients with HIV-1 infection of the central nervous system. *N Engl J Med* 1990;323:418–419.

43. Roos MTL, Lange JMA, Goede REY, et al. Viral phenotype and immune response in primary human immunodeficiency virus type 1 infection. *J Infect Dis* 1992;165:427–432.

44. Ruutu P, Suni J, Oksanen K, Ruutu T. Primary infection with HIV-1 in a severely immunosuppressed patient with acute leukemia. *Scand J Infect Dis* 1987;19:369–372.

45. Samuel D, Castaing D, Adam R, et al. Fatal acute HIV-1 infection with aplastic anaemia, transmitted by liver graft. *Lancet* 1988;i:1221–1222.

46. Scully RE, Mark EJ, McNeely WF, McNeely BU. Case Records of the Massachusetts General Hospital, Case 33—1989. *N Engl J Med* 1989;321:454–463.

47. Sinicco A, Biglino A, Sciandra M, et al. Cytokine network and acute primary HIV-1 infection. *AIDS* 1993;7:1167–1172.

48. Sinicco A, Palestro G, Caramello P, et al. Acute HIV-1 infection, clinical and biological study of 12 patients. *J Acquired Immune Deficiency Syndromes* 1990;3:260–265.

49. Sonnerborg AB, von Stedingk L-V, Hansson L-O, Strannegard OO. Elevated neopterin and beta$_2$-microglobulin levels in blood and cerebrospinal fluid occur early in HIV-1 infection. *AIDS* 1989;3:277–283.

50. Tindall B, Cooper DA. Primary HIV infection. Primary human immunodeficiency virus infection: host responses and intervention strategies. *AIDS* 1991:5;1–14.
51. Tindall B, Carr A, Goldstein D, Cooper DA. Administration of zidovudine during primary HIV-1 infection may be associated with a less vigorous immune response. *AIDS* 1993;7:127–128.
52. Tindall B, Gaines H, Imrie A, et al. Zidovudine in the management of primary HIV infection. *AIDS* 1991;5:477–484.
53. Vendrell J, Heredia C, Pujol M, et al. Guillain-Barré syndrome associated with seroconversion for anti-LAV HTLV-III. *Neurology* 1987;37:544.
54. von Sydow M, Gaines H, Sonnerborg A, Forsgren M, Pehrson PO, Strannegard O. Antigen detection in primary HIV-1 infection. *Br Med J* 1988;296:238–240.
55. von Sydow M, Sonnerborg A, Gaines H, Strannegard T. Interferon-alpha and tumor necrosis factor-alpha in serum of patients in varying stages of HIV-1 infection. *AIDS Res Human Retroviruses* 1991; 7:375–380.
56. Wiselka MJ, Nicholson KG, Ward SC, Flower AJE. Acute infection with human immunodeficiency virus associated with facial nerve palsy and neuralgia. *J Infect* 1987;15:189–194.
57. Wong MC, Suite NA, Labar DR. Seizures in human immunodeficiency virus infection. *Arch Neurol* 1990;47:640–642.
58. Zeman A, Donaghy M. Acute infection with human immunodeficiency virus presenting with neurogenic urinary retention. *Genitourin Med* 1991;67:345–347.
59. Zhu T, Mo H, Wang N, et al. Genotypic and phenotypic characterization of HIV-1 in patients with primary infection. *Science* 1993;261:1179–1181.

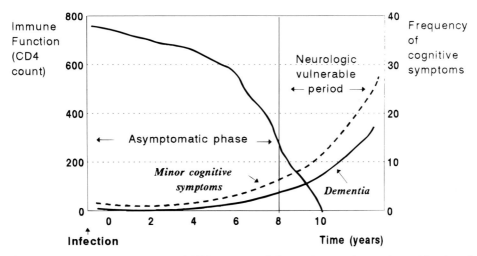

FIG. 1. Approximate frequencies of HIV-associated dementia complex and cognitive impairment and timing relative to systemic disease. Note "vulnerable" period after AIDS.

relatively flat incidence rates in the past few years. On the one hand, antiretrovirals are in widespread use, tending to push down the rates of dementia. On the other hand, people with advanced HIV infection are living longer, with more time in the "vulnerable" period for development of dementia, tending to push up incidence rates. For example, data from the Multicenter AIDS Cohort Study (MACS) show the average survival after the first AIDS-defining illness has increased from 12 months in 1984 to 25 months in 1992 (64). Thus, the pool of AIDS survivors at risk for HIV dementia has increased with lengthening survival times. In contrast to the improved survival after AIDS, survival after diagnosis of HIV dementia has not

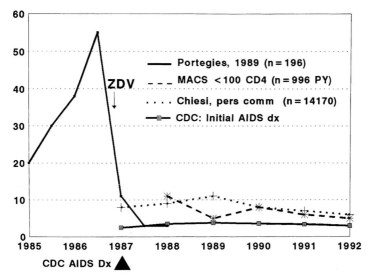

FIG. 2. Composite of incidence data for HIV dementia for several studies. Portegies's data suggest a neuroprotective effect from zidovudine. Recent studies show flat incidence rates.

improved (82). Even though the actual incidence of dementia has remained relatively constant in recent years, because this discrepancy between post-AIDS and postdementia survival has increased, so the number of "dementia-free" AIDS survivors at any point in time has increased. An analogous situation is seen with amyotrophic lateral sclerosis (ALS), which has an incidence similar to multiple sclerosis (MS), 1.8 per 100,000 compared to 3 per 100,000, yet because survival with ALS is very short, prevalence figures are low, whereas because MS does not shorten life span substantially, it is a relatively prevalent disorder. Thus, the projections for numbers of dementia cases tend to underestimate the burden on neurologic and neurodiagnostic services of patients with evolving HIV dementia who die prematurely from their neurologic disease.

Portegies et al. (110) diagnosed HIV dementia in 7.5% (40/536) symptomatic HIV-infected individuals in Amsterdam referred for neurologic evaluation between 1982 and 1992. An identical prevalence of HIV dementia was reported among individuals with AIDS in California from 1989 to 1991 (117). In a multicultural study of neurocognitive disorders in HIV infection organized by the World Health Organization (WHO), the prevalence of dementia was 7% overall in six centers in Thailand, Africa, Germany, and the United States (77), and it did not develop in asymptomatic individuals. These data are comparable to the 7% incidence (after AIDS) and the 15% cumulative prevalence figures from the MACS (84).

In adults, only 3% of AIDS cases present initially with dementia; more typically, dementia develops after constitutional symptoms, immunodeficiency, and systemic opportunistic processes (66,81,96). Identified risk factors for the development of dementia include anemia, low weight, and more constitutional symptoms; i.e., it develops in patients with advanced disease (84). Typically, dementia develops insidiously over a few weeks or months in a patient with advanced immunodeficiency or frank AIDS, although some patients show some insidious cognitive decline before AIDS (Fig. 3) (127).

In children, progressive dementia occurs more commonly than opportunistic infections (37,94). Belman estimates that 62% of children will become demented, with a typical survival of 6 to 24 months (13). Clinical features in children include microcephaly, progressive motor dysfunction, and developmental delay, leading to loss of milestones, with death occurring within the first few years of life. Current serologic techniques may produce a false-positive result in infants because of the presence of maternally derived anti-HIV-1 immunoglobulin G (IgG). Virus isolation or gene amplification techniques [polymerase chain reaction (PCR)] can be helpful in indicating the presence of true infection in an infant.

HIV-ASSOCIATED MINOR COGNITIVE-MOTOR DISORDER

While the incidence and prevalence of frank dementia has been well studied and is clearly delineated now, the frequency and clinical significance of neuropsychologic abnormalities detected earlier in HIV infection remain contentious. The introduction of the American Academy of Neurology definition of "HIV-associated minor cognitive/motor disorder" has in some ways hindered rather than helped this field because it lends a concrete terminology to a group of vague symptoms and signs that probably have heterogeneous etiologies. Because of the vague nature of this entity, reliable estimates of its incidence and prevalence are not yet available, nor has its natural

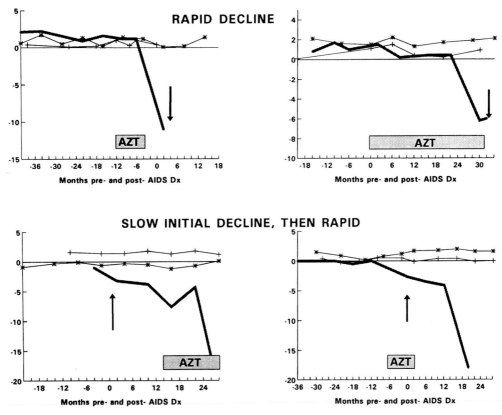

FIG. 3. Patterns of psychomotor decline in four cases of HIV dementia. Note period of relative cognitive stability before AIDS with only slight decline until development of dementia (onset indicated by arrow). The asterisks and minuses indicate patterns in HIV-positive and HIV-negative controls (prepared by O. Selnes). (From Harrison MJG, McArthur JC. *AIDS and neurology.* Churchill Livingstone; 1995.)

history or significance been characterized. Our clinical experience suggests that it is even more common than HIV dementia, although the precise relationship of these two disorders is not understood. A number of observations within prospective studies indicate that minor cognitive-motor disorder may remain stable for many months or years, even without antiretroviral therapy. Mayeux et al. (80) have found that minor cognitive impairment is a marker for reduced survival, and it is likely that, at least in some individuals, evolving neuropsychologic deficits reflect incipient dementia.

Neuropsychologic Studies in Asymptomatic HIV Infection

Many groups of investigators (both in the United States and abroad) have used neuropsychologic test batteries in asymptomatic HIV seropositive individuals to probe for "early" HIV-associated cognitive deficits. Some general statements may be made. First, while some studies have detected a higher frequency of neuropsychologic test abnormalities than seronegative controls, none has shown that these cognitive "deficits" are progressive, or indicative of the later development of clinical

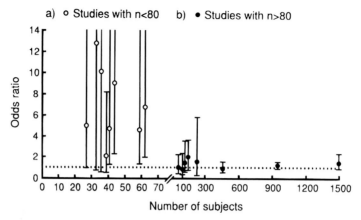

FIG. 4. Relationship between sample size and likelihood of finding statistical significance between HIV seropostiives and seronegatives. (From Newman S, Harrison M. Neuropsychological testing of HIV-infected subjects in the literature. *AIDS 1995;9:1211–1220.*)

dementia. The clinical significance of new cognitive symptoms or test impairment in asymptomatic HIV infection is uncertain because the reported neuropsychologic abnormalities do not necessarily progress and may reflect the effects of low education, age, and alcohol and drug use. Second, most of the studies which indicate a higher frequency of abnormalities have used extensive batteries in relatively small numbers of subjects. By contrast, large studies, in general, have failed to detect differences. Newman and Harrison show a peculiar inverse relationship between the size of the study and the likelihood of detecting a difference in neuropsychologic performance (Fig. 4) (99). For example, among several hundred asymptomatic HIV-1 seropositive men without AIDS or constitutional symptoms in the MACS, the prevalence of HIV dementia was less than 1% (1 in 270 HIV seropositives), and overall the frequency of neuropsychologic impairment was not significantly higher in medically healthy HIV seropositives than in HIV-1 seronegative controls (83). Similar results have been described in injecting drug users (121). These results stand in contrast to other, smaller studies which have demonstrated differences in the frequency of neuropsychologic test abnormalities and which we reviewed in Chapter 15. The 1992 WHO report on neuropsychiatric aspects of HIV-1 infection concluded that ''there is no evidence for an increase of clinically significant neuropsychiatric abnormalities in CDC Groups II or III HIV seropositive (i.e. asymptomatic) individuals as compared to HIV-1 seronegative controls'' (149). More direct evidence comes from several longitudinal studies with data extending over several years. For example, from longitudinal neuropsychologic evaluation both in the MACS and also from a cohort of injecting drug users, we found no evidence for cognitive decline during the asymptomatic phase of infection (Fig. 5, Table 1) (128,129). In a prolonged longitudinal study within the MACS (126), we examined changes in cognitive function before and after development of clinical AIDS or a CD4+ count less than 200/mm^3. The study population included participants either with clinical AIDS ($n = 52$) or who had at least one measurement of CD4+ count less than 200/mm^3 ($n = 57$) and who had at least four separate neuropsychologic evaluations—two or more before and two or more after the diagnosis of AIDS. A group of subjects who developed HIV dementia ($n = 29$) was also included for comparison. The neuropsychologic test

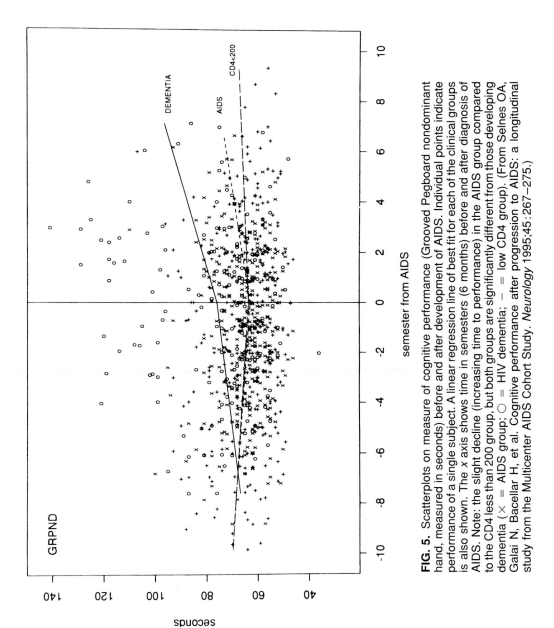

FIG. 5. Scatterplots on measure of cognitive performance (Grooved Pegboard nondominant hand, measured in seconds) before and after development of AIDS. Individual points indicate performance of a single subject. A linear regression line of best fit for each of the clinical groups is also shown. The x axis shows time in semesters (6 months) before and after diagnosis of AIDS. Note: the slight decline (increasing time to performance) in the AIDS group compared to the CD4 less than 200 group, but both groups are significantly different from those developing dementia (× = AIDS group; ○ = HIV dementia; — = low CD4 group). (From Selnes OA, Galai N, Bacellar H, et al. Cognitive performance after progression to AIDS: a longitudinal study from the Multicenter AIDS Cohort Study. *Neurology* 1995;45:267–275.)

TABLE 1. *Longitudinal neuropsychologic studies in asymptomatic HIV[a] infection*

Study	Year	Cohort	Follow-up (months)	Number of cases	Number of controls
Selnes et al.	1990	Homosexuals	18	238	170
Saykin et al.	1991	Homosexuals	18	21	21
Gastaut et al.	1990	Homosexuals	6–18	50	8
Selnes et al.	1992	Injecting drug users	12	37	69
Helmsteadter et al.	1992	Hemophiliacs	20	62	—[b]
Whitt et al.	1992	Hemophiliacs	24	25	25
Robertson et al.	1992	Homosexuals	24	118	0
Karlsen et al.	1993	Homosexuals	24	36	
Selnes et al.	1992	Injecting drug users	36	19	40

[a] Human immunodeficiency virus.
[b] No controls.

battery included measure of attention, memory, constructional abilities, and psychomotor speed. Before AIDS, the dementia group showed significant decline only on measures of psychomotor speed. For all other measures, there was no evidence of decline in performance before AIDS in the other groups. The group with clinical AIDS showed significant decline on psychomotor speed after the development of AIDS, but no decline on the other cognitive measures. The group with CD4+ count less than 200 did not show significant decline on any of the cognitive measures after the development of AIDS (defined by CD4+ count less than 200). Sensory neuropathy was associated with a significant decline in performance on measures of psychomotor speed. Antiretroviral therapy was not associated with any measurable changes in neuropsychologic performance (Fig. 5). These results are consistent with our previous studies showing no significant decline in cognitive function before AIDS, unless overt dementia develops, and no decline in immune-suppressed subjects without AIDS-defining illnesses (129). Stern et al. (135), in another large longitudinal study, showed poorer memory in HIV seropositive individuals and attenuation of practice effect in measures of language and attention, but not in more typically affected domains. They also showed an association between mortality and more rapid cognitive progression.

Neuropsychologic Studies in Symptomatic HIV Infection

Relatively few prospective studies of subjects with symptomatic HIV disease have been published. Marder et al. (78) reported that neurologic signs (specifically extrapyramidal and release signs) were more likely to develop over time in HIV seropositive individuals with mild to moderate CD4+ counts (baseline CD4+ count 407) than seronegatives. These neurologic signs appeared to be markers for cognitive impairment. In subjects who have developed clinical AIDS, there is a mild decline in fine motor skills, which may be related to the development of subclinical or clinical sensory neuropathy or to cerebral involvement, but no significant change in other cognitive domains. Results of a prospective study (35) of patients with AIDS-related complex (ARC) followed for 6 months to 2 years are consistent with the findings from the Selnes study. The performance of 15 ARC patients who progressed to AIDS was compared to a group of ARC patients who did not develop AIDS. There was a trend toward greater impairment among the progressers; however, there were few statistically significant differences between the two groups, and the area in which both progressers (to AIDS) and nonprogressers showed some degree of impairment was primarily motor function. Another study (133) examined longitudinal changes in cognition in a group of methadone-maintained patients and found significant decline in psychomotor speed over a 4-year period of follow-up. Only 12 patients had symptomatic HIV disease, however, limiting the interpretation of this study.

Overall, it appears that frank dementia is rare during the asymptomatic phase of HIV infection, and reports of frequent neuropsychologic abnormalities may reflect other confounding factors rather than direct effects of HIV infection. Particularly important confounds include premorbid neurologic disease, including head injury, substance abuse, and learning disorders. The effects of fatigue, anxiety, age, and education on the interpretation of neuropsychologic performance are critical. So how can we reconcile the biology of HIV infection—early CNS infection—with the apparent lack of CNS disease until much later in the infection. Presumably, cerebral reserve is sufficient to accommodate the small amounts of replicating virus present in the CNS during the asymptomatic phase of infection. It is not until later, when immunodeficiency is more advanced, that replication of HIV in the brain increases rapidly, with macrophage activation and the triggering of the neuron-damaging cascade of pathophysiologic events (see Chapter 4).

CLINICAL FEATURES OF HIV-ASSOCIATED DEMENTIA COMPLEX

The clinical features of HIV dementia were first described by Snider et al. (134) and then defined in greater detail by Navia et al. (98). Though there is some variability among patients, the syndrome is sufficiently stereotypic to be relatively easily recognized, particularly in a patient who is well known to the observer. In adults, the clinical manifestations of HIV dementia suggest predominantly subcortical involvement, at least initially (98). In a large personal series of 299 patients with HIV dementia evaluated at Johns Hopkins University, the four commonest presenting symptoms were memory impairment, gait difficulty, mental slowing, and depressive symptoms (principally withdrawal and lack of interest) (Fig. 6). Although a typical presentation includes prominent apathy, memory loss, cognitive slowing, and social withdrawal, some variability in presentation has been reported. Occasionally agitation or mania may be the initial manifestation (98). Generalized seizures can also occur as a manifestation of HIV dementia; however, they are usually not refractory and, in many cases, may be triggered by medications or illicit drugs (58).

The early symptoms are often subtle and may be confused with psychiatric complaints or overlooked (Table 2). In fact, in the busy setting of a large HIV clinic, particularly with multiple providers, early dementia is usually missed unless active screening procedures are in place. Typical symptoms described by the patient include increasing forgetfulness, difficulty with concentration, loss of libido, apathy, inertia, and waning interest in work and hobbies resulting in social withdrawal. Patients complain of losing track of conversation and the plots of books and films and of taking longer to complete more complex daily tasks. Impaired short-term memory causes difficulty with remembering appointments, medications, and telephone numbers. Motor complaints include poor handwriting, insecure balance, and a tendency

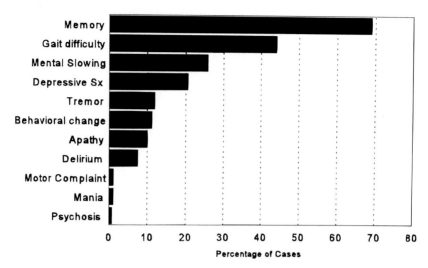

FIG. 6. Presenting symptoms in HIV dementia (Johns Hopkins University, *n* = 299).

to drop things easily. Gait difficulty is a relatively early symptom and may be similar to the impairment of postural reflexes in patients with other extrapyramidal diseases, including Parkinson's and Huntington's. Arendt et al. (5) examined postural control using static posturography and postural reflexes and confirmed the frequency of postural abnormalities in HIV-associated dementia. Friends and partners report shifts in personality with apathy, irritability, social withdrawal, and blunting of emotional responsiveness.

Neurologic examination is often normal in the early stages of HIV dementia, although there may be demonstrable impairments of rapid eye and limb movements and diffuse hyperreflexia (Fig. 7). Arendt et al. (4) have applied motor recording techniques to assess motor function in HIV dementia. Some patients showed a Parkinsonian-type tremor with a test of "most rapid contractions" (isometric index finger extension). These findings correspond to slowing of rapid repetitive movements (for example, thumb-finger tapping) on simple bedside testing. Eye movement abnormalities, including disturbances of both saccadic and smooth pursuit function, appear frequently in HIV dementia (30,91). As HIV dementia progresses, increased tone develops, particularly in the lower extremities, and is usually associated with tremor, clonus, frontal release signs, and hyperactive reflexes. Some of these signs may reflect the effects of an accompanying HIV-related myelopathy (105) and a peripheral neuropathy may develop concurrently. Focal neurologic signs should point to CNS opportunistic processes rather than HIV dementia. Retinal "cotton-wool" spots occur

TABLE 2. *Differential diagnosis of early HIV-associated dementia complex*

Bereavement	Recreational drugs
Depression	Medication
Anxiety	Metabolic encephalopathy
Alcohol	

From Harrison MJG, McArthur JC. *AIDS and neurology.* Churchill Livingstone; 1995.

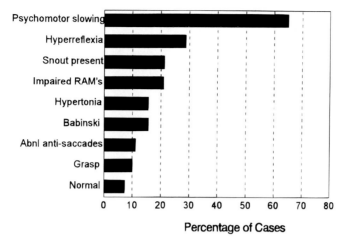

FIG. 7. Presenting signs of HIV dementia (Johns Hopkins University, *n* = 299).

in 60% of patients with AIDS but are not pathognomonic for HIV dementia (108). Myoclonus is not a feature, but generalized seizures may occur (58). Terminally, the patient is bed bound, incontinent, abulic, or mute, with decorticate posturing.

Price and Brew (114) have devised a staging system for HIV dementia that is widely used in both clinical and research areas (Table 3). The scale combines function impact of both cerebral and spinal cord dysfunction, however, I (J. C. M.) have found it more useful to grade the two areas separately because myelopathy can be accompanied by minimal or no dementia and vice versa. Thus, in practice, a severely demented patient with only mild myelopathy would be characterized as Memorial Sloan Kettering 3 (MSK 3; Dementia) MSK 1 (myelopathy). The subclinical stage 0.5, a stage when neurocognitive deficits may be present but frank dementia is not apparent, corresponds to the AAN terminology HIV-associated minor cognitive-motor impairment. This clinical staging system correlates well with performance on psychomotor speed measures and is useful to track progression and response to therapy.

With advancing dementia, new learning and memory deteriorate, there is a further slowing of mental processing, and some language impairment, dysnomia, reduced spontaneity, and abulia become more obvious (see Table 4). The later phases of the syndrome are characterized by global impairment with severe psychomotor retardation and mutism.

Neuropsychologic Involvement in HIV Dementia

Neuropsychologic features of HIV dementia reflect the prominence of subcortical involvement initially and are characterized by (a) memory loss characterized by impaired retrieval, (b) impaired manipulation of acquired knowledge, and (c) a general slowing of psychomotor speed and thought processes (Table 5). Neuropsychologic testing adds to the neurologic evaluation of suspected HIV dementia by quantifying the severity of cognitive impairment and defining the patterns of involvement. For example, attention, concentration, and language are usually not affected in HIV dementia, at least initially, fitting with the subcortical pattern of involvement. Mem-

TABLE 3. *Severity scales of dementia and myelopathy.*

Stage	Dementia	Myelopathy
0	Normal mental and motor function. Neurologic signs are within the normal age-appropriate spectrum.	Normal
0.5	Equivocal or subclinical: Absent, minimal, or equivocal symptoms *without impairment of work or capacity to perform (ADL).*[a] Exam may be normal or mildly abnormal; signs may include reflex changes (e.g., generalized increase in deep tendon reflexes with active jaw jerk, snout or glabellar sign) or mildly slowed ocular movements, but without clear slowing of extremity movements or loss of their dexterity or strength.	
1	Mild: Able to perform all but the more demanding aspects of work or ADL but with unequivocal evidence (symptoms or signs including performance on neuropsychologic testing) of intellectual or motor impairment. The abnormal motor signs usually include slow or clumsy movements of extremities.	Tandem gait may be impaired, but the patient can walk without assistance
2	Moderate: Able to perform basic activities of self-care at home but cannot work or maintain more demanding aspects of daily life (e.g., maintain finances, read text more complex than a tabloid newspaper)	Ambulatory, but may require single prop (e.g., cane)
3	Severe: Major intellectual incapacity (cannot follow news or personal events, cannot sustain complex conversation, considerable slowing of all output) or motor disbility	Cannot walk unassisted, requiring walker or personal support, usually with slowing and clumsiness of arms as well
4	End stage: Nearly vegetative. Intellectual and social comprehension and output are at a rudimentary level. Nearly or absolutely mute.	Paraparetic or paraplegic with double incontinence

Modified from Price RW, Brew BJ. The AIDS dementia complex. *J Infect Dis* 1988;158:1079–1083.
[a] Activities of daily living.

TABLE 4. *Late features of HIV dementia*

Global cognitive impairment	Spastic weakness
Mutism	Decorticate posture
Abulia	Ataxia
Severe psychomotor retardation	Myoclonus
Reduced insight/denial	Seizures
Hallucinations	

From Harrison MJG, McArthur JC. *AIDS and neurology.* Churchill Livingstone; 1995.

TABLE 5. *Cognitive domains most affected in early HIV dementia*

Psychomotor speed
Verbal and visual memory (retrieval rather than recognition)
Complex sequencing
Mental flexibility
Visual construction

From Harrison MJG, McArthur JC. *AIDS and neurology.* Churchill Livingstone; 1995.

ory impairments, both verbal and nonverbal, and deficits in psychomotor speed are characteristic of HIV dementia and are typically more severe than deficits in other cognitive domains (Fig. 8A–F, Table 5). Neuropsychologic testing should be an adjunct to the neurologic exam, not a replacement, and abnormalities on neuropsychologic testing are not necessarily specific. The influence of premorbid conditions,

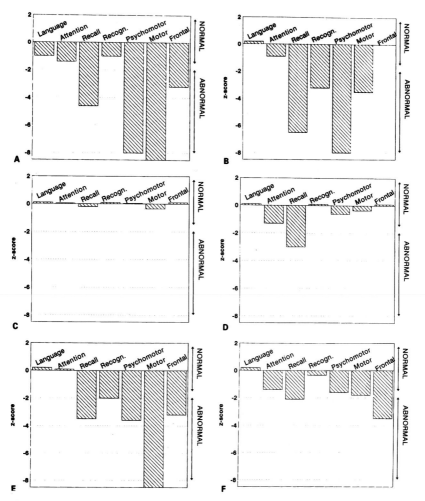

FIG. 8. A: A typical neuropsychologic profile from a 53-year-old homosexual man with moderate HIV dementia. Vertical axis indicates *Z*-score performance standard deviation units (note relatively preserved language, attention and recognition memory, but severely impaired recall memory and tests of psychomotor speed). **B:** Neuropsychologic profile from a 64-year-old homosexual male with HIV dementia and a history of heavy alcohol use. Note the difference in profiles with greater impairment of recognition memory than in the typical HIV dementia patient and less impairment on Grooved Pegboard. **C, D:** Neuropsychologic profiles from a patient with cognitive symptoms and major affective disorder before (C) and after (D) treatment. Note relative impairment of attention and concentration compared with psychomotor performance and improvement in all domains with antidepressant therapy. **E:** Profile from a patient with HIV dementia. **F:** Profile from a patient with HIV dementia and prominent frontal lobe dysfunction. (From Harrison MJG, McArthur JC. *AIDS and neurology.* Churchill Livingstone; 1995.)

including previous head trauma, learning disability, as well as the effects of systemic illness and substance abuse need to be considered carefully when interpreting results from cross-sectional neuropsychologic testing. Age and education are particularly critical variables which influence neuropsychologic performance independently. Because of the variability in performance related to education, age, stress of chronic disease, etc., the preferred method should be to assess change in neuropsychologic performance over time. The documentation of decline in two or more cognitive domains provides the most reliable evidence that there has been a change in cognitive abilities, since the expectation would be that performance should actually improve secondary to practice effects. When longitudinal assessments are not possible, the interpretation of cross-sectional neuropsychologic findings should take into account not only whether there is evidence of impairment, but also whether the pattern of impairment is consistent with what is known about HIV dementia. For these reasons, the most useful tests for screening for HIV dementia are those which examine psychomotor speed—Trailmaking, Grooved Pegboard, Symbol-Digit. The National Institute of Mental Health (NIMH) has proposed a battery for neuropsychologic assessment of AIDS-related cognitive changes (22). The proposed battery includes 25 different neuropsychologic tests covering 10 separate cognitive domains. The battery requires approximately 7 to 9 hours for administration. While this battery is well-suited to documenting the full range of neuropsychologic deficits associated with HIV infection, in general, it is impractical for longitudinal assessment and poorly tolerated in patients with advanced HIV infection. Selnes and Miller (125) described the development of a neuropsychologic test battery within the MACS. The choice of specific screening measures used were motivated by several concerns: (a) the tests were required to be sensitive to a wide range of impairments; (b) the tests needed to be robust to the effect of serial repetition; (c) the test battery needed to include tests already demonstrated to be sensitive to HIV-related changes in cognition; and (d) the overall test battery should be short. Selnes and Miller used a multistage approach to derive a brief neuropsychologic assessment battery sensitive to the effects of HIV infection. First, analysis of variance was used to identify measures that discriminated performance of patients with AIDS from those of seronegative controls. Second, factor analysis was used to identify major areas of cognitive function using data from the available neuropsychologic measures. The results agreed with previous investigators, identifying motor performance, speed of processing, and abstraction as the main areas of early cognitive deficits in patients with symptomatic HIV disease (104). Symptomatic HIV seropositive subjects performed worse than seronegative controls on measures of simple reaction time and choice reaction time, measures of divided attention and abstract, and measures of motor skills. Using factor analyses, Selnes and Miller combined all of the measures that theoretically ''probe'' a specific cognitive function. Table 6 represents the neuropsychologic test battery that is currently used in the MACS. The battery is brief and sensitive to the earliest symptoms of HIV-induced cognitive impairment. Standardized and familiar tests, such as Folstein's Minimental State Exam (MMSE), are not particularly useful for screening for HIV dementia, principally because the tests do not encompass timed tasks. Power et al. (113) have developed a modification of the MMSE, the HIV Dementia Scale (HDS). This 5-minute test instrument includes a measure of mental flexibility, the antisaccades test, timed alphabet, timed construction, and four-item recall. Its sensitivity is superior to the MMSE and it can be easily administered as a screening battery and used in the setting of an HIV clinic to provide baseline and follow-up

TABLE 6. *A short battery appropriate for evaluating suspected dementia cases*

Trailing tests; parts A and B
Grooved pegboard; dominant and nondominant hand
Symbol-digit modalities: raw score, paired recall
Rey Auditory Learning Verbal Test: trials 1–5, interference, recall after interference, delayed recall, delayed recognition
Rey Osterreith Complex Figure Test: copy, immediate recall, delayed recall
Stroop Color Interference Test
California Computerized Assessment Package (CalCap): simple reaction time, choice reaction time, sequential reaction time

cognitive data. Figure 9 shows the HDS. An alternative testing device is the Mental Alternation Test, a verbal version of the Trailmaking Test. One advantage is that it can be used in visually impaired patients or those unable to use paper and pencil. Jones et al. (145) showed that it could be administered in approximately 60 seconds and had a high sensitivity and specificity for abnormal performance on the Trailmaking Test Part B. As yet, this test has not been validated in a sample of dementia patients.

For monitoring treatment effects in patients with established dementia, a shorter battery has been developed by Sidtis, Price, and the AIDS Clinical Trials Neurology Group which measures treatment response well, is robust, and relatively resistant to practice effects (131). The "Micro" battery includes four tests—Timed Gait, Grooved Pegboard dominant hand, Digit-Symbol, and Finger Tapping nondominant. The "Macro" battery consists of 10 measures—WAIS-R Vocabulary, Timed Gait, Grooved Pegboard dominant and nondominant, Trailmaking Test A and B, Digit-Symbol, Finger Tapping dominant and nondominant, Rey Auditory Verbal Learning Test, and Profile of Mood State. Conversion of raw scores with age- and education-specific norms to units of standard deviation or *z scores* is recommended and allows for the easy comparison of scores between individuals. In trials of HIV dementia (132), a composite score representing the average of the sum of z scores from all completed neuropsychologic tests has provided a single measure of neuropsychologic function. This summary score correlates well with the clinical severity of HIV dementia, as judged by the MSK stage (131).

These neuropsychologic features fit with the pattern of subcortical dementia as encountered in extrapyramidal diseases, including Huntington's and Parkinson, progressive supranuclear palsy, and normal pressure hydrocephalus. Imaging data support this premise with evidence of a correlation between measured atrophy of the caudate region in HIV dementia (6,32). Hestad et al. (54) found significant correlation between caudate region atrophy as measured by enlargement of the bicaudate ratio (BCR) and impaired performance on several measures of neurocognitive performance, including Grooved Pegboard, Verbal Fluency, and Trailmaking Test. This suggests that subcortical damage and, particularly caudate region atrophy, underlies the subcortical pattern of neuropsychologic impairment (Fig. 10).

Course of Dementia

Without treatment, the dementia is rapidly progressive, with a mean survival of about 6 months, about half the average survival of nondemented AIDS patients (81,118). Unfortunately, survival times after diagnosis of HIV dementia have re-

HIV DEMENTIA SCALE

Max Score	Score	
		MEMORY - REGISTRATION
		Give four words to recall (dog, hat, green, peach) - 1 second to say each. Then ask the patient all 4 after you have said them.
4	( )	**ATTENTION**
		Anti-saccadic eye movements: 20 (twenty) commands.
		_____errors of 20 trials
		≤3 errors = 4; 4 errors = 3; 5 errors = 2; 6 errors = 1; >6 errors = 0
6	( )	**PSYCHOMOTOR SPEED**
		Ask patient to write the alphabet in upper case letters horizontally across the page (use back of this form) and record time: _____ seconds.
		≤21 sec = 6; 21.1 - 24 sec = 5; 24.1 - 27 sec = 4; 27.1 - 30 sec = 3; 30.1 - 33 sec = 2; 33.1 - 36 sec = 1; >36 sec = 0
4	( )	**MEMORY - RECALL**
		Ask for 4 words from Registration above. Give 1 point for each correct. For words not recalled, prompt with a "semantic" clue, as follows: animal (dog); piece of clothing (hat), color (green), fruit (peach). Give 1/2 point for each correct after prompting.
2	( )	**CONSTRUCTION**
		Copy the cube below; record time: ____ seconds.
		<25 sec = 2; 25 - 35 sec = 1; >35 sec = 0

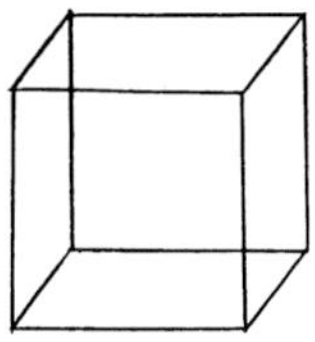

TOTAL SCORE: _____/16

Department of Neurology
Johns Hopkins University

FIG. 9. The HIV Dementia Scale. (From Harrison MJG, McArthur JC. *AIDS and neurology.* Churchill Livingstone; 1995, and Power C, Selnes OA, Grim JA, McArthur JC. *J Aids* 1995;8: 273–278.)

mained dismal, with no significant increase over the past 6 years, despite the more widespread use of antiretrovirals, nutritional supplements, and prophylactic treatments for systemic and CNS opportunistic infections (Fig. 11). The progression of HIV dementia can be quite variable, some patients having a "typical" progression with worsening neurologic deficits over 3 to 6 months, while others remain only mildly demented and cognitively stable right up to death (Fig. 12). A subset of individuals with HIV dementia have prolonged survival, sometimes for several years. While, in general, these individuals have higher CD4+ counts and slower immunologic decline, the determinants of prolonged survival with dementia remain unknown.

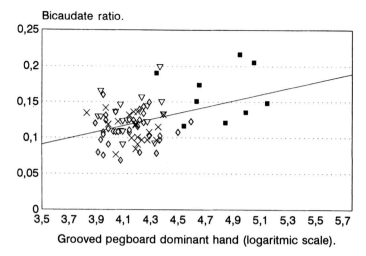

FIG. 10. Scatterplot of Grooved Pegboard dominant hand (logarithmic scale) and bicaudate ratio. (From Hestad K, McArthur JH, Dal Pan GJ, et al. Regional brain atrophy in HIV-1 infection: association with specific neuropsychological test performance. *Acta Neurol Scand* 1993; 88:112–118.)

The cause of this variability is uncertain, but it may depend on the degree of immuno-deficiency or the CNS effects of antiretroviral therapy. In one analysis based on 60 prospectively evaluated patients with dementia from Johns Hopkins University, rapid progression of cognitive deficits was associated with risk factors of receiving blood products or injection drug use, CD4+ count less than 200 at onset of dementia, magnetic resonance imaging (MRI) atrophy, and increased cerebrospinal fluid (CSF) tumor necrosis factor alpha (TNF-α). No differences in any other demographic features, clinical features of dementia, patterns of AIDS-defining illnesses, or antiret-roviral exposure were identified (Table 7) (88). Analysis of 40 autopsies from these 60 patients showed no differences in the frequency of multinucleated giant cells, myelin pallor, vacuolar myelopathy, or the abundance of immunostaining for viral antigens (gp41) or activated macrophages (HAM-56) (44).

Vacuolar Myelopathy and HIV Dementia

Spinal cord syndromes are discussed in Chapter 8. Although vacuolar myelopathy (NM) was originally included as part of the AIDS dementia complex because of the frequent coexistence of dementia and vacuolar myelopathy, it appears that VM can develop and progress as a discrete syndrome without dementia. Although rare as an initial presentation of AIDS, several well-documented patients have developed VM as their initial AIDS-defining illness (81). Pathologically, there are similarities with the pathology of HIV dementia—both show intense macrophage infiltration and activation with cytokine production within the tissue. One difference, however, is that multinucleated giant cells are relatively uncommon in the cord, even though PCR techniques can demonstrate HIV RNA within infiltrating macrophages (S. Wes-selingh, personal communication). Clinically affecting 5% to 10% of AIDS patients, the clinical expression of VM underestimates its frequency because VM can be detected at autopsy in up to 47% of adult AIDS patients (31). The syndrome is rarer

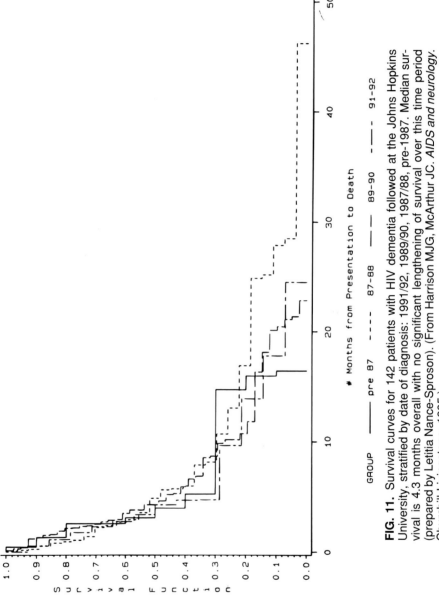

FIG. 11. Survival curves for 142 patients with HIV dementia followed at the Johns Hopkins University, stratified by date of diagnosis: 1991/92, 1989/90, 1987/88, pre-1987. Median survival is 4.3 months overall with no significant lengthening of survival over this time period (prepared by Letitia Nance-Sproson). (From Harrison MJG, McArthur JC. *AIDS and neurology.* Churchill Livingstone; 1995.)

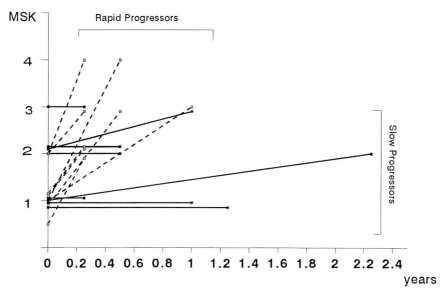

FIG. 12. Variability in progression with HIV dementia. "Rapid progressers" had a survival of 3 to 6 months, while "slow progressers" maintained cognitive stability for many months.

in children, occurring in only about 3%. The approach to evaluation and therapy for a patient with a predominantly myelopathic syndrome is discussed in Chapter 8.

DIAGNOSIS

In the early stages of HIV dementia, diagnosis is particularly difficult because the initial symptoms can be confused with depression, anxiety disorders, or the effects of psychoactive substances (see Table 2). The differential diagnosis of complaints of poor concentration and lapses in memory in the early stages of HIV dementia includes the effects of bereavement, anxiety, sensitivity to medications, recreational drugs, and toxic confusional states, for example, related to the hypoxia of *Pneumo-cystis carinii* pneumonia. Certain medications are particularly common causes of cognitive symptoms. These include tricyclic antidepressants, anxiolytics, hypnotics, narcotic analgesics, and muscle relaxants. Often, detailed historical information from

TABLE 7. *HIV dementia: comparison of rapid versus slow progressers (n = 30)*

	Rapid	Slow	P Value
Median survival (months)	4.1 ± 2.6	11.9 ± 12.4	0.0015*
CD4<200/mm³	93%	67%	0.09
Age	41 ± 10	39 ± 7	0.36
Homosexual risk	42%	86%	0.002*
Blood/IDU	38%	14%	0.06
MSK scores	1.1 ± 0.40	1.2 ± 0.49	NS
MRI atrophy	65%	35%	0.10
CSF TNF-α	4 ± 3.5	0	0.03*

IDU, intravenous drug users; MSK, Memorial Sloan Kettering; MRI, magnetic resonance imaging; CSF, cerebrospinal fluid; TNF-α, tumor necrosis factor alpha.

TABLE 8. *Clinical features useful for diagnosis of HIV-1-related dementia*

HIV-1 seropositivity (Western blot confirmation)
History of *progressive* cognitive/behavioral decline with apathy, memory loss, and slowed mental processing
Neurologic exam: diffuse CNS signs, including slowed rapid eye/limb movements, hyperreflexia, hypertonia, and release signs
Neuropsychologic assessment: progressive deterioration on serial testing in at least two areas, including motor speed, nonverbal memory, and frontal lobe
CSF analysis: elevated $\beta 2$ microglobulin, nonspecific abnormalities of immunoglobulin G and protein, exclusion of CMV[a] encephalitis, neurosyphilis, tuberculosis, and cryptococcal meningitis
Imaging studies: diffuse cerebral atrophy with ill-defined white matter hyperintensities on MRI, exclusion of opportunistic processes
Absence of major psychiatric disorder or intoxication
Absence of metabolic derangement, e.g., hypoxia, sepsis
Absence of active CNS opportunistic processes

[a] Cytomegalovirus.

friends, family, or co-workers is helpful and psychiatric consultation may be indicated. Differentiation from infections such as CMV encephalitis, cerebral toxoplasmosis, neurosyphilis, and cryptococcal or tuberculous meningitis is critical. Although relatively uncommon in the United States, tuberculous meningitis and cryptococcal meningitis are extremely prevalent in the developing world and can easily be confused with dementia. Table 8 lists features that may be helpful in establishing the diagnosis of HIV dementia. Table 9 indicates the clinical features which distinguish HIV dementia from other CNS processes. In the United States, one frequent CNS opportunistic infection which is easily mistaken for HIV dementia is CMV encephalitis. This presents in about 10% of all patients with AIDS as a rapidly developing encephalopathy (67). Distinguishing features from HIV dementia include more rapid onset, with frequent delirium and cranial nerve deficits; coexisting CMV infection (retinitis, colitis, etc.) in 60%; hyponatremia reflecting CMV adrenalitis in 80%; and in half, periventricular abnormalities on MRI consistent with a periventriculitis (57).

Cerebrospinal Fluid

The majority of patients with HIV dementia will have CSF abnormalities; however, a similar frequency of CSF abnormalities is found in neurologically normal HIV carriers. At present, no single CSF test or combination of tests can reliably diagnose HIV dementia; however, a completely normal CSF profile, with no abnormalities

TABLE 9. *Common brain diseases complicating AIDS: clinical differentiation*

Disorder	Course	Alert	Fever/HA	Focal exam
HIV dementia	weeks to months	NL	0	0
Toxoplasmosis	<2 weeks	↓	+	+ + +
1° Lymphoma	2–8 weeks	↓ or NL	0	+
PML	weeks to months	NL	0	+ +
Cryptococcus	<2 weeks	↓	+ + +	0
CMV encephalitis	<2 weeks	↓ or NL	+	0

Modified from Price RW. American Academy of Neurology (AAN) Annual Course #347. Infections of the nervous system. AAN; May 5, 1990.
HA, headache; NL, normal; PML, progressive multifocal leukoencephalopathy.

of protein or IgG points away from the diagnosis. Lumbar puncture is important to exclude opportunistic infections (OIs) in the patient with suspected HIV dementia, particularly in areas with high rates of neurosyphilis, tuberculosis (TB), or cryptococcosis, but in a typical case of dementia, one may rely on serologic screening for cryptococcal antigen and syphilis. The CSF should be examined for CMV PCR in a rapidly developing encephalopathy when CMV encephalitis is suspected. The CSF is usually acellular but may show a mild lymphocytic pleocytosis with proportions of CD4 and CD8 lymphocytes that parallel peripheral blood (87). Elevated total protein is found in about 65% of cases and increased total IgG fraction in up to 80% (81). Oligoclonal bands are found in up to 35%, but myelin basic protein is usually not elevated. Intrathecal synthesis (ITS) of anti-HIV-1 IgG is not specific since ITS can be detected in up to 45% of neurologically normal HIV carriers (141). Markers of immune activation in the CSF such as neopterin, quinolinic acid, and $\beta 2$ microglobulin are frequently elevated, although they are nonspecific and can also be elevated with OIs (16,17,55). A wide range of immune activation markers, including prostaglandin, cytokines, and platelet activating factor, have been shown to be increased in CSF (42). Most of these assays are not available in the clinical setting. The $\beta 2$ microglobulin is a stable immune activation marker which can be easily measured commercially by enzyme-linked immunosorbent assay (ELISA) or radioimmunoassay (RISA). In cases of suspected mild dementia, elevation of CSF $\beta 2$ microglobulin levels can be useful diagnostically to distinguish an evolving dementia from other causes of cognitive symptoms. Thus, a CSF $\beta 2$ microglobulin concentration above 3.8 mg/L, in the absence of CNS opportunistic infections, has a positive predictive value for dementia of 88% (86). Other markers of immune activation, such as elevated prostaglandin-E2 (49), neopterin (16), and quinolinic acid (55) levels are also often elevated in HIV dementia, but at this point remain research tools. In a research setting, serial CSF analysis has shown that a rising CSF $\beta 2$ microglobulin correlates with the evolution of HIV dementia, whereas stable or persistently low CSF $\beta 2$ microglobulin is found in individuals who remain cognitively intact (Fig. 13)

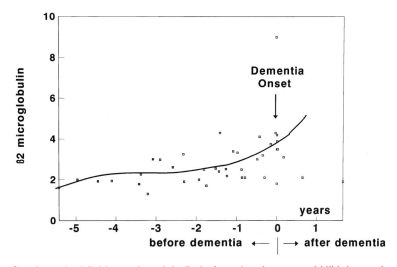

FIG. 13. Cerebrospinal fluid $\beta 2$ microglobulin before development of HIV dementia. Note the gradual rise in the 18 months before dementia onset. (From Harrison MJG, McArthur JC. *AIDS and neurology.* Churchill Livingstone; 1995.)

(95). Unfortunately this rise is not consistent enough for serial measurements of CSF $\beta 2$ microglobulin to be a clinically useful predictor of dementia.

The frequent spinal fluid abnormalities in the early stages of infection and the neuropathologic abnormalities in over 90% of patients dying with AIDS suggest that viral invasion of the nervous system occurs in the majority of HIV-1-infected patients, yet not all develop progressive dementia. Differences in neurotropism and neurovirulence or in rates of replication among strains of HIV-1 may be important in explaining this discrepancy.

Imaging Studies

Imaging studies are critical in the evaluation of suspected HIV dementia to exclude opportunistic processes. Radiologic features of HIV dementia include both central and cortical atrophy and white matter rarefaction. In children, calcifications of the basal ganglia are commonly seen on computed tomography (CT) scan. Central atrophy can often be observed to progress in parallel with clinical deterioration. Magnetic resonance imaging demonstrates white matter abnormalities in HIV dementia which appear as ill-defined areas of increased signal intensity on T2-weighted images (73,115). These often evolve from small ill-defined hyperintensities seen in deep white matter in patients with early HIV dementia to more diffuse abnormalities in severely demented individuals (Fig. 14). Generally, MRI is superior to CT scan in identifying the white matter changes. For example, Portegies et al. (110) detected white matter abnormalities on MRI in 73%, but in only 35% on CT. Table 10 contrasts the different radiologic patterns. Care needs to be taken in interpreting MRIs, particularly early in HIV infection, because several studies have shown that discrete focal white matter hyperintensities are quite common in neurologically normal individuals with or without HIV infection and probably have no pathologic significance (85).

Quantitative MRI studies have shown that selective caudate region atrophy occurs in HIV dementia (7,32) as well as in other basal ganglia structures and posterior cortex (6). A generalized loss of white matter occurs in HIV infection and is more severe in demented individuals. Proton magnetic resonance spectroscopy (MRS) has been used to study HIV dementia and it appears that it may be sensitive to changes in brain cellular oxidative metabolism or in neuronal markers such as N-acetyl aspartate (NAA) in areas that appear normal on standard MRI (90). This is particularly relevant with the recent observations of neuronal loss in cortical areas (38,79). We have demonstrated extensive metabolic changes in HIV dementia (Fig. 15) with reduced levels of NAA, a neuronal marker, and increased levels of choline, possibly reflecting astrocytosis in white matter regions (11). Recently, longitudinal changes in MRS have been shown to correlate with progression of dementia in a small group of patients, and it is possible that MRS may be a useful measure for assessing treatment efficacy (89). At this point, MRS remains a research tool, and its clinical utility remains to be determined.

Both single positron emission computed tomography (SPECT) and positron emission tomography (PET) have been used in small numbers of individuals with HIV dementia. Using PET, Rottenberg and colleagues demonstrated subcortical hypermetabolism in the early stages of HIV dementia, with later progression to cortical and subcortical hypometabolism (119). Normalization of PET abnormalities (150) and SPECT (138) has also been shown with administration of antivirals. With SPECT,

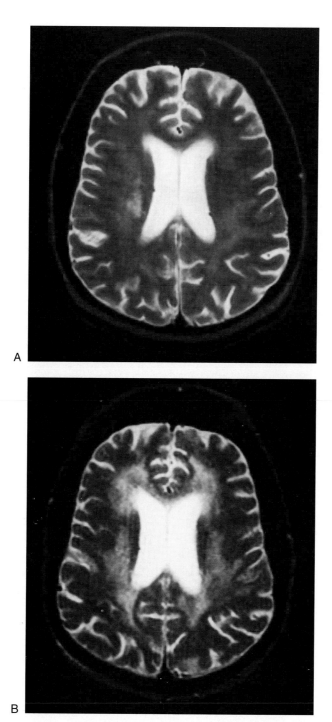

FIG. 14. Magnetic resonance imaging abnormalities in dementia. Evolving white matter hyper-intensities in HIV dementia (scans 10 months apart), mild white matter hyperintensity, cerebralatrophy **(A)**; severe central and moderate cortical atrophy in HIV dementia **(B)**.

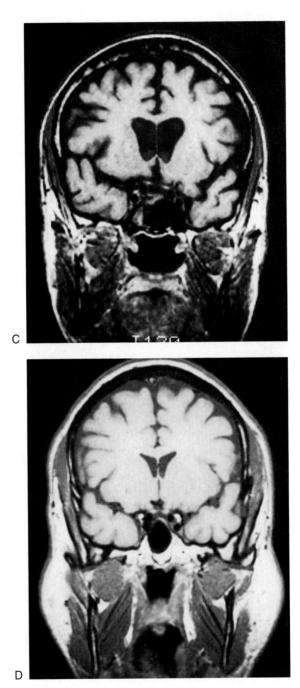

FIG. 14. *Continued.* **(C)**, compared to age-matched nondemented control **(D)**.

TABLE 10. *Radiologic pattern of HIV-related CNS disease*

Disorder	Number of lesions	Pattern	Enhancement	Location
HIV encephalitis	diffuse	Ill-defined	0	Deep white
Toxoplasmosis	1 to many	Ring mass	+ +	Basal ganglia
1° lymphoma	1 to several	Solid mass	+ + +	Periventricular
PML	1 to several	No mass	0	Subcortical white
Cryptococcus	1 to many	Punctate	0	Basal ganglia
CMV encephalitis	1 to several	Confluent	+ +	Periventricular

Modified from Price RW. American Academy of Neurology (AAN) Annual Course #347. Infections of the nervous system. AAN; May 5, 1990.

abnormalities in cerebral blood flow have been identified in most individuals with HIV dementia and in neurologically normal HIV-1 carriers, raising the possibility that SPECT might be a useful predictive tool (70). It appears, however, that some of these changes may be mimicked by the effects of cocaine (50), and so the usefulness of PET or SPECT in detection of HIV dementia or in assessing treatment effects remains to be determined.

Electrophysiology

Minor electroencephalogram (EEG) abnormalities have been reported in asymptomatic HIV seropositives (69), but not confirmed by the MACS using conventional (101) or quantitative EEG (100). Parisi et al. (102) carried out a prospective EEG study on asymptomatic HIV seropositives. Twenty-two of 40 with an EEG abnormality developed signs of CNS involvement, compared to 2 of 37 with normal records. Computer-analyzed EEG and brain mapping techniques have been studied to only a limited extent in established dementia, and the clinical utility of these sophisticated techniques remains uncertain (10,62).

The EEG has not been systematically studied in either the diagnosis or staging of HIV dementia. In the late stages of HIV dementia a diffuse slowing with low amplitudes is frequently noted (51,98); however, in less advanced stages of dementia the EEG may be normal in 50% of patients (81). The specificity of the EEG in differentiating psychiatric disorders from early dementia is uncertain and in general neither standard EEG nor computerized spectral analysis adds little information.

Event-related potentials (ERPs) have been used with mixed results by a number of investigators to probe the cerebral effects of CNS HIV infection. Some studies (116) suggest that auditory ERPs are the most sensitive for detecting subclinical CNS involvement, while others show more frequent abnormalities of somatosensory ERPs (63). A number of other studies are difficult to interpret because of small numbers of subjects, limited clinical characterization of neurologic deficits, or failure to take into account confounding influences of premorbid neurologic disease or substance abuse. Connolly et al. (27), in a longitudinal study of long-latency event-related potentials, showed no physiologic evidence of dysfunction during the asymptomatic stages of HIV infection. Messenheimer et al. (92) found delays in the latency of several components of ERPs in individuals with advanced HIV infection, and Iragui et al. (61), using a battery of evoked potentials, found that one or more evoked potentials were abnormal in 14% of asymptomatic carriers and 43% of subjects with

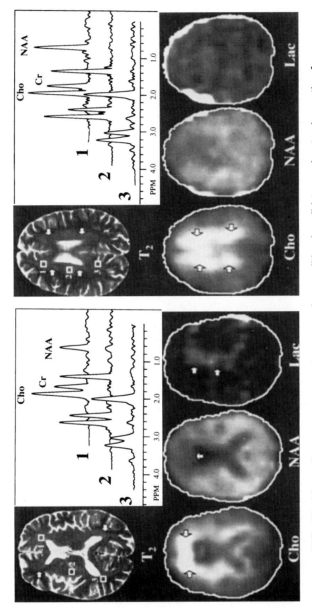

FIG. 15. Magnetic resonance spectroscopy abnormalities in mild to moderate dementia. **A:** T2-weighted MRI, representative spectra from selected voxels, and Cho, NAA, and Lac images from section 2 of the spectroscopic imaging sequence. **B:** T2-weighted MRI, representative spectra from selected voxels, and Cho, NAA, and Lac images from section 3 of the spectroscopic imaging sequence. Arrows = areas of abnormal signal intensity. (From Barker PB, Lee RR, McArthur JC. AIDS dementia complex: evaluation with proton MR spectroscopic imaging. *Radiology* 1995;195;58–64.)

ARC/AIDS, compared to only 2% of HIV seronegative controls. Koralnik et al. (69) also found an increased frequency of electrophysiologic abnormalities in asymptomatic HIV seropositives. Arendt et al. (3) are the only group to have used cognitive ERPs in patients with frank dementia. In 33 patients, clinical symptoms and time-dependent psychometric abilities correlated with N2 and P3 latency prolongations and with a generalized slowing of the alpha rhythm, suggesting involvement of both cortical and subcortical structures in HIV dementia. In a small number of subjects, Schroeder et al. (124) found a delay of P3 peak latencies and reduced P3 amplitudes in all seropositives, including asymptomatic HIV seropositives when compared to seronegative controls. The specificity and significance of these findings and their predictive value for development of frank dementia remain uncertain (9). In an individual patient, none of these studies has been shown to have diagnostic or prognostic utility and none of these measures has been shown to be useful in following treatment response.

PATHOLOGIC FEATURES

These are described in detail in Chapter 18. The clinical, radiologic, and pathologic features of HIV dementia suggest a predominantly subcortical pattern of neurocognitive deficits, with prominent leukoencephalopathy, but recent radiologic and pathologic studies have demonstrated involvement of the cortex with neuronal loss (38,43,79,147). Because of the absence of multinucleated giant cells (MNGCs) or diffuse myelin pallor in 50% of demented individuals, indirect mechanisms of neuronal damage are probably important, including local cytokine release and other toxic substances from activated macrophages or from neurotoxic effects of HIV proteins.

Despite the wealth of pathologic descriptions, most studies have not used prospective clinical information to provide an accurate clinical-pathologic correlation. The relationship of any of these pathologic changes to the clinical features of progressive dementia in AIDS remains unclear. There have been only a few studies specifically addressing clinical-neuropathologic correlation in AIDS dementia in which the clinical diagnosis of AIDS dementia was based on prospective patient identification. The original description of the "AIDS dementia complex" involved a retrospective chart review and correlated neuropathologic changes with the presence or absence of dementia (97). A correlation was found between the presence of MNGCs, myelin pallor, and the severity of dementia. However, not all patients with dementia showed these changes. We recently completed a prospective analysis of HIV dementia and found that only 25% of cases with HIV dementia had MNGCs, and 50% showed neither MNGCs nor white matter pallor (45). The brains of these clinically characterized patients were immunocytochemically stained for viral antigens (gp41) and macrophage activation (HAM-56) (44). A highly significant correlation between the abundance of activated macrophage/microglia staining and the severity of dementia was found. A significant association between the abundance of macrophage staining and the presence of diffuse myelin pallor or multinucleated giant cells in severely demented patients was also demonstrated. Staining for viral antigens (gp41) showed only a trend for patients with more severe dementia to have more abundant gp41 immunoreactivity. In fact, several nondemented patients showed abundant gp41 immunoreactivity and several severely demented patients showed little to no gp41 immunoreactivity. Immunopositive cells staining for gp41 were found in the majority of cases from both demented and nondemented groups (Fig. 16). In contrast to previous analyses (48), we found no association between gp41 or HAM-56 immunostaining and antiretroviral use. We also found no association between gp41 or HAM-56 abundance and the length of survival after AIDS, arguing against the hypothesis that viral burden or macrophage and microglial activation increases directly as a function of the duration of immunosuppression. These data suggest that the presence of productive HIV-infected cells within the brain as identified by immunostaining for gp41 is nearly universal in patients dying with AIDS but that this is not specific for the clinical syndrome of HIV dementia. These data are a strong confirmation of the importance of indirect mechanisms (as discussed in Chapter 4), probably triggered by HIV infection in the brain, in the pathogenesis of HIV-associated dementia. It seems likely that the presence of HIV within the brain is necessary but not sufficient to cause HIV dementia. These data are consistent with Petito's study of vacuolar myelopathy in which she found that HIV antigen and DNA correlated with macrophage infiltration and not vacuolar myelopathy (106).

It appears likely that after productive HIV infection within the CNS there is an activation of macrophages and microglia with the release of cytokines into the brain parenchyma. The cytokines may play a number of roles, including the amplification of HIV replication, stimulation of astrocytosis, and via autocrine feedback loops, additional production of cytokines and arachidonic acid metabolites. Activated astrocytes may play a role in modulating and amplifying the release of neurotoxic substances. Stimulation of the N-methyl-d-aspartate (NMDA) with ingress of calcium may be the final common pathway for neuronal damage.

Viral Load and HIV Dementia

Although, up to now, the relationship between systemic HIV load and neurologic decline has not been defined fully, evidence is beginning to appear that systemic viral load probably plays and important role in ''driving'' the development of cognitive dysfunction. Several virologic measures have been used to assess HIV load, including p24 antigen in blood and CSF, limiting dilution cultures, determination of plasma viremia, and quantitative PCR to detect HIV proviral DNA or RNA transcripts. Studies of systemic viral load have demonstrated that increasing systemic HIV load, assessed by p24 antigen (1,39,71,76,103), plasma viremia (28), or the ratio of genomic RNA to viral DNA sequences (93), correlates with increasing stage of HIV infection, is associated with progression to AIDS in HIV seropositives, and generally portends a poor prognosis. To date, similar correlations of HIV load with neurologic symptoms or dementia have been limited. In postmortem brain, using Southern blot analysis, Shaw et al. (130) demonstrated more viral DNA in brain than in lymph nodes or spleen. By contrast, Vazeux et al. (142) found HIV antigen in only three of nine children with histologic findings of HIV encephalitis, although all had HIV detectable by PCR within the brain. Studies of HIV load in the CSF have been equally confusing. Goswami et al. (46) used PCR to detect HIV sequences in CSF and found positive PCR in 95% of HIV-infected patients with neurologic disease but only 20% of patients without. By contrast, Steuler et al. (136) found proviral DNA in a higher proportion of CSF cells than in peripheral blood mononuclear cells, although there was no correlation with neurologic disease. Buffet et al. (20) found that neither HIV isolation nor p24 antigen detection in CSF were associated with

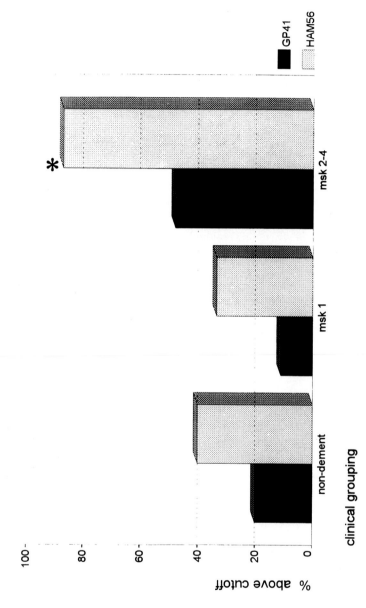

FIG. 16. Frequency of "abundant" immunostaining within the clinical groups. For gp41 the cutoff was >3/6, and for HAM-56 >4/6. Differences among the groups were significant for HAM-56 (p = 0.01) but not for gp41 (p = 0.066).

cognitive symptoms. Other studies of CSF p24 antigen have also shown conflicting results. In early studies, p24 antigen was detected in CSF in only about 50% of patients with dementia (47,111). However, using acid hydrolysis to increase the assay sensitivity, Royal et al. (120) detected p24 antigen in CSF in two-thirds of patients with severe dementia (MSK 2 through 4). Further work is needed to define the relationship between systemic HIV burden and neurologic disease. The conflicting results may reflect technical differences, or more likely, the fact that productive HIV infection in the body may be sequestered in lymphoid tissue, so sampling the blood does not directly assess total body burden of HIV.

Host Factors in HIV Dementia

To date, epidemiologic studies have not defined any specific host factors which clearly predispose to HIV dementia. In the MACS analysis (84), apart from age, no specific demographic factors correlated with an increased hazard of dementia. However, with the demonstration that there is overproduction of certain cytokines such as TNF, within the brains of patients with HIV dementia, genetic factors may play a role in determining progression to dementia. The gene coding for TNF-α lies within the major histocompatibility complex (MHC) on chromosome 6, and several studies have suggested that the level of TNF production (14) and rapid progression to AIDS are linked to the MHC (41). There is an association between certain haplotypes and an increased risk of progression to AIDS (68). It is plausible that a particular haplotype might be associated with an overproduction of TNF-α or other macrophage activating cytokines, such as interleukin 12 (IL-12) or macrophage colony stimulating factor (MCSF).

Entry of infected monocytes into the brain appears to depend on the expression of certain adhesion molecules on the capillary endothelium. Monocytes only adhere in the presence of VCAM-1, an endothelial adhesion molecule of the immunoglobulin supergene family. Sasseville et al. (122) found that VCAM-1 was only expressed in SIV-infected macaques with encephalitis, and not in those without, suggesting that expression of adhesion molecules may determine the entry of infected macrophages. The expression of the adhesion molecules may also vary among humans, thus providing another area in which host factors determine the development of neurologic disease.

HIV Tropism and HIV Dementia

Because not all HIV-infected patients, even in the very last stages of AIDS, become demented, it has been suggested that there may be specific neurotropic or neurovirulent strains of HIV. Several aspects of the biology of HIV are important in this regard, including its neuroinvasiveness (ability to invade the nervous system), neurotropism (ability to infect cells in the brain parenchyma), and neurovirulence (ability to cause neural damage). The V3 envelope region of HIV is an important determinant of cell tropism, and several groups have shown that specific sequences within this region affect tropism for lymphocytes and macrophages (25,146). In general, most isolates of HIV derived from brain grow more readily in cultured macrophages than lymphocytes. Watkins et al. (144) have shown that macrophage-tropic strains grow more readily in primary cultures of human microglia. Sequential studies with SIV-infected macaques have shown that lymphocyte-tropic SIV produces no brain infection. However, serial intracerebral inoculation induces envelope mutations, changing the lymphocyte-tropic strain into a macrophage-tropic strain, which is capable of producing encephalitis. Desrosiers et al. (34) have shown that macrophage tropism is a prerequisite for productive infection within the brain (neurotropism) but that not all macrophage-tropic strains are equally neurotropic.

Another area of the HIV genome which may have relevance for neurotropism is the long terminal repeat (LTR). Corboy et al. (29) suggested that LTR sequences may affect tropism for specific CNS cells. Because the LTR controls transcription activity, it is possible that sequence differences in an LTR may play a role in the productivity of HIV infection within the brain and thus affect the neurovirulence of a particular HIV strain.

We recently showed that there were specific sequence differences in brain-derived HIV-1 clones from demented patients, suggesting that there may be neurovirulent strains of HIV-1 (112). One hypothesis linking these observations is that specific mutations in the dominant HIV strain in an infected person may lead to the emergence of macrophage-tropic quasi-species. The emergence of macrophage-tropic strains which are also neurotropic leads to the development of productive HIV infection within the brain and subsequently to encephalitis.

Nutritional and Vitamin Deficiencies

A relative or absolute deficiency of vitamin B_{12} has been proposed as a cofactor in the neurologic impairment associated with HIV infection. Herbert et al. (53) found that up to 50% of patients with HIV infection had subtle evidence of impaired absorption of B_{12}. Serum levels and Schilling tests might be normal, but low levels of serum holotranscobalamin II implied impending deficiency. The changes were attributed to gastric changes due to HIV and opportunistic infections. Beach et al. (12) found low serum B_{12} in 25% of asymptomatic HIV-infected individuals and further showed some relationship between such findings and performance on some cognitive tests. The hypothesis is that poor delivery of B_{12} to nervous tissue where glial cells only have receptors for holotranscobalamin leads to or aggravates dysfunction through impaired methyl group transfer and buildup of homocysteine (52). However, patients with HIV infection, even with neurologic signs ($n = 18$), had normal CSF levels of methylmalonic acid (MMA), which is normally low in pernicious anemia (139). There is as yet no clear indication to prescribe regular B_{12} injections in the absence of pathologically low serum levels.

TREATMENT OF HIV DEMENTIA

Despite the unresolved questions in pathogenesis, antiretroviral agents are currently used in the treatment of HIV dementia. Five antiretroviral agents are currently licensed in the United States—ZDV (Retrovir), didanosine (ddl, Videx), dideoxycytidine (ddC, Hivid), stavudine (d4T, Zerit), and lamuvidine (3TC). All are nucleoside analogues that act by inhibiting reverse transcriptase, an enzyme critical in HIV's life cycle. An important point is that these agents act at a preintegration site in the replicative life cycle of HIV and are less likely to be effective in cells with a slow turnover rate, including macrophages and microglia. This has important implications for infection in the CNS, where these are principal targets. The nucleoside analogues are only active against replicating HIV and not latent provirus. Differing toxicities are seen with each: ZDV—anemia, myopathy; ddl—pancreatitis, neuropathy; ddC—stomatitis, neuropathy; d4T—neuropathy. The frequency of neuropathy is about 20% with ddC and 10% to 15% with ddl and d4T. The nucleoside analogues are only active against replicating HIV, not latent provirus. *In vitro* resistance can develop to all of them within 6 to 12 months of use, although the clinical significance of this is uncertain.

Neuroprotective Effects of Antiretrovirals

More widespread and earlier use of ZDV may have reduced the incidence of HIV dementia; a drop in the incidence of HIV dementia from 53% before ZDV was available to 10% has been reported (109). Whether this represents a true prophylactic effect or an attenuation of the neurologic disease is unclear. More recent studies have shown stable incidence rates in the past few years and have not shown any definite neuroprotective effects of antiretrovirals (8). Evidence from the multicenter licensing trial (40) of ZDV in patients with AIDS or ARC suggests that this drug improves neuropsychologic function even without frank dementia (123). Although this study excluded patients with frank dementia, a proportion had measurable neuropsychologic deficits. The ZDV-treated patients showed significant improvements in cognitive performance, particularly in measures of psychomotor speed, which was sustained for the 16 weeks of the study. Unfortunately, the study was concluded after only 16 weeks, so the long-term effects of antiretrovirals on cognition are not yet known.

Treatment of Established Dementia

Early open-label studies with ZDV in demented individuals showed promising improvements in clinical functioning, neuropsychologic performance, and, in one case, normalization of PET scans (150). The optimal dose of ZDV for treatment of HIV dementia has not been determined. Most of the studies above used doses of 1,000 to 1,500 mg daily; however, the recommended dose of ZDV for general use has now been reduced to 600 mg because this dose has equivalent efficacy in preventing systemic infections (143). Children treated with intravenous ZDV showed dramatic improvements in neuropsychologic performance and, in some cases, reversal of cerebral atrophy (33,107). Improvements in adaptive behavior have also been demonstrated in encephalopathic children (148). Animal experiments with murine retrovirus infections have better viral inhibition with continuous infusion of ZDV than with intermittent bolus therapy (15).

Data from the only placebo-controlled trial of ZDV in HIV dementia have suggested that the greatest neurocognitive improvement is seen with very high doses of ZDV, around 2,000 mg daily (132). The effect was modest, however, and no change in clinical severity of dementia was demonstrated. Whether significant improvement can be induced with lower doses remains to be proven, although experience with open-label use of ZDV suggests that cognitive function be improved with doses of 800 to 1,000 mg, particularly in an ZDV-naive patient. Our current practice for treatment of established dementia is to start ZDV at 1,000 mg daily, or if ZDV is already in use, to increase the dose. Blood counts should be checked regularly

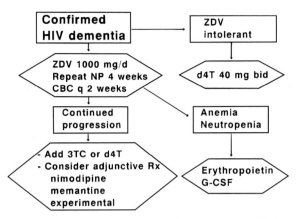

FIG. 17. Algorithm for assessment and treatment of HIV dementia.

(Fig. 17), and anemia or neutropenia can be controlled by dose reduction or the use of the hematopoietic growth factors, erythropoietin (Procrit) or granulocyte colony stimulating factor (GCSF) (Neupogen).

In patients who develop HIV dementia and are ZDV intolerant, substitution of d4T 40 mg b.i.d. is appropriate, although as yet, there is no definite proof of its efficacy. There is very little information about the CNS efficacy of the other dideoxy-nucleosides, and CNS penetrance of ddI and ddC is limited—about 20%, compared to about 50% with ZDV or d4T. Didanosine has been shown to improve IQ scores in children where plasma concentration of ddI correlated both with IQ improvement and decline in p24 antigen (21). In adults, there is only very limited information about the therapeutic effects of ddI, d4T, or ddC for dementia (151).

In our own open-label studies and also in studies by Portegies et al. (110), it has been observed that dementia can be reversed with antiretroviral therapy but that the duration of treatment response varies and, for unexplained reasons, some individuals fail to respond (Fig. 18). Whether this is because of irreversible neuronal loss or the

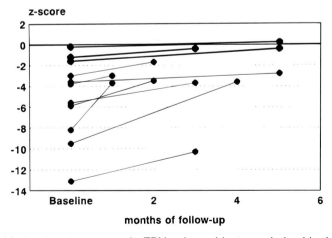

FIG. 18. Variable treatment response in ZDV naive subjects, as judged by improvement in psychomotor speed. Note that some individuals with very severe impairment may improve dramatically.

development of resistance to antiretroviral agents is uncertain. Few studies have examined why some demented patients respond and others fail to, and there has been little study of patterns of response for longer than a few months of treatment. Tartaglione et al. (137) noted neurologic improvement in most patients with mild neurologic abnormalities but no relationship between treatment response and CSF ZDV concentration, cumulative ZDV dose, or HIV isolation from CSF. Most observations of treatment response have relied on changes in neuropsychologic or neurologic testing. Other outcome measures may be helpful, particularly in the research setting. For example, several studies have shown improvements in markers of immune activation in the CSF (16,55). Neurophysiologic measurements may improve with ZDV treatment (2), and several studies have shown improvements in MRI white matter hyperintensities (personal observation; Post et al.) (138), cerebral atrophy (107), or PET scans (36).

In an open-label study of 30 patients with HIV dementia, Tozzi et al. (138) observed improvements in clinical severity in 50% after 1 month of therapy, and 83% after 6 months, using doses of 500 to 1,000 mg/day. Survival was predicted by clinical severity at entry, and 8 patients who had initially responded showed deterioration after 6 to 12 months. Interestingly, MRI white matter hyperintensities improved in 6 of 13 patients, and SPECT scans showed reductions in uptake deficits in 9 of 13. This study is one of the most comprehensive to date and shows that, at least for patients with mild to moderate HIV dementia, clinical improvements can be sustained for several months.

Several autopsy series have suggested a beneficial effect from the use of antiretrovirals by observing reductions in the frequency of multinucleated giant cells with antiretroviral use (45,48,140). In contrast, in prospectively studied patients at autopsy, we found no correlation between immunocytochemical scores for HIV gp41 or macrophage activation and the length of antiretroviral use. This discrepancy could reflect differences in the timing of discontinuation of antiretrovirals. For example, discontinuation of antiretrovirals in the weeks just prior to death might be associated with a ''preterminal'' rebound in the production of HIV in the brain. Recent studies of the kinetics of HIV replication suggest that the replicative cycle of HIV-1 is very short, so even a few weeks off antiretrovirals might change tissue levels of HIV and gp41 immunostaining considerably (56).

Another large group of ''adjunctive'' agents have been developed based on advances in our understanding of the pathophysiologic mechanisms of HIV dementia. Some of these are reviewed in Chapter 4, Pathophysiology. It seems likely that, in the future, effective and sustained treatment of established dementia will require both antiretroviral and agents targeting neuron-damaging mechanisms. Several experimental treatments have been tried in dementia or trials are planned.

One agent, a synthetic pentapeptide ''peptide T'' (18), may be effective in treating HIV dementia by blocking the actions of TNF-α. This agent is currently under study in the United States in a large placebo-controlled trial. Alternative treatments currently being explored include calcium channel antagonists, such as nimodipine, which may block viral protein induced neurotoxicity (74). In the recently completed AIDS Clinical Trials Group (ACTG) protocol 162, a phase I double-blind, placebo-controlled trial, patients with AIDS dementia were randomized to receive nimodipine, 60 mg 5 times daily, or nimodipine, 30 mg t.i.d., or placebo, with antiretrovirals. In this study, nimodipine was well tolerated and there was some improvement in neurocognitive performance (the study was not powered to be an efficacy trial).

TABLE 11. *Potential novel treatments for HIV dementia*

Antiretrovirals	Calcium channel blockers
Nucleoside RTI	Nimodipine
Nonnucleoside RTI	Glutamate/NMDA
Protease inhibitors	Memantine
Cytokine blockers	Gabapentin
Pentoxifylline	Antioxidants
Thalidomide	OPC14117
Peptide T	Thioctic acid
NHDG	

RTI, reverse transcriptase inhibitor; NMDA, N-methyl-d-aspartate; NHDG, nordihydroguiaretic acid.

Although efficacy data are not yet available, nimodipine is a licensed drug (but very expensive) and can be prescribed for the patient with progressive dementia. Other potential agents are listed in Table 11 and include cytokine antagonists and antioxidants. Pilot trials of the latter class of agents are underway in the United States. In the future, potentially neuron-protective agents, such as memantine, which block NMDA receptors may be proven as useful adjunctive therapy (75).

Symptomatic treatment is an important adjunct to antiviral treatment. Patients with HIV dementia are extremely susceptible to the adverse effects of psychoactive drugs, so hypnotics and anxiolytics should be avoided. Small doses of neuroleptics, such as haloperidol (Haldol), 0.5 mg b.i.d. to t.i.d., may be needed in the agitated or combative patient; however, patients with HIV dementia appear to have neuroleptic sensitivity. Hriso et al. (60) found extrapyramidal symptoms were 2.5 times as high among patients with AIDS and suggested that they were more susceptible to extrapyramidal symptoms than psychotic patients without AIDS. If marked depressive symptoms are present, tricyclic antidepressants or fluoxetine (Prozac) can be tried in doses 25% to 50% of the usual dose. Full doses of tricyclics may precipitate delirium, and serum levels should be monitored frequently. In patients with progressive dementia, medicolegal issues should be discussed at any early stage before the dementia becomes too severe: establishing a power of attorney, completion of a living will, and arrangement for the dispersal of assets.

FUTURE PROJECTIONS

It is estimated that HIV dementia occurs in 20% of individuals with advanced HIV disease. With an estimated one million individuals already infected in the United States alone, we can anticipate an annual incidence of HIV dementia of 10,000 cases, similar to the annual incidence of multiple sclerosis. In young Americans HIV has become the leading cause of dementia and places tremendous burdens on caregivers, families, and neurologic services. With the advances in our understanding of the pathophysiologic mechanisms and the rapid initiation of trials of novel neurologic therapies, we are optimistic that the outlook for preventing and treating dementia is brighter now than at any time during the epidemic.

ACKNOWLEDGMENTS

We are grateful to the many patients and research volunteers who have contributed to our studies and to our many colleagues at Johns Hopkins for their advice and support. We acknowledge the work of the AIDS Service and the medical and pathology house staff. Our studies are supported by the National Institutes of Health, grants NS 26643, AI 35042, and RR 00722, and by the Charles A. Dana Foundation. Some of this chapter was modified from *AIDS and Neurology,* by MJG Harrison and JC McArthur, Churchill-Livingstone, Edinburgh, 1995.

REFERENCES

1. Allain JP, Laurian Y, Paul DA, et al. Long-term evaluation of HIV antigen and antibodies to p24 and gp41 in patients with hemophilia. Potential clinical importance. *N Engl J Med* 1987;317: 1114–1121.
2. Arendt G, Hefter H, Hilperath F, von Giesen HJ, Strohmeyer G, Freund HJ. Motor analysis predicts progression in HIV-associated brain disease. *J Neurol Sci* 1994;123:180–185.
3. Arendt G, Hefter H, Jablonowski H. Acoustically evoked event-related potentials in HIV-associated dementia. *EEG Clin Neurophysiol* 1993;86:152–160.
4. Arendt G, Hefter H, Neuen-Jacob E, et al. Electrophysiological motor testing, MRI findings and clinical course in AIDS patients with dementia. *J Neurol* 1993;240:439–445.
5. Arendt G, Maecker H-P, Purrmann J, Homberg V. Control of posture in patients with neurologically asymptomatic HIV infection and patients with beginning HIV-1-related encephalopathy. *Arch Neurol* 1994;51:1232–1235.
6. Aylward EH, Brettschneider PD, McArthur JC, et al. MRI grey matter volume reductions in HIV-1 dementia. *Am J Psychiatr* 1995;152(7):987–994.
7. Aylward EH, Henderer JD, McArthur JC, et al. Reduced basal ganglia volume in HIV-1-associated dementia: results from quantitative neuroimaging. *Neurology* 1993;43:2099–2104.
8. Bacellar H, Munoz A, Miller EN, et al. Temporal trends in the incidence of HIV-1 related neurologic diseases: Multicenter AIDS Cohort Study, 1985–1992. *Neurology* 1994;44:1892–1900.
9. Baldeweg T, Lovett E. Psychophysiology and neurophysiology of HIV infection. *Int Rev Psychiatr* 1991;3:331–342.
10. Baldeweg T, Gruzelier JH, Stygall J, et al. Detection of subclinical motor dysfunctions in early symptomatic HIV infection with topographical EEG. *Int J Psychophysiol* 1993;15:227–238.
11. Barker PB, Lee RR, McArthur JC. AIDS dementia complex: evaluation with proton MR spectroscopic imaging. *Radiology* 1995;195:58–64.
12. Beach RS, Morgan R, Wilkie F, et al. Plasma vitamin B12 level as a potential cofactor in studies of human immunodeficiency virus type-1-related cognitive changes. *Arch Neurol* 1992;49:501–506.
13. Belman AL, Diamond G, Dickson D, et al. Pediatric acquired immunodeficiency syndrome. Neurologic syndromes [published erratum appears in *Am J Dis Child* 1988;142(5):507]. *Am J Dis Child* 1988;142:29–35.
14. Bendtzen K, Morling N, Fomsgaard A, et al. Association between HLA-DR2 and production of tumour necrosis factor alpha and interleukin 1 by mononuclear cells activated by lipopolysaccharide. *Scand J Immunol* 1988;28:599–606.
15. Bilello JA, Eiseman JL, Standiford HC, Drusano GL. Impact of dosing schedule upon suppression of a retrovirus in a murine model of AIDS encephalopathy. *Antimicrob Agents Chemother* 1994; 38:628–631.
16. Brew BJ, Bhalla RB, Paul M, et al. Cerebrospinal fluid neopterin in human immunodeficiency virus type-1 infection. *Ann Neurol* 1990;28:556–560.
17. Brew BJ, Bhalla RB, Paul M, et al. Cerebrospinal fluid β2 microglobulin in patients with AIDS dementia complex: an expanded series including response to zidovudine treatment. *AIDS* 1992;6: 461–465.
18. Bridge TP, Heseltine PNR, Parker ES, et al. Results of extended peptide T administration in AIDS and ARC patients. *Psychopharmacol Bull* 1991;27:237–245.
19. Britton CB, Marquardt MD, Koppel B, Garvey G, Miller JR. Neurological complications of the gay immunosuppressed syndrome: clinical and pathological features. *Ann Neurol* 1982;12:80.
20. Buffet R, Agut H, Chieze F, et al. Virological markers in the cerebrospinal fluid from HIV-1 infected individuals. *AIDS* 1991;5:1419–1424.
21. Butler KM, Husson RN, Balis RM, et al. Dideoxyinosine in children with symptomatic human immunodeficiency virus infection. *N Engl J Med* 1991;324:137–144.
22. Butters N, Grant I, Haxby J, et al. Assessment of AIDS-related cognitive changes: recommendations of the NIMH Workshop on Neuropsychological Assessment Approaches. *J Clin Exp Neuropsychol* 1990;12:963–978.
23. Catalan J, Thornton S. Whatever happened to HIV dementia? *Int J STD AIDS* 1993;4:1–4.
24. Centers for Disease Control. Revision of the CDC surveillance case definition for acquired immunodeficiency syndrome. *MMWR Morb Mortal Wkly Rep* 1987;36(Suppl 1S):3S–15S.

25. Cheng-Mayer C, Shioda T, Levy JA. Host range, replicative, and cytopathic properties of human immunodeficiency virus type 1 are determined by very few amino acid changes in tat and gp 120. *J Virol* 1991;65:6931–6941.

26. Chiesi A, Agresti MG, Dally LG, et al. Decrease in notifications of AIDS dementia complex in 1989–1990 in Italy: possible role of the early treatment with zidovudine. *Medicina* 1990;10:415–416.

27. Connolly S, Manji H, McAllister RH, et al. Long-latency event-related potentials in asymptomatic human immunodeficiency virus type 1 infection. *Ann Neurol* 1994;35:189–196.

28. Coombs RW, Collier AC, Allain JP, et al. Plasma viremia in human immunodeficiency virus infection. *N Engl J Med* 1989;321:1626–1631.

29. Corboy JR, Buzy JM, Zink MC, Clements JE. Expression directed from HIV long terminal repeats in the central nervous system of transgenic mice. *Science* 1992;258:1804–1808.

30. Currie J, Benson E, Ramsden B, Perdices M, Cooper D. Eye movement abnormalities as a predictor of the acquired immunodeficiency syndrome dementia complex. *Arch Neurol* 1988;45:949–953.

31. Dal Pan GJ, Glass JD, McArthur JC. Clinicopathological correlations of HIV-1-associated vacuolar myelopathy: an autopsy-based case-control study. *Neurology* 1994;44:2159–2164.

32. Dal Pan GJ, McArthur JH, Aylward E, et al. Patterns of cerebral atrophy in HIV-1 infected individuals: results of a quantitative MRI analysis. *Neurology* 1992;42:2125–2130.

33. DeCarli C, Fugate L, Falloon J, et al. Brain growth and cognitive improvement in children with human immunodeficiency virus-induced encephalopathy after 6 months of continuous zidovudine therapy. *J AIDS* 1991;4:585–592.

34. Desrosiers RC, Hansen-Moosa A, Mori K, et al. Macrophage-tropic variants of SIV are associated with specific AIDS-related lesions but are not essential for the development of AIDS. *Am J Pathol* 1991;139:29–35.

35. Dunbar N, Perdices M, Grunseit A, Cooper DA. Changes in neuropsychological performance of AIDS-related complex patients who progress to AIDS. *AIDS* 1992;6:691–700.

36. Ell PJ, Costa DC, Harrison M. Imaging cerebral damage in HIV infection (letter). *Lancet* 1987;2: 569–570.

37. Epstein LG, Sharer LR, Joshi VV, Fojas MM, Koenigsberger MR, Oleske JM. Progressive encephalopathy in children with acquired immune deficiency syndrome. *Ann Neurol* 1985;17:488–496.

38. Everall IP, Luthert PJ, Lantos PL. Neuronal loss in the frontal cortex in HIV infection. *Lancet* 1991; 337:1119–1121.

39. Farzadegan H, Chmiel JS, Odaka N, et al. Association of antibody to human immunodeficiency virus type 1 core protein (p24), CD4- lymphocyte number, and AIDS-free time. *J Infect Dis* 1992; 166:1217–1222.

40. Fischl MA, Richman DD, Grieco MH, et al. The efficacy of azidothymidine (AZT) in the treatment of patients with AIDS and AIDS-related complex. *N Engl J Med* 1987;317:185–191.

41. French M, Abraham L, Mallal S, Delgi-Espositi M, Dawkins R. MHC genes and HIV. *Today's Life Sci* 1992;32–36.

41a. Gastaut JL, Bolgert F, Brunet D, et al. Early intellectual impairment in HIV seropositive patients. A longitudinal study (abstract). *Neuro and Neuropsychol Complications of HIV Infect* 1990;1:95.

42. Gelbard HA, Nottet HSLM, Swindells S, et al. Platelet activating factor. A candidate human immunodeficiency virus type 1-induced neurotoxin. *J Virol* 1994;68:4628–4635.

43. Gelman BB, Guinto FC. Morphometry, histopathology, and tomography of cerebral atrophy in the acquired immunodeficiency syndrome. *Ann Neurol* 1992;32:31–40.

44. Glass JD, Fedor H, Wesselingh SL, McArthur JC. Immunocytochemical quantitation of HIV in the brain: correlations with HIV-associated dementia. *Ann Neurol* 1995;38:755–762.

45. Glass JD, Wesselingh SL, Selnes OA, McArthur JC. Clinical-neuropathologic correlation in HIV-associated dementia. *Neurology* 1993;43:2230–2237.

46. Goswami KK, Miller RF, Harrison MJ, Hamel DJ, Daniels RS, Tedder RS. Expression of HIV-1 in the cerebrospinal fluid detected by the polymerase chain reaction and its correlation with central nervous system disease. *J AIDS* 1991;5:797–803.

47. Goudsmit J, de Wolf F, Paul DA, et al. Expression of human immunodeficiency virus antigen (HIV-Ag) in serum and cerebrospinal fluid during acute and chronic infection. *Lancet* 1986;2: 177–180.

48. Gray F, Belec L, Keohane C, et al. Zidovudine therapy and HIV encephalitis: a 10-year neuropathological survey. *AIDS* 1994;8:489–493.

49. Griffin DE, Wesselingh SL, McArthur JC. Elevated central nervous system prostaglandins in HIV-associated dementia. *Ann Neurol* 1994;35:592–597.

50. Handelsman L, Aronson M, Maurer G, et al. Neuropsychological and neurological manifestations of HIV-1 dementia in drug users. *J Neuropsychiatr Clin Neurosci* 1992;4:21–28.

51. Harden CL, Daras M, Tuchman AJ, Koppel BS. Low amplitudee EEG's in demented AIDS patients. *EEG Clin Neurophysiol* 1993;87:54–56.

51a. Helmstaedter C, Hartmann A, Niese C, Brackman HH, Sass R. Stage-independence and individual outcome of neuro-cognitive deficits in HIV. A follow-up study of 62 HIV-positive hemophilic patients. *Nervenarzt* 1992;63:88–94.

52. Herbert V. Vitamin B12 deficiency neuropsychiatric damage in acquired immunodeficiency syndrome (letter). *Arch Neurol* 1993;50:569.
53. Herbert V, Fong W, Gulle V, Stopler T. Low holotranscobalamin II is the earliest serum marker for subnormal vitamin B12 (cobalamin) absorption in patients with AIDS. *Am J Hematol* 1990;34:132–139.
54. Hestad K, McArthur JH, Dal Pan GJ, et al. Regional atrophy in HIV-1 infection: association with specific neuropsychological test performance. *Acta Neurol Scand* 1993;88:112–118.
55. Heyes MP, Brew BJ, Martin A, et al. Quinolinic acid in cerebrospinal fluid and serum in HIV-1 infection: relationship to clinical and neurologic status. *Ann Neurol* 1991;29:202–209.
56. Ho DD, Neumann AU, Perelson AS, Chen W, Leonard JM, Markowitz M. Rapid turnover of plasma virions and CD4 lymphocytes in HIV-1 infection. *Nature* 1995;373:123–126.
57. Holland NR, Power C, Mathews VP, Glass JD, Forman M, McArthur JC. CMV encephalitis in acquired immunodeficiency syndrome (AIDS). *Neurology* 1994;44:507–514.
58. Holtzman DM, Kaku DA, So YT. New-onset seizures associated with human immunodeficiency virus infection: causation and clinical features in 100 cases. *Am J Med* 1989;87:173–177.
59. Horowitz SL, Benson DF, Gottlieb MS, Davos I, Bentson JR. Neurological complications of gay-related immunodeficiency disorder. *Ann Neurol* 1982;12:80.
60. Hriso E, Kuhn T, Masdeu JC, Grundman M. Extrapyramidal symptoms due to dopamine-blocking agents in patients with AIDS encephalopathy. *Am J Psychiatry* 1991;148:1558–1561.
61. Iragui VJ, Kalmijn J, Thal LJ, et al. Neurological dysfunction in asymptomatic HIV-1 infected men. Evidence from evoked potentials. *EEG Clin Neurophysiol* 1994;92:1–10.
62. Itil TM, Ferracuti S, Freedman AM, Sherer C, Mehta P, Itil KZ. Computer-analyzed EEG (CEEG) and dynamic brain mapping in AIDS and HIV-related syndrome: a pilot study. *Clin Electroencephalogr* 1990;21:140–144.
63. Jabbari B, Coats M, Salazar A, Martin A, Scherokman B, Laws WA. Longitudinal study of EEG and evoked potentials in neurologically asymptomatic HIV-infected subjects. *EEG Clin Neurophysiol* 1993;86:145–151.
64. Jacobson LP, Kirby AJ, Polk S, et al. Changes in survival after acquired immunodeficiency syndrome (AIDS): 1984–1991. *Am J Epidemiol* 1993;138:952–964.
65. Janssen RS, Cornblath DR, Epstein LG, et al. Nomenclature and research case definitions for neurological manifestations of human immunodeficiency virus type-1 (HIV-1) infection. Report of a Working Group of the American Academy of Neurology AIDS Task Force. *Neurology* 1991;41:778–785.
66. Janssen RS, Nwanyanwu OC, Selik RM, Stehr-Green JK. Epidemiology of human immunodeficiency virus encephalopathy in the United States. *Neurology* 1992;42:1472–1476.
67. Kalayjian RC, Cohen ML, Bonomo RA, Flanigan TP. Cytomegalovirus ventriculoencephalitis in AIDS. *Medicine (Baltimore)* 1993;72:67–77.
67a. Karlsen NR, Reinvang I, Froland SS. A follow-up study of neuropsychological function in asymptomatic HIV-infected patients. *Acta Neurol Scand* 1993;87:83–87.
68. Kaslow R, Duquesnoy R, VanRaden M, et al. A1, Cw7, B8, DR3 HLA antigen combination associated with rapid decline of T-helper lymphocytes in HIV-1 infection. A report from the Multicenter AIDS Cohort Study. *Lancet* 1990;335:927–930.
69. Koralnik IJ, Beaumanoir A, Hausler R, et al. A controlled study of early neurologic abnormalities in men with asymptomatic human immunodeficiency virus infection. *N Engl J Med* 1990;323:864–870.
70. LaFrance N, Pearlson GD, Schaerf FW, et al. I-123 IMP-SPECT in HIV-related dementia. *Adv Functional Imag* 1988;1:9–15.
71. Lange JM, Paul DA, Huisman HG, et al. Persistent HIV antigenaemia and decline of HIV core antibodies associated with transition to AIDS. *Br Med J* 1986;293:1459–1462.
72. Levy RM, Bredesen DE, Rosenblum ML. Neurological manifestations of the acquired immunodeficiency syndrome (AIDS): experience at UCSF and review of the literature. *J Neurosurg* 1985;62:475–495.
73. Levy RM, Rosenbloom S, Perrett LV. Neuroradiologic findings in AIDS: a review of 200 cases. *Am J Roengenol* 1986;147:977–983.
74. Lipton SA. HIV-related neurotoxicity. *Brain Pathol* 1991;1:193–199.
75. Lipton SA, Gendelman HE. Dementia associated with the acquired immunodeficiency syndrome. *N Engl J Med* 1995;332:934–940.
76. MacDonell KB, Chmiel JS, Poggensee L, Wu S, Phair JP. Predicting progression to AIDS: combined usefulness of CD4 lymphocyte counts and p24 antigenemia. *Am J Med* 1990;89:706–712.
77. Maj M, Janssen R, Satz P, et al. The World Health Organization's cross-cultural study on neuropsychiatric aspects of infection with the human immunodeficiency virus 1 (HIV-1). *Br J Psychiatry* 1991;159:351–356.
78. Marder K, Liu X, Stern Y, et al. Neurologic signs and symptoms in a cohort of homosexual men followed for 4.5 years. *Neurology* 1995;45:261–267.

79. Masliah E, Achim CL, Ge N, Deteresa R, Terry RD, Wiley CA. Spectrum of human immunodeficiency virus-associated neocortical damage. *Ann Neurol* 1992;32:321–329.
80. Mayeux R, Stern Y, Tang MX, et al. Mortality risks in gay men with human immunodeficiency virus infection and cognitive impairment. *Neurology* 1993;43:176–182.
81. McArthur JC. Neurologic manifestations of AIDS. *Medicine (Baltimore)* 1987;66:407–437.
82. McArthur JC, Harrison MJG. HIV-associated dementia. In: Appel S, ed. *Current neurology.* Chicago: Mosby-Year Book; 1994.
83. McArthur JC, Cohen BA, Selnes OA, et al. Low prevalence of neurological and neuropsychological abnormalities in otherwise healthy HIV-1-infected individuals: results from the Multicenter AIDS Cohort Study. *Ann Neurol* 1989;26:601–611.
84. McArthur JC, Hoover DR, Bacellar H, et al. Dementia in AIDS patients: incidence and risk factors. *Neurology* 1993;43:2245–2252.
85. McArthur JC, Kumar AJ, Johnson DW, et al. Incidental white matter hyperintensities on magnetic resonance imaging in HIV-1 infection. Multicenter AIDS Cohort Study. *J AIDS* 1990;3:252–259.
86. McArthur JC, Nance-Sproson TE, Griffin DE, et al. The diagnostic utility of elevation in cerebrospinal fluid β2 microglobulin in HIV-1 dementia. *Neurology* 1992;42:1707–1712.
87. McArthur JC, Sipos E, Cornblath DR, et al. Identification of mononuclear cells in CSF of patients with HIV infection. *Neurology* 1989;39:66–70.
88. McArthur JC, Skolasky R, Dal Pan G, Glass J, Selnes OA. Variation in clinical progression with HIV-associated dementia. In: *Neuroscience of HIV infection: basic and clinical frontiers.* Vancouver, British Columbia, August 2–5, 1994.
89. McConnell JR, Swindells S, Ong CS, et al. Prospective utility of cerebral proton magnetic resonance spectroscopy in monitoring HIV infection and its associated neurological impairment. *AIDS Res Hum Retroviruses* 1994;10:977–982.
90. Menon DK, Baudouin CJ, Tomlinson D, Hoyle C. Proton MR spectroscopy and imaging of the brain in AIDS: evidence of neuronal loss in regions that appear normal with imaging. *J Comput Assist Tomogr* 1990;14:882–885.
91. Merrill PT, Paige GD, Abrams RA, Jacoby RG, Clifford DB. Ocular motor abnormalities in human immunodeficiency virus infection. *Ann Neurol* 1991;30:130–138.
92. Messenheimer JA, Robertson KR, Wilkins JW, Kalkowski JC, Hall CD. Event-related potentials in human immunodeficiency virus infection. A prospective study. *Arch Neurol* 1992;49:396–400.
93. Michael NL, Vahey M, Burke DS, Redfield RR. Viral DNA and mRNA expression correlate with the stage of human immunodeficiency virus (HIV) type 1 infection in humans: evidence for viral replication in all stages of HIV disease. *J Virol* 1992;66:310–316.
94. Mintz M, Epstein LG, Koenigsberger MR. Neurological manifestations of acquired immunodeficiency syndrome in children. *Int Pediatrics* 1989;4:161–171.
95. Nance-Sproson T, McArthur JC, Selnes OA, Griffin DE. Predictive value and temporal trends in cerebrospinal fluid abnormalities during HIV infection. *Neurology* 1993;43(Suppl):A265(abst).
96. Navia BA, Price RW. The acquired immunodeficiency syndrome dementia complex as the presenting or sole manifestation of human immunodeficiency virus infection. *Arch Neurol* 1987;44:65–69.
97. Navia BA, Cho ES, Petito CK, Price RW. The AIDS dementia complex: II. Neuropathology. *Ann Neurol* 1986;19:525–535.
98. Navia BA, Jordan BD, Price RW. The AIDS dementia complex: I. Clinical features. *Ann Neurol* 1986;19:517–524.
99. Newman SP, Lunn S, Harrison MJG. Do asymptomatic HIV-seropositive individuals show cognitive deficit? *AIDS* 1995;9:1211–1220.
100. Newton TF, Leuchter AF, Miller EN, Weiner H. Quantitative EEG in patients with AIDS and asymptomatic HIV infection. *Clin Electroencephalogr* 1994;25:18–25.
101. Nuwer MR, Miller EN, Visscher BR, et al. Asymptomatic HIV infection does not cause EEG abnormalities: results from the Multicenter AIDS Cohort Study (MACS). *Neurology* 1992;42:1214–1219.
102. Parisi A, Strosselli M, Di Perri G, et al. Electroencephalography in the early diagnosis of HIV-related subacute encephalitis: analysis of 185 patients. *Clin Electroencephalogr* 1989;20:1–5.
103. Paul DA, Falk LA, Kessler HA, et al. Correlation of serum HIV antigen and antibody with clinical status in HIV-infected patients. *J Med Virol* 1987;22:357–363.
104. Perry S. Organic mental disorders caused by HIV: update on early diagnosis and treatment. *Am J Psychiatry* 1990;147:696–710.
105. Petito CK, Navia BA, Cho ES, Jordan BD, George DC, Price RW. Vacuolar myelopathy pathologically resembling subacute combined degeneration in patients with the acquired immunodeficiency syndrome. *N Engl J Med* 1985;312:874–879.
106. Petito CK, Vecchio D, Chen YT. HIV antigen and DNA in AIDS spinal cords correlate with macrophage infiltration but not with vacuolar myelopathy. *J Neuropathol Exp Neurol* 1994;53:86–94.
107. Pizzo PA, Eddy J, Falloon J, et al. Effect of continuous intravenous infusion of zidovudine (AZT) in children with symptomatic HIV infection. *N Engl J Med* 1988;319:889–896.

108. Pomerantz RJ, Kuritzkes DR, de la Monte SM, et al. Infection of the retina by human immunodeficiency virus type 1. *N Engl J Med* 1987;317:1643–1647.

109. Portegies P, de Gans J, Lange JM, et al. Declining incidence of AIDS dementia complex after introduction of zidovudine treatment [published erratum appears in *BMJ* 19894;299(6708):1141]. *Br Med J* 1989;299:819–821.

110. Portegies P, Enting RH, de Gans J, et al. Presentation and course of AIDS dementia complex: ten years of follow-up in Amsterdam, the Netherlands. *AIDS* 1993;7:669–675.

111. Portegies P, Epstein LG, Hung ST, de Gans J, Goudsmit J. Human immunodeficiency virus type 1 antigen in cerebrospinal fluid. Correlation with clinical neurologic status. *Arch Neurol* 1989;46: 261–264.

112. Power C, McArthur JC, Johnson RT, et al. Demented and non-demented patients with AIDS differ in brain-derived human immunodeficiency virus type 1 envelope sequences. *J Virol* 1994;68: 4643–4649.

113. Power C, Selnes OA, Grim JA, McArthur JC. The HIV Dementia Scale: a rapid screening test. *J AIDS* 1995;8:273–278.

114. Price RW, Brew BJ. The AIDS dementia complex. *J Infect Dis* 1988;158:1079–1083.

115. Price RW, Navia BA. Infections in AIDS and in other immunosuppressed patients. In: Kennedy PGE, Johnson RT, eds. *Infections of the nervous system.* London: Butterworths; 1987.

116. Ragazzoni A, Grippo A, Ghidini P, et al. Electrophysiological study of neurologically asymptomatic HIV-1 seropositive patients. *Acta Neurol Scand* 1993;87:47–51.

117. Reardon J, Singleton J, Wilson MJ, Alderete E. Epidemiology of HIV encephalopathy (HIV-E): reported frequencies in California, 1988–1991. *VII International Conference on AIDS/III STD World Congress,* 1992;POC 4009 (abstr).

117a. Robertson KR, Wilkins J, Robertson W, Hall CD. Neuropsychological changes in HIV seropositive subjects over time: one and two year follow-up (abstract). Neuroscience of HIV Infection: *Basic and Clin Frontiers* 1992;1992:1:129.

118. Rothenberg R, Woelfel M, Stoneburner R, Milberg J, Parker R, Truman B. Survival with the acquired immunodeficiency syndrome: experience with 5833 cases in New York City. *N Engl J Med* 1987; 317:1297–1302.

119. Rottenberg DA, Moeller JR, Strother SC, et al. The metabolic pathology of the AIDS dementia complex. *Ann Neurol* 1987;22:700–706.

120. Royal W, Selnes OA, Concha M, Nance-Sproson TE, McArthur JC. Cerebrospinal fluid HIV-1 p24 antigen levels in HIV-1-related dementia. *Ann Neurol* 1994;36:32–39.

121. Royal W, Updike M, Selnes OA, et al. HIV-1 infection and nervous system abnormalities among a cohort of intravenous drug users. *Neurology* 1991;41:1905–1910.

122. Sasseville VG, Newman W, Brodie SJ, Hesterberg P, Pauley D, Ringler DJ. Monocyte adhesion to endothelium in simian immunodeficiency virus-induced AIDS encephalitis is mediated by vascular cell adhesion molecule-1/alpha 4 beta 1 integrin interactions. *Am J Pathol* 1994;144:27–40.

122a. Saykin AJ, Janssen RS, Sprehn GC, Kaplan JE, Spira TJ, O'Connor B. Longitudinal evaluation of neuropsychological function in homosexual men with HIV infection: 18-month follow-up. *J Neuropsychiatry* 1991;3:286–298.

123. Schmitt FA, Bigley JW, McKinnis R, et al. Neuropsychological outcome of zidovudine (AZT) treatment of patients with AIDS and AIDS-related complex. *N Engl J Med* 1988;319:1573–1578.

124. Schroeder MM, Handelsman L, Torres L, et al. Early and late cognitive event-related potentials mark stages of HIV-1 infection in the drug-user risk group. *Biol Psychiatry* 1994;35:54–69.

125. Selnes OA, Miller EN. Development of a screening battery for HIV-related cognitive impairment: the MACS experience. In: Grant I,d Martin A, eds. *Neuropsychology of HIV infection: current research and new directions.* New York: Oxford University Press; 1995.

126. Selnes OA, Galai N, Bacellar H, et al. Cognitive performance after progression to AIDS: a longitudinal study from the Multicenter AIDS Cohort Study. *Neurology* 1995;45:267–275.

127. Selnes OA, McArthur JC, Gordon B, Miller EN, McArthur JH, Saah A. Patterns of cognitive decline in incident HIV-dementia: longitudinal observations from the Multicenter AIDS Cohort Study (abstract 497P). *Neurology* 1991;41(Suppl 1):252.

128. Selnes OA, McArthur JC, Royal W, et al. HIV-1 infection and intravenous drug use: longitudinal neuropsychological evaluation of asymptomatic subjects. *Neurology* 1992;42:1924–1930.

129. Selnes OA, Miller E, McArthur JC, et al. HIV-1 infection: no evidence of cognitive decline during the asymptomatic stages. *Neurology* 1990;40:204–208.

130. Shaw GM, Harper ME, Hahn BH, et al. HTLV-III infection in brains of children and adults with AIDS encephalopathy. *Science* 1985;227:177–182.

131. Sidtis JJ. Evaluation of the AIDS dementia complex in adults. In: Price RW, Perry SW, eds. *HIV, AIDS and the brain.* New York: Raven Press; 1994;273–287.

132. Sidtis JJ, Gatsonis C, Price RW, et al. Zidovudine treatment of the AIDS dementia complex: results of a placebo-controlled trial. *Ann Neurol* 1993;33:343–349.

133. Silberstein CH, O'Dowd MA, Chartock P, et al. A prospective four-year follow-up of neuropsycho-

logical function in HIV seropositive and seronegative methadone-maintained patients. *General Hospital Psychiatry* 1993;15:351–359.

134. Snider WD, Simpson DM, Nielsen S, Gold JW, Metroka CE, Posner JB. Neurological complications of acquired immune deficiency syndrome: analysis of 50 patients. *Ann Neurol* 1983;14:403–418.

135. Stern Y, Liu X, Marder K, et al. Neuropsychological changes in a prospectively followed cohort of homosexual and bisexual men with and without HIV infection. *Neurology* 1995;45:467–472.

136. Steuler H, Munzinger S, Wildemann B, Storch-Hagenlocher B. Quantitation of HIV-1 proviral DNA in cells from cerebrospinal fluid. *J AIDS* 1992;5:405–408.

137. Tartaglione TA, Collier AC, Coombs RW, et al. Acquired immunodeficiency syndrome: cerebrospinal fluid findings in patients before and during long-term oral zidovudine therapy. *Arch Neurol* 1991;48:695–699.

138. Tozzi V, Narciso P, Galgani S, et al. Effects of zidovudine in 30 patients with mild to end-stage AIDS dementia complex. *AIDS* 1993;7:683–692.

139. Trimble KC, Goggins MG, Molloy AM, Mulcahy F, Scott JM, Weir DG. Vitamin-B12 deficiency is not a cause of HIV-associated neuropathy. *AIDS* 1993;7:1132–1133.

140. Vago L, Castagna A, Lazzarin A, Trabattoni G, Cinque P, Costanzi G. Reduced frequency of HIV-induced brain lesions in AIDS patients treated with zidovudine. *J AIDS* 1993;6:42–45.

141. Van Wielink G, McArthur JC, Moench T, Farzadegan H, Johnson RT, Saah A. Intrathecal synthesis of anti-HIV-IgG: correlation with increasing duration of HIV-1 infection. *Neurology* 1990;40:816–819.

142. Vazeux R, Lacroix-Ciaudo C, Blanche S, et al. Low levels of human immunodeficiency virus replication in the brain tissue of children with severe acquired immunodeficiency syndrome encephalopathy. *Am J Pathol* 1992;140:137–144.

143. Volberding PA, Lagakos SW, Koch MA, et al. Zidovudine in asymptomatic human immunodeficiency virus infection. A controlled trial in persons with fewer than 500 CD4-positive cells per cubic millimeter. *N Engl J Med* 1990;322:941–949.

144. Watkins BA, Dorn HH, Kelly WB, et al. Specific tropism of HIV-1 for microglial cells in primary human brain cultures. *Science* 1990;249:549–553.

145. Weis S, Haug H, Budka H. Astroglial changes in the cerebral cortex of AIDS brains: a morphometric and immunohistochemical investigation. *Neuropathol Appl Neurobiol* 1993;19:329–335.

146. Westervelt P, Gendelman HE, Ratner L. Identification of a determinant within the human immunodeficiency virus 1 surface envelope glycoprotein critical for productive infection of primary monocytes. *Proc Natl Acad Sci USA* 1991;88:3097–3101.

146a. Whitt JK, Hooper SR, Tennison MB, Robertson WT, Gold SH, Burchinal M, Wells R, McMillan C, Whaley RA, Combest J. Neuropsychologic functioning of human immunodeficiency virus-infected children with hemophilia. *J Pediatr* 1993;122:52–59.

147. Wiley CA, Masliah E, Morey M, et al. Neocortical damage during HIV infection. *Ann Neurol* 1991;29:651–657.

148. Wolters PL, Brouwers P, Moss HA, Pizzo PA. Adaptive behavior of children with symptomatic HIV infection before and after zidovudine therapy. *J Pediatr Psychol* 1994;19:47–61.

149. World Health Organization (WHO). *Report on the consultation on the neuropsychiatric aspects of HIV infection.* Geneva: WHO; 1988.

150. Yarchoan R, Berg G, Brouwers P, et al. Response of human-immunodeficiency-virus-associated neurological disease to 3'-azido-3'-deoxythymidine. *Lancet* 1987;1:132–135.

151. Yarchoan R, Pluda JM, Thomas RV, et al. Long-term toxicity/activity profile of 2',3'-dideoxyinosine in AIDS and AIDS-related complex. *Lancet* 1990;336:526–529.

AIDS and the Nervous System, Second Edition,
edited by J. R. Berger and R. M. Levy.
Lippincott-Raven Publishers, Philadelphia © 1997.

22

Progressive Multifocal Leukoencephalopathy

°Joseph R. Berger, †Bruno V. Gallo, and †Mauricio Concha

°Department of Neurology, University of Kentucky Medical Center, Lexington, Kentucky 40536–2226; and †Department of Neurology, Jackson Memorial Hospital, Miami, Florida 33136

As a consequence of acquired immunodeficiency syndrome (AIDS), progressive multifocal leukoencephalopathy (PML), a formerly rare disease, is seen with increasing frequency. Crystallized as a distinct entity by Aström, Mancall, and Richardson in 1958 (7), the syndrome was identified chiefly on the basis of its unique pathological features of demyelination, abnormal oligodendroglial nuclei, and giant astrocytes. In 1965, electron microscopic studies suggested the presence of viral particles morphologically typical of the papovaviruses in the brains of patients dying of PML (185), and in 1971, the causative agent, JC virus (JCV) (after the initials of the patient from whom it was first isolated), was cultivated and identified (12).

Aström, Mancall, and Richardson, in their review of the literature, discovered prior descriptions of this entity dating to as early as 1930 (60). Hallervorden (60), a V. C. German pathologist, in a monograph titled "Eignnartige und nicht rubriziebare prozess" ("Unique and Non-Classifiable Process"), published the first recognized description of this entity, describing two patients, one with tuberculosis and the other without recognized underlying systemic disease, who exhibited multifocal neurological symptoms associated with discrete areas of demyelination accompanied by bizarre enlarged astrocytes (60). He did not, however, identify the third histopathological hallmark of PML, namely, the enlarged oligodendroglial nuclei. Hallervorden wisely expressed the opinion that this disease, similar to so many other rare diseases, was often excluded from "comprehensive surveys as worthless curiosities" (60). However, he correctly asserted that the value of these unusual cases was often in uncovering unexpected relationships, as proved clearly to be the case with PML.

By 1984, a comprehensive review of PML found only a total of 230 reported cases in the literature (25), of which 69 cases were pathologically confirmed and 40 cases both virologically and pathologically confirmed. In this series, only 2 of the 230 cases were associated with AIDS (13,105). This number represented 3.0% of all cases in which an underlying disease was identified (25). Progressive multifocal leukoencephalopathy occurring in association with AIDS had been initially reported within 1 year (105) of the first description of AIDS in 1981 (56,102,138). Since then, this formerly rare disease has become remarkably common.

ETIOLOGY AND PATHOGENESIS

Progressive multifocal leukoencephalopathy is a demyelinating disease of the central nervous system (CNS) that results from infection of oligodendrocytes with JCV, a papovavirus. Electron microscopic studies initially provided evidence of a viral etiology demonstrating papovavirus-like particles in the nuclei of abnormal oligodendrocytes (139,184,185). Approximately a decade after its initial clinical and pathological description (7,28,120,130) viral isolation subsequently confirmed this observation. In 1971, Padgett et al. (120) isolated a human polyomavirus (double-stranded DNA containing virus with an icosahedral symmetry) from long-term cultures comprised chiefly of glial cells. The virus's ability to cause hemagglutination of human type O erythrocytes allowed for the determination of antibody in patients. Probably JCV is the only cause of PML. In only three cases (111,121,167) has another papovavirus, SV40, been implicated and a third papovavirus, BK virus, has not been neuropathogenic. The cases attributed to SV40 have not been well characterized and, in some instances, reexamination of these brain tissues by *in situ* DNA hybridization has revealed JCV, not SV40 (146).

After two decades of investigation, we are beginning to understand the pathogenesis of PML for two reasons. First, there has been an increased incidence of PML due to AIDS and, consequently, more opportunity to study the disease. Second, there has been development of highly sensitive molecular techniques which allow detection of very few copies of a viral genome, including advances in *in situ* hybridization and amplification of viral genomes using polymerase chain reaction (PCR) (6,64,65,70,89,155,158,173). Application of these techniques to tissues available from PML patients has focused recent investigations on determining mechanisms of viral multiplication (89,90,93), cellular control over viral gene expression (4,149), and delivery of virus to the CNS (71,173). Information now forthcoming helps explain how the etiologic virus, JCV, can be such a widespread infectious agent in the population by antibody measures yet target such a highly specialized cell in the nervous system, the myelinating oligodendrocyte.

BIOLOGY OF JCV

The JCV belongs to the genus *Polyomavirus* in the family Papovaviridae. The JCV has a simple DNA genome of 5.1 kilobases in a double-stranded, supercoiled form, encapsulated in an icosahedral protein structure measuring 40 nm in diameter. The DNA codes for one nonstructural but multifunctional protein (T) and three capsid proteins (VP1, VP2, VP3). The T protein is a DNA binding protein and is responsible for initiation of viral DNA replication and transcription of the capsid proteins. In certain rodent and nonhuman primate cells, JCV T protein expression is consistent with a malignant transformation or tumor induction, particularly of astroglial cells into astrocytomas (87,88,97,119,170,184). Another nonstructural protein, t, from the same DNA strand as the T protein accounts for the cellular splicing. It is not considered important for pathogenicity. The region located between the two coding sequences of the genome contains the signals for DNA replication as well as for promotion and enhancement of transcription (47,48) and is termed the regulatory region. This region is believed to be responsible for the cellular tropism of JCV (78,162). It also demonstrates the most sequence variability resulting from deletions and rearrangements perhaps acquired during propagation in brain or in extraneural host tissues (37,100).

The JCV does not infect neurons in PML brain tissue or in cultures from either human adult or fetal brain but does infect both oligodendrocytes and astrocytes (3,95,179). There is a glial specific host range for transcription of JCV as evidenced by experiments using infectious clones of viral DNA (48,101). Other studies using recombinant DNA constructs of the viral regulatory sequences linked to a reporter gene confirmed the human glial cell as a specific host (74). Unlike many other human viral pathogens, susceptibility to JCV infection is not associated with viral attachment to specific cell receptors and penetration but is controlled by cell-type-specific factors for transcription and species-specific factors for replication (44). Experiments have concentrated on identifying nuclear DNA binding proteins that selectively interacted with the regulatory region of the genome to explain the neurotropism of JCV for glial cells. Such proteins are likely to bind specific cis-acting nucleotide base pairs (np) for control of JCV transcription. It appears that there are proteins that positively regulate JCV expression and those which block expression in a cell-type-specific manner. Glial cell susceptibility to JCV infection may be determined by the presence of specific members of a family of transcription proteins that are only present in permissive cells. Cells that are not permissive to JCV infection probably do not have these same protein factors and/or have other proteins that bind the JCV regulatory sequences and block transcription (4,149).

The increased incidence of PML in AIDS patients has suggested a direct interaction between JCV and human immunodeficiency virus 1 (HIV-1). It is clear that the JCV T protein can transactivate the HIV-1 long terminal repeat (LTR) units and that the reverse, the transactivator protein of HIV-1, *tat*, can increase transcription from the JCV regulatory region (52). To date there are no clear data showing that both HIV-1 and JCV infect the same cells in AIDS patients with PML. The white matter lesions from such patients' brain tissue frequently are quite distinct but could also be in close proximity (176). The HIV-1 *tat* protein has been shown to diffuse in cell cultures and can be taken up by neighboring cells (46,63). Whether a similar mechanism for distribution of *tat* to JCV-infected cells occurs *in vivo* remains to be observed or tested. Direct or indirect interactions between these two viruses may take place outside the nervous system before entry to the brain. The most likely location for this to take place would be cells of the immune system. The HIV-1 chiefly infects macrophages, monocytes, and T and B lymphocytes. In addition to glial cells, JCV has been found in uroepithelial cells in the urinary tract (12,43) and recently in B lymphocytes in bone marrow and spleen (71) and in peripheral blood lymphocytes (158,159). Further studies of potential viral interactions at the molecular level are underway in several laboratories.

The mechanism by which JCV enters the brain and initiates infection remains the subject of study. Current evidence implicates viral latency in lymphocytes in bone marrow or other lymphoid tissues which can be activated during immune suppression and enter the peripheral blood (94). Circulating infected lymphocytes may be able to cross the blood-brain barrier and pass infection to astrocytes at the border of vessels, which in turn augments infection through multiplication to eventually infect oligodendrocytes. Using *in situ* DNA hybridization, JCV-infected cells are frequently found near blood vessels in the brain, in B lymphocytes in bone marrow (71) and in brain (93). Using PCR technology with a series of paired primers representative of three regions of the viral genome to eliminate possible nonspecific amplification of closely related DNA sequences over 90% of patients with biopsy-proven PML had JCV DNA in peripheral blood lymphocytes (PBLs) (158). The number of cases of PML with viral DNA in their PBL circulation is now greater, but the percentage remains at approximately 95%. The JCV DNA has also been demonstrated in the peripheral circulation of significant numbers of immunocompromised patients without PML. The group whose immune systems may be compromised through immunosuppressive therapies or other diseases would be considered at risk for the development of PML.

Approximately 5% to 10% of the population excrete JCV in urine as detected by either PCR or virus isolation, including pregnant women, older individuals, and some organ transplant patients (6,30,45,109), suggesting the kidney as the site of viral latency. The DNA sequence of the regulatory region from kidney or urine in these individuals is markedly different from the sequence found in the brain of PML patients (180). Since the regulatory DNA sequence chiefly governs infectivity of JCV, a number of JCV isolates or clones of DNA have been examined. The most prominent DNA sequence arrangement found related to kidney has been described as an archetype sequence (181). The archetype sequence contains 187 nucleotide pairs with no tandem repeats but does contain the origin of viral replication, the TATA sequence as an RNA start site and other inserts that probably serve as a functional binding site for the Sp1 DNA transcription factor (22,66). To convert the archetype sequence to that most often found in PML brain tissue, however, would require deletions, substitutions, and duplications (156,180). Currently there is no evidence for any biological activity for the archetype sequence or virus isolates that contain these sequences. Several regulatory region sequences have been identified from JCV DNA in peripheral blood of PML patients that are not related to the archetype but closely related to sequences found in PML brain (158). Further examination of the distribution and importance of the archetype sequence is needed to understand its role in the pathogenesis of PML. However, the existence of many variations of the DNA sequence of the regulatory region of JCV highlights the genome diversity of JCV. Several regions within the regulatory sequences have been identified that are always represented and thought to be critical for viral multiplication and pathogenicity (66,100,158,181). Lymphocytes, particularly B cells, may harbor JCV in a latent state and, upon activation, may carry virus to the brain. Several human B cell lines were described as permissive for JCV multiplication and possessed DNA binding proteins that recognized the same sequences on the JCV genome as the highly permissive human glial cells (8).

ASSOCIATION WITH AIDS

The incidence of PML in conditions associated with cellular immunodeficiency *(vide infra)* other than AIDS is difficult to assess but, as suggested by Stoner et al. (147), does not appear to approach the 4% to 5% incidence observed with HIV-1 infection. This apparent increased incidence of PML with HIV-1 infection may be the result of a combination of cellular immunodeficiency and CNS inflammation resulting from HIV-1 infection. The cellular immunosuppression leads to the expression of JCV in B lymphocytes, and the HIV-1-associated CNS inflammation results in a facilitation of the entry of these cells into the CNS and the activation of JCV replication. Subsequent infection of glial cells by JCV leads to the development of PML.

Early after HIV-1 infection, and often long before the development of significant immunosuppression, there is evidence of HIV-1 infection of the CNS, including recovery of HIV-1 from the CSF (67), intrathecal synthesis of antibody to HIV-1 (129), and abnormalities of cerebrospinal fluid (CSF) (41,68,99). The HIV-1 has been demonstrated by PCR in the brain of a patient dying within 15 days of infection (33). Viral cultures (67,86) and immunostaining (171) and *in situ* hybridization (137) confirm the presence of HIV-1 infection in the brain. The infection of the CNS with HIV-1 has been postulated to result from a trafficking into the brain of HIV-1-infected monocytes/macrophages which then establish residence within the brain (80). There is some evidence showing an activated state of cellular and humoral immunity in the HIV-1-infected CNS despite a coexistent systemic immunodeficiency. Cells expressing major histocompatibility (MHC) class I and class II antigens, the prerequisite for antigen presentation to the immunocompetent T cells, are relatively increased in CNS tissue derived from AIDS patients compared to normal CNS tissue (160,164). B cell activation in the CNS compartment, perhaps, in part, a response to increased levels of interleukin-6 (IL-6, B cell stimulatory factor 2) (49), is evidenced by the intra-blood-brain barrier production of antibodies to HIV-1 antigens (129). Although the predominant cell types comprising cellular infiltrates observed in the tissue of HIV-1 encephalitis are macrophages and microglia (84,110,160), some T cells and B cells have been demonstrated by immunohistochemical technique (160,164). In addition, several cytokines have been demonstrated in CNS tissue from AIDS patients using immunohistochemical techniques: tumor necrosis factor alpha (TNF-α) (160,183), IL-1-β, IL-6, and interferon-γ (160).

The migration of B cells into nonlymphoid tissues has been less well characterized than the selective homing of B lymphocytes to the various lymphoid organs (peripheral lymph nodes, Peyer's patches). The mechanism of B cell entry into the brain may result from both selective homing and less specific mechanisms. Cytokines released from macrophages and T cells may be chemotactic for B cells (115), increase the adherence of endothelial cells for B cells (29), or alter the blood-brain barrier to allow passage of a variety of inflammatory cells into the brain parenchyma (23). Tumor necrosis factor alpha, IL-1, IL-4, and γ-interferon, cytokines produced by macrophages and other inflammatory cells, e.g., T cells (39), have been demonstrated to increase the adhesion of vascular endothelium for B lymphocytes (19,29,126). The overall environment of "immune activation" which has been described in the CNS (160) will possibly result in the chemoattraction, enhanced adhesion of B cells to brain endothelia, and activation of B cells latently infected by JCV. The increased B cell adhesion to brain endothelia is likely to result from elaboration of IL-1 and TNF-α described in the brains of HIV-1-infected individuals. The stimulation of B cells (79,143) is possibly mediated by IL-6, IL-4 (B cell stimulatory factor 1), and other substances, such as transforming growth factor beta (TGF-β), a cytokine with potent chemotactic activity which has been demonstrated immunohistochemically in CNS tissue from patients with AIDS (166). The adhesion of circulating lymphocytes to target tissue vasculature precedes their subsequent migration into the organ. Under physiological conditions, lymphocyte traffic into the brain is limited. It is possible that the entry of JCV-infected B lymphocytes into the brain is facilitated by an upregulation of adhesive molecules on brain endothelial cells in response to HIV-1 infection of the CNS. It is possible that JCV-antigen-specific lymphocytes appear in the CNS early, rarely migrating far from the vasculature. Because monocytes and astrocytes can present antigen *in situ*, it is at this site that the antigen-specific B cells are further activated, most likely in an antigen-specific manner. The cytokines secreted locally by microglial cells and monocytes activate the endothelium and surrounding perivascular cells, leading to the expression of adhesion molecules. For example, due to the expression of an avidly binding form of lymphocyte function antigen (LFA-1), activated B cells are preferentially recruited to tissue expressing intercellular adhesion molecule (ICAM-1) or other ligands and present in PML. Astrocytes in culture, and maybe *in vivo* as well, express ICAM, particularly human fetal astrocytes in culture. Lesions of PML, similar to those of multiple sclerosis and experimental allergic encephalitis (EAE), are centered on blood vessels and are formed by a specific subset of inflammatory cells.

EPIDEMIOLOGY OF JCV INFECTION

Ten percent of children ages 1 to 5 years demonstrate antibody to JCV. By age 10, 40% to 60% of the population also exhibit antibodies (151,168,169). By middle adulthood 80% to 90% have immunoglobulin G (IgG) antibodies against JCV and seroconversion rates exceed 90% in some urban areas (168). By adulthood, this number escalates sevenfold (168) (Fig. 1). No disease is convincingly associated with acute infection, despite Blake and colleagues' report of a 13-year-old girl with meningoencephalitis attributed to acute JCV infection (20). In their report, acute infection in this patient was identified by a rise of IgM titers to JCV, not by viral

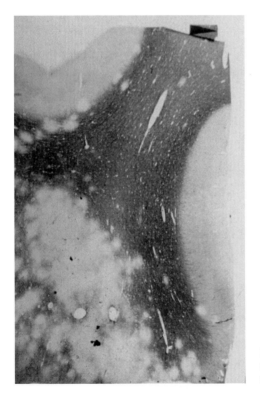

FIG. 1. Gross pathology. Demyelination evident on hematoxylin-eosin and luxol fast blue stain.

isolation (20). It is remarkable the overwhelming majority of people who have antibodies to JCV by adulthood, indicating prior exposure to virus, yet the occurrence of PML in the absence of cellular immunodeficiency is never encountered. It is a minority of persons with underlying impairment of cellular immunodeficiency who will ultimately acquire the disease, suggesting that the presence of JCV and immunodeficiency are not solely adequate conditions for the development of PML.

The male-to-female ratio of PML approximated 1:1 prior to the AIDS epidemic. By 1987, secondary to AIDS, this was transformed to a ratio of 5:1 (69). However, we suspect that the changing pattern of infection with increasing numbers of women infected with HIV and ultimately affected by AIDS will return this ratio toward parity. Additionally, PML, instead of affecting chiefly elderly individuals (25), as was observed in studies prior to AIDS epidemic, has become a disease of the young and middle-age populations affected by AIDS; the greatest incidence being in people 20 to 50 years of age (69). Progressive multifocal leukoencephalopathy is rarely observed in the immunosuppressed child, primarily the result of the lower percentages of children who have been exposed to JCV. Nevertheless, despite its rarity in this age group, it has been described in both HIV-infected children (18,64,65) and in those with other causes of immunodeficiency (73).

Shah postulated that the spread of JCV is via respiratory means. In individuals who have become immunosuppressed, it is the high prevalence of antibodies in adult populations and the rarity of PML in children that support the contention that PML is the consequence of a reactivation of JCV. As a result of acute infection, high titers of IgM antibody that are specific for JCV would be anticipated in patients with PML. Nonetheless, antibody studies show that the sera of only 1 of 21 patients with PML had IgM specific for JCV, while 20 of 21 had IgG antibody specific for JCV (117). But since many of these patients were studied late in the course of their disease, some investigators have argued that the latter study does not exclude the possibility of PML resulting from acute JCV infection (53).

Evidence of prior infection is facilitated by the ability of JCV to cause hemagglutination of type O erythrocytes. Seroconversion rates to JCV have exceeded 90% in some urban areas (168). The high prevalence of antibodies in the adult population and the rarity of PML in children support the contention that PML is the consequence of reactivation of JCV in individuals who become immunosuppressed.

HOST FACTORS AND UNDERLYING DISEASES

Despite AIDS being the most common underlying illness implicated with PML, in some communities where AIDS is not prevalent, lymphoproliferative diseases remain the most frequent cause (25). Since 1981, when AIDS first became recognizable, increasing numbers of individuals with PML have been identified. It is estimated to occur in association with AIDS in 55% to 85% of all current cases (94). The overwhelming majority of people have antibodies to JCV by adulthood and have been rarely described to have disease in the absence of underlying cellular immunosuppression. It is rarely observed in childhood.

Lymphocyte proliferation to mitogen reveals a blunted response in patients with PML in *in vitro* studies (177). In PML, the lymphocyte production of leukocyte migration inhibitory factor in response to JCV antigens is absent, while the production of this factor is normal in unaffected patients. This suggests that a specific deficiency in cellular immune response to JCV antigen may be superimposed on generalized cellular immunodeficiency.

The patients described in the seminal description of PML (7) had either chronic lymphocytic leukemia or lymphoma, and until the early part of the last decade, most patients with PML had lymphoproliferative disorders as the underlying cause of their immunosuppression. In a review of 69 pathologically confirmed cases and 40 virologically and pathologically confirmed cases of PML in 1984, Brooks and Walker found (25) that lymphoproliferative disease was the underlying illness in 62.2%, myeloproliferative diseases in 6.5%, carcinomatous disease in 2.2%, and acquired immunodeficiency chiefly due to autoimmune and immunosuppressive therapy, but as well a result of AIDS, in 10.9%. And 5.6% of cases had no underlying disease. In this series, PML was associated with AIDS in approximately 30% of the cases and with acquired causes of immunodeficiency in only 3.0% of total cases. Figures regarding how frequently each of these illnesses or conditions of immunological compromise is complicated by PML are relatively unavailable. Renal and other organ transplantations are conceivably the most severe states of prolonged cellular immunodeficiency, yet PML was not mentioned as a complication in two recent reviews (61,182). Divakar et al. did not observe PML in a study of 36 long-term survivors of renal transplantation (36). And PML was cited as only affecting 1 patient in a study of 21 patients who were preselected because of the development of neurological complications following bone marrow transplantation (35). Yearly, at the University of Miami/Jackson Memorial Hospital Medical Center, approximately 100 patients undergo renal transplant and 50 patients undergo other major organ (predominantly liver) transplants. For the years 1981–1994 we have observed no cases of clinically suspected or pathologically confirmed PML among this group.

Indeed, AIDS has greatly changed the frequency with which PML is observed. An estimated prevalence of 0.3% of PML was observed in a study among patients with AIDS in the San Francisco Bay area (55). This finding suggested that PML in HIV-infected patients was underestimated by as much as 50% (55). The incidence of this disease is substantially higher and probably approaches 4% to 5% in developed countries. In a study by Holman et al. (69) on the epidemiology of PML in the United States, mortality data indicated that 0.72% of persons with AIDS reported to the Centers for Disease Control (CDC) from 1981 through June 1990 had PML. Nevertheless, relying on reported mortality data to estimate the rate of PML or other diseases associated with AIDS is likely to be misleading (108). Other studies indicate that the rate of PML in AIDS is substantially higher. In a retrospective, hospital-based, clinical study (15), PML occurred in approximately 4% of patients hospitalized with AIDS. More recent analysis of this experience indicates little change in that rate. Autopsy series have revealed a similar rate. In a combined series of seven neuropathological studies comprising a total of 926 patients with AIDS (83), 4.0% had PML. Correspondingly, a neuropathology series from Switzerland detected PML in more than 7% of their patients dying with AIDS (85). However, estimating incidence from these studies also has drawbacks due to selection bias. A pathological study performed on 548 consecutive, unselected autopsies performed on patients with AIDS by the Broward County (Florida) Medical Examiner (L. Tate, personal communication, November 1991) revealed that 29 (5.3%) had PML confirmed at autopsy. HIV-1 has changed the demography of PML as well as increased its prevalence, and instead of affecting chiefly elderly individuals (25), it has become a disease of persons between the ages of 20 and 50 years. Interestingly, despite its rarity in younger age groups, it is also observed in HIV-1-infected children (18).

High-risk groups (gay and bisexual men) may possibly exhibit PML more commonly than other high-risk groups (parenteral drug abusers). Whether this is decisive information remains to be shown. Notwithstanding, there appears to be an increased frequency of PML since the inception of the AIDS epidemic, and it is a virtual certainty that as survival in the face of severe cellular immunosuppression is prolonged, this fundamental observation will hold true.

PATHOLOGY

The cardinal feature, macroscopically, of PML is demyelination. Demyelination may be unifocal and rare but typically occurs as a multifocal process. Lesions occur anywhere in the white matter, but a predilection for the parieto-occipital regions has been noted. Not infrequently it is found to involve the grey matter (165) and the cerebellum, brainstem, and in peculiar cases the spinal cord (10,82,165). An autopsy series of 21 cases showed 17 PML foci in infratentorial structures: 13 cases in cerebellum, 13 cases in brainstem, and 10 cases in both regions (82). The size of lesions range from 1 mm to several centimeters (7,131), and larger lesions are normally the result of coalescence of multiple smaller ones.

Multifocal demyelination, hyperchromatic, enlarged oligodendroglial nuclei, and enlarged bizarre astrocytes with lobulated hyperchromatic nuclei are triad histopathological hallmarks of PML (7,131). Bizarre astrocytes may be seen to undergo mitosis (Fig. 2) and appear malignant. The JCV can be shown in the nucleus of the oligodendroglial cells under electron microscopic examination. The virions appear singly or in dense crystalline arrays and measure 28 to 45 nm in diameter (184,185). Less frequently, the virions are detected in reactive astrocytes and are uncommonly observed in macrophages that are engaged in removing the affected oligodendrocytes

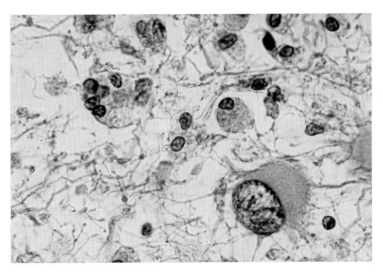

FIG. 2. Microscopic. Enlarged bizarre astrocytes from region of demyelination that is in the process of mitosis.

(103,104). Virions are generally not seen in the large, bizarre astrocytes (104). *In situ* hybridization for JCV antigen allows for detection of the virion in the infected cells.

CLINICAL DISEASE

Signs and Symptoms

Emphasis needs to be placed on the focal features of this disease, particularly those that are apparent on clinical examination. The presentation of the AIDS patient with PML does not appear to be substantially different from that of patients with PML complicating other immunosuppressive conditions (15,81). And the clinical hallmark is indeed the presence of focal neurological disease associated with radiographic evidence of white matter disease in the absence of mass effect.

The most common presentations are cognitive abnormalities, weakness, and visual deficits, each occurring as a heralding manifestation in approximately one-third of patients (25) (Table 1). Weakness is typically a hemiparesis, but monoparesis, hemiplegia, and quadriparesis may be observed. Eighty percent of patients complain of weakness at the time of diagnosis (25). Other noticeable motor disturbances observed include limb and trunk ataxia resulting most often from cerebellar involvement and is detected in as many as 10% of patients. On occasion, the ataxia may be the result of severe impairment in position sense (sensory ataxia). Extrapyramidal disease, at least at onset, is rare. However, bradykinesia and rigidity may be detected in a substantial minority of patients with advanced disease (131,132). Dystonia and severe dysarthria have been observed as a consequence of lesions in the basal ganglia (141). Not unexpectedly, lesions due to PML in the basal ganglia are primarily a reflection

TABLE 1. *Comparison of the initial neurologic manifestations of PML[a] in patients with and without AIDS:[b] a summary of three clinical series[c]*

| | AIDS-related PML | | | | |
| | Berger 1996[d] (N = 64) | von Einsiedel et al.,[e] no. (N = 15) | Total (N = 79) | | Brook et al.,[f] % (N = 107)[g] |
Manifestation			No.	%	
Cognitive deficits	22	6	28	35.4	36.1
Mono- or hemiparesis	43	9	52	65.8	33.3
Sensory deficits	14	1	15	19.0	5.8
Visual deficits	16	3	19	24.1	33.3
Speech deficits	28	8	36	45.6	17.3
Limb incoordination	4	6	10	12.7	13.0
Headache	9	1	10	12.7	7.2
Vertigo	3	1	4	5.1	4.3
Seizures	5	3	8	10.1	5.8

[a] Progressive multifocal leucoencephalopathy.
[b] Acquired immunodeficiency syndrome.
[c] Refs. 15, 25, 82.
[d] Ref. Berger J. personal observation of 64 pathologically proven cases of PML.
[e] Ref. 165.
[f] Ref. 25.
[g] Percentage of cases in pathologically confirmed cases.

of involvement of medullated fibers coursing through this region rather than involvement of the deep gray matter (175).

Neuro-ophthalmic symptoms occur in 50% of patients with PML and are the presenting manifestation in 30% to 45% (9,25). Most commonly the visual deficits are homonymous hemianopsia or quadrantanopsia due to lesions of the optic radiations (9). These patients may develop cortical blindness with progression of the disease. Indeed, cortical blindness is present at the time of diagnosis in 5% to 8% (25). Other ophthalmic manifestations include optic aphasia, alexia without agraphia, and, on rare occasion, ocular motor abnormalities (9); the latter occurs as a result of demyelinating lesions in the brainstem. Visual blurring without further specification has also been described. Although optic atrophy has been reported as a consequence of PML (25), it has never been confirmed histopathologically (9). In several reported cases, coexistent diseases could explain the optic nerve involvement (9,62).

The spectrum of cognitive changes noted is substantial. The mental impairments of PML are often more rapidly advancing and typically occur in conjunction with focal neurological deficits, in contrast to the slowly evolving, global dementia of HIV-related cognitive/motor disorder (e.g., AIDS dementia complex or HIV encephalopathy). Abnormalities seen are memory impairment, personality and behavioral changes, motor impersistence, dyslexia, dyscalculia, and the alien hand syndrome. Rarely will a global dementia occurring in the absence of focal neurological disease present as the initial manifestation of PML. Disturbances of language that may be observed include both dysarthria and aphasia (Table 2).

Less frequently observed are the sensory disturbances. They are distinctly less common than the impairment of strength or visual function. Ten to twenty percent of patients will exhibit a sensory deficit (25). Rarer still are the clinical manifestations of headache, seizures, and vertigo. Seizures may be seen and have been logically attributed to lesions affecting the cortical grey matter (82). Our data suggests that AIDS-related PML cases present more frequently with hemiparesis and speech deficits (aphasia and dysarthria) than non-AIDS-associated PML. We should use caution in the interpretation of this data, which were based on autopsy results and the clustering of reports with very small sample sizes.

Prognosis

In patients with other underlying diseases, as in patients with AIDS, PML usually progresses relentlessly to death within a mean of 4 months (15). Although, rare individuals with recovery of their clinical and radiographic manifestations have been reported (14). The explanation of this recovery remains a conundrum, but 5 of approximately 50 personally observed (J. Berger) HIV-1-infected patients with biopsy-proven PML have been observed to exhibit both neurological recovery and survival in excess of 1 year. These patients represent approximately 7% of the total number of patients seen to date with PML complicating AIDS. Generally, when compared to the group of patients with a typical course of PML, the individuals with neurological improvement and prolonged survival more often had PML as the initial manifestation of AIDS, were systemically healthier, and had higher CD4 T-lymphocyte counts (CD4+ counts). Furthermore, cerebellar and brainstem disease was not observed in this group. Enhancement of the lesions, a rare phenomenon with PML, was seen more often on radiographic imaging, and inflammatory infiltrates were frequently

TABLE 2. *Signs and symptoms of PML: percent of cases in pathologically confirmed cases[a]*

Signs and symptoms	Sign or symptom present at onset	New sign or symptom present at time of diagnosis[b]
Mental deficits	36.1 (37.5)	27.5 (20.0)
Decreased attention only	2.9 —	0.0
Decreased memory only	4.3 (2.5)	0.0
Confusion only	7.2 (12.5)	2.9 (7.5)
Personality change	10.1 (20.0)	0.0
Dementia	11.6 (2.5)	24.6 (12.5)
Speech deficits	17.3 (15.0)	10.1 (10.0)
Dysarthria	7.2 —	1.4
Dysphasia/aphasia	10.1 (15.0)	8.7 (10.0)
Visual deficits	34.7 (45.0)	11.6 (12.5)
Visual blurring	7.2 —	0.0
Diplopia	1.4 (2.5)	0.0
Homonymous hemianopia	23.2 (42.5)	5.8 (5.0)
Cortical blindness	2.9 —	5.8 (7.5)
Optic atrophy	0.0 —	1.4
Motor weakness	33.3 (20.0)	85.4 (75.0)
Mono- or hemiparesis	33.3 (20.0)	68.1 (60.0)
Mono- or hemiplegia	0.0 —	13.0 (15.0)
Quadriplegia	0.0 —	4.3
Tone alterations	2.8 —	8.6
Bradykinesia/akinesia	1.4 —	1.4
Rigidity/parkinsonism	1.4 —	7.2
Sensory deficits	5.8 (5.0)	11.6 (5.0)
Face, arm numbness	5.8 (5.0)	0.0
Hemisensory deficit	0.0 —	11.6 (5.0)
Incoordination	13.0 (10.0)	18.8
Arm, leg ataxia	10.1 (7.5)	15.9
Cerebellar dysarthria	2.9 (2.5)	2.9
Miscellaneous	17.3 (7.5)	8.6
Headache	7.2 (5.0)	0.0
Vertigo	4.3 —	0.0
Seizures	5.8 (2.5)	7.2
Coma	0.0 —	1.4
No presenting signs or symptoms	1.4 —	1.4

From Brooks DL, Walker DL. Progressive multifocal leukoencephalopathy. *Neurol Clin* 1984;2:299–313.
[a] Numbers in parentheses are percent of cases in virologically and pathologically confirmed cases.
[b] Signs or symptoms not present at onset, which developed during progression of disease.

observed on histopathological study. One of these patients remained neurologically well 8 years after the initial diagnosis of PML despite the subsequent development of tuberculosis pericarditis and lymphoma (14), and another previously described (14) had no evidence of demyelination of PML at autopsy nearly 3 years after her initial diagnosis and biopsy. Nevertheless, more than 80% succumb within 1 year from the time of diagnosis (15,25,82,165).

Radiographic Imaging

Radiographic imaging provides us with our strongest support in diagnosing PML, but presently confirmation requires brain biopsy. Affecting the white matter, generally not enhancing with contrast, and exhibiting no mass effect, the hypodense lesions of PML on computed tomography (CT) of the brain reveal (Fig. 3) areas that may have a "scalloped" appearance as a result of the subcortical arcuate fibers lying directly beneath the cortex (175). Cranial magnetic resonance imaging (MRI) shows a hyperintense lesion on T2-weighted images in the affected regions (Fig. 4). As with CT scan, contrast enhancement is an exception. However, contrast enhancement has been observed with both brain imaging techniques in approximately 5% to 10% of pathologically confirmed cases of PML (175). The enhancement observed is typically faint and peripheral. The lesions of PML in AIDS have a predilection for the frontal and parieto-occipital lobes but may occur virtually anywhere. In a review of 47 cases of biopsy or autopsy-proven PML, we found involvement of the basal ganglia, external capsule, and posterior fossa structures (cerebellum and brainstem) (175). One-third of our patients had involvement of the posterior fossa and in 5% to 10% of patients the disease activity was isolated to these structures (14,175).

Other disorders may cause white matter disease in association with HIV infection. Demyelination observed with HIV-associated cognitive/motor disorder (ADC) may be radiographically indistinguishable from that of PML. Clinically, however, PML is associated with focal neurological disease and is much more rapidly progressive. Radiographic distinctions include a greater propensity of lesions to involve the subcortical white matter, its hypointensity on T1-weighted images (T1WIs), and its rare enhancement (175). Cytomegalovirus (CMV) may also cause demyelinating lesions. Typically these lesions are located in the periventricular white matter and centrum semiovale (21) where subependymal enhancement is also observed as a consequence of CMV infection (148).

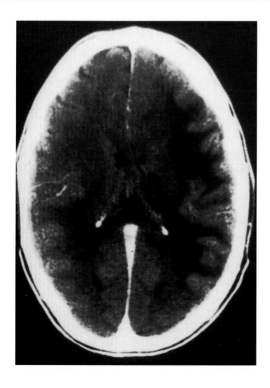

FIG. 3. Computed tomography scan. Extensive hypodense abnormality of the left hemisphere and less severe lesion in the posterior regions of the right hemisphere.

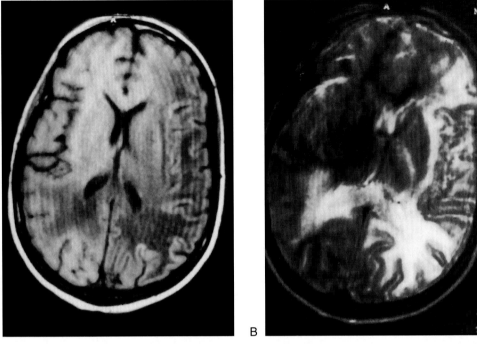

A   B

FIG. 4. A, B: Magnetic resonance image. The T1-weighted image shows hypointense signal of the left hemisphere and posterior region of the right hemisphere. The T2-weighted image shows hyperintense signal abnormalities in the same regions.

Cerebrospinal Fluid and Other Studies

All CSF specimens are nondiagnostic and generally reflect the abnormalities that one expects to observe in the face of HIV-1 infection with the exception of PCR for the JCV. The CSF protein may be slightly elevated, and myelin basic protein may be detected as a consequence of PML, again a reflection of an acute demyelination. A mononuclear pleocytosis (<20 cells/mm^3), a borderline low glucose (99,113), and an elevated protein (<65 mg/dL) may be noted.

We have found the CSF to be positive for JCV by PCR in approximately 30% of confirmed cases. However, others have found significantly higher rates (172). Until very recently the confirmation relied exclusively on typical histopathological changes and detections of JCV in brain samples from biopsies or at autopsy. The JCV can be detected by electron microscopy or isolated in cell cultures, viral antigens detected by immunocytochemistry, and viral DNA detected by *in situ* hybridization or PCR (107,120,158,185). With the advent of these techniques invasive procedures may no longer be required. Recent application of the PCR to CSF samples is promising in establishing the diagnosis premortem with less invasive procedures (i.e., brain biopsy) (173). Two early encouraging reports were able to detect JCV DNA with 100% specificity in more than three-fourths of CSF samples from patients with PML (54,107). Gibson and colleagues detected JCV DNA in 10 of 13 CSF samples in patients with confirmed PML, while no amplification was obtained in 42 CSF samples from patients without PML (54). In a second study, CSF samples from 12 AIDS patients were examined by PCR. Interestingly, all nine samples from patients with

TABLE 3. *JC virus detection by PCR[a] in cerebrospinal fluid from PML*

Groups	Moret et al.[b] Number	Total	Gibson et al.[c] Number	Total	Weber et al.[d] Number	Total	McGuire et al.[e] Number	Total	Aksamit et al.[f] Number	Total
PML										
AIDS	9	9	10	13	23	28	24	26*	11	23
Other	–	–	–	–	–	–	–	–	20	28
Total	9	9	10	13	23	28	24	26*	31	51
Control	0	3	0	41	0	82	10	114	1	170
AIDS	0	5	–	–	–	–	1	16**	0	249
Other	0	8	0	41	0	82	11	130	1	419
Total										

[a] Polymerase chain reaction.
[b] Sensitivity 100%; specificity 100%. Ref. 107.
[c] Sensitivity 76%; specificity 100%. Ref. 54.
[d] Sensitivity 82%; specificity 100%. Ref. 172.
[e] Sensitivity 92%; specificity 92%. Ref. 92a.
[f] Sensitivity 61%; specificity 99%. Ref. 2.
[g] Defined as human immunodeficiency virus (HIV) infected patients.
[h] Positive sample was from a patient with chronic lymphocytic leukemia and unexplained hemiparesis.

PML diagnosis amplified JCV DNA products; 5 five controls and the AIDS patients without PML did not show amplification (107). These and other reports of PCR amplification in CSF are summarized in Table 3. Based on a series of 110 CSF samples, 28 PML cases and 82 controls, Weber et al. reported 82% sensitivity and a 100% specificity for the diagnosis of PML with PCR (72). Aksamit et al. reported an overall sensitivity of 61% and a specificity of 99% in a large sample size—470 CSF samples (32). False-positive samples might depend on the stage of the disease or on the technical variation, such as set of primers and amount of CSF analyzed (54,72,107). Despite these variations and the limited clinical experience with this technique thus far, PCR is likely to prove a sensitive and highly specific diagnostic tool for confirming PML. It may even reduce the need for brain biopsy to establish the diagnosis if larger and more intensive studies are executed.

Serum antibodies are not helpful in the establishment of the diagnosis, since 80% or more of the population show seropositivity to antibodies against JCVs by adulthood (151). The electroencephalogram may show focal slowing but, like other studies, is also nondiagnostic.

DIFFERENTIAL DIAGNOSIS

There can be no question that the large increase in the incidence of PML in the last decade has been chiefly due to the AIDS epidemic, and therefore it is no surprise to find the majority of PML cases presenting in AIDS patients. Clinicians will continue to find themselves faced with HIV-infected patients who have cognitive impairment and a cranial MRI showing "hyperintense signal abnormalities on T2-weighted image (T2WI) characteristic of PML" due to the HIV dementia (AIDS dementia complex). It is these white matter lesions detected on MRI that frequently lead to the incorrect diagnosis of PML. The HIV dementia may be the initial manifestation of AIDS in up to 3.0% of adult AIDS patients (72,91), has an estimated annual incidence of close to 7%, and will affect one-third or more of AIDS patients before their death (91).

Cardinal features of an insidiously progressive psychomotor slowing, impaired memory, and apathy are highly suspicious signs (91,124). Early complaints of forgetfulness, difficulty concentrating and manipulating complex tasks, problems reading, general slowness, headache, and fatigue are classic. Because of the advanced degree of immunosuppression, AIDS patients with HIV dementia or PML generally exhibit similar constitutional features, including wasting, global alopecia, oral thrush and hairy leukoplakia, seborrheic dermatitis, and generalized lymphadenopathy. Patients with HIV dementia commonly have slow mental processing (bradyphrenia), abnormalities of saccadic and pursuit eye movements, diminished facial expression, low-volume, poorly articulated speech, impaired coordination and balance, postural tremor, poor dexterity, and a slow, clumsy gait. Unlike PML, focal neurological findings are uncharacteristic and suggest an alternative diagnosis. Cerebrospinal fluid examination is most valuable in eliminating the possibility of other disorders. Pathological examination reveals brain atrophy and meningeal fibrosis with the common histopathological feature of white matter pallor, associated with an astrocytic reaction chiefly distributed perivascularly in periventricular and central white matter (112). There is no evidence of myelin breakdown or loss of myelin basic protein. Multinucleate giant cells secondary to virus-induced macrophage fusion is the pathological hallmark of the disease (136). Other pathological features include microglial nodules, diffuse astrocytosis, and perivascular mononuclear inflammation (112).

Cerebral atrophy is the most common abnormality on CT in HIV dementia. However, low-density white matter abnormalities are also frequently observed. Computed tomography scan is quite helpful in ruling out focal mass lesions as a cause of a patient's altered mental status (17). The MRI will show large areas of white matter lesions, observed diffusely over a large area, typically in the centrum semiovale and periventricular white matter (114,123). Less commonly, localized involvement with ill-defined margins (patchy) or small foci less than 1 cm in diameter (punctate) are observed (114). These white matter abnormalities are frequently mistaken for PML, and the history, clinical findings, and to a lesser extent CSF parameters are quite helpful in distinguishing between the two disorders (Table 4) (57,134). The clinician needs to be mindful that these conditions are not mutually exclusive and that both conditions may coexist in the same patient.

Human immunodeficiency virus dementia and PML are not the only disorders of

TABLE 4. *Distinguishing HIV dementia from PML*

Characteristics	HIV Dementia	PML
Clinical		
Dementia	Prominent	Rare
Progression	Usually slow (months)	Usually rapid (weeks)
Focal neurologic findings	Unusual	Characteristic
Radiographic		
Subcortical involvement	Infrequent	Characteristic
Intensity on T-1 weighted image	Isointense	Hypointense
Enhancement	No	Faint and peripheral (5–10%)
Infratentorial lesions	No	Often (30% or more)
Cerebrospinal fluid		
Surrogate markers	Commonly increased	No correlation with disease
p24 antigen	Commonly increased	No correlation with disease
Myelin basic protein	Negative	May be present
JCV PCR amplification	Negative	Often positive (60% or more)

white matter occurring in AIDS in the absence of mass-producing lesions. Incidental white matter abnormalities are not uncommonly observed in HIV-infected individuals and do not appear to have any clinical significance (77). Among the disorders in the radiographic differential diagnosis, an acute, diffuse, rapidly fatal leukoencephalopathy has been reported. Others include (a) an HIV-associated granulomatous angiitis, (b) a multifocal necrotizing leukoencephalopathy with a predilection for the pons, (c) a relapsing and remitting illness clinically indistinguishable from multiple sclerosis, and (d) CMV ventriculoencephalitis and other viral opportunistic infections (114,123).

TREATMENT

Effective therapy of PML, whether specific antiviral therapy directed at the JCV or attempts to enhance cellular immunity, remains elusive. The treatment remains frustrating without any unequivocally successful modality. A variety of anecdotal reports and small series have resulted in a number of treatment regimens being proposed (Table 5). No randomized, double-blind therapeutic regimen has yet been conducted. However, the observation that PML may remain stable for long periods of time or even remit in the rare patient (14,42,75,118,125,140,145) clearly indicates that the illness, as any disease, is potentially treatable. Though, as expected, the anecdotal reports highlight their own inadequacies and emphasize their deficiency. The rarity of PML prior to the AIDS epidemic precluded practical therapeutic trials.

Nucleoside analogues exhibit established efficacy in the treatment of some viral diseases. Their mechanism of action is the interference with the synthesis of DNA. Several nucleoside analogues have been used in the treatment of PML with varying degrees of anecdotal success. Early experience with *cytosine arabinoside (ARA-C, cytarabine)*, a drug chiefly used in the treatment of myeloproliferative disorders, has been mixed (11,31,27). Bauer et al. (11) reported rapid and sustained improvement in neurological symptoms with ARA-C administered intravenously as 60 mg/m^2/day

TABLE 5. *Therapies for PML*

Nucleoside analogues
Cytosine arabinoside
Adenine arabinoside
Iododeoxyuridine
Zidovudine
Immunomodulatory agents
Alpha interferon
Beta interferon
Transfer factor
Levamisole
Tilorone
Other
Camptothecin and analogues
Topotecan
Corticosteroids
Heparin
Antisense oligonucleotides (proposed)

Adapted from Major ED, Ameniya K, Tornatore C, Houff S, Berger JO. Pathogenesis and molecular biology of progressive multifocal leucoencephalopathy, the JC virus-induced demyelinating disease of the human brain. *Clin Microbiol Rev* 1992;5:49–73.

and intrathecally as 10 mg/m^2. The patient described by Marriott et al. (98) showed more delayed, but similarly sustained, improvement following ARA-C 2 mg/kg/day on 5 consecutive days every 3 weeks. Similar anecdotal reports of various degrees of improvement have been reported by others (26,31,116,121,122,133). These regimens employed either intrathecal and/or intravenous administration of ARA-C. A study of intrathecal ARA-C administered as 10 mg/m^2 daily for 3 days with repeat dosing at variable intervals in 26 AIDS patients with PML revealed a salutory effect of 60% that was sustained in 50% for up to 2 years and was transient (<6 months) in the remainder (24). The reports of ARA-C efficacy in PML need to be tempered by the reports of its lack of benefit. Some case reports suggest a total lack of efficacy of cytosine arabinoside administered either solely intravenously (27,142) or in combination with intrathecal therapy (163). Clearly the most efficient way to administer the drug remains to be determined. Simultaneous intrathecal and intravenous administration would hypothetically address the systemic viral reservoir and prevent reinfection while treating the CNS infection. Unfortunately ARA-C is quite toxic to the bone marrow, particularly when administered concomitantly with antiretrovirals. This adverse effect would require the use of erythropoietin and granulocyte colony stimulating factor. The intrathecal administration avoids the bone marrow toxicity while not reaching certain affected areas of the brain that are more effectively treated with systemic administration.

At the present time, an ongoing AIDS Clinical Trials Group study is comparing high-dose antiretroviral therapy to high-dose antiretroviral therapy and intravenous ARA-C or intrathecal ARA-C in patients with AIDS-associated PML. In motivated patients with biopsy-proven disease, we have employed intravenous ARA-C at 2 mg/kg daily for 5 days every 2 weeks and intrathecal ARA-C at 80 mg/m^2 monthly. This regimen is quite toxic, particularly when administered with antiretrovirals and must be used cautiously. Approximately 50% of patients are intolerant to the therapy and did not appear to be effective (Berger JR, personal observation).

Adenine arabinoside (ARA-A, vidarabine), an adenine analogue, has been used in four patients with PML and chronic lymphocytic leukemia (127,178), the rationale for its use being its potentially less toxic side effects when compared to ARA-C. In doses of 20 mg/kg/day for 14 days (127,178) there was no response and all patients progressed.

5-Iodo-2'-deoxyuridine, a timidine analogue, has been used by intraventricular route through an Ommaya reservoir (2 mg/kg every 12 hours for 21 days, followed by 28 more days) with no improvement and severe toxicity evidenced by periventricular necrosis and gliosis in the dependent occipital horns (127,178).

Other nucleoside analogues do not appear to have had the same success as ARA-C in the treatment of PML. Wolinsky et al. (178) noted the failure of a 14-day course of ARA-A 20 mg/kg/day in two patients with PML. Similar failures of adenosine arabinoside therapy in the treatment of PML have also been described (127,167). Tarsy et al. (153) had no success with a combination of prednisone and intrathecal idoxuridine (5-iodo-2'-deoxyuridine) 2 mg/kg/12 h.

The antineoplastic drug camptothecin, a DNA topoisomerase I inhibitor, was used by Kerr and colleagues in certain studies and has shown some efficacy. It has been demonstrated to block JCV replication *in vitro* by means of pulsed doses employed in amounts that were nontoxic to cells (77).

Because of their antiviral activity, presumably the result of their ability to stimulate natural killer (NK) cells (161), interferons have been proposed as potential therapeutic agents in the treatment of PML. Alpha interferon has established efficacy in the treatment of other papovavirus-related diseases (174). In an open-label trial of the safety and efficacy of recombinant α-interferon 2A administered as 3 million units subcutaneously daily with a gradual increment (typically by 3 million units every third day) in the treatment of HIV-associated PML, 2 of 17 patients had survival extending greater than 1 year (16). No patient had a dramatic reversal in neurological function. In one patient, combined therapy of intravenous adenine arabinoside and β-interferon (154) showed no efficacy. However, intrathecal β-interferon 1 million units weekly for a total of 19 weeks and, thereafter, monthly was associated with modest improvement in her clinical picture and MRI (154).

The clinical observations regarding the potential efficacy of ARA-C in PML is supported by the recently acquired *in vitro* data on human fetal brain tissue infected with JCV. Major and colleagues have determined that cytosine b-D arabinofuranoside at a concentration of 25 μg/mL of culture effectively suppresses JCV replication. Whether this *in vitro* data can be translated into effective therapy remains to be determined.

Zidovudine (ZDV) and other antiretrovirals have been proposed as adjunctive therapy for AIDS-associated PML. One patient has been described with an apparent response to ZDV (32) and other investigators have commented on similar cases. In theory, the down regulation of HIV *tat* may decrease the transactivation of JCV. Zidovudine at 1,000 mg or more daily should be attempted in light of its superior ability to cross the blood-brain barrier (BBB).

The rationale for the use of low dose *heparin sulfate* as an adjunct in the treatment of PML is based on the model of the pathogenesis of PML suggested by Houff et al. (71). They postulate that PML is the result of activated JCV-infected B lymphocytes crossing the BBB and initiating new areas of neuroglial infection throughout the course of the disease. Heparin sulfate has been shown to prevent activated lymphocytes from crossing the BBB in animal models by stripping the lymphocyte glycoprotein cell surface receptors for cerebrovascular endothelial cells. This therapy has no demonstrated efficacy in established disease and is theoretically of value only as a means of prophylaxis.

Other agents, either alone or in combination with nucleoside analogues, have been tried in the treatment of PML. Tarsy et al. (153) administered prednisone in combination with idoxuridine and Van Horn et al. (163) administered corticosteroids, adrenocorticotrophin, and transfer factor with cytosine arabinoside without success. Theoretically, recovery of the underlying immunological disorder should be associated with recovery from PML. Selhorst et al. (135) reported a stabilization of the neurological deficits in a patient treated with tilorone, an immune enhancer. Conversely, Dawson et al. (34) noted no improvement following the cessation of immunosuppressive therapy in a patient with PML and myasthenia gravis. A recent report (32) suggests that PML occurring in association with HIV infection may respond to ZDV. A dramatic improvement followed the administration of ZDV 200 mg every 4 hours, and worsening followed a reduction in dose to 200 mg every 8 hours. A return to prior higher ZDV doses resulted in neurological stability (32). Zidovudine may effect levels of the tat protein that have been demonstrated to transactivate JCV (150). In our experience, ZDV use in AIDS-associated PML, even in high doses (1000 mg/day) has been devoid of benefit.

Finally, increased understanding of the molecular biology of the JCV and new technologies will result in innovative strategies. One possibility is the use of antisense oligonucleotides. An antisense oligonucleotide that is properly designed with a specific complementary base sequence that binds selectively to a targeted region of messenger RNA (mRNA) can prevent that translation of the mRNA into protein. Antisense oligonucleotide directed to JCV T antigen may reduce the viral expression by 80% (Khalili, personal communication, 1994). Targeting transcription sites is difficult due to the changes that occur in the viral cycle. Antisense oligonucleotides may also be designed to inhibit genes via triplex formation between the synthetic oligonucleotides and the double-helical DNA (2). Genetic manipulation or certain proteins that bind to a purine-rich domain may also result in inhibition of transcription and down regulate viral expression (Khalili, personal communication, 1994).

REFERENCES

1. Ahmed S, Rappaport J, Tada H, Kerr D, Khalili K. A nuclear protein derived from brain cells stimulates transcription of the human neurotropic virus promoter, JCVE, in vitro. *J Biol Chem* 1990; 265:13899–13905.
2. Aksamit AJ, Kost S. PCR detection of JC virus in PML and control CSF. 1994. Presented at *Neuroscience of HIV infection. Basic and Clinical Frontiers*, Vancouver, Aug 2–5, 1994.
3. Aksamit AJ, Proper J. JC virus replicates in primary adult astrocytes in culture. *Ann Neurol* 1988; 24:471.
4. Amemiya K, Traub R, Durham L, Major EO. Adjacent nuclear factor-1 and activator protein binding sites in the enhancer of the neurotropic JC virus. *J Biol Chem* 1992;267:14204–14211.
5. Amemiya K, Traub R, Durham L, Major EO. Interaction of a nuclear factor-1-like protein with the regulatory region of the human polyomavirus JC virus. *J Biol Chem* 1989;264:7025–7032.
6. Arthur RR, Dagostin S, Shah K. 1989. Detection of BK virus and JC virus in urine and brain tissue by the polymerase chain reaction. *J Clin Microbiol* 1989;27:1174–1179.
7. Aström KE, Mancall EL, Richardson EP Jr. Progressive multifocal leukoencephalopathy: a hitherto unrecognized complication of chronic lymphocytic leukemia and lymphoma. *Brain* 1958;81:93–111.
8. Atwood W, Amemiya K, Traub R, Harms J, Major EO. Interactions of the human polyomavirus, JCV, with human B lymphocytes. *Virology* 1992;190(2):716–723.
9. Bachman DM, Mark AS. [Personal communication].
10. Bauer W, Chamberlin W, Horenstein S. Spinal demyelination in progressive multifocal leukoencephalopathy. *Neurology* 1969;19:287.
11. Bauer WR, Turci AP Jr, Johnson KP. Progressive multifocal leuko encephalopathy and cytarabine. *JAMA* 1973;226:174–6.
12. Beckman A, Shah KV. Propagation and primary isolation of JCV and BKV in urinary epithelial cell cultures. In: Sever JL, Madden D, eds. *Polyomaviruses and human neurological diseases.* New York: Alan R Liss; 1983:3–14.
13. Bedri J, Weinstein W, Degregorio P, et al. Progressive multifocal leukoencephalopathy in acquired immunodeficiency syndrome. *N Engl J Med* 1983;309:492–493.
14. Berger JR, Mucke L. Prolonged survival and partial recovery in AIDS-associated progressive multifocal leukoencephalopathy. *Neurology* 1988;38:1060–1065.
15. Berger JR, Kaszovitz B, Post MJ, Dickinson G. Progressive multifocal leukoencephalopathy associated with human immunodeficiency virus infection. A review of the literature with a report of sixteen cases. *Ann Intern Med* 1987;107:78–87.
16. Berger JR, Pall L, McArthur J, et al. A pilot study of recombinant alpha 2A interferon in the treatment of AIDS-related progressive multifocalcal leukoencephalopathy. *Neuorlogy* 1992;42 (Suppl 3):257(abst).
17. Berger JR, Post MJD, Levy RM. AIDS. In: Greenberg JO, ed. *Neuroimaging: a companion to Adams and Victor's Principles of neurology.* New York: McGraw-Hill; 1994.
18. Berger JR, Scott S, Albrecht J, Belman AL, Tornatore C, Major E. Progressive multifocal leukoencephalopathy in HIV-infected children. *AIDS* 1992;2:837–841.
19. Bevilacqua MP, Pober JS, Wheeler ME, Cotran RS, Gimbrone MA. Interleukin-1 acts on cultured human vascular endothelium to increase the adhesion of polymorphonuclear leukocytes, monocytes, and related leukocyte cell lines. *J Clin Invest* 1985;76:2003–2011.
20. Blake K, Pillay D, Knowles W, Brown DWG, Griffiths PD, Taylor B. JC virus associated meningoencephalitis in an immunocompetent girl. *Arch Dis Child* 1992;67:956–957.
21. Bowen BC, Post MJD. Intracranial infections. In: Atlas SW, ed. *Magnetic resonance imaging of the brain and spine.* New York: Raven; 1991:501–538.
22. Briggs M, Kadonaga J, Bell S, Tjian R. Purification and biochemical charaacterization of the promoter specific transaction factor, Sp1. *Science* 1986;234:47–52.

23. Brightman MW, Reese TS. Junctions between intimately apposed cell membranes in the vertebrate brain. *J Cell Biol* 1969;40:648–677.

24. Britton CB, Romagnoli M, Sisti M, Powers JM. Progressive multifocal leukoencephalopathy and response to intrathecal ARA-C in 26 patients. *The Proceedings of the Fourth Neuroscience of HIV Infection Conference*, Amsterdam, July 14–17, 1992, p. 40(abst).

25. Brooks BR, Walker DL. Progressive multifocal leukoencephalopathy. *Neurol Clin* 1984;2:299–313.

26. Buckman R, Wiltshaw E. Progressive multifocal leukoencephalopathy successfully treated with cytosine arabinoside. *Br J Haematol* 1976;34:153–154.

27. Castleman B, Scully RE, McNeely BJ. Weekly clinicopathological exercises, case 19—1972. *N Engl J Med* 1972;286:1047–1054.

28. Cavanaugh JB, Greenbaum D, Marshall A, Rubinstein L. Cerebral demyelination associated with disorders of the reticuloendothelial system. *Lancet* 1959;2:524–529.

29. Cavender DE, Haskard DO, Joseph B, Ziff M. Interleukin 1 increases the binding of human B and T lymphocytes to endothelial cell monolayers. *J Immunol* 1986;136:203–207.

30. Coleman DV, Wolfendale MR, Daniel DA, et al. A prospective study of human polyomavirus infection in pregnancy. *J Infect Dis* 1980;142:1–8.

31. Conomy JP, Beard NS, Matsumoto H, Roessmann U. Cytarabine treatment of progressive multifocal leukoencephalopathy. *JAMA* 1974;229:1313–1316.

32. Conway B, Halliday WC, Brunham RC. Human immunodeficiency virus-associated progressive multifocal leukoencephalopathy: apparent response to 3′-azido-3′-deoxythymidine. *Rev Infect Dis* 1990;12:479–482.

33. Davis L, Hjelle BL, Miller VE, et al. Early viral invasion of brain in iatrogenic human immunodeficiency virus infection. *Ann Neurol* 1991;30:314(abst).

34. Dawson DM. Progressive multifocal leukoencephalopathy in myasthenia gravis. *Ann Neurol* 1982;11:218–219.

35. Diener HC, Ehninger G, Schmidt H, Stab U, Majer K, Marquardt B. Neurological complications after bone marrow transplantation. *Nervenarzt* 1991;62:2221–2225.

36. Divakar D, Bailey RR, Lynn KL, Robson RA. Long term complications following renal transplantation. *New Zealand Med J* 1991;104:352–354.

37. Dorries K. Progressive multifocal leukoencephalopathy: analysis of JC virus DNA from brain and kidney tissue. *Virus Res* 1984;1:25–38.

38. Dorries K, Loeber G, Meixensbarger J. Association of polyomaviruses JC, SV40, and BK with human brain tumors. *Virology* 1987;160:268–270.

39. Durum SK, Oppenheim JJ. Macrophage-derived mediators: interleukin 1, tumor necrosis factor, interleukin 6, interferon, and related cytokines. In: Paul WE, ed. *Fundamental immunology*. 2nd ed. New York: Raven Press; 1989:639–661.

40. Dynan W, Tjian R. 1985. Control of eukaryotic RNA synthesis by sequence specific DNA binding proteins. *Nature* 1985;316:774–778.

41. Elovaara I, Iivanainen M, Valle S-L, Suni J, Tervo T, Lahdevirta J. CSF protein and cellular profiles in various stages of HIV infection related to neurological manifestations. *J Neurol Sci* 1987;78:331–342.

42. Embry JR, Silva FG, Helderman JH, Peters PC, Sagalowsky AI. Long term survival and late development of bladder cancer in renal transplant patient with progressive multifocal leukoencephalopathy. *J Urol* 1988;139:580–581.

43. Fareed GC, Takemoto KK, Gimbrone MA. Interaction of simian virus 40 and human papovaviruses, BK and JC, with human endothelial cells. In: Schlessinger D, ed. *Microbiology*.Washington, DC: American Society for Microbiology; 1978:427–431.

44. Feigenbaum L, Khalili K, Major EO, Khoury G. Regulation of the host range of human papovavirus JCV. *Proc Natl Acad Sci USA* 1987;84:3695–3698.

45. Flaegstad T, Sundsfjord A, Arthur RR, Pedersen M, Traavik T, Subramani S. Amplification and sequencing of the control regions of BK and JC virus from human urine by polymerase chain reaction. *Virology* 1991;180:553–560.

46. Frankel AD, Pabo CO. Cellular uptake of the tat protein from human immunodeficiency virus. *Cell* 1988;55:1189–1193.

47. Frisque R, Bream G, Cannella M. Human polyomavirus JC virus genome. *J Virol* 1984;51:458–469.

48. Frisque RJ, Martin JD, Padgett BL, Walker DL. Infectivity of the DNA from four isolates of JCV. *J Virol* 1979;32:476–482.

49. Gallo P, Frei K, Rordorf C, Lazdins J, Tavolato B, Fontana A. Human immunodeficiency virus type 1 (HIV-1) infection of the central nervous system: an evaluation of cytokines in cerebrospinal fluid. *J Neuroimmunol* 1989;23:109–116.

50. Gardner S, MacKenzie E, Smith C, Porter A. Prospective study of the human polyomaviruses BK and JC and cytomegalovirus in renal transplant recipients. *J Clin Pathol* 1984;37:578–586.

51. Gardner SD, Field AM, Coleman DV, Hulme B. New human papovavirus (BK) isolated from urine after renal transplantation. *Lancet* 1971;i:1253–1257.

52. Gendelman H, Phelps W, Feigenbaum L, et al. Trans-activation of the human immunodeficiency virus long terminal repeat by DNA viruses. *Proc Natl Acad Sci USA* 1986;83:9759–9763.
53. Gibson PE, Field AM, Gardner SD, et al. Occurrence of IgM antibodies against BK and JC polyomaviruses during pregnancy. *J Clin Pathol* 1981;34:674–679.
54. Gibson PE, Knowles WA, Hand JF, Brown DWG. Detection of JC virus DNA in the cerebrospinal fluid of patients with progressive multifocal leukoencephalopathy. *J Med Virol* 1993;39:278–281.
55. Gillespie SM, Chang Y, Lemp G, et al. Progressive multifocal leukoencephalopathy in persons infected with human immunodeficiency virus, San Francisco, 1981–1989. *Ann Neurol* 1991;30:597–604.
56. Gottlieb MS, Schroff R, Schranker HM, et al. *Pneumocystis carinii* pneumonia and mucosal candidiasis in previously healthy homosexual men. *N Engl J Med* 1981;305:1425–1431.
57. Griffin DE, McArthur JC, Cornblath DR. Neopterin and interferon-gamma in serum and cerebrospinal fluid of patients with HIV associated neurological disease. *Neurology* 1991;41:69–74.
58. Gruss P, Khoury G. The SV 40 tandem repeats as an element of the early promoter. *Proc Natl Acad Sci USA* 1981;78:943–947.
59. Hadler NM. Antisense oligonucleotide therapies: are they the "magic bullets"? *Ann Intern Med* 1994;120:161–164.
60. Hallervorden J. Eigennartige und nicht rubriziebare Prozesse. In: Bumke O, ed. *Handbuch der Geiteskranheiten*, vol 2: *Die Anatomie der Psychosen*. Berlin: Springer; 1930:1063–1107.
61. Harmon WE. Opportunistic infections in children following renal transplantation. *Pediatr Nephrol* 1991;5:118–125.
62. Headington JT, Umiker WO. Progressive multifocal leukoencephalopathy. a case report. *Neurology* 1962;12:434–439.
63. Helland D, Welles J, Caputo A, Haseltine W. Transcellular transactivation by the human immunodeficiency virus type 1 tat protein. *J Virol* 1991;65:4547–4549.
64. Henson J, Rosenblum M, Armstrong R, Furneaux H. Amplication of JC virus DNA from brain and cerebrospinal fluid of patients with progressive multifocal leukoencephalopathy. *Neurology* 1991;41:1967–1971.
65. Henson J, Rosenblum M, Furneaux H. A potential diagnostic test for PML: PCR analysis of JC Virus DNA. *Neurology* 1991;41(Suppl):338.
66. Henson J, Saffer J, Furneaux H. The transcription factor Sp1 binds to the glial specific JC virus promotor and is selectively expressed in glial cells in human brain. *Ann Neurol* 1992;32:72–77.
67. Ho DD, Rota TR, Schooley RT, et al. Isolation of HTLV-III from cerebrospinal fluid and neural tissues of patients with neurological syndromes related to the acquired immunodeficiency syndrome. *N Eng J Med* 1985;313:1493–1497.
68. Hollander H. Cerebrospinal fluid normalities and abnormalities in individuals infected with human immunodeficiency virus. *J Infect Dis* 1988;158:855–858.
69. Holman RC, Janssen RS, Buehler JW, Zelasky MT, Hooper WC. Epidemiology of progressive multifocal leukoencephalopathy in the United States: analysis of national mortality and AIDS surveillance data. *Neurology* 1991;41:1733–1736.
70. Houff SA, Katz D, Kufta C, Major EO. A rapid method for in situ hybridization for viral DNA in brain biopsies from patients with acquired immunodeficiency syndrome (AIDS). *AIDS* 1989;3:843–845.
71. Houff SA, Major EO, Katz D, et al. Involvement of JC virus-infected mononuclear cells from the bone marrow and spleen in the pathogenesis of progressive multifocal leukoencephalopathy. *N Engl J Med* 1988;318:301–305.
72. Janssen RS, Nwanyanwu OC, Selik RM, Stehr-Green JK. Epidemiology of human immunodeficiency virus encephalopathy in the United States. *Neurology* 1992;42:1472–1476.
73. Katz DA, Berger JR, Hamilton B, Major EO, Donovan MJ. Progressive multifocal leukoencephalopathy complicating Wiskott-Aldrich Syndrome. Report of a case and review of the literature of progressive multifocal leukoencephalopathy with other inherited immunodeficiency states. *Arch Neurol* 1994;51:422–426.
74. Kenney SV, Natarajan T, Strike D, Khoury G, Saltzman NP. JC virus enhancer-promoter active in human brain cells. *Science* 1984;226:1337–1339.
75. Kepes JJ, Chou SM, Price LW Jr. Progressive multifocal leukoence phalopathy with 10 year survival in a patient with nontropical sprue: report of a case with unusual light and electron microscopic features. *Neurology* 1975;25:1006–1012.
76. Kerr D, Khalili K. A recombinant cDNA derived from human brain encodes a DNA binding protein that stimulates transcription of the human neurotropic virus JCV. *J Biol Chem* 1991;286:15876–15881.
77. Kerr DA, Chang CF, Gordon J, Bjornsit M, Khalili K. Inhibition of human neurotropic virus (JCV) DNA replication in glial cells by camptothecin. *Virology* 1993;196:612–618.
78. Khalili E, Rappaport J, Khoury G. Nuclear factors in human brain cells bind specifically to the JCV regulatory region. *EMBO J* 1988;7:1205–1210.
79. Kishimoto T. The biology of interleukin-6. *Blood* 1989;74:1–10.

80. Koenig S, Gendelman HE, Orenstein JM, et al. Detection of AIDS virus in macrophages in brain tissue from AIDS patients with encephalopathy. *Science* 1986;233:1089–1093.
81. Krupp LB, Lipton RB, Swerdlow ML, Leeds NE, Llena J. Progressive multifocal leukoencephalopathy: clinical and radiographic features. *Ann Neurol* 1985;17:344–349.
82. Kuchelmeister K, Gullotta F, Bergmann M. Progressive multifocal leukoencephalopathy (PML) in the acquired immunodeficiency syndrome (AIDS). A neuropathological autopsy study of 21 cases. *Pathol Res Pract* 1993;189:163–173.
83. Kure K, Lyman WD, Weidenheim KM, Dickson DW. Cellular localization of an HIV-1 antigen in subacute AIDS encephalitis using an improved double labeling immunohistochemical method. *Am J Pathol* 1990;136:1085–1092.
84. Kure K, Llena JF, Lyman WD, et al. Human immunodeficiency virus-1 infection of the nervous system: an autopsy study of 268 adult, pediatric and fetal brains. *Hum Pathol* 1991;22:700–710.
85. Lang W, Miklossy J, Deruaz JP, et al. Neuropathology of the acquired immune deficiency syndrome (AIDS): a report of 135 consecutive autopsy cases from Switzerland. *Acta Neuropathol* 1989;77:379–390.
86. Levy JA, Shimabukuro J, Hollander H, Mills J, Kaminsky L. Isolation of AIDS associated retroviruses from cerebrospinal fluid and brain of patients with neurological symptoms. *Lancet* 1985;ii:586–588.
87. London WT, Houff SA, McKeever PE, et al. Viral-induced astrocytomas in squirrel monkeys. *Prog Clin Biol Res* 1982;105:227–237.
88. London WT, Houff SA, Madden DL, et al. Brain tumors in owl monkeys inoculated with a human polyomavirus (JC virus). *Science* 1978;201:1246–1249.
89. Lynch KJ, Frisque RJ. Factors contributing to the restricted DNA replicating activity of JC virus. *Virology* 1991;180:306–317.
90. Lynch KJ, Frisque RJ. Identification of critical elements with the JC virus DNA replication origin. *J Virol* 1990;64:5812–5822.
91. McArthur JC, Hoover DR, Bacellar H, Miller EN, et al. Dementia in AIDS patients: incidence and risk factors. *Neurology* 1993;43:2245–2252.
92. McArthur JC, Kumar AJ, Johnson DW, et al. Incidental white matter hyperintensities on magnetic resonance imaging in HIV-1 infection. *J AIDS* 1990;3:252–259.
92a. McGuire D, Barhite S, Hollander H, Miles M. PCR-based assay of JC virus DNA in spinal fluid of HIV-Infected patients: high sensitivity and specificity for PML. Presented at *Neuroscience of HIV Infection: Basic and Clinical Frontiers*, Vancouver, Aug. 2–5, 1994.
93. Major EO, Amemiya K, Elder G, Houff SA. Glial cells of the human developing brain and B cells of the immune system share a common DNA binding factor for recognition of the regulatory sequences of the human polyomavirus, JCV. *J Neurosci Res* 1990;27:461–471.
94. Major EO, Amemiya K, Tornatore C, Houff S, Berger J. Pathogenesis and molecular biology of progressive multifocal leukoencephalopathy, the JC virus-induced demyelinating disease of the human brain. *Clin Microbiol Rev* 1992;5:49–73.
95. Major EO, Vacante DA. Human fetal astrocytes in culture support the growth of the neurotropic human polyomavirus, JCV. *J Neuropathol Exp Neurol* 1989;48:425–436.
96. Major EO, Vacante DA, Houff S. Human papovaviruses: JC virus, progressive multifocal leukoencephalopathy, and model systems for tumors of the central nervous system. In: Spector S, Bendinelli M, Friedman H, eds. *Neuropathogenic viruses and immunity*. New York: Plenum; 1992:207–229.
97. Major EO, Vacante DA, Traub TG, London WT, Sever JL. Owl monkey astrocytoma cells in culture spontaneously produce infectious JC Virus which demonstrates altered biological properties. *J Virol* 1987;53:306–311.
98. Marriott PJ, O'Brien MD, MacKenzie IC, et al. Progressive multifocal leukoencephalopathy: remission with cytarabine. *J Neurol Neurosurg Psychiatry* 1975;38:205–209.
99. Marshall DW, Brey RL, Cahill WT, Houk RW, Zajac RA, Boswell RN. Spectrum of cerebrospinal fluid findings in various stages of human immunodeficiency virus infection. *Arch Neurol* 1988;45:954–958.
100. Martin JD, King DM, Slauch JM, Frisque RJ. Differences in regulatory sequences of naturally occurring JC virus variants. *J Virol* 1985;53:306–311.
101. Martin JD, Padgett BL, Walker DL. Characterization of tissue culture induced heterogenicity in DNAs of independent isolates of JC virus. *J Gen Virol* 1983;64:2271–2280.
102. Masur H, Michelis MA, Greene JB, et al. An outbreak of community-acquired *Pneumocystis carinii* pneumonia: initial manifestation of cellular immune dysfunction. *N Engl J Med* 1981;305:1439–1444.
103. Mazlo M, Herndon RM. Progressive multifocal leukoencephalopathy: ultrastructural findings in two brain biopsies. *Neuropathol Appl Neurobiol* 1977;3:323–339.
104. Mazlo M, Tariska I. Are astrocytes infected in progressive multifocal leukoencephalopathy. *Acta Neuropathol (Berl)* 1982;56:45–51.

105. Miller JR, Barrett RE, Britton CB, et al. Progressive multifocal leukoencephalopathy in a male homosexual with T-cell immune deficiency. *N Engl J Med* 1982;307:1436–1438.
106. Miyamura T, Jikuya H, Soeda E, Yoshiike K. Genomic structure of human polyomavirus JC: nucleotide sequence of the region containing replication origin and small T antigen gene. *J Virol* 1983; 45:73–79.
107. Moret H, Guichard M, Matheron S, et al. Virological diagnosis of progressive multifocal leukoencephalopathy: detection of JC Virus DNA in cerebrospinal fluid and brain tissue of AIDS patients. *J Clin Microbiol* 1993;31:3310–3313.
108. Moriyama IM. Problems in measurement of accuracy of cause-of-death statistics. *Am J Public Health* 1989;79:1349–1350.
109. Myers C, Frisque RJ, Arthur RR. Direct isolation and characterization of JC virus from urine samples of renal and bone marrow transplant patients. *J Virol* 1989;63:4445–4449.
110. Nandi A, Dos G, Salzman NP. Characterization of a surrogate TATA box promoter that regulates in vitro transcription of the simian virus 40 major late gene. *Mol Cell Biol* 1985;5:591–594.
111. Narayan O, Penney JB, Johnson RT, Herndon RM, Weiner LP. Etiology of progressive multifocal leukoencephalopathy. Identification of papovavirus. *N Engl J Med* 1973;289:1278–1282.
112. Navia BA, Cho ES, Petito CK, Price RW. The AIDS dementia complex. II. Neuropathology. *Ann Neurol* 1986;19:525–535.
113. Navia BA, Jordan BD, Price RW. The AIDS dementia complex: I. Clinical features. *Ann Neurol* 1986;19:517–524.
114. Olsen WL, Longo FM, Mills CM, Norman D. White matter disease in AIDS. Findings at MR imaging. *Radiology* 1988;169:445–448.
115. Oppenheim JJ. Lymphokines. In: Oppenheim JJ, Rosenstreich DL, Potter M, eds. *Cellular functions in immunity and inflammation.* New York: Elsevier/North Holland; 1981:259–282.
116. O'Riordan T, Daly PA, Hutchinson M, Shattock AG, Gardner SD. Progressive multifocal leukoencephalopathy—remission with cytarabine. *J Infect* 1990;20:51–54.
117. Padgett BL, Walker DL. Virologic and serologic studies of progressive multifocal leukoencephalopathy In: Sever J, Madden DL, eds. *Polyomaviruses and human neurological disease.* New York: Alan R Liss; 1983.
118. Padgett BL, Walker DL. Virologic and serologic studies of progressive multifocal leukoencephalopathy. *Prog Clin Biol Res* 1983;105:107–117.
119. Padgett BL, Walker DL, ZuRhein GM, JN Varakis. Differential neurooncogenicity of strains of JC virus, a human polyoma virus, in newborn Syrian hamsters. *Cancer Res* 1977;37:718–720.
120. Padgett BL, ZuRhein GM, Walker DL, Echroade RJ, Dessel BH. Cultivation of papova-like virus from human brain with progressive multifocal leukoencephalopathy. *Lancet* 1971;1:1257–1260.
121. Peters ACB, Versteeg J, Bots GTA, et al. Progressive multifocal leukoencephalopathy: immunofluorescent demonstration of SV40 antigen in CSF cells and response to cytarabine therapy. *Arch Neurol* 1980;37:497–501.
122. Portegies P, Algra PR, Hollar CEM, et al. Response to cytarabine in progressive multifocal leucoencephalopathy in AIDS. *Lancet* 1991;337:680–681.
123. Post MJD, Tate LG, Quencer RM, et al. CT, MR and pathology in HIV encephalitis and meningitis. *Am J Roentgenol* 1988;151:449–454.
124. Price RW, Brew BJ. The AIDS dementia complex. *J Infect Dis* 1988;158:1079–1083.
125. Price RW, Nielsen S, Horten B, Rubino M, Padgett B, Walker D. Progressive multifocal leukoencephalopathy: a burnt-out case. *Ann Neurol* 1983;13:485–490.
126. Pryce G, Male DK, Sarkar C. Control of lymphocyte migration into brain: selective interactions of lymphocyte subpopulation with brain endothelium. *Immunology* 1991;72:393–398.
127. Rand KH, Johnson KP, Rubenstein LJ, et al. Adenine arabinoside in the treatment of progressive multifocal leukoencephalopathy: use of virus containing cells in the urine to assess response to therapy. *Ann Neurol* 1977;1:458–462.
128. Remenick J, Radonovich M, Brady J. Human immunodeficiency virus tat transactivation: induction of a tissue specific enhancer in a non-permissive cell line. *J Virol* 1991;65:5641–5646.
129. Resnick L, Berger JR, Shapshak P, Tourtellotte WW. Early penetration of the blood-brain-barrier by HIV. *Neurology* 1988;38:9–14.
130. Richardson EP Jr. Progressive multifocal leukoencephalopathy. *N Engl J Med* 1961;265:815–823.
131. Richardson EP Jr. Progressive multifocal leukoencephalopathy. In: Vinken PJ, Bruyn GW, eds. *Handbook of clinical neurology,* vol 9. *Multiple sclerosis and other demyelinating diseases.* New York: Elsevier/North Holland; 1970:485–499.
132. Richardson EP Jr. Our evolving understanding of progressive multifocal leukoencephalopathy. *Ann NY Acad Sci* 1974:230:358–364.
133. Rockwell D, Ruben FL, Winkelstein A, et al. Absence of immune deficiencies in a case of progressive multifocal leukoencephalopathy. *Am J Med* 1976;61:433–436.
134. Royal W III Jr, Selnes OA, Concha M, Nance-Spronson TE, McArthur JC. Cerebrospinal fluid human immunodeficiency virus type 1 (HIV-1) p24 antigen levels in HIV-1-related dementia. *Ann Neurol* 1994;36:32–39.

135. Selhorst JB, Ducy KF, Thomas JM, et al. Remission and immunologicaal reversals. *Neurology* 1978; 28:337(abst).
136. Sharer LR. Pathology of HIV-1 infection of the central nervous system. A review. *J Neuropathol Exp Neurol* 1992;51:3–11.
137. Shaw GM, Harper ME, Hahn BH, et al. HTLV-III infection in brains of children and adults with AIDS encephalopathy. *Science* 1985;227:177–182.
138. Siegal FP, Lopez C, Hammer GS, et al. Severe acquired immunodeficiency in male homosexuals manifested by chronic perianal ulcerative Herpes simplex lesions. *N Engl J Med* 1981;305: 1439–1444.
139. Silverman L, Rubinstein LJ. Electron microscopic observation on a case of progressive multifocal leukoencephalopathy. *Acta Neuropathol (Berl)* 1965;5:215–224.
140. Sima AAF, Finkelstein SD, McLachlan DR. Multiple malignant astrocytomas in a patient with spontaneous progressive multifocal leukoencephalopathy. *Ann Neurol* 1983;14:183–188.
141. Singer C, Berger JR, Bowen BC, Bruce JH, Weiner WJ. Akinetic-rigid sydnrome in a 13 year old female with HIV related progressive multifocal leukoencephalopathy. *Movement Disorders* 1993; 8:113–116.
142. Smith CR, Sima AAF, Salit IE, Gentili F. Progressive multifocal leukoencephalopathy: failure of cytarabine therapy. *Neurology* 1982;32:200–203.
143. Snapper CM, Findelman FD. Regulation of IgG1 and IgE production by interleukin 4. *Immunol Rev* 1988;102:51–75.
144. Sock E, Wegner M, Grumnt F. DNA replication of human polyomavirus JC is stimulated by NF-1 in vivo. *Virology* 1991;182:298–308.
145. Stam FC. Multifocal leukoencephalopathy with slow progression and very long survival. *Psychiatr Neurol Neurochir* 1966;69:453–459.
146. Stoner G, Ryschkewitsch C. Evidence of JC virus in two progressive multifocal leukoencephalopathy (PML) brains previously reported to be infected with SC40. *J Neuropathol Exp Neurol* 1991;50: 342.
147. Stoner GL, Ryschkewitsch CF, Walker DL, Webster HD. JC papovavirus large tumor (T)-antigen expression in brain tissue of acquired immune deficiency syndrome (AIDS) and non-AIDS patients with progressive multifocal leukoencephalopathy. *Proc Natl Acad Sci USA* 1986;23:2271–2275.
148. Sze G, Zimmermann RD. The magnetic resonance imaging of infectious and inflammatory disease. *Radiol Clin North Am* 1988;26:839–859.
149. Tada H, Lashgari M, Rappaport J, Khalili K. Cell type-specific expression of JC virus early promoter by positive and negative regulation. *J Virol* 1989;63:463–466.
150. Tada H, Rappaport J, Lashgari M, Amini S, Wong-Staal F, Khalili K. Trans-activation of the JC virus late promoter by the tat protein of type 1 human immunodeficiency virus in glial cells. *Proc Natl Acad Sci USA* 1990;87:3479–3483.
151. Taguchi F, Kajioka J, Miyamura T. Prevalence rate and age of acquisition of antibodies aganist JC virus and BK virus in human sera. *Microbiol Immunol* 1982;26:1057–1064.
152. Tamura T, Inoue T, Nagata K, Mikoshiba K. 1988. Enhancer of human polyoma JC virus contains nuclear factor 1-binding sequences; analysis using mouse brain nuclear extracts. *Biochem Biophys Res Commun* 1988;157:419–425.
153. Tarsy D, Holden EM, Segarra JM, et al. 5-iodo-2′-deoxyuridine (IUDR): NSC-39661) given intraventricularly in the treatment of progressive multifocal leukoencephalopathy. *Cancer Chemothery Repts* 1973;57(Pt 1):73–78.
154. Tashiro K, Doi S, Moriwaka F, Nomura M. Progressive multifocal leucoencephalopathy with magnetic resonance imaging verification and therapeutic trials with interferon. *J Neurol* 1987;234: 427–429.
155. Telenti A, Aksamit AJ, Proper J, Smith TF. Detection of JC virus DNA by polymerase chain reaction in patients with progressive multifocal leukoencephalopathy. *J Infect Dis* 1990;162:858–861.
156. Tominaga T, Yogo Y, Kitamura T, Aso Y. Persistence of archetypal JC virus DNA in normal renal tissue derived from tumor bearing patients. *Virology* 1992;186:736–741.
157. Tooze J. Human papovaviruses. In: Tooze J, ed. *Molecular biology of tumor viruses*, vol 2: *DNA tumor viruses*. Cold Spring Harbor, NY: Cold Spring Harbor Laboratory; 1980:205–296.
158. Tornatore C, Berger JR, Houff S, et al. Detection of JC virus DNA in peripheral lymphocytes from patients with and without progressive multifocal leukoencephalopathy. *Ann Neurol* 1992;31: 454–462.
159. Tornatore C, Berger J, Winfield D, LaVoie L, Major E. Detection of JC viral genome in the lymphocytes of non-PML HIV positive patients: association with B cell lymphopenia. Paper presented at the American Academy of Neurology Meeting, San Diego, May 1992.
160. Tyor WR, Glass JD, Griffin JW, et al. Cytokine expression in the brain during the acquired immunodeficiency syndrome. *Ann Neurol* 1992;31:349–360.
161. Tyring SK, Cauda R, Ghanta V, Hiramoto R. Activation of natural killer cell function during interferon-alpha treatment of patients with condyloma acuminatum is predictive of clinical response. *J Biol Reg Homeo Agents* 1988;2:63–66.

162. Vacante DA, R Traub, EO Major. Extension of JC virus host range to monkey cells by insertion of a simian virus 40 enhancer into the JC virus regulatory region. *Virology* 1988;170:353–361.

163. Van Horn G, Bastien FO, Moake JL. Progressive multifocal leuk oencephalopathy: failure of response to transfer factor and cytarabine. *Neurology* 1978;28:794–797.

164. Vazeux R, Brousse N, Jarry A, et al. AIDS subacute encephalitis, identification of HIV-infected cells. *Am J Pathol* 1987;126:403–410.

165. von Einsiedel RW, Fife TD, Aksamit AJ, et al. Progressive multifocal leukoencephalopathy in AIDS: a clinicopathologic study and review of the literature. *J Neurol* 1993;240:391–406.

166. Wahl SM, Allen JV, McCartney-Franscis N, et al. Macrophage- and astrocyte-derived transforming growth factor beta as a mediator of central nervous system dysfunction in acquired immune deficiency syndrome. *J Exp Med* 1991;173:981–991.

167. Walker DL. Progressive multifocal leukoencephalopathy: an opportunistic viral infection of the central nervous system. In: Vinken PJ, Bruyn GW, eds. *Handbook of clinical neurology*, vol 34. Amsterdam: Elsevier/North Holland; 1978:307–329.

168. Walker DL, Padgett BL. The epidemiology of human polyomaviruses. In: Sever JL, Madden D, eds. *Polyomaviruses and human neurological disease*. New York: Alan R Liss; 1983:99–106.

169. Walker DL, Padgett BL. Progressive multifocal leukoencephalopathy. In Fraenkel-Conrat H, Wagner RR, eds. *Comprehensive virology*. New York: Plenum; 1983.

170. Walker DL, Padgett BL, ZuRhein GM, Albert AE, Marsh RF. Human papovarirus (JC): induction of brain tumors in hamsters. *Science* 1973;181:674–676.

171. Ward JM, O'Leary TJ, Baskin GB, et al. Immunohistochemical localization of human and simian immunodeficiency viral antigens in fixed tissue sections. *Am J Pathol* 1987;127:199–205.

172. Weber T, Turner RW, Frye S, et al. Specific diagnosis of progressive multifocal leukoencephalopathy by polymerase chain reaction. *J Infect Dis* 1994;169:1138–1141.

173. Weber T, Turner RW, Ruf B, et al. JC virus detected by polymerase chain reaction in cerebrospinal fluid of AIDS patients with progressive multifocal leukoencephalopathy In: Berger JR, Levy RL, eds. *Neurological and neuropsychological complications of HIV infection. Proceedings from the Satellite Meeting of the International Conference on AIDS.* 1990:100.

174. Weck PK, Buddin DA, Whisnant JK. Interferons in the treatment of genital human papillomavirus infections. *Am J Med* 1988;85:159–164.

175. Whiteman M, Post MJD, Berger JR, Limonte L, Tate LG, Bell M. PML in 47 HIV-patients. *Radiology* 1993;187(1):233–240.

176. Wiley CA, Grafe M, Kennedy C, Nelson JA. Human immunodeficiency virus (HIV) and JC virus in acquired immunodeficiency syndrome (AIDS) patients with progressive multifocal leukoencephalopathy. *Acta Neuropathol* 1988;76:338–346.

177. Willoughby E, Price RW, Padgett BL, Walker DL, Dupont B. Progressive multifocal leukoencephalopathy (PML): in vitro cell-mediated immune responses to mitogens and JC virus. *Neurology* 1980; 30:256–262.

178. Wolinsky JS, Johnson KP, Rand K, Merigan TC. Progressive multifocal leukoencephalopathy: clinical patholgoical correlates and failure of a drug trial in two patients. *Trans Am Neurol Assoc* 1976; 101:81–82.

179. Wroblewska Z, Wellish M, Gilden D. Growth of JC virus in adult human brain cell cultures. *Arch Virol* 1980;65:141–148.

180. Yogo Y, Kitamura T, Sugimoto C, et al. Sequence rearrangement in JC virus DNAs molecularly cloned from immunosuppressed renal transplant patients. *J Virol* 1991;65:2422–2428.

181. Yogo T, Kitamura T, Sugimoto C, et al. Isolation of a possible archetypal JC virus DNA sequence from nonimmunocompromised individuals. *J Virol* 1990;64:3139–3143.

182. Yoshimura N, Oka T. Medical and surgical complications of renal transplantion: diagnosis and management. *Med Clin North Am* 1990;74:1025–1037.

183. Yoshioka M, Nakamura S, Nagano I, Kogure K, Shapshak P. The detection of cytokines in the AIDS brain. Paper presented at the American Academy of Neurology, San Diego, May 5, 1992.

184. ZuRhein GM. Polyoma-like virions in a human demyelinating disease. *Acta Neuro Pathol (Berl)* 1967;8:57–68.

185. ZuRhein GM, Chou SM. Particles resembling papovavirions in human cerebral demyelinating disease. *Science* 1965;148:1477–1479.

AIDS and the Nervous System, Second Edition,
edited by J. R. Berger and R. M. Levy.
Lippincott-Raven Publishers, Philadelphia © 1997.

23

Cytomegalovirus and Other Herpesviruses

°Bruce A. Cohen and †Richard D. Dix

°Department of Neurology, Northwestern University Medical School, Chicago,
Illinois 60611; and †Departments of Ophthalmology, Microbiology and
Immunology and Neurology, University of Miami School of Medicine, Bascom
Palmer Eye Institute, Miami, Florida 33136

The human herpesviruses are among the most common of the opportunistic pathogens in patients with acquired immunodeficiency syndrome (AIDS). Although herpesvirus infections are usually self-limiting in immunocompetent individuals, these unique viruses can reactivate to cause serious progressive disease in individuals immunosuppressed by human immunodeficiency virus 1 (HIV-1). A knowledge of the human herpesviruses and their neuropathological potential is therefore important to both clinicians and scientists who focus their efforts on AIDS related neurological diseases. As many previously fatal opportunistic pathogens become amenable to therapeutic control, it is likely that neurological diseases now associated with herpesvirus infections will become an increasingly frequent clinical problem in the growing AIDS patient population. It is also likely that additional neurological syndromes will be associated with these viruses in future AIDS patients once improvements in diagnostic techniques allow recognition of novel or subtle clinical expressions of these pathogens.

A number of general issues concerning the occurrence of herpesvirus infections in AIDS remain to be resolved. Because of their ubiquitous nature, the mere presence of these viruses is not sufficient to attribute pathological significance. Serological changes in recurrent infection are not commonly seen in AIDS patients, and culture techniques of body fluids and tissues have limited reliability, considerations that have stimulated development of new diagnostic approaches to increase sensitivity and specificity. Once diagnosed, the ability of current therapeutic regimens that rely exclusively on antiviral chemotherapy to eradicate virus from the nervous system have been inadequate, due in part to the emergence of resistant virus strains. This observation has prompted examination of alternative treatment modalities such as immune-based therapies. Finally, the potential role of herpesviruses as pathogenic cofactors that serve to accelerate the evolution of AIDS is actively being explored. The potential disruption of cellular functions and the implications for perturbing neuronal relationships make herpesviruses plausible contributors to the pathophysiology of progressive encephalopathy in AIDS.

TABLE 1. *The human herpesvirus*

Subfamily	Virus	Tropism
Alpha-herpesvirus	Herpes simplex virus type 1, herpes simplex virus type 2, varicella-zoster virus	Sensory ganglia
Beta-herpesvirus	Cytomegalovirus, human herpesvirus 6, human herpesvirus 7	Secretory glands, kidneys, T-lymphocytes, monocytes/macrophages
Gamma-herpesvirus	Epstein-Barr virus	B-lymphocytes

OVERVIEW OF THE HUMAN HERPESVIRUSES

Members of the family Herpesviridae are relatively large, enveloped, DNA-containing viruses that are highly disseminated in nature. Of the nearly 100 herpesviruses identified in a variety of species, seven have been recognized so far in humans: herpes simplex virus type 1 (HSV-1), herpes simplex virus type 2 (HSV-2), varicella-zoster virus (VZV), cytomegalovirus (CMV), Epstein-Barr virus (EBV), human herpesvirus 6 (HHV-6), and human herpesvirus 7 (HHV-7) (311). As with all herpesviruses, the human herpesviruses have been classified into one of three distinct subfamilies on the basis of biological properties (Table 1).

HSV-1, HSV-2, and VZV are classified as alpha-herpesviruses, a subfamily of viruses that exhibit a variable host range, relatively short reproductive cycle, rapid spread and efficient destruction of tissue culture cells, and the capacity to establish latent infections primarily, but not exclusively, in sensory ganglia. In comparison, CMV is classified as a beta-herpesvirus on the basis of restricted host range, relatively long reproductive cycle, slow progression of infection in tissue culture with infected cells becoming enlarged (cytomegalia), and the capacity to become latent in secretory glands, lymphoreticular cells, kidneys, and probably other tissues and organs. HHV-6 and HHV-7 are also classified as beta-herpesviruses. Finally, EBV is a member of the gamma-herpesvirus subfamily. Members of this subfamily exhibit limited host range and replicate in lymphoblastoid cells *in vitro*, although productive infection has also been recognized in epithelioid and fibroblastic cells. In addition, viruses of this group are specific for either T or B lymphocytes, with latent virus frequently found in lymphoid tissue. Thus, at least on the basis of classification, HSV-1, HSV-2, and VZV are considered to be neurotropic viruses, whereas the other human herpesviruses are considered to be lymphotropic to various extents.

CYTOMEGALOVIRUS

Epidemiology and Pathogenesis

Human CMV is a ubiquitous human herpesvirus that is acquired throughout life. Approximately 1% of infants are infected *in utero* and excrete virus at birth (356) and 50% to 80% of adults in the United States are seropositive for CMV by age 50 (95,136). Sexual promiscuity contributes to higher rates of infection; Drew and coworkers (96) reported that over 90% of young, sexually active, homosexual men have serological evidence of CMV infection. The major routes of transmission appear to be oral and respiratory, although sexual contact is an important means of transmission (53). Multiple blood transfusions and organ transplants (32,244) are also potential sources of infection.

Primary infection in young healthy adults is usually asymptomatic but may result in a mononucleosis-like syndrome associated with mild but transient immune suppression (196). Viremia lasting weeks to months accompanies primary infection (195,196), and infectious virus may be recovered from the pharynx and urine at the onset of disease, although viruria may persist for a year or more. Following clearance of virus by humoral and cell-mediated immune responses (302), CMV establishes lifelong persistent or latent infections with potential for reactivation. A molecular marker for CMV latency has not yet been identified. Reservoirs for persistence or latency have been incompletely identified but include salivary glands, kidney (renal tubular epithelial cells), spleen, and possibly lung as well as peripheral blood cells [CD4+ T lymphocytes (CD4+ counts) and monocytes/macrophages] (5,20,347). Targets of CMV infection within tissues and organs appear to be fibroblasts, epithelial cells, and endothelial cells. Thus, endothelial cells and monocytes/macrophages may be involved in hematogenous spread of CMV, while fibroblasts and epithelial cells play a role in virus distribution within the tissue or organ. It is noteworthy that numerous strains of CMV have been recognized by DNA restriction enzyme analysis of clinical isolates (166) which may vary in pathogenicity and sensitivity to antiviral drugs (375).

Dissemination of CMV During AIDS

Of the human herpesviruses, CMV is the major cause of morbidity in AIDS patients (235,286,300) and is frequently the cause of death (235). These observations correlate with an extremely high seroprevalence rate among HIV-1-infected populations which often approaches 100% (96,299,300). Serological studies suggest that the presence of CMV in AIDS patients correlates with more rapid progression of disease (386). As HIV-1-induced immune dysregulation progresses, rates of isolation of CMV from urine and blood increase (64), presumably due to progressive depletion of CMV-specific cell-mediated immune responses (110,313,301). However, despite evidence of increasing CMV replication with progressive HIV-1-induced immune dysregulation, morbidity directly due to CMV infection is rarely observed until there is a significant decline in absolute CD4+ counts (386).

In most AIDS cases, CMV is widely disseminated throughout the body, a pattern of infection not dissimilar to that seen in other immunocompromised patient populations (e.g., bone marrow transplant and cancer patients) (156). It is therefore not surprising that a wide spectrum of clinical manifestations of CMV infection has been observed in AIDS patients. These include CMV infection of the lungs, adrenal glands, gastrointestinal tract, liver, eye, and central and peripheral nervous systems (2,26,33,36,58,60,75,104,141,192,237,239,249,254,278,286,304,337,373). In contrast to other patient populations, however, the pattern of CMV infection in some tissues, including the central nervous system (CNS), is more fulminant in AIDS (263).

Neuropathology of CMV Infection

A number of autopsy series have identified CMV infection of CNS tissues in up to 42% of AIDS cases depending in part on criteria and methodology. Morgello and colleagues (254) described five types of lesions in 30 patients. The most common finding was the presence of disseminated microglial nodules found more commonly in deep gray structures but also seen in white matter. However, classic CMV inclusion-bearing cells (cytomegalocytes) (Fig. 1) were seen rarely within the nodules (Fig. 2), occurring in only 6.5%. In comparison, isolated cytomegalocytes were seen in one-half of the cases in basal ganglia, brainstem, cortical gray matter, and, in 10 patients, in capillary endothelia. No inflammatory reaction was associated with the presence of cytomegalocytes. Three additional patterns of neuropathology were observed each in approximately 10% of the cases. These included focal parenchymal necrosis characterized by macrophage infiltration and cytomegalocytes; ventriculitis characterized by hemorrhagic necrosis, cytomegalocytes, and acute and chronic inflammatory infiltration; and radiculomyelitis characterized by superficial meningitis extending into nerve roots and spinal cord. All cell types were apparently involved, including neurons, astrocytes, and endothelia, the latter suggested as a portal of entry to the CNS. In 29 of the 30 cases, systemic CMV disease was present.

Using immunohistochemical staining and in situ hybridization techniques, Wiley and Nelson (399) detected CMV-specific antigens and DNA in one-third of a series of 93 autopsied brains from AIDS patients. Two distinct patterns of localization were identified: (i) diffuse microglial nodules and (ii) microinfarctions containing numerous cytomegalocytes, some of which were found within the endothelia of small blood vessels. The initial focus of infection was ventricular ependymitis in approximately 10% of the cases.

Vinters and colleagues (378) identified 31 cases of CMV infection in an autopsy series of 160 AIDS patients using light microscopy for detection of CMV-specific pathology. Systemic CMV disease was present in 84% of the cases. Diffuse mi-

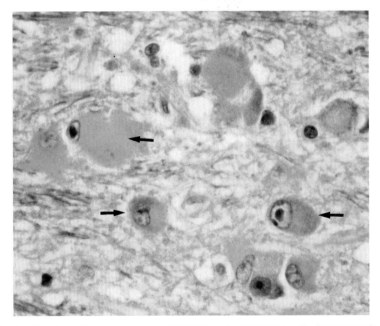

FIG. 1. Typical "owl eye" appearance of CMV inclusion-bearing cells (cytomegalocytes) *(arrows)*, ×400. (Courtesy of Betty Ann Brody, Department of Pathology-Neuropathology, Northwestern University Medical School, Chicago, IL.).

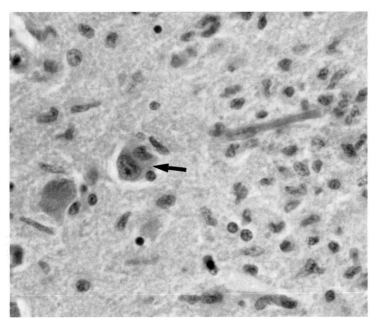

FIG. 2. Microglial nodule with associated cytomegalocyte *(arrow)*, ×250. (Courtesy of Betty Ann Brody, Department of Pathology-Neuropathology, Northwestern University Medical School, Chicago, IL.)

croglial nodules were observed in 29 of 31 cases, some associated with cytomegalocytes. Less frequently found were leptomeningitis, necrotizing ventricular ependymitis with choroid plexus involvement, vasculitis, radiculomyelitis, and focal necrosis or infarction. Concurrent neuropathology was noted in a significant number of their cases; multinucleated giant cells characteristic of HIV-1 encephalopathy were detected in 22% of the cases and CNS lymphoma was present in 16%.

The pathological features of CMV infection of peripheral nervous system (PNS) structures have also attracted considerable interest. Grafe and Wiley (140) identified CMV cytomegalocytes in Schwann cells of four of seven AIDS patients with inflammatory radiculopathy or neuropathy. Similarly, Said and colleagues (323) described multifocal necrosis with polymorphonuclear and mononuclear inflammatory infiltrates localized around endoneurial capillaries and associated with CMV cytomegalocytes in nerve biopsies of four patients with progressive sensorimotor neuropathies. Electron microscopic studies identified herpesvirus-like particles in monocytes/macrophages, endoneurial fibroblasts, and endothelial cells, but not Schwann cells. Roullet and colleagues (318) described similar features and additionally found necrotizing arteritis in one case.

Several authors have described pathological features of a CMV-associated ascending polyradiculopathy syndrome in AIDS patients. These include Cowdry type A inclusions in Schwann cells, focal necrosis in peripheral nerve segments and evidence of demyelination with relative axonal sparing (36), dorsal root ganglioneuritis and leptomeningitis involving superficial regions of CNS parenchyma and cranial nerves (373), and severe inflammatory necrotizing radiculitis characterized by perineurial and endoneurial infiltration by polymorphonuclear leukocytes and lymphocytes, segmental thrombosis of inflamed vessels, and cytomegalocytes in Schwann cells and some endothelial cells (28,104,237,249,258).

The pathological picture emerging from these reports is of a spectrum of infection in CNS tissues ranging from severe necrosis to isolated CMV-infected cells of little apparent pathological significance. Application of more sensitive methods of detection, particularly *in situ* hybridization techniques, has succeeded in identifying CMV-specific molecules in morphologically normal cells (400) and microglial nodules lacking cytomegalocytes (2), suggesting latent, abortive, or a semipermissive infection of neural cells. While CMV-specific inclusions are most commonly detected in what appear to be neurons and astrocytes, they can also be found in apparent oligodendrocytes, vascular endothelia, ependyma, and leptomeninges. On the basis of preliminary neuropathological and serological findings, CMV was suspected initially as the etiological agent of AIDS-associated subacute encephalopathy (111,202,258,259,266,304,350,379,388).

In comparison with CNS pathology, CMV infection of the PNS is associated with a more active inflammatory response involving polymorphonuclear and mononuclear cells, often in association with meningitis. In most instances, disseminated CMV disease is found concomitant with PNS infection.

Pathogenesis of CMV Encephalitis

Little information is available regarding the pathogenic events associated with CMV encephalitis in HIV-1-infected individuals, due in part to the species specificity of human CMV. A glial nodule encephalitis in guinea pigs produced by CMV has been described which has several neuropathological features similar to those of AIDS patients with CMV encephalitis (38–40) and may prove useful in the elucidation of the evolution of neurological disease in humans.

Dissemination of CMV in patients with AIDS supports the hypothesis that virus spreads from extraneural sites of CMV infection (e.g., salivary glands, kidneys, lungs) to CNS tissues by hematogenous routes, probably carried by monocytes/macrophages which are known to harbor virus. A similar Trojan Horse hypothesis has been postulated for HIV-1 infection of the CNS (198). Dissemination of CMV through the cerebrospinal fluid (CSF) has also been suggested (254,400) to explain the apparent ventriculofugal spread of virus from the ventricular walls to the brain parenchyma in some AIDS patients.

CMV-specific molecules have been detected in neurons, astrocytes, oligodendrocytes, ependyma, choroid plexus, endothelia, and cells of the leptomeninges in brains of AIDS patients at autopsy (333). The neurotropic nature of human CMV is being explored *in vitro* using a number of cell culture systems. Human neural cell aggregate cultures established from fetal CNS tissues have been shown to be permissive for human CMV infection (232,295,296); McCarthy and co-workers (232) have used this culture system to demonstrate that CMV strains may differ in their neurotropic properties. Monolayer cultures of primary astrocytes, neuroblastoma cell lines (SK-N-MC and SY5Y), astrocytoma/glioblastoma cell lines (U373-MG and Hs 683), and undifferentiated glioblastoma cell lines (A172 and T98G) (158,177,288) have also been used to explore susceptibility to human CMV infection. Cultures of primary astrocytes, U373-MG, Hs683, and SY5Y are fully permissive for CMV infection while A172 cells are completely nonpermissive for CMV gene expression, and CMV replication in T98G and SK-N-MC cell lines is restricted at the level of some early gene products. Since most of the cell lines used in these studies are transformed and not primary cells recovered from fetal or adult CNS tissue, additional work must be done using primary cultures of astrocytes, oligodendrocytes, and microglia of unquestionable purity (i.e., without contaminating fibroblasts) to explore more fully the permissiveness of neural cells for CMV infection.

By what mechanism does CMV infection cause tissue necrosis in the setting of AIDS? It is unlikely that T cell-dependent immunological reactions such as delayed hypersensitivity and cytotoxic T-lymphocyte activity participate in tissue destruction since HIV-1 infection directly affects these immune effectors (316). Natural killer cells also display depressed cytotoxic capabilities in HIV-1-infected individuals. Tissue necrosis may be a direct consequence of virus replication leading to cytopathology and cell death or be cytokine mediated. Tumor necrosis factor alpha (TNF-α) is an important mediator in inflammatory and immune reactions involved in tissue injury (377). Increased TNF-α production has been observed in liver transplant patients with CMV disease (370), and TNF-α transcripts have been found to be abundantly present in the colonic mucosa from AIDS patients with CMV colitis (349). Evidence for involvement of TNF-α in the pathogenesis of CMV disease has been presented recently by Haagmans and co-workers (145) using a rat model. In addition to TNF-α (100), the immediate early genes of CMV have also been shown in fibroblasts to upregulate expression of other cytokines, including transforming growth factor beta (247), interleukin-6 (3), interleukin-1 (173), and interleukin-2 (125), a regulatory cytokine that restores cytotoxic capabilities of natural killer cells recovered from HIV-1-infected patients (315).

CMV Encephalitis

Clinical Features

A number of case reports of CMV encephalitis in patients with AIDS have appeared in the literature. However, despite several autopsy series that document a high frequency of CMV-specific neuropathological findings within CNS tissues of AIDS patients, the diagnosis of CMV encephalitis prior to death remains difficult since the infection can occur without apparent neurological sequelae or may present with nonspecific clinical symptoms (378). The presence of additional opportunistic pathogens may also obscure the diagnosis. A variety of presentations have been described in AIDS patients.

Most often, CMV encephalitis presents as a subacutely progressive diffuse encephalopathy evolving over several weeks and characterized by confusion and impaired sensorium, with variably associated cranial neuropathies, ataxia, and motor weakness (121,163,188,339). Alternatively the presentation may result in focal neurological symptoms corresponding to the location of discrete parenchymal lesions (102,241,364), which may progress to a more diffuse encephalitis (121,278). Signs of meningitis may be present (102,121) but are often absent (163,188). A single case presenting with fatal subarachnoid hemorrhage due to CMV vasculitis has been described (153). Median survivals following neurological presentation in small series are about a month (163,188).

Imaging studies are often nonspecific in patients with diffuse encephalopathic

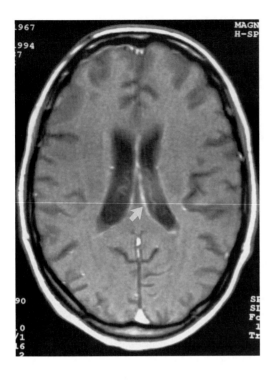

FIG. 3. An MRI following gadolinium infusion showing periventricular enhancement *(arrow)* in an AIDS patient with CMV encephalitis.

features (163). When present, periventricular ependymal enhancement (188) (Fig. 3) or meningeal enhancement (163) (Fig. 4) may suggest the diagnosis, though these findings are nonspecific in themselves. Progressive ventricular enlargement may be seen on serial studies (188).

The CSF may be normal or show nonspecific protein elevation (121,163,364). However, CSF may reveal a variable pleocytosis with mononuclear, polymorphonuclear, or mixed character and hypoglycorrhachia (102,188).

Most patients with CMV encephalitis have multiorgan involvement (163,188,339), although this has not universally been the case (121,364). Extraneurological involvement may precede CMV encephalitis, which may develop despite antiviral therapy directed at CMV (188,339) or may be discovered as a result of neurological presentation.

Diagnosis

The preceding description illustrates the difficulty in establishing a premortem clinical diagnosis of CMV encephalitis in patients with AIDS due to variability in clinical signs, symptoms, CSF formulas, and imaging patterns. Kalayjian and colleagues (188) have offered some useful clinical clues for patients with ventriculitis, suggesting the combination of encephalitis, cranial neuropathies, nystagmus, CSF inflammation with polymorphonuclear leukocytes and hypoglycorrhachia, and progressive ventriculomegaly characterize this condition. However, these features do not pertain to all cases of AIDS-associated CMV encephalitis. Significant polymorphonuclear CSF pleocytosis may be helpful when present, but changes in the cellular and protein contents of the CSF are not specific for CMV encephalitis, and, more

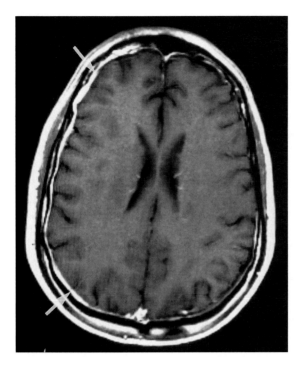

FIG. 4. An MRI following gadolinium infusion showing meningeal enhancement *(arrows)* in an AIDS patient with CMV encephalitis.

commonly, CSF pleocytosis is lacking. Efforts have therefore focused on identification of CMV-specific changes in the CSF to identify a diagnostic procedure that is sensitive and specific for CMV infection of the CNS.

Dix and colleagues (83), in a retrospective study, examined the frequency with which herpesviruses were recovered from CSF of 58 homosexual men immunocompromised with either Hodgkin's disease or AIDS. Four (6.9%) CSF samples yielded either CMV, VZV, or HSV-1 upon culture, three of which came from patients with the AIDS dementia complex or ascending myelitis. The fourth was free of neurological illness. Dix and colleagues (87) then investigated, in a prospective fashion, the potential diagnostic importance of CSF virus culture in 259 individuals who either were asymptomatic or suffered from encephalopathy, myelopathy, and/or peripheral neuropathy. CMV, HSV-1, HSV-2, adenovirus, and presumptive enteroviruses were detected in CSF samples of only 15 (5.6%) of the participants. There was no correlation between detection of an opportunistic virus within CSF and the presence or future development of neurological disease.

The same patient population was used by Tahseen and co-workers (366) to investigate the frequency of detectable CMV-specific immunoglobulin G (IgG) within matched serum and CSF samples of these HIV-1-infected individuals. A high percentage of these individuals, 96% (183 of 191) and 100% (99 of 99) of patients who were asymptomatic or symptomatic for neurological disease, respectively, had serum IgG to CMV. Surprisingly, IgG to CMV was detected in matched CSF samples from 22% (41 of 183) of asymptomatic patients and 29% (25 of 85) of patients with neurological illness. Approximately 80% of the CMV-positive CSF samples from asymptomatic patients had elevated total IgG contents and IgG-albumin indices of greater than 0.70, indicative of intrathecal antibody synthesis and suggestive of a possible smouldering, subclinical CMV infection of the CNS. Only 1 of 10 HIV-1-negative control participants had a CSF sample that was positive for CMV IgG, whereas 50% (5 of 10) of these individuals were CMV seropositive. Whether the presence of CMV-specific IgG within CSF samples of HIV-1-infected individuals will be of diagnostic value for AIDS-related CMV infection of the CNS remains to be determined.

Several recent retrospective studies suggest that the polymerase chain reaction (PCR) amplification technique to detect CMV-specific DNA in CSF samples may be a highly sensitive and specific diagnostic test for CMV infection of the CNS. Cinque and colleagues (55) and Wolf and Spector (403) demonstrated a high degree of specificity and sensitivity for this technique by correlating neuropathological evidence of CMV infection with the presence of CMV DNA in CSF samples by PCR. Control populations included AIDS patients with active systemic but not neurological CMV infection as well as individuals lacking any evidence of active CMV-related disease. Gozlan and associates (139) obtained similar results in a population with more limited pathological assessment. A contrasting view has been offered by Achim and colleagues (2), who retrospectively analyzed stored samples obtained from AIDS patients at autopsy. Their results challenge the specificity of CSF PCR for neurological CMV infection, though tissue samples from spinal cord and nerve roots were limited, leaving possible sources of neurological CMV infection unevaluated.

A very recent study by Revello and associates (306) has evaluated a technique for detecting the lower matrix protein, pp65, of human CMV in polymorphonuclear leukocytes from CSF in three patients with polyradiculomyelitis and one with encephalitis. Analysis of the samples for CMV DNA by PCR was also performed. The protein pp65 was detected in 9 of 10 CSF samples containing CMV DNA by PCR analysis and none of the 17 samples in which CMV DNA was not detected. When leukocytes are present in CSF, this technique may provide a more rapid means of detecting CMV.

At the time of this writing, CSF PCR appears to be the most sensitive technique short of biopsy for determining the presence of CMV neurological infection, though refined data on its specificity and sensitivity await prospective studies. Similarly, the value of serial CSF PCR analysis as a marker for the course of neurological CMV infection is in need of future evaluation. Definitive diagnosis of CMV encephalitis at present therefore remains based on neuropathological confirmation.

Necrotizing Myelitis

Necrotizing myelitis attributable to CMV in AIDS patients has been reported by a number of authors (144,323,373,378). Clinical features include paraplegia, urinary retention, and hypesthesia typical of myelopathy. Diagnosis may be facilitated by CSF pleocytosis, hypoglycorrhachia, and viral isolation (373) or by the emergence of acute CMV infection in extraneural tissues (144,323). In addition to necrotizing myelitis, neuropathological features may include meningoradiculitis, ventricular ependymitis, and microvascular thrombosis (378).

Polyradiculomyelitis

Cytomegalovirus polyradiculomyelitis (PRAM) in patients with AIDS presents subacutely with paresthesias or pain, progressive hypotonic weakness, areflexia, and variable sensory deficits ascending from the lower extremities to involve spinal cord, upper extremities, and cranial nerves in some patients (28,36,60,104,237,249,373). Urinary retention is an early feature of PRAM, and loss of rectal sphincter control is common; weakness and sphincter dysfunction are the predominant symptomatic complaints. The CSF findings include polymorphonuclear or mixed pleocytosis, prominent protein elevation, and variable degrees of hypoglycorrhachia, which contribute to a characteristic (though not pathognomonic) clinical picture. Most AIDS patients with CMV PRAM have preceding or concurrent systemic CMV disease, though in one case, PRAM was the initial presentation of AIDS (237).

Magnetic resonance imaging (MRI) analysis using gadolinium has demonstrated leptomeningeal enhancement of lumbar nerve roots or conus medullaris in some AIDS patients with PRAM (Fig. 5) (26,367). Neuroimaging examination to exclude compressive myelopathy is essential in the evaluation of an AIDS patient presenting with this clinical picture.

Electrophysiological studies typically demonstrate features of an axonal neuropathy. Miller and colleagues (249) described acute denervation changes with the appearance of widespread fibrillations and positive sharp waves within 2 weeks of presentation, and declining amplitudes and areas of serial evoked sensory and compound muscle action potentials. Others have reported modest (28) to marked slowing and absent or prolonged F waves (33).

Diagnosis of CMV-associated polyradiculomyelitis requires the exclusion of similar clinical presentations due to syphilis, lymphomatous meningitis, toxoplasmosis, cryptococcus, other herpesviruses, or bacterial meningitis. Cytomegalovirus can be

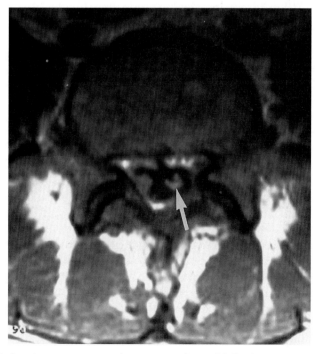

FIG. 5. An MRI showing nerve root enhancement *(arrow)* following gadolinium infusion in an AIDS patient with CMV polyradiculomyelitis.

cultured from CSF of some patients. Clifford and colleagues (58) described an AIDS patient with PRAM in whom PCR amplification of CMV DNA in a CSF sample confirmed a clinical diagnosis in the absence of a positive CSF culture. Additional studies have affirmed the potential value of PCR amplification techniques in the diagnosis of CMV-associated PRAM (55,139,403). Immunohistochemical staining of CSF cells for CMV-specific proteins has also been used diagnostically (239,306).

Peripheral Neuropathy

Numerous serological and epidemiological surveys have attempted to link CMV infection in adults to Guillain-Barré syndrome, an acute inflammatory demyelinating polyradiculopathy. Cytomegalovirus has never been recovered by direct culture of peripheral nerve in such cases; thus, activation of the virus in patients with Guillain-Barré syndrome may reflect an indirect immune response or an epiphenomenon. A chronic inflammatory demyelinating polyradiculoneuropathy characterized by limb weakness of insidious onset sometimes involving the trunk and cranial nerves has also been recognized in association with CMV infection on the basis of its clinical course, prognosis, and association with previous virus infection (101,151). The CSF may or may not show pleocytosis, but the protein content is usually elevated.

A progressive distal symmetric neuropathy associated with AIDS was first reported by Snider and colleagues (350). Sural nerve was normal in the one patient biopsied. Lipkin and co-workers (224) reported 12 homosexual men with persistent generalized lymphadenopathy who developed chronic inflammatory polyneuropathy. The symptoms were multifocal in 9 patients and distal and symmetric in 3. Nerve biopsy in 5 patients showed axonal degeneration and chronic perivascular inflammation without evidence of vasculitis. Dix and Bredesen (81) evaluated two AIDS patients with chronic inflammatory polyradiculoneuropathy at autopsy showing evidence of widely disseminated CMV disease in both. Cytomegalocytes were present in cells of dorsal root ganglia and were accompanied by mononuclear and polymorphonuclear infiltration, neuronophagia, and perineurial edema. Cytomegalovirus was recovered from cultures of femoral nerve of one patient.

A gradually progressive multifocal motor and sensory axonal neuropathy associated with endoneurial CMV infection and inflammatory changes ranging from an occasional cytomegalocyte to severe necrosis was described by Said and colleagues (323). Their patients developed paresthesiae and dysesthesiae with subsequent weakness and sensory and reflex loss which evolved over several months in two patients. Extraneural CMV disease was or became apparent in all patients during the course of their neurological illness. Histopathological features of nerve biopsy specimens included multiple foci of endoneurial necrosis with mononuclear and polymorphonuclear inflammatory infiltrates containing cytomegalocytes localized around endoneurial capillaries. A similar patient was described by Robert and associates (310). Small and colleagues (348) described a patient with predominantly motor polyneuropathy who developed hoarseness and dysphagia as a result of laryngeal nerve paralysis. Autopsy revealed extensive CMV infection in nerve roots and dorsal root ganglia at cervical, thoracic, and lumbar levels as well as in the superior and recurrent laryngeal nerves on the affected side.

Roullet and colleagues (318) recently described a series of 15 patients with CMV multifocal neuropathy, characterizing the salient features. The syndrome consists of an asymmetric sensorimotor neuropathy usually presenting with paresthesias and dysesthesias in a patchy distribution, followed within weeks by progressive motor impairment involving both upper and lower extremities which overshadows the sensory symptoms. Electrophysiological studies are compatible with an axonal neuropathy revealing diminished compound motor and sensory amplitudes, absent or delayed F-wave responses, and normal or mildly slowed nerve conduction velocities with variable degrees of denervation.

Cytomegalovirus viremia was detected in three-fourths of these patients at the onset of neurological symptoms while CSF was normal or revealed only increased protein in two-thirds. Two individuals who had a polymorphonuclear pleocytosis also had positive cultures of CSF for CMV. Of ten patients whose CSF was evaluated by PCR, nine had CMV DNA detected.

The composite clinical picture that emerges from these reports is of a progressive multifocal mononeuropathy multiplex, usually asymmetric, which has both motor and sensory components although motor features predominate. Neurogenic atrophy may be a prominent feature. CMV-associated PRAM may evolve later in the course of multifocal neuropathy, and sphincter involvement may be present if sacral radiculitis or myelitis develops. Cerebrospinal fluid studies show increased protein content, but may be normal unless PRAM develops. CSF analysis for CMV DNA by PCR appears to be a sensitive diagnostic measure. Cytomegalovirus mutifocal neuropathy can be distinguished from the more common distal painful sensory neuropathy of AIDS by the degree of motor involvement and asymmetry. The latter syndrome is of unknown etiology at the present time, although Fuller and colleagues (122) have suggested a CMV dorsal root ganglionitis as an etiology while noting a temporal association between the onset of neurological symptoms and systemic CMV disease.

Antiviral Treatment

Ganciclovir

Ganciclovir [9-(1,3-dihydroxy-2-propoxymethyl)-guanine] is an acyclic nucleoside analogue of acyclovir whose mechanism of action is dependent initially upon intracellular phosphorylation to ganciclovir-monophosphate by a virus-specific phosphotransferase (251), followed by additional phosphorylation to ganciclovir-triphosphate by cellular kinases. Levels of active ganciclovir-triphosphate are approximately 10 times higher in infected cells than in uninfected cells, imparting some measure of selectivity to the drug (243). In its active form, ganciclovir appears to block viral DNA synthesis by inhibiting the binding of deoxyguanosine triphosphate to DNA polymerase (411). Unlike acyclovir, however, it does not have the additional action of DNA chain termination.

Clinical studies have shown that ganciclovir is effective for treatment of AIDS-related CMV disease, especially retinitis and colitis (14,52,63,116,213,250,276). Due to the chronic nature of CMV infections during AIDS, ganciclovir treatment must be prolonged. Associated toxicity is primarily hematological; neutropenia is encountered in over 40% of patients treated, and approximately 20% will develop thrombocytopenia (63,411). The hematological toxicity of ganciclovir is exacerbated by simultaneous treatment with zidovudine (161). Prolonged use of ganciclovir can lead to the emergence of CMV strains that are resistant to the drug (112). The mechanism by which resistance develops is unclear, but resistance has been mapped on the CMV genome to the gene for the phosphotransferase responsible for initial phosphorylation of ganciclovir to its monophosphate derivative (251). Ganciclovir is virostatic in its action and fails to clear virus from infected tissues; thus, if the drug is discontinued, active virus replication can resume.

Foscarnet

Foscarnet (trisodium phosphonoformate) is an alternative antiviral drug for treating CMV infections in AIDS patients. This pyrophosphate analogue resembles ganciclovir in its mechanism of action by reversibly inhibiting the DNA polymerase of the virus. Unlike ganciclovir, however, it is also active against the reverse transcriptase of retroviruses (269). Several small clinical trials have shown therapeutic efficacy of foscarnet in the treatment of CMV retinitis (114,176,218,275), with initial response and ability to sustain disease remission comparable to ganciclovir. Unfortunately, it too is a virostatic agent. A multicenter clinical trial that directly compared the two antiviral drugs demonstrated that, while both agents exhibit equivalent efficacy against CMV retinitis, patients treated with foscarnet have a longer median survival time (362), a finding that may reflect its antiretrovirus activity (269). Foscarnet is active against ganciclovir-resistant strains of CMV (369).

Foscarnet exhibits toxicity characterized by a reversible decline in renal function in 20% to 25% of patients (114,115,176,218,275,369). Additional toxicities include anemia, paresthesias, seizures, and genital ulcers. While foscarnet alone rarely causes significant neutropenia, a decline in granulocyte count may also be anticipated in patients treated concurrently with zidovudine (275).

Acyclovir

Acyclovir is an acyclic analogue of guanosine whose mechanism of action is dependent upon a herpesvirus-specified thymidine kinase (TK) for phosphorylation to its monophosphate form prior to further phosphorylation by cellular kinases (392) (see below, Herpes Simplex Virus). Although CMV does not have a TK, acyclovir nonetheless exhibits low-level *in vitro* activity against the virus, and two clinical trials have demonstrated that intravenous and oral acyclovir therapy results in a delay in the onset of CMV shedding in recipients of renal allografts (19,246). However, acyclovir has less *in vitro* activity against CMV than has ganciclovir (392).

Treatment of CMV Neurological Disease

Reported experience in treating CMV neurological disease in AIDS patients with antivirals has been limited to isolated case reports, in part due to difficulties in antemortem diagnosis. While the optimal regimen of antiviral therapy is unknown at the present time, some clinical experience suggests efficacy of these agents in anecdotal instances. Price and associates (291) described an AIDS patient with acute meningoencephalitis, ventriculitis, CSF pleocytosis and hypoglycorrhachia, and isolation of CMV from CSF. After 2 weeks of induction therapy with ganciclovir, ventricular enhancement resolved and CSF pleocytosis and hypoglycorrhachia improved; however, the patient remained encephalopathic until his death 4 months later. Autopsy was not performed precluding neuropathological confirmation of a diagnosis of CMV encephalitis. In contrast, Sullivan and colleagues (364) reported an AIDS patient with biopsy-proven focal CMV encephalitis who appeared to respond successfully to treatment with ganciclovir.

Additional case reports have suggested an inability of ganciclovir therapy alone to modify the clinical course of CMV encephalitis (188,339). These observations suggest either the emergence of resistant virus strains or limited efficacy of the antiviral agents in the therapeutic regimens used. Peter and colleagues (281) successfully used alternating ganciclovir and foscarnet therapy in an AIDS patient with CMV neurological disease who apparently failed to respond to ganciclovir therapy alone. Another possible treatment option is combination therapy with foscarnet and ganciclovir despite failure with either drug alone. Dieterich and associates (80) suggest that response rates are similar to standard therapy with single agents, although myelosuppression of the combined regimen was also increased. Enting and collegues (109) added foscarnet to the regimen of a patient on maintenance ganciclovir for CMV retinitis who presented with CMV meningoencephalitis and obtained an initial clinical response which was not maintained, however, when doses were subsequently lowered.

Results are somewhat more encouraging using antiviral drugs to treat AIDS patients with CMV-associated PRAM and multifocal neuropathy. Several reports have noted clinical improvement of PRAM following institution of ganciclovir, usually when instituted early in the course of neurological disease (60,75,141,192,249,378). In other instances, however, clinical disease has progressed despite ganciclovir therapy (60,175). Little information exists regarding the therapeutic efficacy of foscarnet to treat CMV-associated PRAM. Jacobsen and colleagues (175) observed only modest and temporary clinical improvement following foscarnet treatment of an AIDS patient after ganciclovir therapy failed to halt progression of neurological disease; extensive necrotizing CMV encephalomyelitis was found at autopsy. A similar case was described by De Gans and associates (75). Cohen and colleagues (60) also described an AIDS patient with PRAM from whom a documented ganciclovir-resistant strain of CMV was recovered from a CSF sample during treatment. Although improvement in CSF pleocytosis was observed when placed on foscarnet therapy, he died of pneumonia shortly thereafter without clinical neurological improvement. Less information is available regarding the therapeutic efficacy of antivirals on CMV polyneuropathy during AIDS, although Said and associates (323) described one patient who appeared to respond well to ganciclovir therapy. Roullet and colleagues (318) obtained an initial response to therapy in 14 of 15 patients in their series. Relapse of neuropathy occurred in 3 and CNS CMV infection in 4 during follow-up in spite of maintenance therapy. Of 12 patients followed to death, 9 died of CMV infection.

Thus, it would appear as though antiviral chemotherapy is effective in at least some cases of CMV neurological disease in patients with AIDS. Patients can be treated with the usual induction dose of drug for 14 to 21 days, followed by a reduced maintenance dose. Assessment of the response to antiviral treatment should probably be done through examination of serial CSF samples and clinical evaluations. Cohen and associates (60) have suggested monitoring CSF pleocytosis and hypoglycorrhachia as indicators of possible antiviral resistance in AIDS patients with CMV-associated PRAM. As PCR amplification procedures become more widely available, detection and, perhaps, quantification of CMV-specific DNA in CSF samples may prove to be a useful therapeutic marker. Controlled clinical trials are needed to establish the optimal protocols for the available agents.

Immune-Based Therapies

Traditional antiviral chemotherapy has provided some benefit in the treatment of CMV disease during AIDS. Nevertheless, the results have been limited given the significant toxicities associated with the antivirals, the emergence of drug-resistant strains, and the virostatic nature of available agents. A live vaccine to prevent CMV infection prophylactically remains controversial, although two attenuated vaccines have been developed that are now in clinical trials (5,287). An alternate approach may be the use of immune-based therapies either in place of or as an adjunct to antiviral chemotherapy.

Passive transfer of antibodies is the most widely used and oldest form of immunotherapy. An active area of clinical investigation has focused on the use of CMV hyperimmune globulin for prevention and treatment of CMV infections in bone marrow transplant patients (42,65,245,272,351,402) with some encouraging results (106,303).

Adoptive transfer of specific immune effector cell populations represents another form of immunotherapy. Following primary CMV infection, immunocompetent individuals develop a strong cell-mediated immune response to the virus (307,338). Riddell and co-workers (308) generated CMV-specific CD8- cytotoxic T-lymphocyte (CTL) clones from three CMV seropositive bone marrow donors and then administered them to the bone marrow transplant recipients. After the first T cell infusion, weak CMV-specific CD8- class I major histocompatibility complex (MHC) restricted CTL responses were detected in each of the three recipients which were augmented with subsequent infusions of CTL clones, equivalent to or greater than that observed in the immunocompetent bone marrow donors. The adoptively transferred CD8- CTL immunity persisted for at least 1 month, demonstrating that large numbers of clonally derived T cells with defined antigen specificity can be generated and adoptively transferred without toxicity to selectively reconstitute immune responses in humans.

Cytokine immunotherapy in the treatment of AIDS patients has also received considerable attention (353), stimulated by the observation of Clerici and Shearer (57) that as HIV-1 infection progresses to AIDS, there is a distinct shift in overall cytokine production from a pattern that promotes cellular immunity, mediated by CD4 + -dependent delayed hypersensitivity responses (Th1-type response), to one that promotes humoral immunity, especially IgE production (Th2-type response). It has been hypothesized that reversal of the HIV-1-induced Th1/Th2 cytokine shift by cytokine immunotherapy will restore cell-mediated immune responses, thereby reducing morbidity and mortality associated with opportunistic pathogens including CMV. Clinical trials using interleukin-2 (IL-2) therapy alone or in combination with zidovudine are in progress (353). A mouse model of retrovirus-induced murine immunodeficiency (MAIDS) (181) that also displays a Th1/Th2 cytokine shift (124,189) may be useful in evaluating cytokine immunotherapy, especially immunotherapy oriented toward AIDS-related CMV retinitis (84,85).

The efficacy of combination immunotherapy using adoptive transfer of activated (phytohemagglutinin and recombinant IL-2) autologous CD8 T cells followed by low-dose continuous IL-2 infusion has recently been investigated by Klimas and co-workers (197), although CMV disease was not assessed. Nevertheless, this phase I clinical trial suggests that combination immunotherapy involving adoptive transfer of immune effector cells and immunoregulatory cytokines may be a viable therapeutic strategy to manage AIDS-related CMV disease, especially as an adjunct to traditional antiviral chemotherapy.

VARICELLA-ZOSTER VIRUS

Epidemiology and Pathogenesis

Two distinct clinical syndromes in humans are caused by VZV: varicella (chickenpox) and herpes zoster (shingles) (126). The annual national incidence of varicella has been estimated to be 1,500 per 100,000 of the population (289). Restriction enzyme analysis has shown no detectable difference between matched virus isolates obtained during distinct episodes of chickenpox and shingles, suggesting that both syndromes are caused by the same virus (172).

The pathogenesis of varicella or herpes zoster in immunocompetent patients is not completely understood. In children, VZV infects the mucosa of the upper respiratory tract and oropharynx, which results in an asymptomatic primary viremia. A secondary viremia during which virus replicates within blood mononuclear cells (132) is associated with prodromal symptoms that progress to focal cutaneous and mucosal lesions characteristic of the disease. Virus is ultimately cleared from the blood following stimulation of VZV-specific humoral and cell-mediated immune responses during the secondary viremia (168). Cellular immune responses and possibly interferon are apparently required to limit VZV infection (9), as antibody response to VZV does not correlate with the severity of varicella (135,387).

During primary infection, VZV spreads centripetally by neural routes from the skin and mucosal lesions to the corresponding sensory ganglia via the contiguous sensory nerve endings and sensory nerve fibers, although the virus may seed the ganglia hematogenously. In the ganglia, it establishes a persistent or latent infection without replication or cell damage. *In situ* hybridization has localized VZV-specific nucleic acid to either neuronal cells (134,171) or surrounding satellite cells (360). Reactivated virus may travel centrifugally down the sensory nerves to the skin and produce the clusters of vesicles along the dermatome that are the hallmark of herpes zoster.

Neurological complications of VZV infection have been recognized clinically in patients with varicella and in those with herpes zoster. Varicella-zoster virus is presumed to cause a spectrum of neurological illnesses, including cranial and peripheral nerve palsies, transverse myelitis, ascending myelitis, encephalitis, leukoencephalopathy, and a contralateral hemiplegia due to cerebral vasculitis associated with herpes zoster ophthalmicus (130).

Segmental Herpes Zoster

An underlying decline in immune competence, especially VZV-specific cell-mediated immunity, is common to most patients with segmental herpes zoster. The age-adjusted risk of herpes zoster in the HIV-1-infected population has been found to be 17 times higher when compared with a control homosexual population (44), although the risk of herpes zoster is not predictive of more rapid progression of HIV infection. The frequency of herpes zoster radiculitis in HIV-1-infected individuals appears to range from 2% to 4% (220,231). The clinical picture of segmental herpes zoster in both HIV-1-infected and uninfected individuals, is a cutaneous eruption characterized by pain and vesicles on an erythematous base in a pattern reflecting involvement of one or several dermatomes. The trunk is most frequently affected, followed by the face and extremities with areas supplied by the trigeminal nerve (especially the ophthalmic division) and thoracic ganglia (T3-L2) most commonly involved. On occasion, the immune response prevents the formation of cutaneous lesions; thus, severe ganglionitis associated with neuralgia may occur in the absence of vesicles. Cutaneous dissemination may follow segmental herpes zoster, suggesting an associated viremia (126) and VZV-specific DNA has been detected in circulating mononuclear cells during herpes zoster (131). VZV DNA has also been detected by PCR analysis in peripheral blood mononuclear cells of the elderly, even in the absence of recent herpes zoster (78).

Acyclovir treatment of immunocompromised patients has been associated with significant improvements in the rate of healing and the severity of acute pain of herpes zoster (27,148,170,255,405). The effect of acyclovir on postherpetic neuralgia has been less clear-cut. Three studies that compared a 7- to 10-day regimen of oral acyclovir therapy (4 g/day) with placebo reported a lower incidence of prolonged pain in the acyclovir-treated patients (148,170,255). Other studies have found no benefit on prolonged pain in patients who received intravenous or oral acyclovir (27,404,405).

Herpes zoster ophthalmicus may be complicated by a contralateral hemiparesis that results from infarction in the distribution of the larger branches of the circle of Willis ipsilateral to the site of radiculitis. The vascular occlusions may be thrombotic without vasculitis (103) or may be associated with necrotizing angiitis (155,120). In some cases, granulomatous angiitis occurs with inflammatory cells positive for VZV-specific antigens (120,412). Several case reports of herpes zoster ophthalmicus complicated by contralateral hemiparesis in HIV-1-infected patients have appeared in the literature (50,285,319,412). The hemiparesis occurred from 2 to 13 months following onset of herpes zoster ophthalmicus with variable clinical recovery, sometimes despite therapy with acyclovir. Rousseau and colleagues described one patient in whom oral acyclovir therapy (3 g/day) appeared to stabilize recurrent herpes zoster that was associated with MRI findings suggestive of silent ischemic infarction over a 22-month period. A second patient with VZV retinitis, and later ataxia due to a brainstem infarction, also appeared to stabilize following treatment with oral acyclovir, although he subsequently developed encephalitis after the dosage of acyclovir was reduced to 2 g/day (319). While these cases might encourage the use of long-term acyclovir maintenance therapy for HIV-1-infected patients with herpes zoster, a report of four AIDS patients who developed acyclovir-resistant dermatological herpes zoster 12 to 20 months following institution of oral acyclovir therapy could argue against this treatment strategy (174).

Herpes Zoster Encephalitis

Pathogenesis

Encephalitis attributed to herpes zoster may appear within weeks of VZV cutaneous lesions or, on occasion, before, usually resolving completely (178). Evidence that VZV is directly responsible for the CNS disorders in patients with herpes zoster encephalitis has been largely circumstantial. Cowdry A intranuclear inclusions and herpesvirus-like particles have been identified in neural tissues by histopathological analysis or electron microscopy (162,165,233). Elevated titers of antibodies to VZV in the CSF have also been reported in some patients (129,178,240). Successful recovery of VZV from CSF (7,129,178,270) and CNS tissues (162,233,267) has been documented, although this appears to be a rare event due to extreme lability of VZV in culture. On the basis of clinical findings at least three pathogenic mechanisms for the evolution of VZV encephalitis can be postulated. These include (i) a virus-induced autoimmune hypersensitivity reaction against CNS antigens, (ii) retrograde spread of virus from sensory ganglia along related neural pathways to the CNS, and (iii) hematogenous dissemination of virus to the CNS. The latter two mechanisms are not mutually exclusive.

Occurrence in AIDS

Given the ubiquitous nature of VZV and the strong association between herpes zoster and defects in cell-mediated immunity in other immunocompromised patient populations, surprisingly few neurological complications associated with VZV infection have been reported in patients with AIDS. In one neuropathological study, herpes zoster encephalitis was found in only 2% (3 of 153) of AIDS patients at autopsy (282).

Subacute encephalitis has been attributed to VZV in a number of AIDS patients on the basis of clinical or neuropathological features (62,133,142,253,322,350). The clinical features reflect a progressive encephalopathy with lethargy, confusion, and variable focal findings, including cranial neuropathies (62,142,322,350). Cutaneous VZV lesions were usually apparent within months of the onset of encephalopathy and a number of patients had recurrent VZV radiculitis at differing levels (133,142,253), though Morello and colleagues pathologically documented a case in the absence of any history or features of radicular VZV (253). Though most of the described cases have been subacute, Gilden and colleagues described a patient who followed an 18-month course of progressive cognitive and motor deterioration with VZV necrotizing encephalitis found at autopsy (133).

Neuropathological features reflect a necrotizing leukoencephalitis with multifocal distribution (253,322). Cowdry type A intranuclear inclusions can be found in astrocytes, oligodendrocytes, and neurons (322) and VZV-specific antigens and DNA can be detected within the lesions (133,253,322). Adjacent vessels may show proliferative changes (253) and involved thoracic spinal cord segments show similar necrosis (253,322).

Spread of VZV to the CNS may occur by either hematogenous or neutral routes. Evidence for the latter was convincingly presented by Rosenblum and colleagues, who demonstrated a restricted spread to the ipsilateral dorsal-lateral medulla in a patient with VZV opthalmicus who died of a CNS lymphoma within a month (317).

The composite clinical picture of herpes zoster encephalitis in a setting of HIV-1-induced immunosupression appears to be a leukoencephalitis usually of subacute duration with similarities to progressive multifocal leukoencephalopathy in temporal course and, to some extent, localization. A noninflammatory proliferative vasculopathy may be present, resulting in bland infarctions which contribute to the necrosis. A prior history of herpes zoster radiculitis is commonly present, although it may be temporally remote. While a history of recurrence of herpes zoster at different dermatomal levels or cutaneous VZV dissemination may provide diagnostic clues, it is noteworthy that at least two cases of AIDS-related herpes zoster encephalitis have been documented in which there was no history of cutaneous zoster (142,253).

Diagnosis of herpes zoster encephalitis presently rests on the basis of neuropathological findings at the time of biopsy or autopsy. In contrast to patients immunocompromised for reasons other than HIV-1 infection, CSF samples of AIDS patients with herpes zoster encephalitis usually show elevated protein content, but in the absence of pleocytosis. Although VZV has been recovered successfully from CSF samples of AIDS patients with neurological disease (81,83), this is an uncommon occurrence (81,87). Cerebrospinal cultures can be negative for detectable infectious VZV even though CNS tissue is infected with virus, as evidenced by the presence of virus-specific antigens and nucleic acid (322). The successful use of PCR techniques for detection of VZV-specific DNA within CSF samples of patients with herpes zoster meningitis (345) offers hope for a sensitive and specific noninvasive diagnostic procedure that may be forthcoming in the near future. Recently, DeAngelis and colleagues (73) described radiological features of three patients with encephalopathy who had subcortical lesions which progressed to involve adjacent cortical areas with prominent enhancement. Brain biopsy in two patients failed to reveal a diagnosis, but postmortem examination revealed zoster as the etiology. The authors suggest the radiological picture may be characteristic for zoster encephalitis.

Little information is available regarding antiviral therapy for herpes zoster encephalitis in the setting of AIDS. Both vidarabine (adenine arabinoside or Ara-A) and acyclovir prevent dissemination of VZV in immunosuppressed children with varicella (292,393) and in immunosuppressed patients with herpes zoster (18,41,397). A prospective, randomized trial showed that acyclovir was superior to vidarabine in the treatment of VZV infections in severely immunocompromised patients (343). Cole and colleagues treated one AIDS patient with vidarabine with subsequent neurological improvement (62); however, treatment of radicular VZV with either vidarabine or acyclovir has failed to prevent subsequent encephalitis (62,322).

It is possible that treatment will alter the natural history of the disease in this patient population, but optimal drug dosage as well as duration of therapy (including possible maintenance therapy) have yet to be determined. Moreover, the distinct possibility that acyclovir-resistant strains of VZV (13,174) will emerge must be considered. Thus, as in CMV encephalitis, alternative antiviral drugs and therapeutic strategies may need to be considered for successful management of VZV encephalitis during AIDS.

Herpes Zoster Myelitis

Most patients who develop herpes zoster myelitis are immunocompromised for various reasons (130). With the exception of temporal pattern, the clinical features of herpes zoster myelitis in AIDS patients do not appear to be different from those in patients who are immunosuppressed for reasons other than HIV-1 infection. Myelitis associated with herpes zoster results from centripetal extension following cutaneous eruptions. This complication occurs in less than 1% of patients. Subacute progression of motor weakness, sensory deficits, and sphincter disturbances in varying combinations evolve over weeks, usually beginning within a 3-week period following the rash (130). In HIV-1-infected patients, however, the interval between time of cutaneous herpes zoster and onset of myelitis may be measured in months (77). Neuropathological examination typically reveals a dorsal root ganglionitis associated with hemorrhagic necrosis, thrombosis and vasculitis, posterior nerve root inflammation with hemorrhagic necrosis in severe cases, and a demyelinating or necrotizing myelitis predominating in the posterior horns. Evidence for VZV infection has been provided by detection of Cowdry type A intranuclear inclusion bodies in oligodendrocytes and astrocytes (77,130,162) and recovery of virus from white matter of affected spinal cord tissue (162). Although little information is available regarding the efficacy of antiviral therapy, transient clinical response to acyclovir therapy was observed in one patient with herpes zoster myelitis (77).

HERPES SIMPLEX VIRUS

Epidemiology and Pathogenesis

The prevalence of antibodies to HSV generally increases with age and correlates with socioeconomic status and sexual activity (67,391). Usually, HSV-1 is acquired through nonsexual activities during early childhood, whereas HSV-2 is usually not acquired until commencement of sexual activity. Corey (67) has observed that while the incidence of HSV-1 infection may be declining in some populations (e.g., middle-class whites in Western industrialized nations), the incidence of sexually transmitted HSV-2 infection may be increasing in our society. Antibodies to HSV-2 have been detected in greater than 75% of female prostitutes, 50% to 60% of adults in lower socioeconomic groups, and 10% to 20% of adults in higher socioeconomic groups and are virtually nonexistent in nuns (391). Serological evidence of HSV-2 infection among sexually active heterosexual and homosexual men has been found to be as high as 70% and 90%, respectively, in some areas of the United States. Irrespective of sexual preference, the number of sexual contacts correlates directly with the acquisition of HSV-2 infection (260). The prevalence of HSV-2 infection is not a trivial matter with respect to AIDS; HSV-2 infection, by nature of being an ulcerative disease, correlates with acquisition of HIV-1 (164,357).

Herpes simplex virus is transmitted through personal, intimate contact. Infection is usually acquired from virus shed at a mucosal surface or other peripheral site. Following virus replication at the site of primary infection, either an intact virion or a nonenveloped capsid is transmitted by retrograde axonal flow via neurons of the peripheral nervous system to the sensory ganglia where latency is established after another round of virus replication (391). Hematogenous virus spread seldom occurs in adults, although isolated cases of viremia have been reported (68,262). Latent HSV-1 has been recovered from human trigeminal, superior cervical, and vagus ganglia (23,25,383,384) and from human trigeminal nerve roots (385). Latent HSV-2 has been recovered from human sacral ganglia (21). While neither infectious virus nor virus particles may be detected in latently infected ganglia, virus-specific RNA (latency active transcript, or LAT) that maps to the ICP0 region of the genome has been identified in human trigeminal ganglia (69). In a fraction of neurons harboring latent HSV, the virus is thought to periodically reactivate. To date, no gene or sequence tested has been identified as being essential for maintenance of latency (312).

Virus may be reactivated by various stimuli, including mechanical trauma, exposure to cold, wind, and sunlight, menstruation, emotional stress, and hormonal intake. The molecular basis of reactivation and the order in which virus genes are induced is not known (312). Once reactivated, virus may travel by axonal transport to the corresponding dermatome and produce lesions on ocular, oral, genital, or cutaneous sites. In patients with normal immune systems, recurrent HSV infections usually remain localized and heal within 1 to 2 weeks. In patients receiving immunosuppressive therapy and those with severe burns or hematological malignancies, recurrences are frequently more serious, require longer to heal, and may become disseminated (226). Although immunosuppression has been associated with increased severity of reactivated infections, the rate of reactivation is apparently not affected. Thus, defects of immune function, in general, and cell-mediated immunity, in particular, appear to play a major role in reactivated HSV infection.

No two epidemiologically unrelated HSV-1 or HSV-2 isolates are identical (46). Literally thousands of strains of either type of virus may therefore be present within the human population. Clinical isolates of HSV-1 and HSV-2 can be fingerprinted by DNA cleavage patterns, which has proven valuable in tracing the transmission of individual virus strains from one person to the next and in identifying multiple virus isolates from a single patient.

HSV Encephalitis

Herpes simplex virus may produce an acute hemorrhagic necrotizing encephalitis in immunologically normal adults (184,389,395,396,398) with predilection for the subfrontal and medial temporal lobes (261), suggesting that HSV may reach the CNS via the olfactory tracts (180). Alternatively, encephalitis may result from virus residing in trigeminal ganglia where it produces recurrent oral and ocular infection (71). Paired isolates from patients with HSV encephalitis and oral herpetic lesions may or may not show identity (394). Recurrent HSV encephalitis has been described (72,82).

The typical clinical features include headache, fever, and variable combinations of seizures, behavioral and cognitive changes, focal signs, and ultimately obtundation. Diagnosis may be facilitated by electroencephalography and imaging studies (184,234,261,398). Periodic spike, sharp-wave, or spike-wave patterns or localized slow-wave activity may be seen on the electronencephalogram (EEG). Imaging may show density changes with or without enhancing or hemorrhagic components. The preferred imaging technique is MRI because of its increased sensitivity for the classical regions of involvement. The CSF is nonspecific, typically showing a lymphocytic-mononuclear pleocytosis, often some erythrocytes, increased protein and, variable hypoglycorrhachia. HSV-specific antigens (205) and, later, antibodies (234) and oligoclonal bands may be found in CSF. HSV-1 may be recovered from CSF (86), and the use of PCR techniques to detect HSV-1 DNA has been shown to enhance diagnosis (12,294,320), though specificity of PCR is still being evaluated (391). The clinical picture may be seen in a number of other conditions (390); therefore definitive diagnosis requires recovery of HSV or demonstration of specific viral presence in tissue obtained by biopsy.

In AIDS patients, HSV encephalitis may present with these typical clinical features (81,368). In other instances HSV-1 has been found in conjunction with CMV in AIDS patients with encephalitis (206,208,277) who have not displayed the typical clinical features of either disease. Chronic encephalitis attributed to HSV has been reported (325), as has possible spontaneous recovery in untreated individuasls (193). Together these reports suggest that immunosuppression may modify disease course and presentation and that interactions between herpes viruses in the setting of AIDS may be important. A number of observations suggest that clinical and neuropathological features of HSV encephalitis may depend on cell-mediated immune responses (10,72,82,152,290,325,352). Alteration of typical neuropathological features has been demonstrated in an immunosuppressed setting (290,325). The CSF may contain elevated levels of cytokine IL-6 and interferon gamma early in the course followed by later increases of soluble IL-2 receptor, CD8 antigen, and TNF-α (10). Animal models for HSV encephalitis (6,22,35,167,168,225,372) are available, and some evidence of CD8-mediated cytotoxicity has been reported (168).

HSV-2 has occasional been implicated as the cause of encephalitis in immunosuppressed (223,365) and immunologically normal (261,271) individuals. HSV-2 has been presumed to cause encephalitis on the basis of temporal association with herpes genitalis and response to therapy in the setting of AIDS (236) and has been demonstrated pathologically by Dix and colleagues (Fig. 6) (88).

Acyclovir is the current antiviral agent of choice for HSV encephalitis because of its more benign side effects when compared to vidarabine (389). Relapse may occur despite therapy and demonstrated viral sensitivity (376). Progression of disease despite appropriate antiviral therapy may occur, suggesting the potential for emergent HSV resistance to these agents (368).

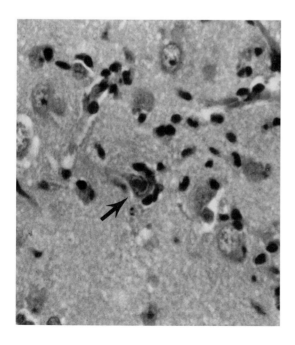

FIG. 6. Cowdry A-type intranuclear inclusion *(arrow)* in the biopsy specimen of a patient with culture-proven HSV-2 encephalitis, ×200.

In summary, these case reports suggest that herpes simplex encephalitis in the AIDS patient population can be atypical in several respects. First, AIDS-related HSV-1 infection of the CNS has been associated with concurrent CMV infection. It is intriguing to speculate that dual herpesvirus infection is synergistic and enhances overall pathogenicity. Second, HSV-1 infection is not always confined to the subfrontal and medial temporal lobes of the brain, as is usually the case in immunocompetent patients (Fig. 7A,B). Focal or panencephalitis may occur during AIDS, with evidence of active viral infection found not only in the subfrontal and medial temporal lobes but also in the cerebellum, brainstem, and subependymal region as well. Third, HSV-2 rather than HSV-1 may be the cause of some cases of encephalitic disease in adult AIDS patients. Finally, a wide spectrum of clinical neurological disease may be associated with HSV infection of the CNS during AIDS, including acute disease which may lead to coma and death within days of onset of clinical symptoms, subacute disease during which clinical symptoms progress slowly over weeks to months, and subclinical disease which remains asymptomatic.

The latter observation may provide important insights into the pathophysiology of herpes simplex encephalitis in the immunocompetent adult. It has generally been assumed that a strong immune response (both humoral and cell-mediated immunity) serves to reduce the spread of virus within the CNS during HSV infection and thereby reduces the extent and severity of tissue destruction and associated clinical symptoms. However, the observation that some AIDS patients with HSV infection of the CNS exhibit less severe neuropathological findings and a more chronic disease course suggests that herpes simplex encephalitis in the immunocompetent adult is an immunopathological disease, probably mediated by cellular immunity (e.g., CD4 + -dependent delayed hypersensitivity and/or CD8- T-lymphocyte cytotoxicity). In the AIDS patient, where such cellular immunity is impaired due to HIV-induced immune dysregulation and immunodeficiency, destruction of CNS tissue infected with HSV-1 would be due primarily to virus-induced cytopathology and cytokine-mediated inflammation involving macrophages and neutrophils. Thus, the extent of neuropathology in the AIDS patient due to HSV-1 infection might depend on the degree of HIV-1-induced immunosuppression in that individual.

HSV Meningitis

Herpes simplex meningitis is most commonly due to HSV-2 (68), often temporally associated with herpes genitalis (67,68). On occasion, HSV-1 has been recovered in patients with aseptic meningitis (49,149,154,257,407). Clinical and CSF findings are nonspecific, comprising headache, fever, lymphocytic pleocytosis, elevated protein, and moderate hypoglycorrhachia. HSV-2 may also be isolated from CSF. Polymerase chain reaction analysis may reveal HSV-2 DNA in the absence of viral isolation (61,284). In the nonimmunosuppressed individual, HSV-2 meningitis is often self-limited, though it may be recurrent. In the AIDS patient, the meningitis may become apparent due to associated encephalitis, myelitis, or radiculitis.

HSV Myelitis and Radiculitis

Herpes genitalis has been associated with urinary retention and lumbosacral radiculitis (48). Paresthesiae and neuralgic pain in the perineum and lower extremities,

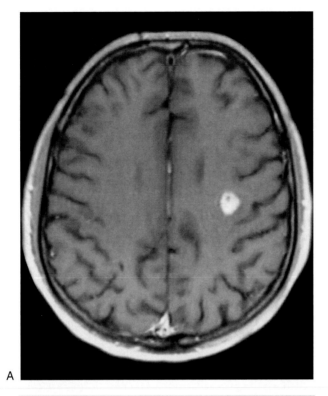

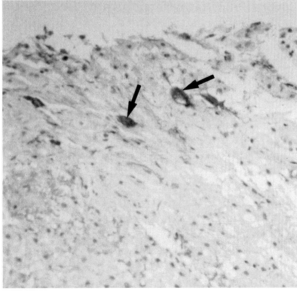

FIG. 7. A: An MRI showing focal herpes simplex encephalitis in an AIDS patient. **B:** Stereotactic biopsy specimen from lesion showing positive staining for HSV-1-specific antigens *(arrows)* by the immunoperoxidase procedure, ×250. (Courtesy of Betty Ann Brody, Department of Pathology-Neuropathology, Northwestern University Medical School, Chicago, IL.)

associated with a vesicular eruption from which virus can be cultured in the acute stages, is typical in cases with neurological involvement. This clinical picture may be complicated by meningitis and an ascending myelitis (68,401), which may also occur in the absence of vesicular lesions (31,194). Histopathological examination of spinal cord has revealed a necrotizing myelitis involving both gray and white matter regions (194,401). HSV-2 involvement has been confirmed by the identification of virus-specific antigens in spinal cord, chronically inflamed peripheral nerves, and dorsal root ganglia using immunohistochemical staining techniques (401).

In the AIDS patient population, isolated case reports of HSV-2 myelitis may be confounded by simultaneous CMV infection (373). Brittan and co-workers (43) described an AIDS patient with perianal HSV-2 infection and CMV retinitis who developed a slowly progressive thoracic myelopathy which evolved over a 4- to 5- month period. Histopathological analysis of the spinal cord showed thoracic myelitis with recent hemorrhages and cells bearing Cowdry type A intranuclear inclusions in the region of myelomalacia. Inclusion-bearing cells and arteritis involving the anterior spinal artery were also seen. Immunohistochemical staining revealed HSV-2 antigens in cells of most spinal cord regions, with only a small focus of cells positive for CMV antigens.

Antiviral Treatment

Acyclovir [9-(2-hydroxyethoxymethyl) guanine] is the initial antiviral drug of choice for treatment of neurological disease associated with HSV-1 or HSV-2 infection (389,391). Its mechanism of action is dependent upon a virus-specified TK that phosphorylates acyclovir to its monophosphate derivative. Acyclovir monophosphate is phosphorylated further by cellular kinases to acyclovir triphosphate, which binds to virus-induced DNA polymerase, and acts as a DNA chain terminator (392). Since acyclovir is taken up selectively by virus-infected cells, the concentration of acyclovir triphosphate is 40 to 100 times higher in infected cells than in uninfected cells (105,329). In addition, virus-induced DNA polymerase exhibits a 10- to 30-fold greater affinity for acyclovir triphosphate than do cellular polymerases (105,329). For these reasons, the drug exhibits low toxicity for uninfected cells and is therefore well tolerated clinically.

Treatment of HSV infections in AIDS patients is becoming more complex as acyclovir-resistant strains of virus emerge (113,123,392). Resistance to the antiviral can develop through mutations in one of two virus genes that encode for either TK or DNA polymerase (59,70,210). The TK mutants either fail to produce the enzyme (TK-deficient mutants) or synthesize an enzyme that is unable to phosphorylate acyclovir (altered substrate specificity) (92). Although virus mutants that exhibit resistance by all mechanisms can be produced experimentally, clinical acyclovir-resistant isolates are almost universally deficient in TK. Early *in vivo* studies of TK-deficient mutants showed them to have reduced neurovirulence in mice and they did not readily establish latent infections in sensory ganglia (117). Erlich and co-workers (113) reported a series of 12 AIDS patients from whom acyclovir-resistant HSV strains were isolated. All proved to be TK deficient, and all were found to be sensitive to vidarabine and foscarnet, antiviral drugs that do not require virus TK for activation. Such agents offer alternative anti-HSV therapy in AIDS patients (53,324).

EPSTEIN-BARR VIRUS

Epidemiology and Pathogenesis

Epstein-Barr virus is the etiological agent of infectious mononucleosis. In addition, the virus has been associated with African Burkitt's lymphoma, nasopharyngeal carcinoma, and lymphoproliferative diseases associated with immunodeficiency disorders or with immunosuppression after organ transplantation (221,248). Limited morbidity data suggest that the rate of infectious mononucleosis in the general population of the United States is 48 persons per 100,000 people per year, although this rate increases to approximately 840 per 100,000 people per year among college students (248).

Early in the course of primary infection, EBV infects B lymphocytes where the virus does not usually replicate but instead establishes latent infection. As a consequence of host immune responses, the number of latently infected lymphocytes in peripheral blood falls to 1 in 1 million cells during the months after primary EBV infection (221,248) and remains at this level throughout the lifetime of the patient. Two EBV genotypes circulate in most human populations (327,414). Both types of EBV have been identified in patients with AIDS (341).

Neurological Complications

Central nervous system complications in patients with infectious mononucleosis of EBV origin include meningoencephalitis, acute cerebellar ataxia, transverse myelitis, ascending myelitis, and acute psychosis (30,76,94,138,143,185,212,321,335,346). Although infectious mononucleosis is a common disease, serious neurological complications are infrequent, with estimates ranging from 0.7% to 5.5% in a series of 144 hospitalized patients (346). However, since most individuals with infectious mononucleosis do not require hospitalization, the true prevalence of neurological complications is probably closer to the lower estimate.

Epstein-Barr virus encephalitis usually presents at the time of other clinical manifestations of infectious mononucleosis but can present before or after onset of systemic disease (143). Clinical symptoms of EBV encephalitis are not different from other diffuse viral encephalitides and may be marked by delirium, psychosis, and visual distortion (147,209,346). Outcome is usually good, although residual neurological sequelae occur in 8% to 12% of cases and some fatalities have been reported. Occasional neuropathological analysis of fatal cases of EBV encephalitis have noted hemorrhage in gray matter of the brain and spinal cord, marked perivascular and pericellular edema, cranial nuclear degeneration with mononuclear infiltration, Purkinje cell degeneration, lymphocytic meningitis, and perivascular cuffing and infiltration of cranial and spinal nerve roots (89,138). Although CSF antibody studies are generally unrevealing, antibody to EBV capsid antigen has been reported in CSF of patients with encephalitis (89,182,330) and acute cerebellar ataxia (138). Additional CSF findings vary from normal to mild mononuclear pleocytosis with or without an increased protein content (207,209,346,413). Isolation of EBV from the CSF has also been reported (147). How the virus reaches the brain has not yet been adequately explained. Passage of EBV-infected B lymphocytes across the blood-brain barrier during acute illness seems a likely possibility because such cells and EBV-specific antibodies have been detected in the CSF of a patient with infectious mononucleosis and encephalitis (330).

A number of cranial neuropathy syndromes have been associated with EBV infection, the most common being Bell's palsy (143,335,346). Virtually all other cranial nerves have been reported to be involved in occasional cases (138). Epstein-Barr virus infection has been associated with acute inflammatory polyradiculitis (Guillain-Barré syndrome) (93,346), acute brachial plexopathy (138), and isolated cases of autonomic neuropathy (406).

Epstein-Barr virus infection is quite common in patients with AIDS; Quinnan and co-workers (300) diagnosed EBV infection in 33 of 34 AIDS patients. It is perhaps surprising that, at this writing, EBV has not been implicated in nonneoplastic neurological complications of AIDS. However, many of the symptoms noted above are nonspecific and have been reported in HIV-1-infected patients. It is therefore possible that some of these occurrences could be related to EBV infections since polyclonal B cell activation and hypergammaglobulinemia are commonly seen in connection with HIV-1-induced immune dysregulation prior to profound immunodeficiency (207).

Neoplastic Conditions

Epstein-Barr virus infection has been associated with a Burkitt's-like lymphoma in patients with AIDS (309,411). Of more significance in the setting of HIV-1-induced immunodeficiency is the evolving recognition of an association between EBV infection and primary CNS lymphoma, the most common brain tumor found in AIDS. A detailed discussion of CNS lymphoma in the AIDS patient population is found elsewhere in this monograph (see Chapter 28); only the relationship between EBV and CNS lymphoma is considered here.

Epstein-Barr virus has been shown to induce multifocal large-cell lymphomas in nonhuman primates, with individual tumors in each animal arising from different B cell clones (56). The clinical association of EBV with primary CNS lymphoma was first made by Hochberg and colleagues (160), who detected EBV-specific DNA in the tumor of an immunocompetent patient. Others have reported lymphoma of the brain associated with EBV infection in AIDS (190,314). The association between EBV and AIDS-related CNS lymphoma has been confirmed in several subsequent reports that examined series of AIDS patients with primary CNS lymphoma and found evidence of EBV in 50% to 100% (230,252,344).

The mechanism whereby EBV contributes to the pathogenesis of primary CNS lymphomas in the setting of AIDS remains unclear. HIV-1-induced immune dysregulation contributes to an increased frequency of circulating EBV-positive B lymphocytes that are capable of *in vitro* proliferation (34). Similarly, a decline in absolute CD4+ numbers has been associated with an increase in IgG to EBV capsid antigen and a concomitant decrease in antibody to EBV nuclear antigen in a series of 56 HIV-1-infected patients (300). Thus, progressive failure of immune surveillance caused by HIV-1 infection may allow reactivation of latent EBV and increased systemic EBV infection. However, whether EBV infection is directly responsible for the oncogenesis of primary CNS lymphomas or acts as a cofactor is not known (274). It is also intriguing to speculate that HIV-1 infection of EBV-infected B lymphocytes is another important cofactor in increasing tumorigenicity within the CNS (216).

HERPESVIRUSES AS COFACTORS IN AIDS

The average interval between HIV-1 infection of an adult and development of clinical AIDS is measured in years. Moreover, the incubation period may vary greatly among HIV-1-infected individuals. The basis for such prolonged and variable periods of clinical latency is unclear, but several contributing factors have been proposed. These include genetic susceptibility of the host, variations in HIV-1 strain virulence and pathogenicity, extent of virus mutation after infection, and amount and route of initial HIV-1 inoculation (215). Other viruses, however, may also play a role in determining the rate of progression of HIV-1-related disease by serving as infectious cofactors that modulate HIV-1 replication and contribute to immune dysregulation. In addition to their roles as opportunistic pathogens in the setting of HIV-1 infection, it has been suggested that human herpesviruses might play important roles as cofactors in facilitating the progression of HIV-1 infection (127,204,214,337). Herpesviruses are important immunomodulating agents; e.g., primary CMV infection causes a mild but transient suppression of cellular immunity (309). In addition, studies at the cellular and molecular levels have provided intriguing evidence that several human herpesviruses, including HSV-1 (256,257,273,380), CMV (157,159,340,354), EBV (191), and HHV-6 (79,108,128,382), may promote HIV-1 replication through effects on the tat gene product. Moreover, this synergism is bidirectional since HIV-1 replication will promote replication of several human herpesviruses (127,214,238,337).

With respect to neurological disease in AIDS, considerable attention has focused on the interaction between CMV and HIV-1. A body of evidence suggests that CMV may play an important cofactor role in the pathogenesis of HIV-1 disease in several ways. First, the immunosuppressive effects of CMV itself may facilitate the spread of HIV-1. Second, CMV infection of the brain may attract monocytes latently infected with HIV-1 into the CNS and induce their differentiation into macrophages, leading to activation of the retrovirus. Finally, *in vitro* studies have shown that coinfection of cultures of lymphoblastoid cells, monocytes, or primary astrocytes with CMV and HIV-1 results in enhanced HIV-1 replication due to *trans* activation of the retrovirus LTR promoter (159,214,238,340,354). The HIV-1 *trans* activator *tat* gene, when introduced into cells infected with CMV, also enhances expression of CMV genes (157). More recent work, however, suggests that coinfection is considerably more complex than previously thought, and the positive or negative effects of CMV on HIV-1 replication in brain-derived cells correlate with permissiveness of the cells for each virus (177,354). These *in vitro* findings have important clinical implications since double-labeling *in situ* techniques have shown that CMV and HIV-1 can coinfect the same cell in the CNS of AIDS patients (29,264). While the temporal course of the evolution of CMV and HIV-1 within the CNS is unknown, the common simultaneous occurrence of both viruses within the brains of AIDS patients suggests that *in vivo* interaction between them may play an important role in the overall pathogenesis of AIDS-related encephalitis or other neurological disorders.

CONCLUSIONS

The human herpesviruses are ubiquitous in the general population, infecting most individuals early in life. With normal immune functions, these viruses are usually

TABLE 2. *Neurologic syndromes associated with herpesviruses in AIDS*

Cytomegalovirus
  Encephalitis
  Myelitis
  Radiculitis
  Peripheral neuritis
  Vasculitis
Varicella-zoster virus
  Encephalitis
  Myelitis
  Radiculitis
  Vasculitis
Herpes simplex virus
  Encephalitis (types 1 and 2)
  Myelitis (type 2)
  Radiculitis (type 2)
Epstein-Barr virus
  Primary CNS lymphoma

AIDS, acquired immunodeficiency syndrome; CNS, central nervous system.

well controlled, often remaining clinically silent for the lifetime of the host. However, when immune surveillance is compromised by HIV-1 infection, they can become important pathogens which exhibit a wide spectrum of neuroinvasiveness and neuro-virulence whose true scope is still being defined (Table 2). Decreased inflammatory responses in combination with limitations in diagnostic techniques may obscure some of the clinical variants of these opportunistic infections in patients with AIDS. A paucity of treatment options and the lack of established markers for therapeutic efficacy, coupled with the genetic mutability of these viruses in response to antivirals, currently limits effective clinical responses to both acute and chronic neurological manifestations of these unique pathogens.

The ability of CMV and HIV-1 to coinfect the same cell in the CNS has been demonstrated, suggesting that other members of the human herpesvirus family may share this capability. It is therefore possible that intracellular interactions between herpesviruses and HIV-1 are important in the evolution of neurological syndromes attributed at the present time to HIV-1 alone, an important consideration in understanding the pathogenesis of neurological complications of AIDS.

It is clear to us that further investigation into the role of herpesviruses both as opportunistic pathogens and as potential cofactors in HIV-1 pathogenesis is an increasingly important focus in the understanding and management of neurological complications of AIDS. We anticipate a prolific expansion of information on these viruses and hope the material in this chapter provides the reader with a perspective with which to better evaluate these reports as they continue to appear in the literature.

ACKNOWLEDGMENTS

We thank Scott Cousins, Charles Wood, Micheline McCarthy, Joseph Berger, Robert Keane, and Gordon Dickinson for helpful discussions and Rosemary Ortiz for her assistance in preparation of this manuscript. This work was supported in part by the National Institutes of Health, grants EY10568 (to R. D. D.) and NO 1 A1 32535 (to B.C.).

REFERENCES

1. Ablashi DV, Balachandran N, Josephs SF, et al. Genomic polymorphism, growth properties, and immunological variations in human herpesvirus-6 isolates. *Virology* 1991;184:545–552.
2. Achim CL, Nagra R, Wang R, Nelson JA, Wiley C. Detection of cytomegalovirus in cerebrospinal fluid autopsy specimens from AIDS patients. *J Infect Dis* 1994;169:623–627.
3. Admirand JH, Bruening E, Ilia A, Yamboliev W, Gerthoffer W, St. Joer S. Induction of interleukin-6 and activation of MAP kinases by human cytomegalovirus. Abstract 343. Presented at the Nineteenth International Herpesvirus Workshop, Vancouver, 1994.
4. Akashi K, Yoshito E, Sumiyoshi Y. Brief report: severe infectious mononucleosis-like syndrome and primary human herpesvirus 6 infection in an adult. *N Engl J Med* 1993;329:168–171.
5. Alford CA, Britt WJ. Cytomegalovirus. In: Roizman B, Whitley RJ, Lopez C, eds. *The human herpesviruses.* New York: Raven; 1993:227–256.
6. Altmann DM, Blyth WA. Protection from herpes simplex virus-induced neuropathology in mice showing delayed hypersensitivity tolerance. *J Gen Virol* 1985;66:1297–1303.
7. Andiman WA, White-Greenwald M, Tinghitella T. Zoster encephalitis. *Am J Med* 1982;73:769–772.
8. Andiman WA, Eastman R, Martin K, et al. Opportunistic lymphoproliferation associated with Epstein-Barr viral DNA in infants and children with AIDS. *Lancet* 1985;338:1390–1393.
9. Arvin AM, Koropchak CM, Williams BRG, Grumet FC, Foung SKH. Early immune response in healthy and immunocompromised subjects with primary varicella-zoster virus infection. *J Infect Dis* 1986;154:422–429.
10. Aurelius E, Andersson B, Forsgren M, Sköldenberg B, Strannegård Ö. Cytokines and other markers of intrathecal immune response in patients with herpes simplex encephalitis. *J Infect Dis* 1994;170: 678–681.
11. Aurelius E, Johansson B, Sköldenberg B, Forsgren M. Encephalitis in immunocompetent patients due to herpes simplex virus type 1 or 2 as determined by type-specific polymerase chain reaction and antibody assays of cerebrospinal fluid. *J Med Virol* 1993;39:179–186.
12. Aurelius E. Johansson B, Skoldenberg B, Staland A, Forsgren M. Rapid diagnosis of herpes simplex encephalitis by nested polymerase chain reaction assay of cerebrospinal fluid. *Lancet* 1991;337: 189–192.
13. Averett ER, Pahwa S, Swenson P, Stanat SC, Biron KK. Varicella zoster virus clinical isolate resistant to acyclovir. In: *Proceedings of the Eighty-Seventh Annual Meeting of the American Society of Microbiology.* No. A94. Washington, DC: American Society for Microbiology; 1987.
14. Bach MC, Bagwell SP, Knapp NP, Davis KM, Hedstrom PS. 9-(1,3-Dihydroxy-2-propoxymethyl) guanine for cytomegalovirus infections in patients with the acquired immunodeficiency syndrome. *Ann Intern Med* 1985;103:381–382.
15. Bale JF Jr. Human cytomegalovirus infection and disorders of the nervous system. *Arch Neurol* 1984;41:310–320.
16. Bale JF Jr, Jordan MC. Cytomegalovirus. In: McKendall RR, ed. *Handbook of clinical neurology: viral disease,* vol 12. Elsevier: Amsterdam; 1989:263–279.
17. Bale JF Jr, Rote NS, Bloomer LC. Guillain-Barré like polyneuropathy after renal transplant: possible association with cytomegalovirus infection. *Arch Neurol* 1980;37;784.
18. Balfour HH Jr, Bean B, Laskin OL. Acyclovir halts progression of herpes zoster in immunocompromised patients. *N Engl J Med* 1983;308:1448–1453.
19. Balfour HH, Chace BA, Stapleton JT, Simmone RL, Fryd DS. A randomized placebo-controlled trial of oral acyclovir for the prevention of cytomegalovirus disease in recipients of renal allografts. *N Engl J Med* 1989;320:1381–1387.
20. Balthesen M, Messerle M, Reddehase MJ. Lungs are a major organ site of cytomegalovirus latency and recurrence. *J Virol* 1993;67:5360–5366.
21. Baringer JR. Recovery of herpes simplex virus from human sacral ganglions. *N Engl J Med* 1974; 291:828–830.
22. Baringer JR. Neurobiology of herpesviruses, workshop summary. In: Nahmias AJ, Dowdle WR, Schinazi RF, eds. *The human herpesviruses.* New York: Elsevier; 1981:567.
23. Baringer JR, Swoveland P. Recovery of herpes simplex virus from human trigeminal ganglions. *N Engl J Med* 1973;288:648–650.
24. Barza M, Pauker SG. The decision to biopsy, treat, or wait in suspected herpes encephalitis. *Ann Intern Med* 1980;92:641–649.
25. Bastian FO, Rabson AS, Yee CL, Tralka TS. Herpes simplex hominis: isolation from human trigeminal ganglion. *Science* 1972;178:306–307.
26. Bazan C, Jackson C, Jinkins JR, Barohn RJ. Gadolinium-enhanced MRI in a case of cytomegalovirus polyradiculopathy. *Neurology* 1991;41:1522–1523.
27. Bean B, Braun C, Balfour HH Jr. Acyclovir therapy for acute herpes zoster. *Lancet* 1982;2:118–121.
28. Behar R, Wiley C, McCutchan JA. Cytomegalovirus polyradiculoneuropathy in acquired immune deficiency syndrome. *Neurology* 1987;37:557–561.

29. Belec L, Gray F, Mikol J, et al. Cytomegalovirus (CMV) encephalomyeloradiculitis and human immunodeficiency virus (HIV) encephalitis: presence of HIV and CMV co-infected multinucleated giant cells. *Acta Neuropathol* 1990;81:99–104.

30. Bennett DR, Peters HA. Acute cerebellar syndrome secondary to infectious mononucleosis in a fifty-two year old man. *Ann Intern Med* 1961;55:147–149.

31. Bergstrom J, Vahlne A, Alestig K. Primary and recurrent herpes simples virus type 2 induced meningitis. *J Infect Dis* 1990;162:322–330.

32. Betts RF. The relationship of epidemiology and treatment factors to infection and allograft survival in renal transplantation. In: Plotkins SA, Michelson S, Pagano JS, Rapp F, eds. *CMV: pathogenesis and prevention of human infection.* New York: Liss; 1984:87–100.

33. Beydoun SR. Misdiagnosis of cytomegalovirus polyradiculopathy coexisting with HIV neuropathy. *Muscle Nerve* 1991;14:575–576.

34. Birx DL, Redfield RR, Tosato G. Defective regulation of Epstein-Barr virus infection in patients with acquired immunodeficiency syndrome (AIDS) or AIDS-related disorders. *N Engl J Med* 1986; 314:874–879.23

35. Bishop SA, Hill TJ. Herpes simplex virus infection and damage in the central nervous system: immunomodulation with adjuvant, cyclophosphamide, and cyclosporin A. *Arch Virol* 1991;116: 57–62.

36. Bishopric G, Bruner J, Butler J. Guillain-Barré syndrome with cytomegalovirus infection of peripheral nerves. *Arch Pathol Lab Med* 1985;109:1106–1108.

37. Black D, Stewart J, Melmed C. Sacral nerve dysfunction plus generalized polyneuropathy in herpes simplex genitalis. *Ann Neurol* 1983;14:692.

38. Booss J, Kim JH. Cytomegalovirus encephalitis: Neuropathological comparison of the guinea pig model with the opportunistic infection in AIDS. *Yale J Biol Med* 1989;62:187–195.

39. Booss J, Dann PR, Griffith BP, Kim JH. Glial nodule encephalitis in guinea pigs: serial observations following cytomegalovirus infection. *Acta Neuropathol (Berlin)* 1988;75:465–473.

40. Booss J, Dann PR, Griffith BP, Kim JH. Host defense response to cytomegalovirus in the central nervous system. Prominence of the monocyte. *Am J Pathol* 1989;134:71–78.

41. Bowman RV, Lythall DA, DeWytt C. A case of herpes zoster associated encephalitis treated with acyclovir. *Aust NZ J Med* 1985;15:43–44.

42. Bowden RA, Sayers M, Flournoy N. Cytomegalovirus immune globulin and seronegative blood products to prevent primary cytomegalovirus infection after marrow transplantation. *N Engl J Med* 1986;314:1006–1010.

43. Britton CB, Mesa-Tejada R, Fenoglio CM, et al. A new complication of AIDS: thoracic myelitis caused by herpes simplex virus. *Neurology* 1985;35:1071–1074.

44. Buchbinder S, Katz MH, Hessol N. Herpes zoster and human immunodeficiency virus infection. *J Infect Dis* 1992;166:1153–1156.

45. Buchbinder A, Josephs SF, Ablashi DV. Polymerase chain reaction amplification and in situ hybridization for the detection of human B lymphotropic virus. *J Virol Methods* 1988;21:133–140.

46. Buchman TG, Simpson T, Nosal C, Roizman B. The structure of herpes simplex virus DNA and its application to molecular epidemiology. *Ann NY Acad Sci* 1980;354:279–290.

47. Buchwald, Cheney PR, Peterson DL. A chronic illness characterized by fatigue, neurological and immunological disorders, and active human herpesvirus type 6 infection. *Ann Intern Med* 1992; 116:103–113.

48. Caplan LR, Kleeman FJ, Berg S. Urinary retention probably secondary to herpes genitalis. *N Engl J Med* 1977;297:920–921.

49. Cappel R, Klastersky J. Herpetic meningitis (type 1) in a case of acute leukemia. *Arch Neurol* 1973; 28:415–416.

50. Carneiro AV, Ferro J, Figueiredo C, et al. Herpes zoster and contralateral hemiplegia in an African patient infected with HIV-1. *Acta Med Portug* 1991;4:91–92.

51. Carrigan DR, Drobyski WR, Russler SK, Tapper MA, Knox KK, Ash RC. Interstitial pneumonia associated with human herpesvirus-6 infection after marrow transplantation. *Lancet* 1991;338: 147–149.

52. Chachoua A, Dieterich D, Krasinski K, et al. 9-(1,3-Dihydroxy-2-propoxymethyl) guanine (ganciclovir) in the treatment of cytomegalovirus gastrointestinal disease with the acquired immunodeficiency syndrome. *Ann Intern Med* 1987;107:133–137

53. Chatis PA, Miller CH, Schrager LE, Crumpacker CS. Successful treatment with foscarnet of an acyclovir-resistant mucocutaneous infection with herpes simplex virus in a patient with acquired immunodeficiency syndrome. *N Engl J Med* 1989;320:297–300.

54. Chin W, Magoffin R, Frierson JG, Lennette EH. Cytomegalovirus infection: a case with meningoencephalitis. *JAMA* 1973;225:740–741.

55. Cinque P, Vago L, Brytting M, et al. Cytomegalovirus infection of the central nervous system in patients with AIDS: diagnosis by DNA amplification from cerebrospinal fluid. *J Infect Dis* 1992; 166:1408–1411.

56. Cleary ML, Epstein MA, Finerty S. Individual tumors of multifocal EB virus-induced malignant lymphomas in tamarins arise from different B cell clones. *Science* 1985;228:722–724.

57. Clerici M, Shearer GM. The Th1 to Th2 shift is a critical step in the etiology of HIV infection. *Immunol Today* 1993;14:107–111.

58. Clifford DB, Buller RS, Mohammed S, et al. Use of polymerase chain reaction to demonstrate cytomegalovirus DNA in CSF of patients with human immunodeficiency virus infection. *Neurology* 1993;43:75–79.

59. Coen DM, Schaffer PA. Two distinct loci confer resistance to acycloguanosine in herpes simplex virus type 1. *Proc Natl Acad Sci USA* 1980;77:2265–2269.

60. Cohen BA, McArthur JC, Grohman S, Patterson B, Glass J. Neurological prognosis of cytomegalovirus polyradiculomyelopathy in AIDS. *Neurology* 1993;43:493–499.

61. Cohen BA, Rowley AH, Long CM. Herpes simplex type 2 in a patient with Mollaret's meningitis: demonstration by polymerase chain reaction. *Ann Neurol* 1994;35:112–116.

62. Cole EL, Meisler DM, Calabiese LH, Holland GN, Mondino BJ, Conant MA. Herpes zoster ophthalmicus and acquired immune deficiency syndrome. *Arch Ophthalmol* 1984;102:1027–1029.

63. Collaborative DHPG Treatment Study Group. Treatment of serious cytomegalovirus infections with 9-(1,3-dihydroxy-2-propoxymethyl)guanine in patients with AIDS and other immunodeficiencies. *N Engl J Med* 1986;314:801–805.

64. Collier AC, Meyers JD, Corey L, Murphy VL, Roberts PL, Handsfield HH. Cytomegalovirus infection in homosexual men: relationship to sexual practices, antibody to human immunodeficiency virus, and cell-mediated immunity. *Am J Med* 1987;82:593–601.

65. Condie RM, O Reilly RJ. Prevention of cytomegalovirus infection in bone marrow transplant recipients by prophylaxis with an intravenous, hyperimmune cytomegalovirus globulin. In: Plotkin SA, Michelson S, Pagano JS, Rapp F, eds. *CMV: pathogenesis and prevention of human infection.* New York: Liss; 1984:327–344.

66. Cone RW, Hackman RC, Huang M-L W. Human herpesvirus 6 in lung tissue from patients with pneumonitis after bone marrow transplantation. *N Engl J Med* 1993;329:156–161.

67. Corey L. Genital herpes. In: Holmes KK, Mardh P-A, Sparling RF, Wiesner PJ, Cates W Jr, Lemon SM, Stamm W, eds. *Sexually transmitted diseases.* 2nd ed. New York: McGraw-Hill; 1990:391–414.

68. Craig CP, Nahmias AJ. Different patterns of neurological involvement with herpes simplex virus types 1 and 2: isolation of herpes simplex virus type 2 from the buffy coat of two adults with meningitis. *J Infect Dis* 1973;127:365–372.

69. Croen KD, Ostrove JM, Dragovic LJ, Smialek JE, Straus SE. Latent herpes simplex virus in human trigeminal ganglia. Detection of an immediate early gene anti-sense transcript by in situ hybridization. *N Engl J Med* 1987;317:1427–1432.

70. Darby G, Field HJ, Salisbury SA. Altered substrate specificity of herpes simplex virus: thymidine kinase confers acyclovir resistance. *Nature* 1981;289:81–83.

71. Davis LE, Johnson RD. An explanation for the localization of herpes simplex encephalitis? *Ann Neurol* 1979;5:2–5.

72. Davis LE, McLaren LC. Relapsing herpes simplex encephalitis following antiviral therapy. *Ann Neurol* 1983;13:191–195.

73. DeAngelis L, Weaver S, Rosenblum M. Herpes varicella zoster (HVZ) encephalitis in immunocompromised patients. *Neurology* 1994;44(Suppl 2):A332.

74. DeAngelis LM, Wong E, Rosenblum M, Furneaux H. Epstein-Barr virus in acquired immune deficiency syndrome (AIDS) and non-AIDS primary central nervous system lymphoma. *Cancer* 1992; 70:1607–1611.

75. De Gans J, Portegies P, Tiessens G. Therapy for cytomegalovirus polyradiculomyelitis in patients with AIDS: treatment with ganciclovir. *AIDS* 1990;40:421–425.

76. Demey HE, Martin JJ, Leus RM, Moeremans CJ, Bossaert LL. Coma as a presenting sign of Epstein-Barr encephalitis. *Arch Intern Med* 1988;148:1459–1461.

77. Devinsky O, Cho E-S, Petito CK, Price RW. Herpes zoster myelitis. *Brain* 1991;114:1181–1196.

78. Devlin ME, Gilden DH, Mahalingam R, Dueland AN, Cohrs R. Peripheral blood mononuclear cells of the elderly contain varicella-zoster virus DNA. *J Infect Dis* 1992;165:619–622.

79. Di Luca D, Secchiero P, Bovenzi P, et al. Reciprocal in vitro interactions between human herpesvirus-6 and HIV-1 Tat. *AIDS* 1991;5:1095–1098.

80. Dieterich DT, Poles MA, Lew EA. Concurrent use of ganciclovir and foscarnet to treat cytomegalovirus infection in AIDS patients. *J Infect Dis* 1993;167:1184–1188.

81. Dix RD, Bredesen DE. Opportunistic viral infections in acquired immunodeficiency syndrome. In: Rosenblum ML, Levy RM, Bredesen DE, eds. *AIDS and the nervous system.* New York: Raven; 1988:221–262.

82. Dix RD, Baringer JR, Panitch HS, Rosenberg SH, Hagendorn J. Whaley J. Recurrent herpes simplex encephalitis: recovery of virus after Ara-A treatment. *Ann Neurol* 1983;13:196–200.

83. Dix RD, Bredesen DE, Erlich KS, Mills J. Recovery of herpesviruses from cerebrospinal fluid of immunodeficient homosexual men. *Ann Neurol* 985;18:611–614.

84. Dix RD, Cray C, Cousins SW. Mice immunosuppressed by murine retrovirus infection (MAIDS) are susceptible to cytomegalovirus retinitis. *Curr Eye Res* 1994;13:587–595.
85. Dix RD, Cray C, Cousins SW. Cytomegalovirus retinitis: current issues and future directions. *Regional Immunol [in press]*.
86. Dix RD, Lukes S, Pulliam L, Baringer JR. DNA restriction enzyme analysis of viruses isolated from cerebrospinal fluid and brain-biopsy tissue is a patient with herpes simplex encephalitis. *N Engl J Med* 1983;308:1424.
87. Dix RD, McCarthy M, Berger JR. Diagnostic value for culture of cerebrospinal fluid from HIV-1-infected individuals for opportunistic viruses: a prospective study. *AIDS* 1994;8:307–312.
88. Dix RD, Waitzman DM, Follansbee S, et al. Herpes simplex virus type 2 encephalitis in two homosexual men with persistent lymphadenopathy. *Ann Neurol* 1985;17:203–206.
89. Dolgopol VR, Husson GS. Infectious mononucleosis with neurological complications. Report of a fatal case. *Arch Intern Med* 1984;83:179–183.
90. Donaghy M, Gray JA, Squier W. Recurrent Guillain-Barré syndrome after multiple exposures to cytomegalovirus. *Am J Med* 1989;87:339–341.
91. Dorfman LF. Cytomegalovirus encephalitis in adults. *Neurology* 1973;23:136–144.
92. Dorsky DI, Crumpacker CS. Drugs five years later: acyclovir. *Ann Intern Med* 1987;107:859–874.
93. Dowling PC, Cook SD. Role of infection in Guillain-Barré syndrome: laboratory confirmation of herpesviruses in 41 cases. *Ann Neurol* 1981;9(Suppl):44–55.
94. Dowling MD, Van Slyek EJ. Cerebellar disease in infectious mononucleosis. *Arch Neurol* 1966;15:270–274.
95. Drew WL. Cytomegalovirus infection in patients with AIDS. *J Infect Dis* 1988;158:449–456.
96. Drew WL, Mintz L, Miner RC, Sands M, Ketterer B. Prevalence of cytomegalovirus infection in homosexual men. *J Infect Dis* 1981;143:188–192.
97. Drobyski WR, Knox K, Majewski D, Carrigan DR. Brief report: fatal encephalitis due to variant B human herpesvirus-6 infection in a bone marrow-transplant recipient. *N Engl J Med* 1994;330:1356–1360.
98. Dubedat S, Kappagoda N. Hepatitis due to human herpesvirus-6. *Lancet* 1989;1:1463–1464.
99. Duchowny M, Caplan L, Siber G. Cytomegalovirus infection of the adult nervous system. *Ann Neurol* 1979;5:458–461.
100. Duncombe AS, Meager A, Prentice HG, et al. g-Interferon and tumor necrosis factor production after bone marrow transplantation is augmented by exposure to marrow fibroblasts infected with cytomegalovirus. *Blood* 1990;76:1046–1053.
101. Dyck JD, Daube J, O Brien P, et al. Plasma exchange in chronic inflammatory demyelinating polyradiculoneuropathy. *N Engl J Med* 1986;314:461–465.
102. Edwards RH, Messing R, McKendall RR. Cytomegalovirus meningoencephalitis in a homosexual man with Kaposi's sarcoma: isolation of CMV from CSF cells. *Neurology* 1985;35:560–562.
103. Eidelberg D, Sotrel A, Horoupian DS, et al. Thrombotic cerebral vasculopathy associated with herpes zoster. *Ann Neurol* 1986;19:7–14.
104. Eidelberg D, Sotrel A, Vogel H. Progressive polyradiculopathy in acquired immune deficiency syndrome. *Neurology* 1986;36:912–916.
105. Elion GB, Furman PA, Fyfe JA, de Miranda P, Beauchamp L, Schaeffer HJ. Selectivity of action of an anti-herpetic agent, 9-(2-hydroxyethoxymethyl) guanine. *Proc Natl Acad Sci USA* 1977;74:5716–5720.
106. Emanuel D, Cunningham I, Elysee KJ. Cytomegalovirus pneumonia after bone marrow transplantation successfully treated with the combination of ganciclovir and high-dose intravenous immune globulin. *Ann Intern Med* 1988;109:777–782.
107. Englund JA, Zimmerman ME, Swierkosz EM. Herpes simplex virus resistant to acyclovir. A study in a tertiary care center. *Ann Intern Med* 1990;112:416–422.
108. Ensoli B, Lusso P, Schachter F. Human herpes virus-6 increases HIV-1 expression in co-infected T cells via nuclear factors binding to the HIV-1 enhancer. *EMBO J* 1989;8:3019–3027.
109. Enting R, DeGans J, Reiss P, Jansen C, Portegies P. Ganciclovir/foscarnet for cytomegalovirus meningoencephalitis in AIDS (Letter). *Lancet* 1992;340:559–560.
110. Epstein JS, Frederick WR, Rook AH, et al. Selective defects in cytomegalovirus and mitogen-induced lymphocyte proliferation and interferon release in patients with acquired immunodeficiency syndrome. *J Infect Dis* 1985;152:727–733.
111. Epstein LG, Sharer LR, Joshi VV, Fojas MM, Koenigsberger MR, Oleske JM. Progressive encephalopathy in children with acquired immune deficiency syndrome. *Ann Neurol* 1985;17:488–496.
112. Erice A, Chou S, Biron KK, Stanat SC, Balvour HH, Jordan MC. Progressive disease due to ganciclovir-resistant cytomegalovirus in immunocompromised patients. *N Engl J Med* 1989;320:289–293.
113. Erlich KS, Mills J, Chatis P. Acyclovir-resistant herpes simplex virus infections in patients with the acquired immunodeficiency syndrome. *N Engl J Med* 1989;320:293–296.
114. Fanning MM, Read SE, Benson M. Foscarnet therapy of cytomegalovirus retinitis in AIDS. *J Acquired Immune Deficiency Syndrome* 1990;3:472–479.

115. Farese RV, Schambelan M, Hollander H, Stringari S, Jacobson MA. Nephrogenic diabetes insipidus associated with foscarnet treatment of cytomegalovirus retinitis. *Ann Intern Med* 1990;112:955–956.

116. Felsenstein D, D'Amico DJ, Hirsch MS, et al. Treatment of cytomegalovirus retinitis with 9-(2-hydroxy-1-(hydroxymethyl)ethoxymethyl)guanine. *Ann Intern Med* 1985;103:377–380.

117. Field HJ, Darby G. Pathogenicity in mice of strains of herpes simplex virus which are resistant to acyclovir in vitro and in vivo. *Antimicrob Agent Chemother* 1980;17:209–216.

118. Flamand L, Stefanescu I, Ablashi DV, Menezes J. Activation of the Epstein-Barr virus replication cycle by human herpesvirus 6. *J Virol* 1993;67:6768–6777.

119. Fleisher GR. Epstein-Barr virus. In: Belshe RB, ed. *Textbook of human virology.* Littleton, NH: PSG Publishing; 1984:853–886.

120. Fukumoto S, Kinjo M, Hokamura K. Subarachnoid hemorrhage and granulomatous angiitis of the basilar artery: demonstration of the varicella-zoster-virus in the basilar artery lesions. *Stroke* 1986; 17:1024–1028.

121. Fuller GN, Guiloff RJ, Scaravilli F, Harcourt-Webster JN. Combined HIV-CMV encephalitis presenting with brainstem signs. *J Neurol Neurosurg Psychiatry* 1989;52:975–979.

122. Fuller GN, Jacobs JM, Guiloff RJ. Association of painful peripheral neuropathy in AIDS with cytomegalovirus infection. *Lancet* 1989;2:937–941.

123. Gateley A, Gander RM, Johnson PC. Herpes simplex virus type 2 meningoencephalitis resistant to acyclovir in a patient with AIDS. *J Infect Dis* 1990;161:711–715.

124. Gazzinelli RT, Makino M, Chattopadhyay SK, et al. CD4- subset regulation in viral infection preferential activation of Th2 cells during progression of retrovirus-induced immunodeficiency in mice. *J Immunol* 1992;148:182–188.

125. Geist LJ, Monick MM, Stindki MF, Hunninghake GW. The immediate early genes of human cytomegalovirus upregulate expression of the interleukin-2 and interleukin-2 receptor genes. *Am J Respir Cell Mol Biol* 1991;5:292–296.

126. Gelb LD. Varicella-zoster virus. Clinical aspects. In: Roizman B, Whitley RJ, Lopez C, eds. *The human herpesviruses.* New York: Raven; 1993:281–308.

127. Gendelman HE, Phelps W, Feigenbaum L. Trans-activation of the human immunodeficiency virus long terminal repeat sequence by DNA viruses. *Proc Natl Acad Sci USA* 1986;83:9759–9763.

128. Geng Y, Chandran B, Josephs SF, Wood C. Identification and characterization of a human herpesvirus 6 gene segment that trans activates the human immunodeficiency virus type 1 promoter. *J Virol* 1992;66:1564–1570.

129. Gershon A, Steinberg S, Greensberg S, Taber L. Varicella-zoster-associated encephalitis: detection of specific antibody in cerebrospinal fluid. *J Clin Microbiol* 1980;12:764–767.

130. Gilden DH, Vafai A. Varicella zoster. In: McKendall RR, ed. *Handbook of clinical neurology,* vol 12: *Viral disease.* Amsterdam: Elsevier; 1989:229–247.

131. Gilden DH, Devlin H, Wellish M, et al. Persistence of varicella-zoster virus DNA in blood mononuclear cells of patients with varicella or zoster. *Virus Genes* 1989;2:299–305.

132. Gilden DH, Hayward AR, Krupp J, Hunter-Laszlo M, Huff JC, Vafai A. Varicella-zoster virus infection of human mononuclear cells. *Virus Res* 1987;7:117–129.

133. Gilden DH, Murray RS, Wellish M, Kleinshmidt-Demasters BK, Vafai A. Chronic progressive varicella-zoster virus encephalitis in an AIDS patient. *Neurology* 1988;38:1150–1153.

134. Gilden DH, Vafai A, Shtram Y, Becker Y, Devlin M, Wellish M. Varicella-zoster virus DNA in human sensory ganglia. *Nature* 1983;306;478–480.

135. Gold E. Serological and virus-isolation studies of patients with varicella or herpes-zoster infection. *N Engl J Med* 1966;274:181–185.

136. Gold E, Nankervis GA. Cytomegalovirus. In: Evans AS, ed. *Viral infections of humans: epidemiology and control.* New York: Plenum; 1982:167–186.

137. Gopal MR, Thompson BJ, Fox J, Tedder RS, Honess RW. Detection by PCR of HHV-6 and EBV DNA in blood and oropharynx of healthy adults and HIV-seropositives. *Lancet* 1990;1:1598–1599.

138. Gotlieb-Stematsky T, Arlazoroff A. Epstein-Barr virus. In: McKendall RR, ed. *Handbook of clinical neurology.* Amsterdam: Elsevier; 1989:248–261.

139. Gozlan J, Salord JM, Roullet E, et al. Rapid detection of cytomegalovirus DNA in cerebrospinal fluid of AIDS patients with neurologica disorders. *J Infect Dis* 1992;166:1416–1421.

140. Grafe MR, Wiley CA. Spinal cord and peripheral nerve pathology in AIDS: the roles of cytomegalovirus and human immunodeficiency virus. *Ann Neurol* 1989;25:561–566.

141. Graveleau P, Perol R, Chapman A. Regression of cauda equina syndrome in AIDS patient being treated with ganciclovir (Letter) *Lancet* 1989;2:511–512.

142. Gray F, Mohr M, Rozenberg F, et al. Varicella-zoster virus encephalitis in acquired immunodeficiency syndrome: report of four cases. *Neuropathol Appl Neurobiol* 1992;18:502–514.

143. Grose C, Henle W, Henle G, Feorino PM. Primary Epstein-Barr virus infections in acute neurologica disease. *N Engl J Med* 1975;292:392–395.

144. Güngör T, Funk M, Linde R, et al. Cytomegalovirus myelitis in perinatally acquired HIV. *Arch Dis Child* 1993;68:399–401.

145. Haagmans B, Stals FS, van der Meide PH, Bruggeman CA, Horzinek MC, Schijns VECJ. Tumor

necrosis factor alpha promotes replication and pathogenicity of rat cytomegalovirus. *J Virol* 1994; 68:2297–2304.

146. Hall CB, Long CE, Schnabel KC, et al. Human herpesvirus-6 infection in children. A prospective study of complications and reactivation. *N Engl J Med* 1994;331:432–438.

147. Halsted CC, Chang RS. Infectious mononucleosis and encephalitis: recovery of EB virus from spinal fluid. *Pediatrics* 1979;64:257–258.

148. Harding SP, Porter SM. Oral acyclovir in herpes zoster ophthalmicus. *Curr Eye Res* 1991;10(Suppl): 177–182.

149. Harford CG, Wellinghoff W, Weinstein RA. Isolation of herpes simplex virus from the cerebrospinal fluid in viral meningitis. *Neurology* 1975;25:198–200.

150. Harnett GB, Farr TJ, Pietroboni GR, Bucens MR. Frequent shedding of human herpesvirus 6 in saliva. *J Med Virol* 1990;30:128–130.

151. Hart IK, Kennedy PGE. Guillain-Barré syndrome associated with cytomegalovirus infection. *Quart J Med* 1988;253:425–430.

152. Hatson JR, Pedley TA. The neurological complications of cardiac transplantation. *Brain* 1976;99: 673–694.

153. Hawley DA, Schaefer JF, Schulz DM, Muller J. Cytomegalovirus encephalitis in acquired immuno-deficiency syndrome. *Am J Clin Pathol* 1983;80:874–877.

154. Heller M, Dix RD, Baringer JR, Schachter J, Conte JE Jr. Herpetic proctitis and meningitis: recovery of two strains of herpes simplex virus type 1 from cerebrospinal fluid. *J Infect Dis* 1982;146: 584–588.

155. Hilt DC, Buchholz D, Krumholz A, Weiss H, Wolinsky J. Herpes zoster ophthalmicus and delayed contralateral hemiparesis caused by cerebral angiitis: diagnosis and management approaches. *Ann Neurol* 1983;4:543–553.

156. Ho M. *Cytomegalovirus biology and infection.* 2nd ed. New York: Plenum; 1991.

157. Ho W-Z, Harouse JM, Rando RF, Gonczol E. Srinivasan A, Plotkin SA. Reciprocal enhancement of gene expression and viral replication between human cytomegalovirus and human immunodeficiency virus type 1. *J Gen Virol* 1990;71:97–103.

158. Ho W-Z, Long L, Douglas ST. Human cytomegalovirus infection and trans-activation of HIV-1 LTR in human brain-derived cells. *J AIDS* 1991;4:1098–1106.

159. Ho W-Z, Song L, Douglas ST. Human cytomegalovirus infection and trans-activation of HIV-1 LTR in human brain-derived cells. *J Acquired Immune Deficiency Syndromes* 1991;4:1098–1106.

160. Hochberg FH, Miller G, Schooley RT. Central nervous system lymphoma related to Epstein-Barr virus. *N Engl J Med* 1983;309:745–748.

161. Hochster H, Dietrich D, Bozzette S, et al. Toxicity of combined ganciclovir and zidovudine for cytomegalovirus disease associated with AIDS: an AIDS Clinical Trials Group study. *Ann Intern Med* 1990;133:111–117.

162. Hogan EL, Krigman MR. Herpes zoster myelitis: evidence for viral invasion of spinal cord. *Arch Neurol* 1973;29:309–313.

163. Holland NR, Power C, Matthews VP, Glass JD, Forman M, McArthur JC. Cytomegalovirus encepha-litis in acquired immunodeficiency syndrome (AIDS). *Neurology* 1994;44:507–514.

164. Hook E, Cannon R, Nahmias AL, et al. Herpes simplex virus infection as a risk for human immunode-ficiency virus infection in heterosexuals. *J Infect Dis* 1992;165:251–255.

165. Horton B, Price RW, Jimenez D. Multifocal varicella-zoster leukoencephalitis temporally remote from herpes zoster. *Ann Neurol* 1981;9:251–266.

166. Huang ES, Alford CA, Reynolds DW, Stagno S, Pass RF. Molecular epidemiology of cytomegalovi-rus infections in women and their infants. *N Engl J Med* 1980;303:958–962.

167. Huang L-M, Lee C-Y, Lin K-H, et al. Human herpesvirus-6 associated with fatal haemophagocytic syndrome. *Lancet* 1990;336:60–61.

168. Hudson SJ, Streilein JW. Functional cytotoxic T cells are associated with focal lesions of the brains of SJL mice with experimental herpes simplex encephalitis. *J Immunol* 1994;152:5540–5547.

169. Hudson SJ, Dix RD, Streilein JW. Induction of encephalitis in SJL mice by intranasal infection with herpes simplex virus type 1: a possible model of herpes simplex encephalitis in humans. *J Infect Dis* 1991;163:720–727.

170. Huff JC, Bean B, Balfour HH Jr. Therapy of herpes zoster with oral acyclovir. *Am J Med* 1988; 85(Suppl 2A):84–89.

171. Hyman RW, Ecker JR, Tenser RB. Varicella-zoster virus RNA in human trigeminal ganglia. *Lancet* 1983;2:814–816.

172. Ilyid JP, Oakes JE, Hyman RW, Rapp F. Comparison of the DNAs of vaicella-zoster viruses isolated from clinical cases of varicella and herpes zoster. *Virology* 1977;82:345–352.

173. Iwamoto GK, Monick MM, Clark BD, Auron PE, Stinski MF, Hunninghake GW. Modulation of interleukin 1 beta gene expression by the immediate early genes of human cytomegalovirus. *J Clin Invest* 1990;85:1853–1857.

174. Jacobson MA, Berger TG, Fikrig S. Acyclovir resistant varicella zoster virus infection after chronic

oral acyclovir therapy in patients with the acquired immunodeficiency syndrome (AIDS). *Ann Intern Med* 1990;112:187–191.

175. Jacobson MA, Mills J, Rush J. Failure of antiviral therapy for acquired immunodeficiency syndrome-related cytomegalovirus myelitis. *Arch Neurol* 1988;45:1090–1092.

176. Jacobson MA, O Donnell JJ, Mills JF. Foscarnet treatment of cytomegalovirus retinitis in patients with the acquired immunodeficiency syndrome. *Antimicrob Agents Chemother* 1989;33:736–741.

177. Jault FM, Spector SA, Spector DH. The effects of cytomegalovirus on human immunodeficiency virus replication in brain-derived cells correlate with permissiveness of the cells for each virus. *J Virol* 1994;68:959–973.

178. Jemskck J, Greenberg SB, Taber L, Harvey D, Gershon A, Couch RB. Herpes zoster-associated encephalitis: clinicopathological report of 12 cases and review of the literature. *Medicine* 1983;62:81–97.

179. Johnson RT. *Viral infections of the nervous system.* New York: Raven; 1982.

180. Johnson RT, Mims CA. Pathogenesis of viral infections of the nervous system. *N Engl J Med* 1968;278:23–30.

181. Jolicoeur P. Murine acquired immunodeficiency syndrome (MAIDS): an animal model to study the AIDS pathogenesis. *FASEB J* 1991;5:2398–2405.

182. Joncas JH, Chicoine L, Thivierge R, Bertrand M. Epstein-Barr virus antibodies in the cerebrospinal fluid. A case of infectious mononucleosis with encephalitis. *Am J Dis Child* 1974;127:282–285.

183. Josephs SF, Buchbinder A, Streicher A. Detection of human B-lymphotrophic virus (human herpesvirus-6) sequences in B cell lymphoma tissue of three patients. *Leukemia* 1988;2:132–135.

184. Jubelt B, Friedmann A, Gordan SR, Harter DH. Herpes simplex virus encephalitis: a review and update. In: Yahr MD, ed. *H. Houston Merritt Memorial Volume.* New York: Raven Press; 1983:177–201.

185. Junker AK, Roland EH, Hahn G. Transverse myelitis and Epstein-Barr virus infection with delayed antibody responses. *Neurology* 1991;41:1523–1524.

186. Kabins S, Keller R, Peitchel RT, Ali MK. Acute idiopathic polyneuritis caused by cytomegalovirus. *Arch Intern Med* 1976;136:100–101.

187. Kabins S, Keller R, Naragi S, Peitchel R. Viral ascending radiculomyelitis with severe hypoglycorrhachia. *Arch Intern Med* 1976;136:933–935.

188. Kalayjian RC, Cohen ML, Bonomo RA, Flanigan TP. Cytomegalovirus ventriculoencephalitis in AIDS. *Medicine* 1993;72:67–77.

189. Kanagawa O, Vaupel BA, Gayama S, Koehler G, Kopt M. Resistance of mice deficient in IL-4 to retrovirus-induced immunodeficiency syndrome (MAIDS). *Science* 1993;262:240–242.

190. Katz BZ, Andiman WA, Eastman R, Martin K, Miller G. Infection with two genotypes of Epstein-Barr virus in an infant with AIDS and lymphoma of the central nervous system. *J Infect Dis* 1986;153:601–604.

191. Kenney S, Kamine J, Markovitz D, Fenrick R, Pagano J. An Epstein-Barr virus immediate early gene product trans-activates gene expression from the human immunodeficiency virus long terminal repeat. *Proc Natl Acad Sci USA* 1988;85:1652–1656.

192. Kim YS, Hollander H. Polyradiculopathy due to cytomegalovirus: report of two cases in which improvement occurred after prolonged therapy and review of the literature. *Clin Infect Dis* 1993;17:32–37.

193. Klapper PE, Cleator GM, Longson M. Mild forms of herpes encephalitis. *J Neurol Neurosurg Psychiatry* 1984;47:1247–1250.

194. Klastersky J, Carpel R, Snoeck JM, Flament J, Thiry L. Ascending myelitis in association with herpes simplex virus. *N Engl J Med* 1972;287:182–184.

195. Klemola E. Cytomegalovirus infection in previously healthy adults. *Ann Intern Med* 1973;79:267–268.

196. Klemola E, von Essen R, Wager O. Cytomegalovirus mononucleosis in previously healthy adults. *Ann Intern Med* 1969;79:267–268.

197. Klimas N, Patarca R, Walling J, et al. Clinical and immunological changes in AIDS patients following adoptive transfer with activated autologous CD8 T cells and interleukin-2 infusion. *AIDS* 1994;8:1073–1081.

198. Koenig S, Gendelman HE, Orenstein JM. Detection of AIDS virus in macrophages in brain tissue from AIDS patients with encephalopathy. *Science* 1986;233:1089–1093.

199. Kondo K, Hayakawa Y, Mori H. Detection by polymerase chain reaction amplification of human herpesvirus 6 DNA in peripheral blood of patients with exanthem subitum. *J Clin Microbiol* 1990;28:970–974.

200. Kondo K, Kondo T, Okuno T, Takahashi M, Yamanishi K. Latent human herpesvirus 6 infection of human monocytes/macrophages. *J Gen Virol* 1991;72:1401–1408.

201. Kondo K, Nagafuji H, Hata A, Tomomori C, Yamanishi K. Association of human herpesvirus 6 infection of the central nervous system with recurrence of febrile convulsion. *J Infect Dis* 1993;167:1197–1200.

202. Koppel BS, Wormser GP, Tuchman AJ, Maayan S, Hewlett D Jr, Daras M. Central nervous system

involvement in patients with acquired immune deficiency syndrome (AIDS). *Acta Neurol Scand* 1985;71:337–353.

203. Knox KK, Carrigan DR. Disseminated active HHV-6 infections in patients with AIDS. *Lancet* 1994; 343:577–578.
204. Kung H-J, Wood C. *Interactions between retroviruses and herpesviruses.* River Edge, NJ: World Scientific Publishing; 1994.
205. Lakeman FD, Koga J, Whitley RJ, NIAID Collaborative Antiviral Study Group. Detection of antigen to herpes simplex virus in cerebrospinal fluid from patients with herpes simplex encephalitis. *J Infect Dis* 1987;155:1172–1175.
206. Lakin OL, Stahl-Bayliss CM, Morgello S. Concomitant herpes simplex virus type 1 and cytomegalovirus ventriculoencephalitis in acquired immunodeficiency syndrome. *Arch Neurol* 1987;44: 843–847.
207. Lane HC, Masur H, Edgar LC, Whalen G. Rook AH, Fauci AS. Abnormalities of B cell activation and immunoregulation in patients with the acquired immunodeficiency syndrome. *N Engl J Med* 1983;309:453–458.
208. Lang W, Miklossy J, Dervaz JP. Neuropathology of the acquired immune deficiency syndrome (AIDS): a report of 135 consecutive autopsy cases from Switzerland. *Acta Neuropathol* 1989;77: 379–390.
209. Lange BJ, Berman PH, Bender J. Encephalitis in infectious mononucleosis: diagnostic considerations. *Pediatrics* 1976;58:877–880.
210. Larder BA, Darby S. Selection and characterization of acyclovir-resistant herpes simplex virus type 1 mutants inducing altered DNA polymerase activities. *Virology* 1985;146:262–271.
211. Larsen JK, Melgaard B. Simultaneous neuroinfection with cytomegalovirus and herpes simplex virus in an immunocompetent adult. *J Intern Med* 1989;226:59–61.
212. Lascelles RG, Longson M, Johnson PJ, Chiang A. Infectious mononucleosis presenting as acute cerebellar syndrome. *Lancet* 1973;2:707–709.
213. Laskin OL, Cederberg DM, Mills J, for the Ganciclovir Study Group. Ganciclovir for the treatment and suppression of serious infections caused by cytomegalovirus. *Am J Med* 1987;83:201–207
214. Laurence J. Molecular interactions among herpesviruses and human immunodeficiency viruses. *J Infect Dis* 1990;162:338–346.
215. Laurence J. Viral cofactors in the pathogenesis of HIV disease. In: Wormser GP, ed. *AIDS and other manifestations of HIV infection.* 2nd ed. New York: Raven; 1992:77–83.
216. Laurence J, Astrin SM. Human immunodeficiency virus induction of malignant transformation in human B lymphocytes. *Proc Natl Acad Sci USA* 1991;88:7635–7639.
217. Lawrence GL, Chee M, Craxton MA, Gompels UA, Honess RW, Barrell BG. Human herpesvirus 6 is closely related to human cytomegalovirus. *J Virol* 1990;64:287–299.
218. Lehoang P, Girard B, Robinet M. Foscarnet in the treatment of cytomegalovirus retinitis in acquired immune deficiency syndrome. *Ophthalmology* 1989;96:865–874.
219. Levy JA, Ferro F, Greenspan D, Lennette ET. Frequent isolation of HHV-6 from saliva and high seroprevalence of the virus in the population. *Lancet* 1990;335:1047–1050.
220. Levy RM, Bredeson DE, Rosenblum ML. Neurological manifestations of the acquired immunodeficiency syndrome (AIDS): experience of UCSF and review of the literature. *J Neurosurg* 1985;62: 475–495.
221. Liebowitz D, Kieff E. Epstein-Barr virus. In: Roizman B, Whitley RJ, Lopez C, eds. *The human herpesviruses.* New York: Raven; 1993:107–172.
222. Linneman CC Jr, Dunn CR, First MR, Alvira M, Schiff GM. Late onset of fatal cytomegalovirus infection after renal transplantation. Primary or reactivation infection? *Arch Intern Med* 1978;138: 1247–1250.
223. Linneman CC Jr, First MR, Alvira MM, Alexander JW, Schiff GM. Herpesvirus hominis type 2 meningoencephalitis following renal transplantation. *Am J Med* 1976;61:703–708.
224. Lipkin WI, Parry G, Kiprov D, Abrams D. Inflammatory neuropathy in homosexual men with lymphadenopathy. *Neurology* 1985;35:1479–1483.
225. Lohler J. Immunopathological reactions in viral infections of the central nervous system. *J Neuroimmunol* 1988;20:181–185.
226. Lopez C. Natural resistance mechanisms against herpesviruses in health and disease. In: Rouse BT, Lopez C, eds. *Immunobiology of herpes simplex virus infection.* Boca Raton, FL: CRC Press; 1984: 45–69.
227. Lopez C. Human herpesviruses 6 and 7. Molecular biology and clinical aspects. In: Roizman B, Whitley RJ, Lopez C, eds. *The human herpesviruses.* New York: Raven; 1993:309–316.
228. Lusso P. Target cells for infection. In: Ablashi DV, Krueger GRF, Salahuddin SZ, eds. *Human herpesvirus-6.* New York: Elsevier; 1992:25–36.
229. Lusso P, Malnati MS, Garzino-Demo A, Crowley RW, Long EO, Gallo RC. Infection of natural killer cells by human herpesvirus 6. *Nature* 1993;362:458–462.
230. MacMahon EME, Glass JD, Hayward SD. Epstein-Barr virus in AIDS-related primary central nervous system lymphoma. *Lancet* 1991;338:969–973.

231. McArthur JC. Neurological manifestations of AIDS. *Medicine* 1987;66:407–437.
232. McCarthy M, Resnick L, Taub F, Stewart RV, Dix RD. Infection of human neural cell aggregate cultures with a clinical isolate of cytomegalovirus. *J Neuropathol Exp Neurol* 1991;50:441–450.
233. McCormick WF, Rodnitzky RL, Schochet SS, McKee AP. Varicella-zoster encephalomyelitis: a morphological and virological study. *Arch Neurol* 1969;21:559–570.
234. McKendall RR. Herpes simplex. In: McKendall RR, ed. *Handbook of clinical neurology,* vol. 12: *Viral disease.* Amsterdam: Elsevier; 1989:207–227.
235. Macher AM, Reichert CM, Straus SE, et al. Death in the AIDS patient: role of cytomegalovirus. *N Engl J Med* 1983;309:1454.
236. Madhoun ZT, DuBois DB, Rosenthal J, Findlay JC, Aron DC. Central diabetes insipidus: a complication of herpes simplex type 2 encephalitis in a patient with AIDS. *Am J Med* 1991;90:658–659.
237. Mahieux F, Gray F, Fenelon G. Acute myeloradiculitis due to cytomegalovirus as the initial manifestation of AIDS. *J Neurol Neurosurg Psychiatry* 1989;52:270–274.
238. Manion DJ, Hirsch MS. Bidirectional interactions between human immunodeficiency virus and cytomegalovirus. In: Kung H-J, Wood C, eds. *Interactions between retroviruses and herpesviruses.* River Edge, NJ: World Scientific Publishing; 1994:45–64.
239. Marmaduke DP, Brandt JT, Theil KS. Rapid diagnosis of cytomegalovirus in the cerebrospinal fluid of a patient with AIDS-associated polyradiculopathy. *Arch Pathol Lab Med* 1991;115:1154–1157.
240. Martinez-Martin P, Garcia-Saiz A, Rapin JL, Echevarria JM. Intrathecal synthesis of IgG antibodies to varicella-zoster virus in two cases of acute aseptic meningitis syndrome with no cutaneous lesions. *J Med Virol* 1985;16:201–209.
241. Masdeu JC, Small CB, Weiss L, et al. Multifocal cytomegalovirus encephalitis in AIDS. *Ann Neurol* 1988;23:97–99.
242. Mateos-Mora M, Ratzan KR. Acute viral encephalitis. In: Schlossberg D, ed. *Infections of the nervous system.* New York: Springer-Verlag; 1990:105–134.
243. Matthew T, Boechme R. Antiviral activity and mechanism of action of ganciclovir. *Rev Infect Dis* 1988;10:S490–494.
244. Meyers JD. Cytomegalovirus infection following marrow transplantation: risk, treatment, and prevention. In: Plotkins SA, Michelson S, Pagano JS, Rapp F, eds. *CMV: pathogenesis and prevention.*
245. Meyers JD, Leszczynski J, Zaia JA. Prevention of cytomegalovirus infection by cytomegalovirus immune globulin after marrow transplantation. *Ann Intern Med* 1983;98:442–446.
246. Meyers JD, Reed EC, Shepp DH. Acyclovir for prevention of cytomegalovirus infection and disease in allogeneic marrow transplantation. *N Engl J Med* 1988;318:70–75.
247. Michelson S, Alcami J, Kim S-J, et al. Human cytomegalovirus infection induces transcription and secretions of transforming growth factor beta-1. *J Virol* 1994;68:5730–5737.
248. Miller G. Epstein-Barr virus. In: Fields BN, Knipe DM, Chanock RM, Hirsch MS, Melnick JL, Monath TP, Roizman B, eds. *Virology.* New York: Raven; 1990:1921–1958.
249. Miller RG, Storey JR, Greco CM. Ganciclovir in the treatment of progressive AIDS-related polyradiculopathy. *Neurology* 1990;40:569–574.
250. Mills J, Jacobson MA, O Donnell JJ, Cederberg D, Holland GN. Treatment of cytomegalovirus retinitis in patients with AIDS. *Rev Infect Dis* 1988;10:S522–527.
251. Mocarski ES Jr. Cytomegalovirus biology and replication. In: Roizman B, Whitley RJ, Lopez C, eds. *The human herpesviruses.* New York: Raven; 1993:173–227.
252. Morgello S. Epstein-Barr and human immunodeficiency viruses in acquired immunodeficiency syndrome related primary central nervous system lymphoma. *Am J Pathol* 1992;141:441–450.
253. Morgello S, Block GA, Price RW, Petito CK. Varicella-zoster virus leukoencephalitis and cerebral vasculopathy. *Arch Pathol Lab Med* 1988;112:173–177.
254. Morgello S, Cho ES, Nielsen S. Cytomegalovirus encephalitis in patients with acquired immunodeficiency syndrome. *Hum Pathol* 1987;18:289–297.
255. Morton P, Thomson AN. Oral acyclovir in the treatment of herpes zoster in general practice. *N Z Med J* 1989;102:93–95.
256. Mosca JD, Bednarik DP, Raj NBK. Activation of human immunodeficiency virus by herpesvirus infection: identification of a region within the long terminal repeat that responds to a trans-acting factor encoded by herpes simplex virus 1. *Proc Natl Acad Sci USA* 1987;84:7408–7412.
257. Mosca JD, Bednarik DP, Raj NBK, et al. Herpes simplex virus type-1 can reactivate transcription of latent human immunodeficiency virus. *Nature* 1987;325:67–70.
258. Moskowitz LB, Gregorious JB, Hensley JT, Berger JR. Cytomegalovirus induced demyelination associated with acquired immune deficiency syndrome. *Arch Pathol Lab Med* 1984;108:873–877.
259. Moskowitz LB, Hensley GT, Chan JC, Gregorios J, Conley FK. The neuropathology of acquired immune deficiency syndrome. *Arch Pathol Lab Med* 1984;108:867–872.
260. Nahmias AJ, Lee FK, Beckman-Nahmias S. Sero-epidemiological and sociological patterns of herpes simplex virus infection in the world. *Scand J Infect Dis* 1990;69:19–36.
261. Nahmias AJ, Whitley RJ, Visintine AF, Takei Y, Alford DA Jr. Herpes simplex virus encephalitis: laboratory evaluations and their diagnostic significance. *J Infect Dis* 1982;145:829–836.

262. Naragi S, Jackson GG, Jonasson OM. Viremia with herpes simplex type 1 in adults: four nonfatal cases, one with features of chicken pox. *Ann Intern Med* 1976;85:165–169.

263. Nelson JA, Ghazal P, Wiley CA. Role of opportunistic viral infections in AIDS. *AIDS* 1990;4:1–10.

264. Nelson JA, Reynolds-Kohler C, Oldstone MBA, Wiley CA. HIV and HCMV coinfect brain cells in patients with AIDS. *Virology* 1988;165:286–290.

265. Niederman JC, Liu C-R, Kaplan MH, Brown NA. Clinical and serological features of human herpesvirus-6 infection in three adults. *Lancet* 1988;2:817–819.

266. Nielsen SL, Petito CK, Urmacher CD, Posner JB. Subacute encephalitis in acquired immune deficiency syndrome: a postmortem study. *Am J Clin Pathol* 1984;82:678–682.

267. Norris FH Jr, Leonards R, Calanchini PR, Calder CD. Herpes-zoster meningoencephalitis. *J Infect Dis* 1970;122:335–337.

268. Oates JK, Greenhouse PRDH. Retention of urine in anogenital herpetic infection. *Lancet* 1978;1:691–692.

269. Oberg B. Antiviral effects of phosphonoformate (PFA, foscarnet sodium). *Pharmacol Ther* 1983;19:387–415.

270. O'Donnell P, Pula TP, Sellman M, Camenga DL. Recurrent herpes zoster encephalitis, a complication of systemic lupus erythematosus. *Arch Neurol* 1981;38:49–51.

271. Ommen KJ, Johnson PC, Ray CG. Herpes simplex type 2 virus encephalitis presenting as psychosis. *Am J Med* 1982;73:445–448.

272. O'Reilly RJ, Reich L, Gold J, Condie RM. A randomized trial of intravenous hyper-immune globulin for the prevention of cytomegalovirus following marrow transplantation: preliminary results. *Transplant Proc* 1983;15:1405–1413.

273. Ostrove JM, Leonard J, Weck KE, Rabson AB, Gendelman HE. Activation of the human immunodeficiency virus by herpes simplex virus type 1. *J Virol* 1987;61:3726–3732.

274. Pagano JS. Epstein-Barr virus: culprit or consort? *N Engl J Med* 1992;327:1750–1751.

275. Palestine AG, Polis MA, De Smet MD. A randomized controlled trial of foscarnet in the treatment of cytomegalovirus retinitis in patients with AIDS. *Ann Intern Med* 1991;115:665–673.

276. Palestine AG, Stevens G Jr, Lane HC. Treatment of cytomegalovirus retinitis with dihydroxy propoxymethyl guanine. *Am J Ophthalmol* 1986;101:95–101.

277. Pepose JS, Hilborne LH, Cancilla PA, Foos RY. Concurrent herpes simplex and cytomegalovirus retinitis and encephalitis in the acquired immune deficiency syndrome (AIDS). *Ophthalmology* 1984;91:1669–1677.

278. Pepose JS, Holland GN, Nestor MS, Cochran AJ, Foos RY. Acquired immune deficiency syndrome. Pathogenic mechanisms of ocular disease. *Ophthalmology* 1985;92:472–484.

279. Pellett PH, Black JB, Yamamoto M. Human herpesvirus 6: the virus and the search for its role as a human pathogen. *Adv Virus Res* 1992;41:1–52.

280. Perham TGM, Caul EO, Clarke SKR, Gibson AGF. Cytomegalovirus meningoencephalitis. *Br Med J* 1971;2:50.

281. Peter M, Timm U, Schürmann D. Combined and alternating ganciclovir and foscarnet in acute and maintenance therapy of human immunodeficiency virus-related cytomegalovirus encephalitis refractory to ganciclovir alone. *Clin Investig* 1992;70:456–458.

282. Petito CK, Cho E-S, Lemann W, Navia BA, Price RW. Neuropathology of acquired immunodeficiency syndrome (AIDS): an autopsy review. *J Neuropathol Exp Neurol* 1986;45:635–646.

283. Phillips CA, Fanning WL, Gump DW, Phillips CF. Cytomegalovirus encephalitis in immunologically normal adults: successful treatment with vidarabine. *JAMA* 1977;238:2299–2300.

284. Picard FJ, Dekaban GA, Silva J, Rice GPA. Mollaret's meningitis associated with herpes simplex type 2 infection. *Neurology* 1993;43:1722–1727.

285. Pillai S, Mahmood MA, Limaye SR. Herpes zoster ophthalmicus, contralateral hemiplegia, and recurrent ocular toxoplasmosis in a patient with acquired immune deficiency syndrome-related complex. *J Clin Neurol Ophthalmol* 1989;9:229–233.

286. Pillay D, Lipman MCI, Lee CA, Johnson MA, Griffiths PD, McLaughlin JE. A clinico-pathological audit of opportunistic viral infections in HIV-infected patients. *AIDS* 1993;7:969–974.

287. Plotkin SA. Vaccines for varicella-zoster virus and cytomegalovirus: recent progress. *Science* 1994;265:1383–1385.

288. Poland SD, Costello P, Dekaban GA, Rice GPA. Cytomegalovirus in the brain in vitro infection of human brain-derived cells. *J Infect Dis* 1990;162:1252–1262.

289. Preblud SR. Varicella: complications and costs. *Pediatrics* 1986;78:728–735.

290. Price R, Chernik NL, Horta-Barbosa L, Posner JB. Herpes simplex encephalitis in an anergic patient. *Am J Med* 1973;54:222–227.

291. Price TA, Digioia RA, Simon GL. Ganciclovir treatment of cytomegalovirus ventriculitis in a patient infected with human immunodeficiency virus. *Clin Infect Dis* 1992;15:606–608.

292. Prober CG, Kirk LE, Keeney RE. Acyclovir therapy of chickenpox in immunosuppressed children—a collaborative study. *J Pediatr* 1982;101:622–625.

293. Pruksananonda P, Hall CB, Insel RA. Primary human herpesvirus 6 infection in young children. *N Engl J Med* 1992;326:1445–1450.

294. Puchhammer-Stockl E, Popow-Kraupp T, Heinz FX, Mandl CW, Kunz C. Establishment of PCR for the early diagnosis of herpes simplex encephalitis. *J Med Virol* 1990;32:77–82.
295. Pulliam L. Cytomegalovirus preferentially infects monocyte derived macrophage/microglial cell in human brain cultures: neuropathology differs between strains. *J Neuropathol Exp Neurol* 1991;50: 432–440.
296. Pulliam L, Berens ME, Rosenblum ML. A normal human brain cell aggregate model for neurological studies. *J Neurosci Res* 1988;21:521–530.
297. Qavi HB, Green MT, SeGall GK, Lewis DE, Hollinger FB. Transcriptional activity of HIV-1 and HHV-6 in retinal lesions from AIDS patients. *Invest Ophthalmol Vis Sci* 1992;33:2759–2767.
298. Quesnel A, Pozzetto B, Touraine F. Antibodies to Epstein-Barr virus and cytomegalovirus in relation to CD4 cell number in human immunodeficiency virus 1 infection. *J Med Virol* 1992;36:60–64.
299. Quinn TC, Piot P, McCormick JB, et al. Serological and immunological studies in patients with AIDS in North America and Africa: the potential role of infectious agents as cofactors in human immunodeficiency virus infection. *JAMA* 1987;257:2617–2621.
300. Quinnan GV, Masur H, Rook AH. Herpesvirus infections in the acquired immune deficiency syndrome. *JAMA* 1984;252:72–77.
301. Quinnan GV, Siegel JP, Epstein JS, Manischewitz JF, Barnes S, Wells MA. Mechanisms of T-cell functional deficiency in the acquired immunodeficiency syndrome. *Ann Intern Med* 1985;103: 710–714.
302. Rasmussen L. Immune response to human cytomegalovirus infection. *Curr Top Microbiol Immunol* 1990;154:221–254.
303. Reed EC, Raleigh BA, Dandiker PS, Lilleby KE, Meyers JD. Treatment of cytomegalovirus pneumonia with ganciclovir and intravenous cytomegalovirus immunoglobulin in patients with bone marrow transplants. *Ann Intern Med* 1988;783:785.
304. Reichert CM, O Leary TJ, Levens DL, Simrell CR, Macher AM. Autopsy pathology in the acquired immune deficiency syndrome. *Am J Pathol* 1983;112:357–382.
305. Reusser P, Riddell SR, Meyers JD, Greenberg PD. Cytotoxic T-lymphocyte response to cytomegalovirus after human allogeneic bone marrow transplantation: pattern of recovery and correlation with cytomegalovirus infection and disease. *Blood* 1991;78:1373–1380.
306. Revello MG, Percivalle E, Sarasini A, et al. Diagnosis of human cytomegalovirus infection of the nervous system by pp65 detection in polymorphonuclear leukocytes of cerebrospinal fluid from AIDS patients. *J Infect Dis* 1994;170:1275–1279.
307. Riddell SR, Rabin M, Geballe AP, Britt WJ, Greenberg PD. Class I-MHC restricted cytotoxic T-lymphocyte recognition of cells infected with human cytomegalovirus does not require endogenous viral gene expression. *J Immunol* 1991;146:2795–2804.
308. Riddell SR, Watanabe KS, Goodrich JM, Mi CR, Agha ME, Greenberg PD. Restoration of viral immunity in immunodeficient humans by the adoptive transfer of T cell clones. *Science* 1992;257: 238–240.
309. Rinaldo CR, Carney WP, Richter B, Black S, Hirsch MS. Mechanisms of immunosuppression in cytomegalovirus mononucleosis. *J Infect Dis* 1980;141:488–495.
310. Robert ME, Geraghty JJ III, Miles SA, et al. Severe neuropathy in a patient with acquired immune deficiency syndrome (AIDS). *Acta Neuropathol* 1989;79:255–261.
311. Roizman B. The family Herpesviridae. A brief introduction. In: Roizman B, Whitley RJ, Lopez C, eds. *The human herpesviruses.* New York: Raven; 1993:1–10.
312. Roizman B, Sears AE. Herpes simplex viruses and their replication. In: Roizman B, Whitley RJ, Lopez C, eds. *The human herpesviruses.* New York: Raven; 1993:11–68.
313. Rook AH, Manischewitz JF, Frederick WR, et al. Deficiency, HLA-restricted, cytomegalovirus-specific cytotoxic T cells and natural killer cells in patients with the acquired immunodeficiency syndrome. *J Infect Dis* 1985;152:627–630.
314. Rosenberg NL, Hochberg FH, Miller G, Kleinschmidt-DeMasters BK. Primary central nervous system lymphoma related to Epstein-Barr virus in a patient with acquired immunodeficiency syndrome. *Ann Neurol* 1986;20:98–102.
315. Rosenberg ZF, Fauci AS. Immunology of AIDS: approaches to understanding the immunopathogenesis of HIV infection. *Res Clin Lab* 1989;19:189–196.
316. Rosenberg ZF, Fauci AS. Immunopathogenesis of HIV infection. In: DeVita VT Jr, Hellman S, Rosenberg SA, eds. *AIDS etiology, diagnosis, treatment and prevention.* 3rd ed. Philadelphia: Lippincott; 1992:61–76.
317. Rosenblum MK. Bulbar encephalitis complicating trigeminal zoster in the acquired immune deficiency syndrome. *Hum Pathol* 1989;20:292–295.
318. Roullet E, Assuerus V, Gozlan J, et al. Cytomegalovirus multifocal neuropathy in AIDS: analysis of 15 consecutive cases. *Neurology* 1994;44:2174–2182.
319. Rousseau F, Perronne C, Raguin G, et al. Necrotizing retinitis and cerebral vasculitis due to varicella-zoster virus in patients infected with the human immunodeficiency virus. *Clin Infect Dis* 1993;17: 943–944.

320. Rowley AH, Whitley RJ, Lakeman FD, Wolinsky SM. Rapid detection of herpes-simplex-virus DNA in cerebrospinal fluid of patients with herpes simplex encephalitis. *Lancet* 1990;335:440–441.

321. Russell J, Fisher M, Zivin J, Sullivan J, Drachman DA. Status epilepticus and Epstein-Barr virus encephalopathy. *Arch Neurol* 1985;42:789–792.

322. Ryder JW, Croen K, Kleinshmidt-Demasters BK. Progressive encephalitis three months after resolution of cutaneous zoster in a patient with AIDS. *Ann Neurol* 1986;19:182–188.

323. Said G, Lacroix C, Chemovilli P. Cytomegalovirus neuropathy in acquired immunodeficiency syndrome: a clinical and pathological study. *Ann Neurol* 1991;29:139–146.

324. Safrin S, Crumpacker C, Chatis P. A controlled trial comparing foscarnet with vidarabine for acyclovir-resistant muco-cutaneous herpes simplex in the acquired immunodeficiency syndrome. *N Engl J Med* 1991;325:551–555.

325. Sage JI, Weinstein MP, Miller DC. Chronic encephalitis possibly due to herpes simplex virus: two cases. *Neurology* 1985;35:1470–1472.

326. Salahuddin SZ, Ablaski DW, Markham PD, et al. Isolation of a new virus, HBLV, in patients with lymphoproliferative disorders. *Science* 1986;234:596–601.

327. Sample J, Young L, Martin B, Chatman T, Kieff E, Rickinson A. Epstein-Barr virus types 1 and 2 differ in their ENA-3A, EBNA-3B and EBNA-3C genes. *J Virol* 1990;64:4084–4092.

328. Saxinger C, Polesky H, Eby N. Antibody reactivity with HBLV (HHV-6) in U.S. populations. *J Virol Methods* 1988;21:199–208.

329. Schaeffer HJ, Beauchamp L, deMiranda P, Elion GB, Baver DJ, Collins P. 9-(2-Hydroxyethoxy-methyl) guanine activity against viruses of the herpes group. *Nature* 1978;272:583–585.

330. Schiff JA, Schaefer JA, Robinson JE. Epstein-Barr virus in cerebrospinal fluid during infectious mononucleosis encephalitis. *Yale J Biol Med* 1982;55:59–63.

331. Schirmer EC, Wyatt LS, Yamanishi K, Rodriguez WJ. Differentiation between two distinct classes of viruses now classified as human herpesvirus 6. *Proc Natl Acad Sci USA* 1991;88:5922–5926.

332. Schlitt M, Lakeman AD, Wilson ER, To A, Harsh GR III, Whitley RJ. A rabbit model of focal herpes simplex encephalitis. *J Infect Dis* 1986;153:732–735.

333. Schmidbauer M, Budka H, Vlrick W, Ambros P. Cytomegalovirus (CMV) disease of the brain in AIDS and connatal infection: a comparative study by histology, immunocytochemistry and in situ DNA hybridization. *Acta Neuropathol* 1989;79:286–293.

334. Schneck SA. Neuropathological features of human organ transplantation. *J Neuropathol Exp Neurol* 1965;24:415–429.

335. Schnell RG, Dyck PJ, Walter EJ, et al. Infectious mononucleosis: neurological and EEG findings. *Medicine* 1966;45:51–63.

336. Schober R, Herman MM. Neuropathology of cardiac transplantation. *Lancet* 1973;1:962–967.

337. Schooley RT. Herpesvirus infection in individuals with HIV infection. In: DeVita VT Jr, Hellman S, Rosenberg SA, eds. *AIDS. Etiology, diagnosis, treatment and prevention*. 3rd ed. Philadelphia: Lippincott; 1992:193–207.

338. Schrier RD, Oldstone MBA. Recent clinical isolates of cytomegalovirus suppress human cytomegalovirus-specific human leukocyte antigen-restricted cytotoxic T-lymphocyte activity. *J Virol* 1986;59:127–131.

339. Schwarz TF, Loeschke K, Hanus I. CMV encephalitis during ganciclovir therapy of CMV retinitis. *Infection* 1990;18:289–290.

340. Scolnik PR, Kosloff BR, Hirsch MS. Bidirectional interactions between human immunodeficiency virus type 1 and cytomegalovirus. *J Infect Dis* 1988;157:508–513.

341. Scully TB, Apolloni A, Hurren L, Moss DJ, Cooper DA. Coinfection with A- and B-type Epstein-Barr virus in human immunodeficiency virus-positive subjects. *J Infect Dis* 1990;162:643–648.

342. Segondy M, Astruc J, Atoui N. Herpesvirus 6 infection in young children. *N Engl J Med* 1992;327:1099.

343. Shepp DH, Dandliker PS, Meyers JD. Treatment of varicella-zoster virus infection in severely immunocompromised patients. A randomized comparison of acyclovir and vidarabine. *N Engl J Med* 1986;314:208–212.

344. Shiramizu B, Herndier B, Meeker T, Kaplan L, McGrath M. Molecular and immunophenotypic characterization of AIDS-associated Epstein-Barr virus-negative, polyclonal lymphomas. *J Clin Oncol* 1992;10:383–389.

345. Shoji H, Honda Y, Murai I. Detection of varicella-zoster virus DNA by polymerase chain reaction in cerebrospinal fluid of patients with herpes zoster meningitis. *J Neurol* 1992;239:69–70.

346. Silverstein A, Steinberg G, Nathanson M. Nervous system involvement in infectious mononucleosis. *Arch Neurol* 1972;26:356–358.

347. Sissons JGP, Borysiewicz LK, Rodgers B, Scott D. Cytomegalovirus—its cellular immunology and biology. *Immunol Today* 1986;7:57–61.

348. Small PM, McPhaul LW, Sooy CD. Cytomegalovirus infection of the laryngeal nerve presenting as hoarseness in patients with acquired immunodeficiency syndrome. *Am J Med* 1989;86:108–110.

349. Smith PD, Saini SS, Raffeld M, Manischewitz JF, Wahl SM. Cytomegalovirus induction of tumor necrosis factor-a by human monocytes and mucosal macrophages. *J Clin Invest* 1992;90:1642–1648.

350. Snider WD, Simpson DM, Nielson S, Gold JWM, Metroka CE, Posner JB. Neurological complications of acquired immune deficiency syndrome: analysis of 50 patients. *Ann Neurol* 1983;14: 403–418.
351. Snydman DR. Prevention of cytomegalovirus disease with intravenous immune globulin. *Trans Proc* 1991;23:20–25.
352. Sobel RA, Collins AB, Colvin RB, Bhan AK. The in situ cellular response in acute herpes simplex encephalitis. *Am J Pathol* 1986;125:332–338.
353. Spector S, Hadden JW. Immunotherapy for AIDS. Status and prospects. In: Wormser GP, ed. *AIDS and other manifestations of HIV infection.*, 2nd ed. New York: Raven; 1992:625–632.
354. Spector DH, Koval V, Jault FM, Lathey J, Spector SA. Positive and negative effects of human cytomegalovirus on HIV replication. In: Kung H-J, Wood C, eds. *Interactions between retroviruses and herpesviruses.* River Edge, NJ: World Scientific Publishing; 1994:65–89.
355. Spitzer PG, Tarsy D, Eliopoulos GM. Acute transverse myelitis during disseminated cytomegalovirus infection in a renal transplant recipient. *Transplantation* 1987;44:151–153.
356. Stagno S, Pass RF, Dworsky ME, Alford CA. Maternal cytomegalovirus infection and perinatal transmission. In: Knox GE, ed. *Clinical obstetrics and gynecology.* Philadelphia: Lippincott; 1982: 563–576.
357. Stamm W, Handsfield HH, Rompalo A, Ashley R, Roberts P, Corey L. The association between genital ulcer disease and acquisition of HIV infection in homosexual men. *JAMA* 1988;260: 1449–1450.
358. Steel JG, Dix RD, Baringer JR. Isolation of herpes simplex virus type 1 in recurrent (Mollaret) meningitis. *Ann Neurol* 1982;11:17–21.
359. Steeper TA, Horwitz CA, Ablashi DV, et al. The spectrum of clinical and laboratory findings resulting from human herpesvirus-6 (HHV-6) in patients with mononucleosis-like illness not resulting from Epstein-Barr virus or cytomegalovirus. *Am J Clin Pathol* 1990;93:776–783.
360. Straus SE. Clinical and biological differences between recurrent herpes simplex virus and varicella-zoster virus infections. *JAMA* 1989;262:3455–3458.
361. Stroop WG, Schaefer DC. Production of encephalitis restricted to the temporal lobes by experimental reactivation of herpes simplex virus. *J Infect Dis* 1986;153:721–731.
362. Studies of Ocular Complications of AIDS Research Group in Collaboration with the AIDS Clinical Trials Group. Mortality in patients with acquired immunodeficiency syndrome treated with either foscarnet or ganciclovir for cytomegalovirus retinitis. *N Engl J Med* 1992;326:213–220.
363. Suga S, Yoshikawa T, Asano Y. Clinical and virological analyses of 21 infants with exanthem subitum (roseola infantum) and central nervous system complications. *Ann Neurol* 1993;33:597–603.
364. Sullivan WM, Kelley GG, O'Connor PG. Hypopituitarism associated with a hypothalamic CMV infection in a patient with AIDS. *Am J Med* 1992;92:221–223.
365. Sutton AL, Smithwick EM, Seligman SJ, Kim DS. Fatal disseminated herpesvirus hominis type 2 infection in an adult with associated thymic dysplasia. *Am J Med* 1974;56:545–553.
366. Tahseen N, Chuang EL, Berger JR, Dix RD. Detection of cytomegalovirus-specific antibody within cerebrospinal fluid of asymptomatic HIV-infected individuals is associated with intrathecal antibody synthesis. *Invest Ophthal Vis Sci* 1992;33(Suppl):247.
367. Talpos D, Tien RD, Hesselink JR. Magnetic resonance imaging of AIDS-related polyradiculopathy. *Neurology* 1991;41:1995–1997.
368. Tan SV, Guiloff RJ, Scaravilli F. Herpes simplex type 1 in acquired immunodeficiency syndrome. *Ann Neurol* 1993;34:619–622.
369. Teich SA, Cheung TW, Friedman AH. Systemic antiviral drugs used in ophthalmology. *Surv Ophthalmol* 1992;37:19–53.
370. Tilg H, Vogel W, Herold M, Aulitzky WE, Huber C. Cachexia and tumor necrosis factor-a in cytomegalovirus infection. *J Clin Pathol* 1991;44:519–520.
371. Torelli G, Marasca R, Luppi M. Human herpesvirus-6 in human lymphomas: identification of specific sequences in Hodgkin's lymphomas by the polymerase chain reaction. *Blood* 1991;77:2251–2258.
372. Townsend JJ, Baringer JR. Morphology of central nervous system disease in immunosuppressed mice after peripheral herpes simplex virus inoculation. *Lab Invest* 1979;40:178–182.
373. Tucker T, Dix RD, Katzen C, Davis RL, Schmidley JW. Cytomegalovirus and herpes simplex virus ascending myelitis in a patient with acquired immune deficiency syndrome. *Ann Neurol* 1985;18: 74–79.
374. Tyler KL, Gross RA, Cascino GD. Unusual viral causes of transverse myelitis: hepatitis A virus and cytomegalovirus. *Neurology* 1986;36:855–858.
375. Tyms AS, Taylor DL, Parkin JM. Cytomegalovirus and the acquired immunodeficiency syndrome. *J Antimicrob Chemother* 1989;23(Suppl A):89–105.
376. Van Landingham KE, Marsteller HB, Ross GW, Hayden FG. Relapse of herpes simplex encephalitis after conventional acyclovir therapy. *JAMA* 1988;259:1051–1053.
377. Vassalli P. The pathophysiology of tumor necrosis factors. *Annu Rev Immunol* 1992;10:411–452.
378. Vinters HV, Kwok MK, Ho HW, et al. Cytomegalovirus in the nervous system of patients with the acquired immune deficiency syndrome. *Brain* 1989;112:245–268.

379. Vital C, Vital A, Vignoly B, Dupon M, Lacut JY. Cytomegalovirus encephalitis in a patient with acquired immunodeficiency syndrome. *Arch Pathol Lab Med* 1985;109:105–106.
380. Vlach J, Pitha PM. Interactions between herpes simplex virus type 1 and human immunodeficiency virus type 1. In: Kung H-J, Wood C, eds. *Interactions between retroviruses and herpesviruses.* River Edge, NJ: World Scientific Publishing; 1994:36–44.
381. Walker RE, Lane HC. Interferon-a in HIV infection. In: DeVita VT Jr, Hellman S, Rosenberg SA, eds. *AIDS Etiology, diagnosis, treatment, and prevention.* 3rd ed. Philadelphia: Lippincott; 1992: 395–406.
382. Wang J, Jones C, Norcross M, Bohnlein E, Razzaque A. Identification and characterization of a human herpesvirus 6 gene segment capable of transactivating the human immunodeficiency virus type 1 long terminal repeat in an Sp1 binding site-dependent manner. *J Virol* 1994;68:1706–1713.
383. Warren KG, Brown SM, Wroblewska Z, Gilden D, Koprowski H, Subak-Sharpe J. Isolation of latent herpes simplex virus from superior cervical and vagus ganglions of human beings. *N Engl J Med* 1978;298:1068–1069.
384. Warren KG, Devlin M, Gilden DH. Isolation of herpes simplex virus from human trigeminal ganglia, including ganglia from one patient with multiple sclerosis. *Lancet* 1977;2:637–639.
385. Warren KG, Marausyk RG, Lewis ME, Jeffrey VM. Recovery of latent herpes simplex virus from human trigeminal nerve roots. *Arch Virol* 1982;73:85–89.
386. Webster A, Cook DG, Emery VEC, et al. Cytomegalovirus infection and progression towards AIDS in hemophiliacs with human immunodeficiency virus infection. *Lancet* 1989;ii:63–66.
387. Weigle KA, Grose C. Molecular dissection of the humoral immune response to individual varicella-zoster viral proteins during chickenpox, quiescence, reinfection, and reactivation. *J Infect Dis* 1984; 149:741–749.
388. Welch K, Finbeiner W, Alpers CE, et al. Autopsy findings in the acquired immune deficiency syndrome. *JAMA* 1984;252:1152–1159.
389. Whitley RJ, Alford CA Jr, Hirsch MS, et al. Vidarabine versus acyclovir therapy in herpes simplex encephalitis. *N Engl J Med* 1986;314:144–149.
390. Whitley RJ, Cobbs CG, Alford CA. Diseases that mimic herpes simplex encephalitis. *JAMA* 1989; 262:234–239.
391. Whitley RJ, Gnann JW Jr. The epidemiology and clinical manifestations of herpes simplex virus infections. In: Roizman B, Whitley RJ, Lopez C, eds. *The human herpesviruses.* New York: Raven; 1993:69–107.
392. Whitley RJ, Gnann JW Jr. Antiviral therapy. In: Roizman B, Whitley RJ, Lopez C, eds. *The human herpesviruses.* New York: Raven; 1993:329–348.
393. Whitley RJ, Hilty M, Haynes R, et al. Vidarabine therapy of varicella in immunosuppressed patients. *J Pediatr* 1982;101:125–131.
394. Whitley RJ, Lakeman AD, Nahmias A, Roizman B. DNA restriction-enzyme analysis of herpes simplex isolates obtained from patients with encephalitis. *N Engl J Med* 1982;307:1060–1062.
395. Whitley RJ, Schlitt M. Encephalitis caused by herpesviruses including B virus. In: Scheld WM, Whitley RJ, Durack DT, eds. *Infections of the central nervous system.* New York: Raven; 1991: 41–86.
396. Whitley RJ, Soong SJ, Hirsch MS, et al. Herpes simplex virus encephalitis: vidarabine therapy and diagnostic problems. *N Engl J Med* 1981;304:488–498.
397. Whitley RJ, Soong SJ, Dolin R, Betts R, Linneman C Jr, Alford CA Jr. Early vidarabine therapy to control the complications of herpes zoster in immunosuppressed patients. *N Engl J Med* 1982; 307:971–975.
398. Whitley RJ, Soong SJ, Linneman C Jr, Chien L, Pazin G, Alford CA. Herpes simplex encephalitis—clinical assessment. *JAMA* 1982;247:317–320.
399. Wiley CA, Nelson JA. Role of human immunodeficiency virus and cytomegalovirus in AIDS encephalitis. *Am J Pathol* 1988;133:73–81.
400. Wiley CA, Schrier RD, Denaro FJ. Localization of cytomegalovirus proteins and genome during fulminant central nervous system infection in an AIDS patient. *J Neuropathol Exp Neurol* 1986; 45:127–139.
401. Wiley CA, Van Patten PD, Carpenter PM, Powell HC, Thal LJ. Acute ascending necrotizing myelopathy caused by herpes simplex virus type 2. *Neurology* 1987;37:1791–1794.
402. Winston DJ, Ho WG, Lin CH. Intravenous immune globulin for prevention of cytomegalovirus infection and interstitial pneumonia after bone marrow transplantation. *Ann Intern Med* 1987;106: 12–18.
403. Wolf DG, Spector SA. Diagnosis of human cytomegalovirus central nervous system disease in AIDS patients by DNA amplification from cerebrospinal fluid. *J Infect Dis* 1992;166:1412–1415.
404. Wood MJ, Johson RW, McKendrick MW, Taylor J, Mandal BK, Crooks J. A randomized trial of acyclovir for 7 days or 21 days with and without prednisolone for treatment of acute herpes zoster. *N Engl J Med* 1994;330:896–900.
405. Wood MJ, Ogan PH, McKendrick MW, Care CD, McGill JI, Webb EM. Efficacy of oral acyclovir treatment of acute herpes zoster. *Am J Med* 1988;85(Suppl 2A):79–83.

406. Yahr MD, Frontera AT. Acute autonomic neuropathy. Its occurrence in infectious mononucleosis. *Arch Neurol* 1975;32:132–133.
407. Yamamoto LJ, Tedder DG, Ashley R, Levin MJ. Herpes simplex virus type 1 DNA in cerebrospinal fluid of a patient with Mollaret's meningitis. *N Engl J Med* 1992;325:1082–1084.
408. Yamanishi K, Okuno T, Skhiroki K. Identification of human herpesvirus-6 as a causal agent for exanthem subitum. *Lancet* 1988;1:1065–1067.
409. Yanagi K, Harada S, Ban F, Oya A, Okabe N, Tobinai K. High prevalence of antibody to human herpesvirus-6 and decrease in titer with increase in age in Japan. *J Infect Dis* 1990;161:153–154.
410. Yanagisaw N, Toyokura Y, Shiraki B. Double encephalitis with herpes simplex virus and cytomegalovirus in an adult. *Acta Neuropathol (Berlin)* 1975;33:153–164.
411. Yarrish RL. Cytomegalovirus infection in AIDS. In: Wormer GP, ed. *AIDS and other manifestations of HIV infection.* 2nd ed. New York: Raven; 1992:249–268.
412. Zaraspe-Yoo E, Miletich R, Tourtellotte WW. Herpes zoster ophthalmicus with contralateral hemiplegia in a patient with autoimmune deficiency syndrome (AIDS). *Neurology* 1984:34(Suppl 1):229.
413. Zeigler JL, Drew WL, Miner L. Outbreak of Burkitt's lymphoma in homosexual men. *Lancet* 1982;2:631–633.
414. Zimber U, Aldinger HK, Lenoir GM, et al. Geographic prevalence of two Epstein-Barr virus types. *Virology* 1986;154:56–66.

AIDS and the Nervous System, Second Edition,
edited by J. R. Berger and R. M. Levy.
Lippincott-Raven Publishers, Philadelphia © 1997.

24

Toxoplasmosis

Peter Mariuz, Elizabeth Bosler, and Benjamin J. Luft

*Department of Medicine, State University of New York at Stony Brook,
Stony Brook, New York 11794*

Toxoplasma gondii is a ubiquitous, obligate intracellular protozoan found throughout the world. For patients with the acquired immunodeficiency syndrome (AIDS), it is the most common cause of focal central nervous system (CNS) infection (66). This organism poses many diagnostic and therapeutic challenges for clinicians treating human immunodeficiency virus (HIV) infected patients. To appreciate the complexity of these challenges, it is necessary to understand the life cycle of *T. gondii*, the epidemiology and the pathogenesis of toxoplasmosis, as well as the currently recommended treatment regimens. Although *T. gondii* can infect any mammalian cell, our focus will be on disease involving the nervous system.

HISTORICAL BACKGROUND

In 1928, *T. gondii* was first described by Nicolle and Manceaux, and in the same year it was identified as the causative agent of a significant zoonosis in rabbits (89). The organism was first isolated from a human by Jamku (55), and in 1937, several authors established *T. gondii* as a cause of congenital neonatal encephalitis (93,114,130). Only with the development in 1948 of a reliable serological test to detect antitoxoplasma antibody (Sabin-Feldman dye test) could the wide spectrum of clinical manifestations and the ubiquitous nature of the infection throughout the world be fully appreciated (113). The life cycle of *T. gondii* was not established until 1969, when it was shown that *T. gondii* is a coccidian and the definitive host is the cat (36). Recognized since 1968 and 1978, respectively, as a cause of encephalitis in immunocompromised patients with malignancy or organ transplant recipients (79,112,126), only with the advent of AIDS is toxoplasmosis, particularly toxoplasmic encephalitis (TE), occurring in epidemic proportions (76).

As for the name *Toxoplasma gondii*, toxoplasma is derived from the Greek word for arc, *toxon*, which refers to the bow shape of the tachyzoite; gondii comes from the name of the North African rodent, *Ctenodactylus gondi*, from which Nicolle and Manceaux first isolated the organism.

LIFE CYCLE

In the life cycle of *T. gondii*, three different forms must be considered; oocysts, tachyzoites, and tissue cysts (125). The cat is the definitive host for *T. gondii* (127).

In this animal, the organism undergoes its complete life cycle, which is comprised of two stages; an enteroepithelial (intraintestinal), sexual stage which results in the production of oocysts, and an extraintestinal, asexual stage, which results in the production of tissue cysts. Oocyst production, therefore, takes place only in cats while the extraintestinal stage takes place both in cats and intermediate hosts, including man. Cats become infected by ingesting infectious (sporulated) oocysts from fecally contaminated food and/or water or tissue cysts in the tissues of infected intermediate hosts (5). After enzymatic degradation in the gut, the infective stages (bradyzoites from tissue cysts; sporozoites from oocysts) are liberated and as tachyzoites (the rapidly proliferating form) infect the intestinal epithelium with subsequent spread to other organs. Only in the gut of the cat will the sexual cycle take place, producing oocysts which are shed into the environment where sporulation occurs. After sporulation the oocysts are infectious for intermediate hosts (30). This maturation process is more rapid at warm temperatures, and under favorable conditions (e.g., in warm moist soil), oocysts may remain infectious for over 1 year. Millions of oocysts are excreted in the feces of the cat each day for approximately 1 to 3 weeks after the acute infection. One possible route of human infection is ingestion of food or beverages contaminated with sporulated oocysts from soil or cat litter boxes.

The asexual, extraintestinal stage which takes place both in cats and intermediate hosts occurs when tachyzoites, after infecting the gut mucosa, invade the bloodstream and lymphatics and disseminate widely throughout the body, causing tissue injury and disease. The tachyzoite is an obligate intracellular parasite capable of infecting every kind of mammalian cell. It replicates within vacuoles in the host cell until 8 to 16 organisms accumulate, at which time the cell lyses. Contiguous cells are then infected. These events continue until an adequate host immune response takes place. The tachyzoite cannot survive the digestive juices of the stomach (54) but can be involved in transmission of toxoplasmosis via blood product transfusions and laboratory accidents (88,117).

Tissue cysts are formed in various tissues by replicating tachyzoites. The exact mechanism of cyst formation is not known. While protective immunity against the tachyzoite has been postulated to be the impetus for cyst formation, it may not fully explain this phenomena. Even in tissue culture systems devoid of antibody or immune cells, cyst formation takes place (56). Cyst formation has also been noted during progressive fatal encephalitis of infected immunosuppressed mice (37). Tachyzoites may form pseudocysts, which are present in host cells for prolonged periods of time without forming true tissue cysts. Tissue cysts vary in size and may contain several thousand bradyzoites. The tissue cyst is characteristic of chronic infection but can be found as early as 6 to 12 days after acute infection (33). Tissue cysts are most commonly found in the brain, heart, and striated muscle. However, any organ may become chronically infected. The wall of the mature tissue cyst is believed to be formed by a combination of host and parasitic components (69). The presence of host material may explain, in part, the absence of inflammation around tissue cysts. To date it is uncertain whether cysts reside solely inside host cells or if they can persist extracellularly (33,96,118). There is evidence from animal models that cysts rupture periodically, releasing the bradyzoites, which then develop ``daughter'' cysts (64). These recurrent episodes of asymptomatic, active infection could be responsible for the lifelong persistence of antibodies and cell-mediated immunity to toxoplasmosis. Furthermore, the spontaneous rupture of cysts may be the initial event in the development of encephalitis, for example, in immunosuppressed patients unable to contain the infectious process.

In the AIDS patient with TE, the tachyzoite is the form of *T. gondii* responsible for the destructive necrotizing process (37). Even within these lesions the tissue cyst can be found. This form of *T. gondii* probably persists in infected host tissues for the life of the host. Tissue cysts are associated with the transmission of *T. gondii* since they persist in tissues of chronically infected animals, which may be ingested by carnivores, including humans. Undercooked lamb and pork have been implicated as the source of several outbreaks of toxoplasmosis (30,60). Undercooked beef, however, probably plays a small role in the transmission of toxoplasmosis (30). The tissue cyst is important in the transmission of infection in organ transplantation (79,110,112). Heart transplant recipients, seronegative for toxoplasma antibody and receiving a heart from a seropositive donor, have a high incidence of developing disseminated toxoplasmosis (112).

EPIDEMIOLOGY

In patients with AIDS, over 95% of TE is due to reactivation of a chronic (latent) infection. The incidence of TE is directly proportional to the prevalence of antibodies to *T. gondii* in any given population. In the United States 10% to 40% of adults with AIDS are latently infected, and it is estimated that 30% of these patients will develop TE (73). Toxoplasmic encephalitis occurs more frequently in blacks and Hispanics and more frequently in heterosexual males as compared to homosexual males. There are significant differences in the incidence of TE in different geographic locations in the United States. It occurs three times more frequently in Florida than in other states (104). However, these regional differences in the incidence rates of TE probably reflect the ethnic population differences for the prevalence of toxoplasma seropositivity (42,70,104,107).

In Africa, Haiti, Europe, and Latin America, where the incidence of latent infection is much higher, the total number of individuals with AIDS who develop TE will be three to four times higher than in the United States. Also, a greater proportion (>30%) of seropositive patients from these regions may develop TE. For example, in a study from Austria, 47% of AIDS patients seropositive for *T. gondii* developed TE (132). In Europe and Africa, it is estimated that 25% to 50% of seropositive patients with AIDS will ultimately develop TE (14,100). The reasons for this increased propensity to develop TE in countries other than the United States have not been elucidated. It remains unclear why only 30% to 50% of AIDS patients latently infected with *T. gondii* develop TE once they become severely immunocompromised. However, host factors (e.g., genetic predisposition) or variation in virulence among different strains of *T. gondii* may play a role (27,84,121).

For most HIV-infected patients, TE develops when the CD4 + -T lymphocyte count (CD4 + count) falls below $100/mm^3$ (26). When *T. gondii*-seropositive, HIV-infected patients were followed prospectively, 7% and 21% of those with CD4+ counts between 100 and $200/mm^3$ developed TE by 12 and 18 months, respectively, whereas 22% and 40%, respectively, developed TE over the same time period when CD4+ counts were below $100/mm^3$ (41,67,79). In these studies over 80% of *T. gondii*-seropositive, AIDS patients developed TE when CD4+ counts were less than $100/mm^3$.

PATHOGENESIS

The pathogenesis of toxoplasmosis in the immunocompromised patient depends on several host factors, including (a) the time of acquisition of the infection (acute versus chronic), (b) the nature (cellular versus humoral immunity), and (c) the severity of the underlying immunocompromising illness and whether it is reversible. Initially the human host becomes acutely infected by ingesting raw or undercooked meat containing the tissue cysts or foods or beverages contaminated with oocysts. Infected individuals will remain seropositive and viable tissue cysts will remain in various organs for the remainder of the life of the host. The depletion of CD4+ T lymphocytes and macrophage dysfunction appear to predispose patients to reactivation of chronic latent toxoplasmosis. Thus, in patients with AIDS, the tissue cysts rupture and the organism multiplies unimpeded by host immunity to give rise to a focal infection usually limited to the brain (37). In the brain, this infection evolves into a focal necrotizing encephalitis. In contrast, outside of the CNS, host immunity is usually still effective in controlling infection to a degree. This may explain the prominence of CNS manifestations in such patients (111). Isolation of *T. gondii* from the blood of up to 38% of AIDS patients with TE suggests that hematogenous spread from the brain, from sites outside the CNS, or from both also occur (26,65,123).

Newly acquired toxoplasmosis manifested either as disseminated disease in the seronegative, HIV-infected patient with significant immunosuppression (CD4 cells $<200/mm^3$) or as asymptomatic seroconversion of antitoxoplasma antibody titers have been reported. In France, a prospective study of seronegative HIV-infected patients showed a seroconversion rate of 5.5% during a median observation period of 28 months (94). It is important that seronegative patients be educated on how to prevent themselves from becoming infected. The utility of repeat serological studies in seronegative patients at risk for developing acute toxoplasmosis, however, has not been established.

PATHOLOGY

The histopathological changes associated with toxoplasmosis in AIDS patients are variable depending upon the pathogenesis of the infection (acute versus chronic), the CD4+ count, and the length of specific therapy. In the brain, the histopathological changes vary from a well-localized, indolent, granulomatous process to a widely diffuse, necrotizing encephalitis (40,62,120,122). Necrotizing lesions are not dependent on the host's inflammatory response as severe necrotizing processes may occur with minimal or no inflammation. This suggests that unimpeded proliferation of tachyzoites cause lysis and destruction of infected cells. The lesions may be unifocal or multifocal and may vary in size from microscopic (53) to involvement of almost an entire cerebral hemisphere (87). Both the white and grey matter as well as every part of the CNS may be affected. There is a propensity for *T. gondii* to localize in the basal ganglia, thalamus, and corticomedullary junction; white matter may be involved also (104,128). The pituitary gland undergoes changes either as a focal area of infection or as part of an extensive encephalitic process (75,86). The leptomeninges are usually spared except as part of a localized reaction to an underlying cortical process. Focal areas of encephalitis separated by normal brain tissue are seen most commonly.

Post et al. (104) described three histopathological zones of focal TE in AIDS patients: (a) the central zone, containing necrotic amorphous material with few, if any, identifiable organisms; (b) the intermediate zone with engorged blood vessels showing spotty necrosis and containing numerous free extracellular and intracellular tachyzoites but rarely cysts as well as perivascular cuffing by round cells and endothelial cell hyperplasia with frank vasculitis; and (c) the outer zone, where necrosis is rare, vascular lesions are minimal, and tissue cysts predominate.

These histopathological abnormalities have been clarified further by correlating the pathology with the chronicity of infection and amount of chemotherapy (87). In biopsy or autopsy specimens from untreated patients, the lesions were poorly demarcated areas of necrosis surrounded by acute and chronic inflammatory cells, reactive astrocytes, and macrophages. Prominent vascular proliferation with endothelial hyperplasia and frank vasculitis was noted. In patients treated for 2 weeks or longer, the lesions were well-demarcated areas of central necrosis surrounded by a thin rim of tightly packed lipid-laden macrophages. Cysts and tachyzoites were identified adjacent to the organizing abscess in only three of seven patients studied. In patients treated for 4 or more weeks, chronic abscesses were observed. These were small, cystic spaces containing a few lipid-laden and hemosiderin-containing macrophages with surrounding gliosis. Rarely, cysts were noted in adjacent brain tissue.

A diffuse form of TE has been described. Macroscopically the brain appears normal while microglial nodules, without abscess formation, mostly involving the grey matter were noted. These microglial nodules contained cysts and free tachyzoites demonstrated by immunoperoxidase staining (44). Occasionally, the cellular response to toxoplasma can be so intense and atypical that it can mimic an intracerebral lymphoma (75,77,104,129). The differential diagnosis can be particularly difficult when only small amounts of tissue are available such as in needle biopsy specimens. Such cases can be resolved with careful immunohistochemical staining.

Since *T. gondii* can infect any type of cell, there are many reports of pathological changes in a variety of organs and tissues, including lungs, heart, eyes, testes, skeletal muscle, bone marrow, gastrointestinal tract, liver, pancreas, lymph nodes, thyroid, kidney, skin, prostate, ovary, and adrenals (6,10,11,23,24,45,95,111,118). The histopathological findings vary from organ to organ and the reader is referred to the individual reports for further detail.

CLINICAL MANIFESTATIONS

Toxoplasmosis in the AIDS patient is most frequently manifested by TE, usually alone, or less frequently, as part of a multiorgan infection. Isolated organ involvement without CNS disease is uncommon. The clinical manifestations of TE are protean and include signs and symptoms of focal or generalized neurological dysfunction or, more commonly, a mixture of both, depending on the number, size, and location of the lesions (Table 1). Cerebral edema, vasculitis, and hemorrhage which can occur concomitantly with active infection also contribute to the disease process (15,18,31). Toxoplasmic encephalitis most frequently presents (50% to 89%) with a subacute onset of focal neurological deficits, with or without evidence of generalized cerebral dysfunction. Less often (15% to 25%), seizures may be the initial manifestation. Occasionally, signs and symptoms of generalized cerebral dysfunction dominate the presentation of TE and patients develop focal neurological deficits as the infection

TABLE 1. *Clinical abnormalities of TE in patients with AIDS*

Focal cerebral, cerebellar, and brainstem dysfunction	Generalized cerebral dysfunction	Neuropsychiatric abnormalities	Other abnormalities
Hemiparesis	Lethargy	Dementia	Panhypopituitarism
Hemiplegia	Confusion	Anxiety	Diabetes insipidus
Dysphasia	Coma	Personality changes	Syndrome of inappropriate antidiuretic hormone
Aphasia	Decreased recent memory	Psychosis	Hydrocephalus
Movement disorders: hemichorea hemiballismus	Global cognitive impairment similar to AIDS dementia		
Seizures	Decreased attention		
Ataxia	Slowed verbal responses		
Diplopia	Slowed motor responses		
Visual field deficits			
Cranial nerve palsies			
Cerebellar tremor			
Parkinsonian symptoms			
Thalamic syndrome			
Hemisensory loss			
Headache (severe, localized)			
Intractable hiccups			

References: 3, 9, 14, 31, 37, 45, 48, 69, 70, 72, 74, 85, 86, 89, 102, 107, 114, 123.
TE, toxoplasmic encephalitis; AIDS, acquired immunodeficiency syndrome.

progresses. The clinical presentation varies from an insidious process evolving over several weeks to a more acute, at times, fulminant, course. Abnormalities associated with focal cerebral, cerebellar, and brainstem dysfunction include hemiplegia, hemiparesis, dysphasia, aphasia, movement disorders (hemichorea and hemiballismus), seizures, ataxia, diplopia, visual field deficits, cranial nerve palsies, cerebellar tremor, parkinsonian symptoms, thalamic syndrome, hemisensory loss, severe localized headache, and intractable hiccups (14,32,38,46,49,71,73,75,79,87,103,108,115). The focal neurological deficits may at first be subtle and transient and with time evolve to persistent focal deficits (128). These findings correlate with the anatomic location of focal encephalitis. The most frequent focal neurological deficits are hemiparesis and speech disorders. Abnormalities attributable to generalized cerebral dysfunction include lethargy, confusion, coma, and global cognitive impairment similar to AIDS-related dementia, with decreased recent memory, decreased attention, and slowed verbal and motor responses (14,32,46,49,71,73,75,78,87,103,108,115,124). Neuropsychiatric abnormalities including dementia, anxiety, personality changes, and psychosis can dominate the clinical picture (3,87). Panhypopituitarism, diabetes insipidus, and the syndrome of inappropriate antidiuretic hormone (SIADH) secretion also occur (49,75,86,87). Hydrocephalus as the sole manifestation of TE has been described (9,90).

Other symptoms associated with TE include headache which can be focal, generalized, and unremitting. Fever is variably present, noted in 1 of 15 (7%) patients in one series (83) but in 15 of 27 (56%) patients in another series (87). Toxoplasmic encephalitis is predominantly intra-axial so that significant meningeal involvement is rare; thus signs and symptoms of meningeal irritation are unusual, and examination of cerebrospinal fluid (CSF) is unrewarding in the majority of cases except to exclude other diseases. Isolated toxoplasmic myelitis involving the cervical, thoracic, and lumbosacral spine has been reported (47,50,85,102). Clinical manifestations include isolated upper or lower extremity sensory or motor deficits, bladder and bowel dysfunction, and back pain. Conus medularis syndrome has also been described (59,92).

Patients may also develop a diffuse encephalitis (44), manifested by rapidly progressive, fatal, generalized, cerebral dysfunction without focal neurological deficits or focal lesions on neuroradiographic study. Macroscopically, the brain appeared normal in three of four cases, while numerous scattered (hence the term *diffuse*) microglial nodules, mainly involving the gray matter, most with central *T. gondii* cysts or free tachyzoites, were noted on microscopic examination. This appears to be a form of TE unique to AIDS patients. An autopsy study of 55 cases of TE revealed diffuse encephalitis without focal lesions as the sole manifestation in 7 patients (61). One case of diffuse TE, diagnosed by isolation of *T. gondii* from the CSF using tissue culture, was reported (12). Computed tomography (CT) scans of the brain are frequently negative in these cases, thus underestimating the incidence of TE. It is important to note that microglial nodules per se are not specific for toxoplasmosis and are observed as the result of numerous other pathological processes, including cytomegalovirus encephalitis, HIV encephalitis, and cerebral lymphoma (82).

DIAGNOSIS

Clinically, serological tests for the diagnosis of toxoplasmosis in AIDS patients are useful only to identify individuals at risk for development of TE and as support for the diagnosis of TE in AIDS patients with focal brain lesions. Many serological tests are available and can detect different classes of antibodies, e.g., IgM, IgG, IgA, and IgE. It is important to be aware that the results from these tests vary considerably in different laboratories. Commercial kits are equally poor and give unacceptable false-positive and false-negative results. Reference laboratories are available for confirmation of conflicting results.

The Sabin-Feldman dye test is the accepted standard for the measurement of IgG antibodies, which have been shown to be higher in AIDS patients with TE than those without TE (43,114). The IgG titers usually appear 1 to 2 two weeks after infection, reach levels of 1:1,000 by 6 to 8 weeks, then gradually decrease over months and years (103). Low titers (1:65) may persist throughout life. The immunofluorescence assay (IFA), which is used more commonly than the dye test, measures the same IgG antibodies. However, commercially available kits are poorly standardized, and the results must be used within the context of the clinical setting.

Almost 100% of AIDS patients with TE will have detectable IgG by dye test or IFA (28,65,123). However, the level of the titer can be variable and is unimportant in diagnosis. Variable IgG levels have been noted in patients with toxoplasmosis infections other than TE (51,52,65). Patients with TE rarely show a significant rise in antibody titer over time. Simply, the presence of antibodies in the serum of HIV-infected individuals identifies a patient at risk for development of TE. The absence of these antibodies strongly suggests an alternative etiology for patients presenting with neurological signs and symptom.

Agglutination tests, although commercially available, are of limited value due to high false-positives as the result of nonspecific agglutination. Techniques to reduce this false-positive rate have been developed (29), but the test is still considered to be less useful than the dye test and IFA. Indirect hemagglutination assay (IHA) and complement fixation (CF) detect antibodies produced later than those detected by the dye test and IFA, but these tests are not currently recommended for AIDS patients.

Immunoglobulin M antibodies occur within the first 2 weeks after infection but do not persist as long as IgG antibodies. The enzyme-linked immunosorbent assay (ELISA) is more sensitive and specific than IFA, but both tests report high false-positive results. The IgM and IgA antibodies detected by ELISA are rarely observed in AIDS patients. However, the immunosorbent agglutination assay (ISAGA) appears to have less false-positive results than ELISA and has been useful for detecting IgM and IgE antibodies in AIDS patients with TE (99,103). There is no single serological test that is accurate enough to be recommended for use diagnostically. However, when several tests are performed as a panel, diagnosis is more reliable.

Magnetic resonance imaging (MRI) is a more sensitive neuroimaging procedure than CT for the demonstration of focal CNS lesions. Even if CT scanning is unremarkable in a clinical setting consistent with TE, multiple lesions may be detected on MRI (19). The presence of multiple lesions on CT or MRI greatly increases the probability of TE versus other causes of focal CNS disease. The probability of a CNS lymphoma is higher or equal to TE in the presence of a solitary lesion.

The current standard of care allows for the treatment of TE to be initiated upon presumptive diagnosis when a characteristic neuroradiographic abnormality is noted on CT or MRI scan (74) (Figs. 1 and 2). The clinical diagnosis is made as a result of clinical and radiographic response to specific therapy because patients may have similar symptoms due to lesions of other etiologies. This clinical practice has evolved with the appearance of AIDS because of (a) the inability to biopsy all lesions, (b) the morbidity associated with brain biopsy, and (c) the reluctance of many neurosurgeons to perform brain biopsy. The practice of presumptive therapy for patients with a characteristic finding on CT or MRI and a positive serology for *Toxoplasma* is widely accepted. With the use of these criteria, the predictive value in one study was 80% (21). However, for patient populations such as intravenous drug abusers in whom other CNS processes are more prevalent, the predictive value of a positive serology for *Toxoplasma* may be diminished (7). In addition, with the widespread use of anti-pneumocystis prophylaxis, which is also effective against *Toxoplasma*, the predictive value of these indicators may be further diminished.

Guidelines for establishing a diagnosis on the basis of empiric therapy requires that a therapeutic response be demonstrated. Recently, we demonstrated that greater than 50% of patients enrolled in a prospective treatment trial showed a quantifiable clinical improvement by day 5 of therapy and more than 70% showed clinical improvement by day 7 (78). Furthermore, for greater than 90% of responding patients, more than half of their signs and symptoms that were abnormal at baseline clearly improved by day 14 of therapy. In contrast, for all patients who ultimately failed to respond to therapy or who had lymphoma, their baseline signs and symptoms worsened and new abnormalities appeared by day 10 of therapy. A more rapid time to empiric diagnosis will allow the appropriate initiation of therapy in the patient without TE.

Headache and seizures were not reliable indicators of therapeutic efficacy (78). Focal cortical abnormalities (motor strength, speech, and language) improved slowly

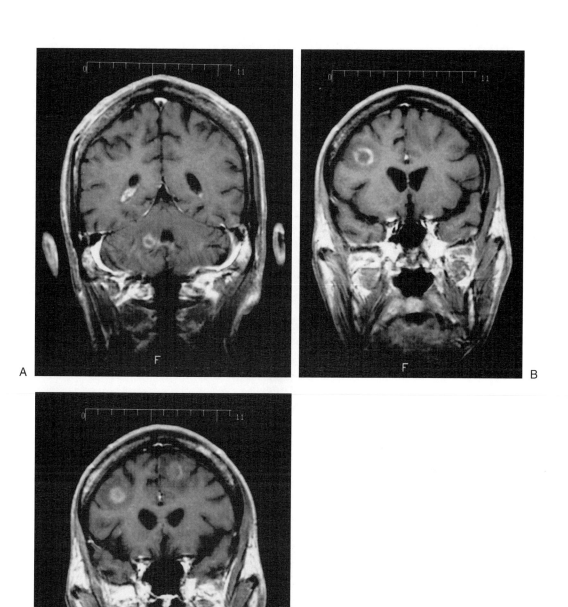

FIG. 1. An MRI with contrast. Multiple ring-enhancing lesions at presentation.

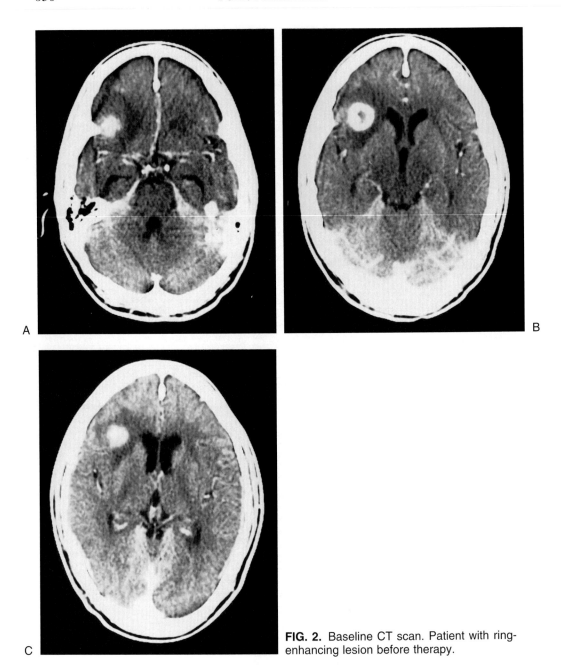

FIG. 2. Baseline CT scan. Patient with ring-enhancing lesion before therapy.

and often incompletely. Conversely, all patients not responding to therapy had progression of baseline abnormalities or developed new ones within the first 10 days of therapy. Of the patients with a neurological response, 91% had a detectable radiological response within 6 weeks of starting therapy. Corticosteroids were used only when there was evidence of increased intracranial pressure and had no effect on the time to clinical response or on survival. The use of corticosteroids may complicate the interpretation of empiric therapy because clinical and radiographic improvement may be related to reduced cerebral edema and the anti-inflammatory effects of corticosteroids. Some CNS lymphomas are steroid sensitive. Brain biopsy should be considered in the following settings: (a) patients whose baseline abnormalities (except headache and seizures) do not improve within the first 10 to 14 days of therapy or whose condition deteriorates early in the course of therapy; (b) patients with solitary CNS lesions on CT or MRI, and (c) those receiving trimethoprim-sulfamethoxazole for *Pneumocystis carinii* pneumonia (PCP) prophylaxis. The absence of a response to therapy does not always exclude TE because concurrent disease processes, e.g., other infections or lymphoma, may be present. In a few patients, TE continues despite optimal therapy resulting in death.

TREATMENT

Acute

Acute therapy should be administered for at least 3 weeks; 6 weeks or more is indicated in severely ill patients and when a complete clinical and/or radiological response has not been achieved (Table 2, Fig. 3). To date, the combination of pyrimethamine and sulfadiazine (P/S) remains the mainstay of treatment for toxoplasmosis. This combination is also the standard of comparison for most experimental regimens. Pyrimethamine, a dihydrofolate inhibitor, and sulfadiazine, a competitive inhibitor of tetrahydropteroate synthetase, synergistically and sequentially block the tachyzoites' folic acid metabolism while having no effect on the cyst form. Oral folinic acid is added to this regimen to preclude the hematological toxicity associated with antifolate agents. At low doses, 10 to 20 mg/day, folinic acid does not appear to affect the activity of this regimen. A clinical response with this combination has been reported in 68% to 95% of patients with TE (48,72,109). Unfortunately, high toxicity rates lead to early discontinuation of therapy in up to 40% of patients. Adverse effects of pyrimethamine are commonly dose-related cytopenia and rash. Whereas, adverse effects of sulfadiazine include rash, nausea, cytopenia, nephrotoxicity including crystalluria, hematuria, radiolucent stones, interstitial nephritis, and renal failure. Sulfadiazine-induced encephalopathy has been described and is difficult to differentiate from underlying TE (106,131). However, sulfa-induced encephalopathy will resolve upon discontinuation of the drug. Patients experiencing a sulfa-related rash during acute therapy may use sulfadiazine at a lower dose for maintenance therapy. Aside from the high incidence of adverse reactions, other problems have been reported in association with this treatment regimen, including early mortality rate [within the first 3 weeks of therapy of almost 20% of patients (73,97)], residual neurological dysfunction (71), inactivity against the tissue cyst, and erratic serum levels for pyrimethamine which necessitates the use of a loading dose (80). Clearly alternative treatment regimens are needed.

Clindamycin, a lincosamide antibiotic, is the primary alternative agent for TE (78,80). Its mode of action against *T. gondii* probably involves inhibition of protein synthesis (8,98). It is well absorbed from the gut and has excellent tissue penetration, but the concentrations reached in the CSF and brain tissue are erratic (25). The combination of oral pyrimethamine and oral or parenteral clindamycin (P/C) seems comparable in efficacy to P/S (26,57,78), and it is the recommended alternative regimen for the sulfa-intolerant patient. Again the incidence of adverse events is

TABLE 2. *Overview of drugs currently used for treatment of TE in patients with AIDS*

Antimicrobial	Mode of action	Metabolism	Adverse effects	Recommended dose (immunocompromised)
Pyrimethamine (Daraprim), oral	Inhibits folic acid synthesis	Readily absorbed by gut; hepatic metabolism, lipid soluble	Cytopenias and rash GI intolerance	Acute: loading dose 100–200 mg; then 50–75 mg daily; 3–6 weeks; with folinic acid (leucovorin) orally: 10–20 mg per day Maintenance: 25–50 mg per day; with folinic acid orally: 10–20) mg per day
Sulfadiazine or trisulfa-pyrimidine, oral	Inhibits folic acid synthesis; acts synergistically and sequentially with pyrimethamine	Readily absorbed by gut; penetrates blood-brain barrier; some hepatic metabolism	GI intolerance, rash (Stevens-Johnson syndrome), cytopenias, nephrolithiasis, crystalluria, interstitial nephritis, encephalop-athy	Acute: 4–6 g per day; 3–6 weeks Maintenance: 4 g per day in 4 equally divided doses
Clindamycin, oral and IV	Unknown; possibly inhibition of protein synthesis	Readily absorbed by gut; excellent tissue penetration	GI intolerance, rash, pseudo-membranous colitis	Acute: 600 mg every 6 h; 3–6 weeks Maintenance: same
Atovaquone[b] (Mepron), oral	Inhibition of *de novo* pyrimidine biosynthesis	Suspension has better bioavailability than old tablet formulation; improved if taken with food, particularly fatty foods	Rash, elevated liver function tests	Acute: 1,500 mg 2 times per day; 3–6 weeks Maintenance: same
Azithromycin[b] (Zithromax), oral	Unknown; possibly inhibition of protein synthesis	Readily absorbed by gut; high intracellular levels	GI intolerance	Acute: 1,250–1,500 mg per day; 3–6 weeks Maintenance: same
Clarithromycin[b] (Biaxin), oral	Unknown; possibly inhibition of protein synthesis	Readily absorbed by gut; high tissue levels	GI intolerance; hearing loss; elevated liver function tests	Acute: 1 g per day in 2 equally divided doses; 3–6 weeks Maintenance: same

[a] Gastrointestinal.
[b] Alternative/investigational drugs for treatment of TE in patients with AIDS.

high, including nausea, vomiting, diarrhea, rash, neutropenia, and pseudomembra-nous colitis. Myopathy with typical electromyographic abnormalities and elevated creatinine phosphokinase levels have been reported (22). A consensus panel of experts has recommended a dose of 600 mg orally or intravenously every 6 hours (107). Higher doses (1,200 mg every 6 hours) also have been used successfully (26).

Atovaquone, a hydroxynaphthoquinone, appears to be a promising agent for the treatment of TE because of its excellent *in vitro* and *in vivo* activity against *Tox-oplasma* (2). This drug, at a dose of 750 mg four times per day, is well tolerated in the AIDS patient (63). However, despite reports of a 66% to 75% initial response

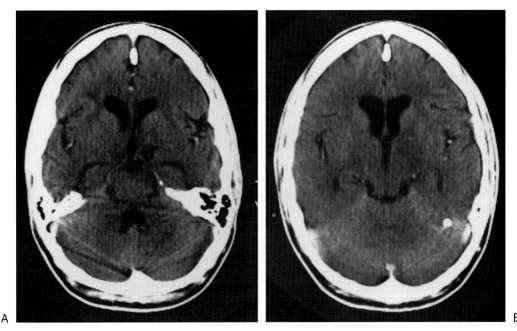

A   B

FIG. 3. Six-week CT scan. Patient shown in Fig. 2 after 6 weeks of therapy; no lesions.

rate, over 50% of patients relapse when atovaquone is used alone for acute and maintenance therapy (63). A large, international, multicentered AIDS Clinical Trials Group (ACTG) study was initiated in July 1994 to evaluate a new, better absorbed formulation of atovaquone in combination with each of the following companion agents: pyrimethamine, sulfadiazine, or clarithromycin. At present, we recommend the use of atovaquone in combination with pyrimethamine pending the results of this clinical trial. The new macrolide antibiotics, azithromycin, roxithromycin, and clarithromycin have been tested in animal models (1,16,17,68). A recently completed ACTG-sponsored study of azithromycin and pyrimethamine for the treatment of TE suggested that azithromycin (1,200 to 1,500 mg/day) in conjunction with pyrimethamine (50 to 75 mg/day) may have some role as alternative therapy, but further studies are necessary (B. J. Luft, personal communication). Also, clarithromycin shows promise in combination with pyrimethamine, but again more research with this combination is needed (34). Neither of these agents should be used alone for the treatment of toxoplasmosis.

Even though the same chemotherapeutic regimens are used for treatment of extraneural toxoplasmosis, data on the optimal length and outcome of chemotherapy are limited. The information available on the treatment of ocular and pulmonary toxoplasmosis suggests that these forms of infection are responsive to treatment (39,52,91,101,105).

Maintenance and Prophylaxis

Surviving tissue cysts reinitiate TE and the other manifestations of reactivated, latent toxoplasmosis in up to 80% of AIDS patients when suppressive therapy is discontinued (21,97). Chronic suppressive (maintenance) therapy becomes necessary when the chemotherapeutic agents used during acute therapy are ineffective against the tissue cyst form and an adequate cell-mediated immune response is not reestablished. There are no standard recommendations for maintenance therapy at this time. A regimen of pyrimethamine (25 to 50 mg) and sulfadiazine (2 to 4 g) daily is recommended (31,35). Pyrimethamine with clindamycin (1,200 to 2,400 mg/day in divided doses) is an alternative for the sulfa-intolerant patient (107). Because of the high rate of relapse documented with the lower dose of clindamycin, we tend to use the higher dose as long as tolerated. Other agents under study for maintenance therapy include fansidar and dapsone.

Primary chemoprophylaxis is an attractive therapeutic option for the subpopulation of AIDS patients at risk for developing acute reactivation of latent toxoplasmosis, i.e., those HIV-infected patients who are seropositive for antitoxoplasma antibodies and have CD4+ counts below $100/mm^3$. It appears from retrospective studies that oral trimethoprim-sulfamethoxazole has efficacy in the prevention of TE in patients who are able to tolerate therapy (13). Unfortunately, prospective randomized trials have not been performed to determine the optimal regimen which would be necessary to prevent both TE and PCP. Dapsone alone appears to be ineffective as chemoprophylaxis for TE. However, when dapsone was combined with pyrimethamine, it seemed to be highly efficacious (41). In a randomized double-blind trial, pyrimethamine (50 mg with 15 mg of folinic acid three times per week) did not significantly reduce the incidence of TE as compared to a placebo group in an intent-to-treat analysis (65a). However, for patients who tolerated pyrimethamine therapy, the incidence of TE was low. An open study of oral pyrimethamine (50 mg daily) with oral folinic acid (50 mg twice weekly) as prophylaxis for TE showed favorable results (4). However, toxicities limited the use of this drug to only 59% of the 44 patients enrolled.

The standard for maintenance therapy has not been conclusively established. We need further prospective, placebo-controlled, double-blind, randomized trials in order to determine the optimal drug and dosing regimens. In conclusion, we must highlight the need for alternative drugs for the treatment of toxoplasmosis in the AIDS patient due to the high incidence of adverse events with currently available agents.

REFERENCES

1. Araujo FG, Guptill DR, Remington JS. Azithromycin. A macrolide antibiotic with potent activity against *Toxoplasma gondii*. *Antimicrob Agents Chemother* 1988;22:755–757.
2. Araujo FG, Huskinson J, Remington JS. Remarkable in vitro and in vivo activity of the hydroxynapthoquinone (566C80) against tachyzoites and cysts of *T. gondii*. *Antimicrob Agents Chemother* 1991; 35:293–999.
3. Arendt G, Hefter H, Figge C, et al. Two cases of cerebral toxoplasmosis in AIDS patients mimicking HIV-related dementia. *J Neurol* 1991;238:439–442.
4. Bachmeyer C, Gorin I, Deleuze J, et al. Pyrimethamine as primary prophylaxis of toxoplasmic encephalitis in patients infected with human immunodeficiency virus: open study. *Clin Infect Dis* 1991;18:479–480.
5. Benson MW, Takajuji ET, Lewon SM, et al. Oocyst transmitted toxoplasmosis associated with the ingestion of contaminated water. *N Engl J Med* 1982;307:666.
6. Bergin C, Murphy M, Lyons D, et al. Toxoplasma pneumonitis: fatal presentation of disseminated toxoplasmosis in a patient with AIDS. *Eur Respir J* 1992;5:1013.
7. Bishburg E, Eng RH, Slim J, et al. Brain lesions in patients with the acquired immunodeficiency syndrome. *Arch Intern Med* 1989;149:541–543.
8. Blais J, Tardif C, Chamberland S. Effect of clindamycin on intracellular replication, protein synthesis, and infectivity of *Toxoplasma gondii*. *Antimicrob Agents Chemother* 1993;37:2571–2577.

9. Bourgonin PM, Melancon D, Carpenter S, et al. Hydrocephalus and prominence of the choroid plexus: an unusual computed tomographic presentation of cerebral toxoplasmosis. *Can Assoc Radiol J* 1992;43:55–59.

10. Brion JP, Pelloux H, Le Marc hadour F, et al. Acute toxoplasmic hepatitis in a patient with AIDS. *Clin Infect Dis* 1992;15:183.

11. Calico I, Cabaclero E, Martinez O, et al. Isolation of *T. gondii* from immunocompromised patients using tissue culture. *Infections* 1991;19:340.

12. Caramello P, Forno B, Lucchini A, et al. Toxoplasmosis diffuse encephalitis diagnosed by isolation of *Toxoplasma gondii* in cell culture. In: *Programs and Abstracts of the XI International Conference on AIDS,* Berlin, Germany, June 6–11, 1993 (abst).

13. Carr A, Tindall B, Brew BJ, et al. Low-dose trimethoprim-sulfamethoxazole prophylaxis for toxoplasmic encephalitis in patients with AIDS. *Ann Intern Med* 1992;117:106–111.

14. Carrazana EJ, Rossitch EJ, Samuels MA. Parkinsonian symptoms in a patient with AIDS and cerebral toxoplasmosis. *J Neurol Neurosurg Psychiatry* 1989;52:1445–1446.

15. Casado-Naranjo I, Lopez-Trigo J, Ferrandiz A, et al. Hemorrhagic abssess in a patient with acquired immunodeficiency syndrome. *Neuroradiology* 1989;31:289.

16. Chang HR, Pechere JC. Activity of roxithromycin against *Toxoplasma gondii* in murine models. *J Antimicrob Chemother* 1987;20:69–74.

17. Chang HR, Rudareanu FC, Pechere JC. Activity of A-56268 (TE-031), a new macrolide, against *Toxoplasma gondii* in mice. *J Antimicrob Chemother* 1988;22:359–361.

18. Chaudhari AB, Singh A, Jindal S, et al. Hemorrhage in cerebral toxoplasmosis: a report on a patient wth acquired immunodeficiency syndrome. *S Afr Med J* 1989;76:272–274.

19. Ciricillo SF, Rosenblum ML. Use of CT and MR imaging to distinguish intracranial lesions and to define the need for biopsy in AIDS patients. *J Neuro Surg* 1990;73:720–724.

20. Clumeck M, Sonnet J, Taelman H, et al. Acquired immunodeficiency syndrome in African patients. *N Engl J Med* 1984;310:492–497.

21. Cohn J, McMeeking A, Cohen W, et al. Evaluation of the policy of empirical treatment of suspected toxoplasmic encephalitis in patients with the acquired immunodeficiency syndrome. *Am J Med* 1989;86:521–527.

22. Coppola S, Angarano G, Monno A, et al. Adverse effects of clindamycin in the treatment of cerebral toxoplasmosis in AIDS patients. In: *VII International Conference on AIDS,* Florence, Italy, June 16–21, 1991, No. 265 (abst).

23. Corbett E. Clinicopathology conference: polymyositis and a thalamic mass. *Va Med* 1992;119:42.

24. Crider SR, Horstman WG, Massey GS. Toxoplasma orchitis: report of a case and review of the literature. *Am J Med* 1988;85:421.

25. Danneman B, Israelski DM, Remington JS. Treatment of toxoplasmic encephalitis with intravenous clindamycin. *Arch Intern Med* 1988;148:2477–2482.

26. Danneman B, McCutchan JA, Israelski D, et al. Treatment of toxoplasmic encephalitis in patients with AIDS, a randomized trial comparing pyrimethamine plus clindamycin to pyrimethamine plus sulfadiazine. *Ann Intern Med* 1992;116:33–43.

27. Darde ML, Bouteille B, Pestre-Alexandre M. Isoenzymatic characterization of seven strains of *Toxoplasma gondii* by isoelectrofocusing in polyacrylamide gels. *Am J Trop Med Hyg* 1988;39:551–558.

28. Derouin F, Mazeron MC, Garin YJF. Comparative study of tissue culture and mouse inoculation methods for demonstration of *Toxoplasma gondii. J Clin Microbiol* 1989;25:1597–1600.

29. Desmonts G, Remington JS. Direct agglutination test for diagnosis of toxoplasma infection: method for increasing sensitivity and specificity. *J Clin Microbiol*1980;11:562–568.

30. Dubey JP, Miller NL, Frenkel JK. The *Toxoplasma gondii* oocyst from cat feces. *J Exp Med* 1970;133:636–640.

31. Engstrom JW, Lowenstein DH, Bredesen DE. Cerebral infarctions and transient neurological deficits with the acquired immunodeficiency syndrome. *Am J Med* 1989;86:528.

32. Farkash AE, Maccabee PJ, Sher JH. CNS toxoplasmosis in acquired immunodeficiency syndrome: a clinical-pathological-radiological review of 12 cases. *J Neurol Neurosurg Psychiatry* 1986;49:744–748.

33. Ferguson DJ, Hutchinson WM. An ultrastructural study of the early development and tissue cyst formation of *Toxoplasma gondii* in brains of mice. *Parasitol Res.* 1987;73:483–491.

34. Fernandez-Martin J, Leport C, Morlat P, et al. Pyrimethamine/clarithromycin combination therapy of acute toxoplasma in patients with AIDS. *Antimicrob Agents Chemother* 1991;35:2049–2052.

35. Fong IW, Glazer S, Fletcher D, et al. Recurrence of CNS toxoplasmosis in AIDS patients on chronic suppressive treatment. In: *VIII International Conference on AIDS*, Amsterdam, The Netherlands, July 19–24, 1992, No. B115 (abst).

36. Frenkel JK. Pursuing Toxoplasma. *J Infect Dis* 1970;122:553–556.

37. Frenkel JK, Nelson BM, Arias-Stelle J. Immunosuppression and toxoplasmic encephalitis: clinical and experimental aspects. *Hum Pathol* 1975;6:97–111.

38. Friedland JS. Hiccups, toxoplasmosis and AIDS. *Clin Infect Dis* 1994;18:835.

39. Friedman AH, Orellana J, Gaggiuso DJ, Teich SA. Ocular toxoplasmosis in AIDS patients. *Trans Am Opthalmol Soc* 1990;88:63–66.
40. Ghatak NR, Sawyer DR. A morphological study of opportunistic cerebral toxoplasmosis. *ACTA Neuropathol* 1978;42:217–226.
41. Girard PM, Landeman R, Gaudebout C, et al. Dapsone-pyrimethamine compared with aerosolized pentamidine as primary prophylaxis against pneumocystis carinii pneumonia and toxoplasmosis in HIV infection. *New Eng J Med* 1993;328:1514–1520.
42. Glatt AE. *Toxoplasma gondii* serologies in patients with human immunodeficiency virus infection. *Infect Dis Clin Pract* 1992;1:237.
43. Grant IH, Gold JWM, Rosenblum M, et al. *Toxoplasma gondii* serology in HIV-infected patients: the development of central nervous toxoplasmosis. *AIDS* 1990;4:319–521.
44. Gray F, Gherardi R, Wingate E, et al. Diffuse encephalitic cerebral toxoplasmosis in AIDS. Report of four cases. *J Neurol* 1989;236:273–277.
45. Groll A, Schneider M, Althoff PH, et al. Morphological and clinical significance of AIDS-related lesions in the adrenals and pituitary. *Dtsch Med Wochenschr* 1990;115:483.
46. Hamed LM, Schatz NJ, Galetta SL. Brainstem ocular motility defects and AIDS. *Am J Ophtalmol* 1988;106:437–442.
47. Harris TM, Smith R, Bognanno JR, et al. Toxoplasmic myelitis in AIDS gadolinium-enhanced MR. *J Comput Assist Tomogr* 1990,14:809–811.
48. Haverkos HW. Assessment of therapy for toxoplasmic encephalitis. The TE study group. *Am J Med* 1987;82:907–914.
49. Helweg-Larsen S, Jakobsen J, Boeser F, Artier-Siberg P. Neurological complications and comcomitants of AIDS. *ACTA Neurol Scand* 1986;74:467–474.
50. Herskovitz S, Siegel SE, Schneider AT, et al. Spinal cord toxoplasmosis in AIDS. *Neurology* 1989; 39:1552–1553.
51. Hofflin GN, Remington JS. Tissue culture isolation of *Toxoplasma* from blood of a patient with AIDS. *Arch Intern Med* 1985;145:925–926.
52. Holland GN, Engstrom RE Jr, Glasgow B, et al. Ocular toxoplasmosis in patients with the acquired immunodeficiency syndrome. *Am J Opthalmol* 1988;106:653–667.
53. Hooper AD. Acquired toxoplasmosis: report of a case with autopsy findings. *Am Arch Pathol* 1957; 64:1–6.
54. Jacobs L, Remington JS, Melton NL. The resistance of the encysted form of *Toxoplasma gondii*. *J Parasitol* 1960;46:11–15.
55. Jamku J. Pathogenesa a patrologicka anatomie tak mazvameho vrozemeho kolobomu zlute sdvrny v oku morualme velikem a mikropthalmickeu S malezeu parazitu V sitmici. *Cesk Parasitol* 1929; 6:9.
56. Jones TC, Bierz KA, Erb D. In vitro cultivation of *Toxoplasma gondii* cysts in astrocytes in the presence of gamma interferon. *Infect Immun* 1986;51:147–152.
57. Katlama C. Evaluation of the efficacy and safety of clindamycin plus pyrimethamine for induction and maintenance of TE in AIDS. *Eur J Clin Microbiol Infect Dis* 1992;10:189–191.
58. Kaufman HE, Geisler PH. The hematological toxicity of pyrimethamine in man. *Arch Ophtholmol* 1960;64:140–146.
59. Kayser C, Campbell R, Sartorius C, et al. Toxoplasmosis of the conus medularis in a patient with hemophilia A-associated AIDS. *J Neurosurg* 1990;73:951–953.
60. Kean BH. Clinical toxoplasmosis: fifty years. *Trans R Soc Trop Med Hyg* 1972;66:549.
61. Khuong MA, Matherson S, Marche C, et al. Diffuse toxoplasmic encephalitis without abscess in AIDS patients. In: *Program and Abstracts of the Interscience Congress of Antimicrobial Agents and CHemotherapy,* Atlanta, GA, October 21–24, 1990 (abst 1157).
62. Koeze TH, Klinger GH. Acquired toxoplasmosis. *Arch Neurol* 1964;11:191–196.
63. Kovacs JA. Efficacy of atovaquone in treatment of toxoplasmosis in patients with AIDS. *Lancet* 1992;340:637–638.
64. Lainson R. Observations on the development and nature of pseudocysts and cysts of *Toxoplasma gondii*. *Trans R Soc Trop Med Hyg* 1985;12:221.
65. Lavareda De Souza S, Maslo C, Depouy-Camet J, et al. PCR in blood for diagnosis of toxoplasmosis in AIDS patients. In: *Third European Conference on the Clinical Aspects and Treatment of HIV Infection,* Paris, 1992 (abst 045).
65a. Leport C, Chêne G, Morlat P, et al. Pyrimethamine for primary prophylaxis of toxoplasmic encephalitis in patients with human immunodeficiency virus infection: A double blind, randomized trial. *J Infect Dis* 1996;173:91–97.
66. Levy RM, Bredesen DE, Rosenblum ML. Neurological manifestations of the acquired immunodeficiency syndrome (AIDS): experience at UCSF and review of the literature. *J Neurosurg* 1985;62: 475–495.
67. Levy RM, Janssen RS, Bush TJ, Rosenblum ML. Neuroepidemiology of acquired immunodeficiency syndrome. *J Acquired Immune Defic Syndr* 1988;1:31–40.

68. Luft BJ. In vivo and in vitro activity of roxithromycin against *Toxoplasma gondii* in mice. *Eur J Clin Microbiol* 1987;6:479–481.

69. Luft BJ. *Toxoplasma gondii*. In: Walzer PD, Gertz RM, eds. *Parasitic infections in the compromised host*. New York: Marcel Dekker; 1989:179.

70. Luft BJ, Castro KG. An overview of the problem of toxoplasmosis and pneumocystosis in AIDS in the USA: implication from future therapeutic trials. *Eur J Clin Microbiol Infect Dis* 1991;10: 178–181.

71. Luft BJ, Hafner R. Toxoplasmic encephalitis [Editorial]. *AIDS* 1990;4:593–595.

72. Luft BJ, Remington JS. Toxoplasmosis of the central nervous system. In: Remington JS, Swartz WM, eds. *Current clinical topics in Infectious Diseases*. New York: McGraw-Hill; 1985:315.

73. Luft BJ, Remington JS. AIDS commentary: toxoplasmic encephalitis. *J Infect Dis* 1988;157:1–6.

74. Luft BJ, Remington JS. Toxoplasmic encephalitis in AIDS. *Clin Infect Dis* 1992;15:211–222.

75. Luft BJ, Brooks RG, Conley FK, et al. Toxoplasmic encephalitis in patients with the acquired immunodeficiency syndrome (AIDS) and other immunocompromising diseases. *JAMA* 1984;252: 913–917.

76. Luft BJ, Conely TK, Remington JS, et al. Outbreak of CNS toxoplasmosis in Western Europe and North America. *Lancet* 1983;1:781–784.

77. Luft BJ, Fromowitz F, Peress N, et al. Immunohistochemical and in situ hybridization analysis of cellular infiltrate occurring in toxoplasmic encephalitis and AIDS. In: *Programs and Abstracts of the IV International Conference on AIDS*, 1988:395 (abst).

78. Luft BJ, Hafner R, Korzun AH, et al. Toxoplasmic encephalitis in patients with the acquired immunodeficiency syndrome. *N Engl J Med* 1993;329:995–1000.

79. Luft BJ, Naot Y, Araujo FG, et al. Primary and reactivated *Toxoplasma* infection in patients with cardiac transplants: clinical spectrum and problems in diagnosis in a defined population. *Ann Intern Med* 1983;99:27–31.

80. Mariuz P, Luft BJ. New therapeutic approaches to toxoplasmic encephalitis. *Curr Opin Infect Dis* 1991;826–833.

81. Matheron S, Dournon E, Garakhanian S, et al. Prevalence of toxoplasmosis in 365 AIDS and ARC patients before and during zidovudine treatment. In: *VI International Conference on AIDS*, San Francisco, CA, June 20–24, 1990;476 (abst).

82. Mathiessen L, Caberousse F, Marche C, et al. Morphology and etiology of microglial nodules in 27 AIDS autopsy cases. *Clin Neuropathol* 1988;7:187–189.

83. McArthur JC. Neurological manifestations of AIDS. *Medicine, Baltimore* 1987;66:407–37.

84. Mcleod R, Skamene E, Brown CR, et al. Genetic regulation of early survival and cyst number after perioral *Toxoplasma gondii* infection of AxB/BxA recombinant inbred and B/O congenic mice. *J Immunol* 1989;143:3031–3034.

85. Mehren M, Burns PJ, Mamani F, et al. Toxoplasmic myelitis mimicking intramedullary spinal cord tumor. *Neurology* 1988;38:1648–1650.

86. Milligan SA, Katz MS, Craven PC, et al. Toxoplasmosis presenting as panhypopituitarism in a patient with the acquired immunodeficiency syndrome. *Am J Med* 1984;77:760–764.

87. Navia BA, Petito CK, Gold JWM, et al. Cerebral toxoplasmosis complicating the acquired immunodeficiency syndrome: clinical and neuropathological findings in 27 patients. *Ann Neur* 1989;19: 224–228.

88. Neu HC. Toxoplasmosis transmitted at autopsy. *JAMA* 1967;202:284–287.

89. Nicolle C, Manceaux L. Sur un protozaire nouveau de *gondi Toxoplasma*. *Arch Inst Pasteur (Tnnis)* 1929;2:9079.

90. Nolla-Sallas J, Ricart C, Ohlaberringue F, et al. Hydrocephalus: an unusual CT presentation of cerebral toxoplasmosis in a patient with the acquired immunodeficiency syndrome. *Eur Neurol* 1987;27:130.

91. Oksenhendler E, Cadranel J, Sarafati C, et al. *Toxoplasma gondii* pneumonia in patients with the acquired immunodeficiency syndrome. *Am J Med* 1990;88:5-18N–21N.

92. Overhage JM, Greist A, Brown DR. Conus medullaris syndrome resulting from *Toxoplasma gondii* infection in a patient with the acquired immunodeficiency syndrome. *Am J Med* 1990;89:814–815.

93. Paige BH, Cowen D, Wolf A. Toxoplasmic encephalitis. Further observations of infantile toxoplasmosis: intrauterine inception of the disease: visceral manifestations. *Am J Dis Child* 1942;63: 474–477.

94. Partisani M, Candolfi H, Demautort, et al. Seroprevalence of latent *T. gondii* infection in HIV infected individuals and long-term follow-up of *Toxoplasma* seronegative subjects. In: *Programs and Abstracts of the VII International Conference on AIDS*, Florence, Italy, 1991 (abst Wb 2294).

95. Pauwels A, Meyohas MC, Eliaszewicz M, et al. *Toxoplasma* colitis in the acquired immunodeficiency syndrome. *Am J Gastroenterol* 1992;87:518.;

96. Pavesio C, Chiappino M, Setzer P, Nichols B. *Toxoplasma gondii:* differentiation and death of bradyzoites. *Parasitol Res* 1992;78:109.

97. Pedrol E, Gonzalez-Clementz JM, Gatell JM, et al. Central nervous toxoplasmosis on AIDS patients: efficacy of an intermittent maintenance therapy. *AIDS* 1990;4:511–517.

98. Pfefferkorn ER, Hothnagel RF, Borotz SE. Parasiticidal effects of clindamycin on *Toxoplasma gondii* grown in cultured cells and selection of a drug-resistant mutant. *Antimicrob Agents Chemother* 1992;36:1091–1096.
99. Pinon JM, Toubas D, Marx C, et al. Detection of specific immunoglobulin E in patients with toxoplasmosis. *J Clin MIcrobiol* 1990;28:1739–1743.
100. Pohl HD, Eichenlaub D. Toxoplasmosis of the CNS in AIDS patients. In: *Program of Berlin Symposium: HIV and the nervous system.* Berlin, Germany: 1987.
101. Pomeroy C, Felice GA. Pulmonary toxoplasmosis: a review. *Clin Infect Dis* 1992;14:863–870.
102. Poon TP, Tchertkoff V, Pares GF, et al. Spinal cord *Toxoplasma* lesion in AIDS: MRI findings. *J Comput Assist Tomogr* 1992;16(5):817–819.
103. Porter SB, Sande M. Toxoplasmosis of the central nervous system in the acquired immunodeficiency syndrome. *N Engl J Med* 1992;327:1643–1648.
104. Post MJ, Chan JC, Hensely GT, et al. Toxoplasmosis encephalitis in Haitian adults with the acquired immunodeficiency syndrome: a clinical pathological CT correlation. *Am J Roengenol* 1983;4:155–162.
105. Rabaud C, May TH, Amiel C, et al. Pulmonary toxoplasmosis in patients infected with human immunodeficiency virus: a French nationwide survey, 1990–1992. In: *Programs and Abstracts of the IX International Conference on AIDS,* Berlin, Germany, June 6–11, 1993 (abst WS-B14-4).
106. Reboli AC, Mandler HD. Encephalopathy and psychosis associated with sulfadiazine in two patients with AIDS and toxoplasmosis. *Clin Infect Dis* 1992;15:556–557.
107. Remington JS, Desmonts G. Toxoplasmosis. In: Remington JS, Klein JD, eds. *Infectious diseases of the fetus and newborn infants.* 3rd ed. Philadelphia: Saunders; 1990:89.
108. Renold C, Sugar A, Chave J-D, et al. *Toxoplasma* encephalitis in patients with the acquired immuodeficiency syndrome. *Medicine* 1992;71:224–239.
109. Roldan ED, Moskowitz L, Hemsley GT. Pathology of the heart in acquired immunodeficiency syndrome. *Arch Pathol Lab Med* 1987;111:943–946.
110. Rose AC, Vys CJ, Novitsky D, et al. Toxoplasmosis of donor and recipient hearts after heterotopic cardiac transplantation. *Arch Pathol Lab Med* 1987;107:368.
111. Ruskin J, Remington JS. Toxoplasmosis in the compromised host. *Ann Intern Med* 1976;84:193–198.
112. Ryning FW, Mcleod R, Maddox JC, et al. Probable transmission of *Toxoplasma gondii* by organ transplantation. *Ann Intern Med* 1979;90:47–49.
113. Sabin A, Feldman HA. Dyes as microchemical indicators of a new immunity phenomenon affecting a protozoan parasite *(Toxoplasma). Science* 1948;108:660–662.
114. Sabin A, Olitski P. *Toxoplasma* and obligate intravellular parasitism. *Science* 1937;85:336–339.
115. Sanchez-Ramos JR, Factor SA, Weiner WJ, et al. Hemichorea-hemibalismus associated with acquired immunodeficiency syndrome and cerebral toxoplasmosis. *Mov Disord* 1989;4:226–273.
116. Sibley LD, Boothroyd J. Virulent strains of *Toxoplasma gondii* comprise a single clonal lineage. *Nature* 1992;359:982–985.
117. Siegel SE, Lunde MN, Gelderman AH, et al. Transmission of toxoplasmosis by leukocyte transfusion. *Blood* 1971;37:388–394.
118. Sims TA, Hay J, Talbot IC. An electron microscope and immunohistochemical study of the intracellular location of toxoplasma tissue cysts within the brains of mice with congenital toxoplasmosis. *Br J Exp Pathol* 1989;70:317–325.
119. Smart PE, Weinfeld A, Thompson ME, et al. Toxoplasmosis of the stomach: a cause of antral narrowing. *Radiology* 1990:17;369.
120. Strittmatler C, Lang W, Wiestler OD, Kleihues P. The changing pattern of human immunodeficiency virus associated cerebral toxoplasmosis: a study of 46 postmortem cases. *ACTA Neuropathol* 1992;83:475–481.
121. Suzuki Y, Joh K, Onellanea MA, et al. A gene(s) within the H-2D region determines the development of toxoplasmic encephalitis in mice. *Immunology* 1991;74:732–739.
122. Tavolato B. *Toxoplasma* encephalitis in the adult. *Acta Neurol (Napoli)* 1978;33:321–328.
123. Tirard V, Neil G, Rosenblum M, et al. Diagnosis of toxoplasmosis in patients with AIDS by isolation of the parasite from the blood. *N Engl J Med* 1991;324:632.
124. Tolge CF, Factor SA. Focal dystonia secondary to cerebral toxoplasmosis in a *Toxoplasma gondii. J Parasitol* 1960;46:11–15.
125. Vandervaaj D. Formation, growth and multiplication of *Toxoplasma gondii. Trans R Soc Trop George Med* 1959;11:345.
126. Vietzke WM, Gelderman AH, Grimley, Valsamis MP. Toxoplasmosis complicating malignancy. *Cancer* 1968;21:816–827.
127. Wallace GD. The role of the cat in the natural history of *Toxoplasma gondii. Am J Trop Med Hyg* 1973;22:313–321.
128. Wanke C, Tuazon CV, Kovacs C, et. al. Toxoplasmic encephalitis in patients with the acquired immunodeficiency syndrome. Diagnosis and response to therapy. *Am J Trop Med Hyg* 1987;36:509.

129. Whelan MA, Krichelt II, Handler M, et al. Neuroradiological findings in AIDS: a review of 200 cases. *Am J Neuroradiol* 1986;147:977–983.
130. Wolf A, Cowen D. Granulomatous encephalomyelitis due to encephalitozoan (encephalitozoic encephalomyelitis). A new protozoan disease of man. *Bull Neurol Inst NY* 1937;6:306.
131. Young CL. Acute encephalopathy associated with sulfadiazine in a patient with AIDS-related complex [Letter]. *J Infect Dis* 1989;160:163–164.
132. Zangerle R, Allenberger F, Pohl P, et al. High risk of developing toxoplasmic encephalitis in AIDS patients seropositive for *Toxoplasma gondii*. *Med Microbiol Immunol* 1991;180:59–66.

AIDS and the Nervous System, Second Edition,
edited by J. R. Berger and R. M. Levy.
Lippincott-Raven Publishers, Philadelphia © 1997.

25

Cryptococcal Meningitis

°†Victor E. Mulanovich and °Michael S. Saag

°†Department of Medicine, †Division of Infectious Diseases, The University of
Alabama at Birmingham, Birmingham, Alabama 35294

Cryptococcosis is the most common systemic fungal infection associated with AIDS worldwide, except for certain areas endemic for histoplasmosis or coccidioidomycosis. The organism is inhaled and dissemination occurs with predilection for the central nervous system (CNS). Basic concepts of its microbiology, epidemiology, and immunopathogenesis give a better understanding of the disease and its clinical presentation. The diagnosis of cryptococcal meningitis requires appropriate interpretation of the neuroimaging and cerebrospinal fluid (CSF) findings. Cryptococcal antigen testing in serum and CSF is an invaluable aid for rapid diagnosis when properly performed.

Over the last decade, clinical trials have tested amphotericin B, flucytosine, and the newer azoles in different doses and combinations. We summarize the results and discuss the current recommendations for initial and maintenance therapy. Elevated intracranial pressure (ICP) appears to be an important contributor to morbidity and mortality. Current information on its significance and management is presented.

THE ORGANISM

Cryptococcus neoformans is an encapsulated yeast that measures 4 to 6 μm in diameter surrounded by a capsule that is 1 to 30 μm. A perfect form or sexual stage can be produced *in vitro*; however, it has not been found in nature. Thus, the asexual, yeast form is considered the primary infectious agent. Most isolates grow readily on bacterial or fungal media within a week after inoculation. Occasionally, 3 to 4 weeks is required for growth; therefore, all plates should be held for 1 month before declaring the culture negative. The organism is differentiated from nonpathogenic cryptococcal species by its ability to grow at 37°C and to convert phenolic compounds to melanin, producing dark colonies when incubated in niger seed extract or similar media. Its ability to produce urease helps in the rapid identification of the organism (36).

Glucuronoxylomannan is the predominant capsular polysaccharide and is the principal antigenic domain. On the basis of its antigenic variability, four serotypes have been delineated. Serotypes A and D are classified as *C. neoformans* var. *neoformans* and serotypes B and C are classified as *C. neoformans* var. *gattii*. Human infection caused by cryptococci other than *C. neoformans* has been reported, especially *Cryptococcus albidus* and *Cryptococcus laurentii*, but these are of doubtful clinical significance (28).

Cryptococcus neoformans var. *neoformans* exists, most likely, in common grass or cereal that birds, and pigeons in particular, eat. The organism does not cause infection in birds, but the droppings from pigeons and soil contaminated with avian droppings are important sources of infection in humans. *Eucaliptus camaldulensis* (the Red River Gum Tree), which is indigenous in Australia but has been extensively exported to other tropical and subtropical areas of the world, is the host for var. *gattii* and is probably released into the surrounding environment in the flowering season (18,28).

EPIDEMIOLOGY

Cryptococcus neoformans var. *neoformans* is the most frequent cause of infection worldwide, accounting for close to 100% of the clinical isolates from Europe and Japan and more than 85% of the isolates in the United States (excluding Southern California), Canada, and Argentina. *Cryptococcus neoformans* var. *gattii* is more frequent in tropical and subtropical regions of Australia, Brazil, Southeast Asia, Central Africa and Southern California and, in the pre-acquired immunodeficiency syndrome (AIDS) era, constituted 35% to 100% of all clinical isolates (27). With the advent of the AIDS epidemic the percentage of cases caused by var. *gattii* has decreased significantly, due in large part to its tendency to infect immunocompetent hosts. Most cases in AIDS patients are caused by var. *neoformans* (43,48). Rozen-baum et al. (45) studied *Cryptococcus* isolates from Brazil in both immunocompetent and immunocompromised patients. Among 12 immunocompetent patients, 7 (58.3%) were infected with var. *gattii* compared to 65 of 66 (98.5%) patients with AIDS who were infected by var. *neoformans*. Very few examples of var. *gattii* infecting AIDS patients have been reported (33,45).

Cryptococcal disease occurs in 1.9% to 11.6% of patients with AIDS in the United States (5,6,15,19,54) and is the first opportunistic infection in 40% to 75% (6,26,46,54). Cryptococcosis is the fourth most common cause of life-threatening opportunistic disease after *Pneumocystis carinii*, cytomegalovirus, and mycobacterial disease (26). Along with *Toxoplasma gondii*, CNS lymphoma, and human immuno-deficiency virus (HIV) itself, it is one of the four most common causes of neurological disease in AIDS patients and is the most common cause of meningeal infection.

IMMUNOLOGY AND PATHOGENESIS

Unencapsulated or partially encapsulated yeasts released to the environment are inhaled and deposited in the small airways. In the immunocompetent host, a granulo-matous response producing a primary complex, similar but less exuberant than the one found in primary tuberculosis, usually controls the infection. If the immune response is defective, proliferation and extrapulmonary dissemination follow. Whether primary infection or reactivation leads to disseminated disease in the immu-nocompromised host is still unclear.

Cryptococcus neoformans produces no toxins and evokes very little inflamatory response. Its main virulence factor is the capsular polysaccharide. Acapsular mutants have substantially reduced virulence. Regulation of capsule production is an adaptive process. The unencapsulated state promotes growth, mating, and penetration into the small airways. In the host, the larger capsule provides resistance to phagocytosis.

Severely immunodeficient patients may exert little selective pressure for capsule production. Some AIDS patients have variants with small capsules that later produce large capsules when innoculated into animals. The carbon dioxide tension found in mammalian tissues may also be a stimulus for capsule production. The polysaccharide has also been shown to induce T-suppressor cell activity in experimental animals, which may depress T-cell-dependent functions such as induction of macrophage response to yeast cells. Antibody plays a role in the phagocytosis and killing of cryptococci, but its clinical significance is uncertain (35). Cellular immunity is essential for control of the infection, which is why persons with HIV infection or lymphoreticular malignancies or those using corticosteroids are particularly prone to develop disseminated disease (36).

CLINICAL MANIFESTATIONS

The course of cryptococcal meningitis is usually subacute, with a median time from onset of symptoms to diagnosis of 30 days (54). The onset is generally insidious, although cases of acute disease occur on occasion. Headache and fever are the most common manifestations. More specific symptoms of meningeal involvement such as stiff neck, photophobia, nausea, and vomiting are present in only 20% to 40% of patients. The lack of specific symptoms along with the prolonged and often fluctuant course of disease frequently cause a delay in diagnosis. Table 1 lists the most common symptoms.

Altered mental status is the most common predictor of poor outcome and is present in 20% to 30% of patients. Papilledema is found in less than 10% of patients and seizures in 4% to 9%. Thirteen of 89 (15%) patients in one series had focal deficits

TABLE 1. *Clinical and ancillary findings in patients with cryptococcal meningitis with and without AIDS (percentage of patients at presentation)*

	Non-AIDS		AIDS		
Finding	Ref. 47	Ref. 54	Ref. 5	Ref. 6	Ref. 46
Clinical					
Headache	87	81	73	67	92
Fever	60	88	65	62	78
Nausea, vomiting	53	—	42	1	8
Altered mental status	52	19	28	—	27
Stiff neck	50	31	22	—	30
Visual disturbances	33	—	—	—	30
Cranial nerve palsies	32	—	—	—	6
Papilledema	28	—	—	—	6
Malaise	—	38	76	—	—
Photophobia	—	19	18	—	6
Seizures	15	8	4	9	—
Cerebrospinal fluid					
WBC > 20 cells/mm^3	97	31	21	13	—
Glucose < 60% serum level	75	65	24	17	—
Protein > 45 mg/dL	90	61	55	35	—
Positive India ink	60	72	74	88	77
Opening pressure > 200 mm H$_2$O	65	62	66	—	—

Modified from Lapidus W, Saag M. Cryptococcal meningitis. In: Johnson S, Johnson FN, Powderly WB, Van't Wout JW, eds. *The antifungal agents: fluconzaole.* Lancashire, England: Marius; 1992:137.
AIDS, acquired immunodeficiency syndrome; WBC, white blood cell count.

on neurological exam, while computed tomography (CT) of the head showed focal lesions in 6 (7%) patients (5).

The occurrence of concomitant extraneural disease in patients with cryptococcal meningitis ranges between 20% and 60% (5,6,19,26,46) and may often lead to the diagnosis of meningitis. The most frequent site of extraneural culture isolation is the blood, which is positive in 50% to 64% of cases (19,46). Even though the lungs are the portal of entry, symptoms of pulmonary disease occur in only 20% to 30% of patients (5,6,46). Raised and sometimes umbilicated skin lesions resembling molluscum contagiosum have been reported in 7% of patients, presenting on occasion as an isolated symptom and, thus, the only clue to the diagnosis (6). Other sites of involvement include the oral cavity, eyes, bone marrow, liver, spleen, lymph nodes, pericardium, mediastinum, and genitourinary tract, which is believed to provide a reservoir for *C. neoformans* that may lead to relapsing disease (29).

DIAGNOSIS

Cryptoccocal meningitis should be suspected in the HIV-infected patient who presents with fever and/or headache, particularly with a CD4+ count below 100/mm^3. Owing to the array of clinical symptoms, which may present alone or in variable combinations, a low treshold to initiate the diagnostic work-up will result in more rapid diagnosis and hopefully improve overall outcome. In patients who present with extraneural cryptococcosis it is mandatory to exclude meningeal involvement. The conventional diagnostic approach is to obtain a brain-imaging scan to exclude mass effect and other CNS processes. Once noncommunicating hydrocephalus and mass effect is ruled out, a lumbar puncture should be performed.

Brain-Imaging Studies

There are no specific radiological findings of cryptococcal disease. Table 2 lists common CT findings in several series. The CT of the head is normal or shows cerebral atrophy (presumably due to HIV infection) in 75% to 90% of the cases. Nonenhancing and contrast-enhancing lesions, presenting as either nodular or ringlike patterns, are described in 8% to 15% of patients. Hydrocephalus and diffuse cerebral edema are less common. Some cases of concomitant cerebral toxoplasmosis (6) and CNS lymphoma (31) have been reported, so CT follow-up to assess response to

TABLE 2. *Percentage of cerebral CT findings in patients with CNS cryptococcosis reported in different series*

CT findings	Ref. 54, $n = 13$	Ref. 5, $n = 58$	Ref. 6, $n = 37$	Ref. 37,[a] $n = 35$	Ref. 44, $n = 40$
Normal	69	71	81	43	65
Atrophy	8	17	—	34	12.5
Mass lesions	15	10	8	11	7.5
Hydrocephalus	—	—	—	9	—
Cerebral edema	—	—	3	3	10
Other	8	2	8	—	10

[a] Only 80% of the patients had AIDS.
CT, computed tomography; CNS, central nervous system.

therapy of mass lesions or biopsy of highly suspicious lesions are important considerations. Magnetic resonance imaging (MRI) is more sensitive for detection of cryptococcomas and dilated perivascular spaces, but its clinical utility is less well defined (31).

Cerebrospinal Fluid Analysis

Patients with non-AIDS-related cryptococcal meningitis almost always have abnormal CSF findings, including elevation of the white blood cell count ($>20/mm^3$), protein (>45 mg/dL), and CSF opening pressure (>200 mm of water), along with a decreased CSF glucose ($<50\%$ of serum glucose level) (47). In contrast, up to 59% of patients with AIDS-related cryptococcal meningitis have normal CSF chemistry and cell count (6). However, the opening pressure is elevated in greater than 60% (Table 1). Although the exact mechanism of elevated ICP is uncertain, the large number of yeast cells and/or free polysaccharide antigen have been postulated to occlude the channels and valves of the subarachnoid villi and the lymphatic pathways, thereby interfering with CSF reabsorption. The lack of ventricular dilatation is probably due to the coexistence of cerebral edema and diffuse parenchymal cryptococcal infiltration (Fig. 1) (11). Measurement of the opening pressure is essential for prognostic evaluation as well as clinical management.

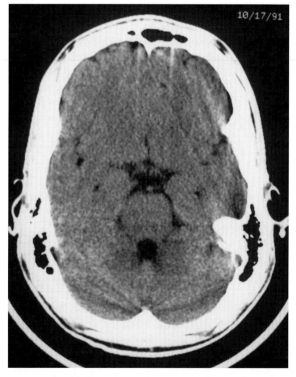

FIG. 1. Computed tomography (CT) scan from a patient with AIDS-related cryptococcal meningitis and elevated intracranial pressure (>550 mm of water) that demonstrates the association of normal to small ventricles and absence of radiological hydrocephalus, which is typical of this disease. (Reprinted with permission from Ennis DM, Saag MS. Cryptococcal meningitis in AIDS. *Hosp Pract* 1993;28:101.

Fortunately, in view of the relative normality of the CSF in this patient population, more specific diagnostic tests which have a high diagnostic yield are readily available. India ink preparations are positive in 72% to 88% of patients, although this test must be performed by experienced technicians in order to minimize false-positive results due to artifacts. Positive results in non-AIDS patients are less frequent, occurring in up to 60% of patients. Although this test provides the advantage of rapid diagnosis, it should be confirmed with CSF cryptococcal antigen test and culture.

Cryptococcal Antigen Test

The cryptococcal antigen (CRAG) test is routinely performed on both the CSF and serum. In patients with AIDS-related crytococcal meningitis, the sensitivity of the CSF CRAG test is 91% to 100% (5,6,26,54), with titers that range from positive only when undiluted to 1:64,000 (6). Patients with cryptococcal meningitis without AIDS tend to have lower CSF CRAG titers, with a median titer of 1 to 128 (17). In contrast, 39% to 48% of AIDS patients have titers greater than or equal to 1 to 1,024 (5,6).

Serum CRAG has a sensitivity of 94% to 100% in HIV-infected patients with cryptococcal meningitis (5,6,26,54), with titers ranging from 1:1 to 1:1,000,000 (6). Generally, the serum CRAG is at least one tube dilution higher than the CSF titer (54). The serum cryptococcal antigen test is occasionally used as a screening test when cryptococcal meningitis is suspected: a negative result suggests the diagnosis is unlikely; a positive result requires evaluation for meningeal disease.

False-positive CRAG tests have been reported in patients with a positive rheumatoid factor, although different laboratory techniques and reagents can correct this problem. Contamination of the CSF sample with trace amounts of surface condensation from agar present on the platinum wire inoculating loop was noted to produce weak false-positive reactions (22). A bone marrow transplant patient with disseminated *Trichosporon beigelii* had a serum CRAG positive at 1 to 2,560 (32); fortunately, this infection is extremely uncommon. Conversely, false-negative results have been reported in the CSF of up to 9% of patients (5). The most common cause of false-negative tests is the presence of a large number of organisms resulting in impaired cross-linking. This "prozone phenomena" may be corrected by diluting the specimen (21).

The use of serum CRAG for routine screening of HIV-positive patients is controversial, but it is currently not recommended in the United States. In Zaire, where the prevalence of cryptococcal disease among AIDS patients approaches 30%, a recent study demonstrated a positive serum CRAG in 55 of 450 (12%) HIV-positive patients, with meningitis being documented in 66% (13). In contrast, a study in Denmark, where the prevalence of cryptococcal disease is only 0.8%, evaluated 334 HIV-infected patients and revealed none of them to have a positive serum antigen (23). Another study from London, where the prevalence is 4.5%, detected a positive serum antigen in 17 of 828 (2%) HIV-positive patients with fever. Of note, 16 of those 17 antigen positive patients also had headache and meningismus, thus requiring a lumbar puncture anyway (34). In addition to its limited value as a screening test, a recently published review of the data from two large prospective studies on acute treatment (46) and maintenance therapy (41) for cryptococcal meningitis in patients with AIDS demonstrated no correlation between changes in serum CRAG titers obtained during acute or suppressive therapy and outcome. In contrast, increasing CSF CRAG titers during acute and suppressive therapy were associated with treatment failure and relapse, respectively. However, a considerable number of patients who failed to respond to acute therapy or relapsed during suppressive therapy had declining titers in the CSF. Thus, the prognostic value of antigen monitoring during acute or maintenance therapy for cryptococcal meningitis in patients with AIDS is limited (39).

Cerebrospinal Fluid Culture

A positive CSF culture is the definitive diagnostic test for cryptococcal meningitis and the main entry criteria in published studies. Being the gold standard, its sensitivity approaches, by definition, 100%

In patients with extraneural disease or cryptococcomas, histology can yield a presumptive diagnosis, to be later confirmed by cultures. As mentioned earlier, obtaining CSF to rule out meningeal involvement is crucial in these patients.

PROGNOSTIC FACTORS AND OUTCOME

Cryptococcal meningitis is associated with significant morbidity and mortality, even if aggressively treated. The mortality in non-AIDS patients has been reported to be as high as 20% to 30% (14,17), with up to 40% of those considered cured having residual neurological sequelae such as decreased mental function, significant visual loss, cranial nerve palsies, and/or significant motor impairment. In one series, 10% of the patients required shunting procedures for management of increased ICP (14). In patients with AIDS the reported mortality during initial therapy is 10% to 25%, and in historical studies, the 12-month survival rate is 30% to 60% (38).

Many studies have evaluated factors associated with poor outcome (mainly treatment failure and mortality) in both AIDS and non-AIDS patients. The most important pretreatment factor associated with poor prognosis is abnormal mental status (lethargy, obtundation, or coma) at presentation (17,46). Indicators of a high burden of organisms, such as a positive India ink (14,46), serum CRAG greater than 1 to 32 dilutions in non-AIDS patients (17) or CSF CRAG greater than 1 to 1,024 dilutions in patients with AIDS (46), and the presence of positive extrameningeal cultures all suggest a poor response. Evidence of a poor inflamatory response, such as having less than 20 white blood cells per cubic milliliter of CSF, also predicts poor outcome (14,17,46). Increased intracranial opening pressure is significantly associated with early death in patients without AIDS (14). The importance of this association in patients with AIDS is currently being investigated. Interestingly, AIDS patients with nonmeningeal disseminated cryptococcosis did not have a better outcome (5).

INITIAL THERAPY

The standard initial therapy for patients with cryptococcal meningitis without AIDS is amphotericin B (AMB), 0.5 to 1.0 mg/kg/d, plus flucytosine (5FC), 150 mg/kg/d in four divided doses, administered for 6 weeks (16,17). The initial studies in patients with AIDS-related cryptococcal meningitis evaluated the use of AMB alone or in combination with 5FC, with controversy surrounding the use of 5FC because of its frequent toxicity. With the introduction of the triazole antifungal agents, several treatment options became available. The following is a summary of clinical data reported over the last decade.

Amphotericin B

Amphotericin B alone or in combination with flucytosine has been evaluated in numerous studies. In 1985 Kovacs and colleagues reported success in 10 of 24 (42%) patients who received 0.3 to 0.6 mg/kg/d of AMB with or without 150 mg/kg/d of 5FC. Nine patients (38%) died during the first 4 weeks. Seven of 20 patients who received 5FC (35%) had to have therapy stopped because of toxicity (26). Zuger et al, in 1986, evaluated 24 patients treated with AMB (0.4 to 0.6 mg/kg/d) alone or with 5FC. Eighteen of 24 (75%) patients survived the course of treatment and 5FC was discontinued in 4 of 11 patients (36%) due to adverse reactions (54). In 1989, Chuck and Sande presented a retrospective review of 89 cases of AIDS-associated cryptococcal meningitis. All patients received 6 weeks of AMB (average dose 0.48 mg/kg/d) and 49 also received 5FC, 75 to 100 mg/kg/d. Overall, survival at 6 weeks was 79%. Flucytosine had to be stopped in 53% of the patients because of side effects. Of note, the median survival was higher in the group that received 5FC compared to those who did not (186 vs. 144 days, respectively), but the difference was not statistically significant (5).

Amphotericin B is generally well tolerated in AIDS patients. The most significant adverse effect is renal toxicity, which usually requires dose adjustment but rarely discontinuation. The use of higher doses of AMB, in the range of 0.7 to 1.0 mg/kg/d, is now being advocated by leading authorities (1,16,38). Supporting evidence comes from two studies. Larsen et al., in 1990, reported on 6 patients treated with AMB, 0.7 mg/kg/d, and 5FC, 150 mg/kg/d, all of whom were CSF culture negative with a mean time of 16 days. Elevation of serum creatinine occurred in 5 of 6 (83%) patients receiving AMB but only 2 required to have it withheld briefly (30). In 1992, White and co-workers treated 26 patients with 1.0 mg/kg/d of AMB plus 5FC, 100 mg/kg/d. Seventy-eight percent of patients were cured or improved 6 months after diagnosis. Median overall survival was 9 months (53).

Flucytosine has not been shown to significantly improve the outcome of AIDS patients as it has in non-AIDS-related cryptococcal meningitis. When administered at standard doses of 150 mg/kg/d, discontinuation of the drug because of toxicity, mostly leukopenia, occurs in 35% to 53% of patients (5,26,53,54). In most studies, blood levels have not been routinely followed. Currently, lower doses (100 mg/kg/d) are generally recommended and blood levels should be monitored, mantaining the levels between 50 and 100 μg/mL, in order to minimize toxicity (1,16,38).

Fluconazole

Early small studies indicated favorable results with oral fluconazole therapy. Stern et al. treated 5 patients with cryptococcal meningitis with 50 to 200 mg/d of fluconazole, including 3 patients who previously failed AMB. Clinical improvement and sterilization of the CSF was noted in 4 of the 5 patients (50). Larsen and colleagues had less encouraging results. Fluconazole treatment (400 mg/d) for 10 weeks produced clinical improvement and negative CSF cultures in 6 of 14 patients (43%), with 4 deaths over the study period. Five of the 14 patients with less severe disease fared better, with 4 of them becoming CSF culture negative (30).

The effectiveness of fluconazole was compared to AMB with or without 5FC in a clinical trial performed by the Mycosis Study Group (MSG) and the AIDS Clinical Trials Group (ACTG), in conjunction with Pfizer Central Research (46). Among the 194 patients evaluated, 131 received a loading dose of 400 mg of fluconazole followed by 200 mg/d that could be doubled after 2 weeks if there was clinical deterioration or the CSF cultures were still positive, and 63 patients received AMB, median dose 0.45 mg/kg/d. All patients were followed for 10 weeks. Succesful outcome was defined as clinical improvement and two consecutive negative CSF cultures. Forty percent (25 of 63) of the AMB-treated group and 34% (44 of 131) of the fluconazole recipients were succesfully treated according to this definition. There was no statistically significant difference between the two groups ($p = 0.39$). Overall, 67% of the patients on the AMB arm and 60% of those treated with fluconazole had clinical improvement ($p = 0.40$).

A large number of patients in each treatment arm, 27% of AMB recipients and 26% of fluconazole recipients, had so-called quiescent disease, defined as clinical improvement but persistent CSF culture positivity at the end of treatment. Overall mortality was similar in both groups (14% in the AMB group versus 18% in the fluconazole group; $p = 0.48$); however, early deaths (within the first 2 weeks of study) were more common in the fluconazole group (15% vs. 8%, $p = 0.25$). Fluconazole recipients also required more time to become culture negative (a median of 64 days versus 42 days for AMB), which is similar to the time to negative culture noted in the report by Larsen et al. (30).

The low overall response rate to standard treatment in the MSG/ACTG study might be explained by the use of lower doses of AMB, by the use of 5FC in only 9 of 63 patients (14%), or by the use of a stricter definition of succesful treatment than used in previous studies. In addition, the population may have presented with more advanced disease, with 27% of the patients having altered sensorium at baseline. These considerations, along with anecdotal data from smaller studies, have led many authorities to recommend higher dose AMB, with or without 5FC, as first-line treatment.

The use of fluconazole in the treatment of ''less severe'' cryptococcal meningitis has not been thoroughly investigated. A low mortality risk group was retrospectively defined in the MSG/ACTG study (Table 3), but comparative treatment trials have not been completed.

TABLE 3. *Pretreatment factors predicting outcome*

Pretreatment factors associated with a low risk of death while receiving therapy:
1. Normal mental status
2. CSF CRAG equal to or less than 1:1024.
3. CSF WBC equal to or greater than 20 mm^{-3}
Pretreatment factors predictive of treatment failure:
1. Positive India ink stain
2. Visual abnormalities (blurred vision, photophobia, diplopia or papilledema)
3. Age < 35 years
4. Absence of zidovudine therapy

CSF, cerebrospinal fluid; CRAG, cryptococcal antigen.

The use of fluconazole (400 mg/d) in combination with flucytosine (150 mg/kg/d) was evaluated in 32 patients by the California Collaborative Treatment Group (25) with clinical success in 20 of 32 (63%) and culture conversion from positive to negative in 24 of the 32 (75%) patients at 10 weeks. The median time to conversion was 23 days and overall mortality was 13%. Flucytosine had to be stopped because of toxicity in 28% of patients. This combination is currently being tested by the MSG in non-AIDS patients with cryptococcal meningitis.

The use of higher doses of fluconazole (800 mg/d for a mean of 4.5 months) in AIDS patients who did not respond to conventional therapy with fluconazole or AMB converted cultures to negative in six of eight patients, with three later dying of cryptococcal meningitis (2). Fluconazole has generally been well tolerated and rarely needs to be discontinued because of adverse effects (46). Drug interactions might be a more important factor, especially with anticonvulsants, rifampin or rifabutin, and clarithromycin (8).

Itraconazole

In a study by Denning and collaborators (12), 33 patients with cryptococcosis were treated with itraconazole, 200 mg twice a day. Ten of the 14 (71%) patients with AIDS-related cryptococcal meningitis had both clinical and mycological response. Less encouraging results were obtained by de Gans et al. (10), who compared the same dose of itraconazole versus AMB plus 5FC. A complete response was found in 5 of 12 (42%) itraconazole recipients by 6 weeks; the remaining 7 patients had only partial responses. In contrast, all 10 patients who received AMB (0.3 mg/kg/d) and 5FC (150 mg/kg/d) had a complete response.

Drug interactions are more of a concern with itraconazole than with fluconazole. Concomitant use of itraconazole with anticonvulsants or rifampin derivatives results in accelerated metabolism of itraconazole and subtherapeutic drug levels. Antacid or H-2-receptor antagonist use interferes with absorption of itraconazole from the gastrointestinal tract (8).

Newer Preparations of Amphotericin B

Amphotericin B–colloidal dispersion, liposomal AMB, and AMB-lipid complex are novel formulations of AMB designed to deliver greater doses of the parent compound with reduced toxicity. Coker et al. recently presented the results of a multicenter European trial of liposomal AMB (7). In that study, 12 of 18 (67%) patients with AIDS-related cryptococcal meningitis had a complete microbiological response (defined as negative CSF cultures for 2 successive weeks), with 2 additional patients having clinical improvement. The toxicity was minimal and included increases in serum creatinine and transaminases, along with hypokalemia, none of which required discontinuation of the study drug. The use of these and other investigational drugs are currently restricted to clinical trials or as compassionate-use therapy.

Most investigators currently recommend the regimen presently being employed in the MSG 17/ACTG 159 study, namely an aggressive "induction" phase with high-dose AMB (0.7 to 0.8 mg/kg/d) with or without 5FC (100 mg/kg/d) for 2 weeks, followed by a "consolidation" phase of 8 weeks with fluconazole, 400 mg/d. The use of itraconazole, 200 mg twice a day, remains investigational, although this drug may be used in patients who are unable to take fluconazole (16,20,38).

MANAGEMENT OF INCREASED INTRACRANIAL PRESSURE

Diamond and Bennett (14) demonstrated that patients with non-AIDS-related cryptococcal meningitis who died less than 4 weeks after diagnosis had significantly higher mean opening CSF pressures (315 versus 209 mm of water) than those who were cured ($p < 0.01$). Increased ICP occurs in more than 60% of AIDS patients with cryptococcal meningitis (see Table 1), usually in the form of communicating hydrocephalus without radiological evidence of enlarged ventricles or cerebral edema in most cases (see Table 2). In fact, the majority of patients with increased ICP have normal or small ventricles. Its role in morbidity and mortality among AIDS patients has not been systematically evaluated.

The use of CSF drainage by serial lumbar punctures with subsequent improvement of mental status and cranial nerve abnormalities has been the subject of anecdotal reports by several investigators. Denning and co-workers reported three patients with opening pressures (OPs) ranging from 500 to 577 mm of water with impaired cognitive function, papilledema, cranial nerve palsies, and impaired vision with normal cerebral imaging studies who responded to serial lumbar punctures. A ventriculoperitoneal shunt was required in one of these cases (11).

Van Gemert and Vermeulen reported the case of an unconscious patient who underwent three lumbar punctures with an OP greather than 800 mm of water, with consciousness improving during the procedure. He finally had an external lumbar CSF drainage system placed (100 to 185 mL/d of CSF) with return to baseline mental status and resolution of his facial nerve palsy (52).

In the large MSG 8A/ACTG 059 trial previously discussed (46), the OP was measured in only 30% of patients, and careful documentation of pressure management was not recorded. Nevertheless, we know of one patient who required 53 lumbar punctures in 60 days for management of increased ICP (unpublished observation). For patients with communicating hydrocephalus, serial lumbar punctures provide the best mechanism for relieving the neurological complications of increased ICP. Ten to 20 cc can be safely removed with each tap. Some recommend draining enough CSF to reduce the OP by 50%; others prefer to decrease it to less than 100 mm of water. The true benefit is most likely due to CSF leakage through the puncture defect in the dura over time. These recommendations have not been properly evaluated; however, the ongoing MSG 17/ACTG 159 trial is addressing this issue. When serial lumbar punctures are not sufficient to control the symptoms of increased ICP, placement of a lumbar drain or ventriculostomy may be indicated temporarily. The placement of a ventriculoperitoneal shunt to achieve long-term symptom control is necessary on occasion.

Drug therapy for pressure management has been proposed by some investigators. Dexamethasone was used in at least four patients in the MSG 8A/ACTG 59 study with variable results (unpublished observation). Johnston et al. reported the use of acetazolamide, a diuretic that inhibits carbonic anhydrase, thus reducing CSF production in the choroid plexus. Two AIDS patients with cryptococcal meningitis and OP above 400 mm of water, requiring lumbar punctures every other day, were given acetazolamide (250 mg twice a day) with subsequent sustained reduction of the OP to less than 200 mm of water (24). However, it remains unclear whether the succesful reduction in pressure was due to acetazolamide or the serial taps. The use of these two medications is still controversial and is not recommended on a routine basis.

MAINTENANCE THERAPY

After successful initial therapy, 27% to 58% of AIDS patients with cryptococcal meningitis will relapse if no suppressive therapy is administered, usually within the first 6 months (3,5,54). These relapses are caused by failure to completely eradicate *C. neoformans,* especially in "sanctuary sites" such as the urinary tract. Spitzer et al. demonstrated that isolates cultured from the same patient on recurrent episodes were genetically similar and distinguishable from those obtained from other patients (49). These organisms generally did not possess an increase in antibiotic resistance relative to the initial isolates (4). However, one case of AMB-resistant *C. neoformans* has been described (40). Maintenance therapy is aimed at suppressing the multiplication of the residual organisms, which the debilitated immune system is unable to suppress.

Zuger et al. reported no relapses at 6 months in 7 patients who received AMB, 100 mg weekly, compared with 4 of 8 patients on no maintenance therapy (54). Chuck and Sande (5) found that median survival was significantly better ($p < 0.004$) among patients receiving suppressive therapy with either ketoconazole (238 days) or AMB (280 days) compared with those receiving no treatment (141 days). Clark reported a 7% relapse rate (2 of 27 patients) among patients receiving AMB maintenance therapy (50 to 120 mg/week) as opposed to 3 of 8 (38%) relapses in untreated patients (6).

The use of fluconazole as maintenance therapy was evaluated in 14 patients by Stern (50), 13 of whom remained CSF culture-negative for a mean of 25 weeks. Sugar and Saunders had only 1 of 19 patients receiving fluconazole therapy relapse in 6 months (51). A larger, placebo-controlled study by the California Collaborative Treatment Group reported a 37% (10 of 27) recurrence of cryptococcal infection at any site in the placebo group (mean follow-up of 117 days), versus 3% (1 of 34 patients) in the fluconazole group (mean follow-up of 164 days). Fifteen percent of placebo recipients had recurrent cryptococcal meningitis, compared to no cases of meningitis in the fluconazole group (3).

To establish whether daily fluconazole, 200 mg orally, and weekly AMB, 1 mg/kg intravenously, were equivalent maintenance regimens, the MSG and the ACTG conducted a multicenter, randomized trial that evaluated 189 patients with AIDS who had been succesfully treated for cryptococcal meningitis (Table 4). With a mean follow-up of 286 days, relapses occurred in 14 of 78 patients in the AMB arm (18%),

TABLE 4. *Approach to the management of cryptococcal meningitis in patients with AIDS*

Therapy	Recommended approach	Alternative approach
Initial	AMB (0.5–1 mg/kg/d IV) plus 5FC (100 mg/kg/d) for 6 weeks or 1.5–2 gm of AMB	Fluconazole 400 mg/d PO
Increased ICP	Serial lumbar punctures	VP shunt or lumbar drain[a]
Maintenance	Fluconazole, 200 mg/d PO	AMB, 1 mg/kg/week IV

[a] If increased ICP is severe and/or persistent despite appropriate management.
AMB, amphotericin B; 5FC, flucytosine; ICP, intracranial pressure; VP, ventriculoperitoneal.

versus only 2 of the 111 (2%) patients assigned to the fluconazole arm ($p < 0.001$). Drug-related toxicities and bacterial infections (mainly catheter related and bacteremia) were more common in the AMB group, resulting in discontinuation of the study drug in 15% of the AMB group, compared to 5% of the fluconazole group (41). Of note, in these two large prospective studies with intense follow-up including regularly scheduled serum cryptococcal antigen testing (42) and CSF cultures, the patients who relapsed each presented with clinically evident disease. This suggests that regular clinical monitoring of the signs and symptoms of disease is sufficient to detect relapse in the majority of patients (3,42).

The role of itraconazole, 200 mg/d, was reported by de Gans et al., with two relapses reported in nine patients treated succesfully with AMB (10). An ongoing study of the Mycosis Study Group (MSG 25) is currently comparing itraconazole versus fluconazole. It should be completed by the winter of 1995. Thus far, fluconazole at a dose of 200 mg/d is considered the treatment of choice for maintenance therapy after initial therapy of cryptococcal meningitis in patients with AIDS.

REFERENCES

1. Armstrong D. Treatment of opportunistic fungal infections. *Clin Infect Dis* 1993;16:1–9.
2. Berry AJ, Rinaldi MG, Graybill JR. Use of high-dose fluconazole as salvage therapy for cryptococcal meningitis in patients with AIDS. *Antimicrob Agents Chemother* 1992;36:690–692.
3. Bozzette SA, Larsen RA, Chiu J, et al. A placebo-controlled trial of maintenance therapy with fluconazole after treatment of cryptococcal meningitis in the acquired immunodeficiency syndrome. *N Engl J Med* 1991;324:580–584.
4. Casadevall A, Spitzer ED, Webb D, Rinaldi MG. Susceptibilities of serial *Cryptococcus neoformans* isolates from patients with recurrent cryptococcal meningitis to amphotericin B and fluconazole. *Antimicrob Agents Chemother* 1993;37:1383–1386.
5. Chuck SL, Sande MA. Infections with *Cryptococcus neoformans* on the acquired immunodeficiency sydrome. *N Engl J Med* 1989;321:794–799.
6. Clark RA, Greer D, Atkinson W, Valainis GT, Hyslop N. Spectrum of *Cryptococcus neoformans* infection in 68 patients infected with human immunodeficiency virus. *Rev Infect Dis* 1990;12: 768–777.
7. Coker RJ, Viviani M, Gazzard BG, et al. Treatment of cryptococcosis with liposomal amphotericin B (AmBisome) in 23 patients with AIDS. *AIDS* 1993;7:829–835.
8. Como JA, Dismukes WE. Oral azole drugs as systemic antifungal therapy. *N Engl J Med* 1993;330: 263–272.
9. Currie BP, Freundlich LF, Soto MA, Casadevall A. False-negative cerebrospinal fluid cryptococcal latex agglutination tests for patients with culture-positive cryptococcal meningitis. *J Clin Microbiol* 1993;31:2519–2522.
10. de Gans J, Portegies P, Tiessens G. Itraconazole compared with amphotericin B plus flucytosine in AIDS patients with cryptococcal meningitis. *AIDS* 1992;6:185–190.
11. Denning DW, Armstrong RW, Lewis BH, Stevens DA. Elevated cerebrospinal fluid pressures in patients with cryptococcal meningitis and acquired immunodeficiency syndrome. *Am J Med* 1991; 91:267–272.
12. Denning DW, Tucker RM, Hanson LH, Hamilton JR, Stevens DA. Itraconazole therapy for cryptococcal meningitis and cryptococcosis. *Arch Intern Med* 1989;149:2301–2308.
13. Desmet P, Kayembe KD, De Vroey C. The value of cryptococcal serum antigen screening among HIV-positive/AIDS patients in Kinshasa, Zaire. *AIDS* 1989;3:77–78.
14. Diamond RD, Bennett JE. Prognostic factors in cryptococcal meningitis: a study of 111 cases. *Ann Intern Med* 1974;80:176–181.
15. Dismukes WE. Cryptococcal meningitis in patients with AIDS. *J Infect Dis* 1988;157:624–628.
16. Dismukes WE. Management of cryptococcosis. *Clin Infect Dis* 1993;17(Suppl 2):S507–512.
17. Dismukes WE, Cloud G, Gallis HA, et al. Treatment of cryptococcal meningitis with combination of amphotericin B and flucytosine for four as compared with six weeks. *N Engl J Med* 1987;317: 334–341.
18. Ellis DH, Pfeiffer TJ. Ecology, life cycle, and infectious propagule of *Cryptococcus neoformans*. *Lancet* 1990;336:923–925.

19. Eng RHK, Bishburg E, Smith SM, Kapila R. Cryptococcal infections in patients with acquired immunodeficiency syndrome. *Am J Med* 1986;81:19–23.
20. Ennis DM, Saag MS. Cryptococcal meningitis in AIDS. *Hosp Pract* 1993;28:99–112.
21. Hamilton JR, Noble A, Denning DW, Stevens DA. Performance of cryptococcus latex agglutination kits on serum and cerebrospinal fluid specimens of AIDS patients before and after pronase treatment. *J Clin Microbiol* 1991;29:333–339.
22. Heelan JS, Corpus L, Kessimian N. False-positive reactions in the latex agglutination test for *Cryptococcus neoformans* antigen. *J Clin Microbiol* 1991;29:1260–1261.
23. Hoffmann S, Stenderup J, Mathiesen LR. Low yield of screening for cryptococcal antigen by latex agglutination assay on serum and cerebrospinal fluid from Danish patients with AIDS or ARC. *Scand J Infect Dis* 1991;23:697–702.
24. Johnston SRD, Corbett EL, Foster O, Ash S, Cohen J. Raised intracranial pressure and visual complications in AIDS patients with cryptococcal meningitis. *J Infect* 1992;24:185–189.
25. Jones BE, Larsen RA, Bozzette S, et al. A phase II trial of fluconazole plus flucytosine for cryptococcal meningitis (abstract W.B. 2337). *Seventh International Conference on AIDS. Science challenging AIDS.* Rome: Instituto Superiore di Sanita; 1991:266.
26. Kovacs JA, Kovacs AA, Polis M, et al. Cryptococcosis in the acquired immunodeficiency syndrome. *Ann Intern Med* 1985;103:533–538.
27. Kwon-Chung KJ, Bennett JE. Epidemiological differences between the two varieties of *Cryptococcus neoformans*. *Am J Epidemiol* 1984;120:123–130.
28. Kwon-Chung KJ, Bennett JE. *Medical mycology.* Pittsburgh: Lea & Febiger, 1992.
29. Larsen RA, Bozzette S, McCutchan JA, et al. Persistent *Cryptococcus neoformans* infection of the prostate after successful treatment of meningitis. *Ann Intern Med* 1989;111:125–128.
30. Larsen RA, Leal MAE, Chan LS. Fluconazole compared with amphotericin B plus flucytosine for cryptococcal meningitis in AIDS: a randomized trial. *Ann Intern Med* 1990;113:183–187.
31. Mathews VP, Alo PL, Glass JD, Kumar AJ, McArthur JC. AIDS-related CNS cryptococcosis: radiological-pathological correlation. *Am J Neuroradiol* 1992;13:1477–1486.
32. McManus EJ, Jones JM. Detection of *Trichosporon beigelii* antigen cross-reactive with *Cryptococcus neoformans* capsular polysaccharide in serum from a patient with disseminated *Trichosporon* infection. *J Clin Microbiol* 1985;21:681–685.
33. Muyembe Tamfum JJ, Mupapa Kibadi D, Nganda L, et al. Cryptococcosis caused by *Cryptococcus neoformans* var. *gattii*. A case associated with acquired immunodeficiency syndrome (AIDS) in Kinshasa, Zaire. *Med Trop* 1992;52:435–438.
34. Nelson MR, Bower M, Smith D, Reed C, Shanson D, Gazzard B. The value of serum cryptococcal antigen in the diagnosis of cryptococcal infection in patients infected with human immunodeficiency virus. *J Infect* 1990;21:175–181.
35. Patterson TF, Andriole VT. Current concepts in cryptococcosis. *Eur J Clin Microbiol Infect Dis* 1989;8:457–465.
36. Perfect JR. Cryptococcosis. *Infect Dis Clin North Am* 1989;3:77–102.
37. Popovich MJ, Arthur RH, Helmer E. CT of intracranial cryptococcosis. *AJR Am J Roentgenol* 1990;154:603–606.
38. Powderly WG. Cryptococcal meningitis and AIDS. *Clin Infect Dis* 1993;17:837–842.
39. Powderly WG, Cloud GA, Dismukes WE, Saag MS. Measurement of cryptococcal antigen in serum and cerebrospinal fluid: value in the management of AIDS-associated cryptococcal meningitis. *Clin Infect Dis* 1994;18:789–792.
40. Powderly WG, Keath EJ, Sokol-Anderson M, Kitz D, Russell Little J, Kobayashi G. Amphotericin B-resistant *Cryptococcus neoformans* in a patient with AIDS. *Infect Dis Clin Pract* 1994:314–316.
41. Powderly WG, Saag MS, Cloud GA, et al. A controlled trial of fluconazole versus amphotericin B to prevent relapse of cryptococcal meningitis in patients with the acquired immunodeficiency syndrome. *N Engl J Med* 1992;326:793–798.
42. Powderly WG, Saag MS, Cloud GA, Dismukes WE. Letter. *N Engl J Med* 1992;327:566.
43. Rinaldi MG, Drutz DJ, Howell A, et al. Serotypes of *Cryptococcus neoformans* in patients with AIDS. *J Infect Dis* 1986;153:642.
44. Rozenbaum R, Rios AJ. Clinical epidemiological study of 171 cases of cryptococcosis. *Clin Infect Dis* 1994;18:369–380.
45. Rozenbaum R, Rios AJ, Wanke B, et al. *Cryptococcus neoformans* varieties as agents of cryptococcosis in Brazil. *Mycopathologia* 1992;119;133–136.
46. Saag MS, Powderly WG, Cloud GA, et al. Comparison of amphotericin B with fluconazole in the treatment of acute AIDS-associated cryptococcal meningitis. *N Engl J Med* 1992;326:83–89.
47. Sabetta JR, Andriole VT. Cryptococcal infection of the central nervous system. *Med Clin North Am* 1985;69:333–344.
48. Shimizu RY, Howard DH, Clancy MN. The variety of *Cryptococcus neoformans* in patients with AIDS. *J Infect Dis* 1986;154:1042.
49. Spitzer ED, Spitzer SG, Freundlich LF, Casadevall A. Persistence of initial infection in recurrent *Cryptococcus neoformans* meningitis. *Lancet* 1993;341:595–596.

50. Stern JJ, Hartman BJ, Sharkey P, et al. Oral fluconazole therapy for patients with acquired immunode-ficiency syndrome and cryptococcosis: experience with 22 patients. *Am J Med* 1988;85:477–480.
51. Sugar AM, Saunders C. Oral fluconazole as suppressive therapy of disseminated cryptococcosis in patients with acquired immunodeficiency syndrome. *Am J Med* 1988;85:481–489.
52. van Gemert HMA, Vermeulen M. Treatment of impaired consciousness with lumbar punctures in a patient with cryptococcal meningitis and AIDS. *Clin Neurol Neurosurg* 1991;93:257–258.
53. White M, Cirrincione C, Blevins A, Armstrong D. Cryptococcal meningitis: outcome in patients with AIDS and patients with neoplastic disease. *J Infect Dis* 1992;165:960–963.
54. Zuger A, Louie E, Holzman RS, Simberkoff MS, Rahal JJ. Cryptococcal disease in patients with the acquired immunodeficiency syndrome. Diagnostic features and outcome of treatment. *Ann Intern Med* 1986;104:234–240.

AIDS and the Nervous System, Second Edition,
edited by J. R. Berger and R. M. Levy.
Lippincott-Raven Publishers, Philadelphia © 1997.

26

Syphilis, Human Immunodeficiency Virus, and the Nervous System

Christina M. Marra

Departments of Neurology and Medicine, University of Washington School of Medicine, Harborview Medical Center, Seattle, Washington 98104-2499

Despite centuries of study of syphilis and neurosyphilis, many gaps persist in our understanding of the clinical manifestations and host response to these serious infections. The advent of human immunodeficiency virus type 1 (HIV-1) infection and its interactions with syphilis have emphasized this lack of knowledge. Recent observations that HIV-infected patients with syphilis may have more severe clinical manifestations of early disease, may not develop "normal" antibody responses to infection with *Treponema pallidum*, and may be more likely to relapse with neurosyphilis after standard therapy for early syphilis have prompted reevaluation of current diagnostic and treatment strategies. This chapter will critically review the literature concerning alterations in clinical manifestations and therapeutic response of syphilis in HIV-infected individuals.

EARLY SYPHILIS AND HIV

Over the last 10 years, a number of case reports have suggested that the clinical course of syphilis is altered in patients also infected with HIV. These have included uncommon ocular manifestations (22,78), unusual rashes (10,23), delayed healing after therapy for secondary syphilis (21), lues maligna (10,15,77,85), gumma (14,26,33,47), osteitis (44), and pneumonitis (17). Cases of secondary syphilis (35,81,83) or ocular syphilis (26,31,54) with nonreactive serological tests have also been described. In two instances, serological tests became reactive 20 days (35) and 3 months (81) after presentation; follow-up serological tests were not reported in the remainder.

Extrapolation of these findings to all patients with concurrent HIV and syphilis is difficult. Case reports may represent biased reporting of unusual findings. Without denominator data it is impossible to determine what proportion of HIV-infected patients with syphilis actually experience these "atypical" clinical manifestations. On the other hand, all patients with atypical findings may not be appropriately diagnosed. Because serum nontreponemal tests are commonly used to screen for syphilis, patients with nonreactive tests would not be further investigated for evidence of syphilis, and thus cases of "seronegative" syphilis could be missed. Nonetheless, comparison with data collected in the pre-HIV era show that seronegative secondary syphilis was estimated to occur in about 3% of cases (79) and that atypical clinical manifestations of syphilis described in recent case reports were well recognized at the turn of the century (80).

Cross-sectional and longitudinal studies may yield more information. A retrospective series of patients attending Baltimore sexually transmitted diseases clinics showed that HIV-infected patients with first-episode secondary syphilis had higher serum Rapid Plasma Reagin (RPR) test titers than corresponding HIV-uninfected patients (39). In a second study, the same authors confirmed their earlier serological findings and also observed that HIV-infected patients were more likely to present with secondary syphilis and were more likely to have concomitant chancres (40). A prospective study could avoid potential differences in health-care-seeking behavior that cannot be excluded in a retrospective study. Such a study of injection drug users showed no difference in stage or clinical manifestations of syphilis at presentation in HIV-infected compared to HIV-uninfected subjects and showed higher median serum nontreponemal titers only in HIV-infected subjects with a prior history of syphilis (25). Another ongoing prospective study has shown that serum RPR titers at presentation are higher in HIV-infected compared to HIV-uninfected patients with syphilis but that this difference does not reach statistical significance (73). The observation that serum nontreponemal test titers may be higher in HIV-infected patients has sparked the suggestion that seronegative early syphilis may simply reflect the presence of a prozone phenomenon (43); however, this possibility was excluded in several of the reported cases.

Data from animal models support the contention that differences in the clinical and serological response to syphilis do occur in the setting of concomitant retroviral infection. In a rabbit model, syphilitic cutaneous lesions were more severe in HIV-infected animals compared to controls (87), despite lack of demonstrable immunodeficiency. In a macaque model, chancres persisted longer and a serum Venereal Disease Research Laboratory (VDRL) test was more often nonreactive in simian immunodeficiency virus (SIV) infected animals compared to controls (49,52).

Taken together, data from animal and human studies suggest that nonreactive serological tests for syphilis should not exclude the diagnosis of syphilis in cases where clinical suspicion is high. In these instances, repeat serological testing with exclusion of a prozone phenomenon, identification of *T. pallidum* in clinical specimens by dark-field microscopy, fluorescent antibody staining, or polymerase chain reaction (PCR), and biopsy with histological examination should be pursued.

NEUROSYPHILIS AND HIV

Early Central Nervous System Invasion

It has been long recognized that *T. pallidum* invades the central nervous system (CNS) early in the course of infection. Investigators in the first half of this century showed that as many as 70% of patients with secondary syphilis had cerebrospinal fluid (CSF) pleocytosis, elevated protein or globulin concentration, or a reactive CSF Wasserman test (57,72,89), and *T. pallidum* could be demonstrated in CSF by rabbit inoculation in 15% of patients with untreated early syphilis who had no other CSF abnormality (12). Serial observations suggested that, even without therapy, organisms were cleared from the CSF in 70% of individuals by the time the rash of secondary syphilis resolved (72). Several workers showed that patients with the most abnormal CSF (62) or with persistence of CSF abnormalities for 6 months or more (30) had the highest likelihood of developing symptomatic neurosyphilis, and that patients with normal CSF were at low risk for subsequent development of neurosyphilis (38,63).

A prospective study performed at the University of Washington (48) confirmed the high frequency of CSF abnormalities in early syphilis. In this study, 40% of patients with untreated primary and secondary syphilis had CSF pleocytosis. The CSF-VDRL was reactive in 24% of patients with secondary, but no patients with primary syphilis. *Treponema pallidum* was recovered from 30% of CSF samples, one-third of which were otherwise normal. Importantly, this study showed that CSF-VDRL reactivity and identification of *T. pallidum* in CSF were equally common in HIV-infected compared to HIV-uninfected patients. Cerebrospinal fluid pleocytosis was more common in HIV-infected patients, an observation that has been made in HIV-infected subjects without syphilis (2). Similarly, a prospective multicenter study of early syphilis in HIV-infected and HIV-uninfected individuals showed that HIV-infected subjects were more likely to have CSF pleocytosis but equally likely to have a reactive CSF-VDRL or elevated protein concentration (73). Thus, syphilitic involvement of the CNS is equally likely in HIV-infected and HIV-uninfected individuals.

Clinical Manifestations of Neurosyphilis

Neurosyphilis has been traditionally divided into meningeal and parenchymal forms. The meningeal forms include asymptomatic and symptomatic meningitis and meningovasculitis. The parenchymal forms include tabes dorsalis and general paresis. Uncommon forms of neurosyphilis such as myelitis and gumma may be either meningeal or parenchymal. Generally, the meningeal forms occur early (weeks to months) after infection, and the parenchymal forms occur late (years to decades) after infection (Fig. 1). The clinical findings for the major forms of neurosyphilis are outlined in Table 1.

Several investigators have described development of neurosyphilis in HIV-infected patients (reviewed in 67, 68; 16, 27, 76). Most reports describe patients with early neurosyphilis, including symptomatic meningitis or meningovasculitis with stroke, often occurring in combination with syphilitic ocular disease (45). Uncommon but previously well-recognized manifestations have also been described in patients with HIV, including CNS gumma (6) (Fig. 2) and gummatous meningovascular neurosyphilis (64,65). Most cases of neurosyphilis in HIV-infected individuals have been similar in terms of clinical manifestations and estimated time of development after primary syphilis to cases reported in the pre-HIV era (55).

Because most descriptions come from individual cases or small series, it is hard to know whether neurosyphilis is more common in HIV-infected compared to HIV-uninfected individuals. In the 1940s, Merritt and co-workers (55) found asymptomatic neurosyphilis in 9.5% of 2,263 patients examined in the neurosyphilis outpatient department of the Boston City Hospital. This number is likely an underestimation because the majority (90%) of patients were seen more than 5 years after primary infection. The proportion with early symptomatic neurosyphilis (meningeal and meningovascular) was estimated at 0.5% to 3%, and late symptomatic neurosyphilis

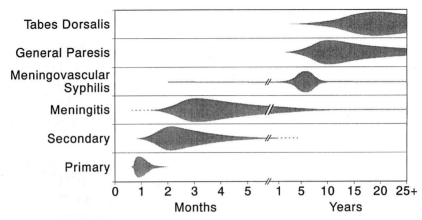

FIG. 1. Time course of the clinical manifestations of syphilis. Neurosyphilis can occur at any time after primary infection, but meningeal and meningovascular disease are more common early in the course of the disease, while paresis and tabes are more common late in disease. (Reproduced with permission from Hook EW III, Marra CM. Acquired syphilis in adults. *N Engl J Med* 1992;326:1060–1069.)

(general paresis and tabes dorsalis) at 5 % to 9% (55). Studies of the proportion of HIV-infected patients with asymptomatic neurosyphilis defined by reactive serum serological tests and reactive CSF-VDRL tests give estimates ranging from 2% to 54% (18,36,91), and estimates of the frequency of symptomatic neurosyphilis range from 5.7% to 12.5% (5,8). It is difficult to compare proportions between current and past studies given differences in criteria for diagnosis of neurosyphilis and in patient acquisition, and it is thus difficult to determine whether the numbers of cases of neurosyphilis in HIV-infected individuals are more than would be expected. Even prior to the recognition of HIV, late neurosyphilis was believed to be declining compared to early disease, perhaps due to the widespread availability of antibiotics for unrelated conditions (9,90). Nonetheless, a retrospective study of hospitalized patients at the University of Miami identified equal numbers of cases of CSF-VDRL reactive neurosyphilis in HIV-infected and HIV-uninfected patients over 64 months,

TABLE 1. *Clinical findings in neurosyphilis*

Asymptomatic neurosyphilis: Defined by CSF abnormalities (white blood cells, protein concentration, and CSF VDRL) alone. Treatment prevents progression to symptomatic neurosyphilis.

Meningeal neurosyphilis: Clinical findings include headache, stiff neck, nausea, and vomiting. Complications may include cranial nerve involvement and hydrocephalus. Treatment results in clinical improvement.

Meningovascular neurosyphilis: Clinical findings are consistent with stroke, usually in the distribution of the middle cerebral artery. Symptoms of meningitis may also be present. Therapy usually results in clinical improvement, although residual deficits are common.

General paresis: Early clinical findings include forgetfulness and personality changes, and psychiatric symptoms may develop. Dementia ensues, often accompanied by pupillary abnormalities, hypotonia, and intention tremor. Treatment may halt progression of the disease but does not usually result in clinical improvement.

Tabes dorsalis: Clinical findings include sensory loss, ataxia, lancinating pains, and bowel and bladder dysfunction. Treatment may halt progression of the disease but does not usually result in clinical improvement.

CSF, cerebrospinal fluid; VDRL, Venereal Disease Research Laboratory.

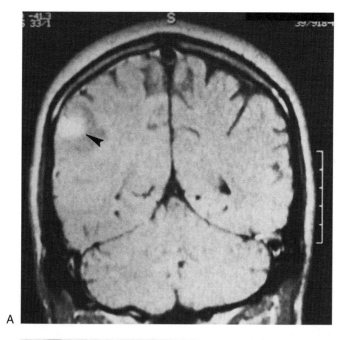

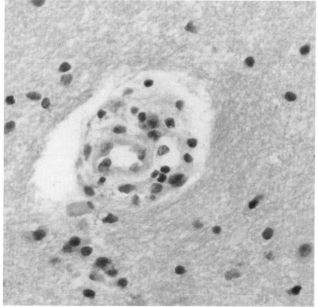

FIG. 2. **A:** Cerebral gumma in an HIV-infected patient. Coronal gadolinium enhanced cranial magnetic resonance scan shows an enhancing nodule in the right parietal cortex with surrounding edema. **B:** Endarteritis obliterans with perivascular and parenchymal infiltration of lymphocytes and plasma cells in the gumma (hematoxylin and esoin × 150). (Reproduced with permission from Berger JR, Waskin H, Pall L, Hensley G, Ihmedian I, Post MJD. Syphilitic cerebral gumma with HIV infection. *Neurology* 1992;42:1282–1287.)

but showed that syphilitic meningitis was more common in HIV-infected patients without acquired immunodeficiency syndrome (AIDS) compared to those who were HIV-uninfected (46).

Neurorelapse

In the preantibiotic era, CSF was routinely examined 6 months after initiating nonpenicillin therapy for early syphilis, and the results of this examination were used to determine the duration of therapy (59). With the availability of penicillin for early syphilis, several authors demonstrated that CSF abnormalities were uncommon 6 months or more after treatment with 2.4 or 4.8 million units (MU) of intramuscular (IM) penicillin (1,3), and the practice of routine CSF examination in early syphilis became uncommon. Despite subsequent observations that doses of benzathine penicillin G as high as 14.4 MU (58) do not reliably achieve treponemacidal penicillin levels in CSF and that virulent *T. pallidum* could be recovered from CSF after treatment with 2.4, 4.8, and 10.8 MU of benzathine penicillin G (48,86), the issue of routine CSF evaluation for patients with early syphilis has only reemerged since the advent of HIV.

In contrast to the experience in HIV-uninfected persons, a striking feature of cases of neurosyphilis in HIV-infected individuals is the frequency of prior therapy for early syphilis (67,68). In a review of 42 HIV-infected patients with neurosyphilis (68), 16 (38%) had been previously treated with penicillin for syphilis, and 5 developed neurosyphilis within 6 months of treatment. A recent report describes development of symptomatic neurosyphilis 18 months after therapy with 7.2 MU benzathine penicillin in a HIV-2-infected individual (75). Although reinfection cannot be excluded in all cases, the short duration between treatment for early syphilis and development of neurosyphilis in many cases make this explanation less likely.

Ocular disease frequently coexists with neurosyphilis in HIV-infected patients. Ocular manifestations were seen in 5 (42%) of 12 patients with AIDS and neurosyphilis in a retrospective study (45) and was significantly more common in HIV-infected patients studied at the University of Miami (46). In a series of 9 HIV-infected patients with ocular syphilis, the CSF-VDRL test was reactive in 4 (67%) of 7 that agreed to lumbar puncture (54).

In the preantibiotic era, meningeal neurosyphilis was more commonly seen as a manifestation of relapse in patients who had been inadequately or incompletely treated for early syphilis (56). Similarly, uveitis occurred more commonly as a form of relapse in patients inadequately treated for early syphilis and was often accompanied by meningitis (61). Moore (60,61) contended that limited therapy was able to eradicate all organisms except those that remained in privileged sites such as the CNS or the eye and led to attenuation of the immune response. The organisms remaining in these sites were then able to multiply and produce disease. A parallel can be made to the HIV-infected patient treated with benzathine penicillin for early syphilis. This treatment does not achieve treponemacidal levels in the CSF and presumably in the eye. This does not appear to pose a significant problem for the immunocompetent host whose immune system is able to clear or contain remaining organisms. However, because of impaired cell-mediated immunity, the HIV-infected patient is less able to eradicate persisting organisms and remains at risk for development of symptomatic neurosyphilis or ocular disease. A prospective study performed at the University of Washington supports this contention. Seven patients with *T. pallidum* isolated from CSF before therapy for secondary syphilis had repeat CSF examinations after therapy (48). Four of the seven patients received a single dose of 2.4 MU of benzathine penicillin. Three of these four required retreatment for neurosyphilis because of persistence of *T. pallidum* in CSF of two and worsening of CSF parameters in the third. Two of these patients were HIV infected, and a third became HIV seropositive during follow-up. The only patient cured by a single dose of benzathine penicillin was not infected with HIV. Neurosyphilis in HIV-infected patients seems to be less common in the United Kingdom (70) and the Netherlands (19), where therapy for early syphilis consists of three doses of 2.4 MU IM benzathine penicillin G or 10 to 14 days of 0.6 to 0.9 MU/day IM procaine penicillin. This observation adds further support to the theory that HIV-infected patients suffer neurorelapse because of the combination of inadequate therapy and cellular immunodeficiency.

Diagnosis of Neurosyphilis

The diagnosis of symptomatic neurosyphilis is based on clinical evidence and is supported by CSF abnormalities such as pleocytosis, elevated protein, and a reactive CSF-VDRL. The diagnosis of asymptomatic neurosyphilis is based solely on CSF abnormalities. Mild CSF mononuclear pleocytosis (10 to 400 cells/μL) is characteristic of neurosyphilis, and higher cell counts are seen in early compared to late disease (55). Mild elevations in CSF protein (45 to 200 mg/dL) are also common, with higher values in early neurosyphilis (55). The CSF-VDRL test is considered to be the "gold standard" test. However, the reported sensitivity of the CSF-VDRL test depends upon the diagnostic criteria chosen to define neurosyphilis in a given study; the generally accepted sensitivity today is 30% to 70% (32). The CSF-VDRL test is very specific, but false-negative tests are common and false-positive results may be obtained when the CSF is visibly blood tinged (13,41). Thus, a reactive CSF-VDRL establishes the diagnosis of neurosyphilis, but a nonreactive test does not exclude it.

The low sensitivity of the CSF-VDRL test is especially difficult in patients with HIV infection, in whom mild CSF pleocytosis or elevated protein are common in patients without syphilis (2). In this population, demonstration of an elevated *T. pallidum* hemagglutination (TPHA) index [defined as the CSF microhemagglutination–*T. pallidum* (MHA-TP) titer divided by 1,000 times the ratio of CSF to serum albumin] may support the diagnosis of neurosyphilis, although it may not be elevated in instances where the CSF-VDRL test is reactive (84). Conversely, the absence of CSF treponemal antibodies measured by the MHA-TP or fluorescent treponemal antibody absorption (FTA-ABS) test can be used to exclude the diagnosis of neurosyphilis (53).

To date, no case of CSF-VDRL reactive neurosyphilis has been described in an HIV-infected patient with nonreactive serum VDRL or RPR. This observation may reflect an ascertainment bias; patients with nonreactive or low-titer reactive serum VDRL or RPR may not be offered lumbar puncture as often as those with detectable or high titers. Several small series of HIV-infected patients have shown that, compared to individuals with CSF pleocytosis and elevated protein but nonreactive CSF-VDRL, CSF-VDRL reactivity is associated with higher serum VDRL or RPR titers

(18,36,91). In the University of Miami series of patients with neurosyphilis defined by a reactive CSF-VDRL (46), serum RPR titers ranged from 1:4 to 1:4,096 and were similar in HIV-infected and HIV-uninfected patients. A report of two HIV-infected patients with symptomatic meningeal neurosyphilis, in whom the CSF-VDRL became reactive 12 days and 3 months after starting therapy for neurosyphilis (20), is reminiscent of the cases of delayed seroconversion in secondary syphilis (35,81) and remind us that, as in patients who are not infected with HIV, a nonreactive CSF VDRL does not exclude the diagnosis of neurosyphilis in patients also infected with HIV. A suggested algorithm for the laboratory diagnosis of neurosyphilis in patients infected with HIV is shown in Fig. 3.

Therapy for Neurosyphilis

The penicillin regimens recommended by the Centers for Disease Control (11) for treatment of neurosyphilis are outlined in Table 2. No alternative drugs have been well studied, and patients with a history of penicillin allergy should be skin tested and desensitized if necessary. Experimental regimens using high-dose oral amoxicillin with probenecid (66), high-dose oral doxycycline (88), or IM or intravenous (IV) ceftriaxone (18,37,51) have not been studied prospectively and should not be considered as acceptable therapy. In a retrospective study of therapy for neurosyphilis, latent syphilis, and presumed latent syphilis (many of whom were eventually diagnosed with neurosyphilis) in patients also infected with HIV, a 23% failure rate for ceftriaxone was demonstrated using serological criteria for cure (18). A recent report describes continued CSF abnormality after 2 weeks of intravenous ceftriaxone therapy in an HIV-uninfected patient with a brainstem gumma. The CSF subsequently became normal after 3 weeks of high-dose intravenous penicillin (34).

Response to Therapy for Neurosyphilis

Serum Nontreponemal Antibody Titers

Little information is available to guide decisions regarding adequacy or inadequacy of therapy for neurosyphilis. Romanowski and co-workers (74) conducted a careful retrospective study of serological response to currently accepted treatment for infectious syphilis. None of these patients had neurosyphilis, and all were presumed to be HIV uninfected. They found that serum RPR titers declined fourfold at 6 months and eightfold at 12 months after treatment for primary and secondary syphilis and fourfold at 12 months after therapy for early latent syphilis. The RPR titers dropped more rapidly in patients with higher pretreatment values and more slowly in those with a prior history of syphilis. A retrospective study from New York suggested that therapy for primary syphilis in HIV-infected patients was significantly less likely to result in "appropriate" declines in titer, a trend also seen in secondary syphilis (82). In contrast, a prospective study of injection drug users found no difference in serological response to therapy between HIV-infected and HIV-uninfected patients; however, more HIV-infected patients received higher than recommended doses of penicillin (25). Interestingly, a multicenter study of conventional therapy for early syphilis (2.4 MU IM benzathine penicillin G) versus enhanced therapy (conventional therapy plus amoxicillin, 2 g by mouth three times per day, with probenecid, 500

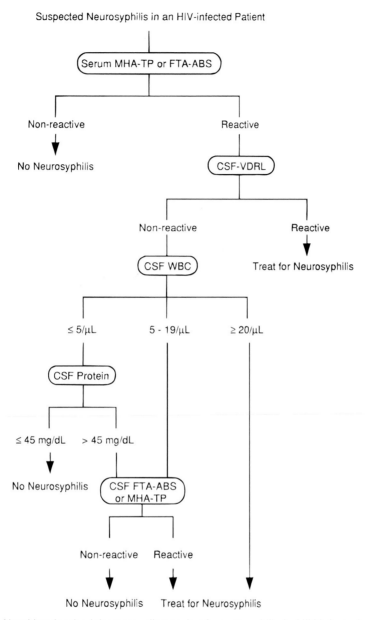

FIG. 3. Algorithm for the laboratory diagnosis of neurosyphilis in HIV-infected patients.

TABLE 2. *Centers for Disease Control and Prevention-recommended regimens for treatment of neurosyphilis*

Aqueous crystalline penicillin G, 2–4 million units intravenously every 4 h for 10–14 days
or
Procaine penicillin, 2.4 million units intramuscularly once daily, plus probenecid, 500 mg by mouth four times a day, both for 10–14 days

Some experts recommend following therary for neurosyphilis with intramuscular benzathine penicillin G, 2.4 million units weekly for 3 weeks.

mg by mouth three times per day for 14 days) showed a trend toward better serological response (as defined by decline in titer) in both HIV-infected and HIV-uninfected patients after enhanced therapy (73). This observation raises further concerns about the adequacy of benzathine penicillin therapy in both HIV-infected and HIV-uninfected patients.

Few studies have examined serological response after therapy for latent and neurosyphilis. The CDC guidelines (11) state that after therapy for latent syphilis serum nontreponemal titers should not increase fourfold, or a pretreatment titer of $\geq 1:32$ should decline fourfold at 12 to 24 months. In a Brazilian study of 62 presumed HIV-uninfected patients with symptomatic neurosyphilis treated with 5 MU IV penicillin G every 6 hours for 15 to 30 days ($n = 55$) or 4 MU IV every 4 hours for 20 days ($n = 7$), serum Wassermann was still reactive in 10 of 11 (91%) patients 2 years after therapy (69).

In the pre-HIV era, serum nontreponemal titer did not always reflect activity of CNS disease (29). This observation has been recently exemplified in case reports of HIV-infected (7) and at-risk (4) individuals treated for early syphilis who had appropriate initial declines in serum nontreponemal antibody titers despite subsequent development of symptomatic neurosyphilis.

Serum Treponemal Antibodies

Treponemal antibody tests, such as the MHA-TP and FTA-ABS, generally remain reactive after therapy and are considered to be good indicators of prior syphilis. However, seroreversion of these tests to nonreactive has been observed, usually in patients with first-episode primary syphilis (74). Haas and co-workers (28) showed that seroreversion of serum FTA-ABS or MHA-TP after therapy was more common in HIV-infected (13 of 90,14.4%) than HIV-uninfected (0 of 19) patients, and was increasingly common with more advanced immunosuppression. Similar reports have followed (42,71). In contrast, a prospective study showed that loss of serum treponemal test reactivity was equally likely among HIV-infected and HIV-uninfected patients and did not correlate with stage of syphilis or degree of immunosuppression (25). It is important to emphasize that all reports of loss of treponemal test reactivity have occurred in individuals who had been treated for syphilis. No series has suggested such a high proportion of nonreactive treponemal tests in patients with active syphilis.

CSF Parameters

The CDC guidelines (11) recommend that CSF cell count, if initially elevated, should decline by 6 months after neurosyphilis therapy and should normalize by 2 years. No guidance is provided concerning the expected rate of normalization of elevated CSF protein concentration or reactive CSF-VDRL. In the study from Brazil (69), CSF cell counts were normal in 23 of 27 patients (85%) at 3 to 6 months after therapy, but CSF protein was normal in only 13 of 29 (45%). The CSF Wassermann was still reactive in 9 of 10 patients (90%) 19 to 24 months after treatment (69). In a retrospective study of 16 HIV-infected and 14 HIV-uninfected patients with neurosyphilis treated with either CDC-recommended penicillin regimen, CSF cells and protein were normal in 95% of patients by 8 months, and CSF-VDRL became nonreactive in 95% of patients at 10 months after therapy. Time to normalization of CSF white blood cell count was longer in HIV-infected compared to HIV-uninfected patients, but time to normalization of protein level and CSF-VDRL reactivity was similar in the groups (50).

Clinical Parameters

Although it has never been extensively studied, high-dose IV penicillin is assumed to be effective therapy for neurosyphilis in HIV-infected patients. As discussed above, it can be difficult to define failure of therapy based on serum or CSF criteria because standards have not been established. Development of new neurological abnormalities after therapy may be a more unequivocal indication of failure. Feraru et al. (20) described an HIV-infected patient that developed syphilitic polyradiculopathy 7 weeks after a 9-day course of 24 MU/day IV aqueous penicillin G. Katz and co-workers (46) describe two HIV-infected patients who developed progressive neurological symptoms and worsening CSF parameters 4 and 6 months after treatment with high-dose IV aqueous penicillin G. In a study of seven HIV-infected patients with symptomatic neurosyphilis treated with high-dose IV penicillin, two failed therapy based on increases in serum RPR and worsening CSF parameters (including CSF VDRL reactivity), and one failed clinically with meningovascular syphilis 6 months after therapy (24). These reports suggest that, similar to therapy for early syphilis in HIV-infected patients, therapy for neurosyphilis in this population is less likely to be successful based on clinical and laboratory criteria.

CONCLUSIONS AND RECOMMENDATIONS

Much of the information on interactions between HIV and syphilis is based upon case reports and retrospective series. Despite the limitations of such data, there is compelling evidence that neurosyphilis and ocular syphilis are more likely to develop in HIV-infected persons after standard therapy for early syphilis. Combined with results from animal models, case reports give weight to the contention that HIV-infected patients with syphilis may have more severe cutaneous manifestations of early syphilis and sometimes may not develop a "normal" antibody response to early infection. In addition, accumulating evidence suggests that, as in therapy for early syphilis, standard therapy for neurosyphilis may not be sufficient for cure in HIV-infected patients.

Until more definitive studies can be performed, the following recommendations are offered:

1. All patients infected with HIV who have evidence of current or prior syphilis should undergo CSF examination. Patients with CSF pleocytosis or a reactive CSF-VDRL should be treated for neurosyphilis. In equivocal cases, nonreactivity of CSF treponemal tests can be used to exclude the diagnosis of neurosyphilis (Fig. 3).

2. The serum VDRL or RPR should be considered to be an imperfect screening test. Patients with nonreactive serum nontreponemal tests but clinical findings suggestive of cutaneous, ocular, or neurological syphilis should undergo intensive investigation. This includes repeat serological tests with exclusion of a prozone phenomenon, identification of *T. pallidum* in clinical specimens by dark-field micros-

copy, immunofluorescence staining or PCR, and biopsy with histological examination.

3. After treatment for neurosyphilis in HIV-infected patients, serum nontreponemal tests should be obtained monthly for the first 3 months and then every 3 to 6 months until nonreactive or repeatedly reactive at a titer of $\leq 1:8$. The CSF should be reexamined at 3 months after therapy and every 6 months thereafter until normal.

Criteria for retreatment include a fourfold increase in serum nontreponemal titer, worsening of CSF pleocytosis at 6 months or later, increase in CSF-VDRL titer, worsening of existing neurological symptoms or signs, or development of new neurological symptoms or signs.

ACKNOWLEDGMENTS

This work was supported in part by a grant from the National Institute of Neurological Diseases and Stroke (NS 01529). The author thanks Sheila A. Lukehart for valuable assistance in preparing this chapter.

REFERENCES

1. Altshuler L, Karpinos BD, Leifer W, Ozog JJ. Efficacy of penicillin treatment of early syphilis in the army. *Am J Syph* 1949;33:126–138.
2. Appleman ME, Marshall DW, Brey RL, et al. Cerebrospinal fluid abnormalities in patients without AIDS who are seropositive for the human immunodeficiency virus. *J Infect Dis* 1988;158:193–199.
3. Bauer TJ, Price EV, Cutler JC. Spinal fluid examinations among patients with primary or secondary syphilis. *Am J Syph* 1952;36:309–318.
4. Bayne LL, Schmidley JW, Goodin DS. Acute syphilitic meningitis. Its occurrence after clinical and serological cure of secondary syphilis with penicillin G. *Arch Neurol* 1986;43:137–138.
5. Berger JR. Neurosyphilis in human immunodeficiency virus type 1-seropositive individuals. A prospective study. *Arch Neurol* 1991;48:700–702.
6. Berger JR, Waskin H, Pall L, Hensley G, Ihmedian I, Post MJD. Syphilitic cerebral gumma with HIV infection. *Neurology* 1992;42:1282–1287.
7. Berry CD, Hooton TM, Collier AC, Lukehart SA. Neurological relapse after benzathine penicillin therapy for secondary syphilis in a patient with HIV infection. *N Engl J Med* 1987;316:1587–1589.
8. Brandon WR, Boulos LM, Morse A. Determining the prevalence of neurosyphilis in a cohort co-infected with HIV. *Int J STD AIDS* 1993;4:99–101.
9. Burke JM, Schaberg DR. Neurosyphilis in the antibiotic era. *Neurology* 1985;35:1368–1371.
10. Caumes E, Janier M, Janssen F, Feyeux C, Vignon-Pennamen MD, Morel P. Acquired syphilis during human immunodeficiency virus infection. 6 cases. *Presse Med* 1990;19:369–371.
11. Centers for Disease Control and Prevention. 1993 Sexually transmitted diseases treatment guidelines. *Morb Mortal Wkly Rep* 1993;42:27–46.
12. Chesney AM, Kemp JE. Incidence of *Spirochaeta pallida* in cerebrospinal fluid during early stage of syphilis. *JAMA* 1924;83:1725–1728.
13. Davis LE, Sperry S. The CSF-FTA test and the significance of blood contamination. *Ann Neurol* 1979;6:68–69.
14. Dawson S, Evans BA, Lawrence AG. Benign tertiary syphilis and HIV infection. *AIDS* 1988;2:315–316.
15. De Rie MA, Mekkes JR, Cohen EB, Hulsebosch HJ. Syphilis maligna: a HIV-related problem? *Br J Dermatol* 1991;125:390–391.
16. DiNubile MJ, Baxter JD, Mirsen TR. Acute syphilitic meningitis in a man with seropositivity for human immunodeficiency virus infection and normal numbers of CD4 lymphocytes. *Arch Intern Med* 1992;152:1324–1326.
17. Dooley DP, Tomski S. Syphilitic pneumonitis in an HIV-infected patient. *Chest* 1994;105:629–631.
18. Dowell ME, Ross PG, Musher DM, Cate TR, Baughn RE. Response of latent syphilis or neurosyphilis to ceftriaxone therapy in persons infected with human immunodeficiency virus. *Am J Med* 1992;93:481–488.
19. Esselink R, Enting R, Portegies P. Low-frequency of neurosyphilis in HIV-infected individuals (Letter). *Lancet* 1993;341:571.

20. Feraru ER, Aronow HA, Lipton RB. Neurosyphilis in AIDS patients: initial CSF VDRL may be negative. *Neurology* 1990;40:541–543.
21. Frederick WR, Delapenha R, Barnes S, Olopenia L, Saxinger C, Greaves W. Secondary syphilis and HIV infection. In: *Abstracts of the 28th Interscience Conference Antimicrobial Agents Chemotherapy*. Washington DC: American Society for Microbiology; 1988:320(abst).
22. Gass JD, Braunstein RA, Chenoweth RG. Acute syphilitic posterior placoid chorioretinitis. *Ophthalmology* 1990;97:1288–1297.
23. Glover RA, Piaquadio DJ, Kern S, Cockerell CJ. An unusual presentation of secondary syphilis in a patient with human immunodeficiency virus infection. A case report and review of the literature. *Arch Dermatol* 1992;128:530–534.
24. Gordon SM, Eaton ME, George R, et al. Response of symptomatic neurosyphilis to high-dose intravenous penicillin G in patients with human immunodeficiency virus infection. *N Engl J Med* 1994; 331:1469–1473.
25. Gourevich MN, Selwyn PA, Davenny K, et al. Effects of HIV infection on the serological manifestations and response to treatment of syphilis in intravenous drug users. *Ann Intern Med* 1993;118: 350–355.
26. Gregory N, Sanchez M, Buchness MR. The spectrum of syphilis in patients with human immunodeficiency virus infection. *J Am Acad Dermatol* 1990;22:1061–1067.
27. Gue J-W, Wang S-J, Lin Y-Y, Liao K-K, Wong W-W. Neurosyphilis presenting as tabes dorsalis in a HIV carrier. *Chin Med J* 1993;51:389–391.
28. Haas JS, Bolan G, Larsen SA, Clement MJ, Bacchetti P, Moss AR. Sensitivity of treponemal tests for detecting prior treated syphilis during human immunodeficiency virus infection. *J Infect Dis* 1990; 162:862–866.
29. Hahn RD, Clark EG, Felsovanyi A, Keisselbach M, Koteen H, Potter R. Asymptomatic neurosyphilis: prognosis. *Am J Syph Gonorrhea Vener Dis* 1946;30:513–548.
30. Hahn RD, Cutler JC, Curtis AC, et al. Penicillin treatment of asymptomatic central nervous system syphilis. II. Results of therapy as measured by laboratory findings. *Arch Dermatol* 1956;74:367–377.
31. Halperin LS. Neuroretinitis due to seronegative syphilis associated with human immunodeficiency virus. *J Clin Neuro-ophthalmol* 1992;12(3):171–172.
32. Hart G. Syphilis tests in diagnostic and therapeutic decision making. *Ann Intern Med* 1986;104: 368–376.
33. Hay PE, Tam FWK, Kitchen VS, Horner S, Bridger J, Weber J. Gummatous lesions in men infected with human immunodeficiency virus and syphilis. *Genitourin Med* 1990;66:374–379.
34. Herrold JM. A syphilitic cerebral gumma manifesting as a brain-stem mass lesion that responded to corticosteroid monotherapy. *Mayo Clin Proc* 1994;69:960–961.
35. Hicks CB, Benson PM, Lupton GP, Tramont EC. Seronegative secondary syphilis in a patient infected with the human immunodeficiency virus (HIV) with Kaposi sarcoma. A diagnostic dilemma. *Ann Intern Med* 1987;107:492–495.
36. Holtom PD, Larsen RA, Leal ME, Leedom JM. Prevalence of neurosyphilis in human immunodeficiency virus-infected patients with latent syphilis. *Am J Med* 1992;93:9–12.
37. Hook EW III, Baker-Zander SA, Moskovitz BL, Lukehart SA, Handsfield HH. Ceftriaxone therapy for asymptomatic neurosyphilis. Case report and western blot analysis of serum and cerebrospinal fluid IgG response to therapy. *Sex Transm Dis* 1986;13:185–188.
38. Hopkins HH. Prognostic import of a negative spinal fluid in early and in latent syphilis. *Arch Derm Syphilol* 1931;24:404–408.
39. Hutchinson CM, Rompalo AM, Reichart CA, Hook EW III. Characteristics of patients with syphilis attending Baltimore STD clinics. Multiple high-risk subgroups and interactions with human immunodeficiency virus infection. *Arch Intern Med* 1991;151:511–516.
40. Hutchinson CM, Hook EW III, Shepherd M, Verley J, Rompalo AM. Altered clinical presentation of early syphilis in patients with human immunodeficiency virus infection. *Ann Intern Med* 1994; 121:94–99.
41. Izzat NN, Bartruff JK, Glicksman JM, Holder WR, Knox JM. Validity of the VDRL test on cerebrospinal fluid contaminated by blood. *Br J Vener Dis* 1971;47:162–164.
42. Johnson PDR, Graves SR, Stewart L, Warren R, Dwyer B, Lucas CR. Specific syphilis serological tests may become negative in HIV infection. *AIDS* 1991;5:419–423.
43. Jurado RL, Campbell J, Martin PD. Prozone phenomenon in secondary syphilis. Has its time arrived? *Arch Intern Med* 1993;153:2496–2498.
44. Kastner RJ, Malone JL, Decker CF. Syphilitic osteitis in a patient with secondary syphilis and concurrent human immunodeficiency virus infection. *Clin Infect Dis* 1994;18:250–252.
45. Katz DA, Berger JR. Neurosyphilis in acquired immunodeficiency syndrome. *Arch Neurol* 1989;46: 895–898.
46. Katz DA, Berger JR, Duncan RC. Neurosyphilis. A comparative study of the effects of infection with human immunodeficiency virus. *Arch Neurol* 1993;50:243–249.
47. Kearns G, Pogrel MA, Honda G. Intraoral tertiary syphilis (gumma) in a human immunodeficiency virus-positive man: a case report. *J Oral Maxillofac Surg* 1993;51:85–88.

48. Lukehart SA, Hook EW III, Baker-Zander SA, Collier AC, Critchlow CW, Handsfield HH. Invasion of the central nervous system by *Treponema pallidum*: implications for diagnosis and therapy. *Ann Intern Med* 1988;109:855–862.
49. Marra CM, Handsfield HH, Kuller L, Morton WR, Lukehart SA. Alterations in the course of experimental syphilis associated with concurrent simian immunodeficiency virus infection. *J Infect Dis* 1992;165:1020–1025.
50. Marra CM, Longstreth WT Jr, Lukehart SA. Resolution of CSF abnormalities in neurosyphilis: influence of stage and HIV infection. *Neurology* 1992;42(Suppl 3):212(abst).
51. Marra CM, Slatter V, Tartaglione TA, Baker-Zander SA, Lukehart SA. Evaluation of aqueous penicillin G and ceftriaxone for experimental neurosyphilis [Letter]. *J Infect Dis* 1992;165:396–397.
52. Marra CM, Kuller L, Shaffer JM, Morton WR, Lukehart SA. The impact of SIV on the immunological response to syphilis. *Paper presented at IXth International Conference on AIDS IVth STD World Congress*, Berlin, Germany, June 7–11, 1993.
53. Marra CM, Critchlow CW, Hook EW III, Collier AC, Lukehart SA. Cerebrospinal fluid treponemal antibodies in untreated early syphilis. *Arch Neurol* 1995;52:68–72..
54. McLeish WM, Pulido JS, Holland S, Culbertson WW, Winward K. The ocular manifestations of syphilis in the human immunodeficiency virus type 1-infected host. *Ophthalmology* 1990;97:196–203.
55. Merritt HH, Adams RD, Solomon HC. *Neurosyphilis*. New York: Oxford; 1946.
56. Merritt HH, Moore M. Acute syphilitic meningitis. *Medicine (Baltimore)* 1935;14:119–183.
57. Mills CH. Routine examination of the cerebrospinal fluid in syphilis: its value in regard to more accurate knowledge, prognosis and treatment. *BMJ* 1927;2:527–532.
58. Mohr JA, Griffiths W, Jackson R, Saadah H, Bird P, Riddle J. Neurosyphilis and penicillin levels in cerebrospinal fluid. *JAMA* 1976;236:2208–2209.
59. Moore JE. Studies in asymptomatic neurosyphilis II. The classification, treatment, and prognosis of early asymptomatic neurosyphilis. *Bull Johns Hopkins Hosp* 1922;33:231–246.
60. Moore JE. The relation of neurorecurrences to late syphilis. A clinical study of eighty-one cases. *Arch Neurol Psychiatry* 1929;21:117–136.
61. Moore JE, Gieske M. Syphilitic iritis. A study of 249 patients. *Am J Ophthalmol* 1931;14:110–126.
62. Moore JE, Hopkins HH. Asymptomatic neurosyphilis VI. The prognosis of early and late asymptomatic neurosyphilis. *JAMA* 1930;95:1637–1641.
63. Moore JE, Kemp JE. The treatment of early syphilis II. Clinical results in 402 patients. *Bull Johns Hopkins Hosp* 1926;39:16–35.
64. Morgello S, Laufer H. Quaternary neurosyphilis (Letter). *New Engl J Med* 1988;319:1549–1550.
65. Morgello S, Laufer H. Quaternary neurosyphilis in a Haitian man with human immunodeficiency virus infection. *Hum Pathol* 1989;20:808–811.
66. Morrison RE, Harrison SM, Tramont EC. Oral amoxycillin, an alternative treatment for neurosyphilis. *Genitourin Med* 1985;61:359–362.
67. Musher DM, Hamill RJ, Baughn RE. Effect of human immunodeficiency virus (HIV) infection on the course of syphilis and on the response to treatment. *Ann Intern Med* 1990;113:872–881.
68. Musher DM. Syphilis, neurosyphilis, penicillin, and AIDS. *J Infect Dis* 1991;163:1201–1206.
69. Nitrini R, Spina-França A. Penicilinoterapia intravenosa em altas doses na neurossífilis. Estudo de 62 casos. II. Avaliç o do líqüido cefalorraqueano. *Arquivos de Neuro-psiquiatria* 1987;45:231–241.
70. O'Farrell N, Thin RN. Neurosyphilis and HIV (Letter). *Lancet* 1993;341:1224.
71. Puppin D, Janier M, Strazzi S, Morel P. HIV infection and loss of treponemal test reactivity (Letter). *Acta Derm Venereol Stockh* 1992;72:313.
72. Ravaut P. Le liquide céphalo-rachidien des syphiliques en période secondaire. *Ann Dermatol Syphiligr* 1903;4:537–554.
73. Rolfs R, Gold M, Hackett K, et al. Treatment of early syphilis in HIV-infected and HIV-uninfected patients—preliminary report of the Syphilis & HIV Study Group (abstract PO-B11-1534). *Paper presented at IXth International Conference on AIDS IVth STD World Congress*, Berlin, Germany, June 7–11, 1993.
74. Romanowski B, Sutherland R, Fick GH, Mooney D, Love EJ. Serological response to treatment of infectious syphilis. *Ann Intern Med* 1991;114:1005–1009.
75. Savall R, Cabré M, Grifol M. Neurosyphilis and human immunodeficiency virus type 2 infection (Letter). *Arch Neurol* 1992;49:440.
76. Savall R, Valls F, Cabré M. Syphilis and HIV infection (Letter). *Genitourin Med* 1991;67:353.
77. Shulkin D, Tripoli L, Abell E. Lues maligna in a patient with human immunodeficiency virus infection. *Am J Med* 1988;85:425–427.
78. Smith JL, Byrne SF, Cambron CR. Syphiloma/gumma of the optic nerve and human immunodeficiency virus seropositivity. *J Clin Neuroophthalmol* 1990;10:175–184.
79. Sparling PF. Diagnosis and treatment of syphilis. *N Engl J Med* 1971;284;642–653.
80. Stokes JH, Beerman H, Ingraham NR. Modern clinical syphilology. *Diagnosis, treatment, case study*. Philadelphia: WB Saunders; 1944.
81. Strobel M, Beauclair Ph, Lacave J. Seronegative syphilis in AIDS (Letter). *Presse Med* 1989;18:1440.

82. Telzak EE, Zweig Greenberg MS, Harrison J, Stoneburner RL, Schultz S. Syphilis treatment response in HIV-infected individuals. *AIDS* 1991;5:591–595.
83. Tikjøb G, Russel M, Petersen CS, Gerstoft J, Kobayashi T. Seronegative secondary syphilis in a patient with AIDS: identification of *Treponema pallidum* in biopsy specimen. *J Am Acad Dermatol* 1991;24:506–508.
84. Tomberlin MG, Holtom PD, Owens JL, Larsen RA. Evaluation of neurosyphilis in human immunodeficiency virus-infected individuals. *Clin Infect Dis* 1994;18:288–294.
85. Tosca A, Stavropoulos PG, Hatziolou E, et al. Malignant syphilis in HIV-infected patients. *Int J Dermatol* 1990;29:575–577.
86. Tramont EC. Persistence of *Treponema pallidum* following penicillin therapy. Report of two cases. *JAMA* 1976;236:2206–2207.
87. Tseng CK, Hughes MA, Hsu P-L, Mahoney S, Duvic M, Sell S. Syphilis superinfection activates expression of human immunodeficiency virus 1 in latently infected rabbits. *Am J Pathol* 1991;138:1149–1164.
88. Whiteside Yim C, Flynn NM, Fitzgerald FT. Penetration of oral doxycycline into the cerebrospinal fluid of patients with latent or neurosyphilis. *Antimicrob Agents Chemother* 1985;28:347–348.
89. Wile UJ, Stokes JH. A study of the spinal fluid with reference to involvement of the nervous system in secondary syphilis. *J Cutan Dis* 1914;32:607–623.
90. Wolters EC. Neurosyphilis: a changing diagnostic problem? *Eur Neurol* 1987;26:23–28.
91. Zisfein J, DiPietro D, Lugo-Torres O. CSF Venereal Disease Research Laboratory in neurologically asymptomatic HIV-infected patients with serological evidence for syphilis. *Ann Neurol* 1993;34:283(abst).

AIDS and the Nervous System, Second Edition,
edited by J. R. Berger and R. M. Levy.
Lippincott-Raven Publishers, Philadelphia © 1997.

27

Other Opportunistic Infections

Harry Hollander

University of California, San Francisco, California 94143

Since the early series of neurological complications described the prevalence of common opportunistic infections (50,53,78), numerous clinical and pathological reports have documented other nervous system infections in human immunodeficiency virus (HIV) infected individuals. Many of these reports are anecdotal, and some of the secondary infections almost certainly represent a chance occurrence in an HIV-infected patient. The other problem in discerning the role of HIV is that some individuals have had other risk factors for unusual infections such as injection drug use. Nevertheless, enough data exist to conclude that many of the infections discussed in this chapter are truly associated with HIV infection. In the nervous system, opportunism is manifested by a higher incidence of neurological involvement than in other hosts and/or a presentation of clinical illness that is modified by the immunodeficiency of HIV. Unlike toxoplasmosis and progressive multifocal leukoencephalopathy (PML), where neurological problems occur in isolation, many of the less common infections present with significant simultaneous extraneural involvement. Table 1 reviews the organ system involvement of these infections. Table 2 summarizes current therapeutic options.

VIRAL INFECTION

In postmortem studies, opportunistic viral infections are common in patients dying of acquired immunodeficiency syndrome (AIDS) related complications. Cytomegalovirus (CMV) is the most common infection, occurring up to 66% of the time and causing widespread organ system involvement. Other herpesviruses, JC virus, and adenovirus may also be found at a much lower frequency (64). In neuropathological series, CMV is also the most common postmortem finding, with a frequency of infection of approximately 25% (63). In comparison, histological evidence of other viral infections is found in fewer than 7% of brains.

Herpes Simplex

Although there have been case reports of myelitis due to herpes simplex virus (HSV) (34), encephalitis may be a more common central nervous sytem (CNS) complication in HIV-infected adults. Levy et al. suggested that HSV encephalitis occurred in approximately 3% of patients with neurological complications, or, by

TABLE 1. *Extraneural manifestations of uncommon CNS infections*

Finding	Organism
Skin lesions	Herpesviruses
	Nocardia species
	Bartonella (formerly *Rochalimaea*) species
	Blastomyces dermatiditis
	Sporothrix schenckii
Pulmonary infiltrates	*Nocardia* species
	Mycobacterium tuberculosis
	Mycobacterium kansasii
	Coccidioides imitis
	Histoplasma capsulatum
	B. dermatiditis
	Aspergillus species
Hepatosplenomegaly	*Bartonella* species
	M. tuberculosis
	Mycobacterium avium complex
	H. capsulatum
Cardiomyopathy	*Trypanosoma cruzi*
Arthritis	*S. schenckii*
Lytic bone lesions	*Bartonella* species

extrapolation, in about 1% of all patients with advanced HIV disease that they studied (50). This is a higher frequency than has been reported in other premortem series. In general, the clinical presentation of HSV encephalitis in HIV-coinfected patients cannot be differentiated from that seen in seronegative adults, but several anecdotes suggest that a more fulminant course may be seen with HIV coinfection. While most cases have been caused by HSV-1, several cases of HSV-2 encephalitis have also been reported. One unique feature seen in several cases is HSV and CMV coinfection leading to an intense ventriculitis; this subset of patients may have more cranial nerve findings than usual (46,58). As in seronegative patients, diagnosis of HSV encephalitis may be difficult without brain biopsy. The small number of reported cases does not allow definitive conclusions about the CSF profile, but the sensitivity of CSF viral culture appears to be low. Small series using polymerase chain reaction (PCR) assays show an improved sensitivity of 75% to 100%, but few HIV-seropositive cases have been studied (7,55,83). One radiological report suggests that typical temporal lobe enhancement may be less common in the setting of HIV coinfection (85). Since imaging studies and cerebrospinal fluid (CSF) diagnostic tests are imperfect, clinicians are faced with difficult choices regarding brain biopsy versus empiric therapy in individuals who present with a febrile encephalopathy in the setting of HIV infection. An additional complicating factor is the recent documentation of HSV encephalitis caused by an acyclovir-resistant strain of HSV (26).

Varicella-Zoster Virus

Dermatomal Herpes zoster infection is strongly correlated with HIV infection (13). By the time HIV causes advanced immunodeficiency, approximately 25% of infected individuals will have had at least one bout of cutaneous zoster (28). In the context of this high prevalence of disease, neurological complications of zoster remain quite uncommon and probably occur at a significantly lower rate than in other immunocompromised hosts. The reasons for this are unknown. In contrast, ocular complications

TABLE 2. *Therapy of less common neurologic infections*

Organism/Syndrome	Therapy
Herpes simplex encephalitis	Acyclovir, 10 mg/kg i.v. q8h, 10–14 days[a]
Herpes zoster encephalitis/myelitis	Acyclovir, 10 mg/kg i.v. q8h, 10–14 days
Adenovirus encephalitis	None known
Bacterial meningitis	Empirically, ampicillin, 2 g i.v. q4–6 h, plus a third-generation cephalosporin (e.g., cefotaxime), 2 g i.v. q4h, then narrow regimen based upon isolates and sensitivities, 10–14 days[b]
Nocardia brain abscess	Trimethoprim, 5 mg/kg i.v. q12h, plus sulfamethoxazole, 25 mg/kg i.v. q12h (fixed combination), 4–6 weeks, followed by maintenance trimethoprim, 160 mg, plus sulfamethoxazole, 800 mg, p.o., q12h indefinitely[c]
Cerebral bacillary angiomatosis	Clarithromycin, 500–1000 mg p.o. q12h, with/without rifampin, 600 mg p.o. q.d. (optimum regimen and duration of therapy unknown)
Mycobacterium tuberculosis meniningitis or mass lesion	Isoniazid, 300–600 mg p.o. q.d., plus rifampin, 600 mg p.o. q.d., plus ethambutol, 15–25 mg/kg p.o. q.d., plus pyrazinamide, 25 mg/kg p.o. q.d., pending sensitivities for at least 12 months
Mycobacterium kansasii brain abscess or meningitis	Isoniazid, 300 p.o. q.d., plus rifampin, 600 mg p.o., q.d., plus ethambutol, 15–25 mg/kg p.o. a.d., pending sensitivities for a 9-month total course
Mycobacterium avium complex meningitis	Consider clarithromycin, 500–1000 mg p.o. q12h, plus ethambutol, 15 mg/kg p.o. q.d., plus rifampin, 600 mg p.o. q.d., plus ciprofloxacin, 500–750 mg p.o. q12h, indefinitely[e]
CNS histoplasmosis	Amphotericin-B, 0.6–0.8 mg/kg i.v. q.d. to a total dose of 2.0–2.5 g, then maintenance with itraconazole, 200–400 mg p.o. q.d., indefinitely
Coccidioides meningitis	Amphotericin-B, 0.6 mg/kg i.v. q.d. to a total dose of at 2.5 g, then maintenance with weekly amphotericin, 1 mg/kg i.v., or fluconazole, 200 mg p.o. q.d., indefinitely[f]
CNS aspergillosis	Amphotericin-B, 0.8–1.0 mg/kg i.v. q.d. (optimum duration of therapy unknown)[g]
Strongyloides hyperinfection syndrome	Thiabendazole, 25 mg/kg p.o. q.d. for 3–7 days, plus broad-spectrum antibiotics i.v. for secondary bacterial infection (e.g., meningitis, pneumonia)
Trypanosoma cruzi encephalitis or mass lesion	Benznidazole, 5 mg/kg p.o. q.d. for 30 days[h]

[a] If herpes simplex virus encephalitis occurs despite chronic acyclovir prophylaxis, consider foscarnet, 40 mg/kg i.v. q8h as an alternative.

[b] For *Listeria*, add gentamicin, 1 mg/kg i.v. q8h, to ampicillin. Pneumococci must be tested for penicillin resistance.

[c] In patients intolerant of this regimen, imipenem, minocycline, and third-generation cephalosporins are in general the most active alternative agents, but susceptibility testing should be done if possible.

[d] If multidrug-resistant *M. tuberculosis* is suspected, consider adding at least two of the following—ofloxacin, cycloserine, streptomycin, or ethionamide. The role of adjunctive corticosteroids is unclear in the setting of human immunodeficiency virus (HIV) infection. Many tuberculomas need neurosurgical evacuation.

[e] Efficacy in CNS disease is unknown.

[f] High risk patients may need the addition of intraventricular amphotericin-B 1–5 mg weekly to control disease. Some selected low risk patients may be treated with fluconazole 200–400 mg p.o. q12 hr.

[g] Addition of rifampin, 600 mg p.o. q.d., is advocated by some investigators but clinically unproven. Consider adjunctive filgrastim (GCSF) if absolute neurophil count is <500 mm^{-3}.

[h] Not available in United States.

of cervicofacial zoster are common. Retrospective series suggest that acute retinal necrosis occurs as a sequela of ophthalmic zoster 20% of the time. This complication is also seen at a lower frequency when zoster occurs in more distant dermatomes (39,71).

Radiculitis secondary to zoster and/or postherpetic neuralgia are commonly represented in large series of neurological complications (50,53) and account for a significant percentage of HIV-seropositive patients who present for evaluation of pain (76).

The CNS complications of zoster are rare in this setting; encephalitis is the most common of these complications. Clinically, this entity is pleomorphic, with both acute and chronic zoster encephalitis described (27,35,70). The temporal relationship to dermatomal zoster has also varied. Cases have occurred in the absence of cutaneous lesions, but most have occurred contemporaneously with skin lesions, or days to months after the resolution of lesions. Pathologically, multifocal necrosis, demyelination, and intranuclear Cowdry type A inclusions are seen. Another histological feature noted in several cases is a vasculopathy involving medium-sized leptomeningeal vessels associated with areas of cortical and subcortical infarction. This histology is identical to the isolated vasculopathy that causes contralateral hemiplegia after ophthalmic zoster, a previously recognized syndrome which has also been described in at least one HIV-infected individual (15). Other reported CNS complications of zoster include optic neuritis, cranial nerve palsies, aseptic meningitis, and myelitis (8,17,40,88).

Diagnosis of CNS zoster remains problematic using traditional noninvasive techniques. It is very rare to culture the virus from CSF (19). Preliminary studies suggest that PCR assays will increase the sensitivity (65,75). However, even with this technology, two of five patients with zoster-associated meningitis had false-negative results, and the sensitivity for encephalitis may be even lower. Since active viral replication contributes to some neurological complications of zoster, antiviral therapy is appropriate, although the efficacy is unknown. When neuropathology suggests predominantly a parainfectious immune-mediated process, the benefit of antivirals is doubtful, and the role of immunosuppressive agents in these immunocompromised patients is unknown.

Adenovirus

Finally, adenovirus has been described as an uncommon cause of encephalitis in HIV-infected adults and children (5,86). There were no clinical or radiographic features that differentiated these cases from other secondary viral encephalitides.

BACTERIAL INFECTION

Pneumococcus

Pyogenic bacterial infections have been increasingly noted over the course of the HIV epidemic, and these infections may precede the onset of severe immunodeficiency (89). Invasive disease, particularly pneumonia, caused by *Pneumococcus* and *Haemophilus infuenzae*, occurs much more commonly in HIV-seropositive individuals than in seronegative, age-matched controls (72,81). Futhermore, in the case of pneumococcal pneumonia, HIV-infected patients with this complication have a rate of bacteremia that exceeds 50% (66). It is therefore somewhat surprising that bacterial meningitis remains a very rare event in this population. In one African study, HIV serostatus did not correlate with the risk of meningitis in a cohort of patients with serious pneumococcal disease (60). However, in this series, the small number of patients with pneumococcal meningitis and HIV infection had a significantly higher mortality than HIV-seronegative controls with meningitis. Pneumococcal brain abscess has also been described (68), but the combined anecdotal data do not support a claim of a higher incidence of CNS complications when HIV-infected individuals develop serious infections with encapsulated pathogens.

Listeria

Neurological infections may also be caused by nonpyogenic bacteria. *Listeria monocytogenes* infection is markedly increased in prevalence in HIV-infected individuals. In a population-based study, there was a 60- to 120-fold increase in disease frequency compared to the control metropolitan population (44). Listeriosis can precede the diagnosis of other opportunistic infections, but most cases occur in people with advanced HIV disease. Approximately half of HIV-infected patients with listeriosis will have CNS complications. Of these patients, meningitis is found in 90% and brain abscess in the remainder (10). *Listeria* meningitis has a higher rate of brainstem involvement and cranial neuropathies than other bacterial meningitides. As in other immunocompromised hosts, the mortality from *Listeria* meningitis is approximately 30%.

Salmonella and Other Bacteria

Salmonella infection in HIV-infected individuals is often accompanied by bacteremia (49,57). *Salmonella* meningitis and brain abscess have been reported and probably occur as a result of bacteremia (24,74). *Nocardia* is a classic opportunistic pathogen in individuals with defective cellular mediated immunity, but until recently, it was not commonly reported in individuals with HIV infection. Since 1990, there have been several reports of intracerebral mass lesions caused by *Nocardia*, usually accompanied by pleuropulmonary or disseminated disease (41,43,45,46). Therapy is complicated by the high frequency of adverse reactions to trimethoprim-sulfamethoxazole in HIV-infected patients.

Finally, there has been one report of intracerebral mass lesions caused by *Bartonella* (fomerly *Rochalimaea*), the etiological genus of cutaneous bacillary angiomatosis (80). Since the histology of this vascular lesion may be confused with that of Kaposi's sarcoma (KS), it is interesting to speculate about whether the rare reported cases of "intracerebral KS" actually represent misdiagnosed bacillary angiomatosis. In addition to the presence of large numbers of bacilli on Warthin-Starry staining, lesions of bacillary angiomatosis have several histological features which differentiate it from KS. These include the presence of clusters of neutrophils, basophilic granular material, and histiocytoid rather than spindle-shaped endothelial cells.

MYCOBACTERIAL INFECTION

Tuberculosis has become an increasingly common problem in HIV-infected persons, and extrapulmonary involvement is seen in 60% of cases (77). In patients with HIV-related tuberculosis, positive CSF cultures are obtained 3% to 10% of the time (9,77). Given the difficulty of culturing this organism from CSF, this implies an even higher rate of CNS involvement. Tuberculous meningitis is the most common CNS complication and typically presents as a subacute meningitis. Headache and fever are noted in the majority of cases, with encephalopathy also common, particularly if there is elevated intracranial pressure. Cranial nerve abnormalities and frank meningeal signs are less common. The CSF formula usually demonstrates a lymphocytic pleocytosis with a total cell count in the range of 200 to 500/mm^3; hypoglycorrhachia is also commonly observed. Two large series suggest that the clinical presentation, overall CSF profile, and prognosis are identical in patients with and without HIV infection (9,20), although these authors and others note that a significant minority of patients with HIV-related CNS tuberculosis may present with acellular CSF (47). The only difference betweeen seropositive and seronegative patients is an increased incidence of intracerebral mass lesions in the HIV-infected group (60% versus 14%) (20). However, not all of these mass lesions were proven to be tuberculous, and the presence of lesions did not correlate with focal neurological findings or mortality.

Isolated CNS tuberculomas may present without concomitant tuberculous meningitis. Their characteristics on cerebral imaging studies have varied; some appear as ring-enhancing lesions while others are hypodense and nonenhancing (1,12,52). Medical therapy alone has been successful in a few of the reported cases. Spinal cord tuberculoma has also been reported (54). Paradoxical expansion of intracranial tuberculomas occurs commonly during antituberculous therapy and may be accompanied by neurological deterioration (2). Adjunctive corticosteroids appear to ameliorate this reaction, which probably occurs when lysis of organisms causes an inflammatory response.

Finally, anecdotal evidence suggests that CNS tuberculosis may be more common when initial antituberculous therapy has failed, when there is a relapse of disease, or when multidrug-resistant organisms cause disease (21,59). Diagnosis of CNS tuberculosis is still difficult because of the lack of rapid diagnostic tests. Polymerase chain reaction based techniques are being studied for this purpose. Thus, therapy is most often begun empirically and should be aggressive, with at least four drugs initiated, especially in regions such as New York City and Miami, which have a high incidence of drug resistance (22,27). Apart from their usage in the setting of an enlarging tuberculoma, there are no data regarding glucocorticoids in the treatment of tuberculous meningitis uncomplicated by a mass lesion. Prednisone is routinely used in patients with moderate to severe *Pneumocystis carinii* pneumonia and does not seem to cause a short-term increase in other opportunistic infections, but how to translate these observations into recommendations for tuberculous meningitis is unclear.

Nontuberculous mycobacterial CNS infections have also been described. *Mycobacterium avium* complex has been isolated from CSF, usually in patients with widely disseminated infection. The significance is unclear since the patients generally did not have signs and symptoms of meningitis, although a mild lymphocytic pleocytosis was often present (42). Cases of *Mycobacterium kansasii* brain abscess and meningitis have also been described, with or without concurrent pulmonary infection with this organism (11,31).

FUNGAL INFECTION

In addition to cryptococcal meningitis, other CNS fungal infections have been increasingly reported. Most commonly, these are complications of the endemic fungal infections, but nonendemic mycoses have also been described.

Histoplasmosis

Disseminated histoplasmosis is a common complication of HIV disease in the midwestern United States, occurring in over 25% of patients with advanced HIV disease (87). Since this diagnosis may occur years to decades after exposure, a detailed travel history is an important component of the evaluation of an HIV-infected individual with unexplained CNS disease. Central nervous system involvement occurs in 5% to 20% of cases and portends a poor prognosis, with a mortality rate of over 60% (4,87). In these patients, *Histoplasma capsulatum* may produce meningitis, brain abcesses, or both (4,14). The diagnosis of *Histoplasma* meningitis is hampered by nonspecific CSF findings, a low rate of positive cultures from CSF, and insensitive serological tests; however, the diagnostic yield can be improved by utilizing a *Histoplasma* polysaccharide antigen assay (87). The majority of the patients have other organ system involvement, and the presence of diffuse, reticulonodular pulmonary infiltrates should prompt consideration of histoplasmosis, as well as other fungal and mycobacterial diseases. In one case, *Histoplasma* meningitis persisted as an isolated sequela of otherwise successfully treated disseminated disease (84).

Coccidioidomycosis

Coccidioidomycosis is another common mycosis in HIV-infected people residing in desert southwestern regions of the United States and northern Mexico. Analogous to histoplasmosis, the longitudinal incidence of this complication exceeds 25% in the endemic area over the course of HIV disease (3). Most cases occur when the CD4 + count has fallen below 200 cells/mm^3. Approximately 12% of patients with HIV-associated coccidioidomycosis have been diagnosed with coccidioidal meningitis, an incidence of CNS disease that is much higher than in HIV-seronegative adults with coccidioidomycosis (23). The HIV seropositivity does not seem to influence the clinical presentation, CSF findings, or response to therapy (25). There is no evidence that race and sex are important determinants of disseminated disease in HIV-infected individuals with coccidioidomycosis. Unlike CNS histoplasmosis, the majority of HIV-infected patients with coccidioidal meningitis will have disease limited to the CNS. Diagnosis depends either upon the isolation of *Coccidiodes imitis* from CSF or positive complement fixation serologies in CSF and serum. In the setting of HIV infection, false-negative serum complement fixation titers may occur, although this phenomenon is much more common with isolated pulmonary disease (23).

Blastomycosis

Blastomycosis, an infection predominantly seen in the southeastern United States, can also behave aggressively when there is HIV coinfection. Blastomycosis is usually a late complication, with most patients having had prior AIDS-defining opportunistic illnesses. Approximately half of the cases described have disseminated disease; of these, 40% have had meningitis, diagnosed by culturing *Blastomyces dermatiditis* from CSF (37,61). The number of reported cases is small, and mortality is high, whether or not CNS involvement is present.

Sporotrichosis

The other dimorphic yeast that may rarely cause CNS complications in these immunocompromised hosts is *Sporothrix schenckii*. This organism is a ubiquitous soil pathogen, and cases have been described in diverse geographical areas. With advanced HIV disease, a subacute or chonic meningitis may occur as part of a syndrome of disseminated sporotrichosis. Other clinical findings include cutaneous lesions, endophthalmitis, and a polyarticular arthritis. In the few cases that have been described, the outcome was poor (38,62).

Aspergillosis

Finally, aspergillosis has become an increasingly important opportunistic infection in patients with very advanced HIV disease and CD4+ counts of 50 cells/mm^3 or less (18,51). Pulmonary infiltrates are the most common manifestation, but dissemination or direct extension with CNS involvement have also been seen. A single brain abscess is the most typical CNS lesion, but other patterns of involvement have included basilar meningitis secondary to *Aspergillus* sinusitis and spinal epidural abscess (16,30,33). There is no convincing evidence of an association between HIV infection and other invasive opportunistic molds such as *Rhizopus* or *Pseudallescheria* species.

PARASITIC INFECTION

With the exception of CNS toxoplasmosis, parasitic CNS infections are quite uncommon. Most appear in the literature as isolated case reports. Examples of these unusual complications include reports of amebic meningoencephalitis caused by *Acanthamoeba* or leptomyxid amebas (6,32), gram-negative bacterial meningitis secondary to the *Strongyloides* hyperinfection syndrome (36,56), and neurocysticercosis (82).

There has been a cluster of reports regarding unusual CNS manifestations of Chagas' disease in HIV-infected individuals from areas endemic for *Trypanosoma cruzi* (29,67,69,79). These cases presumably represent reactivation of trypanosomal infection, as several occurred years after individuals had left the endemic area. Presentations have included encephalitis, meningoencephalitis, and intracerebral mass lesions. At least one of the reported cases responded to medical therapy (67).

CONCLUSIONS

While the major opportunistic pathogens continue to account for the majority of CNS infections in an HIV-infected cohort, a wide array of less common agents is causing increasing neurological morbidity and mortality. Human immunodeficiency virus coinfection can strikingly increase the incidence of CNS involvement by infections such as tuberculosis and histoplasmosis. A thorough travel history is now essential in HIV-infected individuals presenting with new neurological problems, since geographically limited endemic infections have become more common explanations for these problems. Consideration of unusual infections is extremely important since many of them are treatable (see Table 2) and because they may entirely mimic the clinical and radiographic manifestations of more common opportunistic processes.

REFERENCES

1. Abos J, Graus F, Miro JM, et al. Intracranial tuberculomas in patients with AIDS. *AIDS* 1991;5: 461–462.
2. Afghani B, Liberman JM. Paradoxical enlargement or development of intracranial tuberculomas during therapy: case report and review. *Clin Infect Dis* 1994;19:1092–1099.
3. Ampel NM, Dols CL, Galgiani JN. Coccidioidomycosis during human immunodeficiency virus infection: results of a prospective study in a coccidioidal endemic area. *Am J Med* 1993;94:235–240.
4. Anaissie E, Fainstein V, Samo T, Bodey GP, Sarosi GA. Central nervous system histoplasmosis. An unappreciated complication of the acquired immunodeficiency syndrome. *Am J Med* 1988;84: 215–217.
5. Anders KH, Park CS, Cornford ME, Vinters HV. Adenovirus encephalitis and widespread ependymitis in a child with AIDS. *Pediatr Neurosurg* 1990–1991;16:316–320.
6. Anzil A, Rao C, Wrzolek M, et al. Amebic meningoencephalitis in a patient with AIDS caused by a newly recognized opportunistic pathogen. *Arch Pathol Lab Med* 1991;115:21–25.
7. Aslanzadeh J, Osmon DR, Wilhelm MP, Espy MJ, Smith TF. A prospective study of the polymerase chain reaction for detection of herpes simplex virus in cerebrospinal fluid submitted to the clinical virology laboratory. *Molec Cell Probes* 1992;6:367–373.
8. Belec L, Gherardi R, Georges AJ, et al. Peripheral facial paralysis and HIV infection: report of four African cases and review of the literature. *J Neuro* 1989;236:411–414.
9. Berenguer J, Moreno S, Laguna F, et al. Tuberculous meningitis in patients infected with the human immunodeficiency virus. *N Engl J Med* 1992;326:668–672.
10. Berenguer J, Solera J, Diaz, et al. Listeriosis in patients infected with human immunodeficiency virus. *Rev Infect Dis* 1991;13:115–119.
11. Bergen GA, Yangco BG, Adelman HM. Central nervous system infection with *Mycobacterium kansasii*. *Ann Intern Med* 1993;118:396.
12. Bishburg E, Sunderam G, Reichman LB, Kapila R. Central nervous system tuberculosis with the acquired immunodeficiency syndrome and its related complex. *Ann Intern Med* 1986;105:210–213.
13. Buchbinder SP, Katz MH, Hessol NA, et al. Herpes zoster and human immunodeficiency virus infection. *J Infect Dis* 1992;166:1153–1156.
14. Burns DK, Risser RC, White CL. The neuropathology of human immunodeficiency virus infection. The Dallas, Texas experience. *Arch Path Lab Med* 1991;115:1112–1124.
15. Carneiro AV, Ferro J, Figueiredo C, et al. Herpes zoster and contralateral hemiplegia in an African patient infected with HIV-1. *Acta Med Portug* 1991;4:91–92.
16. Carrazana EJ, Rossitch E, Morris J. Isolated central nervous system aspergillosis in the acquired immunodeficiency syndrome. *Clin Neuro Neurosurg* 1991;93:227–230.
17. Chretien F, Gray F, Lescs MC, Geny C et al. Acute varicella-zoster virus ventriculitis and meningomyelo-radiculitis in acquired immunodeficiency syndrome. *Acta Neuropath* 1993;86:659–665.
18. Denning DW, Follansbee SE, Scolaro M, et al. Pulmonary aspergillosis in the acquired immunodeficiency syndrome. *New Engl J Med* 1991;324:654–662.
19. Dix RD, Bredesen DE, Erlich KS, Mills J. Recovery of herpesviruses from cerebrospinal fluid of immunodeficient homosexual men. *Ann Neurol* 1985;18:611–614.
20. Dube MP, Holtom PD, Larsen RA. Tuberculous meningitis in patients with and without human immunodeficiency virus infection. *Am J Med* 1992;93:520–524.
21. Fischl MA, Daikos GL, Uttamchandani RB, et al. Clinical presentation and outcome of patients with HIV infection and tuberculosis caused by multi-drug-resistant bacilli. *Ann Intern Med* 1992;117: 184–190.
22. Fischl MA, Uttamchandani RB, Daikos GL, et al. An outbreak of tuberculosis caused by multiple-drug-resistant tubercle bacilli among patients with HIV infection. *Ann Intern Med* 1992;117:177–183.
23. Fish DG, Ampel NM, Galgiani JN, et al. Coccidioidomycosis during human immunodeficiency virus infection. A review of 77 patients. *Medicine* 1990;69:384–391.
24. Fraimow HS, Wormser GP, Coburn KD, Small CB. Salmonella meningitis and infection with HIV. *AIDS* 1990;4:1271–1273.
25. Galgiani JN, Catanzaro A, Cloud GA, et al. Fluconazole therapy for coccidioidal meningitis. The NIAID mycosis study group. *Ann Intern Med* 1993;119:28–35.
26. Gateley A, Gander RM, Johnson PC, et al. Herpes simplex virus type 2 meningoencephalitis resistant to acyclovir in a patient with AIDS. *J Infect Dis* 1990;161:711–715.
27. Gilden DH, Murray RS, Wellish M, Kleinschmidt-DeMasters BK, Vafai A. Chronic progressive varicella-zoster virus encephalitis in an AIDS patient. *Neurology* 1988;38: 1150–1153.

28. Glesby MJ, Moore RD, Chaisson RE. Herpes zoster in patients with advanced human immunodeficiency virus infection treated with zidovudine. *J Infect Dis* 1993:168:1264–1268.

29. Gluckstein D, Ciferri F, Ruskin J. Chagas disease: another cause of cerebral mass in the acquired immunodeficiency syndrome. *Am J Med* 1992;92:429–432.

30. Go BM, Ziring DJ, Kountz DS. Spinal epidural abscess due to *Aspergillus* sp. in a patient with acquired immunodeficiency syndrome. *South Med J* 1993;86:957–960.

31. Gordon SM, Blumberg HM. *Mycobacterium kansasii* brain abscess in a patient with AIDS. *Clin Infect Dis* 1992;14:789–790.

32. Gordon SM, Steinberg JP, DuPuis MH, et al. Culture isolation of *Acanthamoeba* species and leptomyxoid amebas from patients with amebic meningoencephalitis, including two patients with AIDS. *Clin Infect Dis* 1992;15:1024–1030.

33. Gray F, Gherardi R, Keohane C, et al. Pathology of the central nervous system in 40 cases of acquired immune deficiency syndrome (AIDS). *Neuropathol Appl Neurobiol* 1988;14:365–380.

34. Gray F, Gherardi R, Trotot P, Fenelon G, Poirier J. Spinal cord lesions in the acquired immune deficiency syndrome (AIDS). *Neurosurg Rev* 1990;13:189–194.

35. Gray F, Mohr M, Rozenberg F, et al. Varicella-zoster virus encephalitis in acquired immunodeficiency syndrome: report of four cases. *Neuropathol Appl Neurobiol* 1992;18:502–514.

36. Harcourt-Webster JN, Scaravilli F, Darwish AH. Strongyloides stercoralis hyperinfection in an HIV positive patient. *J Clin Pathol* 1991;44:346–348.

37. Harding CV. Blastomycosis and opportunistic infections in patients with acquired immunodeficiency syndrome. An autopsy study. *Arch Pathol Lab Med* 1991;115:1133–1136.

38. Heller HM, Fuhrer J. Disseminated sporotrichosis in patients with AIDS: case report and review of the literature. *AIDS* 1991;5:1243–1246.

39. Hellinger WC, Bolling JP, Smith TF, Campbell RJ. Varicella-zoster virus retinitis in a patient with AIDS-related complex: case report and brief review of the acute retinal necrosis syndrome. *Clin Infect Dis* 1993;17:943–944.

40. Hollander H, Levy JA. Neurological abnormalities and recovery of human immunodeficiency virus from cerebrospinal fluid. *Ann Intern Med* 1987;106:692–695.

41. Idemyor V, Cherubin CE. Pleurocerebral *Nocardia* in a patient with human immunodeficiency virus. *Ann Pharm* 1992;26:188–189.

42. Jacob CN, Henein SS, Heurich AE, Kamholz S. Nontuberculous mycobacterial infection of the central nervous system in patients with AIDS. *South Med J* 1993;86:638–640.

43. Javaly K, Horowitz HW, Wormser GP. Nocardiosis in patients with human immunodeficiency virus infection. Report of 2 cases and review of literature. *Medicine* 1992;71:128–138.

44. Jurado RL, Farley MM, Pereira E, et al. Increased risk of meningitis and bacteremia due to *Listeria monocytogenes* in patients with human immunodeficiency virus infection. *Clin Infect Dis* 1993;17:224–227.

45. Kim J, Minamoto GY, Grieco MH. *Nocardia* infection as a complication of AIDS: report of six cases and review. *Rev Infect Dis* 1991;13:624–629.

46. Kim J, Minamoto GY, Hoy CD, Grieco MH. Presumptive cerebral *Nocardia asteroides* infection in AIDS: treatment with ceftriaxone and minocyline. *Am J Med* 1991;90:656–658.

47. Laguna F, Adrados M, Ortega A, Gonzalez-Lahoz JM. Tuberculous meningitis with acellular cerebrospinal fluid in AIDS patients. *AIDS* 1992;6:1165–1167.

48. Laskin OL, Stahl-Bayliss CM, Morgello S. Concomitant herpes simplex virus type 1 and cytomegalovirus ventriculoencephalitis in acquired immunodeficiency syndrome. *Arch Neurol* 1987;44:843–847.

49. Levine WC, Buehler JW, Bean NH, Tauxe RV. Epidemiology of nontyphoidal *Salmonella* bacteremia during the human immunodeficiency virus epidemic. *J Infect Dis* 1991;164:81–87.

50. Levy RM, Bredesen DE, Rosenblum ML. Neurological manifestations of the acquired immunodeficiency syndrome (AIDS): experience at UCSF and review of the literature. *J Neurosurg* 1985;62:475–495.

51. Lortholary O, Meyohas MC, Dupont B, et al. Invasive aspergillosis in patients with acquired immunodeficiency syndrome: report of 33 cases. French cooperative study group on aspergillosis in AIDS. *Am J Med* 1993;95:177–187.

52. Malasky C, Reichman LB. Long-term follow-up of tuberculoma of the brain in an AIDS patient. *Chest* 1992;101:278–279.

23. McArthur JC. Neurological manifestations of AIDS. *Medicine* 1987;66:407–437.

54. Melhem ER, Wang H. Intramedullary spinal cord tuberculoma in a patient with AIDS. *Am J Neurorad* 1992;13:986–988.

55. Mertens G, Ieven M, Ursi D, et al. Detection of herpes simplex virus in the cerebrospinal fluid of patients with encephalitis using the polymerase chain reaction. *J Neurol Sci* 1993;118:213–216.

56. Morgello S, Soifer FM, Lin CS, Wolfe DE. Central nervous system *Strongyloides stercoralis* in acquired immunodeficiency syndrome: a report of two cases and review of the literature. *Acta Neuropathol* 1993;86:285–288.

57. Nelson MR, Shanson DC, Hawkins DA, Gazzard BG. *Salmonella, Campylobacter* and *Shigella* in HIV-seropositive patients. *AIDS* 1992;6:1495–1498.

58. Nicoll JA, Kinrade E, Love S. PCR-mediated search for herpes simplex virus DNA in sections of brain from patients with multiple sclerosis and other neurological disorders. *J Neurol Sci* 1992;113: 144–151.

59. Nolan CM, et al. Failure of therapy for tuberculosis in human immunodeficiency virus infection. *Am J Med Sci* 1992;304:168–173.

60. Pallangyo K, Hakanson A, Lema L, et al. High HIV seroprevalence and increased HIV-associated mortality among hospitalized patients with deep bacterial infections in Dar es Salaam, Tanzania. *AIDS* 1992;9:971–976.

61. Pappas PG, Pottage JC, Powderly WG, et al. Blastomycosis in patients with the acquired immunodeficiency syndrome. *Ann Intern Med* 1992;116:847–853.

62. Penn CC, Goldstein E, Bartholomew WR. *Sporothrix schenckii* meningitis in a patient with AIDS. *Clin Infect Dis* 1992;15:741–743.

63. Petito CK, Cho ES, Lemann W, Navia BA, Price RW. Neuropathology of acquired immunodeficiency syndrome (AIDS): an autopsy review. *J Neuropathol Exp Neurol* 1986;45:635–646.

64. Pillay D, Lipman MC, Lee CA, et al. A clinico-pathological audit of opportunistic viral infections in HIV-infected patients. *AIDS* 1993;7:969–974.

65. Puchhammer-Stockl E, Popow-Kraupp T, Heinz FX, Mandl CW, Kunz C. Detection of varicella-zoster virus DNA by polymerase chain reaction in the cerebrospinal fluid of patients suffering from neurological complications associated with chicken pox or herpes zoster. *J Clin Microbiol* 1991;29: 1513–1516.

66. Redd SC, Rutherford GW, Sande MA, et al. The role of human immunodeficiency virus infection in pneumococcal bacteremia in San Francisco residents. *J Infect Dis* 1990;162:1012–1017.

67. Rocha A, Ferreira MS, Nishioka SA, et al. *Trypanosoma cruzi* meningoencephalitis and myocarditis in a patient with acquired immunodeficiency syndrome. *Rev Inst Med Trop Sao Paulo* 1993;35: 205–208.

68. Rodriquez Barradas MC, Musher DM, Hamill RJ, et al. Unusual manifestations of pneumococcal infection in human immunodeficiency virus-infected individuals: the past revisited. *Clin Infect Dis* 1992;14:192–199.

69. Rosemberg S, Chaves CJ, Higuchi ML, et al. Fatal meningoencephalitis caused by reactivation of *Trypanosoma cruzi* infection in a patient with AIDS. *Neurology* 1992;42:640–642.

70. Ryder JW, Croen K, Kleinschmidt-DeMasters BK, et al. Progressive encephalitis three months after resolution of cutaneous zoster in a patient with AIDS. *Ann Neurol* 1986;19:182–188.

71. Sellitti TP, Huang AJ, Schiffman J, Davis JL. Association of herpes zoster ophthalmicus with acquired immunodeficiency syndrome and acute retinal necrosis. *Am J Ophthalmol* 1993;116:297–301.

72. Selwyn PA, Feingold AR, Hartel D, et al. Increased risk of bacterial pneumonia in HIV-infected intravenous drug users without AIDS. *AIDS* 1988;4:267–272.

73. Sepkowitz KA, Telzak EE, Recalde S, Armstrong D. Trends in the susceptibility of tuberculosis in New York City, 1987–1991. *Clin Infect Dis* 1994;18:755–759.

74. Sharer LR, Kapila R. Neuropathological observations in acquired immunodeficiency syndrome (AIDS). *Acta Neuropathol* 1985;66:188–198.

75. Shoji H, Honda Y, Murai I, et al. Detection of varicella-zoster virus DNA by polymerase chain reaction in cerebrospinal fluid of patients with herpes zoster meningitis. *J Neuro* 1992;239:69–70.

76. Singer EJ, Zorilla C, Fahy-Chandon B, et al. Painful symptoms reported by ambulatory HIV-infected men in a longitudinal study. *Pain* 1993;54:15–19.

77. Small PM, Schecter GA, Goodman PC, et al. Treatment of tuberculosis in patients with advanced human immunodeficiency virus infection. *N Engl J Med* 1991;324:289–294.

78. Snider WD, Simpson DM, Nielsen S, et al. Neurological complications of acquired immune deficiency syndrome: analysis of 50 patients. *Ann Neurol* 1983;14:403–418.

79. Solari A, Saavedra H, Sepulveda C, et al. Successful treatment of *Trypanosoma cruzi* encephalitis in a patient with hemophilia and AIDS. *Clin Infect Dis* 1993;16:255–259.

80. Spach DH, Panther LA, Thorning DR, et al. Intracerebral bacillary angiomatosis in a patient infected with human immunodeficiency virus. *Ann Intern Med* 1992;116:740–742.

81. Steinhart R, Reingold AL, Taylor F, Anderson G, Wenger JD. Invasive *Haemophilus influenzae* infections in men with HIV infection. *JAMA* 1992;268:3350–3352.

82. Thornton CA, Houston S, Latif AS. Neurocysticercosis and human immunodeficiency virus infection. A possible association. *Arch Neurol* 1992;49:963–965.

83. Troendle-Atkins J, Demmler GJ, Buffone GJ. Rapid diagnosis of herpes simplex virus encephalitis by using the polymerase chain reaction. *J Pediatr* 1993;123:376–380.

84. Weidenheim KM, Nelson SJ, Kure K, et al. Unusual patterns of *Histoplasma capsulatum* meningitis and progressive multifocal leukoencephalopathy in a patient with the acquired immunodeficiency virus. *Hum Pathol* 1992;23:581–586.

85. Weisberg LA, Garcia C, Stazio A. Computerized tomographic diagnostic aspects of acquired immunodeficiency syndrome. *Comp Med Imag Graph* 1988;12:225–236.

86. West TE, Papasian CJ, Park BH, Parker SW. Adenovirus type 2 encephalitis and concurrent Epstein-Barr virus infection in an adult man. *Arch Neurol* 1985;42:815–817.

87. Wheat LJ, Connolly-Stringfield PA, Baker RL, et al. Disseminated histoplasmosis in the acquired immune deficiency syndrome: clinical findings, diagnosis, and treatment, and review of the literature. *Medicine* 1990;69:361–373.
88. Winward KE, Hamed LM, Glaser JS. The spectrum of optic nerve disease in human immunodeficiency virus infection. *Am J Ophthalmol* 1989;107:373–380.
89. Witt DJ, Craven DE, McCabe WR. Bacterial infections in adult patients with the acquired immune deficiency syndrome (AIDS) and AIDS-related complex. *Am J Med* 1987:82:900–906.

AIDS and the Nervous System, Second Edition,
edited by J. R. Berger and R. M. Levy.
Lippincott-Raven Publishers, Philadelphia © 1997.

28

Neoplasms of the Central Nervous System in Acquired Immunodeficiency Syndrome

°Claudia Tellez, °Jamie VonRoenn, and †Robert M. Levy

Departments of °Medicine and †Surgery, Northwestern University Medical School, Chicago, Illinois 60611

Malignant disease is an increasingly frequent complication of human immunodeficiency virus (HIV) infection (68). Both Kaposi's sarcoma (KS) and primary central nervous system lymphoma (PCNSL) were included in the original Centers for Disease Control definition of acquired immunodeficiency syndrome (AIDS) in 1981. In 1985, intermediate- and high-grade non-Hodgkin's lymphoma (NHL) were added as AIDS-defining conditions. These aggressive, frequently extranodal lymphomas increase in incidence with the duration of HIV infection and have a predilection to involve the CNS, both at presentation and as a site of relapse. As the survival for HIV-infected individuals continues to lengthen due to improved antiviral therapy and prophylaxis and treatment for opportunistic infections, the incidence of malignancy in this population is expected to increase.

IMMUNOSUPPRESSION AND LYMPHOMAS

The relationship between immunosuppression and the increased incidence of lymphoma has been well described. Children with congenital immune deficiencies have a 100-fold greater risk for the development of malignant disease than the general population, with nearly half of these tumors being lymphoreticular in origin. The incidence of lymphoma varies with the type of immunosuppression; lymphoma accounts for 66% of the malignancies seen in patients with ataxia telangiectasia, 59% of tumors seen in patients with Wiskott Aldrich and 55% and 31% of the malignancies seen in patients with common variable immunodeficiency and severe combined immunodeficiency, respectively (68).

Similarly, the increased risk of lymphoma in patients with autoimmune diseases varies depending on the underlying disorder. For example, patients with lymphocytic thyroiditis have a risk of lymphoma that is 67-fold that of the general population (30), while the lymphoma risk for patients with Sjögren's syndrome is about 44-fold the risk of the general population (36). The risk of lymphoma is also increased in patients with celiac disease (23), angioimmunoblastic lymphadenopathy (60), rheumatoid arthritis (20), and systemic lupus erythematosus (52).

Lymphoma is the most common malignancy occurring in patients with iatrogenic immunodeficiency (68). Epidemiological studies suggest that the incidence of lymphoma in transplant recipients is up to 50-fold greater than age-matched controls, representing 20% of the malignances in these patients. Interestingly, the incidence of malignancy increases with the length of follow-up after transplantation, with a median latency from transplant to the development of lymphoma of 33 months (69). Recently, the use of cyclosporine in renal transplant recipients has led to an increased incidence of lymphoma with a short median latency of 4 months in 32% of patients (69).

Lymphoma associated with immunosuppression is characteristically a high-grade, B cell neoplasm (15,55) characterized clinically by rapid progression, advanced stage at presentation, and a high incidence of extranodal involvement, including the CNS (70). In transplant recipients with NHL, the most frequently involved extranodal site is the CNS (37%) (70). This is in sharp contrast to the 1% cerebral and 3.7% meningeal involvement expected with NHL in the general population (26).

The incidence of primary CNS lymphoma is also increased in the setting of immune compromise, whether congenital or iatrogenic. In a large study of renal allograft recipients with NHL, the most common single organ site affected was the CNS, which was involved in 56% of the cases (70). Similarly, CNS lymphoma accounts for 31% of the NHLs seen in association with the Wiscott Aldrich syndrome (70).

The immune system plays an integral role in the prevention of carcinogenesis, a process requiring multiple complex interactions. Tumor initiation results from a DNA mutation which gives rise to a malignant cell with an acquired growth advantage. The initiation process in HIV-infected patients may result from a combination of insults including chronic antigenic stimulation from oncogenic viruses, blood-borne antigens, and cytotoxic or immunosuppressive medications. Exposure to conventional carcinogens such as chemicals or ionizing radiation may also occur. In HIV-infected patients, impaired immune surveillance and faulty immune regulation may allow tumor promotion and further clonal expansion. Imbalance in growth and inhibitory factors, loss of reactivity to foreign antigens, inappropriate activation of proto-oncogenes, and inactivation of tumor suppressor genes may all contribute to the unchecked proliferative process.

SYSTEMIC AIDS-RELATED LYMPHOMA WITH CNS INVOLVEMENT

Non-Hodgkin's Lymphoma is one of the most common malignancies seen in the setting of HIV infection. It is estimated that 7% to 10% of all HIV-infected patients will develop NHL during the course of their illness (42). Pluda noted a 19% incidence of NHL in 116 HIV-infected patients treated with antiretroviral therapy for 36 months (72). Reminiscent of systemic lymphoma seen in other immunosuppressed states, HIV-related NHL is an aggressive, high-grade B cell tumor (43). Extranodal disease and advanced stage at presentation are the rule, occurring in 63% to 84% and up to 98% of cases, respectively (34,35,40,43,54). Central nervous system involvement, usually meningeal, occurs in up to 30% of patients (34,35,46) and is not universally associated with bone marrow involvement (46). Other common extranodal sites of involvement include the GI tract, bone marrow, liver, lung, skin, and multiple other organs (40).

The clinical presentation of NHL is quite varied. Up to 75% of patients present with B symptoms, namely, fever, night sweats, or unexplained weight loss in excess of 10% of usual body weight (40). Patients may present with symptoms related to lymphadenopathy or with complaints referable to an organ site of involvement, such as oral or perirectal lesions.

Leptomeningeal involvement is the most frequent manifestation of CNS spread of NHL (39). Commonly, patients present with headaches or signs of meningeal disease such as meningismus or cranial nerve palsies. Up to 17% of patients with meningeal involvement are asymptomatic (46). Local extension to the epidural space may result in spinal cord or cauda equina compression (Fig. 1). Although leptomeningeal involvement has not been clearly documented to adversely affect prognosis, it is a source of significant morbidity (45).

The staging workup for NHL should include computed tomography (CT) scans of the brain, chest, abdomen, and pelvis and a bone marrow aspirate and biopsy. A lumbar puncture with cerebral spinal fluid examination should be performed routinely to rule out meningeal involvement.

The AIDS-related NHLs are B cell tumors with an unusual distribution of histological subtypes. Fifty-six to 78% of patients present with high-grade histological subtypes, evenly distributed between large-cell immunoblastic and small noncleaved histologies (43,44). This is in striking contrast to non-HIV-related NHL in which the small noncleaved histology accounts for 10% or less of all NHLs (55).

Recently, the treatment of non-AIDS-associated lymphoma has focused on dose-intensive chemotherapy, with improved response rates and survival reported in some series (37,57,76). Unfortunately, early trials employing dose-intensive chemotherapy for HIV-associated NHL resulted in lower complete response rates (20% to 30%, compared with about 50% for ''standard'' dose chemotherapy), a high incidence of CNS relapse (greater than 50%), and high rates of opportunistic infection (9,18,62). Trials of standard dose and lower dose chemotherapy, with CNS prophylaxis with intrathecal chemotherapy and growth factor support, yield response rates in the range of 50%, with rates of complicating opportunistic infection of about 20% (46). Prophylaxis with intrathecal methotrexate or cytosine arabinoside to diminish the rate of CNS relapse has been suggested. Although four weekly doses of intrathecal chemotherapy for CNS prophylaxis is generally recommended, the benefit of this therapy for all patients, regardless of histological subtype or presence of bone marrow involvement, is not entirely clear.

PRIMARY CNS LYMPHOMAS

Primary CNS lymphoma accounts for 1% to 1.5% of all primary brain tumors and 1% to 2% of all cases of extranodal NHL (75). Central nervous system lymphoma is often associated with immunosuppression or immunodeficiency (12,14,32). The first reports of PCNSL in HIV-infected patients were published with the initial description of AIDS in 1981 (78). Recently, there has been a dramatic increase in the incidence of PCNSL in association with AIDS. It is estimated that 1% to 2% of all HIV-infected patients will develop PCNSL (10), while in some patient populations, the incidence may be as high as 5%. Primary CNS lymphoma is the most common cause of a CNS mass lesion in HIV-infected children (11) and the second only to toxoplasmosis in HIV-infected adults (10). Primary CNS lymphoma is the AIDS-

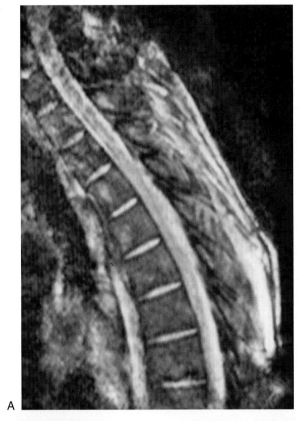

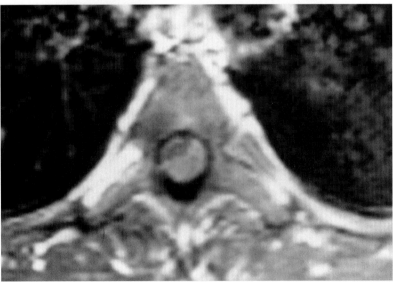

FIG. 1. Epidural metastasis of systemic lymphoma in AIDS. **A:** Midsagittal T2-weighted magnetic resonance imaging (MRI) demonstrating enhancing epidural lesion with spinal cord compression in a patient with acquired immunodeficiency syndrome (AIDS) and subacute paraplegia. **B:** Transaxial T1-weighted MRI demonstrating the epidural lesion filling the spinal canal and compressing the spinal cord ventrally and to the right.

defining illness for 0.5% of HIV-infected patients (33). Due to the large numbers of HIV-infected patients with PCNSL, by 1991 in the United States, AIDS-related PCNSL had become a more common tumor than low-grade astrocytoma and almost as common as meningioma (3).

Pathology

Gross pathological examination of PCNSL reveals a bulky tumor with indistinct borders, often contiguous with meningeal or ventricular surfaces. Most lesions are supratentorial. While solitary lesions occur in one of three of cases, multiple lesions are evident in the majority of cases (3,54,59,64). These lesions are histologically diffuse, with perivascular involvement, high mitotic rates, and variable degrees of necrosis and microglial reaction (64,65) (Fig. 2).

Immunohistochemical studies of PCNSL identify these tumors as B cell in origin. The non-AIDS-related cases often are intermediate- to high-grade histological subtypes while AIDS-related PCNSL is an aggressive histological subtype, large-cell immunoblastic or small, noncleaved cell, in the majority of cases (74,79) (Table 1).

A lymphoproliferative disorder of the CNS of uncertain nature characterized by polyclonal lymphocyte expansion has been reported in association with HIV infection (74,79). This entity presents in a manner identical to PCNSL. Dramatic resolution of this lesion has been noted with treatment with corticosteroids (74,77,79).

Etiological Factors

Epstein-Barr virus (EBV) has been implicated as a causative factor for both systemic and primary CNS lymphoma in association with AIDS or other immunocompromised states. Multiple investigators have identified the incorporation of the EBV genome into the genome of neoplastic cells (2,29). The prevalence of EBV in PCNSL in immunocompromised patients is high. In sharp contrast, there is only one documented case of EBV expression in PCNSL occurring in an immunocompetent patient (4). While EBV is consistently associated with AIDS-related PCNSL, it is identified in fewer than half of the cases of AIDS-related systemic lymphoma (22). The consistent association of EBV expression in PCNSL supports a pathogenic role for EBV in AIDS-related PCNSL (2,22,29).

The prevalence of EBV in AIDS-associated PCNSL has been reported to range between 94% and 100%. The variability can be explained by differences in the processing of the tissue as well as different techniques utilized for detection. *In situ* hybridization of viral RNA transcripts is the most sensitive technique available and can be performed on paraffin-embedded tissues.

Clinical Presentation

Primary CNS lymphoma represents 10% to 20% of all HIV-related NHL (54). Unlike systemic NHL which can occur at any stage of HIV infection, PCNSL typically occurs in profoundly immunocompromised patients with CD4 + -T lymphocyte counts (CD4+ counts) below 50 cells/mm^3 (41). At presentation, patients frequently have a history of prior AIDS-defining opportunistic illness and B symptoms

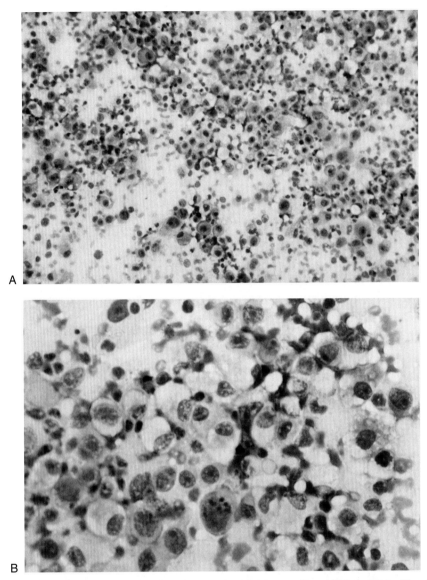

FIG. 2. Cytosmear specimen from a stereotactic brain biopsy of an AIDS patient with primary central nervous system (CNS) lymphoma, showing sheets of large lymphoid cells with immuno-blastic features. **A:** Low power, ×10. **B:** High power, ×40.

TABLE 1. *Pathologic findings in 77 patients with primary CNS lymphoma*

Type of lymphoma	Number of cases	Percent
Large cell, immunoblastic	27	35
Small cell, noncleaved	19	25
Large cell	13	16
Lymphoma not otherwise specified	18	23

TABLE 2. *ECOG performance status scale*

0	Fully active
1	Ambulatory, capable of light work
2	In bed < 50% of time; capable of self-care but not of work activities
3	In bed > 50% of time; capable of limited self-care
4	Completely bedridden

(fever, weight loss, night sweats) (74). The presence of B symptoms may also reflect intercurrent opportunistic infection related to the compromised immune status of this patient population. Patients with AIDS-related PCNSL often have a poor performance status. Remick et al. reported a median ECOG performance status (PS) of 3 in patients with AIDS-related PCNSL, compared to a PS of 1 in the patients with non AIDS-related PCNSL (74; Table 2).

Alteration in the level of consciousness, occurring in 57% of patients, and focal neurological deficits, seen in 38% to 78% of patients, are the most common presenting sign of PCNSL (5,19,71,74,78) (Table 3). Seizures occur in 23% of AIDS patients with PCNSL while cranial nerve deficits are evident in 13%. Signs of increased intracranial pressure are less common (74). The major differences in presentation between AIDS- and non-AIDS-related PCNSL are the high prevalence of B symptoms and the shorter duration of symptoms (days to weeks versus months) for patients with HIV-related tumors (64,74).

Radiological Findings

Although no radiological finding is pathognomonic for PCNSL, some radiological features are suggestive of the diagnosis. A homogeneously enhancing lesion in the central gray matter or corpus callosum is highly suggestive of PCNSL (64). Without contrast, lesions are likely to be hypodense, although they may also be isodense or hyperdense (13,19,74). With contrast enhancement, most lesions will pick up contrast in a diffuse homogeneous pattern (27,31,80) (Fig. 3). Ringlike lesions may occur in 5% to 10% of cases. Most lesions are adjacent to an ependymal or meningeal surface with varying degrees of edema and mass effect. About 50% to 60% of lesions are located peripherally in the hemispheric grey matter or adjacent white matter. Another 25% of the lesions will be found in the deep midline structures of the septum pallucidum, basal ganglia, or corpus callosum (13,64). Uveal, vitreal, and intradural lesions of the spinal cord have also been described (12). Up to 63% of patients with AIDS-related lymphoma will have multiple lesions (3,13,19,50,67,73,74).

In comparing radiological features of PCNSL with those of CNS toxoplasmosis, Gill et al. noted that patients with CNS toxoplasmosis were more likely to have

TABLE 3. *Presenting symptoms in 77 AIDS patients with primary CNS lymphoma*

Symptoms	Number of cases	Percent
Confusion, memory loss, lethargy	44	57
Hemiparesis, sensory loss	29	38
Seizures	18	23
Cranial nerve deficits	13	17

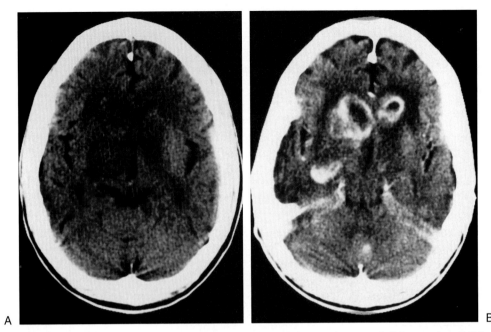

A   B

FIG. 3. Computed tomography (CT) scan of patient with human immunodeficiency virus (HIV) related primary CNS lymphoma. **A:** Precontrast axial CT imaging demonstrates an area of edema in the right basal ganglia, adjacent to the frontal horns of the lateral ventricles. **B:** Postcontrast axial CT scan demonstrates an enhancing mass lesion encasing the frontal horns of the lateral ventricles and involving the right basal ganglia.

multiple, often ''ring-enhancing,'' lesions of smaller size on CT scan (17). The diversity of the radiographic appearance of PCNSL makes diagnosis impossible without tissue confirmation.

A magnetic resonance imaging (MRI) scan, with or without gadolinium enhancement, yields increased sensitivity of detection (8,38,47; Fig. 4) and resolution of the lesions (31). Cerebral angiography is nonspecific. About 60% of these lesions are avascular, while 30% to 40% show a diffuse homogeneous pattern of uptake on angiogram (24,27). Preliminary studies using ^{201}TI single photon emission computed tomography (SPECT) have shown provocative results. O'Malley et al. (63) imaged 13 AIDS patients with intracranial lesions. Among 7 patients prospectively interpreted as having lymphoma, 6 were later shown to have biopsy-proven lymphoma. Six patients prospectively classified as having ''no lymphoma'' were later shown to have toxoplasmosis in 4, progressive multifocal leukoencephalopathy in 1, and venous angioma in 1 patient.

Differential Diagnosis

The differential diagnosis of an intracranial lesion in an HIV-infected patient includes a number of infectious, neoplastic, and ischemic processes. As many conditions may present with similar neurological and radiological findings, tissue biopsy is required to confirm the diagnosis. Most commonly, an abscess caused by *Toxoplasma gondii* must be ruled out. Other less common processes that must be considered

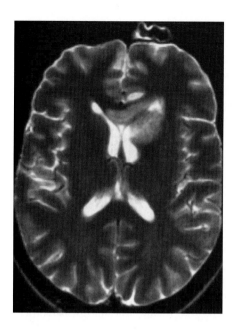

FIG. 4. T2-weighted MRI of patient with HIV-related primary CNS lymphoma. Note the abnormal high T2 intensity around the right frontal horn of the lateral ventricle and extending into the corpus callosum.

include progressive multifocal leukoencephalopathy (PML), fungal, pyogenic, candidal, or herpetic abscesses, infarction with hemorrhage, and metastatic KS (48). In addition, the possibility of some non-HIV-related CNS pathology such as a metastatic or primary malignant brain lesion must be entertained.

Staging

The yield of a systemic work-up in a patient who presents with a CNS lymphoma is unclear. Limited staging has been suggested. This should include a thorough history and physical examination with routine screening laboratory exams and a chest x-ray. The CNS evaluation should include evaluation of the spinal axis to rule out synchronous cord or epidural lesions and a slit-lamp exam to evaluate for ocular invasion, present in up to 7% of patients (12).

Diagnosis

Confirmation of a diagnosis of PCNSL in a patient with an intracranial mass can be obtained utilizing one of three methods: examination of cerebrospinal fluid (CSF), stereotactic brain biopsy, or craniotomy with biopsy. The CSF cytology is diagnostic in only 10% to 30% of all patients with PCNSL. For unclear reasons, the yield from CSF evaluation in patients with AIDS-related PCNSL is somewhat less (19,56,74). Elevated CSF protein and pleocytosis are not uncommon, but are nonspecific. A low CSF glucose level may be seen (5). In addition to cytology, the CSF should be evaluated by immunohistochemistry and for gene rearrangements to increase the diagnostic yield.

Stereotactic brain biopsy performed by an experienced neurosurgeon yields a diagnosis of PCNSL in greater than 95% of cases, with a rate of significant complications of less than 2% (51). This procedure can be used for almost any lesion in the brain, including deep periventricular lesions (6). Craniotomy with surgical resection has a minimally higher diagnostic yield but is associated with greater potential for morbidity and mortality. Furthermore, in patients with other significant medical illnesses and with limited life expectancy, stereotactic brain biopsy allows for local anesthesia and minimal hospitalization and recovery time while craniotomy requires general anesthetic, hospitalization of approximately 1 week, and recovery periods that may last several weeks. The value of a craniotomy for diagnosis is highly controversial (28,53,58,59,81). For diagnostic purposes, the least invasive technique should be performed.

Prognosis and Treatment

In adult HIV-infected patients, cerebral toxoplasmosis is the most frequent cause of a CNS mass lesion. In the presence of positive serum immunoglobulin G (IgG) toxoplasmosis titers and multiple lesions evident on MRI, many clinicians opt to treat patients with intracranial mass lesion(s) empirically for toxoplasmosis (12). Toxoplasmosis generally responds with clear radiographic and clinical improvement within 1 to 2 weeks of initiating therapy. For those patients who fail to respond to a "therapeutic trial" of toxoplasmosis therapy, with negative toxoplasmosis serology, with solitary MRI lesions, or who are in poor neurological condition at presentation, brain biopsy is indicated (see Chapter 24).

The value of surgical resection remains controversial. Although craniotomy with surgical resection has been performed in patients with non-AIDS-related PCNSL, several studies have found no value to surgical resection alone (25,58,59,81). Three small nonrandomized studies suggest that resection followed by radiation therapy is superior to radiation therapy alone in patients with AIDS-related PCNSL with median survival times of 5.5 and 2.0 months, respectively (31,71,79). The surgical experience with AIDS-related PCNSL, however, is very limited and inadequate to suggest a role for surgical resection in the primary management of these patients. Furthermore, the extensive periventricular and frequently multiple lesions of HIV-related PCNSL make gross total surgical resection often impossible.

In general, PCNSL is sensitive to radiation therapy, and complete responses have been observed with a range of radiation therapy doses (12). In our original report (3), we reviewed the response to radiation therapy of 55 patients with AIDS-related PCNSL. Patients were treated with whole brain radiation therapy of 4,000 cGy in 267 Gy/fraction over 3 weeks. Radiological response to radiation therapy, defined as partial or complete resolution of the lesions or stability in the size and number of lesions, was noted in 91% of patients completing this radiation therapy protocol. Ninety percent of patients were stable or improved clinically following radiation therapy. Median survival increased from 27 days (range 8 to 127 days) without radiation therapy to 119 days (range 33 to 380 days) with completion of protocol radiation therapy; cause of death was progression of the PCNSL in 13% of patients receiving protocol radiation therapy, as compared to 77% of patients not so treated.

These data would suggest strongly that radiation therapy is effective in the treatment of AIDS-related PCNSL. Unfortunately, the data are flawed in their uncontrolled, retrospective nature. Furthermore, patients were stratified for purposes of data analysis into those completing protocol radiation therapy and those who did not receive radiation therapy or did not complete planned radiation treatment. Our assumption was that either these latter patients were begun on treatment during a preterminal phase of their illness or that they failed to receive aggressive therapy as a result of therapeutic nihilism. The exclusion falsely suggests that radiation therapy is an effective treatment for AIDS-related PCNSL.

In an attempt to address the shortcomings of this study, we have recently completed a prospective trial of whole brain radiation therapy for the treatment of AIDS-related PCNSL in 25 patients (49). All patients were entered into the study at the time of diagnosis, had good Karnofsky performance scores, and were treated with dexamethasone and external beam radiation therapy, 3,000 to 4,000 cGy over 2 to 3 weeks. Response rates and survival times for patients completing protocol radiation therapy were very much as we had seen in our retrospective study. Radiological and clinical stabilization or improvement were observed in 100% and 84% of the patients, respectively. The mean survival for patients who completed treatment was 184 days (range 63 to 644).

Unfortunately, nine patients progressed rapidly and died before completing radiation therapy, despite their early recruitment and initiation of therapy. This is the patient population improperly excluded from the analysis in the retrospective series. Including the data from these patients, clinical and radiological stabilization or improvement fell to 72% and 83%, respectively, and mean survival fell to 122 days (range 15 to 644). Primary CNS lymphoma was felt to be the cause of death in 40% of all patients. Thus, whole brain irradiation results in an improved neurological status and a modest improvement in survival from 1 to 2 months in untreated patients to 3 to 4 months following radiation therapy (Fig. 5).

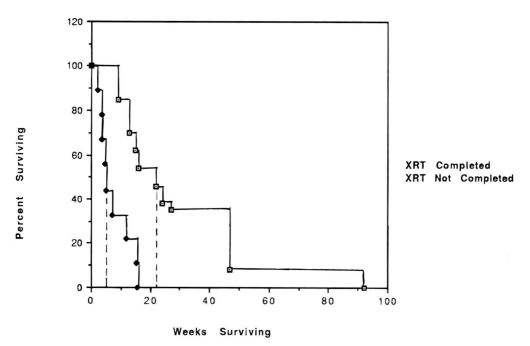

FIG. 5. Kaplan Meier survival curves for AIDS patients with primary CNS lymphoma demonstrating the impact of radiation therapy. •, XRT not completed; ▣, XRT completed.

Clearly, patients with AIDS-related PCNSL have a markedly worse outcome from radiation therapy compared to those with non-AIDS-related PCNSL. The poor outcome for patients with AIDS-related PCNSL may be explained by a number of observations. First, it appears that AIDS-related PCNSL is a histologically aggressive malignancy which may be relatively radioresistant and pathogenetically and biologically different from non-AIDS-related PCNSL (2,4,29,32). In addition, although improved response rates and survival have been reported for non-AIDS-related PCNSL treated with high-dose irradiation (50 to 60 Gy), relatively low dose irradiation is usually administered to patients with AIDS (3,12). Therapeutic nihilism and the theoretical risk of exacerbation of HIV-related encephalopathy by radiation result in the frequent prescription of relatively low dose radiation therapy (74). Spinal irradiation does not appear to impact on survival and may actually increase toxicity.

A variety of chemotherapy regimens have been used for both AIDS-related and non-AIDS-related NHL. Recent studies have suggested a benefit for combined modality therapy for non-AIDS-related PCNSL (7,16,61,66). Gabbai et al. treated 13 patients with three cycles of high-dose methotrexate followed by whole brain irradiation to a total dose of 30 Gy. They reported a 69% complete remission rate and a median survival of more than 27 months (median follow-up 2 years) (16). Neuwelt et al. reported a complete response rate of 81% and a median survival of 44 months in 16 patients treated with blood-brain barrier disruption and cyclophosphamide, methotrexate, and procarbazine followed by whole brain irradiation (61). De Angelis and co-workers treated 32 patients with systemic and intrathecal methotrexate followed by cranial irradiation and concurrent cytosine arabinoside. This resulted in a response rate of 77% with a median survival of 42.5 months (7). The Radiation Therapy Oncology Group (RTOG), in collaboration with the Eastern Cooperative Oncology Group (ECOG) and the North Central Cancer Treatment Group (NCCTG), have treated patients with three cycles of CHOP chemotherapy (cyclophosphamide, adriamycin, vincristine, prednisone) followed by whole brain irradiation. Chemotherapy resulted in a 75% complete response rate with all responses seen after the first cycle of chemotherapy (66). These reports suggest that, at least in the region of brain tumors, the blood-brain barrier is disrupted and chemotherapy may have a role in the treatment of PCNSL. Prospective randomized studies to evaluate the role of chemotherapy for AIDS-related PCNSL are currently underway.

Clinical Course

Systemic dissemination occurs in about 10% of patients with non-AIDS-related PCNSL. Reported sites of involvement include the heart, gastrointestinal tract, epidural space, bone marrow, lymph nodes, testicles, kidneys, lung, and mediastinum. This may become more common in patients with AIDS-related PCNSL as treatment, and hopefully outcome, improves (24,25,74). Local recurrence at the site of previous disease in the brain is common post radiation therapy (12,53).

Autopsy information is scant. Baumgartner et al. published the most complete report of autopsy findings. They noted that for patients treated with radiation therapy (8 of 21) 7 of 8 patients died from opportunistic infections, while for patients who did not receive radiotherapy (13 of 21), progressive lymphoma (10 of 13; 77%) was the most common cause of death (3).

KAPOSI'S SARCOMA

Central nervous system involvement by KS is distinctly unusual (1,21,48). Surgical and autopsy evaluations have identified both single and multiple intraparenchymal brain lesions which grossly appear spongy and hemorrhagic. Cytological examination reveals a proliferation of spindle cells with slitlike blood vessels and an associated network of reticular and collagen fibers (1). The few patients reported have presented with generalized cutaneous KS, usually in association with visceral disease (1,21). In addition, most of these patients were severely immunocompromised. While the CNS tumors appear to be quite radiation sensitive, the few patients reported with CNS involvement by KS have had very short survival, due to the progression of their disseminated KS. A number of these tumors have been discovered at postmortem examination only, underscoring the impression that CNS KS is often an end-stage event for patients with AIDS-related KS.

CONCLUSIONS

Improvements in the treatment of HIV itself and the treatment and prophylaxis of infection have led to prolonged survival of a highly immunocompromised cohort of patients. Thus, the incidence of neoplastic complications will continue to increase. While clinical and radiological evaluation of patients with AIDS-related tumors of the CNS provides important information, definitive diagnosis requires CSF cytological evaluation or brain biopsy. Both radiation therapy and chemotherapy have been used with significant impact on the quality and length of survival, although median survival is still only about 4 months. The challenge is to develop effective and tolerable treatment strategies which can provide palliation as well as further improvements in survival.

REFERENCES

1. Ariza A, Kim JH. Kaposi's sarcoma of the dura mater. *Human Pathol* 1988;19(12):1461–1462.
2. Bashir RM, Haris NL, Hochberg FH, et al. Detection of Epstein-Barr virus in CNS lymphoma in situ hybridization. *Neurology* 1989;39:813–817.
3. Baumgartner JE, Rachlin JR, Beckstead JH, et al. Primary central nervous system lymphoma: natural history and response to radiation therapy in 55 patients with acquired immunodeficiency syndrome. *J Neurosurg* 1990;73:206–211.
4. Bignon YJ, Claveloy P, Ramos F, Jouvet A, et al. Detection of Epstein-Barr virus sequenced in primary brain lymphoma without immunodeficiency. *Neurology* 1991;41:1152–1153.
5. Case records of the Massachusetts General Hospital. *N Engl J Med* 1983;309:359–369.
6. Chappell ET, Guthrie BL, Orenstein J. The role of stereotactic biopsy in the management of HIV-related focal brain lesions. *Neurosurgery* 1992;30:825–829.
7. DeAngelis LM, Yaha Ian J, Thalar HT, et al. Combined modality therapy for primary CNS lymphoma. *J Clin Oncol* 1992;10:635–643.
8. Dina TS. Primary central nervous system lymphoma vs. toxoplasmosis in AIDS. *Radiology* 1991;179:823–828.
9. Dugan M, Subar M, Odajnyk C, et al. Intensive multiagent chemotherapy for AIDS-related diffuse large cell lymphoma. *Blood* 1986;68:124(abstr).
10. Eikin CM, Leon E, Grenell SL, Leeds NE. Intracranial lesions in the acquired immunodeficiency syndrome: radiological (CT) features. *JAMA* 1985;253:393–396
11. Epstein LG, Dicarlo FJ Jr, Joshi VV, et al. Primary lymphoma of the central nervous system in children with acquired immunodeficiency syndrome. *Pediatrics* 1988;82:355–363.
12. Fine HA, Mayer RJ. Primary central nervous system lymphoma. *Ann Intern Med* 1993;119:1093–1104.

13. Formenti SC, Gill PS, Lean E, et al. Primary central nervous system lymphoma in AIDS. Results of radiation therapy. *Cancer* 1989;63:1101–1107.
14. Freeman C, Berg JW, Cutler SJ. Occurrence and prognosis of extranodal lymphomas. *Cancer* 1972; 29:252–260.
15. Frizzera G, Rosai J, Dehner LP, et al. Lymphoreticular disorders in primary immunodeficiency: new findings based on updated histological classification of 35 cases. *Cancer* 1980;46:692.
16. Gabbai AA, Hochberg FH, Linggood RM, et al. High dose methotrexate therapy of non-AIDS primary brain lymphoma. *J Neurosurg* 1989;70:190–194.
17. Gill PS, Graham RA, Boswell W, et al. A comparison of imaging, clinical and pathological aspects of space occupying lesions within the brain in patients with acquired immune deficiency syndrome. *Am J Physiol Imag* 1986;1:134.
18. Gill PS, Levine AM, Krailo M, et al. AIDS-related malignant lymphoma: result of prospective treatment and trials. *J Clin Oncol* 1987;5:1322–1328.
19. Gill PS, Levine AM, Meyer PR, et al. Primary central nervous system lymphoma in homosexual men. Clinical, immunological and pathological features. *Am J Med* 1985;78:742–748.
20. Good AE, Russo RH, Schnitzer B, Weatherbee L. Intracranial histiocytic lymphoma with rheumatoid arthritis. *J Rheumatol* 1978;5:75–78.
21. Gorin FA, Bale JF, Haiks-Mikller M, et al. Kaposi's sarcoma metastatic to the CNS. *Arch Neurol* 1985;42:162–165.
22. Hamilton-Dutoit SJ, Martine R, Josee A, et al. In situ demonstration of Epstein-Barr small RNAs (EBER1) in acquired immunodeficiency syndrome-related lymphomas: correlation with tumor morphology and primary site. *Blood* 1993;82(2):619–624.
23. Harris OD, Cooke WT, Thompson H, et al. Malignancy in adult celiac disease and idiopathic steatorrhea. *Am J Med* 1967;42:899–912.
24. Helle TL, Britt RH, Colby TV. Primary lymphoma of the central nervous system: clinicopathological study of experience at Stanford. *J Neurosurg* 1984;60:94–103.
25. Henry JM, Heffner RR Jr, Dillard SH, et al. Primary malignant lymphomas of the central nervous system. *Cancer* 1974;34:1293–1302.
26. Hermann TS, Hammond N, Jones SE, et al. Involvement of the central nervous system by non-Hodgkin's lymphoma. The Southwest Oncology Group Experience. *Cancer* 1979;43:390–397.
27. Hobson DE, Anderson BA, Carr I, West M. Primary lymphoma of the central nervous system: Manitoba experience and literature review. *Can J Neurol Sci* 1986;13:55–61.
28. Hochberg FH, Miller DC. Primary central nervous system lymphoma. *J Neurosurg* 1988;68:835–853.
29. Hochberg FH, Miller G, Schooley RT, et al. Central nervous system lymphoma related to Epstein-Barr virus. *N Engl J Med* 1983;39:813–817.
30. Holm LE, Blomgren H, Lowhagen T. Cancer risks in patients with chronic lymphocytic thyroiditis. *N Engl J Med* 1985;312:601–604.
31. Jack CR Jr, O'Neill BP, Banks DM, Reese DF. Central nervous system lymphoma: histological types, and CT appearance. *Radiology* 1988;167:211–215.
32. Jellinger K, Raskiewicz TH, Slowik F. Primary malignant lymphoma of the central nervous system in man. *ACTA Neuropathol (Berl)* 1975;6(Suppl):95–102.
33. Jordan BD, Navia BA, Petito C, Cho ES, Price RW. Neurological syndromes complicating AIDS. *Front Radiol Ther Oncol* 1985;19:82–87.
34. Kalter SP, Riggs SA, Cabanillas F, et al. Aggressive NHL in immunocompromised homosexual males. *Blood* 1985;66:655–659.
35. Kaplan LD, Abrams DI, Feigal E, et al. AIDS-associated non-Hodgkin's lymphoma in San Francisco. *JAMA* 1989;261:719–724.
36. Kassan SS, Thomas TL, Moutsopoulos HH, et al. Increased risk of lymphoma in sicca syndrome. *Ann Intern Med* 1978;89:888–892.
37. Klimo P, Connors JM. MACOP B chemotherapy for the treatment of diffuse large cell lymphoma. *Ann Intern Med* 1985;102:596–602.
38. Kupfer MC, Zee CS, Colletti PM, et al. MRI evaluation of AIDS-related encephalopathy: toxoplasmosis vs. lymphoma. *Magn Reson Imag* 1990;8:51–57.
39. Levine AM. AIDS-related malignancies: the emerging epidemic. *J Natl Cancer Inst* 1993;85(17): 1382–1397.
40. Levine AM. AIDS-associated malignant lymphoma. *Med Clin North Am* 1992;76(1):253–268.
41. Levine AM. Acquired immunodeficiency syndrome-related lymphoma. *Blood* 1992;80:8–20.
42. Levine AM. Non-Hodgkin's lymphoma and other malignancies in the acquired immune deficiency syndrome. *Semin Oncol* 1987;14(Suppl):34–39.
43. Levine AM, Gill PS, Meyer PR, et al. Retrovirus and malignant lymphoma in homosexual men. *JAMA* 1985;254:1921.
44. Levine AM, Meyer PR, Begandy M, et al. Development of B cell lymphoma in homosexual men: clinical and immunological findings. *Ann Intern Med* 1984;100:7.
45. Levine AM, Sullivan-Halley J, Pike MC, et al. HIV-related lymphoma: prognostic factors predictive of survival. *Cancer* 1991;68:2466–2472.

46. Levine AM, Wernz JC, Kaplan L, et al. Low dose chemotherapy with CNS prophylaxis and zidovudine maintenance for AIDS-related lymphoma: a prospective multi-institutional trial. *JAMA* 1991;266: 84–88.
47. Levy R, Mills C, Posin J, Moore S, Rosenblum M, Bredesen D. The efficacy and clinical impact of brain imaging in neurologically symptomatic AIDS patients: a prospective CT/MRI study. *J AIDS* 1990;3:461–471.
48. Levy RM, Bredesen DE, Rosenblum ML. Neurological manifestations of the acquired immunodeficiency syndrome (AIDS): experience at UCSF and review of the literature. *J Neurosurg* 1985;62: 476–495.
49. Levy RM, Cohen B, Marymount M, VonRoenn J. Failure of standard therapy for HIV-related primary central nervous system lymphoma (Abstract). *Paper presented at Neuroscience of HIV Infection: Basic and Clinical Frontiers.* Vancouver, British Columbia, Canada, 1994.
50. Levy RM, Pons VG, Rosenblum ML. Central nervous system mass lesions in the acquired immunodeficiency syndrome (AIDS). *J Neurosurg* 1984;61:9–16.
51. Levy RM, Russell E, Yungbluth M, Hidvegi DF, Brody BA, DalCanto MC. Efficacy of image guided stereotactic brain biopsy in neurologically symptomatic acquired immunodeficiency syndrome patients. *Neurosurgery* 1992;30:186–190.
52. Lipsmeyer EA. Development of malignant cerebral lymphoma in a patient with systemic lupus erythematosus treated with immunosuppression. *Arthritis Rheum* 1972;15:183–186.
53. Loeffler JS, Ervin TJ, Mauch P, et al. Primary lymphomas of the central nervous system: patterns of failure and factors that influence survival. *J Clin Oncol* 1985;3:490–494.
54. Lowenthal DA, Straus DJ, Campbell SW, et al. AIDS-related lymphoid neoplasia: the Memorial Hospital experience. *Cancer* 1988;61:2325–2337.
55. Lukes JR, Parker JW, Taylor CR, Tindle BH, Cramer T, Lincoln TL. Immunological aproach to non-Hodgkin's lymphoma and related leukemias. Analysis of the results of multiparameter studies of 425 cases. *Semin Hematol* 1978;15:322–351.
56. McArthur JC. Neurological manifestations of AIDS. *Medicine* 1987;66:407–437.
57. McKelvey EM, Gottlieb JA, Wilson HE, et al. Hydroxyl daunomycin (adriamycin) combination chemotherapy in malignant lymphoma. *Cancer* 1976;38:1484–1493.
58. Mandenhall NP, Thar TL, Agee OF, et al. Computerized tomography scan characteristics and treatment results for 12 cases. *Cancer* 1983;52:1993–2000.
59. Murray K, Kun L, Cox J. Primary malignant lymphoma of the central nervous system: results of treatment of 11 cases and review of the literature. *J Neurosurg* 1986;65:600–607.
60. Nathwan BN, Rappaport H, Moran EM, et al. Malignant lymphoma arising in angioimmunobiostatic lymphadenopathy. *Cancer* 1978;41:578–606.
61. Neuwelt EA, Frenkel EP, Gumarlock MK, et al. Developments in the diagnosis and treatment of primary CNS lymphoma. A prospective series. *Cancer* 1986;58:1609–1620.
62. Odajnyk C, Subar M, Digan M, et al. Clinical features and correlates with immunopathology and molecular biology of a large group of patients with AIDS-associated small non-cleaved cell lymphoma. *Proc Am Soc Hematol* 1986;68:131(abst).
63. O'Malley JP, Ziessman HA, Kumar PN, et al. Diagnosis of intracranial lymphoma in patients with AIDS: value of ^{201}Tl single-photon emission computed tomography. *Am J Roengenol* 1994;163: 417–421.
64. O'Neill BP, Illig JJ. Primary central nervous system lymphoma. *Mayo Clin Proc* 1989;64: 1005—1020.
65. O'Neill BP, Kelly PJ, Earle JD, et al. Computer assisted sterotaxic biopsy for the diagnosis of primary central nervous system lymphoma. *Neurology* 1987;37:1160–1164.
66. O'Neill BP, O'Fallon JR, Brown LD, et al. Primary CNS non-Hodgkin's lymphoma: survival advantage with combined therapy? *Proc ASCO* 1993;(abst 174).
67. Orron DE, Kuhn MJ, Malholtra V, et al. Primary cerebral lymphoma in acquired immunodeficiency syndrome (AIDS) CT manifestations. *Comput Med Imag Graphics* 1989;13:207.
68. Penn I. Principles of tumor immunity: immunocompromised patients. *AIDS Updates* 1990;3:1–4.
69. Penn I. Cancers complicating organ transplantation. *N Engl J Med* 1990;323:1767–1769.
70. Penn I. The occurrence of malignant tumors in immunosuppressed states. *Prog Allergy* 1986;37: 259–300.
71. Pitlik SD, Fainstein V, Bolivar R, et al. Spectrum of central nervous system complications in homosexual men with acquired immune deficiency syndrome. *J Infect Dis* 1983;148:771–772.
72. Pluda JM, Yarchoan R, Jaffe ES, et al. Development of non-Hodgkin's lymphoma in a cohort of patients with severe human immunodeficiency virus (HIV) infection on long-term antiretroviral therapy. *Ann Intern Med* 1990;113:276–282.
73. Post MJ, Kursunogly SJ, Hensley GT, et al. Cranial CT in acquired immunodeficiency syndrome: spectrum of diseases and optimal contrast enhancement technique. *Am J Roentgenol* 1985;145: 929–940.
74. Remick SC, Diamond C, Migiozz JA, et. al. Primary central nervous system lymphoma in patients with and without the acquired immune deficiency syndrome. *Medicine* 1990;69(6):345–360.

75. Rosenblum ML, Levy RM, Bredesen DE, So YT, Wara W, Ziegler JL. Primary central nervous system lymphomas in patients with AIDS. *Ann Neurol* 1988;23(Suppl):513–516.
76. Shipp MA, Harrington DP, Klatt MM, et al. Identification of major prognostic subgroups with large cell lymphoma treated with M-BACOD or m-BACOD. *Ann Intern Med* 1965;104:757–765.
77. Simon J, Jones EL, Trumper MM, Slamon MV. Malignant lymphomas involving the central nervous system. A morphological and immunohistochemical study of 32 cases. *Histopathology* 1987;11: 335–349.
78. Snider WD, Simpson DM, Aronyk KE. Primary lymphoma of the nervous system associated with acquired immunodeficiency syndrome (Letter). *N Engl J Med* 1983;308:45.
79. Song SK, Schwartz IS, Breastone BA. Lymphoproliferative disorder of the central nervous system in AIDS. *Mount Sinai J Med* 1986;53:686–689.
80. Spillane JA, Kendall BE, Moseley IF. Cerebral lymphoma: clinical radiological correlation. *J Neurol Neurosurg Psychiatr* 1982;45:199–208.
81. Woodman R, Shin K, Pineo G. Primary non-Hodgkin's lymphoma of the brain: a review. *Medicine* 1985;64:425–430.

AIDS and the Nervous System, Second Edition,
edited by J. R. Berger and R. M. Levy.
Lippincott-Raven Publishers, Philadelphia © 1997.

29

Hospital Epidemiology and Infection Control

°Gordon Dickinson and †Michael L. Tapper

*°Department of Infectious Diseases and Immunology, University of Miami,
Miami, Florida 33125; and †Department of Medicine, New York University
School of Medicine, and Section of Infectious Diseases, Lennox Hill Hospital,
New York, New York 10021-1883*

The earliest reports of the acquired immunodeficiency syndrome discussed the possibility of an infectious etiology (9,47), and in November of 1982 the Centers for Disease Control issued a precautionary advisory and its first of many recommendations regarding safety precautions for health care workers (12). By the time the human immunodeficiency virus (HIV) was isolated, the major modes of transmission were clearly evident, and the potential for transmission from an infected patient to a health care worker appreciated. A greater understanding of the factors associated with transmission and the pathogenesis of HIV disease has gradually unfolded, although many details remain to be clarified. Additionally, a second serologically distinct strain, designated HIV type 2 to distinguish it from the original isolates, has been identified. The HIV type 2 is found primarily in western Africa and is infrequently seen in the United States. In most respects, its mode of transmission and the pathology it produces are similar to those of HIV type 1.

The HIV epidemic continues to evolve. The number of persons infected is increasing, and there has been a gradual spread to populations not originally considered to be at significant risk for HIV infection. Heterosexually active persons are accounting for a larger percentage of the overall number of cases, and women represent the most rapidly growing subgroup with HIV infection. It is clear that the problem of HIV will be with us for the foreseeable future and that the health care industry must be prepared to cope with the virus in a manner that provides safety for both patients and health care workers with a minimum of inefficiency and cost.

EPIDEMIOLOGY OF HIV INFECTION

The first cases of acquired immunodeficiency syndrome (AIDS) occurred among homosexual men and intravenous drug users, suggesting that the etiology might be an infectious agent (9). Subsequent events have confirmed that HIV is principally transmitted through sexual contact and direct inoculation of blood. Transmission through plasma concentrate infusion (10) and blood transfusion (11) and transmission from infected mothers to their newborn babies were soon reported (13). Transmission via organ transplantation and artificial insemination has also been documented

(19,64,93). Other routes of transmission have not been identified, although biting insects, aerosols, and casual contact have been discussed as possible means of spread. Available data suggest that, except for direct inoculation, sexual intercourse, or perinatal exposure, transmission through casual contact is a very rare event. Although sexual contact between men involving anal penetration appears to carry a particularly high risk for transmission (75,80), heterosexual intercourse accounts for the majority of infections throughout the world and an increasing proportion of infections in the United States (31).

A state-by-state mandatory reporting system in the United States requires that physicians report all patients meeting certain diagnostic criteria to the local public health authorities. These surveillance criteria have been amended several times to conform to changes in our knowledge of the disease caused by HIV infection, but they have provided reasonable continuity of data since the early 1980s. The cumulative number of AIDS cases reported through December 31, 1995, was 349,154 (29). Risk behavior data for the most recent 12 months show that, among adults, male homosexuality (including those homosexuals who also inject drugs) accounted for 47% of cases, intravenous drug use for 26%, and heterosexual intercourse for 11%. These figures reflect a slow but steady increase in the percentage of heterosexually acquired cases. Women accounted for 19% of adult cases. Although a small percentage overall, the numbers of women with AIDS are increasing rapidly. The cumulative data also show considerable geographic variation in rates of AIDS cases per 100,000 population (Table 1). Analysis of cases by ethnicity shows a disproportionately high rate of AIDS among blacks and Hispanics, a finding generally attributed to socioeconomic factors such as limited access to health care and pertinent health education experienced by many members of these groups rather than a racial predisposition.

One disadvantage of the AIDS surveillance program is the inherent delay in detection of newly acquired HIV infections and the failure to identify many patients with asymptomatic infection. The surveillance program is slow to detect shifts and new trends in the epidemic and will always trail the leading edge of the epidemic by years. Additional information about the spread of HIV infection has come from

TABLE 1. *Annual rates of AIDS cases per 100,000 population, by selected metropolitan area with 500,000 or more population, 1995*

Metropolitan area	Annual rate of AIDS
Akron, OH	5.5
Baton Rouge, LA	21.5
Chicago, IL	24.8
Fresno, CA	17.1
Los Angeles, CA	43.7
Miami, FL	117.2
New Orleans, LA	45.2
New York, NY	122.5
Orange County, CA	22.2
Rochester, NY	27.3
San Francisco, CA	129.7
Tampa–St. Petersburg, FL	32.5
Central counties	39.7
Outlyting counties	9.5

Adapted from the HIV/AIDS surveillance report, U.S. HIV and AIDS cases reported through December 1995 year-end edition, vol. 7, no. 2.

serological studies of selected populations (8,36,45,49,60,62,66). These studies are limited by their design and provide data that must then be extrapolated to the general population. The U.S. Public Health Service is now collecting data on HIV infection cases from states which report HIV infection; although in 1995 these included only 28 states, it likely that others also will initiate reporting of HIV seropositive cases.

RATES OF HIV AMONG HOSPITALIZED PATIENTS

As noted above, the rate of HIV infection varies widely from one geographic area to another and, within a given locale, according to high-risk behavior. A multicity study of occult HIV infection performed in 26 hospitals in 1989 found rates of infection ranging from 0.05% to nearly 2% (88). Another study of HIV seroprevalence among patients admitted to 20 hospitals from September of 1989 until November of 1991 found the rates of positivity to range from 0.2% to 14.2% (60). Approximately 68% of these seropositive patients had asymptomatic infection. Studies of HIV infection among persons seen in emergency rooms have found rates as high as 15% among young adults in some locations (45,62). Although the rate of HIV infection among the patients served by the vast majority of hospitals will be low, one cannot assume that it will be zero. The extended period of clinical latency allows HIV infection to remain occult, unrecognized by the infected person or those who care for him or her. As the epidemic spreads into the general population, there will be increasing numbers of infected individuals who do not consider themselves at risk and will be, therefore, unknowingly infected. It is impossible to exclude the presence of HIV based upon patient demographics, and all health care workers must be held to a high standard of infection control practices. Targeting protective precautions to those with known infection will miss many patients.

TRANSMISSION IN THE HEALTH CARE SETTING

Since the first report of HIV infection acquired from a needle stick was published in 1984 (76), there have been a number of published accounts of HIV transmission from patients to health care workers (18,21,77,78,94,99). The Centers for Disease Control and Prevention maintain a registry of health care workers in the United States with documented or possible occupationally acquired HIV infection (Table 2). The majority have been attributed to hollow-bore needle stick injuries. The ubiquitous needle in modern health care is often implicated in percutaneous accidents (59,67,72,81,82,95,100). Suture needle sticks are particularly frequent in procedures in which sutures are placed in areas where the surgeon's visibility is impaired and the needle is guided by finger touch. Hollow-bore needles used for venipuncture or the aspiration of specimens may represent a greater risk because punctures with these needles may inoculate a finite volume of blood or body fluid into the recipient (71). Cuts with glass or scalpels, direct cutaneous exposure, and mucosal splashes have also been implicated in transmission of HIV (18,48). Prospectively collected data of HIV transmission to health care workers experiencing a percutaneous exposure indicate that the risk for a single exposure is approximately 0.3% (52,96). Cutaneous contact with blood is a frequent occurrence in the operating suite and emergency room (44,61,66,81,82,95), and although the risk for transmission appears low, the potential clearly exists. Close contact as occurs between nurses or doctors and their

TABLE 2. *U.S. health care workers[a] with documented and possible occupationally acquired HIV-infection reported through June 1995*

Occupation	Number of cases of documented occupational transmission	Number of cases of possible occupational transmission
Dental worker, including dentist	—	7
Embalmer/morgue technician	—	3
Emergency medical technician/paramedic	—	9
Health aide/attendant	1	12
Housekeeper/maintenance worker	1	7
Laboratory technician, clinical	15	15
Laboratory technician, nonclinical	3	0
Nurse	19	24
Physician, nonsurgical	6	10
Physician, surgical	—	4
Respiratory therapist	1	2
Technician, dialysis	1	2
Technician, surgical	2	1
Technician/therapist, other than those listed above	—	4
Other health care occupations	—	2
Total	49	102

Adapted from the HIV/AIDS surveillance report, U.S. HIV and AIDS cases reported through December 1995 year-end edition, vol. 7, no. 2.

[a] Health-care workers are defined as those persons, including students and trainees, who have worked in a health care, clinical, or HIV laboratory setting at any time since 1978.

[b] Human Immunodeficiency virus.

patients, in the absence of blood exposure, has not been associated with transmission of HIV, an observation in accordance with what is known from epidemiological studies of families with an HIV-infected member. There has been no epidemiological evidence to suggest that HIV is transmitted by the airborne route.

There have been reports of apparent patient-to-patient transmission (7,30,55). The tragic experience of Romania was clearly related to violations of accepted medical practices (55), and the other reports were probably occasioned by breaks in current infection control practices.

PREVENTION OF TRANSMISSION IN THE HEALTH CARE SETTING

Safety in the health care setting, as noted above, was the focus of discussion from early in the epidemic (12), and guidelines have been published and updated periodically (12–17,20,22–23,27). Initially, protective precautions were recommended for persons with AIDS (12,14), but the identification of the causative pathogen and availability of a serological test in 1985 allowed physicians to diagnose clinically asymptomatic infections that also represented potential risks for transmission. There was controversy over the best approach to assure the safety of health care workers. On the one hand, testing of all patients for HIV antibodies with precautions focused on the positive patients was advocated, whereas application of precautions to all patients irrespective of status was considered more appropriate by others. Application of precautions equally to all patients without knowledge of their HIV status, it was argued, would foster complacency and haphazard compliance. On the other hand, instituting precautions only for patients who are HIV antibody positive would miss many who require emergency care before testing could be performed. Also, precautions focused on HIV would not address other blood-borne pathogens. Lastly, widespread testing for HIV raised ethical and legal issues. The consensus leaned toward universality of precautions (42,43) and led the U.S. Public Health Service to recommend that all patients be managed as if they potentially harbored a blood-borne pathogen with potential for transmission (20).

Universal precautions were defined and practice guidelines published by the Centers for Disease Control in August of 1987 (20). These guidelines have been adopted by most medical facilities in the United States. The key concept underlying these guidelines is that all patients are presumed to be potentially infected and that any direct contact with blood, body fluids, or tissues known to harbor HIV is to be prevented. Thus, whenever contact between the health care worker's skin or mucous membranes and blood or body fluids of a patient is anticipated, barrier precautions adequate to prevent such contact are to be employed. Gloves are to be worn whenever a caregiver touches blood, body fluids, mucous membranes, or nonintact skin, handles items or surfaces soiled with blood or body fluids, or performs a procedure such as venipuncture or manipulates a device contaminated with blood or body fluids. Goggles and masks are to be worn if the caregiver performs a procedure likely to generate aerosols of blood or body fluids. Gowns or aprons are indicated if splashes are anticipated. If contamination of skin should occur, the contaminated area is to be washed immediately. The guidelines go on to recommend that all sharp instruments such as needles and scalpels are to be handled with care to avoid injury and that manipulation after use be kept to a minimum. Needles are not to be recapped after use, and all disposable sharps are to be discarded immediately at the site of use in puncture-resistant containers for disposal. Reusable devices are to be transported to the reprocessing area in puncture-resistant containers. To avoid contact with saliva during resuscitation, mouthpieces and ventilation devices should be available in areas where the need for resuscitation is likely to arise. Health care workers with "exudative lesions or weeping dermatitis" should refrain from direct patient contact or handling patient care equipment. The guidelines recognized that pregnant health care workers are not known to be at increased risk, but because of the threat to the fetus should HIV infection of the mother occur, the pregnant worker should be especially familiar with recommended precautions and follow them explicitly.

Protective garb and equipment should be tailored to match the requirements of specialized areas; specific guidelines have been published for hemodialysis units (17) and dental offices (27), for example.

MANAGEMENT OF THE HEALTH CARE WORKER WITH A SIGNIFICANT EXPOSURE

The success of universal precautions is linked to the administrative attention paid to safety in the workplace and the vigor of ongoing education programs (40,50,61,67). In spite of the best of efforts, however, exposure to blood and potentially infectious body fluids is a fact of life in the health care setting for even the most fastidious and careful staff (40,42,44,50,59,66,67,70,72,100). Scrupulous adherence to the precautions described above, fortunately, can greatly minimize the frequency of exposures.

The accidental exposure of a health care worker to blood contaminated with HIV is invariably an emotionally traumatic event, and it should be met immediately with an efficient response that appropriately answers both the physical and emotional needs of the exposed worker. To do this, the hospital should have a program in place before an incident occurs. The health care worker who incurs a percutaneous or mucous membrane exposure should be able immediately to contact employee health office personnel or designees (during after-hours and weekends) who in turn can assess and document the particulars of the incident, provide the health care worker with up-to-date information about the risk for transmission and the preventive options available, and arrange for HIV antibody testing. It is important that all health care workers know about the program and whom to contact when accidents occur. If the source patient is known to be infected with HIV and a significant exposure has occurred, the health care worker should be tested for HIV antibodies at the time of the incident and at 6 weeks, 3 months, and 6 months. The baseline assay is important to document the absence of preexistent infection; otherwise, the employee's rights to workman's compensation and insurance benefits may be jeopardized. The 6-month date for final testing has been selected because nearly all persons infected will sero-convert by that time. To provide an extra degree of certitude and comfort, some centers may choose to offer another test at 12 months, based on the rare instances of delayed seroconversion (39). In actuality, a majority of persons newly infected rapidly develop an antibody response. Horsburgh and co-workers estimated the median time from infection to antibody detection to be 2.1 months, with 95% of patients becoming positive by 5.8 months (58). The suspense of waiting may be so traumatic for the health care worker that other assays are considered. Assays for HIV antigens can demonstrate infection within weeks of onset but are not sufficiently sensitive to detect all infections. Polymerase chain reaction (PCR) assays are not yet commercially available, nor are their sensitivity and specificity fully defined, although they theoretically will detect infection within days of infection. These methods eventually could supplant the serial antibody assays.

Accidents involving the blood or fluids of a patient who has not been evaluated for HIV infection interjects additional uncertainty and complexity into the incident. Rates of HIV infection vary widely throughout the United States, influenced not only by geographic location, but also by demographic features such as age, sex, and socioeconomic status. Fortunately, for most of the country the rate is well below 1%. Still, much anxiety can be avoided if the source patient is known to be antibody negative, and testing will usually provide immense relief for the health care worker. The testing of the source patient raises additional issues, and the hospital should have a defined plan that details the steps to be followed. Even broaching the subject of HIV testing may be unsettling for some patients, and their personal physician should be involved. Therefore, the best scheme is to request permission from the attending physician to approach the source patient. With the attending physician's concurrence and advice, the source patient can be told that an accident occurred and be asked to undergo an HIV assay. Obviously, the patient needs to be counseled fully about the test in accordance with applicable laws and then consent obtained. If the source patient declines, some states allow the staff to test residual blood if it should be available. All patient identifiers are removed from the residual specimen, and it then is tested for HIV antibody and labeled only as needed to link it to the exposed health care worker; the results are recorded only in the employee health records. If no HIV antibodies are detected, the health care worker can be reassured and no further evaluation is necessary.

Many health care workers with an accidental exposure are extremely anxious and worried. Even though no one can offer absolute assurances, in reality the risk is approximately 0.3% (52,96) and in many instances (especially for mucous membrane splashes and superficial skin pricks) virtually nil. A frank discussion of what is known about accidental transmission in which the health care worker has the opportunity to freely question a knowledgeable professional often goes a long way toward allaying the fears that an accident engenders. The need to talk is real, and an expert should be available for immediate consultation and for further discussions on an as-needed basis.

Whereas intuitively it would seem that a drug that interrupts viral replication might prevent infection, the benefit of antiretroviral postexposure prophylaxis is as yet undefined and must be considered an empiric exercise (39,41,51). The inhibitory effect of drugs such as zidovudine on viral replication *in vitro* and *in vivo*, and the observation that administration of zidovudine to pregnant women was protective for their new newborns (28), supports the use of postexposure treatment. On the other hand, well-documented cases of failure of zidovudine to prevent transmission when administered within 1 hour of exposure have been reported (65,69). Experimental studies with animals have been inconclusive (90,97), again showing that transmission may occur despite immediate postexposure treatment toxicity. Although these reports clearly prove that postexposure prophylaxis is not 100% efficacious, one cannot infer that it is without value. Even if the ethical conundrum that a controlled study poses could be solved, the logistical requirements for conduct of a conclusive clinical trial exceed the resources available. With transmission occurring only once in every 250 to 300 exposures, the enrollment needed to detect a 50% effect of treatment would require several thousand subjects. A trial was initiated in 1988, but poor enrollment led to its discontinuation a year later (63). Thus, it is unlikely that an efficacy trial will ever be conducted (see addendum).

Because the currently available antiretrovirals do have a demonstrable effect on HIV replication, it is not unreasonable to make postexposure treatment available. Zidovudine, the first antiretorviral approved for treatment of HIV infection, is the drug most frequently discussed. The optimal dosage and duration of treatment are unknown, although many centers have adopted regimens similar to one of those described by Henderson and Gerberding, e.g., 1,000 mg daily for 4 weeks or 1,200 mg daily for 6 weeks (53).

The decision to take antiretroviral prophylaxis should be made immediately after the accident because the data available suggest that any benefit is likely to be lost if treatment is delayed for more than an hour or two. Prophylaxis is an active response to an emotionally trying event and psychologically may be more satisfying for some than merely waiting to learn the results of serological monitoring. Therefore, a reasonable approach is to have a program established that makes postexposure prophylaxis available to the health care worker, along with information about our understanding of the potential benefit and risks of such prophylaxis. The potential adverse effects of ziodvudine include headache, nausea and vomiting, malaise, and rarely, more serious allergic reactions; fortunately, in the healthy individual these are usually not serious (63,96).

THE HIV-INFECTED HEALTH CARE WORKER

Health care workers with HIV infection were the subject of discussion from early in the epidemic, but the announcement that a dentist in Florida had apparently infected a number of his patients produced widespread consternation and focused attention on the potential risks to patients receiving care from an HIV-infected caregiver (24). An in-depth investigation of the dentist's practice and the patients found to be infected with HIV was launched. The investigation was hindered by the absence of office records—the practice had been sold several years before the study was initiated—and the death of the dentist before the investigation was completed. Ultimately, it was concluded that six of seven of the dentist's patients with HIV infection had acquired the virus from him (25–26,32,79). This conclusion was based both on epidemiological grounds and nucleotide sequence studies of material obtained from the dentist and the patients involved (32,79). Appropriate controls selected from the region strengthened the case for relatedness of the HIV isolates recovered from the dentist and his six patients. What could not be determined was how the transmission occurred. Theories advanced have included volitional acts on the part of the dentist, contamination of dental instruments through self-treatment by the dentist without adequate sterilization before treatment of patients, droplet contamination from the dentist's mouth into the mouth of the patient (the dentist had Kaposi's sarcoma with oral lesions at one point), and inadvertent reuse of syringes and instruments without adequate sterilization. The exact mechanisms will likely never be known.

No other instances of transmission of HIV from an infected health care worker have been identified in the United States, although a number of surgeons and dentists with HIV infection have been investigated (3,4,6,33,37–38,57,68,73,83,85–87,98). The Centers for Disease Control and Prevention continue to compile data about patients of infected health care workers in the United States. As of December 1993, some 22,000 patients of infected health care workers have been identified and tested (84). Although 112 of these patients were found to have HIV infection, high-risk behavior was the probable route of infection for 59, 27 were infected before receiving care, and of the 20 who denied any identified risk behavior, nucleotide sequencing analysis has been completed for 16 and no relatedness has been found.

These look-back studies are all limited to varying degrees. Many patients died before they could be evaluated, some could not be located, and others refused to be tested for HIV infection. The degree of exposure for many patients has been minimal, and it has been difficult to judge the intensity of exposure for many others. The onset of HIV infection in the health care worker has been impossible to pinpoint in most cases, and the level of viremia (viral load)—which presumably is directly related with the potential for transmission (35,56)—at the time of contact cannot be quantified in retrospect.

Comparing HIV to hepatitis B virus (HBV) suggests that the potential for transmission of HIV might vary widely from one health care worker to another (74). Clusters of HBV transmission have occurred, and arguing by analogy, one might reasonably conclude that the same dynamics apply to the health care worker with HIV infection. Thus, multiple look-back studies finding no transmission might not include the occasional efficient transmitter and thereby give a false sense of security. There is, however, a major quantitative difference between HIV and HBV infection. Persons with hepatitis B e antigen (HBeAg) in their serum have up to 10^8 infectious viral particles per milliliter of blood (91); the risk for transmission via a percutaneous exposure is approximately 30% (89). Of the health care workers implicated in clusters of transmission of HBV to patients, all those evaluated have been HBeAg positive (23) and, therefore, highly infectious. Titers of HIV in plasma of HIV-infected persons, on the other hand, are less than 10^5 (and for asymptomatic individuals, 10^2 or less) (35,56) with a risk for transmission via a percutaneous exposure of approximately 0.3% (52,96). At present, there are no data to suggest that one health care worker with HIV infection represents a significantly greater risk to his or her patients than does another with this infection.

Following the initial reports of transmission from the Florida dentist to his patients there was extensive media coverage, and one of the infected patients, a young woman, lobbied a congressional committee to enact strict legislation to prevent a recurrence of her experience. The Centers for Disease Control drafted a set of recommendations that updated earlier guidelines (23). The updated recommendations dealt with testing of health care workers for HIV and HBV and attempted to define which procedures might represent an "increased risk to the patient." Based on experience with HBV transmission from caregivers to patients, certain procedures were considered "exposure prone." These procedures were not enumerated, but the following description was given (23):

> Characteristics of exposure-prone procedures include digital palpation of a needle tip in a body cavity or the simultaneous presence of the health care worker's fingers and a needle or other sharp instrument or object in a poorly visualized or highly confined anatomic site. Performance of exposure-prone procedures presents a recognized risk of percutaneous injury to the health care worker, and—if such an injury occurs—the health care worker's blood is likely to contact the patient's body cavity, subcutaneous tissues, and/or mucous membranes.

The specific six recommendations made were as follows:

1. All health care workers should adhere to universal precautions, including the appropriate use of hand washing, protective barriers, and care in the use and disposal of needles and other sharp instruments. Health care workers who have exudative lesions or weeping dermatitis should refrain from all direct patient care and from handling patient care equipment and devices used in performing invasive procedures until the condition resolves. Health care workers should also comply with current guidelines for disinfection and sterilization of reusable devices used in invasive procedures.

2. Currently available data provide no basis for recommendations to restrict the practice of health care workers infected with HIV or HBV who perform invasive procedures not identified as exposure prone, provided the infected health care workers practice recommended surgical or dental technique and comply with universal precautions and current recommendations for sterilization/disinfection.

3. Exposure-prone procedures should be identified by medical/surgical/dental organizations and institutions at which the procedures are performed.

4. Health care workers who perform exposure-prone procedures should know their HIV antibody status. Health care workers who perform exposure-prone procedures and who do not have serological evidence of immunity to HBV from vaccination or from previous infection should know their HbsAg status and, if that is positive, should also know their HbeAg status.

5. Health care workers who are infected with HIV or HBV (and are HbeAg positive) should not perform exposure-prone procedures unless they have sought counsel

from an expert review panel and been advised under what circumstances, if any, they may continue to perform these procedures (see below). Such circumstances would include notifying prospective patients of the health care worker's seropositivity before they undergo exposure-prone invasive procedures.

6. Mandatory testing of health care workers for HIV antibody, HbsAg, or HbeAg is not recommended. The current assessment of the risk that infected health care workers will transmit HIV or HBV to patients during exposure-prone procedures does not support the diversion of resources that would be required to implement mandatory testing programs. Compliance by health care workers with recommendations can be increased through education, training, and appropriate confidentiality safeguards.

The key elements of these recommendations were recognition that some procedures are exposure prone as currently performed, that the enumeration of these procedures should be made by representative organizations and/or local institutions, that health care workers who perform these procedures should ascertain their own serological status, and that those with positive serological tests should not continue to perform the exposure-prone procedures without the approval of an expert review panel—and then only after informing their prospective patients. It was suggested that the panel include the health care worker's personal physician, an infectious disease specialist with expertise in the epidemiology of HIV and HBV transmission, a professional with expertise in the procedures performed by the health care worker, and a state or local public health official.

Various professional groups and organizations have also issued statements about the HIV-infected health care worker (1,2,5,34,46,92). Most recognize that the potential for transmission is very low and accounts for but a minor fraction of those elements that represent the risk associated with a given invasive procedure. They also note the problematic nature of virtually any mandatory screening program as well as the expense and disruption of normal activity that such a program would entail and that current knowledge does not suggest a need for mandatory screening for HIV and restriction of those found to be infected.

There is clearly a need for further information about all blood-borne pathogens. Ongoing studies of HBV in health care workers suggest that HBV is quite different from HIV. Continued reports of clusters of HBV infection attributed to health care workers clearly show that the health care worker who is HbeAg positive may represent an ongoing risk to his or her patients even if infection control guidelines are scrupulously followed (54). It is likely that new guidelines will be forthcoming that markedly curtail the activities of HbeAg-positive health care workers. Hepatitis C virus transmission is poorly understood, particularly in the health care setting.

SUMMARY

The HIV epidemic will be with us for many years. The number of infected persons will continue to increase, not only because of continued transmission, but also because persons with HIV infection will live longer. All health care professionals must be alert to the presence of HIV as well as other blood-borne pathogens. There is much to be learned about factors that enhance or impede transmission of HIV, but we have the knowledge necessary to prevent nosocomial transmission. Health care professionals should scrupulously observe universal precautions, and those with supervisory responsibilities should be vigilant and energetic in their efforts to maintain a safe work environment for patients and workers alike.

Addendum: Since this chapter was written, a retrospective case control study evaluating factors influencing transmission of HIV to health care workers through percutaneous exposure has shown that post-exposure zidovudine is associated with a reduction in risk of approximately 79% (25a). Unfortunately, this news has been confounded by an increasing frequency of zidovudine-resistant HIV. The optimal regimen in situations in which the source patient has received one or more antiretrovirals is unclear at this time.

ACKNOWLEDGMENTS

We thank Tommie Stapleton and Harvey Kristal for their assistance in the preparation of the chapter.

REFERENCES

1. American Academy of Pediatrics Task Force on Pediatric AIDS. Pediatric guidelines for infection control of human immunodeficiency virus (acquired immunodeficiency virus) in hospitals, medical offices, schools, and other settings. *Pediatrics* 1988;82:801–807.
2. American Medical Association. Ethical issues in the growing AIDS crisis: Council on Ethical and Judicial Affairs. *JAMA* 1988;259:1360–1361.
3. Armstrong FP, Miner JC, Wolfe WH. Investigation of a health-care worker with symptomatic human immunodeficiency virus infection: an epidemiological approach. *Mil Med* 1987;152:414–418.
4. Arnow PM, Chou T, Shapiro R, Sussman EJ. Maintaining confidentiality in a look-back investigation of patients treated by a HIV-infected dentist. *Pub Health Rep* 1993;108:273–278.
5. Association for Practitioners in Infection Control, Society of Hospital Epidemiologists of America. Position paper: "look-back" notifications for HIV/HBV-positive health care workers. *Infect Control Hosp Epidemiol* 1992;13:482–484.
6. Bell DM, Shapiro CN, Culver DH, Martone WJ, Curran JW, Hughes JM. Risk of hepatitis B and human immunodeficiency virus transmission to a patient from an infected surgeon due to percutaneous injury during an invasive procedure. *Infect Agents Dis* 1992;1:263–269.
7. Blank S, Simonds RJ, Weisfuse I, Rudnick J, Chiasson MA, Thomas P. Possible nosocomial transmission of HIV. *Lancet* 1994;344:512–514.
8. Brundage JF, Burke DS, Gardiner LI, et al. Tracking the spread of the HIV infection epidemic among young adults in the United States: results of the first four years of screening among civilian applicants for US military service. *J Acquir Immune Defic Syndr* 1990;3:1168–1180.
9. CDC (Centers for Disease Control). A cluster of Kaposi's Sarcoma and *Pneumocystis carinii* pneumonia among homosexual male residents of Los Angeles and Orange counties, California. *Morb Mortal Wkly Rep* 1982;31:30–37.
10. CDC. *Pneumocystis carinii* pneumonia among persons with hemophilia A. *Morb Mortal Wkly Rep* 1986;31:365–367.
11. CDC. Possible transfusion-associated acquired immune deficiency syndrome (AIDS)—California. *Morb Mortal Wkly Rep* 1982;31:652–654.
12. CDC. Acquired immunodeficiency syndrome: precautions for clinical and laboratory staffs. *Morb Mortal Wkly Rep* 1982;31:577–580.
13. CDC. Unexplained immunodeficiency and opportunistic infections in infants--New York, New Jersey, California. *Morb Mortal Wkly Rep* 1982;31:665–667.
14. CDC. Acquired immunodeficiency syndrome (AIDS): precautions for health-care workers and allied professionals. *Morb Mortal Wkly Rep* 1983;32:450–451.
15. CDC. Summary and recommendations for preventing transmission of infection with human T-lymphotrophic virus type III/lymphadenopathy-associated virus in the workplace. *Morb Mortal Wkly Rep* 1985;34:681–695.
16. CDC. Recommendations for preventing transmission of infection with human T-lymphotrophic virus type III/lymphadenopathy-associated virus during invasive procedures. *Morb Mortal Wkly Rep* 1986;35:221–223.
17. CDC. Recommendations for providing dialysis treatment to patients infected with human T-lymphotropic virus type III/lymphadenopathy-associated virus. *Morb Mortal Wkly Rep* 1986;35:376–383.

18. CDC. Update: human immunodeficiency virus infection in health care workers exposed to blood of infected patients. *Morb Mortal Wkly Rep* 1987;36:285–289.

19. CDC. Human immunodeficiency virus infection transmitted from an organ donor screened for HIV antibody—North Carolina. *Morb Mortal Wkly Rep* 1987;36:306–308.

20. CDC. Recommendations for prevention of HIV transmission in health-care settings. *Morb Mortal Wkly Rep* 1987;36(Suppl 2s):1S–19S.

21. CDC. Update: acquired immunodeficiency syndrome and human immunodeficiency virus infection among health-care workers. *Morb Mortal Wkly Rep* 1988;37:229–234.

22. CDC. Update: universal precautions for preventions of transmission of human immunodeficiency virus, hepatitis B virus, and other blood borne pathogens in health-care settings. *Morb Mortal Wkly Rep* 1988;37:377–382;387–388.

23. CDC. Recommendations for preventing transmission of human immunodeficiency virus and hepatitis B virus to patients during exposure-prone procedures. *Morb Mortal Wkly Rep* 1991;40(RR-8):1–9.

24. CDC. Possible transmission of human immunodeficiency virus to a patient during an invasive dental procedure. *Morb Mortal Wkly Rep* 1990;39:489–493.

25. CDC. Update: transmission of HIV infection during an invasive dental procedure—Florida. *Morb Mortal Wkly Rep* 1991;40:377–381.

25a. CDCP. Case control study of HIV seroconversion in health-care workers after percutaneous exposure to HIV-infected blood—France, United Kingdom, and United States, January 1988–August 1994. *MMWR* 1995;44:929–933.

26. CDCP (Centers for Disease Control and Prevention). Update: investigations of persons treated by HIV-infected health-care workers—United States. *Morb Mortal Wkly Rep* 1993;42:329–331;337.

27. CDC. Recommended infection control practices for dentistry, 1993. *Morb Mortal Wkly Rep* 1993;42(RR-8):1–12.

28. CDC: Zidovudine for the prevention of HIV transmission from mother to infant. *Morb Mortal Wkly Rep* 1994;43:285–287.

29. CDCP. HIV/AIDS Surveillance Report. 1995;7(2):1–39.

30. Chant K, Lowe D, Rubin G, et al. Patient-to-patient transmission of HIV in private surgical consulting rooms (Letter). *Lancet* 1993;342:1548–1549.

31. Chu SY, Berkelman RL, Curran JW. Epidemiology of HIV in the United States. In: DeVita VT Jr, Hellman S, Rosenberg SA, eds. *AIDS: etiology, diagnosis, treatment and prevention.* 3rd ed. Philadelphia: Lippincott; 1992.

32. Ciesielski C, Marianos D, On CY, et al. Transmission of human immunodeficiency virus in a dental practice. *Ann Intern Med* 1992;116:798–805.

33. Comer RW, Mccoy BP, Pashley EL, Myers DR, Zwemer JD. Analyzing dental procedures performed by an HIV-positive dental student. *J Am Dent Assoc* 1992;123:51–54.

34. Committee on Ethics, The American College of Obstetricians and Gynecologists. Human immunodeficiency virus infection: physicians responsibilities. *Obstet Gynecol* 1990;75:1043–1045.

35. Coombs RW, Collier AC, Allain JP, et al. Plasma viremia in human immunodeficiency virus infection. *N Engl J Med* 1989;321:1626–1631.

36. Cowan DN, Brundage JF, Pomerantz RS. The incidence of HIV infection among men in the United States Army Reserve Components, 1985–1991. *AIDS* 1994;8:505–511.

37. Danila RN, Mac Donald KL, Rhame FS, et al. A look-back investigation of patients of an HIV-infected physician: public health implications. *N Engl J Med* 1991;325:1406–1411.

38. Dickinson GM, Morhart RE, Klimas NG, et al. Absence of HIV transmission from an infected dentist to his patients. *JAMA* 1993;269:1802–1806.

39. Fahey BJ, Beekmann SE, Schmitt JM, Fedio JM, Henderson DK. Managing occupational exposures to HIV-I in the healthcare workplace. *Infect Cont Hosp Epidem* 1993;14:405–412.

40. Fahey BJ, Koziol DE, Banks SM, Henderson DK. Frequency of nonparenteral occupational exposures to blood and body fluids before and after universal precautions training. *Am J Med* 1991;90:145–153.

41. Gerberding JL. Is antiretroviral treatment after percutaneous HIV exposure justified? *Ann Intern Med* 1993;118:979–980.

42. Gerberding JL, University of California, San Francisco Task Force on AIDS. Recommended infection-control policies for patients with human immunodeficiency virus infection: an update. *N Engl J Med* 1986;315:1562–1564.

43. Gerberding JL, Henderson DK. Design of rational infection control guidelines for human immunodeficiency virus infection. *J Infect Dis* 1987;156:861–864.

44. Gerberding JL, Littell C, Tarkington A, Brown A, Schecter WP. Risk of exposure of surgical personnel to patients' blood during surgery at San Francisco General Hospital. *N Engl J Med* 1990;322:1788–1793.

45. Gordin FM, Gibert C, Hawley HP, Willoughby A. Prevalence of human immunodeficiency virus and hepatitis B virus in unselected hospital admissions: implications for mandatory testing and universal precautions. *J Infect Dis* 1990;161:14–17.

46. Gostin L. The HIV-infected health care professional: public policy, discrimination, and patient safety. *Arch Intern Med* 1991;151:663–665.
47. Gottlieb MS, Schroff R, Schanker HM, et al. *Pneumocystis carinii* pneumonia and mucosal candidiasis in previously healthy homosexual men. *N Engl J Med* 1981;305:1425–1436.
48. Gurtler LG, Eberle J, Bader L. HIV transmission by needle stick and eczematous lesion—three cases from Germany. *Infect* 1993;21:40–41.
49. Gwinn M, Pappaioanou M, George JR, et al. Prevalence of HIV infection in childbearing women in the United States. *JAMA* 1991;265:1704–1708.
50. Haiduven D, DeMaio T, Stevens D. A five-year study of needlestick injuries: significant reduction associated with communication, education and convenient placement of sharps containers. *Infec Control Hosp Epidemiol* 1992;13:265.
51. Henderson DK. Postexposure chemoprophylaxis for occupational exposure to human immunodeficiency virus type I: current status and prospects for the future. *Am J Med* 1991;91(3B):312S–319S.
52. Henderson DK, Fahey BJ, Willy M, et al. Risk for occupational transmission of human immunodeficiency virus type I (HIV-I) associated with clinical exposures. *Ann Intern Med* 1990;113:740–746.
53. Henderson DK, Gerberding JL. Prophylatic zidovudine after occupational exposure to the human immunodeficiency virus: an interim analysis. *J Infect Dis* 1989;160(2):321–327.
54. Heptonstall J, Collins M, Smith I, Crawshaw SC, Gill ON. Restricting practice of HBeAg positive surgeons. Lessons from hepatitis B outbreaks in England, Wales, and Northern Ireland 1984–1993. *Infect Control Hosp Epidemiol* 1994;15:344(abst).
55. Hersh BS, Poporici F, Apetri RC, et al. Acquired immunodeficiency syndrome in Romania. *Lancet* 1991;338:645–649.
56. Ho DD, Moudgil T, Alam M. Quantitation of human immunodeficiency virus type I in the blood of infected persons. *N Engl J Med* 1989;321:1621–1625.
57. Holmes EC, Zhang LQ, Simmonds P, Rogers AS, Brown AJ. Molecular investigation of human immunodeficiency virus (HIV) infection in a patient of an HIV-infected surgeon. *J Infect Dis* 1993; 167:1411–1414.
58. Horsburgh CR, Ou CY, Jason J, et al. Duration of human immunodeficiency virus infection before detection of antibody. *Lancet* 1989;2:637–641.
59. Jagger J, Hunt EH, Brand-Elnaggar J, Pearson RD. Rates of needle-stick injury by various devices in a university hospital. *N Engl J Med* 1988;319:284–288.
60. Janssen RS, St Louis ME, Satten GA, et al. HIV infection among patients in U.S. acute care hospitals. *N Engl J Med* 1992;327:445–452.
61. Kelen GD, Green GB, Hexter DA, et al. Substantial improvement in compliance with universal precautions in an emergency department following institution of policy. *Arch Intern Med* 1991;151: 2051–2056.
62. Kelen GD, Green GB, Purcell RH, et al. Hepatitis B and hepatitis C in emergency department patients. *N Engl J Med* 1992;326:1399–1404.
63. LaFon SW, Mooney BD, McMullen JP, et al. A double-blind, placebo-controlled study of the safety and efficacy of Retrovir (zidovudine, ZDV) as a chemoprophylactic agent in healthcare workers (Abstract 489). *Programs and Abstracts, presented at the 30th Interscience Conference on Antimicrobial Agents and Chemotherapy, American Society for Microbiology.* Atlanta, Georgia, October 21–24, 1990.
64. L'age-Stehr J, Schwarz A, Ofermann G, et al. HILV-III infection in kidney transplant recipients (Letter). *Lancet* 1985;2:1361–1362.
65. Lange JMA, Boucher CAB, Hollak CEM, et al. Failure of zidovudine prophylaxis after accidental exposure to HIV. *N Engl J Med* 1990;322:1375–1377.
66. Lewandowski C, Ognjan A, Rivers E, et al. Health care worker exposure to HIV-1 and HTLV I-II in critically ill, resuscitated emergency department patients. *Ann Emerg Med* 1992;21:1353–1359.
67. Linnemannn C, Cannon C, Ed Ronde M, et al. Effect of educational programs, rigid sharps containers, and universal precautions on reported needlestick injuries in health care workers. *Infect Control Hosp Epidemiol* 1991;12:214.
68. Longfield JN, Brundage J, Badger G. Look-back investigation after human immunodeficiency virus seroconversion in a pediatric dentist. *J Infect Dis* 1994;169:1–8.
69. Looke DFM, Grove DI. Failed prophylactic zidovudine after needlestick injury (Letter). *Lancet* 1990;335:1280.
70. Marcus R, Culver DH, Bell DM, et al. Risk of human immunodeficiency virus infection among emergency department workers. *Am J Med* 1993;94:363–370.
71. Mast ST, Woolwine JD, Gerberding JL. Efficacy of gloves in reducing blood volumes transferred during simulated needlestick injury. *J Infect Dis* 1993;168:1589–1592.
72. McGeer A, Simor AE, Low DE. Epidemiology of needlestick injuries in house officers. *J Infect Dis* 1990;162:961–964.
73. Mishu B, Schaffner W, Horan J, Wood L, Hutcheson R, McNabb P. A surgeon with AIDS: lack of evidence of transmission to patients. *JAMA* 1990;264:467–470.

74. Mishu B, Schaffner W. HIV-infected surgeons and dentists: looking back and looking forward. *JAMA* 1993;269:1843–1844.
75. Moss AR, Osmond D, Bacchetti P, et al. Risk factors for AIDS and HIV seropositivity in homosexual men. *Am J Epidemiol* 1987;125:1035–1047.
76. Needlestick transmission of HTLV-III from a patient infected in Africa. *Lancet* 1984;2:1376–1377.
77. Neisson-Verant C, Arfi S, Mathez D, et al. HIV infection with seroconversion in a nurse. *Lancet* 1986;2:814.
78. Oskenhendler E, Harzic M, Le Roux JM, et al. HIV infection with seroconversion after a superficial needlestick injury to the finger. *N Engl J Med* 1986;315:582.
79. Ou CY, Ciesielski CA, Myers G, et al. Molecular epidemiology of HIV transmission in a dental practice. *Science* 1992;256:1165–1171.
80. Padian N, Marquis L, Francis DP, et al. Male-to-female transmission of human immunodeficiency virus. *JAMA* 1987;258:788–790.
81. Panlilio A, Foy D, Edwards J, et al. Blood exposures during surgical procedures. *JAMA* 1991;265:1533.
82. Panlilio A, Welch B, Bell D, et al. Blood and amniotic fluid contact sustained by obstetric personnel during deliveries. *Am J Obstet Gynecol* 1992;167:703.
83. Porter JD, Cruikshank JG, Gentle PH, Robinson RG, Gill ON. Management of patients treated by a surgeon with HIV infection. *Lancet* 1990;335:113–114.
84. Robert L, Chamberland M, Marcus R, et al. Update: lookback investigations of patients treated by HIV-infected health care workers (HCWs). *Infect Control Hosp Epidemiol* 1994;15:348(abst 49).
85. Rogers AS, Froggatt JW III, Townsend T, et al. Investigation of potential HIV transmission to the patients of an HIV-infected surgeon. *JAMA* 1993;269:1795–1801.
86. Sacks JJ. AIDS in a surgeon (Letter). *N Engl J Med* 1985;313:1017–1018.
87. Sacks JJ. More on AIDS in a surgeon (Letter). *N Engl J Med* 1986;314:1190.
88. St Louis ME, Rauch KJ, Petersen LR, et al. Seroprevalence rates of human immunodeficiency virus infection at sentinel hospitals in the United States. *N Engl J Med* 1990;323:213–218.
89. Seeff LB, Wright EC, Zimmerman HJ, et al. Type B hepatitis after needle-stick exposure: prevention with hepatitis B immune globulin. *Ann Intern Med* 1978;88:285–293.
90. Shih CC, Kaneshima H, Rabin L, et al. Postexposure prophylaxis with zidovudine suppresses human immunodeficiency virus type I infection in SCID-hu mice in a time-dependent manner. *J Infect Dis* 1991;163:625–627.
91. Shikata T, Karasawa T, Abe K, et al. Hepatitis B e antigen and infectivity of hepatitis B virus. *J Infect Dis* 1977;136:571–576.
92. Speller DEC, Shanson DC, Ayliffe GAJ, Cooke EM. Acquired immune deficiency syndrome: recommendations of a working party of the Hospital Infection Society. *J Hosp Infect* 1990;15:7–34.
93. Stewart GJ, Tyler JPP, Cunninham AL, et al. Transmission of human T-cell lymphotrophic virus type III (HTLV-III) by artificial insemination by donor. *Lancet* 1985;2:581–585.
94. Stricof RL, Morse DL. HTLV-III/LAV seroconversion following a deep intramuscular needle-stick injury. *N Engl J Med* 1986;314:1115.
95. Tokars J, Bell D, Shapiro C, et al. Percutaneous injuries during surgical procedures. *JAMA* 1992;267:2899–2904.
96. Tokars JI, Marcus R, Culver DH, et al. Surveillance of HIV infection and zidovudine use among health care workers after occupational exposure to HIV-infected blood. *Ann Intern Med* 1993;118:913–919.
97. Van Rompay KK, Marthas ML, Ramos RA, et al. Simian immunodeficiency virus (SIV) infection of infant rhesus macaques as a model to test antiretroviral drug prophylaxis and therapy: oral 3'-azido-3'-deoxythymidine prevents SIV infection. *Antimicrob Agents Chemother* 1992;36:2381–2386.
98. von Reyn CF, Gilbert TT, Shaw FE, Parsonnet KC, Abramson JE, Smith MG. Absence of HIV transmission from an infected orthopedic surgeon: a 13-year lookback study. *JAMA* 1993;269:1807–1811.
99. Weiss SH, Saxinger WC, Rechtman D, et al. HTLV-III infection among health care workers: association with needle-stick injuries. *JAMA* 1985;34:575–577.
100. Wong E, Stotka J, Chinchilli V, et al. Are universal precautions effective in reducing the number of occupational exposures among health care workers? A prospective study of physicians on a medical service. *JAMA* 1991;265:1123.

AIDS and the Nervous System, Second Edition,
edited by J. R. Berger and R. M. Levy.
Lippincott-Raven Publishers, Philadelphia © 1997.

30

Algorithms for the Treatment of Acquired Immunodeficiency Syndrome Patients with Neurological Diseases

°Robert M. Levy and †Joseph R. Berger

°Department of Surgery, Northwestern University Medical School, Chicago, Illinois 60611; and †Department of Neurology, University of Kentucky Medical Center, Lexington, Kentucky 40536–2226

Methods of evaluating and treating patients with acquired immunodeficiency syndrome (AIDS) who develop neurological problems have been in a continuous state of evolution. As new diseases are diagnosed and new treatments are made available, algorithms for clinical decision making are bound to change. While the diagnostic and treatment algorithms which arose from the early experience with AIDS have generally proven to be quite vigorous, advances in neuroimaging, changes in the epidemiology of the disease, and increased experience have helped to enrich and refine these recommendations. A working group of the American Academy of Neurology for the evaluation and management of intracranial mass lesions in AIDS has been appointed, and their efforts have further served to improve these treatment algorithms. This chapter describes current recommendations as to how patients with neurological complications related to infection with human immunodeficiency virus (HIV) should be evaluated and managed, with the recognition that these algorithms will continue to evolve as our experience matures. Presented here are algorithms for the diagnosis and management of HIV-infected patients with myopathy, peripheral neuropathy, lumbosacral polyradiculopathy, myelopathy, cranial neuropathy and intracranial space occupying lesions.

MYOPATHY

The approach to the diagnosis and management for patients with HIV-associated myopathy is presented in Fig. 1 and discussed in Chapter 9.

LUMBOSACRAL POLYRADICULOPATHY

The approach to the evaluation of patients with HIV-associated lumbosacral polyradiculopathy is presented in Fig. 3 and discussed in Chapter 7.

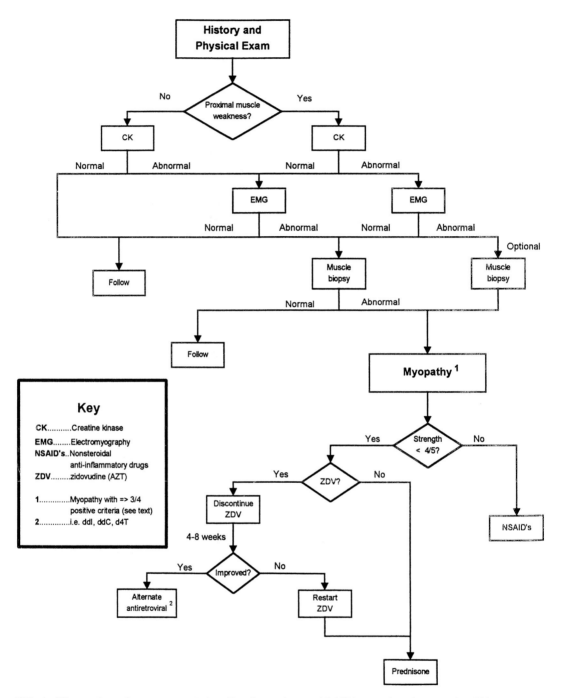

FIG. 1. Diagnosis and management algorithm for patients with HIV-associated myopathy. CK, creatine kinase; EMG, electromyography; NSAIDs, nonsteroidal antiinflammatory drugs; 1, myopathy with >3/4 positive criteria (see text); 2, i.e., ddl, DDC, d4T. (From Simpson and Tagliati, Chapter 9, this volume.)

PERIPHERAL NERVOUS SYSTEM DYSFUNCTION

After the initial neurological examination, patients who present with symptoms of peripheral nerve dysfunction are evaluated (Fig. 2). If the patient is receiving vincristine or other neurotoxic drugs, e.g., the antiretroviral agents ddI and ddC, this treatment is discontinued if possible, and the patient is observed. If there is a radiculitis or radiculomyelitis with a zoster or herpes simplex rash in the corresponding dermatome(s), treatment with acyclovir is instituted because of the high incidence of further complications (such as myelitis and vasculitis) in patients with HIV and herpesvirus infections. If infection with cytomegalovirus (CMV) is suspected, therapy with ganciclovir is initiated immediately while further diagnostic studies are undertaken. If no etiology is apparent, electromyography, nerve conduction studies, and examination of cerebrospinal fluid (CSF) may be considered. The CSF analysis should include the appropriate microbiologic studies, cell count, and glucose and protein determinations. Nerve biopsies are occasionally required to establish a diagnosis.

Before such an extensive evaluation is undertaken, the patient's overall medical condition should be considered. Patients with severe systemic illnesses who have only a mild nondebilitative peripheral neuropathy might not benefit from a detailed work-up of their peripheral neuropathy. If the evaluation described is deemed appropriate and is performed, it is likely that the patient's neuropathy will fit into one of three clinical syndromes. If chronic inflammatory demyelinating polyradiculoneuropathy (CIDP) or mononeuropathy multiplex is diagnosed, plasmapheresis may be undertaken. If distal symmetric peripheral neuropathy (DSPN) is diagnosed, treament of symptoms (such as amitriptyline for pain and ankle-foot orthoses for foot drop) is all that is currently available. If a progressive polyradiculopathy is diagnosed, ganciclovir (DHPG) is considered because of the occasional association of such a radiculopathy with CMV infections; however, neither ganciclovir nor any other therapy has been proven effective for the treatment of progressive polyradiculopathy.

MYELOPATHY

The approach to the evaluation of HIV-infected patients with myelopathic symptoms is presented in Fig. 4 and discussed in Chapter 7.

CRANIAL NEUROPATHY

The first step is to decide if the symptoms are caused by a lesion in the brainstem or other intracerebral location. If a lesion is found or if the diagnosis is unclear, cranial magnetic resonance imaging (MRI) of the brain, with and without gadolinium contrast enhancement, is performed. If MRI is unavailable, computed tomography (CT) with and without nonionic contrast is performed. If these studies demonstrate an abnormality, the patient should be evaluated for central nervous system (CNS) lesions (see below).

If the cranial neuropathy is not caused by intraaxial pathology, the patient is evaluated for the possibility of an associated peripheral neuropathy. In the absence of a peripheral neuropathy, meningoencephalitis is probably the cause of the cranial neuropathy. Subsequent work-up and treatment depend upon the presence of cuta-

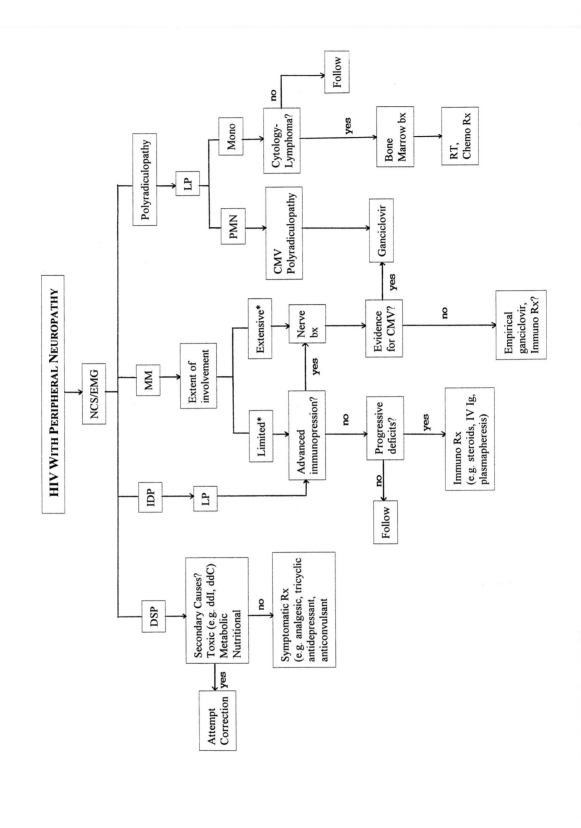

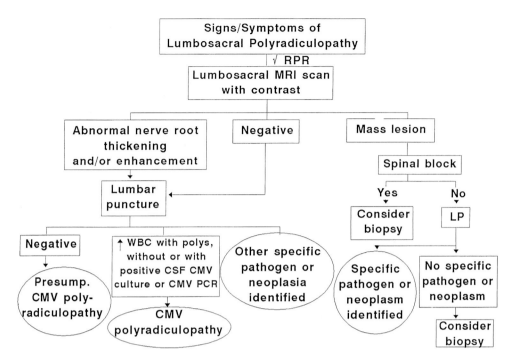

FIG. 3. Evaluation of polyradiculopathy in the HIV-seropositive patient. PCR, polymerase chain reaction. (From Dal Pan et al., Chapter 7, this volume.)

neous lesions and the results of CSF studies. If there is any evidence of varicella-zoster virus (VZV) or herpes simplex virus (HSV) infection, acyclovir is given; DHPG is considered if a CMV infection is diagnosed. If tests for cryptococcal antigen are positive or if India ink staining demonstrates cryptococcal organisms, treatment with amphotericin B and 5-flucytosine or with fluconazole is instituted. The presence of malignant cells in CSF suggests lymphomatous or carcinomatous meningitis and mandates a search for the systemic source of the neoplasm; chemotherapy and radiation therapy are instituted as appropriate. Not infrequently, cranial neuropathies herald an otherwise occult large cell lymphoma (8a) and studies for systemic lymphoma are appropriate when the CSF is unrevealing.

If the cultures from the CSF or other sites are positive, treatment with agents appropriate for the specific causative organism (for example, *Mycobacterium* species or *Coccidioides immitis*) is instituted. If there is a CSF pleocytosis, and all other studies are negative for a specific etiology, it is assumed that the patient has aseptic

FIG. 2. Diagnostic treatment algorithm for patients with peripheral neuropathies associated with HIV infection. NCS, nerve conduction studies; EMG, electromyography; DSP, distal symmetrical polyneuropathy; IDP, inflammatory demyelinating polyneuropathy; MM, mononeuropathy multiplex; LP, lumbar puncture; CMV, cytomegalovirus; IVIG, intravenous immunoglobulin; bx, biopsy; PMN, polymorphonuclear cells; Mono, Mononuclear cells; RT, radiation therapy. (Adapted from Simpson D, Olney R. Peripheral neuropathies associated with human immunodeficiency virus infection. In: Dyck PJ, ed. *Peripheral Neuropathies: New Concepts and Treatments.* Philadelphia: WB Saunders, 1992:685–711, with permission.)

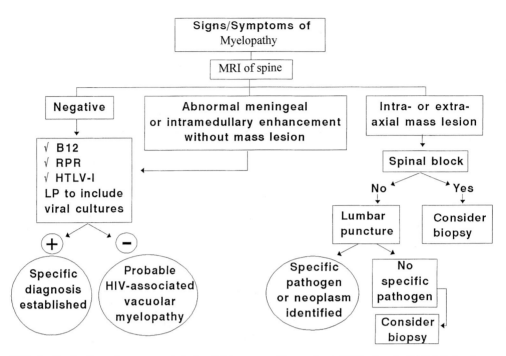

FIG. 4. Evaluation of paraparesis in the HIV-seropositive patient. B12, vitamin B12; LP, lumbar puncture. (From Dal Pan et al., Chapter 7, this volume.)

meningitis due to HIV infection and is observed with that diagnosis in mind. Culture of HIV from CSF does not rule out other causes of cranial neuropathy, as many HIV-infected persons can have positive cultures for HIV associated with systemic HIV infection. If CSF pleocytosis is not present, the patient is followed and repeat evaluations are performed monthly if there is no resolution of the neurological syndrome (Fig. 5).

CENTRAL NERVOUS SYSTEM SYMPTOMS

The presence of an intracranial mass lesion in an HIV-infected person is generally heralded by one or more of the following: headache, seizures, an altered level of consciousness, impaired cognitive function, or focal neurological signs and symptoms. Unfortunately, other equally potential etiologies for these findings in the pres-

→

FIG. 5. Evaluation of cranial neuropathies in the HIV-seropositive patient. (Rosenblum ML, Bredesen DE, Levy RM. Algorithms for the treatment of AIDS patients with neurological diseases. In: Rosenblum ML, Levy RM, Bredesen DE. *AIDS and the nervous system*, New York: Raven Press; 1988; p. 390.) **A:** Acyclovir is recommended because of the high incidence of herpes zoster infections in patients with HIV infection. DHPG (ganciclovir) is currently used for CMV retinitis; efficacy has been shown for progressive polyradiculopathy due to CMV infection. **B;** Culture of HIV from the CSF does not rule out other causes of HIV-related cranial nerve dysfunction. MM, mononeuropathy multiplex; VZV, varicella zoster virus.

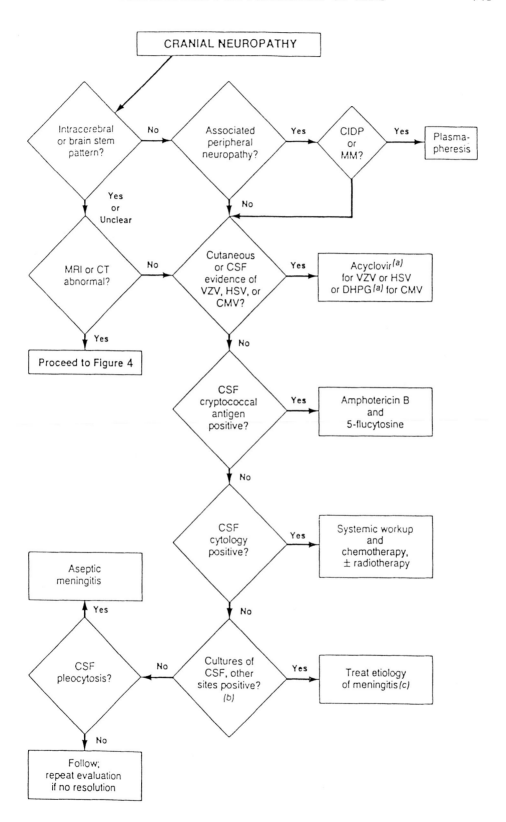

ence of HIV infection include viral meningitis or meningoencephalitis due to HIV or to opportunistic infection with other viruses, such as CMV; bacterial, fungal, or neoplastic meningitis without an accompanying intracerebral mass lesion; metabolic and nutritional disorders; and drug toxicity.

The most sensitive study for the demonstration of an intracranial mass lesion is a cranial MRI performed with and without a contrast agent such as gadolinium. The limited availability of the MRI as well as other considerations (degradation of the image by movement, the time needed to complete the study, and the expense) may preclude its performance. Computed tomography of the head with a double dose (approximately 78 g) of intravenous, iodinated contrast via bolus and drip infusion followed 1 hour later by high-resolution CT scan is a very sensitive technique for detecting these lesions (62). However, its limitations, particularly with respect to the visualization of lesions in the posterior fossa, are well recognized.

Thus, the diagnostic study of choice for the initial evaluation of these patients is cranial MRI, with and without gadolinium contrast enhancement. If MRI is not available, a CT brain scan should be performed; administration of a double dose of contrast material before CT scanning is recommended. Treatment of patients with CNS symptoms depends upon the results of these imaging studies. If the MRI or CT scans are normal or show only diffuse cerebral atrophy, CSF studies are indicated, including cell count, glucose, culture of bacteria, fungi, tuberculous organisms, and viruses; CSF should also be sent for cytology, India ink staining, and cryptococcal antigen studies. If the contrast-enhanced CT scan shows meningeal enhancement, the CSF should be evaluated similarly. If the imaging studies show hydrocephalus, a CSF diversion procedure (usually a ventriculoperitoneal shunt) may be necessary, and CSF should be obtained concurrently.

If a specific disease is diagnosed on the basis of CSF studies, it is treated as described in previous chapters in this text. If no specific etiology is defined and the neurological symptoms persist, both the CSF evaluation and MRI or CT brain scanning may need to be repeated at regular intervals or whenever the patient's neurological condition worsens or new CNS symptoms or signs develop. Repeat studies need not be performed as frequently in patients with progressive neurological deterioration that is consistent with a previous diagnosis of HIV encephalopathy.

The treatment of intracranial space-occupying lesions requires differentiation of lesions that have mass effect and compress brain structures and those that do not. Mass lesions are discussed below. In patients with space-occupying lesions that do not cause mass effect, CSF is obtained and evaluated as described above. These lesions are usually of low density on CT scans and appear as areas of high signal intensity on T2-weighted MRI scans. They are usually located in the white matter but occasionally involve the gray matter as well. The majority of such lesions are caused by progressive multifocal leukoencephalopathy, strokes, and HIV encephalopathy but occasionally are caused by CMV and other viruses. Image-guided stereotactic brain biopsy may be indicated in these cases to definitively establish a diagnosis as a criterion for entry into a therapeutic study or to provide prognostic information, as the natural histories of HIV encephalopathy and PML are quite different.

It is important to consider the possible influence of treatment with corticosteroids in such patients, since corticosteroids can decrease both the mass effect and the contrast enhancement of intracerebral lesions on CT scans. Corticosteroid therapy should be withdrawn as soon as it is clinically reasonable and repeat MRI and/or CT scans obtained (Fig. 6).

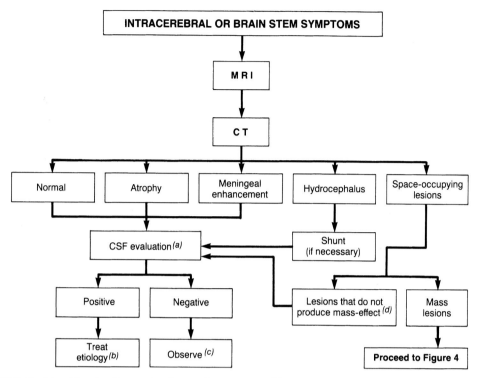

FIG. 6. Algorithm for the evaluation and treatment of intracerebral or brainstem symptoms in patients infected with the human immunodeficiency virus (HIV). [a]Cerebrospinal fluid (CSF) should be analyzed for cells, glucose, bacteria, fungi, tuberculous organisms and viruses. [b]See chapters on specific diseases. [c]If neurological symptoms persist, magnetic resonance imaging (MRI) or computerized tomography (CT) studies and the CSF evaluation are repeated monthly. If significant neurological deterioration occurs or if new symptoms or signs develop, immediate MRI or CT studies are warranted. [d]Space-occupying lesions that do not produce mass effect are usually seen on CT scans as areas of low density that do not enhance after the administration of contrast material; on T2-weighted MRI scans, these lesions are seen as areas of high signal intensity. The majority are due to HIV, CMV, progressive multifocal leukoencephalopathy and strokes.

INTRACRANIAL MASS LESIONS

The proper management of an HIV-infected patient presenting with an intracranial mass lesion requires a working knowledge of the relative frequencies with which the various etiologies of intracranial mass lesions are observed with HIV, the clinical and radiographic manifestations of these mass lesions, the therapeutic options, and the prognosis. There has been considerable controversy regarding the management of these lesions, particularly with respect to when to proceed to a diagnostic brain biopsy. Both quality of life and survival may be affected by the course of action. The magnitude of the problem and the potential economic impact are not insubstantial. As of December 1994, there were estimated to be 1.5 to 2.0 million individuals infected with HIV in the United States.

Toxoplasmosis is the commonest cause of intracerebral mass lesion occurring in association with HIV infection (51,77), generally in advanced stages of immunosuppression (60). In a study from San Francisco, cerebral toxoplasmosis occurred in 4.1% of all patients with AIDS and 28% of AIDS patients with neurological disease symptoms (43). In combined clinicopathological series from Miami (7), it accounted for 40% of all identified neurological illnesses. At autopsy, between 10% (58) and 30% (55) of AIDS patients have cerebral toxoplasmosis. Approximately 25% to 50% of AIDS patients who are seropositive for *Toxoplasma gondii*, an obligate intracellular parasite with worldwide distribution, will ultimately develop toxoplasmosis encephalopathy. Other opportunistic infections resulting in intracranial mass lesions are observed with varying frequency.

The most common brain neoplasm observed in association with HIV infection is primary lymphoma of the central nervous system (PCNSL). As many as 0.6% of AIDS patients present with PCNSL, and PCNSL ultimately develops in 2.0% (44) to nearly 5% (Chapter 28, this volume). Other neoplasms that have been reported in association with HIV infection include gliomas, Kaposi's sarcoma, and metastatic tumor.

The other major cause of HIV-associated intracranial mass lesions is cerebrovascular disease. The reported incidence of cerebrovascular disease in predominantly clinical studies of AIDS patients ranges from 0.5% to 7% (7,21,32,43,51). This incidence is even higher in autopsy studies in which estimates of stroke have varied between 11% and 34% (3,53,70,76). The spectrum of cerebrovascular disease that occurs in association with HIV infection is quite broad and includes both ischemic and hemorrhagic disease (6). In general, ischemic disease is more common than cerebral hemorrhage (6,53), despite the frequency of concomitant thrombocytopenia. Cerebral vasculitis may also complicate HIV infection, occasionally occurring as a consequence of concomitant opportunistic infection, such as herpes zoster (20,54,75,80), syphilis (34), as well as others (6).

Since the majority of intracranial mass lesions in patients with HIV infection are potentially treatable, an aggressive approach to diagnosis is warranted under certain circumstances. The algorithm used in such cases is shown in Fig. 7. If available, MRI scanning with and without the administration of gadolinium should be performed in all patients with intracranial mass lesions.

In light of the high frequency of toxoplasmosis, some centers recommend that solitary lesions unassociated with impending herniation should be treated empirically with an antitoxoplasmosis regimen. In other centers, based upon the infrequency with which patients with toxoplasmosis have solitary lesions on MRI (see below), such patients are referred directly for stereotactic brain biopsy. If a patient is alert or lethargic and stable and the MRI scans show multiple lesions, an empirical trial of antibiotic therapy for toxoplasmosis should be instituted; we recommend a 2- to 3-week course of sulfadiazine (6–8 g per day divided into four equal doses) and pyrimethamine (an initial loading dose of 50–200 mg followed by 50–75 mg/day). Both drugs cross the blood-brain barrier (66). Folinic acid, 5 to 10 mg/day, is needed to diminish bone marrow suppression. If the patient is allergic to either drug or if marked drug-induced toxicity occurs, clindamycin or another alternative anti-*Toxoplasma* drug should be used. Patients are followed weekly with CT or MRI scans during the empirical trial, and if any of the lesions do not respond or if the patient's neurological status worsens at any time, a stereotactic biopsy of the enlarging lesion is performed. If some mass lesions decrease in size despite the appearance or growth of a different mass, anti-*Toxoplasma* therapy should continue for the life of the patient, and the enlarging mass should be biopsied. If corticosteroids are utilized

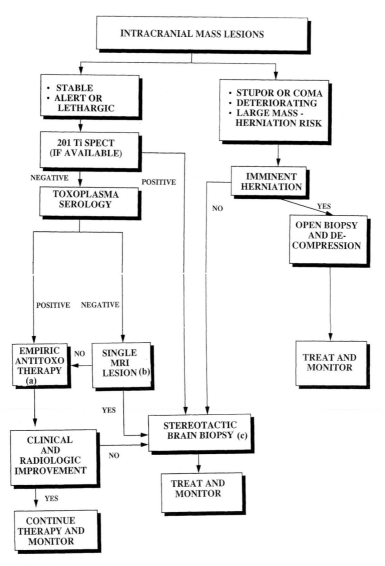

FIG. 7. Algorithm for the evaluation and treatment of intracranial mass lesions in patients infected with human immunodeficiency virus (HIV). **(a)** Three-week course of sulfadiazine and pyrimethamine (see text). **(b)** Because the majority of single mass lesions on magnetic resonance images (MRI) are not caused by Toxoplasma gondii, a biopsy is recommended. **(c)** Stereotactic biopsies are guided by neuroimaging modalities; the only absolute contraindication to stereotactic biopsy is a noncorrectable bleeding diathesis. For a thorough discussion, see text.

during a successful empirical trial, they must be discontinued and CT or MRI scans must demonstrate persistent improvement before it is concluded that the masses were due to toxoplasmosis. If the mass lesions recur during tapering of the corticosteroid dose, a stereotactic biopsy is in order. If the clinical and radiographic assessments indicate a response to antitoxoplasmosis therapy, then it should be continued indefinitely with follow-up radiographic imaging performed every 4 to 6 weeks.

In contrast to adults, opportunistic infections of the CNS, including toxoplasmosis, are rarely observed in children (34). Although toxoplasmosis in HIV-infected children has been anecdotally reported (10), it was not observed in two separate cohorts examined for HIV-associated neurologic disease (5,65). Therefore, in HIV-infected children, proceeding directly to steretactic brain biopsy may be a consideration to eliminate other diagnostic possibilities. Such empiric treatment should be undertaken despite negative serology for toxoplasmosis as these serologies may be negative in the presence of established CNS toxoplasmosis. Thirteen of 80 (16%) patients with clinical toxoplasmosis and 4 of 18 (22%) with pathologically proven toxoplasmosis had undetectable plasma antitoxoplasmosis immunoglobulin G (IgG) antibody titers by indirect immunofluorescence assay (60). Additionally, the prevalence of falsely negative antibody titers for toxoplasmosis may increase with advanced immunosuppression. However, the combination of a negative toxoplasmosis serology and a single lesion on radiographic imaging militates against the presence of *Toxoplasma* encephalopathy. In one large study (60), 28 of 103 (27%) patients with toxoplasmosis had single lesions on CT scan and 3 of 21 (14%) had single lesions on MRI. Another study revealed that 17% of single lesions were toxoplasmosis (13). Therefore, the concomitance of negative toxoplasmosis serology and a single lesion on radiographic imaging is deemed sufficient to warrant the performance of a stereotactic biopsy.

Recently, radionuclide brain scanning has been applied to the evaluation of patients with HIV-associated intracranial mass lesions. Preliminary data using a combination of HMPAO and thallium single photon emission computed tomography (SPECT) appear to demonstrate a high specificity in differentiating infectious lesions from neoplasms. Experience with this technique in 100 patients suggests that it may well be a valuable adjunct in differentiating toxoplasmosis from lymphoma.

If a patient presents stuporous or in coma, with a rapidly deteriorating neurological status, or with a large mass lesion which presents a risk of herniation and death, an immediate biopsy should be considered. The reason for a more aggressive approach in such cases is that the patient might not survive a 3-week trial of anti-*Toxoplasma* therapy if the lesion is not caused by *T. gondii*. The administration of high-dose corticosteroids can occasionally improve neurological status and reduce the mass effect from intracerebral lesions by decreasing cerebral edema and, in the case of CNS lymphomas, the size of the lesion. Finally, if there is an imminent risk of brain herniation, an open biopsy with decompression is indicated.

The diagnostic efficacy of stereotactic brain biopsy has been reported to be as high as 95% (47). The procedure carries a minimal risk of blood loss or infection; the risk of intracerebral hemorrhage may be as high as 6%, with 2% serious morbidity or mortality and 4% minor morbidity resulting from these hemorrhages (47). Most patients require only overnight hospitalization for observation after stereotactic brain biopsy, and costs are roughly one-quarter to one-third those of open craniotomy.

In all cases in which a biopsy is performed, treatment is chosen on the basis of the specific etiology. Rarely, biopsy of a lesion does not yield diagnostic material despite exhaustive pathological analysis; in such cases, a repeat biopsy should be performed to permit a definitive diagnosis. If a patient who has been treated for a mass lesion develops a new mass lesion, a repeat evaluation should be performed because AIDS patients may have muliple intracranial pathologies, either simultaneously or sequentially. A biopsy may be indicated to determine the etiology of the new lesion. The only absolute contraindication to image-guided stereotactic biopsy is a noncorrectable bleeding diathesis. The minimal risk to the patient, particularly when the biopsy is performed under local anesthesia, makes this the most conservative approach under the circumstances described in this algorithm.

REFERENCES

1. Abos J, Graus F, Mirò JM, et al. Intracranial tuberculomas in patients with AIDS (Letter). *AIDS* 1991;5:461–462.
2. Adair JC, Beck AC, Apfelbaum RI, Baringer JR. Nocardial cerebral abscess in the acquired immunodeficiency syndrome. *Arch Neurol* 1987;44:548–550.
3. Anders KH, Guerra W, Tomiyasu U, et al. The neuropathology of AIDS. UCLA experience and review. *Am J Pathol* 1986;124:537–558.
4. Baumgartner JE, Rachlin JR, Beckstead JW, et al. Primary central nervous system lymphoma: natural history and response to radiation therapy in 55 patients with acquired immunodeficiency syndrome. *J Neurosurg* 1990;73:206–211.
5. Belman AL, Diamond G, Dickson D, et al. Pediatric acquired immunodeficiency syndrome: neurological syndromes. *Am J Dis Child* 1988;142:29–35.
6. Berger JR, Harris JO, Gregorios J, Norenberg M. Cerebrovascular disease in AIDS: a case control study. *AIDS* 1990;4:239–244.
7. Berger JR, Moskowitz L, Fischl M, Kelley RE. Neurological disease as the presenting manifestation of acquired immunodeficiency syndrome. *South Med J* 1987;80:683–686.
8. Berger JR, Waskin H, Pall L, Hensley G, Post MJD, Ihmedian I. Syphilitic cerebral gumma with HIV infection. *Neurology* 1992;42:1282–1287.
8a. Berger JR, Flaster M, Schatz N, Droller D, Benedetto P, Poplete R, Post MJD. Cranial neuropathy heralding otherwise occult AIDS-related large cell lymphoma. *J Clin Neurophthalmal* 1993;13:113–118.
9. Bia FJ, Barry M. Parasitic infections of the central nervous system. *Neurol Clin* 1986;4:171–206.
10. Biggemann B, Voit T, Neuen E, et al. Neurological manifestations in three German children with AIDS. *Neuropediatrics* 1987;18:99–106.
11. Bishburg E, Sunderam G, Reichman LB, Kapila R. Central nervous system tuberculosis with the acquired immunodeficiency syndrome and its related complex. *Ann Intern Med* 1986;105:210–213.
12. Carr A, Tindall B, Brew BJ, et al. Low dose trimethoprim-sulfamethoxazole for toxoplasmic encephalitis in patients with AIDS. *Ann Intern Med* 1992;117:106–111.
13. Ciricillo SF, Rosenblum ML. Imaging of solitary lesions in AIDS (Letter). *J Neurosurg* 1991;74:1029.
14. Cryptococcosis in AIDS [editorial]. *Lancet* 1988;25:1434–1436.
15. Cuadrado LM, Guerrero A, Lopez Garcia Asenjo JA, Martin F, Palau E, Urra DG. Cerebral mucormycosis in two cases of acquired immunodeficiency syndrome. *Arch Neurol* 1988;45:109–111.
16. Danneman BR, McCutchan JA, Israelski DM, et al. Treatment of toxoplasmic encephalitis in patients with AIDS: a randomized trial comparing pyrimethamine plus clindamycin to pyrimethamine plus sulfadiazine. *Ann Intern Med* 1992;116:33–43.
17. de Gans J, Portegies P, Reiss P, Troost D, van Gool T, Lange JM. Pyrimethamine alone as maintenance therpay for central nervous system toxoplasma in 38 patients with AIDS. *J AIDS* 1992;5:137–142.
18. de Gans J, Portegies P, Tiessens G, Troost D, Danner SA, Lange JMA. Therapy for cytomegalovirus polyradiculomyelitis in patients with AIDS: treatment with ganciclovir. *AIDS* 1990;4:421–425.
19. DeMent SH, Cox M, Gupta PK. Diagnosis of central nervous system *Toxoplasma gondii* from the cerebrospinal fluid in a patient with acquired immunodeficiency syndrome. *Diagn Cytopathol* 1987;3:148–151.
20. Eidelberg D, Sotrel A, Houtoupian S, Neumann PE, Pumarola-Sune T, Price RW. Thrombotic cerebral vasculopathy associated with herpes zoster. *Ann Neurol* 1986;19:7–14.
21. Engstrom J, Lowenstein DH, Bredesen DE. Cerebral infarctions and transient neurological deficits associated with AIDS. *Neurology* 1988;38(Suppl 1):241.
22. Farkash AE, Maccabee PJ, Sher JH, et al. CNS toxoplasmosis in acquired immunodeficiency syndrome: a clinical-pathological-radiological review of 12 cases. *J Neurol Neurosurg Psychiatry* 1986;49:744–748.
23. Gardner HAR, Martinez AJ, Visvesvara GS, Sotrel A. Granulomatous amebic encephalitis in an AIDS patient. *Neurology* 1991;41:1993–1995.
24. Goldstein JS, Dickson DW, Moser FG, et al. Primary central nervous system lymphoma in acquired immune deficiency syndrome; a clinical and pathological study with results of treatment with radiation. *Cancer* 1991;67:2756–2765.
25. Harris JO, Marquez J, Swerdloff MA. *Listeria* brain abscess in the acquired immunodeficiency syndrome (Letter). *Arch Neurol* 1989;46:250.
26. Haverkos HW. Assessment of therapy for toxoplasma encephalitis. The TE study group. *Am J Med* 1987;82:907–14.

27. Helweg-Larsen S, Jakobsen J, Boesen F, Arlien-S berg P. Neurological complications and concomi-tants of AIDS. *Acta Neurol Scand* 1986;74:467–474.
28. Hochberg FH, Miller DC. Primary central nervous system lymphoma. *J Neurosurg* 1988;68:835–853.
29. Hofflin JM, Remington JS. Tissue culture isolation of *Toxoplasma* from blood of a patient with AIDS. *Arch Intern Med* 1985;145:925–926.
30. Horowitz S, Bentson JR, Benson DF, Pressman P, Gottlieb MS. CNS toxoplasmosis in acquired immunodeficiency syndrome. *Arch Neurol* 1983;40:649–652.
31. Jarvik JG, Hesselink JR, Kennedy C, et al. Acquired immunodeficiency syndrome. Magnetic reso-nance patterns of brain involvement with pathological correlation. *Arch Neurol* 1988;45:731–736.
32. Jordan BD, Navia BA, Petito C, et al. Neurological syndromes complicating AIDS. *Front Radiat Ther Oncol* 1985;19:82–87.
33. Katalama C, De Wit S, Guichard A, et al. Pyrimethamine-clindamycin versus pyrimethamine-sulfadia-zine in toxoplasma encephalitis in AIDS: a randomized, prospective multicenter European study. *Paper presented at VII International Conference on AIDS*, 1991 (abst WB30).
34. Katz D, Berger JR. Neurosyphilis in AIDS. *Arch Neurol* 1989;46:895–901.
35. Keohane C, Gray F. Central nervous system pathology in children with AIDS. *Irish J Med Sci* 1991; 160:277–281.
36. Tuite M, Ketonen L, Kieburtz K, Handy B. Efficacy of gadolinium in MR brain imaging of HIV-infected patients. *AJNR Am Neuroradiol* 1993;14:257–263.
37. Kovacs JA, Dovacs AA, Polis M, et al. Cryptococcosis in the acquired immunodeficiency syndrome. *Ann Intern Med* 1985;103:533–538.
38. Kovacs JA, and the NIAID-Clinical Center Intramural AIDS Program. Efficacy of atovaquone in treatment of toxoplasmosis in patients with AIDS. *Lancet* 1992;340:637–638.
39. Krol G, Becker R, Zimmerman R, et al. Contribution of MRI to the diagnosis of intracranial complica-tions of acquired immune deficiency syndrome. *Neuroradiology* 1986;99–104.
40. Leport C, Raffi F, Matheron B, et al. Treatment of central nervous system toxoplasmosis with pyri-methamine/sulfadiazine combination in 35 patients with the acquired immunodeficiency syndrome: efficacy of long term continuous therapy. *Am J Med* 1988;84:94–100.
41. Leport C, Vilde JL. Katlama C, Regnier B, Matheron S, Saimot AG. Toxoplasmose cerebrale de l'immunodeprime: diagnostic et traitement. *Ann Med Interne* 1987;138:30–33.
42. Levy RM, Berger JR. Neurological critical care in patients with HIV-1 infection. *Critical Care Clin* 1993;9:49–72.
43. Levy RM, Bredesen DE, Rosenblum ML. Neurological manifestations of the acquired immunodefi-ciency syndrome (AIDS): experience at UCSF and review of the literature. *J Neurosurg* 1985;62: 475–495.
44. Levy RM, Janssen RS, Bush TJ, et al. Neuroepidemiology of acquired immunodeficiency sydrome. In: Rosenblum ML, Levy RM, Bredesen DE, eds. *AIDS and the nervous system*. New York: Raven; 1988:13–27.
45. Levy RM, Mills CM, Posin J, et al. The efficacy and clinical impact of brain imaging in neurologically symptomatic AIDS patients: a prospective CT/MRI study. *J AIDS* 1990;3:461–471.
46. Levy RM, Pons VG, Rosenblum ML. Intracerebral mass lesions in the acquired immunodeficiency syndrome (AIDS). *N Engl J Med* 1983;309:1454–1455.
47. Levy RM, Russell E, Yungbluth M, et al. The efficacy of image-guided stereotactic brain biopsy in neurologically symptomatic acquired immunodeficiency syndrome patients. *Neurosurgery* 1992:30: 186–190.
48. Luft BJ, Remington JS. Toxoplasmic encephalitis in AIDS. *Clin Infect Dis* 1992;15:211–222.
49. Luft BJ, Brooks RG, Conley FK, et al. Toxoplasmic encephalitis in patients with acquired immune deficiency syndrome. *JAMA* 1984;252:913–917.
50. Luft BJ, Brooks RG, Conley FK, McCabe RE, Remington JS. Toxoplasmic encephalitis in patients with acquired immune deficiency syndrome. *JAMA* 1984;257:913–917.
51. McArthur JC. Neurological manifestations of AIDS. *Medicine* 1987;66:407–437.
52. MacMahon EME, Glass JD, Hayward SD, et al. Epstein-Barr virus (EBV) in AIDS-related primary central nervous system lymphoma. *Lancet* 1991;338:969–973.
53. Mizusawa H, Hirano A, Llena JF, Shintaku M. Cerebrovascular lesions in acquired immune deficiency syndrome (AIDS). *Acta Neuropathol* 1988;76:451–457.
54. Morgello S, Block GA, Price RW, Petito CK. Varicella-zoster virus leukoencephalitis and cerebral vasculopathy. *Arch Pathol Lab Med* 1988;112:173–177.
55. Moskowitz LB, Hensley GT, Chan JC, et al. The neuropathology of acquired immunodeficiency syndrome. *Arch Pathol Lab Med* 1984;108:867–872.
56. Navia BA, Petito CK, Gold JW, et al. Cerebral toxoplasmosis complicating the acquired immune deficiency syndrome: clinical and neuropathological findings in 27 patients. *Ann Neurol* 1986;19: 224–238.
57. Nolla-Salas J, Ricart C, D'Olhaberriague L, et al. Hydrocephalus: an unusual CT presentation of cerebral toxoplasmosis in a patient with acquired immunodeficiency syndrome. *Eur Neurol* 1987; 27:130–2.

58. Petito CK, Cho ES, Lemann W, et al. Neuropathology of acquired immunodeficiency syndrome (AIDS): an autopsy review. *J Neuropathol Exp Neurol* 1986;45:635–646.
59. Popovich MJ, Arthur RH, Helmer E. CT of intracranial cryptococcosis. *Am J Roengenol* 1990;154: 603–606.
60. Porter SB, Sande MA. Toxoplasmosis of the central nervous system in the acquired immunodeficiency syndrome. *N Engl J Med* 1992;327:1643–1648.
61. Post MJD, Chan JC, Hensley GT, et al. Toxoplasma encephalitis in Haitian adults with acquired immunodeficiency syndrome: a clinical-pathological-CT correlation. *Am J Neuroradiol* 1983;4: 155–162.
62. Post MJD, Kursunoglu SJ, Hensley GT, et al. Cranial CT in acquired immunodeficiency syndrome: spectrum of diseases and optimal contrast enhancement technique. *Am J Neuroradiol* 1985;6:743–754.
63. Post MJD, Sheldon JJ, Hensley GT, et al. Central nervous system disease in acquired immunodeficiency syndrome: prospective correlation using CT, MR imaging and pathological studies. *Radiology* 1986;158:141–148.
64. Potasman I, Resnick L, Luft BJ, Remington JS. Intrathecal production of antibodies against *Toxoplasma gondii* in patients with toxoplasmic encephalitis and the acquired immunodeficiency syndrome (AIDS). *Ann Intern Med* 1988;108:49–51.
65. Remington JS, Vilde JL. Clindamycin for toxoplasma encephalitis in AIDS. *Lancet* 1991;338: 1142–1143.
66. Rolston KV. Treatment of acute toxoplasma with oral clindamycin. *Eur J Clin Microbiol Infect Dis* 1991;10:181–183.
67. Roy S, Geoffroy G, Lapointe N, Michaud J. Neurological findings in HIV-infected children: a review of 49 cases. *Can J Neurol Sci* 1992;19:453–457.
68. Ruskin J, Remington JS. Toxoplasmosis in the compromised host. *Ann Intern Med* 1976;84:193–199.
69. Sahai J, Heimberger T, Collins K, Kaplowitz L, Polk R. Sulfadiazine-induced crystalluria in a patient with acquired immunodeficiency syndrome: a reminder. *Am J Med* 1988;84:791–792.
70. Sharer LP, Kapila R. Neuropathological observations in acquired immune deficiency syndrome. *Acta Neuropathol (Berl)* 1985;66:188–198.
71. So YT, Beckstead JH, Davis RL. Primary central nervous system lymphoma in acquired immune deficiency syndrome: a clinical and pathological study. *Ann Neurol* 1986;20:566–572.
72. Tenant-Flowers M, Boyle MJ, Carey D, et al. Sulphadiazine desensitization in patients with AIDS and crebral toxoplasmosis. *AIDS* 1991;5:311–315.
73. Thornton CA, Houston S, Latif AS. Neuorcysticercosis and human immunodeficiency virus infection: a possible association. *Arch Neurol* 1992;49:963–965.
74. Threlkeld MG, Graves AH, Cobbs CG. Cerebrospinal fluid staining for the diagnosis of toxoplasmosis in patients with the acquired immune deficiency syndrome (Letter). *Am J Med* 1987;83:599–600.
75. Van de Perre P, Bakkers E, Batungwanayo J, et al. Herpes zoster in African patients: an early manifestation of HIV infection. *Scand J Infect Dis* 1988;20:277–282.
76. Vinters HV, Tomiyasu U, Anders KH. Neuropathological complications of infection with the human immunodeficiency virus (HIV). *Prog AIDS Pathol* 1989;1:101–130.
77. Wanke C, Tuazon CU, Kovacs A, et al. Toxoplasma encephalitis in patients with acquired immunodeficiency syndrome: diagnosis and response to therapy. *Am J Trop Med Hyg* 1987;36:509–516.
78. Weiss LM, Udem SA, Tanowitz H, Wittner M. Western blot analysis of the antibody response of patients with AIDS and toxoplasma encephalitis: antigenic diversity among *Toxoplasma* strains. *J Infect Dis* 1988;157:7–13.
79. Woods GL, Goldsmith JC. *Aspergillus* infection of the central nervous system in patients with acquired immunodeficiency syndrome. *Arch Neurol* 1990;47:181–184.
80. Wong B, Gold JWM, Brown AE, et al. Central nervous system toxoplasmosis in homosexual men and parenteral drug abusers. *Ann Intern Med* 1984;100:36–42.
81. Zaraspe-Yoo E, Miletich R, Toutellotte WW. Herpes zoster ophthalmicus with contrealateral hemiplegia in a patient with autoimmune deficiency syndrome (AIDS). *Neurology* 1984;34(Suppl 1); 229(abst).

AIDS and the Nervous System, Second Edition,
edited by J. R. Berger and R. M. Levy.
Lippincott-Raven Publishers, Philadelphia © 1997.

31

Future Therapy of Human Immunodeficiency Virus Related Neurological Disease

°Andrew D. Carr, †Bruce J. Brew, and ‡David A. Cooper

Departments of °†*HIV Medicine and* †*Neurology, St. Vincent's Hospital, and* ‡*National Centre in HIV Epidemiology and Clinical Research, St. Vincent's Hospital, University of New South Wales, Sydney 2010, Australia*

Despite numerous therapeutic and diagnostic advances, the treament of most human immunodeficiency virus (HIV) related neurological diseases either incurs substantial toxicity or has limited efficacy. Future therapeutic advances will obviously depend upon reducing the toxicity of existing drugs or finding new, less toxic, or more effective alternatives. Such advances will not be possible in many instances without better understanding of disease pathogenesis and better diagnostic capabilities. Therapies are often confounded by the lack of sensitive and specific diagnostic tests that are safe, cost-effective, and readily available. For example, the diagnosis of progressive multifocal leukoencephalopathy (PML) or cerebral lymphoma is often hampered by the lack of facilities to perform and interpret brain biopsies. Similarly, acquired immunodeficiency syndrome (AIDS) dementia complex (ADC) is diagnosed solely on clinical grounds. This chapter will focus upon likely future therapies for HIV-related neurological illnesses given current developments in diagnostics, medications, and understanding of disease pathogenesis.

CEREBRAL LYMPHOMA

Conventional therapy for cerebral lymphoma, consisting of radiotherapy and corticosteroids, is usually palliative and of transient benefit. As most patients with cerebral lymphoma have advanced HIV disease, it is unlikely that conventional systemic chemotherapy would be beneficial, given its substantial toxicity, even if adequate blood-brain barrier penetration could be achieved. Intrathecal chemotherapy is also unlikely to be of benefit, except in those rare instances where disease is restricted to the meninges.

Recently, a strong histological association between primary cerebral lymphoma and Epstein-Barr virus (EBV) has been found (11), suggesting that systemic prophylaxis against EBV, if adequately absorbed into the central nervous system, might prevent the development of such lymphomas. To date, high-dose oral acyclovir prophylaxis has not been found to have such benefit, although the statistical power of studies evaluating this were probably limited by patient numbers. Valaciclovir, a proform of acyclovir which achieves greater serum levels by virtue of greater oral absorption, is currently being evaluated for prophylaxis of cytomegalovirus (CMV) disease in patients with advanced HIV disease. As valaciclovir has some *in vitro* activity against EBV, it will be of great interest to see if valaciclovir demonstrates any protective effect on the development of cerebral lymphoma.

TOXOPLASMIC ENCEPHALITIS

Lifelong secondary prophylaxis of toxoplasmosis is mandatory to prevent relapse, usually with pyrimethamine in combination with either sulfadiazine or clindamycin, although pyrimethamine alone is effective in some settings. Whether secondary prophylaxis should be administered as a daily or intermittent regimen is unclear. Primary prophylaxis against toxoplasmic encephalitis has not been widely adopted, unlike primary *Pneumocystis carinii* pneumonia (PCP) prophylaxis. This may be because of the lower prevalence of latent *Toxoplasma gondii* infection in various HIV-infected populations. Nevertheless, the risk of toxoplasmosis in seropositive subjects is 30% to 40% over time, and so primary prophylaxis is an attractive concept (14,24).

Several studies have found trimethoprim-sulfamethoxazole (TMP-SMX) and dapsone-pyrimethamine effective as primary prophylaxis against both toxoplasmic encephalitis and PCP (10,22,28). Which of these therapies is more effective and less toxic is unknown. In the light of these data, an optimal prophylactic regimen against opportunistic infections for patients with advanced HIV disease should prevent both toxoplasmosis and PCP in a single drug regimen to enhance patient acceptance and compliance. Studies of prophylaxis against toxoplasmosis with pyrimethamine have been inconclusive and have not shown efficacy against PCP (22,31). Clindamycin is probably too toxic for regular use as primary toxoplasmosis prophylaxis (32) and offers little protection against PCP. Atovaquone is also undergoing study as combined prophylaxis against PCP and toxoplasmic encephalitis, but its efficacy has been hampered by variable oral absorption. Perhaps surprisingly, there is no report of the efficacy of sulfadiazine-pyrimethamine as primary prophylaxis.

In addition to developing new agents with improved efficacy and less toxicity, some efforts have been made to minimize the toxicity of existing drugs. For example, desensitization to sulfadiazine is effective for improving the tolerance of therapy and secondary prophylaxis in those with prior hypersensitivity (44). Whether use of corticosteroids can be used safely to prevent hypersensitivity to sulfadiazine is unknown. Preliminary studies to minimise sulfonamide hypersensitivity with free-radical scavengers such as glutathione are also in progress.

Therapy for toxoplasmosis consists of pyrimethamine with either sulfadiazine or clindamycin. Other agents with less well-defined roles include atovaquone, azithromycin, clarithromycin, dapsone, or sulfadoxine with pyrimethamine, as well as tetracyclines and TMP-SMX, but most of the data regarding these agents refer to efficacy *in vitro* or in animal models or are anecdotal. Interferon-gamma can augment the efficacy of antimicrobial agents *in vitro* and in murine models of infection but has not been studied in humans (34).

The efficacy and safety of any therapeutic or prophylactic agents will only become better defined when better diagnostic criteria are available. Such criteria should be noninvasive and should not rely on a therapeutic trial which takes at least 10 days. For example, patients seronegative for *T. gondii* and/or receiving TMP-SMX prophylaxis would be less likely to have toxoplasmic encephalitis, even in the presence of appropriate clinical and radiological features; these patients should perhaps be considered for early brain biopsy or alternative therapy. The only additional diagnostic guide on the horizon is isolation of *T. gondii* or its specific DNA from serum (or cerebrospinal fluid (CSF), although lumbar puncture in patients with cerebral mass lesions is unlikely to gain widespread acceptance), but the sensitivity and specificity of this assay are not clear (36).

AIDS DEMENTIA COMPLEX

Only when the pathogenesis of ADC is evident will the most appropriate and specific approaches for its treatment be clear. In particular, is the brain affected or infected by HIV, and if so, at what stage? With this in mind, certain pivotal aspects should be considered. First, subclinical involvement of the nervous system is common throughout the course of HIV-1 infection. For example, various brain-imaging studies have demonstrated abnormalities in asymptomatic HIV-infected patients, whose CSF also often shows a mild mononuclear pleocytosis and elevated protein. However, detection of HIV-specific DNA by PCR of brain tissue from patients with asymptomatic HIV infection is uncommon, suggesting that the brain is not usually infected at an early disease stage. Second, ADC is usually a disease confined to those with CD4+ counts less than 200/mm^3. Third, ADC develops in only some patients with advanced immunodeficiency; most brain-derived viral isolates from patients with HIV encephalitis are macrophage-tropic and HIV will only replicate in microglia if it is macrophage-tropic (19,46). Fourth, the presence and severity of ADC are linked to immune activation within the CSF and brain parenchyma as evidenced by elevated CSF concentrations of beta-2 microglobulin (4), neopterin (5), quinolinic acid (30), interleukin 1 (IL-1) and IL-6 (20), and increased expression of major histocompatibility complex (MHC) I and II (45). Fifth, the pathological and virological features are dominantly subcortical and perivascular in location. The sixth critical point is that productive infection of the brain is confined to cells of the monocyte/macrophage lineage including the microglial cell, with probable restricted infection in astrocytes. Nevertheless, purely virological factors seem unlikely as causative agents for ADC, as the clinical severity or pathology of ADC is often greater than the amount of productive HIV-1 infection found at autopsy (13,45). Thus, productive brain infection appears to be sufficient but not necessary for the development of ADC.

At the cellular level, HIV enters macrophage lineage cells by the CD4 receptor and neural cells by the galactosyl ceramide (29) and possibly other glycolipid receptors. Therefore, antibodies against such receptors might be useful therapeutically, although experience with recombinant soluble CD4 was not encouraging for systemic HIV disease. Also, central nervous system infection by HIV may occur very early following infection (as evidenced by positive CSF culture), and so such antibodies may prevent cell-cell spread but are unlikely to prevent initial infection. If, however, mediators released by neural cells are responsible for ADC (rather than direct infection), such antibodies may have no clinical benefit.

Human immunodeficiency virus replicating within the central nervous system will produce proteins that can injure other cells. For example, gp120 is toxic to rodent neurons (2), although its toxicity requires the presence of an intermediary cell of the macrophage lineage (18). The precise mechanism of neuronal damage is by way of activation of the *N-methyl*-D-aspartate (NMDA) receptor with consequent influx into the cell of calcium and secondary synthesis of nitric oxide in those neurons containing nitric oxide synthetase (15). Therefore, NMDA antagonists may have a role as future therapy of ADC.

Uninfected immune cells produce a variety of toxins aimed at the death of cells supporting HIV infection but which in the process lead to death of normal neural cells. These host-coded toxins are largely produced by macrophage lineage cells and include arachidonic acid metabolites, platelet activating factor, quinolinic acid (an NMDA agonist), and cytokines (4,6,8,23,30). If this were the case, inhibition of cytokine production or activity might be useful, but it remains to be determined whether specific or generalized cytokine inhibition would be beneficial and whether such inhibition is possible without activating other latent infections or even malignancies.

Zidovudine is effective for both therapy and primary prophylaxis of ADC, although the optimal dose for both is unknown (37,38,40,42). However, perhaps only 50% of patients with ADC will respond to zidovudine therapy, there being some evidence to suggest that higher doses are more effective. The explanation for such variation in response is unknown, but it may relate to drug resistance, inadequate penetration across the blood-brain barrier, irreversible brain parenchymal damage, and possibly the nature of a particular strain of virus; for example, the syncytium-inducing virus strain is purported to be relatively insensitive to zidovudine or to develop drug resistance more rapidly (1). Therefore, it is important to determine which patients are at highest risk for failing zidovudine therapy or prophylaxis of ADC, particularly in the absence of zidovudine toxicity.

For practical purposes, patients with ADC should be given the highest tolerable dose of zidovudine. The average time taken to respond to zidovudine appears to be approximately 8 weeks. A response to zidovudine is mirrored in the CSF by a decline in surrogate markers of immune activation, beta-2 microglobulin, neopterin, and quinolinic acid (5,7,30). Whether one or more of these markers can be used to predict response to zidovudine or to determine zidovudine dosages is not known, although such a marker is highly desirable. Other investigation assays yet to be evaluated in the CSF include tumor necrosis factor (TNF), IL-1b, IL-6, and antimyelin basic protein antibodies, all of which have been related to disease pathogenesis.

Therapy for HIV disease in general is tending to use of combination nucleoside inhibitors with the aim of overlapping toxicities, increasing responses, and inhibiting the development of drug resistance. Whether these considerations hold true for ADC is unknown. Because didanosine has less blood-brain barrier penetration than zidovudine, didanosine might be expected to be less effective than zidovudine as monotherapy. Didanosine has, however, been found to improve the neuropsychological deficits of HIV-1-infected children (9), but preliminary data from the Alpha study of didanosine in advanced zidovudine-intolerant patients have not found such a benefit (38). Whether zidovudine and didanosine in combination are more effective than zidovudine monotherapy is unknown. Zalcitabine and 3TC have poor CSF penetration and are unlikely to be useful agents for treatment of ADC.

Some nonnucleoside reverse transcriptase inhibitors (NNRTIs), such as nevirapine and atevirdine, hold promise of both systemic and neurological efficacy by virtue of high penetration across the blood-brain barrier. However, the NNRTIs are associated with rapid development of drug-resistant HIV and so as monotherapy may be effective only in the short term. However, in some settings the doses of NNRTI can be increased so that trough plasma levels are greater than the IC90 of the resistant virus, with resultant continued efficacy. In addition, the induction of resistance to NNRTI may be associated with reversion of zidovudine resistance if zidovudine is administered concurrently, despite maintenance of a zidovudine-resistant genotype. Therefore, combination zidovudine-NNRTI may be effective in those ADC patients with zidovudine-resistant HIV who are able to tolerate zidovudine or even as primary therapy.

Lastly, intrathecal zidovudine through a reservoir with or without systemic antiretroviral cover has been used, particularly where systemic toxicity to zidovudine prevents adequate oral dosing. The utility of such a strategy is still uncertain, but there are data supporting its use (39).

PROGRESSIVE MULTIFOCAL LEUKOENCEPHALOPATHY

Cytosine arabinoside, with or without interferon-alpha, has been found to result occasionally in complete resolution of clinical and radiological abnormalities of PML. However, as is the case for CMV infection of the central nervous system, concurrent zidovudine therapy is difficult because of haematological toxicity. Furthermore, cytosine arabinoside and interferon-alpha have only limited efficacy even if tolerated. A less toxic, more effective (ie. more JC virus-specific) alternative therapy would be of great use. The use of a specific and sensitive PCR-based assay for detection of JC virus in the CSF (21) is likely to reduce the morbidity associated with brain biopsy and current therapy, as only those with definite rather than suspected PML would receive potentially toxic therapy. This is especially important for those patients with very advanced HIV disease.

CYTOMEGALOVIRUS RADICULOMYELOPATHY AND ENCEPHALITIS

Presently, there is no definitive method of making the diagnosis of neurological CMV disease, and a therapeutic trial of ganciclovir or foscarnet therapy is often used. Currently, useful diagnostic information includes antecedent or coexistent CMV organ involvement elsewhere and a CSF polymorphonuclear pleocytosis. The CMV culture from the CSF is cumbersome and slow, but amplification of CMV genome from the CSF by PCR may render a quick and accurate diagnosis (12).

Intravenous ganciclovir at a dose of 5 mg/kg twice daily for 3 weeks is effective in some patients (16). However, as CMV radiculomyelopathy is rare, there has been no controlled study to determine the optimal dose and duration of induction. Furthermore, there has been no comparative study of ganciclovir and foscarnet or an evaluation of both therapies in combination versus monotherapy. Obviously, alternatives are required for those who fail to respond to these therapies because of toxicity or presumed resistance. Ganciclovir may also be beneficial for therapy of CMV encephalitis, but objective data on its efficacy are unavailable.

Trials are currently evaluating CMV hyperimmune globulin and anti-CMV monoclonal antibodies in conjunction with ganciclovir for therapy of CMV retinitis. If these trials show benefit, their study should be extended to central nervous system CMV disease, although the blood-brain penetration of these proteins is not clear.

As mentioned above, valaciclovir is currently being evaluated as primary prophylaxis for CMV disease in patients with CD4+ counts less than $100/mm^3$. This trial arose from several studies which found that acyclovir, 3,200 mg daily, appeared to have a beneficial effect on mortality in such patients but did not reduce the incidence of CMV disease. It is hoped that valaciclovir will achieve higher serum levels and reduce both CMV disease and mortality. Similarly, oral ganciclovir is also being evaluated as primary prophylaxis for CMV disease.

HIV-RELATED NEUROPATHIES

A predominantly sensory neuropathy is the commonest and probably most important of the HIV-related neuropathies. Treatment is purely symptomatic. When pain is prominent, capsaicin cream, low-dose amytriptiline, sodium valproate or desipramine or narcotic analgesics may be beneficial. There are anecdotal reports of the efficacy of peptide T in ameliorating painful neuropathy. Potential mechanisms of action include anti-TNF or anti-pg120 activity, but controlled studies of peptide T have not been promising (D. Simpson, personal communication). It is hoped that current trials of nerve growth factor will demonstrate efficacy. Until the pathogenesis of this neuropathy is known, it is likely that symptomatic treatment rather than specific therapeutic agents will be used. Griffin et al. (26,27) have hypothesised that the neuropathy is due to secretion of cytokines such as TNF-α by activated macrophages infiltrating the involved neurones, although the cause of any such secretion is not known.

A demyelinating neuropathy may occur acutely at seroconversion or chronically at a later stage of HIV disease when there is only mild immunodeficiency (43). Treatment with plasmapheresis is the same as in the non-HIV-infected patients, and response does not seem to be any different. Therapeutic advances are likely to be driven by advances in its treatment in HIV-uninfected patients.

OTHER DISEASES

Vacuolar Myelopathy and Multinucleated Cell Myelitis

Therapy of vacuolar myelopathy will remain problematic until its pathogenesis is made clear. Vacuolar myelopathy would seem unlikely to be due to productive HIV infection per se if one excludes multinucleated cell myelitis, as vacuolar myelopathy can occur in HIV-uninfected patients (33). Another opportunistic infection is conceivable considering that the disorder is so uncommon in children, just as are opportunistic infections in general (41). Anecdotal experience suggests that vacuolar myelopathy does not respond to antiretroviral therapy while multinucleated cell myelitis does. Further data, however, are required.

Seizures

Following an initial seizure for which no underlying cause is identified, there is a high relapse rate. Therefore, indefinite anticonvulsant therapy is essential in such patients. Because approximately 15% of patients will develop hypersensitivity to phenytoin and carbamazepine, useful alternative drugs are clonazepam and sodium valproate. However, the most effective, least toxic therapy is not known. The pathogenesis of such seizures at the moment is entirely conjectural, and so no specific or preventative therapy is available.

Transient Neurological Deficits and Strokes

Transient neurological deficits may develop in the absence of an underlying condition (3,17). Small areas of infarction (35) and cerebral vasculitis due to varicella-zoster virus (25) have been implicated in the development of these deficits. How such a diagnosis should be made is unclear; cerebral angiography may play a role, and amplification of the zoster genome in the CSF by polymerase chain reaction (PCR) may also be helpful. Treatment at the moment is the same as that employed in the HIV-uninfected patient; namely consideration is given to anticoagulation and, where appropriate, acyclovir.

Myopathy

The HIV-associated myopathies are still poorly defined (43) but may be broadly grouped into inflammatory, noninflammatory, and zidovudine induced. For inflammatory myopathy, corticosteroid therapy is often required. The CD4+ count and HIV viral load should be monitored closely, and it may be prudent to consider alternative therapy such as intravenous immunoglobulin. However, there are no data comparing corticosteroids with immunoglobulin. Other immunosuppression is probably contraindicated but has not been trialed. Certainly, when patients are commenced on corticosteroids, appropriate antimicrobial prophylaxis should be commenced for infections such as PCP and tuberculosis.

Noninflammatory myopathy has no known treatment. Zidovudine-induced myopathy is thought to be a mitochondrial myopathy and one of the principal late-onset toxicities of zidovudine. Nevertheless, given the limited alternative antiretroviral agents available, it would be desirable to develop therapy which could prevent or treat this myopathy and allow continuation of zidovudine.

REFERENCES

1. Boucher CA, Lange JMA, Miedema F, et al. HIV-1 biological phenotype and the development of zidovudine resistance in relation to disease progression in asymptomatic individuals during treatment. *AIDS* 1992;6:1259–1264.
2. Brenneman DE, Westbrook GL, Fitzgerald S, et al. Neuronal cell killing by the envelope protein of HIV and its prevention by vasoactive intestinal peptide. *Nature* 1988;335:639–642.
3. Brew BJ, Miller J. Human immunodeficiency virus related transient neurologic deficits and their relationship to AIDS dementia complex. *Am J Med* 1996 (in press).
4. Brew BJ, Bhalla RB, Paul M, et al. Cerebrospinal fluid beta-2 microglobulin in patients with AIDS dementia complex: an expanded series including response to zidovudine treatment. *AIDS* 1992;6: 461–465.
5. Brew BJ, Bhalla RV, Paul M, et al. CSF neopterin in HIV-1 infection. *Ann Neurol* 1990;28:556–560.
6. Kerr SJ, Armati PJ, Brew BJ. Neurocytotoxicity of Quinoline acid in human brain cultues. *J Neuroviral* 1996;1:375–380.
7. Brew BJ, Paul M, Nakajima G, Khan A, Gallardo H, Price RW. Cerebrospinal fluid HIV-1 p24 antigen and culture: sensitivity and specificity for AIDS dementia complex. *J Neurol Neurosurg Psychiatry* 1994;57:784–793.
8. Brew BJ, Corbeil J, Pemberton L, et al. Quinoline acid production by macrophages infected with HIV-1 isolates from patients with and without AIDs dementia complex. *J Neuroviral* 1996;1(5/6): 369–374.

9. Butler KM, Husson RN, Balis FM, et al. Dideoxyinosine in children with symptomatic human immunodeficiency virus infection. *N Engl J Med* 1991;324:137–144.
10. Carr A, Tindall B, Brew B, et al. Low dose trimethoprim-sulfamethoxazole prophylaxis against toxoplasmic encephalitis in patients with AIDS. *Ann Intern Med* 1992;117:106–111.
11. Cinque P, Brytting M, Vago, et al. Epstein Barr virus DNA in cerebrospinal fluid from patients with AIDS-related primary lymphoma of the central nervous system. *Lancet* 1993;342:398–401.
12. Cinque P, Vago L, Brytting M, et al. Cytomegalovirus infection of the central nervous system in patients with AIDS: diagnosis by DNA amplification from cerebrospinal fluid. *J Infect Dis* 1992; 166:1408–1411.
13. Brew BJ, Rosenblum M, Cronin, K, Price RW. The AIDS dementia complex and human immunodeficiency virus type 1 brain infection: clinical-virological correlations. *Ann Neurol* 1995;38:563–570.
14. Danneman BR, Israelski DM, Leoung GS, McGraw T, Mills J, Remington JS. Toxoplasma serology, parasitaemia and antigenaemia in patients at risk for toxoplasmic encephalitis. *AIDS* 1991;5: 1363–1365.
15. Dawson VL, Dawson TM, Uhl GR, Snyder S. Human immunodeficiency virus type 1 coat protein neurotoxicity mediated by nitric oxide in primary cortical cultures. *Proc Natl Acad Sci* 1993;90: 3256–3259.
16. de Gans J, Portegies P, Tiessens G, et al. Therapy for cytomegalovirus polyradiculomyelitis in patients with AIDS: treatment with ganciclovir. *AIDS* 1990;4:421–425.
17. Engstrom JW, Lowenstein DH, Bredesen DE. Cerebral infarctions and transient neurological deficits associated with acquired immunodeficiency syndrome. *Am J Med* 1989;86:528–532.
18. Epstein LG, Gendelman HE. Human immunodeficiency virus type 1 infection of the nervous system: pathogenetic mechanisms. *Ann Neurol* 1993;33:429–436.
19. Brew BJ, Evans L, Byrne C, Pemberton L, Hurren L. The relationship between AIDS dementia complex and the presence of macrophage tropic and non-syncytium inducing isolates of human immunodeficiency virus type 1 in the cerebrospinal fluid. *J Neuroviral* (in press).
20. Gallo P, Frei K, Rordorf C, Lazdins J, Tavolato B, Fontana A. Human immunodeficiency virus type 1 (HIV-1) infection of the central nervous system: an evaluation of cytokines in cerebrospinal fluid. *J Neuroimmunol* 1989;23:109–116.
21. Gibson PE, Knowles, WA, Hand JF, Brown DWG. Detection of JC virus DNA in the cerebrospinal fluid of patients with progressive multifocal leukoencephalopathy. *J Med Virol* 1993;39:278–281.
22. Girard P-M, Landman R, Gaudebout C, et al. Dapsone-pyrimethamine compared with aerosolized pentamidine as primary prophylaxis against *Pneumocystis carinii* pneumonia and toxoplasmosis in HIV infection. *N Engl J Med* 1993;328:1514–1520.
23. Giulian D, Vaca K, Noonan C. Secretion of neurotoxins by mononuclear phagocytes infected with HIV-1. *Science* 1990;250:1593–1596.
24. Grant IH, Gold JWM, Rosenblum M, Niedzwiecki D, Armstrong D. *Toxoplasma gondii* serology in HIV-infected patients: the development of central nervous system toxoplasmosis in AIDS. *AIDS* 1990;4:519–521.
25. Gray F, Belec L, Lescs MC, Chreten F, Ciardi A, Hassine D, Flament-Saillour M, de Truchis P, Clair B, and Scaravilli F. Varicella-zoster virus infection of the central nervous system in the acquired immunodeficiency syndrome. *Brain* 1994;117:987–999.
26. Griffin JW. Peripheral nerve disorders in HIV infection. In: Price RW, Perry SW, eds. *HIV, AIDS, and the brain.* New York: Raven; 1993.
27. Griffin JW, Li CY, Tyor WR, et al. Macrophage phenotypes in peripheral nerves of HIV-1 infected individuals. *Paper presented at Neurological and Neuropsychological Complications of HIV Infection.* Monterey, CA, 1990 (abst Neu-14).
28. Hardy WD, Feinburg J, Finklestein DM, et al. A controlled trial of trimethoprim-sulfamethoxazole or aerosolized pentamidine for secondary prophylaxis of *Pneumocystis carinii* pneumonia in patients with the acquired immunodeficiency syndrome: AIDS Clinical Trials Group protocol 021. *N Engl J Med* 1992;327:1842–1848.
29. Harouse JM, Bhat S, Spitalnik SL, et al. Inhibition of entry of HIV-1 in neural cell lines by antibodies against galactosyl-ceramide. *Science* 1991;253:320–323.
30. Heyes MP, Brew BJ, Martin A, et al. Increased cerebrospinal fluid concentrations of the excitotoxin quinolinic acid in human immunodeficiency virus infection and AIDS dementia complex. *Ann Neurol* 1991;29:202–209.
31. Israelski DM, Remington JS. AIDS-associated toxoplasmosis. In: Sande M, Volberding P, eds. *Medical management of AIDS.* New York: WB Saunders; 1992;319–345.
32. Jacobson MA, Besch CL, Child C, et al. Toxicity of clindamycin as prophylaxis for AIDS-associated toxoplasmic encephalitis. *Lancet* 1992;339:333–334.
33. Kamin SS, Petito CK. Vacuolar myelopathy in immunocompromised non AIDS patients. *J Neuropathol Exp Neurol* 1988;47:385.
34. McCabe RE, Luft BJ, Remington JS. Effect of murine interferon gamma on murine toxoplasmosis. *J Infect Dis* 1984;150:961–962.

35. Mizusawa H, Hirano A, Llena JF, Shintaku M. Cerebrovascular lesions in acquired immune deficiency syndrome (AIDS). *Acta Neuropathol* 1989;76:451–457.
36. Ostergaard L, Nielsen AK, Black FT. DNA amplification on cerebrospinal fluid for diagnosis of cerebral toxoplasmosis among HIV-positive patients with signs or symptoms of neurological disease. *Scand J Infect Dis* 1993;25:227–237.
37. Portegies P, Enting RH, de Gans J, et al. Presentation and course of AIDS dementia complex: 10 years of follow-up in Amsterdam, The Netherlands. *AIDS* 1993;7:669–675.
38. Portegies P, et al. AIDS dementia complex and peripheral neuropathy in zidovudine-intolerant HIV-infected patients treated with didanosine (ddI). *Clin Neuropathol* 1993;12(Suppl 1):S18.
39. Routy JP, et al. Severe AIDS dementia complex treated by intrathecal zidovudine—the French and French-Canadian experience. *Clin Neuropathol* 1993;12(Suppl 1):S19.
40. Schmitt FA, Bigley JW, McKinnis R, et al. Neuropsychological outcome of zidovudine (AZT) treatment of patients with AIDS and AIDS related complex. *N Engl J Med* 1988;319:1573–1578.
41. Sharer LR, Dowling PC, Michaels J, et al. Spinal cord disease in children with HIV-1 infection: a combined molecular biological and neuropathological study. *Neuropathol Appl Neurobiol* 1990;16:317–331.
42. Sidtis JJ, Gatsonis C, Price RW, et al. Zidovudine treatment of the AIDS dementia complex: results of a placebo controlled trial. *Ann Neurol* 1993;33:343–349.
43. Simpson DM, Wolfe DE. Neuromuscular complications of HIV infection and its treatment. *AIDS* 1991;5:917–926.
44. Tenant-Flowers M, Boyle M, Carey D, Marriott D, Cooper DA, Penny R. Sulphadiazine desensitisation in patients with AIDS and cerebral toxoplasmosis. *AIDS* 1991;5:311–315.
45. Tyor W, Glass JD, Griffin JW, et al. Cytokine expression in the brain during the acquired immune deficiency syndrome. *Ann Neurol* 1992;31:349–360.
46. Watkins BA, Dorn HH, Kelly WB, et al. Specific tropism of HIV-1 for microglial cells in primary human brain cultures. *Science* 1990;249:549–553.

Subject Index

Subject Index

Page numbers followed by t refer to tables; page numbers followed by f refer to figures.

ISBN 0-7817-0309-3